Medical Assisting

Medical Assisting:
Administrative and Clinical Competencies

Third Edition

Lucille Keir, CMA-A
Barbara A. Wise, BSN, RN, MA(Ed)
Connie Krebs, CMA-C

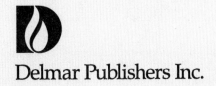

Delmar Publishers Inc.

Notice to the Reader

Publisher does not warrant or guarantee any of the products described herein or perform any independent analysis in connection with any of the product information contained herein. Publisher does not assume, and expressly disclaims, any obligation to obtain and include information other than that provided to it by the manufacturer.

The reader is expressly warned to consider and adopt all safety precautions that might be indicated by the activities described herein and to avoid all potential hazards. By following the instructions contained herein, the reader willingly assumes all risks in connection with such instructions.

The publisher makes no representations or warranties of any kind, including but not limited to, the warranties of fitness for particular purpose or merchantability, nor are any such representations implied with respect to the material set forth herein, and the publisher takes no responsibility with respect to such material. The publisher shall not be liable for any special, consequential or exemplary damages resulting, in whole or in part, from the readers' use of, or reliance upon, this material.

For information, address Delmar Publishers Inc.
3 Columbia Circle Drive
Box 15-015
Albany, New York 12203-5015

Delmar Staff

Administrative Editor: Marion Waldman	Art Supervisor: Judi Orozco
Developmental Editor: Denise Black Gold	Art Coordinator: John Lent
Senior Project Editor: Christopher Chien	Editorial Assistant: Catherine Eads
Senior Production Supervisor: Karen Seebald	Editorial Production Assistant: Lori McDonald

COPYRIGHT © 1993
BY DELMAR PUBLISHERS INC.

10 9 8 7 6   XXX   99 98 97 96 95

Printed in the United States of America
Published simultaneously in Canada
by Nelson Canada
A Division of The Thomson Corporation

Library of Congress Cataloging-in-Publication Data
Keir, Lucille.
    Medical assisting: administrative and clinical competencies/
Lucille Keir, Barbara A. Wise, Connie Krebs. — 3rd ed.
        p. cm.
    Includes bibliographical references and index.
    ISBN 0-8273-5311-1
    1. Medical assistants.   I. Wise, Barbara A.   II. Krebs, Connie.
III. Title.
    (DNLM: 1. Office Management.   2. Physician' Assistants.   W 21.5
    K27m)
R728.8.K44 1993
610.73'7—dc20
DNLM/DC
for Library of Congress   92-49820
                                                 CIP

Table of Contents

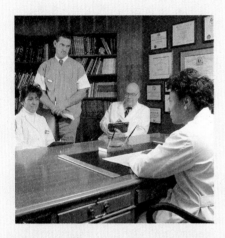

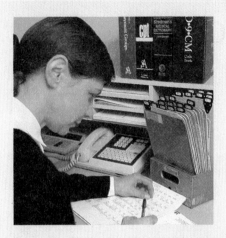

SECTION TWO
The Administrative Assistant

12
Medical Office Management

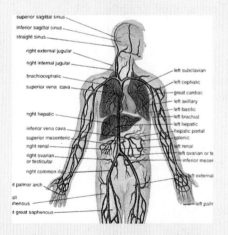

SECTION THREE
Structure and Function of the Body Systems

13
Anatomy and Physiology of the Human Body

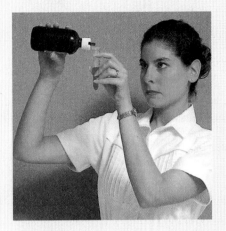

SECTION FOUR

The Clinical Medical Assistant

14

The Medical Assistant as Clinical Assistant

15

Beginning the Database

16
Preparing Patients for Examination

17
Specimen Collection and Laboratory Procedures

18
Diagnostic Tests, X Rays, and Procedures

19
Minor Surgical Procedures

20
Assisting With Medications

21
Medical Emergencies

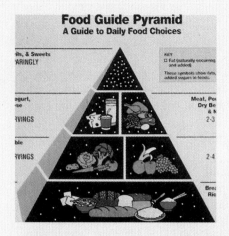

SECTION FIVE
Desired Personal Behavior and Employability Skills

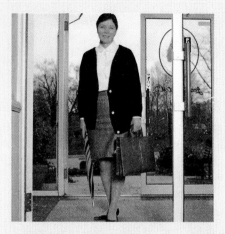

SECTION SIX
A Final Note

Index of Tables

Preface

MEDICAL ASSISTING: Administrative and Clinical Competencies makes available, in a comprehensive text, the current knowledge base, task requirements, and skill development procedures the medical assistant needs to qualify for entry-level employment in a physician's office, a clinic, an HMO, or other appropriate health care setting.

The content of the text is organized to reflect the various responsibilities of the occupation. To support each of these areas, the authors provide thorough, clearly written, and well-illustrated discussions of the major concepts and tasks associated with achieving competency in each responsibility.

It is recognized that medical practice frequently alters the role of the medical assistant. For example, many physicians use laboratory services for the analysis of specimens instead of maintaining the space and equipment required for the medical assistant to accomplish the testing. In addition, geographical location, the type and size of medical practice, the number and types of office employees, and the personal discretion of the physician all tend to affect the role of the medical assistant. The medical assistant who works alone in an office must be able to perform all the supporting functions required by the physician. When employed in a large practice or clinic, however, the medical assistant will often specialize in one function — secretarial, clinical, or managerial. Further differentiation may also occur within these functions, such as a health care insurance specialist. The text has been written to acquaint the reader with all aspects of the medical assistant role.

Throughout the text, the learning required is specified by means of the competency-based unit objectives as well as the terminal performance objectives identified for each procedure. The content includes all introductory-level areas as identified by the *Essentials and Guidelines of an Accredited Educational Program for the Medical Assistant* as revised in 1991. A plan for providing an externship, as required by the Guidelines, is included in the accompanying Instructor's Guide.

The text is designed for use as an introduction to medical assisting in a variety of settings:

- a structured classroom setting, with the expertise of a qualified instructor;
- for individual instruction of students in programs of diversified training, because much of the content and format are appropriate for self-study;
- for on-the-job training in a physician's office, where the text serves as a resource manual.

Major Content Revision for the Third Edition

Extensive changes were made to reflect an increased emphasis on administrative functions, including the latest changes in third-party payments. In the clinical area, technical advances in equipment and procedures are covered, as well as adherence to infectious disease control, which is necessary to quality health care. The anatomy and physiology content also reflects advances in clinical knowledge, diagnosis, and treatment. The use of color photos, combined with an increase in the number and quality of illustrations, improves the total text. The major content changes are summarized as follows:

- *new* — medical/legal/ethical concerns facing health care providers today, and their effect on health care delivery; these are set apart in easily identified sections. Information on durable power of attorney for health care, Right to Die, Miranda Warning Law, and update on living wills.
- *new* — scenarios for medical/legal/ethical concerns.
- *new* — new definition from AAMA for Medical Assistant and new AAMA logo.
- *new* — related health specialty fields information.
- *new* — section on English grammar.
- *new* — examples of math applications.
- *new* — unit on the immune system: includes discussion of allergies, cancer, immunity, lupus erythematosus, chronic fatigue syndrome, rheumatoid arthritis, and expanded information on AIDS.
- *expanded* — interpersonal communications to include sexual harassment and discrimination.
- *expanded* — office computer utilization, added DOS commands, use of FAX, microfiche, copier, word processor, and credit card payments.
- *expanded* — and — updated coverage of Medicare benefits, including new CPT codes reflecting current provisions.
- *expanded* — information on banking, employee forms and benefits, and management responsibilities.
- *expanded* — diseases and disorders, diagnostic tests and treatments in anatomy and physiology chapter. Added content on conception, contraception, pregnancy, labor and delivery.
- *expanded* — discussion of infectious disease control, adding utilization of universal precautions in every clinical procedure as appropriate.
- *expanded* — coverage of communicable diseases, medications and surgical instruments.

- *expanded* — coverage of ECG (EKG), history and data base information including new history form and examination of the eye and ears.
- *expanded* — personal behaviors to include second-hand smoke and added to employability skills information.
- *revised* — laboratory procedure content to reflect CLIA recommendations for POL.
- *revised* — immunization tables.

Supplements

The Student Workbook that accompanies this text provides review questions, vocabulary and skill exercises, forms to complete, puzzles, and other tasks that reinforce the content of the text. The workbook also includes evaluation sheets for measuring performance of the procedures. An Instructor's Guide provides answers to the questions in the workbook and guidelines to the instructor for presenting the content.

Use of the text, reinforced by the Student Workbook and recommendations from the Instructor's Guide, provides for implementation of a complete, competency-based instructional program.

Acknowledgements

John Ross, a very special personal friend, who gave unending encouragement and support as well as computer assistance, photo shooting, and serving as a sounding-board. His contribution and patience was above and beyond all expectations and is gratefully acknowledged.

Carol Watts, practicing CMA, who accepted the challenge to revise Chapters 9, 10, and 11 following the unexpected severe health problems of one of the authors. Her assistance was invaluable.

James C. English, MD, practicing family physician and former instructor in the College of Medicine at The Ohio State University, for reading, identifying, and recommending content to be added or technically updated in Chapter 13, Anatomy and Physiology. His invaluable contribution is truly appreciated.

James B. Soldano, MD, family practice physician who reviewed the content regarding physical examination in Chapter 16.

Jeanne Luddy, retired English teacher, who advised and made contributions to the material on grammar.

Colleen King, RN, of Northwest Family Physicians, who provided in-depth information and assistance with the content on responsibilities involved in the management of a medical practice.

Elaine Glass, MS, RN, OCN, Clinical Nurse Specialist, The Arthur G. James Cancer Hospital and Research Center, who provided technical information and expertise on the immune system and her personal review of the material included in the text.

Diane Hohwald, RN, CNN, Educational Coordinator of Riverside Outpatient Dialysis Center, for providing information, technical assistance, illustrative materials, and her personal review of the content included in the text.

A special appreciation to the following for permitting the use of their offices as sites for many of the photos in this text:

Andrew J. Pultz, MD, and the staff of Metropolitan Family Practice

George A. Huntress, DO, and the staff of Sullivan Family Medical Center

The physicians and staff of Med-Ohio North

Jack Frost, M.D., Plastic Surgery, Arnold, Maryland

Donna Shea, AS, RMA, CMA, CRT: Medical Assisting Instructor, National Education Center, San Bernardino, CA

Ruth Darton, CMA; Medical Assisting Instructor and Consultant, National Education Center, San Bernardino, CA

Adrienne L. Carter-Ward, CMA, RMA, EMT; Instructor Trainer and Medical Assisting Instructor, National Headquarters NEC, San Bernardino, CA

Carol Hinricher; Medical Assisting Instructor, Missoula Technical Center, Missoula, MT

Judy Crissip, CMA-AC; Medical Assisting Instructor and Program Director, Pinellas Technical Education Centers, St. Petersburg, FL

Sally Emery, RN; Medical Assisting Instructor, Aristotle Institute, Westerville, OH

Sharon Pass, RMA (AMT); Medical Assisting Instructor and Program Director, California Paramedical and Technical College, Riverside, CA

Theresa Bowser; Medical Assistant Instructor, Bradford School, Columbus, OH

Wilma J. Stoeckle, CMA; Medical Assistant Instructor, Duff's Business Institute, Pittsburgh, PA

Brenda M. Foster, M.S., CMA; Coordinator, Department of Health Related Professions, Program Director/Medical Assisting, East Tennessee State University, Elizabethton, TN

Linda Scarborough; Instructor, Allied Health Department, Lanier Technical Institute, Oakwood, GA

The authors especially wish to acknowledge and commend the editors and staff of Delmar Publishers Inc. for their encouragement, guidance, recommendations and expertise during the preparation of this edition. Their assistance during the development of the text was most helpful.

Administrative editor — Marion Waldman
Developmental editor — Denise Black Gold
Editorial assistant — Catherine Eads

Dedication

We gratefully acknowledge the support and encouragement of our families, loved ones, and friends throughout the preparation of this edition. We especially recognize the strong friendship and commitment we share for each other, which goes far beyond the pages of this book. Because of our experiences in employment and teaching, we felt a need for this text and we therefore wish to dedicate it to you, the reader, for you are the reason it was written.

A Message to the Learner

You are about to begin a new career in the field of health care. You have decided to become a member of the physician's team to help provide for the needs of the people in your community. You will be expected to be knowledgeable, efficient, and capable of assuming a great deal of responsibility in the performance of your duties.

People go to a physician's office for a variety of reasons. They may desire a general assessment of their health status or they may be injured and need immediate treatment. Often they are very ill and frightened and require assistance with emotional as well as physical problems. The physician must be able to diagnose the reason for their illness or determine the extent of their injury in order to provide the proper treatment or medication. The physician will be better able to concentrate on the needs of the patients if you can be depended upon to carry out your responsibilities. As a medical assistant you will be performing many of the operational tasks necessary for a medical office to function effectively and efficiently as well as assisting the physician to examine and treat the patients.

Purpose of This Text

This text has been written to help you acquire the knowledge and skills needed to work successfully in a medical office. Occasionally, the methods of medical practice or policies where you live will differ from those described in the text. This may affect the tasks you perform or the procedural steps of the skills, but the basic information will be the same.

It is important that you understand the reasons for the procedures you will be performing and that you know how to perform them accurately. Remember, you are working with people's lives. Often you cannot correct mistakes once they have been made, so it is very important that you DO NOT make mistakes. Do not be afraid to ask questions when you do not understand.

Keeping Current

Your training will not end when you have completed this text. There is much information that applies to specific kinds of medical practice or is best learned when the specific employment situation arises. In addition, health care methods change whenever a new drug is developed or a different treatment is proved effective. Occasionally, a new finding will completely change the way to deal with an illness or disease. Consider the changes that nave occurred due to the virus that causes AIDS. Individuals working in health professions have had to change the way they provide care in order to protect themselves and their patients. Workshops, seminars, technical journals, and your employer will become your means of learning additional skills to stay current.

Organization of Text

The text has been organized into sections, chapters, and units. The basic structure is the unit. Units covering similar information are grouped into chapters, which are similarly grouped into the five sections of the text.

Each unit has important features which specify what you are expected to learn.

Objectives. These identify the knowledge or skill you are to develop by studying the material. Recall the objectives as you read the unit. When you have finished, review the objectives and reread portions of the unit until you can accurately respond to all of them. The workbook which accompanies this text has questions, puzzles, diagrams and other activities which will help you acquire the knowledge and skills necessary to meet the objectives and later, become successfully employed as a medical assistant.

Words to Know. These are medical terms and related vocabulary words used in the unit. They are listed separately at the beginning of each unit and highlighted in color at the first significant use within the text. You are expected to be able to include the terms in your personal vocabulary. You will find them listed and defined in the Glossary of the text.

Procedures. These are detailed descriptions of skills required of a medical assistant. They list the actions involved, step-by-step, in a logical sequence. The procedures have been developed from standards of practice that have proven successful. Within each procedure, important points (Key Points) are emphasized.

The procedures also have specific performance criteria called terminal performance objectives. This type of objective identifies exactly what is required to successfully perform the procedure.

Appendix. The Appendix contains medical abbreviations and the prefixes, suffixes, and Latin and Greek words that make up medical terms. Become familiar with this section as quickly as possible. It will help you to define terminology and to understand the language of medicine. Other useful information is also included in the Appendix such as: converting measurements; weights and measures; symbols; and a chart for stain removal.

Other Titles in Delmar's Leading Medical Assisting Series:

- Administrative Medical Assisting, 3rd Edition/Fordney, Follis
- Body Structures and Functions, 8th Edition/Fong, Scott
- Computer Literacy for Health Care Professionals/Anderson
- Computerized Medical Office Management/Johnson, Johnson
- Fundamental Skills for the Clinical Laboratory Professional/Marshall
- Human Anatomy and Physiology in Health and Disease, 3rd Edition/Burke
- Law, Liability, and Ethics for Medical Office Personnel, 2nd Edition/Flight
- Medical Brain Teasers, Puzzles, and Games/Silverman
- Medical Terminology for Health Professionals/Ehrlich
- The Professional Medical Assistant: Clinical Practice/Lindsey, Rayburn
- Therapeutic Communications for Allied Health Professionals/Tamparo, Lindh
- Understanding Medical Insurance/Rowell

Look for Medical Assisting Videos in 1993!

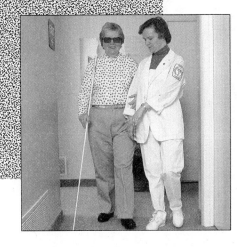

C H A P T E R   1

Your Career as a Medical Assistant

The individual who has a genuine desire to assist in the health care of patients should find the position of medical assistant satisfying in every way. This career offers great variety, normally pleasant surroundings, and an opportunity to advance through improvement of communication, administrative, and clinical skills.

This chapter will introduce you to some of the history of medicine and medical assisting. The medical assistant should have some knowledge of the history of medicine because modern medicine uses terms given to anatomy and physiology many hundreds of years ago. You will also learn of the development of medical assisting as a profession and the opportunities for advancement.

U N I T   1

A Brief History of Medicine and Medical Assisting

OBJECTIVES

Upon completion of the unit, the student will meet the following terminal performance objectives by verifying knowledge of the facts and principles presented through oral and written communication at a level deemed competent.

1. Identify contributions made to the field of medicine by both men and women physicians and nonphysicians.
2. Explain the role of the medical assistant as a member of the health care team.
3. Describe the history and purpose of the American Association of Medical Assistants (AAMA).
4. Spell and define, using the glossary at the back of the text, all the words to know in this unit.

WORDS TO KNOW

anatomic	metabolism
apprenticeships	methodical
aseptic techniques	neurosurgery
celiac	opposition
chemotherapy	ovarian
chloroform	pathological
cystic fibrosis	pernicious anemia
depicted	persecuted
dissected	practitioners
elite	proctoscopy
entity	quackery
ether	pro tem
gangrene	realm
guilds	render
institute	theories

Ancient History

Throughout history, few lives have been more important to the well-being of the world than those of the great

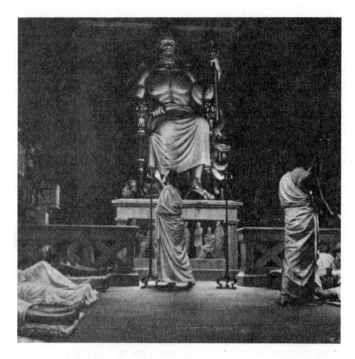

FIGURE 1–1 The temples and cult of Aesculapius (From *Mitchell and Grippando, Nursing Perspectives and Issues, 5th Ed.*, copyright 1993 by Delmar Publishers Inc.)

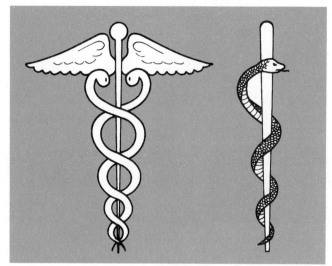

FIGURE 1–2 (Left) Caduceus (Right) Staff of Aesculapius (From *Mitchell and Grippando, Nursing Perspectives and Issues, 5th Ed.*, copyright 1993 by Delmar Publishers Inc.)

physicians and surgeons.

We have proof through findings of skulls and other bones that many thousands of years ago primitive surgeons were performing skull operations and setting broken bones. The formation of new bone covering the edges of the cut or fracture proves the patients survived the procedures. The earliest evidence is found in records of the ancient Egyptians from 3500 B.C. It is believed that the practice of medicine and surgery was closely related to religious rites or to magic. We know that the Egyptians had rules of sanitation because these are recorded on the tombs.

We are more familiar with the laws of Moses, which are described in detail in the Bible. Moses advocated preventive medicine by laws requiring personal cleanliness and sanitary procedures in the preparation and serving of food.

The priests in the temples of Aesculapius, Greek god of healing, used massage, bathing, and exercise in treating patients and sometimes gave iron as a medication. They also depended on the magical power of large, yellow, nonpoisonous serpents, which were trained to lick the wounds of patients who visited the temples. The god of healing was usually depicted holding a staff with a serpent coiled around it, Figure 1–1. This emblem was called the caduceus, Figure 1–2. Today the caduceus is the most recognized symbol of the medical profession, even though the staff of Aesculapius with its single snake is usually considered to be the more appropriate symbol.

The first great physician we can name is the Greek Hippocrates who was born in 460 B.C., Figure 1–3. He placed the practice of medicine in the realm of science, separate from magic and superstition. He is known as the "Father of Medicine." Hippocrates stressed the importance of cleanliness and diet for the well-being of patients. To maintain high standards in the practice of medicine, Hippocrates wrote a set of medical standards known as the Hippocratic oath. To this day, physicians have to swear to that oath. Hippocrates discovered that the course of certain diseases could be traced by listening to the chest of a patient. That knowledge became useful over 2,000 years later when a French physician, Laennec, invented the stethoscope, Figure 1–4.

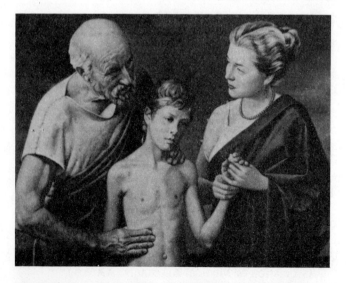

FIGURE 1–3 Hippocrates: medicine becomes a science.

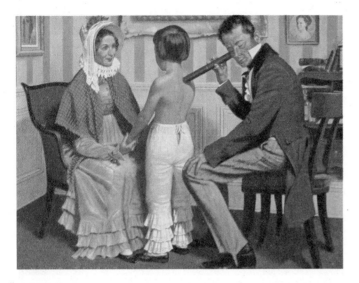

FIGURE 1–4 Laennec and the stethoscope (Courtesy Parke-Davis & Company, copyright 1957)

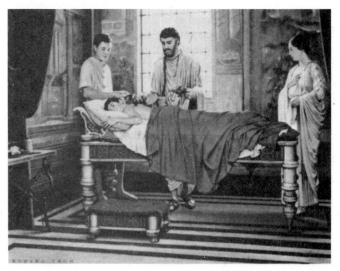

FIGURE 1–5 Galen: influence for forty-five generations (From *Mitchell and Grippando, Nursing Perspectives and Issues, 5th Ed.*, copyright 1993 by Delmar Publishers Inc.)

There was a return to a quackery in medicine following the work of Hippocrates, but then in 130 A.D. Galen was born in Greece, Figure 1–5. He was a serious student of the teachings of Hippocrates. Galen was the first physician of record to use pulse as a measure of the health of a patient, although he did not know that the pulse was affected by the action of the heart. He also believed in the value of physical therapy and preventive medicine.

The early teachings of Hippocrates and Galen were preserved by Arabian physicians, and there are records of a famous medical school established in Salerno, Italy, in 848 A.D. Both men and women were admitted to it and served on its experienced faculty. St. Hildegarde (1099–1179), a German Benedictine abbess, is one of the earliest recorded female physicians. She taught courses to prepare young women as nurses in addition to her practice of medicine.

Modern Medical Pioneers ....

In the year 1514, Andreas Vesalius was born in Brussels. He studied in many of the greatest medical schools and wrote the first detailed studies of anatomy. He is honored by physicians as the founder of modern anatomical study. He introduced many new anatomic terms but named none for himself.

A student of Vesalius, Gabriele Fallopius, gave his own name to the fallopian tubes and also gave the vagina and placenta their present names.

William Harvey was born in England in 1578. He studied medicine in Italian schools and then returned to England to practice and teach. His great contribution was to study the action of the heart. By studying animals, he observed that blood must travel in a circle through action of the heart, but he died not knowing for sure how blood traveled from arteries to veins because he did not have a microscope with which to view the tiny capillaries.

Anton van Leeuwenhoek (1632–1723) was a Dutch draper (a person dealing in cloth) and amateur scientist whose hobby was the grinding of lenses. Through this hobby he discovered how to use a simple biconvex lens and magnify structures that had never before been examined, Figure 1–6, page 4. His work was not carried out along strictly scientific lines, but he did describe his findings of micro-organisms (which he called "tiny little beasties") to the Royal Society in London in 1677.

The practice of medicine in the beginning of the seventeenth century was divided among the members of three guilds: the physicians, the surgeons, and the apothecaries. The physicians were the elite, as they usually possessed a university degree. They preferred studying, teaching, and debating the theories of disease to dealing directly with the sick. They limited their practice to the upper classes. The surgeons were considered inferior to the physicians. They were classified as Surgeons of the Long Robe and the more humble barber-surgeons. Only a few held university degrees. They were trained in hospitals and through apprenticeships. The spelling was originally *chirurgeon,* from the Greek *cheir* meaning *hand* and *ergon* meaning *work*. Barber-surgeons used their razors for opening veins and also for their barbering. Apothecaries were tradesmen and were permitted to charge only for the drugs they prescribed, made up, and sold. They were general practitioners for the masses and learned through apprenticeships.

In the eighteenth century, medical science developed rapidly because of advances in the modern sciences of physics and chemistry, which gave the physicians new

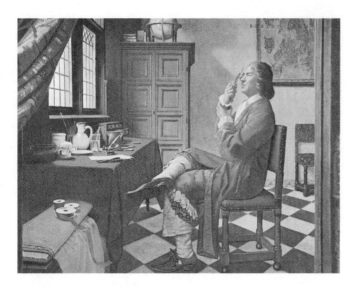

FIGURE 1–6   Leeuwenhoek and his microscope (courtesy Parke-Davis & Company, copyright 1957)

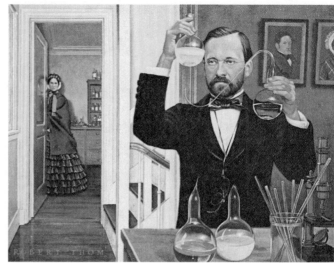

FIGURE 1–7   Pasteur: the chemist who transformed medicine (Courtesy Parke-Davis & company, copyright 1957)

tools and new methods. The brothers William and John Hunter were born in Scotland and studied medicine together. While William became a surgeon in London, John (1728–1793) became an army surgeon. After his army service, John devoted himself to the practice of his profession and to teaching and studying anatomy. He was especially interested in comparing the bodies of animals with one another and with that of man. John Hunter has been called the founder of scientific surgery because his surgical procedures were based on sound pathological findings. In 1778 he introduced artificial feeding by the use of a flexible tube passed into the stomach. His great collection of anatomic and animal specimens is in the museum of the Royal College of Surgeons in London, England.

Edward Jenner was born in England in 1749. He studied under John Hunter. His fame is based on developing a vaccine for smallpox.

Dr. Phillipe Pinel (1755–1826) was the first physician of record to order chains removed from mental patients and institute more humane treatment.

Dr. W.T.G. Morton was practicing medicine in Massachusetts in the mid-1800s when he introduced the use of anesthetic in the form of ether to make his patients more comfortable during surgery. A monument was erected to his memory in the city of Boston after his death. The use of ether stimulated research into safer methods of relieving pain.

Dr. James Simpson of Edinburgh University in Scotland soon began to use chloroform sprinkled on a towel held over the patient's face. It was Oliver Wendell Holmes, both a writer and a physician, who suggested the word *anesthesia*. The word comes from two Greek words which mean *not feeling*.

Louis Pasteur (1822–1895) was born in a small town in France and studied to become a chemist, Figure 1–7.

His motto was "Work, always work." He discovered through his work that the presence of microbes, or bacteria, caused liquids to turn sour. He then found that if these microbes were eliminated the liquids would not turn sour. His name is well known because of the process of pasteurizing, which eliminates dangerous microbes from milk. One of Pasteur's greatest achievements was the discovery of a vaccine to prevent and cure rabies.

Joseph Lister (1827–1912) was born near London, England, Figure 1–8. When he began to practice medicine he was shocked by the number of people who died from infection. He used the knowledge he gained from Pasteur's discoveries to develop ways to keep microbes out of wounds. At first he used carbolic acid on wounds. This process kept out microbes but it also burned the flesh severely and left ugly scars. He then tried carbolic acid spray in the room. He finally determined that the instruments used, the bandages, and the surgeon's hands carried the microbes. He laid the foundation for later aseptic techniques.

Wilhelm Roentgen (1845–1923) was a German physicist who discovered X rays, or roentgen rays as they are called in his honor.

Dr. Elias Metchnikoff (1845–1916) was a Russian Jew who devoted much of his life to studying ways to prolong life. Louis Pasteur invited him to work at the Pasteur Institute and he became the director after Pasteur's death. In 1908 Metchnikoff was awarded the Nobel Prize in medicine for his work on the ways white blood cells protect us from disease.

Early Leaders in American Medicine ....

Thomas Bond was born in Maryland, but since there were no domestic schools or hospitals in which to serve an internship, he studied in France, England, and Scotland at medical schools affiliated with hospitals. These

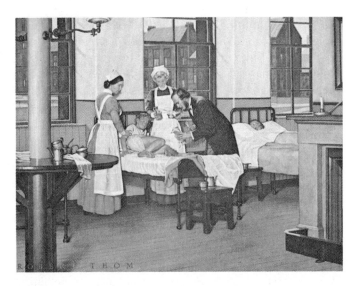

FIGURE 1–8 Lister introduces antisepsis (courtesy Parke-Davis & Company, copyright 1957.)

experiences taught him the value of hospital care for the sick. When he returned to Philadelphia to practice, he tried to secure money from friends to support building a hospital. He made no real progress until he enlisted the help of Benjamin Franklin. Franklin believed in his project and wrote about the proposal in the newspapers. When it was clear the money offerings would not be sufficient, he proposed a bill before the Assembly; the bill passed in May 1751, and the first patients were admitted in 1756. A distinguished Frenchman, M. deWarville, visited the hospital around 1788 and reported it superior to most hospitals he had visited in France. The hospital was clean, and black and white patients were being cared for in the same wards. It was not the first hospital in the American colonies, but it is recognized as the oldest surviving institution for the care of the sick in the United States.

In 1762 William Shippen, Jr., returned to Philadelphia from his study of anatomy under John Hunter in England. He placed an announcement in the *Pennsylvania Gazette* offering a course of anatomical lectures. He had only 10 students for the first course, but following years enrollment climbed as high as 200. During this period in our history it was not unusual for bodies to be stolen from graves so that they could be dissected and studied.

William Beaumont (1785–1853) was a surgeon in the U.S. Army during the War of 1812. In 1822 he treated a young man who was in serious condition because of a bullet wound in his stomach. The treatment was successful and the man regained his health, but the flesh never healed completely. As a result, Dr. Beaumont was able to use the open area as a laboratory to study the action of the stomach. These studies added to our understanding of the digestive process.

Ephraim McDowell (1771–1830) was an American physician who studied at the then most famous medical school in the world, the University of Edinburgh. He practiced medicine in Kentucky and was a skilled surgeon. In the early 1800s Dr. McDowell performed an operation never before recorded. He removed a large ovarian tumor that would otherwise have killed his patient. When neighbors and friends found out he was going to perform the operation they called him a murderer. However, the surgery was successful and the patient lived many more years. McDowell was not recognized for his achievement until years later after he had performed other similar operations. Present-day surgeons still use many of his techniques for this surgery.

At the time Beaumont and McDowell were practicing medicine, the causes of infection were not understood. Many patients developed blood poisoning or gangrene and died from these complications.

Walter Reed (1851–1902) was a Major serving in the U.S. Army in Cuba when he realized the need to find the cause of yellow fever. He was forced to seek out volunteers who were willing to be given the disease. Certainly these people, some of whom died, also made a great contribution to medicine although their names are not remembered. Dr. Reed's work in stamping out yellow fever made it possible to build the Panama Canal.

Theobald Smith (1859–1934), born in Albany, New York, was a professor of bacteriology. He was responsible for the establishment of a department of animal pathology in 1916 near Princeton University. His research laid the foundation for the prevention of diseases like typhoid, diphtheria, and meningitis, which are now prevented by use of vaccines.

Alexis Carrel was born in 1872 in France. He came to the United States after he received his medical degree and became a staff member of the Rockefeller Institute. He discovered, in his study of body tissues, that severed arteries could be joined and again carry on their function. His research work, which was carried out on animals, showed that it is possible to transplant bones and blood vessels and various organs of the body. He was awarded the Nobel Prize in medicine in 1912 for his work in joining blood vessels.

Women in Medicine ....

As mentioned before, there were female doctors in the famous medical school in Salerno, Italy from 1099 to 1179. In England in the sixteenth century women were allowed to practice medicine. Then attitudes toward women changed and they were often persecuted as witches if they tried to cure sickness. In the mid-nineteenth century, still with much opposition, women once again won the right to be trained and to qualify as doctors.

Trotula Platearius (1100 A.D.) was the most famous of the female teachers of medicine at Europe's first medical university at Salerno, Italy. Her specialty was obstetrics and gynecology and her *Diseases of Women* was a major textbook for seven centuries. She married a physician and had two sons who were physicians.

Dr. Elizabeth Garrett Anderson (1836–1917) was the first woman to qualify as a doctor in Britain. A hospital is named after her. In 1872 she opened the New Hospital for Women, staffed entirely by women.

Clara Barton (1821–1912) cared for the wounded in the Civil War. In the course of this work she not only nursed the wounded but recognized the need for support services to meet the emotional and spiritual needs of the soldiers. After the war she worked at locating missing soldiers. She learned of the Red Cross in 1869 when she visited friends in Geneva, Switzerland. In 1881 she formed the American Red Cross and served as its first president.

Elizabeth Blackwell (1821–1910) was the first woman in the United States to qualify as a doctor, Figure 1–9. She was turned down in 1844 by medical schools in Philadelphia and New York but enrolled in a school in Geneva, New York, and was awarded a degree in 1849. Dr. Blackwell, with the help of two other women, also doctors, her sister Emily and Marie Zackrzewska, opened a dispensary and medical college for women in New York in 1853. They opened a hospital exclusively for women in 1857 despite great opposition.

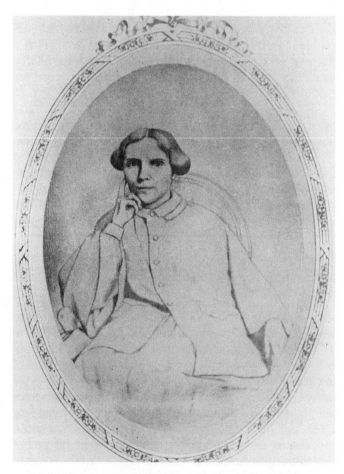

FIGURE 1–9 Elizabeth Blackwell, first woman in United States to qualify as doctor (courtesy Elizabeth Blackwell Center, Riverside Methodist Hospital, Columbus, Ohio)

Florence Nightingale (1820–1910) was the founder of modern nursing. She was born into a wealthy family who were of the opinion that ladies found a suitable husband, were married, and raised children, period. She was greatly influenced by Elizabeth Blackwell, who was a close personal friend. Nightingale studied nursing in Europe and used her knowledge in the Crimean War to care for the wounded and sick. She established a school for nurses in 1860 at St. Thomas Hospital in London.

Dr. Aletta Jacobs (1854–1929) was Holland's first woman physician and opened the world's first birth control clinic in Amsterdam in 1882.

Marie Curie (1867–1934), born Mary A. Sklodowska in Warsaw, Poland, was the first world-famous woman scientist. She discovered the element radium. She won the Nobel Prize in physics with her husband, Pierre, and Henri Becquerel and later won the Nobel Prize herself in the field of chemistry. Her work led directly to the treatment of cancer with radium.

Elsie Strang L'Esperance (1878?–1959) was born in Yorktown, New York. She graduated from Woman's Medical College of the New York Infirmary for Women and Children established by Elizabeth Blackwell. Her concern for the early treatment of cancer led her to establish the Strang Clinic. Her effort represented the first organized attempt to prevent cancer by early diagnosis. The clinic offered complete physical examinations to apparently healthy women to determine the presence of cancer. Major advances were made in the Strang Clinic, including the work of Dr. George Papanicolaou in the diagnosis of cervical cancer. Evaluations of the colon and rectum were also studied through use of **proctoscopy.**

Gerty Theresa Radnitz Cori (1896–1957) was the first American woman to win the Nobel Prize for medicine and physiology. Dr. Cori worked with her husband on the overall process of carbohydrate **metabolism** in the body.

Dorothy Hansine Anderson (1901–1963) was born in Asheville, North Carolina. She was denied a residency in surgery and an appointment in pathology at the University of Rochester because she was a woman. She was accepted as an assistant in pathology at Columbia and in 1930 was appointed to the teaching staff. Her research into **celiac** disease of the pancreas led to the discovery of a previously unrecognized disease **entity** which she called **cystic fibrosis.** She ultimately developed a simple method of diagnosing this disease. She wrote major publications in the 1940s on **chemotherapy** for respiratory tract infections in cystic fibrosis.

Grace Arabell Goldsmith (1904–1975) was born in St. Paul, Minnesota, and received her medical training at Tulane University School of Medicine. Her main interest was nutrition and in the early 1940s she instituted, at Tulane, the first nutrition training for medical students anywhere in the world.

Dorothy Hodgkins was born in 1910 in Egypt of British parents. Her work in analyzing the structure of vitamin B12 as a vital substance in the fight against pernicious anemia won her the Nobel Prize for chemistry in 1964.

Women continue to contribute to the care of patients through determination to prove their abilities.

In 1983, *Ebony* magazine reported only two black women in the United States, Drs. Alexa Canady and M. Deborah Hyde-Rowan, had broken into the field of neurosurgery. They were excellent students and experienced some discouraging remarks from faculty members in medical school. Remarks such as "you don't fully understand" all that is involved in neurosurgery and it is "too difficult a field for a woman" did not stop them from realizing their goals. The women are proud of their accomplishments and say "it shows that black women have the determination, discipline, and dedication to succeed in an area such as neurosurgery."

The Medical Assistant ....

Libraries are filled with books concerning the medical advances of the past 50 years. Research constantly contributes to the welfare of patients. Medical assistants need to be aware of the changes taking place. In 1989 it was reported that 100,000 major organs had been transplanted, mostly in the past 10 to 15 years. It is not unusual now to transplant the heart, heart-lung combinations, liver, kidney, and pancreas. New medications help to cut down the number of rejections. Artificial joints and limbs are commonly replaced.

Ultrasound scanning is a diagnostic technique in which very high frequency sound waves are passed into the body. The reflected echoes are detected and analyzed to build a picture of internal organs or of a fetus in the uterus. The noninvasive procedure is painless and safe.

Medical treatment today is safer and more effective as a result of all the new advances in care. The medical assistant will find that there is always something new to learn.

In a brochure published by the American Association of Medical Assistants (AAMA) entitled "Plan Your Career as a Medical Assistant," a series of questions is listed to help the interested individual decide whether to pursue the career. The questions are:

■ Do you like people?
■ Do you want variety in your work?
■ Can you 'take hold' and get things done?
■ Are you methodical and accurate in what you do?
■ Can you be trusted with confidential information?

If you can answer yes to these questions, you are on the right track.

Medical assistants work in physicians' offices, hospitals, and other medical facilities, performing both administrative and clinical duties under the supervision of a physician. In the early practice of medicine physicians often treated their patients without assistance. Patients came without appointments and waited as long as necessary to see the physician. They paid for their care with food or whatever they had of value. No records were kept or felt to be necessary. It was rare for a patient to file a lawsuit against a physician, who was considered to be a friend in need.

The practice of medicine has changed dramatically. For one thing, it is now necessary to keep extensive records. The services of a receptionist, secretary, bookkeeper, technician, and medical assistant or nurse are essential. The efficiently run medical practice requires absolute attention to detail to protect the reputation of the physician and make it possible to render the best care possible to the patient.

Physicians generally have no specific training in the handling of business matters. Some physicians handle all the business matters. Other physicians will prefer that the experienced professional medical assistant be prepared, with supervision, to discuss fees, arrange collection of accounts, order supplies, and pay the bills. The medical assistant is expected to type letters from dictation and may be required to compose letters as well. The medical assistant who can manage time and keep patients satisfied is well worth the highest salary the physician can pay.

History of American Association of Medical Assistants ....

In 1955, medical assistants from 15 states met in Kansas City, Kansas, and adopted the name American Association of Medical Assistants (AAMA). The representatives elected pro tem officers and made plans for an organizational meeting in 1956. In October 1956, physicians and advisors of the American Medical Association (AMA) met with 250 members of medical assistant societies from 16 states. At this meeting, the AAMA was officially founded with the advice, assistance, and moral support of the AMA. The founder and first president of the American Association of Medical Assistants was Maxine Williams, Figure 1–10, page 8. The primary purpose of the AAMA was to raise the standards of the medical assistant to a more professional level. Physicians realized then, as they do now, that they needed health care professionals to assist them in the multitude of office duties for which nurses had not been trained. They needed help in strengthening the physician-patient relationship. They also needed to attract young people to the profession.

In 1958, a national emblem was selected for use on AAMA stationery and official publications. The new logo for AAMA is seen in Figure 1–11, page 8. In 1978, the AAMA received word from the U.S. Department of Health, Education and Welfare that medical assisting had been formally recognized as an allied health profession

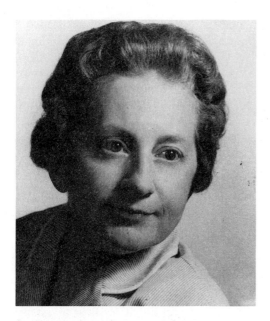

FIGURE 1–10 Maxine Williams, first president of the American Association of Medical Assistants (Courtesy AAMA)

and that its educational programs were eligible for federal funding by the Bureau of Health Manpower.

In February 1991, the AAMA Board of Trustees approved the current definition of medical assisting: "Medical Assisting is a multi-skilled allied health profession whose practitioners work primarily in ambulatory settings, such as medical offices or clinics. Medical assistants function as members of the healthcare delivery team and perform administrative and clinical procedures."

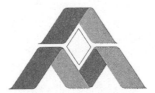

FIGURE 1–11 Logo for American Association of Medical Assistants (Courtesy AAMA)

Occupational Outlook

Physicians are responding to the increasingly complex nature of today's medical care by employing an increasing number of allied health professionals. Data are collected periodically by asking a sample of physicians to identify the number and types of employees in their offices. The current report reflects the recognition of the medical assistant as a major employee category within the medical office. No separate listing was given for such categories as bookkeeper, cashier, file clerk, insurance clerk, and receptionist as had previously been reported by the Bureau of Labor Statistics.

The 1990 edition of *Occupational Projections and Training Data*, published by the United States Department of Labor, Bureau of Labor Statistics, indicated a projected 70% increase in medical assisting. Medical assisting was listed as the fastest growing occupation in

this survey. The occupation of medical secretaries was listed with a 58% projected increase, Table 1–1. In any case, as you can see, you are about to join a large group of health care workers.

TABLE 1–1 U.S. Department of Labor Statistics, April 1990

Occupational Title	1988 Employment	2000 Projected Employment
Medical assistant	149,000	253,000
Medical secretaries	207,000	327,000
Clinical lab technologists and technicians	242,000	288,000
ECG technician	18,000	20,000

(Courtesy R. D. Balthaser, Chairman, Ohio Occupational Information Coordinating Committee)

The medical assistant, as a member of the health care team, is the health care professional who must help make the health care delivery system work for the benefit of all concerned. It is important for the medical assistant to understand the roles of other allied health professionals in the health care profession.

Complete Chapter 1, Unit 1 in the workbook to help you meet the objectives at the beginning of this unit and therefore achieve competency of this subject matter.

UNIT 2

Personal Characteristics

OBJECTIVES

Upon completion of the unit, the student will meet the following terminal performance objectives by verifying knowledge of the facts and principles presented through oral and written communication at a level deemed competent.

1. Discuss the desirable personal characteristics of a medical assistant.
2. Define human relations.
3. Identify methods of maintaining good physical, mental, and emotional health.
4. Spell and define, using the glossary at the back of the text, all the words to know in this unit.

WORDS TO KNOW

adjustments	distinctive	perception
aggressive	intact	project
apprehension	judgment	psychological
authorization	monotone	regimen
contagious		

Desirable Character Traits ·····················

Physicians rank intelligence, dependability, and a pleasant personality as top qualifications for the ideal office assistant. Additional traits that help lead to success are:

- Adaptability
- Empathy
- Enthusiasm
- Friendly attitude
- Genuine liking of people
- Initiative
- Tact
- Willingness to learn
- Discretion
- Good health
- Immaculate appearance
- Pleasant voice and smile

Intelligence

Intelligence is acquired by study of the skills necessary to perform your work. The ability to read and comprehend what is read is essential for a health professional. Use every opportunity you have to expand your knowledge of health care.

Dependability

Dependability is required in many of your duties. Attendance is important because the efficiency of the office in caring for patients decreases when you are absent. You are expected to work without the need of constant supervision. If you do not understand directions, it is essential that you ask for them to be repeated and, if necessary, ask for help. The patient and the physician must be able to trust you at all times.

Pleasant Personality

Personality is of tremendous importance since the medical assistant comes in contact with a constant stream of patients who are not at their best because of illness. Personality can be defined as the sum of mental and moral qualities that make up the distinctive character of an individual. Desirable personality characteristics can be developed if you feel you do not presently possess them. Allen R. Russon, in *Personality Development for Business*, states that "success is ninety percent personality."

Adaptability

In your program of study for becoming a medical assistant you will be given a basic background, but there are always adjustments you must make to fit into each office situation. As you begin employment, you must be careful to find out what is expected. It is only after you are well established in a position that you can suggest what might be better methods of carrying out the work.

Empathy

One of the most important personality traits for a medical assistant, empathy is the ability to put yourself in the patients' place, to know how they feel. Your study of human behavior will help you understand your own behavior as well as that of your patients. Do not confuse empathy with sympathy. Most patients do not want you to feel sorry for them. They simply want you to understand how they feel.

Enthusiasm

If you are enthusiastic about your work you usually look your best, do your best, and people enjoy being around you. You should be careful not to let your enthusiasm appear to be aggressive behavior in your work and patient relationships.

Friendly Attitude and Genuine Liking of People

A friendly attitude will be recognized by the persons you deal with in the office. You should know the names of your patients and use their names in conversation with them. It is extremely important to look directly at your patients. You must also use good judgment and not appear overly friendly. You can create a rewarding working environment if you enjoy working with and for people. This attitude is contagious and people around you usually respond in a positive way. *Human relations* has been defined as the science of dealing with people so that your self-image and theirs remain intact and positive. You have an excellent opportunity to practice this skill as a medical assistant. Courtesy is never out of style. In dealing with all age groups, a simple "please" and "thank you" will go a long way toward communicating your professionalism.

Initiative

A self-starter is a valuable member of a health care team. The physician does not expect always to have to tell you what needs to be done. You should recognize work to be done, even though it may not be your assigned job, and either do the work or offer assistance.

Tact

Tact can be defined as a natural perception of what is right and fitting; quick apprehension of the right thing to say or do in dealing with people in difficult situations. People who are ill are easily upset by things they are told or overhear. For example, you should never be guilty of loud laughter within hearing of patients, who may feel you are laughing at them.

Willingness to Learn

You will find that a willingness to learn advances your professional status. You will also find that your professional skills can always be improved with practice and with new technology. Your knowledge can be expanded by observation, reading, and attending seminars. Physicians recognize the need for continuing education and will often sponsor your attendance at workshops and seminars if you show an interest.

Discretion

You must use good judgment in any discussion regarding your patients. You have access to confidential information that should never be discussed outside of the office. The only exception to this rule would be a possible need to share information with other health professionals if you refer a patient for therapy or treatment. Never give out information about a patient without the patient's written authorization. Keep patient charts and appointment books in an area where the curious cannot look at them. Lock up patient files at night. If you use a computer to make appointments, the screen should be out of the patient's view so that the privacy of other patients is protected.

Good Health

The patients who come into a physician's office gain their first impression of the office from the medical assistant. A neat, attractive assistant has a good psychological effect on everyone who enters the office. To look your best, you must be in good health. You need a balanced regimen of rest, well-balanced meals, exercise, and recreation. As a health professional you are expected to set an example for the patients. If you need medical attention, you should see your own physician without delay.

Immaculate Appearance

Personal cleanliness is the first essential in good grooming. Take a daily bath or shower, use a deodorant or antiperspirant, shampoo your hair at least two or three times a week and more often if it is oily, and brush and floss your teeth regularly. Take special care in the grooming of your hands. Keep a hand cream or lotion at the office to use after washing your hands. Keep your fingernails at a moderate length with colorless or light shades of polish if you are wearing a uniform. Long hair generally should be worn up or at least fastened back out of the face. If you are working with patients, it is generally considered most appropriate to wear a full uniform. The uniform should be clean and free from wrinkles; the

uniform shoes should be clean, with clean shoestrings; and hose should be free from runs or tears. It is good practice to keep an extra clean uniform and pair of hose at the office for emergency use. A stain removal chart is included in the appendix as an aid for you in the care of your uniform. It is recommended the medical assistant wear skin-tone color undergarments; printed patterns usually show through a uniform. The only jewelry suitable with a uniform is a simple chain, wrist watch, and wedding ring. Small earrings may be worn but you may find they tend to get in the way when you answer the telephone. Perfume may be offensive to your patients so it is advisable to use a light fragrance, if any. Mixing scents of soap, hairspray, lotions, and perfume is often offensive. Makeup should be used sparingly.

Good posture can be practiced all the time. The ease with which you move around reflects your poise, and you will experience less fatigue if you practice good posture. You can check your posture by backing up to a wall; if you can place your hand through a space between your lower back and the wall, you need to correct your posture. Focus on extending the spine fully, holding your stomach muscles in, and rolling your buttocks under. Your weight should rest equally on the metatarsals of the feet. Your feet should be several inches apart as you stand. Your shoulder should be relaxed and your ears in a vertical line with your shoulder blades.

Pleasant Voice and Smile

Four characteristics go to make up a pleasing voice; pitch, force, quality, and rate. The pitch of your voice refers to its highness or lowness. If you have a medium pitch you are fortunate because it is generally considered the most pleasing. If you are told your voice sounds high, consider exercises to lower its pitch. Record your voice and listen to it. You can also determine your normal pitch by using a piano for accompaniment. Sing "ah" to find the lowest note you can sing, then sing back up four whole notes. This is your best speaking voice. If you have been speaking above that pitch, practice using the new note as you read aloud. It is unusual to find a need to raise your pitch. Practice at reading aloud will allow you an opportunity to develop variety in your range of pitch. A monotone is not pleasant to listen to.

The force of your voice makes it possible for you to be heard. You generally need little force in office communication. If you find it necessary to increase the intensity of your voice, you will sound less relaxed and you might even be irritating to some patients. You need to project enough to be heard and understood.

The quality of your voice is reflected in the manner in which you pronounce vowels. Relaxation exercises will improve vocal quality. A good relaxation exercise for the jaws is to yawn.

Your speech rate is determined by how long you hold sounds and by pauses between words or phrases. Most of us speak too rapidly. Communication requires understanding and it is extremely hard to understand someone whose words run together and whose enunciation is not clear. Again, you can improve your rate by recording your voice as you read aloud. You can adjust your rate with practice and in doing so improve your communication skills. Practice eliminating "uh" and "er" when you speak. A silent pause while you think is much more pleasant for the listener.

Finally, a genuine smile is a welcome sight to anyone entering the office. It says you acknowledge the individual and are interested in being of service. You may be surprised by how many smiles you receive in return.

Complete Chapter 1, Unit 2, in the workbook to help you meet the objectives at the beginning of this Unit and therefore achieve competency of this subject matter.

U N I T   3
Professionalism

OBJECTIVES ···

Upon completion of the unit, the student will meet the following terminal performance objectives by verifying knowledge of the facts and principles presented through oral and written communication at a level deemed competent.

1. Describe the administrative duties of a medical assistant.
2. Describe the clinical duties of a medical assistant.
3. List areas of employment other than physicians' offices.
4. Describe the possible ways to get approved training.
5. Identify methods of continuing training.
6. Identify the qualifications for and methods of acquiring certification for AAMA (CMA), AAMT, and RMA.
7. Describe methods for revalidation of certification for AAMA (CMA), AAMT, and RMA.
8. Spell and define, using the glossary at the back of the test, all the words to know in this unit.

WORDS TO KNOW ·······································

accreditation	physiology	externship
implications	equivalent	proprietary
autonomous	potential	

Duties of a Medical Assistant ·····················

As you study to become a medical assistant you must be aware that a professional is one trained and skilled in the methods of a profession. In an article in *The Professional Medical Assistant* for January and February of 1987, Barbara Smith defined professionalism as "a state of mind. It is a particular blend of self-esteem, self-confidence, enjoyment of life, respect for the feelings of others, as well as specific knowledge and skills." You must like people. You must like having variety in your work. You must be able to assume responsibility and get things done. You must be methodical and accurate in the work you do. You must be absolutely honest in everything you do. It must be possible to trust you with confidential information. There is no place in the medical office for amateurism. You must develop your skills in communication to ask the necessary questions in making appointments and obtaining medical information. Look directly at your patient with an attitude of caring and a desire to be helpful. Speak clearly and distinctly and use terminology appropriate for the age of the patient. The answers must be accurately recorded. You must look like a professional as described in Unit 2. You must be serious about developing the traits necessary for a successful medical assistant if you do not already possess them.

The duties of a medical assistant vary depending on the size of the office or clinic. In a one-employee office you will have both administrative and clinical duties. In a medium-sized office you might have only administrative or only clinical duties. In a large clinic it is often possible to specialize in one area if you so desire. In any setting you may find yourself helping out in areas other than the one you are regularly assigned to.

All medical assistants need a basic understanding of anatomy, medical terminology, and the legal **implications** of the practice of medicine. Periodically AAMA conducts surveys to determine the competencies necessary for the occupation of medical assisting. This analysis is referred to as the DACUM (**D**evelop **A** **C**urriculum) and identifies areas that should be included in training programs for medical assisting. The 1990 DACUM identified eight general areas of competency. Among the 79 individual skills, 14 were considered advanced and 65 were classified as entry level.

Medical assistants have a wide range of duties in many aspects of a physician's practice. Their business-administrative duties include scheduling and receiving patients; obtaining patient's data; maintaining medical records; typing and transcribing; handling telephone calls, correspondence, reports, and manuscripts; and assuming responsibility for office care, insurance matters, office accounts, fees, and collections.

Their clinical duties may include preparing the patient for examination, obtaining vital signs, taking medical histories, assisting with examinations and treatments, performing routine office laboratory procedures and electrocardiograms, sterilizing instruments and equipment for office procedures, and instructing patients in preparation for radiologic and laboratory examinations.

Modern medical assistants' training serves a vital function in extending the health care potential of the physician. Knowledge of medical terminology, anatomy, and physiology, administrative and clinical assisting skills, and communication skills are all essential. Everyone in the health care profession is involved in the teaching role of helping patients better understand their illness and methods of preventing illness.

Career and Training Opportunities

Training as a medical assistant can be used in many hospital departments, health insurance companies, public health agencies, medical firms, medical schools, and the armed forces, in addition to physicians' offices.

Thirty years ago it was relatively easy to be hired and trained on the job. This still takes place in some offices, but physicians now recognize that office efficiency is dramatically increased with professionally trained personnel.

Vocational schools offer programs for high school students. These graduates are usually fully capable of handling all entry-level duties in a medical office, and many progress rapidly to office manager positions. Instructors might be MAs, registered nurses, licensed practical nurses, or medical technicians; all are medical professionals. The basic medical assistant curriculum is followed, with on-the-job training in the senior year, for which some students are paid.

Many community colleges offer courses leading to a Certificate or Associate Degree. Programs offering a Certificate upon graduation are equivalent to 1 year of training: programs offering an Associate Degree are equivalent to 2 years. Many proprietary schools also train medical assistants. They follow the basic medical assistant curriculum and, in most cases, are taught by professionals with experience as medical assistants. The students serve an externship in an office to complete their training.

American Association of Medical Assistants

The AAMA has established an accreditation program for training programs in medical assisting. Nearly 200 medical assisting programs at the postsecondary level have been accredited by the Committee on Allied Health Education and Accreditation (CAHEA), an autonomous committee of the AMA and an accrediting body sanctioned by the U.S. Department of Education.

Continuing Education

One of the best ways to continue your education is through membership in local, state, and national levels of AAMA. An active member of AAMA must be a Cer-

tified Medical Assistant (CMA) or an individual who was an active member on December 31, 1987 and who maintains continuous active membership. An associate member is one who is not eligible for another category of membership but who is interested in the profession of medical assisting. A student member is one enrolled in a medical assistant program. Student membership may be retained for one dues year after graduation if active or associate membership is not chosen. Physician advisors on all levels often speak before monthly meetings. Physicians offer assistance in paying to attend seminars, workshops, and conventions where topics important to the health professional are shared. Hundreds of educational programs are sponsored by local and state AAMA groups throughout the year. Participants in AAMA-approved workshops can earn Continuing Education Unit (CEU) credit.

As a member of AAMA, you will automatically receive subscriptions to the association's respected publications. *The Professional Medical Assistant*, the bimonthly journal of the AAMA, is devoted to educational articles written by experts in allied health and related fields. In addition, it contains current medical research reports, the latest state and federal health legislative news, education program announcements, and articles offering CEU credit. *The AAMA Network*, the association's quarterly newsletter, contains news of the organization, including board and committee actions and reports on issues important to the profession.

The AAMA offers guided study programs in Law for the Medical Office; Human Relations for the Medical Office; Urinalysis Today; and AIDS Concepts for Medical Assistants. These are professionally designed home study courses that allow medical assistants to learn at their own rate of speed and on their own time. Successful completion of examinations accompanying the guided study courses entitles the medical assistant to CEU credit.

The Maxine Williams Scholarship Fund, named for the first national AAMA president, annually awards several $500 scholarships to students seriously interested in pursuing a career in medical assisting. Scholarships are awarded on the basis of interest, need, and aptitude. Applications are available through the AAMA Executive Office. Completed applications must be postmarked no later than May 1 of the year in which the scholarship will be used.

Certification

The AAMA offers a certification examination designed to evaluate professional competency. Medical assistants, medical assisting educators, and students who successfully complete the examination are entitled to the CMA (Certified Medical Assistant) designation after their names, Figure 1–12. The certification examination is

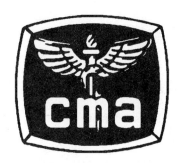

FIGURE 1–12 CMA pin (Courtesy AAMA)

given twice each year at approximately 100 test centers nationwide. The National Board of Medical Examiners serves as educational test consultant and works with the AAMA in preparing the examinations. To be eligible for the certification examination, applicants must meet one of the following requirements. An applicant must be:

- A medical assistant or allied health practitioner who has completed at least 12 months of full-time or 24 months of part-time employment under the supervision of a licensed health care practitioner
- A graduate of a CAHEA-accredited medical assisting program
- A medical assisting instructor in a postsecondary institution approved by a nationally recognized accrediting agency

By mid-1991, approximately 50,000 certificates had been awarded to successful candidates.

Beginning in 1988, certified medical assistants must recertify every five years to demonstrate current knowledge. Recertification reinforces the validity of the CMA credential and helps maintain its continued acceptance by physicians, patients, and other allied health professionals.

The requirement can be met in either of two ways:

- By earning 60 recertification points through continuing education courses or academic credit, with the points distributed equally among the three areas covered in the examination
- By passing the recertification examination

American Association for Medical Transcription

The medical assistant who is employed as a specialist in word processing and machine transcription would benefit from membership in the American Association for Medical Transcription. The association was incorporated in 1978 in Modesto, California. AAMT publishes a bimonthly newsletter and a quarterly journal. State or regional component associations offer members delegate representation at the national convention, and local chapters offer educational opportunities. AAMT has a voluntary certification by examination program. The certification is valid for three years. The member must have accrual of 30 continuing education credits (CECs)

in each three-year cycle for recertification. Recertification may also be accomplished by successfully completing the certification examination again. AAMT has a national convention and offers continuing education programs, workshops, and seminars. AAMT publishes materials specifically for the medical transcription profession.

Registered Medical Assistants

The Registered Medical Assistant (RMA) was established by American Medical Technologists (AMT) in 1972, as a result of a recognized need for certification of medical assistants. Medical assistant training, leading to eligibility to sit for the RMA Certification Examination, may be obtained at a school accredited by the Accrediting Bureau of Health Education Schools (ABHES). Another avenue of eligibility is through the regionally accredited programs in medical assisting. Medical assistants may be eligible by a combination of work and a training program or by verification of five years of work experience without formal training. In 1976, an RMA National Board was organized to allow RMA members (certificants) to operate their own program with continual support and guidance from the AMT. The purpose of the RMA organization is to advance the standards and profession of medical assisting and to promote educational and social advantages for its members. Continuing education is necessary for the medical assistant of today, as this is one of the fastest growing and changing career fields. Through AMTIE (American Medical Technologists Institute for Education) a five-year revalidation process has been developed with the first five-year cycle having been completed in 1987.

Professional Secretaries International® (PSI)®

This organization offers the administrative medical assistant many benefits. PSI® promotes competence and recognition of the professional and represents the interests and welfare of persons working in and preparing for secretarial and related positions. Certified Professional Secretary® (CPS)® is the registered service mark for the rating that has become the recognized standard of measurement of secretarial proficiency. To attain the CPS® rating, a secretary must meet certain education and work experience requirements, and pass the two-day examination. The six-part examination is administered in May and November by the Institute for Certifying Secretaries, a department of PSI®. The CPS® examination has six parts: behavioral science in business, business law, economics and management, accounting, office administration and communication, and office technology.

Complete Chapter 1, Unit 2 in the workbook to help you meet the objectives at the beginning of this unit and therefore achieve competency of this subject matter.

REFERENCES

American Association of Medical Assistants: Medical Assisting Programs; Pride, Partnership, Professionalism. 1989.

American Association of Medical Assistants: Certified Medical Assistants; Healthcare's Most Versatile Professionals. 1989.

American Medical Association.

Encyclopedia of Medicine. Editor: Charles B. Clayman, M.D. New York: Random House, 1989.

Ebony. "Neurosurgery," September 1983, Johnson Publishing Company.

Marks, Geoffrey, and Beatty, William K. *The Story of Medicine in America*, New York: Scribners, 1973.

Mitchell, Paula R., and Grippando, Gloria M., *Nursing Perspectives and Issues*, 5th Ed. Albany: Delmar, 1993.

Peterson, Arlin V., and Allen, Roy C. *The Humanistic Medical Assistant: A Book on Human Relations.* AAMA, 1978.

Raven, Susan, and Weir, Alison. *Women of Achievement.* New York: Harmony, 1981.

Sicherman, Barbara, and Green, Carol Hurd. *Notable American Women: The Modern Period.* Cambridge, MA: Belknap Press, 1980.

U.S. Department of Labor. Occupational Employment Statistics, Washington, DC.

PROFESSIONAL ORGANIZATIONS

American Association of Medical Assistants, 20 North Wacker Drive, Suite 1575, Chicago, IL 60606
(312) 899-1500

American Association for Medical Transcription, 3460 Oakdale Road, Suite M, P.O. Box 576187, Modesto, CA 95355
(209) 551-0883

Professional Secretaries International®, P.O. Box 20404, Kansas City, MO 64195-0404
(816) 891-6600

Registered Medical Assistant of AMT, 710 Higgins Road, Park Ridge, IL 60068
(708) 823-5769

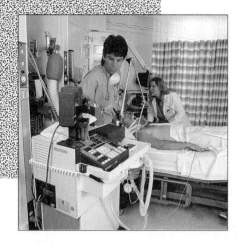

C H A P T E R   2

Overview of Health Care Professions, Medical Specialties, and Other Interests

Ideally, all physicians dedicate their lives to acquiring skills in the art and science of diagnosing and treating disease and maintaining health. Each physician has this same goal. It is, however, impossible for a physician to study in detail every field of medicine. Because of this fact, some physicians become medical specialists. This means that they have chosen to gain expertise in one particular area of medicine. Some doctors additionally have a particular interest that is not a specialty, but is an area they feel worthy of their time and effort and effective in helping their patients toward better health. These areas are viewed as subspecialties or areas of special interest.

Because medical assistants generally are employed by physicians in their offices, they need a basic understanding of the various medical specialties and special interests. The medical assistant who works for a general practitioner may need to initiate contacts with specialists through referrals.

The medical assistant must then be knowledgeable about these areas to help reinforce or clarify the physician's directions to the patient. Moreover, knowing about these various practices will also help the medical assistant to decide in which area to seek employment. Most specialists maintain office practices and have need of medical assistants as general and family practitioners do. Adapting to these special areas after acquiring basic skills and knowledge should be relatively easy. A medical assistant interested in advancement must be willing to put forth the necessary effort.

To help you get familiar with these specialties, Table 2–1 contains basic information concerning each area. You should note that a few specialty practices are not listed in the table. One of those practices is the specialty practice of emergency medicine or traumatic medicine. In this case, the referral may be initiated by the family or general practitioner's office if, when the patient phones in for advice concerning a condition, the patient's symptoms suggest a true emergency or urgency, then referring the patient to an urgent or emergency care center is certainly the procedure. And too,

TABLE 2–1
Medical Specialties

Specialty	Title of Practitioner	Area of Specialization	Types of Patients Seen
Allergy	Allergist	Diagnosing and treating conditions of altered immunological reactivity (allergic reactions)	Adults of all ages, children, both sexes
Anesthesiology	Anesthesiologist	Administering anesthetic agents before and during surgery	Adults of all ages, children, both sexes
Cardiology	Cardiologist	Diagnosing and treating abnormalities, diseases, and disorders of the heart	Adults of all ages, children, both sexes
Chiropractic	Chiropractor. (Chiropractors are not physicians, but they are licensed in their field of practice. They hold the degree of DC, or Doctor of Chiropractic.)	Manipulative treatment of disorders originating from misalignment of the spinal vertebrae	Adults of all ages, children, both sexes
Dentistry	Dentist. (Dentists are not physicians, but they are licensed in their field of practice, which can range from general to highly specialized. They hold the degree of DDS, or Doctor of Dental Surgery.)	Diagnosing and treating diseases and disorders of the teeth and gums	Adults of all ages, children, both sexes
Dermatology	Dermatologist	Diagnosing and treating disorders of the skin	Adults of all ages, children, both sexes
Endocrinology	Endocrinologist	Diagnosing and treating diseases and malfunctions of the glands of internal secretion	Adults of all ages, children, both sexes
Family Practice	Family Practitioner	Similar to general practice in nature, but centering around the family unit	Adults of all ages, infants and children of all ages, both sexes
Gastroenterology	Gastroenterologist	Diagnosing and treating diseases and disorders of the stomach and intestines	Adults of all ages, children, both sexes
Geriatrics	Gerontologist	Diagnosing and treating diseases, disorders, and problems associated with aging	Older adults, both sexes
Gynecology	Gynecologist	Diagnosing and treating diseases and disorders of the female reproductive tract; strong emphasis on preventive measures	Female adolescents and adults
Hematology	Hematologist	Diagnosing and treating diseases and disorders of the blood and blood-forming tissues	Adults of all ages, infants and children, both sexes
Infertility	Infertility Specialist	Diagnosing and treating problems in conceiving and maintaining pregnancy	Married couples who desire to have children but cannot
Internal Medicine	Internist	Diagnosing and treating diseases and disorders of the internal organs	Adults of all ages, children, both sexes
Nephrology	Nephrologist	Diagnosing and treating diseases and disorders of the kidney	Adults, children, both sexes
Neurology	Neurologist	Diagnosing and treating diseases and disorders of the central nervous system	Adults, children, both sexes
Nuclear Medicine	Nuclear Medicine Specialist	Diagnosing and treating diseases with the use of radionuclides (Figure 2–2)	Adults, both sexes
Obstetrics	Obstetrician	Providing direct care to pregnant females during pregnancy, childbirth, and immediately thereafter	Pregnant females
Occupational Medicine	Occupational Medicine Specialist	Diagnosing and treating diseases or conditions arising from occupational circumstances (e.g., chemicals, dust, or gases)	Adults of all ages, both sexes

TABLE 2–1
Medical Specialties (Continued)

Specialty	Title of Practitioner	Area of Specialization	Types of Patients Seen
Oncology	Oncologist	Diagnosing and treating tumors and cancer	Adults of all ages, children, both sexes
Ophthalmology	Ophthalmologist	Diagnosing and treating diseases and disorders of the eye	Adults of all ages, children, both sexes
Optometry	Optometrist (Optometrists are not physicians, but are licensed in their field of practice. They hold the degree of OD, or Doctor of Optometry.)	Measuring the accuracy of vision to determine if corrective lenses are needed	Adults of all ages, children, both sexes
Orthopedics	Orthopedist	Diagnosing and treating disorders and diseases of the bones, muscles, ligaments, and tendons, and fractures of the bones	Adults of all ages, children, both sexes
Otorhinolaryngology	Otorhinolaryngologist (commonly referred to as an ENT Specialist)	Diagnosing and treatment of disorders and diseases of the ear, nose, and throat	Adults of all ages, children, both sexes
Pathology	Pathologist	Analysis of tissue samples to confirm diagnosis	Usually has no direct contact with patients
Pediatrics	Pediatrician	Diagnosing and treating diseases and disorders of children; strong emphasis on preventive measures	Infants, children, and adolescents
Physical Medicine	Physical Medicine Specialist	Diagnosing and treating diseases and disorders with physical agents (physical therapy)	Adults, children, both sexes
Podiatry	Podiatrist (Podiatrists are not physicians, but they are licensed in their field of practice. They hold the degree of DPM, or Doctor of Podiatric Medicine.)	Diagnosing and treating diseases and disorders of the feet	Adults, children, both sexes
Psychiatry	Psychiatrist	Diagnosing and treating pronounced manifestations of emotional problems or mental illness that may have an organic causative factor	Adults of all ages, children, both sexes. (Note: Child Psychiatry is a further specialized field dealing exclusively with children and adolescents.)
Psychology	Psychologist. (Psychologists are not physicians, but they are licensed in their field of practice. They hold the degree of PhD, or Doctor of Philosophy.)	Evaluating and treating emotional problems. These professionals give counseling to individuals, families, and groups	Adults, children, both sexes
Pulmonary Specialties	Pulmonary/Thoracic/Cardiovascular Specialist	Diagnosing and treating diseases and disorders of the chest, lungs, heart, and blood vessels	Adults, both sexes
Radiology	Radiologist	Diagnosing and treating diseases and disorders with roentgen rays (X rays) and other forms of radiant energy	Adults of all ages, children, both sexes
Sports Medicine	Sports Medicine Specialist	Diagnosing and treating injuries sustained in athletic events	Adults, especially young adults (athletes), both sexes
Surgery	Surgeon	Diagnosing and treating diseases, injuries, and deformities by manual or operative methods	Adults of all ages, infants, children, both sexes
Traumatic Medicine	Emergency Physician (commonly referred to as ER or trauma physician since most work in hospital emergency rooms)	Diagnosing and treating acute (traumatic) illnesses and injuries	Adults of all ages, infants, children, both sexes
Urology	Urologist	Diagnosing and treating diseases and disorders of the urinary system of females and genitourinary system of males	Adults of all ages, infants, children

physicians who practice in the specialties of anesthesiology and pathology are usually hospital-based; rarely do they have private practice offices where patients are seen. These specialists work as members of the health care team contributing their expert skills and knowledge in serving patients. More precise knowledge of all these practices will come with experience and further study.

The field of general practice covers perhaps the broadest spectrum. The general practitioner sees all kinds of patients with all kinds of problems. Most can be handled by the general practitioner. If, however, the symptoms of a case suggest a serious or perhaps unknown cause, the patient may be referred to a specialist for further diagnosis and/or treatment, Figure 2–1. When the patient's specific need or problem has been remedied or the recovery plan has been established, the patient returns to the "family doctor" for continued care.

The following pages will introduce you to many fields of medical practice and allied health professions. Because treating patients is a team effort, gaining a basic knowledge of the duties involved in each type of practice will help you better serve the patient. Better communication between colleagues who understand each other leads to more efficient patient care.

U N I T   1

Types of Medical Practice

The Patient

Doctor's Office
Family and General Practitioner

Frequent Referrals	Occasional Referrals
Allergist	**Dentist**
Cardiologist	**Dermatologist**
Gastroenterologist	**Endocrinologist**
Gerontologist	**Infertility Specialist**
Gynecologist	**Nephrologist**
Hematologist	**Nuclear Medicine**
Internist	**Specialist**
Neurologist	**Occupational Medicine**
Obstetrician	**Specialist**
Oncologist	**Physical Medicine**
Ophthalmologist	**Specialist**
Optometrist	**Podiatrist**
Orthopedist	**Psychiatrist**
Otorhinolaryngologist	**Psychologist**
Pediatrician	**Pulmonary/Thoracic/**
Radiologist	**Cardiovascular**
Surgeon	**Specialist**
	Sports Medicine
	Specialist
	Urologist

FIGURE 2–1   Frequency of referrals

OBJECTIVES ....

Upon completion of the unit, the student will meet the following terminal performance objectives by verifying knowledge of the facts and principles presented through oral and written communication at a level deemed competent.

1. Identify the primary medical specialties and give the abbreviations for those that have them.
2. List eight health care professionals with doctoral degrees. Explain who should be called doctor.
3. Name employment possibilities for medical assistants other than with MDs and DOs.
4. Identify and spell correctly the title of each practitioner in each of the specialties.
5. Discuss the educational process of becoming a physician.
6. Spell and define, using the glossary at the back of the text, all the words to know in this unit.

WORDS TO KNOW ....

allergy	internist
anesthesiologist	internship
cardiologist	licensure
chiropractic	maintenance
competency	manifestation
dentist	manipulation therapy
deprivation	misalignment
dermatologist	nephrologist
diplomate	neurologist
doctorates	nuclear medicine
endocrinologist	obstetrician
gastroenterologist	occupational medicine
gerontologist	oncology
gynecologist	ophthalmologist
hematologist	optometrist
immunological	orthopedist
infertility	osteopathy

otorhinolaryngologist
pathologist
pediatrician
perception
podiatrist
practitionerpreventive
proprietorship
psychiatrist
psychologist

psychotherapy
pulmonary
radiologist
radionuclides
residency
surgeon
traumatic
urology

All physicians invest a minimum of nine years in learning how to practice medicine, which is the art and science of the diagnosis, treatment, and prevention of disease, and the maintenance of good health. Until recently, their training, education, and practical experience included a four-year college degree in premed, four years in medical school, and one year of internship. Following this and successful completion of the state board examination for licensure, the person was then considered a general practitioner and was ready to begin a private practice. This license to practice medicine is renewed periodically throughout the physician's life. Today the phrase Postgraduate year following medical school (PGY-1) denotes the internship stage of training. Specialty areas require additional years of study in the particular area of choice. It is usually between two and six years and is commonly known as residency or PGY-2, 3, 4, and so on. After satisfactorily accomplishing all requirements, the physician is awarded a certificate of competency in the specialty area and is recognized as a diplomate of that specialty.

The actual business of practicing medicine may be conducted in several ways. Many physicians prefer to have a solo practice, or sole proprietorship, meaning that the individual alone makes all decisions regarding the practice. Being employed as a medical assistant in this type of office requires that you have both administrative and clinical skills essential for the smooth operation of that practice, especially if you are the only employee.

In a partnership two or more physicians have a legal agreement to share in the total business operation of the practice. In this case, usually two to several medical assistants (or other members of the health care team) are employed to care for patients and conduct business.

A group practice consists of three or more physicians who share a facility for the purpose of practicing medicine. In this legal contract the doctors share expenses, income, equipment, records, and personnel. Many times these practices are a health maintenance organization (HMO) or an independent practice association (IPA) type of practice. You will learn more about these in Chapter 11. Usually several professionals make up the health care team in this setting. Medical assistants, lab technicians, radiology technicians, nurses, physicians assistants, and the physicians work together in providing health care.

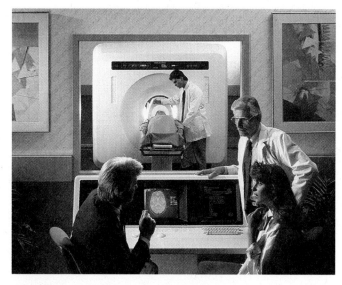

FIGURE 2–2 Magnetic resonance imaging system. The scan is shown on the computer screen on the console in the foreground. (Courtesy of GE Medical Systems)

Subspecialty (S)/
Special Interest (SI) Areas ....

In the following you will be introduced to the subspecialties or special interest areas that branch off from a particular specialty practice. A brief description and definition of each area will give you a basic idea of the roles they play in the health care team. As you learn and study the duties and responsibilities of the medical assistant, you may realize a particular area of interest of your own. When the time comes for your internship and then later for you to begin the job search for gainful employment, you will have a basic understanding of the variety of practices so that you will be better prepared to make a decision of where to apply.

Adolescent Medicine

This area branches from pediatrics and specifically deals with youngsters aged 11 to 20 years, or the years of puberty to maturity. (S)

Acupuncture

This method of treatment originated in the Far East and has been gaining in popularity in western countries since the 1970s. This procedure involves the insertion of fine thin needles into specific sites of the body to alleviate pain or to treat a specific body system or area (its use is still controversial). (SI)

Aerospace Medicine

Physicians who extend their practice of medicine to this area do research in the effects of the environment in space on people. The areas of greatest concern are pathology, physiology, and psychology. (SI)

Alcoholism (Chemical Dependency)

These physicians treat patients who have addiction to alcohol and drugs. (SI)

Allergy and Immunology

An **allergy** is an acquired hypersensitivity a person exhibits to a substance that normally does not cause a reaction. Physicians interested in allergies sometimes combine these areas because they are closely related. **Immunology** is the study of how the body deals with immunity to disease (it is a subspecialty sometimes practiced alone). (S)

Pediatric Allergists

These physicians deal only with treating children who have allergies. (S)

Cardiology (Cardiovascular Disease)

A **cardiologist** is a physician who specializes in treating diseases and disorders of the heart. Because the heart is the center of the circulatory system, a cardiovascular specialist is one who treats only patients with heart and blood vessel problems. (S)

Diabetes

As implied, these physicians have a special interest in treating only patients who have been diagnosed with diabetes. (SI)

Emergency Medicine

Physicians practicing this subspecialty are concerned with the diagnosis and treatment of patients with conditions that have resulted from injury or trauma or from sudden illness. (S)

Preventive Medicine

This branch of medicine deals with the prevention of both mental and physical illness and disease. It is sometimes referred to as General Preventive Medicine (GPM). (S)

Hypertension

A physician who subspecializes in this area treats patients who have high blood pressure (hypertension). (SI)

Hypnosis

This method of treatment is becoming more popular with physicians. This procedure is used mainly in **psychotherapy** in which the patient is induced into a trancelike sleep to help change the memory or the **perception** of something in that person (such as unwanted behavior, i.e., smoking or weight control). Its use in medicine is to help patients deal with pain and stress, which affect their overall health. (SI)

Nutrition

This area of special interest includes patients with disorders or diseases related to how the body utilizes food and drink for growth and maintenance. (SI)

Rheumatology

Physicians in this subspecialty treat inflammatory disorders of the connective tissues and related structures. (S)

Sleep Disorder

As the name implies, physicians who deal with these patients are interested in the various stages of sleep and the effects of sleep **deprivation**. (SI)

Surgery

Most of the subspecialty areas of this branch of medicine and **osteopathy** are listed below:

- Cardiovascular
- Colon (and Rectal)
- Cosmetic (Plastic and Reconstructive)
- Hand
- Head and Neck
- Neurological
- Orthopedic
- Pediatrics
- Spine
- Thoracic
- Urological
- Vascular

With the great strides that medical science achieves, the field of medicine continues to evolve with remarkable new treatments, medications, and discoveries. Being an integral part of the health care team is exciting. New areas of special interest and subspecialties are ever changing with the latest findings. Keeping abreast of these changes by attending ongoing educational programs to increase your knowledge will help you to become not only more confident in your work, but a most valuable medical assistant as well.

A Note Regarding Doctors ....

As you progress in the field of medical assisting, a basic understanding of the frequently misused term *doctor* will be helpful. The term comes from Latin; it means *to teach*. Persons who hold doctoral degrees (*doctorates*) are entitled to be addressed as "Doctor" and to write the initials that stand for their doctorate after their name. The abbreviation "Dr." is the proper way to address a physician or any other type of doctor who has earned this title. In the medical field, the abbreviation "Dr." denotes that the person is qualified to practice medicine. In other fields, it means that the person has achieved the highest academic degree awarded by a college in the particular discipline. The doctors with whom you will be coming into contact include:

- Doctor of Chiropractic (DC)
- Doctor of Dental Medicine (DMD)
- Doctor of Dental Surgery (DDS)
- Doctor of Medicine (MD)
- Doctor of Optometry (OD)
- Doctor of Osteopathy (DO)
- Doctor of Philosophy (PhD)
- Doctor of Podiatric Medicine (DPM)

Doctor of Medicine and Doctor of Osteopathy

One of the areas of greatest confusion is the differentiation between MDs and DOs. Holders of either degree are licensed physicians. The degrees themselves originate from somewhat different schools of thought. (Interestingly enough, it was an MD who founded the osteopathic movement that now produces DOs.) Physicians of both schools must satisfactorily complete board examinations in the state where they wish to practice medicine. In schools of osteopathy, manipulation therapy is an additional skill included in their curriculum. In years past, the scope of practice of DOs was greatly limited by state medical boards. However, in most of the United States today, medical licensing boards permit DOs to perform the same duties as MDs. Should you find employment with either a DO or MD, you will be able to apply the same administrative and clinical knowledge and skills.

Although you are training primarily to assist physicians, with a little adaptation, you could also move into assisting chiropractors, psychologists, or podiatrists. To move into the dental or optometric field would require additional training.

Complete Chapter 2, Unit 1 in the workbook to help you meet the objectives at the beginning of this unit and therefore achieve competency of this subject matter.

UNIT 2

The Health Care Team

OBJECTIVES ......

Upon completion of the unit, the student will meet the following terminal performance objectives by verifying knowledge of the facts and principles presented through oral and written communication at a level deemed competent.

1. List and discuss the allied health care professionals described in this unit.
2. Explain why it is necessary to have a basic understanding of other health care team members.
3. Spell and define, using the glossary at the back of the text, all of the words to know in this unit.

WORDS TO KNOW ......

admissions clerk	paramedic
chiropractor	pharmacist
dental assistant	phlebotomist
dental hygienist	(accessioning tech)
dietitian	physical therapist
electrocardiogram	physician's assistant (PA)
technician (ECG tech)	podiatrist/chiropodist
emergency medical	prophylaxis
technician (EMT)	psychologist
histologist	radiologic technologist
laboratory technician	radiology technician
licensed practical nurse	registered nurse (RN)
(LPN)	respiratory therapy
nurse practitioner	technician
nutritionist	unit clerk
occupational therapist	ultrasound
office manager/business	ventilatory
office manager	X-ray technician

Allied Health Professionals ......

In addition to the physicians you will work with, there are many other health care team professionals for whom you should have a basic understanding and respect for their parts in patient care. Each one performs a specific set of duties for which they were trained. Defined hereafter are the many skilled areas, educational requirements, and primary duties of the most frequently encountered health professionals who cross paths in daily patient care. Many of these members you may not work with directly, but you may have contact with them by telephone or by written communication. Often patients can have several health problems at the same time and cooperation with other members of the health care team to accommodate the patient is vital. Knowing the role each plays in the total health care of patients will enable you to speak more intelligently with others in the medical field and become more efficient at what your role is as the medical assistant.

Admissions Clerk

An admissions clerk in the hospital or medical center has basic medical terminology and administrative medical office skills. Obtaining a basic medical history and other important information from patients when they are admitted is the primary duty of this person. A college degree is desirable, but not essential.

Chiropractor

A **chiropractor** is highly trained and skilled in the mechanical manipulation of the spinal column. The degree of Doctor of Chiropractic, DC, is awarded after the individual completes two years of premedical studies followed by four years of training in an approved chiropractic school.

Dental Assistant

A **dental assistant** helps a dentist in the performance of generalized tasks, including chairside assistance, clerical work, reception, and some radiography and dental laboratory work. The person learns duties in school or on-the-job and becomes certified by taking the national certification examination to become a CDA, Certified Dental Assistant.

Dental Hygienist

A **dental hygienist** is a person with special training to provide dental services under the supervision of the dentist. Services supplied by a dental hygienist include dental *prophylaxis,* radiography, application of medications, and provision of dental education at chairside and in the community.

Electrocardiogram Technician (ECG Tech)

ECG technicians are skilled in performing electrocardiograms and may be employed in medical clinics and hospitals.

Emergency Medical Technician (EMT)

Emergency medical technicians are trained in and responsible for the administration of specialized emergency care and the transportation to a medical facility of victims of acute illness or injury. EMTs have ongoing training following certification and must be recertified every two years.

Histologist

A **histologist** is a medical scientist who specializes in the study of histology, which is the science dealing with the microscopic identification of cells and tissues. Histologists are employed in private laboratories, clinics, and hospitals.

Laboratory Technician

A medical technologist or **laboratory technician** is one who, under the direction of a pathologist or other physician or medical scientist, performs specialized chemical, microscopic, and bacteriologic tests of blood, tissue, and bodily fluids. Those who have successfully completed the examination by the Board of Registry of the American Society of Clinical Pathologists, or a similar professional body, are designated as Certified Medical Technologists.

Nursing

Nursing is the practice in which a nurse assists in the performance of those activities contributing to the health or recovery from illness. The following are specialized areas of nursing:

Nurse Practitioner. A **nurse practitioner** is a **registered nurse (RN)** who, by advanced training and clinical experience in a branch of nursing (they usually hold a Master's degree), has acquired expert knowledge in that special branch of practice. They are employed by physicians in private practice or in clinics.

Registered Nurse. In the United States a registered nurse is defined as a professional nurse who has completed a course of study at a state-approved school of nursing and passed the National Council Licensure Examination (NCLEX-RN). RNs are licensed to practice by individual states. Employment settings for RNs include hospitals, convalescent homes, clinics, and home health care, to name a few.

Licensed Practical Nurse (LPN). Sometimes referred to as licensed vocational nurses, **licensed practical nurses** are trained in basic nursing techniques and direct patient care. They practice under the direct supervision of an RN or a physician and are employed in hospitals and convalescent centers.

Nutritionist

A **nutritionist** studies and applies the principles and science of nutrition (which is the study of food and drink as related to the growth and maintenance of living organisms).

Dietitian. A **dietitian** has specialized training in the nutritional care of groups and individuals and has successfully completed an examination and maintains continuing education requirements of the Commission on Dietetic Registration. This member of the health care team assists patients in regulating their diets. Dietitians are employed in hospitals and clinics.

Occupational Therapist

An **occupational therapist** practices skills of occupational therapy most often in the hospital setting. They may be licensed, registered, certified, or otherwise regulated by law. Occupational therapy is "the use of purposeful activity with individuals who are limited by physical injury or illness, psychosocial dysfunction, developmental or learning disabilities, poverty and cultural differences, or the aging process to maximize independence, prevent disability, and maintain health. The practice encompasses evaluation, treatment, and consultation." (American Occupational Therapy Association)

Office Manager/Business Office Manager

An office manager has managerial skills in the business operations of the medical office or clinic (or hospital). A degree in business administration is most desirable.

Paramedic

Paramedics are also called paramedical personnel and allied health personnel. They act as assistants to physicians or in place of a physician, especially in the military. They are trained in emergency medical procedures and supportive health care tasks.

Pharmacist

A pharmacist is a specialist in formulating and dispensing medications. They are licensed by individual states to practice pharmacy, which is the study of preparing and dispensing drugs. Pharmacists are employed in hospitals, medical centers, and pharmacies. Training consists of two years of postgraduate study in pharmacology.

Phlebotomist

In some areas, the skilled phlebotomists are referred to as accessioning technicians because they are extensively trained in the art of drawing blood for diagnostic laboratory testing. Most often they are lab technicians. They must be nationally certified and are employed in medical clinics, hospitals, and laboratories. (Under the supervision of a physician, the medical assistant who has had instruction, practice on a training arm, and evaluation proving competency in this skill may perform this procedure to obtain blood specimens for analysis.)

Physical Therapist

One licensed to assist in the examination, testing, and treatment of physically disabled or handicapped people and those patients who are going through a physical rehabilitation program following accident, injury, or serious illness through the use of special exercise, application of heat or cold, use of ultrasound therapy, and other techniques is a physical therapist. They qualify by having a BS in physical therapy or getting a special 12-month certificate course after obtaining a BS in a related field.

Physician's Assistant (PA)

A physician's assistant, also called physician's associate, is a person trained in certain aspects of the practice of medicine or osteopathy to provide assistance to the physician. These individuals are trained by physicians and practice under their direct supervision and within the legal license of a physician according to the laws of each state. Training programs vary in length from a few months to two years. They may be nationally certified.

Podiatrist/Chiropodist

Podiatrists and chiropodists are trained to diagnose and treat diseases and disorders of the feet. They may be awarded these degrees: DSC—Doctor of Surgical Chiropody; PodD—Doctor of Podiatry; and with further training, DPM—Doctor of Podiatric Medicine.

Psychologist

Psychologists specialize in the study of the structure and function of the brain and related mental processes. They have a graduate degree in psychology and training in clinical psychology. They provide testing and counseling services to patients with mental and emotional disorders. Psychologists have private practices or may be a part of a group family practice.

Radiology Technician, Radiologic Technologist, X-Ray Technician

An X-ray technician is one who has had specialized training in the various techniques of visualization of the tissues and organs of the body and who under the supervision of a physician radiologist, operates radiologic equipment and assists radiologists and other health professionals. Competence must be proved by the American Registry of Radiologic Technologists.

Respiratory Therapy Technician

Respiratory therapy technicians are graduates of an AMA-approved school designed to qualify persons for the technician certification examination of the National Board for Respiratory Care. These members of the health care team perform procedures of treatment that maintain or improve the ventilatory function of the respiratory tract in patients. The training period for this field is usually a one-year program in a hospital setting, Figure 2–3.

Unit Clerk

A **unit clerk** performs routine clerical and reception tasks in a patient care unit of a hospital. This position requires a self-motivated, mature individual to handle the stress of the hectic pace of coordinating personnel and their duties at the nurses' station. Also called: unit secretary, administrative specialist, ward clerk, or ward secretary. Training is on-the-job or possibly included in a health care program such as medical assisting.

Because medical assistants are the most versatile of all health care workers, it is reasonable for them to seek employment in any of the previously mentioned areas of the medical field. Once these persons have gained basic entry-level skills in medical assisting, they are able to adapt easily to a specialty practice with additional training (the amount of which would obviously depend on the type of practice).

Complete Chapter 2, Unit 2 in the workbook to help you meet the objectives at the beginning of this unit and therefore achieve competency of this subject matter.

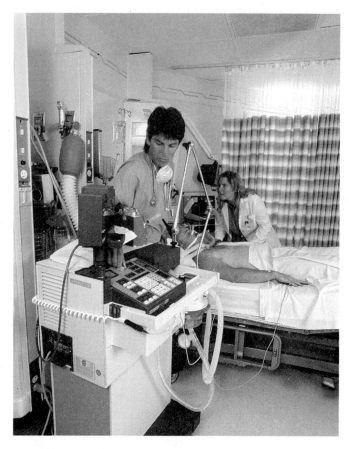

FIGURE 2–3 Respiratory therapist administering breathing treatment to a patient (Courtesy of Puritan Bennett)

REFERENCES

The American Medical Association Family Medical Guide. New York: Random House, 1987.

Diagnostic Tests, Nurse's Ready Reference. Springhouse, PA: Springhouse Corporation, 1991.

Mosby's Medical, Nursing, and Allied Health, 3d ed. St. Louis: C. V. Mosby, 1990.

Reader's Digest Illustrated Encyclopedic Dictionary. Boston: Houghton Mifflin Lexical Databases, 1987.

Sarason, Irwin G. and Sarason, Barbara R. *Abnormal Psychology, The Problem of Maladaptive Behavior,* 5th ed. Englewood Cliffs, NJ: Prentice-Hall, 1987.

Taber, Charles W. *Taber's Cyclopedic Medical Dictionary,* 14th ed. Philadelphia: F. A. Davis, 1983.

Zakus, Sharron. *Mosby's Fundamentals of Medical Assisting: Administrative and Clinical Theory and Technique,* 2d ed. St. Louis: C. V. Mosby, 1990.

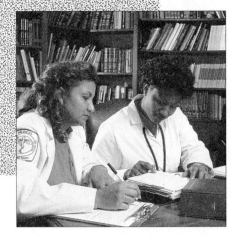

C H A P T E R   3

Basics of Medical Ethics and Medical Law

D uring the past 20 years the numbers of patients bringing lawsuits against physicians has increased dramatically. Medical liability insurance rates have increased so much that physicians in some areas are practicing without liability insurance, although not all states permit this. Laws may be different in different states, but ethical standards are the same in every state. Ethics deal with moral choices and rules of conduct. Both the American Medical Association and the American Association of Medical Assistants have codes of ethics.

UNIT 1
Ethics and Legal Responsibilities

UNIT 2
Professional Liability

U N I T   1

Ethics and Legal Responsibilities

OBJECTIVES ....

Upon completion of this unit, the student will meet the following terminal performance objectives by verifying knowledge of the facts and principles presented through oral and written communication at a level deemed competent.

1. List licensure requirements for physicians.
2. Describe methods of licensure.
3. List exceptions to the need for licensure.
4. Define the components of public and private law.
5. Recognize the differences between ethics and law.
6. Identify areas of medical ethics of particular concern to medical assistants.
7. List the five primary elements of the American Association of Medical Assistants Code of Ethics.
8. Describe the reason diagnostic related groups are causing an ethical issue for physicians.
9. Name one societal group being denied health insurance.
10. List ethical considerations surrounding the life of a fetus.
11. List and define the three categories of medical transplants.

12. Name the most common transplant.
13. Describe a living will.
14. Name four examples of tort law.
15. Define the term *emancipated minor* and give examples.
16. Describe the three parts of the physician-patient contract.
17. Define the terms *implied consent* and *express consent*.
18. Prepare common consent forms used in medical offices.
19. Define the term *privileged communication*.
20. List instances of legally required disclosure.
21. Explain the terms defamation of character, libel, and slander.
22. Describe the conditions for revocation or suspension of a medical license.
23. Spell and define, using the glossary at the back of the text, all the words to know in this unit.

WORDS TO KNOW ....

agent	emancipated minor	peer
assault	enact	reciprocity
battery	endorse	revoke
biennially	explicit	senility
civil	fraudulent	statutes
confidentiality	genetic	surrogate
criminal	insemination	tort
defamation	non compos mentis	

Our founding fathers saw a need for regulation of the practice of medicine and in colonial days medical practice acts were in effect for the protection of citizens. These acts were gradually repealed because it was believed the Constitution gave everyone the right to practice medicine. This resulted in a period of time in the nineteenth century when quackery was common. After a Supreme Court decision in 1899 upheld a state's right to establish qualifications for people wishing to practice medicine, all states soon had once again established medical practice acts. Most state statutes define two basic elements that constitute the practice of medicine. One is diagnosis and the other is the prescribing of treatment. Only a licensed physician can engage in the diagnosis and prescribing of treatment for the physical condition of human beings. In general terms, medical practice acts define the practice of medicine and establish requirements for licensure and grounds for suspending or revoking a license.

Licensure Requirements ....

Licensure requirements are established by each state. A doctor is usually required to:

- be of legal age
- be of good moral character
- have graduated from an approved medical school
- have completed an approved residency program or its equivalent
- be a resident of the state
- have passed the oral and written examinations administered by the Board of Medical Examiners of the state

Physicians who have all of the necessary requirements for licensure may also be licensed by reciprocity or endorsement. A physician who has been licensed in one state and wishes to move to another state may be granted a license by reciprocity if it is determined that the original licensure requirements are equal to the requirements in the new state. Many physicians take the test administered by the National Board of Medical Examiners at the same time they take the first state test. The high standards of the National Board make it possible to obtain a state license by endorsement when the National Board examinations have been successfully passed.

Physicians are required to renew their license annually or biennially. You should be sure the physician has a record of all continuing education units (CEUs) earned since the previous renewal as this is a requirement in many states. Physicians earn CEUs by attending seminars and scientific meetings as well as university courses. The renewal notice will notify the physician of the number of CEUs necessary to renew the license.

There are some exceptions to the rule requiring a current state license to practice medicine. Any physician is free to administer first aid outside the state of residence. Physicians in military service must be licensed to practice medicine in their home states. They do not need to be licensed in the state where they are stationed as long as they practice only on the military base.

The State Board of Medical Examiners provides procedures for revocation or suspension of licensure. In some states the Board has the power to revoke a license and in other states a special review committee has this authority.

A physician may lose the license to practice medicine if convicted of a crime such as murder, rape, violation of narcotic laws, or income tax evasion. A medical license may be revoked for unprofessional conduct. The most usual offenses in this category are betrayal of patient-physician confidence, excessive use of drugs and alcohol, and inappropriate sexual conduct.

A license may be revoked because of proven fraud in the application for a license. In some cases fraudulent diplomas are used. Fraud in the filing of claims for services that were not rendered and fraud in the use of unproven treatments are also grounds for revocation of a license.

Physicians who are found to be incompetent to practice because of senility or mental incapacity may have their license revoked.

Ethical Considerations ....

Whereas laws concern matters enforced through the court system, ethics deal with what is morally right and wrong. The ethical standards established by a profession are administered by peer review, and violation of the standards may result in suspension of membership. The American Medical Association Principles Code of Medical Ethics was revised in 1980 and is reprinted here so that you can see what is expected of a physician.

Physician's Code

Preamble: The medical profession has long subscribed to a body of ethical statements developed primarily for the benefit of the patient. As a member of this profession, a physician must recognize responsibility not only to patients, but also to society, to other health professionals, and to self. The following Principles adopted by the American Medical Association are not laws, but standards of conduct which define the essentials of honorable behavior for the physician.

   I. A physician shall be dedicated to providing competent medical service with compassion and respect for human dignity.

   II. A physician shall deal honestly with patients and colleagues, and strive to expose those physicians deficient in character or competence, or who engage in fraud or deception.

   III. A physician shall respect the law and also recognize a responsibility to seek changes in those requirements which are contrary to the best interests of the patient.

IV. A physician shall respect the rights of patients, of colleagues, and of other health professionals, and shall safeguard patient confidence within the constraints of the law.

V. A physician shall continue to study, apply, and advance scientific knowledge, make relevant information available to patients, colleagues, and the public, obtain consultation, and use the talents of other health professionals when indicated.

VI. A physician shall, in the provision of appropriate patient care, except in emergencies, be free to choose whom to serve, with whom to associate, and the environment in which to provide medical services.

VII. A physician shall recognize a responsibility to participate in activities contributing to an improved community.

(Used with permission of the American Medical Association. From the *American Medical Association Principles of Medical Ethics.* Adopted by the AMA House of Delegates, July 1980.)

Medical Assistant's Code

As an agent of the physician, you too are governed by ethical standards. It must be remembered that the primary objective of the practice of medicine is the welfare of the patient, not the making of a profit. Some offices now notify patients of interest charges on overdue accounts in a brochure introducing the patient to the office practice. The notice of possible interest charge is also included on all billing statements. Some physicians charge for missed appointments and preparing more than one insurance form.

The physician must release patient information when the patient authorizes the release or if the release is required by law. State laws vary regarding release of information. Information that must be reported includes:

- Births and deaths
- Cases of violence such as gunshot wounds, knifings, and poisonings
- Sexually transmitted diseases
- Suspected cases of child abuse
- Cases of contagious, infectious, or communicable diseases

Medical assistants should check with local authorities for the procedures to be followed in making these reports. They need to be aware also of other required local reports. When a physician moves or retires it is important that the original records be kept until the period for filing of liability suits has expired. A copy of the records is provided to a new physician.

The American Association of Medical Assistants Code of Ethics is in many respects similar to that of the American Medical Association.

CODE OF ETHICS
of the American Association of Medical Assistants

The Code of Ethics of AAMA shall set forth principles of ethical and moral conduct as they relate to the medical profession and the particular practice of medical assisting.

Members of AAMA dedicated to the conscientious pursuit of their profession, and thus desiring to merit the high regard of the entire medical profession and the respect of the general public which they do serve, do pledge themselves to strive always to:

A. render service with full respect for the dignity of humanity;
B. respect confidential information obtained through employment unless legally authorized or required by responsible performance of duty to divulge such information;
C. uphold the honor and high principles of the profession and accept its disciplines;
D. seek to continually improve the knowledge and skills of medical assistants for the benefit of patients and professional colleagues;
E. participate in additional service activities aimed toward improving the health and well-being of the community.

MEDICAL ASSISTANT'S CREED

The creed of the American Association of Medical Assistants reads as follows:

I believe in the principles and purposes of the profession.
I endeavor to be more effective.
I aspire to render greater service.
I protect the confidence entrusted to me.
I am dedicated to the care and well-being of all patients.
I am loyal to my physician-employer.
I am true to the ethics of my profession.
I am strengthened by compassion, courage, and faith.

(Copyright by the American Association of Medical Assistants, Inc. Used with permission.)

You will often find it necessary to make decisions based on the professional nature of your employment. Patients can be extremely insistent at times, but you must be firm in carrying out the expectations of your employer and your profession. A patient may, for instance, demand that you call in a prescription for medication when the physician is not immediately available. You have to stand your ground and say that only the physician can give you the orders to do this. You then carefully record on the chart the request of the patient and how it was taken care of. *Never put yourself in the position of practicing medicine.*

The Federal Drug Administration has established five categories, or "schedules," which classify chemical substances with specific regulations as to their use. The states also have laws that further define the use of drugs. It is important for the medical assistant to understand that only the physician can legally prescribe medications. The medical assistant must understand that certain medications cannot be refilled and that restrictions limit the number of times some medications can be refilled. Some drugs require written prescription only to be filled, while others can be called in by telephone.

The United States Department of Justice Drug Enforcement Administration publishes a physician's manual that gives all the information necessary for office personnel to understand the provisions of the Controlled Substances Act. This booklet is free and is furnished on request.

The Drug Enforcement Administration also publishes a *Pharmacist's Manual*, which lists seven recommendations for physicians about the care and security of prescription pads. These will help reduce the number of forged prescription orders:

1. Treat prescription pads like a personal checkbook.
2. Maintain adequate security for prescription pads.
3. Stock only a minimum number of prescription pads.
4. Keep prescription pads in your possession when you are actively using them.
5. Do not leave prescription pads unattended. When not in use, place them in a locked desk or cabinet.
6. Store surplus prescription pads in a locked drawer or in a safe, appropriate place.
7. Report any prescription pad theft to local pharmacies as well as to the state board of pharmacy.

In the practice of medicine it can be difficult to distinguish between legal and ethical issues. The trend in the United States is to demand good health care as a right for everyone. However, not all citizens are willing to finance such a program. The present use of diagnostic related groups (DRGs) in determining the payment hospitals will receive for Medicare patients raises both ethical and legal questions. The problem with the system arises when patients may be discharged too early simply because the hospital will not be paid for more than the DRG-allowed number of days. The physician knows the legal responsibility is to the well-being of the patient, but the hospital must have money to stay in business. The physician wants to stay in good standing with the hospital. In a recent decision in California (Wickline versus State of California), a physician was held liable for releasing a patient too early. In fact, the physician had failed to protest the third party's decision to shorten the patient's recommended hospital stay. In this case, the third party payer was a California Medicare agency called Medi Cal.

Insurance companies are presenting more ethical questions to medical care providers when they refuse insurance to individuals who have acquired immune deficiency syndrome (AIDS) and the AIDS-related complex (ARC).

Many ethical considerations surround the life of a fetus, an infant's birth, and the newborn. New technolo-gies allow us to have more control over birth by detecting *in utero* abnormalities. The improved techniques of artificial insemination bring before the court system the problems associated with surrogate motherhood and paternal responsibility. Many advances have been made in the use of fetal tissue in transplants. Our society must study the ethical and emotional considerations of ending a pregnancy if a serious genetic deficiency is found before birth or allowing the infant to be born handicapped. We seem to have more questions than answers at the present time.

The use of transplants has added another series of ethical problems. Medical transplants are divided into three categories:

- Autograft transplantation of a person's own tissue (can also be used to describe transplant between identical twins)
- Homograft transplantation of tissue from one person to another
- Heterograft transplantation of animal tissue to humans

The blood transfusion is the most common transplant. Nearly all the major organs of the body may be transplanted, and research continues to improve these possibilities.

The Uniform Anatomical Gift Act ....

The Uniform Anatomical Gift Act was passed in 1968. By 1978 it was reported that all 50 states had established some system of organ and tissue donor identification once an individual died. Any person of sound mind and legal age may give any part of the body after death for research or transplant. The family may make this decision for the donor if the donor has not done so while living. The time of death must be determined by a physician who will not be involved in the transplant in any way. No money can be exchanged for making an anatomical donation. Many states allow residents to mark and sign a donor card on the back of the driver's license.

Different ethical problems affect the use of organs from living donors. As the technology of transplantation becomes more readily available, the demand for organs will grow. Human organs should never be sold for profit, but our western ethics are not always followed worldwide. In a book titled *Law, Liability, and Ethics for Medical Office Personnel*, Myrtle Flight discusses the medical community's concern over the sale of human organs for transplant. One source has estimated that by the year 2000, most of the poor in India will learn to survive with only one kidney as the result of the common practice of selling kidneys to wealthy foreigners.

Living Will ....

The health care team will provide a larger percentage of care to geriatric patients as the quality of care extends

Society for the Right to Die

250 West 57th Street/New York, NY 10107

Living Will Declaration

INSTRUCTIONS
Consult this column for help and guidance.

T₀ My Family, Doctors, and All Those Concerned with My Care

I, _____, being of sound mind, make this statement as a directive to be followed if I become unable to participate in decisions regarding my medical care.

This declaration sets forth your directions regarding medical treatment.

If I should be in an incurable or irreversible mental or physical condition with no reasonable expectation of recovery, I direct my attending physician to withhold or withdraw treatment that merely prolongs my dying. I further direct that treatment be limited to measures to keep me comfortable and to relieve pain.

You have the right to refuse treatment you do not want, and you may request the care you do want.

These directions express my legal right to refuse treatment. Therefore I expect my family, doctors, and everyone concerned with my care to regard themselves as legally and morally bound to act in accord with my wishes, and in so doing to be free of any legal liability for having followed my directions.

You may list specific treatment you do <u>not</u> want. For example:

Cardiac resuscitation
Mechanical respiration
Artificial feeding/fluids by tubes

Otherwise, your general statement, top right, will stand for your wishes.

I especially do not want: _____

_____

_____

_____

_____

_____

You may want to add instructions for care you <u>do</u> want—for example, pain medication; or that you prefer to die at home if possible.

Other instructions/comments: _____

_____

_____

_____

Proxy Designation Clause: Should I become unable to communicate my instructions as stated above, I designate the following person to act in my behalf:

Name_____

Address_____

If you want, you can name someone to see that your wishes are carried out, but you do not have to do this.

If the person I have named above is unable to act in my behalf, I authorize the following person to do so:

Name_____

Address_____

Sign and date here in the presence of two adult witnesses, who should also sign.

Signed:_____Date:_____

Witness:_____Witness:_____

Keep the signed original with your personal papers at home. Give signed copies to doctors, family, and proxy. Review your Declaration from time to time; initial and date it to show it still expresses your intent.

FIGURE 3-1 Living will declaration. Choice in Dying makes available legally recognized document forms to residents of states that have enacted right-to-die laws. For people in states that have not enacted right-to-die laws, Choice in Dying supplies Durable Power of Attorney for Health Care forms. (Reprinted by permission of Choice in Dying (formerly Concern for Dying/Society for the Right to Die), 200 Varick Street, New York, New York 10014)

Health Care Proxy

(1) I, _____

hereby appoint _____
(name, home address and telephone number)

as my health care agent to make any and all health care decisions for me, except to the extent that I state otherwise. This proxy shall take effect when and if I become unable to make my own health care decisions.

(2) Optional instructions: I direct my proxy to make health care decisions in accord with my wishes and limitations as stated below, or as he or she otherwise knows. (Attach additional pages if necessary).

_____

_____

(Unless your agent knows your wishes about artificial nutrition and hydration [feeding tubes], your agent will not be allowed to make decisions about artificial nutrition and hydration. See the preceding instructions for samples of language you could use.)

(3) Name of substitute or fill-in proxy if the person I appoint above is unable, unwilling or unavailable to act as my health care agent.

_____
(name, home address and telephone number)

(4) Unless I revoke it, this proxy shall remain in effect indefinitely, or until the date or condition stated below. This proxy shall expire (specific date or conditions, if desired):

_____

(5) Signature _____
Address _____
Date _____

Statement by Witnesses (must be 18 or older)

I declare that the person who signed this document is personally known to me and appears to be of sound mind and acting of his or her own free will. He or she signed (or asked another to sign for him or her) this document in my presence.

Witness 1 _____
Address _____
Witness 2 _____
Address _____

FIGURE 3-2b Durable Power of Attorney for Health Care. (Reprinted by permission of Choice in Dying (formerly Concern for Dying/Society for the Right to Die), 200 Varick Street, New York, New York 10014)

About the Health Care Proxy

This is an important legal form. Before signing this form, you should understand the following facts:

1. This form gives the person you choose as your agent the authority to make all health care decisions for you, except to the extent you say otherwise in this form. "Health care" means any treatment, service or procedure to diagnose or treat your physical or mental condition.

2. Unless you say otherwise, your agent will be allowed to make all health care decisions for you, including decisions to remove or withhold life-sustaining treatment.

3. Unless your agent knows your wishes about artificial nutrition and hydration (nourishment and water provided by a feeding tube), he or she will not be allowed to refuse those measures for you.

4. Your agent will start making decisions for you when doctors decide that you are not able to make health care decisions for yourself.

You may write on this form any information about treatment that you do not desire and/or those treatments that you want to make sure you receive. Your agent must follow your instructions (oral and written) when making decisions for you.

If you want to give your agent written instructions, do so right on the form. For example, you could say:

If I become terminally ill, I don't want to receive the following treatments: . . .

If I am in a coma or unconscious, with no hope of recovery, then I don't want: . . .

If I have brain damage or a brain disease that makes me unable to recognize people or speak and there is no hope that my condition will improve, I don't want: . . .

Examples of medical treatments about which you may wish to give your agent special instructions are listed below. This is not a complete list of the treatments about which you may leave instructions.

- artificial respiration
- artificial nutrition and hydration (nourishment and water provided by feeding tube)
- cardiopulmonary resuscitation (CPR)
- antipsychotic medication
- electric shock therapy
- antibiotics
- psychosurgery
- dialysis
- transplantation
- blood transfusions
- abortion
- sterilization

Talk about choosing an agent with your family and/or close friends. You should discuss this form with a doctor or another health care professional, such as a nurse or social worker, before you sign it to make sure that you understand the types of decisions that may be made for you. You may

also wish to give your doctor a signed copy. You do not need a lawyer to fill out this form.

You can choose any adult (over 18), including a family member, or close friend, to be your agent. If you select a doctor as your agent, he or she may have to choose between acting as your agent or as your attending doctor; a physician cannot do both at the same time. Also, if you are a patient or resident of a hospital, nursing home or mental hygiene facility, there are special restrictions about naming someone who works for that facility as your agent. You should ask staff at the facility to explain those restrictions.

You should tell the person you choose that he or she will be your health care agent. You should discuss your health care wishes and this form with your agent. Be sure to give him or her a signed copy. Your agent cannot be sued for health care decisions made in good faith.

Even after you have signed this form, you have the right to make health care decisions for yourself as long as you are able to do so, and treatment cannot be given to you or stopped if you object. You can cancel the control given to your agent by telling him or her or your health care provider orally or in writing.

Filling Out the Proxy Form

Item (1) Write your name and the name, home address and telephone number of the person you are selecting as your agent.

Item (2) If you have special instructions for your agent, you should write them here. Also, if you wish to limit your agent's authority in any way, you should say so here. If you do not state any limitations, your agent will be allowed to make all health care decisions that you could have made, including the decision to consent to or refuse life-sustaining treatment.

Item (3) You may write the name, home address and telephone number of an alternate agent.

Item (4) This form will remain valid indefinitely unless you set an expiration date or condition for its expiration. This section is optional and should be filled in only if you want the health care proxy to expire.

Item (5) You must sign and date the proxy. If you are unable to sign yourself, you may direct someone else to sign in your presence. Be sure to include your address.

Two witnesses at least 18 years of age must sign your proxy. The person who is appointed agent or alternate agent cannot sign as a witness.

New York State Department of Health

Distributed by Concern for Dying
250 West 57th Street, New York, NY 10107

FIGURE 3-2a Durable Power of Attorney for Health Care. (Reprinted by permission of Choice in Dying (formerly Concern for Dying/Society for the Right to Die), 200 Varick Street, New York, New York 10014)

our life expectancy. It is important that everyone in the office listen to elderly patients and allow them to make decisions regarding a living will, Figure 3–1, page 29. A majority of the states now have laws that define policies on withholding life-sustaining procedures from hopelessly ill patients. The will is signed when the patient is competent and must be witnessed by two individuals. The effect of this will is to protect the wishes of the patient who may become incompetent and thus unable to make rational decisions. The family of the patient and the physician should receive a copy of the document.

Choice in Dying, Inc. now stresses the importance of also completing a Durable Power of Attorney for Health Care, authorized by either your state's statute or some other legal authority. This allows you to appoint another person (known as your agent) to make health care decisions for you if at any time you become unable to make them yourself. It is strongly advised that an individual appoint an agent, assuming there is someone who can be trusted to make the decisions you would make if you could, and who is willing to act for you in this way, Figure 3–2. It may be helpful to record the wishes of a living will and power of attorney on a video tape so there could be no doubt the patient made the statements regarding care.

A new medical "Miranda warning" law approved by Congress and signed by President Bush gives patients legal options for refusing or accepting treatment if they are incapacitated. The law, which took effect in November 1991, applies to hospitals, hospices, nursing homes, health maintenance organizations (HMOs) and other health care facilities that receive money from Medicare and Medicaid programs. Under the law, patients must receive written information explaining their right-to-die options according to their state laws. The law stipulates that hospitals and other providers must note on medical records whether patients have legal directives on treatment. Providers also must have procedures to ensure they comply with a patient's wishes.

Every medical assistant should be trained to use cardiopulmonary resuscitation (CPR). An ethical question arises when the elderly patient does not wish to receive CPR in the event of a cardiopulmonary arrest. The courts have held that individuals have the right to make decisions that affect their own deaths.

Legal Considerations ....

In the United States the laws are divided into the categories of public law and private law. The various branches of public law include criminal law, constitutional law, administrative law, and international law. Criminal law deals with offenses against all citizens. The practice of medicine without a license is an offense under the criminal law. Constitutional law defines the powers of the government and its citizens. Each state has a constitution which defines its powers over matters not covered by the federal government, which are spelled out in the U.S. Constitution. Administrative law is concerned with the powers of government agencies. International law is concerned with agreements and treaties between countries.

The practice of medicine is primarily affected by private law or civil law, specifically by contract law and torts law. The patient-physician relationship is considered a contractual one. A tort is defined as any of a number of actions done by one person or group of persons that cause injury to another. Violations of tort law may be intentional or negligent. The negligent injury, when committed by a physician in the course of professional duties, is commonly referred to as *malpractice*. Intentional torts also result in professional liability suits. Libel and slander are two forms of defamation. Libel refers to written statements, slander to oral remarks. Assault is defined as a deliberate attempt or threat to touch without consent. Another intentional wrong is battery, which is the unauthorized touching of another person. A patient has a right to refuse treatment. Other civil laws govern property ownership, corporations, and inheritance.

The contract between a patient and a physician has three parts. They are the offer, the acceptance, and the consideration. The offer takes place when a competent individual indicates a desire to become a patient. The acceptance takes place when an appointment is given and the physician examines the patient. The consideration is the payment given in exchange for services. When a child is a patient, the parent is expected to pay. A young person is considered to be a minor until reaching full legal age, known as the age of majority. The statutes defining the age of majority vary from state to state. The medical assistant needs to be aware that the rights of minors in medical treatment are changing. More than half of the states allow minors the right to consent to treatment or consultation for pregnancy, contraception, venereal disease, drug abuse, or alcoholism.

An emancipated minor is an individual who is no longer under the care, custody, or supervision of parents. The emancipated minor may be married, in the armed forces, or self-supporting and living apart from parents. An emancipated minor can legally consent to medical care.

An individual who has been judged by the courts to be mentally incompetent must have an appointed guardian. The general legal term for all varieties of mental illness is non compos mentis. The guardian is responsible for both the payment of bills and the care of the patient. In this case the parents are not responsible for payment. When a patient-physician contract is entered into, the physician is responsible for the care of that patient until the physician officially withdraws from the case or the patient discharges the physician.

The contract between the patient and the physician may be either implied or written. An express, or written, contract must be entered into if a third party is to be responsible for payment. If this agreement is not in writ-

```
                        FORM P-2
            CONSENT TO OPERATION, ANESTHETICS, AND
               OTHER MEDICAL SERVICES (ALTERNATE FORM)

                                                      A.M.
                      Date_____Time_____  P.M.
    1. I authorize the performance upon_____
                            (myself or name of patient)
of the following operation_____
                         (state name of operation)
to be performed under the direction of Dr._____
    A. The nature of the operation_____
                              (describe the operation)
_____
_____
    B. The purpose of the operation_____
                              (describe the purpose)
_____
    C. The possible alternative methods of treatment_____
_____
    (describe alternative methods)
    D. The possible consequences of the operation_____
_____
    (describe the possible consequences)
    E. The risks involved_____
_____
    (describe the risks involved)
    F. The possible complications_____
_____
    (describe the possible complications)
    3. I have been advised of the serious nature of the operation and have
been advised that if I desire a further and more detailed explanation of
any of the foregoing or further information about the possible risks or
complications of the above listed operation it will be given to me.
    4. I do not request a further and more detailed listing and explanation
of any of the items listed in paragraph 2.
                      Signed_____
                          (Patient or person authorized
                             to consent for patient)
Witness_____
```

FIGURE 3-3   Consent to operation, anesthetics, and other medical services. (Courtesy American Medical Association)

ing, it is not possible to press for payment. There are also implied consent and express consent agreements between patients and physicians. The fact that the patient has come to see the physician implies consent for treatment. The instances when express consent is required are:

- proposed surgery or other invasive treatments such as cerebrospinal taps
- use of experimental drugs
- use of unusual procedures that may involve high risk

There are exceptions to the rule for surgery. Minor procedures generally involve explanation by the physician and the oral consent of the patient. The notes regarding this conversation need to be entered by the physician in the patient record.

The American Medical Association has developed recommended standardized forms to be used by physicians, Figure 3–3. It will be your responsibility to know what consent forms your employer uses. The physician may wish to develop forms individualized for the practice. It is important that these be explicit as to what is to be done. Experiments have been conducted using a tape recorder to keep a record of the information given the patient before a consent form is signed. These were discussions with patients who had to be told they had can-

cer. Most of these patients had little or no memory of what had been discussed because they were extremely upset by the diagnosis. In some of these cases the patients were certain they were not fully informed, but the replay of the tape proved they had been. The medical assistant should understand that the physician must be legally responsible for obtaining informed consent from a patient. You should not be given that responsibility. Informed consent is necessary to avoid a claim of assault and battery. The law describes this as a threat to make a physical attack on someone and carrying out the attack. You will be expected to prepare consent forms and ideally be present to listen so that you may help determine whether the patient understood before signing the consent form.

If an all-purpose form is used, it is important to cross out the paragraphs that do not apply. You may be asked to sign as a witness. What you say when you ask a patient to sign after the physician has explained the risks is important. A suggested statement is: "If you have no further questions for the doctor and you understand the consent form, will you please sign it?"

If a physician is to treat a patient with unusual or experimental medication, it is best to use a consent to treatment

Form P-22
CONSENT TO TREATMENT

Date _____ Time _____ A.M. / P.M.

I have been informed by Dr. _____ of the nature, risks, possible alternative methods of treatment, possible consequences, and possible complications involved

in the treatment by means of _____

_____

_____

for the relief of _____

_____

Nevertheless, I authorize Dr. _____ to administer such treatment to me.

Signed _____
(Patient or person authorized to consent for patient)

Witness _____

FIGURE 3-4 Consent for treatment. (Courtesy American Medical Association)

Form P-17
REQUEST FOR STERILIZATION

Date _____ Time _____ A.M. / P.M.

We, the undersigned husband and wife, each being more than twenty-one years of age and of sound

mind, request Dr. _____, and assistants of his choice, to per-

form upon _____, the following operation: _____
(name of patient)

_____
(state nature and extent of operation)

It has been explained to us that this operation is intended to result in sterility although this result has not been guaranteed. We understand that a sterile person is NOT capable of becoming a parent.

We voluntarily request the operation and understand that if it proves successful the results will be permanent and it will thereafter be physically impossible for the patient to inseminate, or to conceive or bear children.

Signed _____
(Husband)

Signed _____
(Wife)

Witness _____

Form P-18
REQUEST FOR STERILIZATION
(ALTERNATE FORM)

Date _____ Time _____ A.M. / P.M.

1. I authorize the performance upon myself of the following operation _____

_____
(state name of operation)

to be performed by or under the direction of Dr. _____.

2. It has been explained to me that this operation is intended to result in my sterility, but no such result has been guaranteed.

3. I understand that a sterile person is NOT capable of becoming a parent.

4. I understand that if the operation proves successful the results will be permanent and it will thereafter be physically impossible for me to inseminate, or to conceive or bear children.

5. The nature of this operation, the possible alternative methods of treatment, the risks involved, the possible consequences, the possibility that the operation may be unsuccessful, and the possibility of

complications have been explained to me by Dr. _____ and

by _____.

Signed _____

Witness _____

I have read the above REQUEST FOR STERILIZATION and do hereby consent to the operation under

the terms therein set forth as the spouse of _____.

Signed _____

Date _____ Time _____

FIGURE 3-5 Request for sterilization. (Courtesy American Medical Association)

---

form, Figure 3–4. When a physician is to perform a sterilization procedure, it is preferable to have both husband and wife sign a request for sterilization form, Figure 3–5.

Patients have the right to privacy when they are being examined and treated. Many physicians have arrangements with medical facilities to offer training opportunities for medical students or residents, but the patient has the right to refuse to have observers present. Therefore, physicians may protect themselves by having an authority to admit observers form signed, Figure 3–6, page 34.

Information contained in a patient medical record and information exchanged between a physician and a patient are considered to be privileged communications. Every patient has a legal right to privacy and **confidentiality.** Information disclosed to the health care team must be kept in the strictest confidence, and you must be ever mindful of the legal implications of handling patient's records. Information concerning patients may be given to another member of the health care team, such as a laboratory technician or referring physician, only when it pertains directly to the course of treatment. Another medical office may telephone to inquire about a patient's medical history for diagnostic purposes, to confirm symptoms, or to verify birthdate. In complying with referral appointments or scheduled tests, patients will have given implied consent for necessary information to be transmitted concerning their condition.

Medical information may be given to parties not concerned in the patient's treatment only when the patient has signed a release of information form.

A large number of states have privileged communication statutes that have been **enacted** to offer additional protection to the patient. You will find that curious and well-meaning friends and relatives ask about patients and you must remember to give only information that has been authorized by the patient. Each time a patient authorizes release of information the form must state specifically who is to receive what information covering what time period. This authorization must be kept in the medical record.

All health care providers must be aware of any state regulations governing the reporting of human immunodeficiency virus (HIV) positive tests. At issue is the right of the AIDS patient to confidentiality and the rights of citizens to be protected from accidental exposure to the HIV virus. Such exposure might occur when police, fire, emergency medical personnel, or any medical personnel come into direct contact with the blood or body fluids of a patient whose diagnosis of AIDS is not known to the personnel.

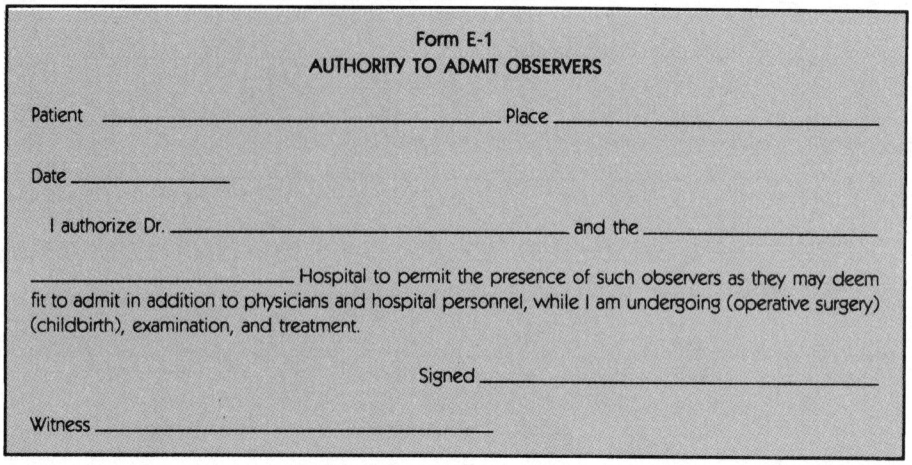
Form E-1
AUTHORITY TO ADMIT OBSERVERS

Patient ______________________ Place ______________________

Date ____________

I authorize Dr. ______________________ and the ______________

______________ Hospital to permit the presence of such observers as they may deem fit to admit in addition to physicians and hospital personnel, while I am undergoing (operative surgery) (childbirth), examination, and treatment.

Signed ______________________

Witness ______________________

FIGURE 3-6 Authority to admit observers. (Courtesy American Medical Association)

In all 50 states, confirmed cases of AIDS constitute a reportable condition either by statute or administrative regulation.

Complete Chapter 3, Unit 1 in the workbook to help you meet the objectives at the beginning of this unit and therefore achieve competency of this subject matter.

UNIT 2

Professional Liability

OBJECTIVES

Upon completion of this unit, the student will meet the following objectives by verifying knowledge of the facts and principles presented through oral and written communication at a level deemed competent.

1. List rights of the physician in providing medical care.
2. List rights of the patient in receiving medical care.
3. Describe the correct procedure for terminating the physician-patient contract.
4. Define and give examples of abandonment.
5. Define and give examples of professional negligence.
6. Give an example of an implied agreement.
7. Describe the precaution that should be observed in giving written instructions to a patient.
8. List the reasons for keeping medical records.
9. Describe who owns medical office records and who has a right to the information in them.
10. List the record keeping necessary to provide legally adequate records.
11. What kinds of notes are not appropriate in a patient chart? Why?
12. Name the six basic principles for preventing unauthorized disclosure of patient information.
13. List six office procedures that cause problems when the physician is involved in a lawsuit.
14. Describe the acceptable method for making changes in medical records.
15. Spell and define, using the glossary at the back of the text, all the words to know in this unit.

WORDS TO KNOW

abandonment	encompass
breach	enumerate
chronological	harmonious
competent	obligate
confrontation	procrastination
criterion	res ipsa loquitur
defamation	respondeat superior
deposition	subpoena duces tecum
doctrine	tort

Physician and Patient Rights

Physicians have the right to determine whom they will accept as patients. Physicians who have been in practice for a long period of time may build up a patient load that is as large as one person can adequately care for. Since a physician must care for all patients accepted, it is not unusual to have to decide to see no new patients. A physician may not, on the other hand, refuse to provide emergency service if assigned to an emergency service, and most physicians will provide emergency service whenever the need exists, since they do not have to continue the patient's treatment. Physicians have the right to decide what types of medicine they wish to practice and where. They have the right to establish their own working hours, to charge for their services, and to take a vacation if they provide names of qualified substitutes to care for their patients while they are unavailable. Physicians have the right to change the location of their office but must notify patients in advance to give them adequate time to make alternate plans for medical care.

Patients have the right to receive care equal to the standards of care in the community as a whole. Patients have the right to choose the physician they wish to receive treatment from. However if a patient becomes a member of an HMO, the right to choose a physician may be restricted to physicians who are members of the chosen HMO. A patient has the right to accept or reject treatment, and to know when treatment is prescribed whether it has side effects, what the prognosis is, what effect the treatment will have on the body, and any alternatives to treatment.

A physician may choose to withdraw from the care of a patient who does not follow instructions for treatment or follow-up appointments or who leaves a hospital against advice. Withdrawal must be by means of a letter sent by certified mail with return receipt requested as proof the letter was received. The return receipt should be filed in the patient record. The letter may state the reason for the withdrawal and needs to state the date the withdrawal will become effective, Figure 3–7. If the patient needs follow-up, the letter should recommend that the patient make an appointment with another physician. It is appropriate to indicate that a copy of the medical records will be sent to the new physician if the patient sends written authorization to do so. The letter should be signed by the physician.

A patient has a right to change physicians. The patient should notify the physician but if this does not take place in a written form the physician may send a letter confirming the dismissal. This letter should also be sent by certified mail, return receipt requested, and a copy of the letter and the receipt should be filed in the patient chart.

A physician who has begun care of a patient must carry through until the patient no longer needs treatment or decides to see a different physician, or the physician has withdrawn from care. A physician who has undertaken care of a patient and is then not available to continue that care may be sued for abandonment unless coverage by some equally qualified physician is provided for. If a patient is admitted to the hospital and the physician does not see the patient right away to check on condition and order treatment, the physician may be charged with abandonment. If a physician is ill, the office staff must refer patients who need care to other qualified physicians who will care for them.

Physicians are not obligated to provide follow-up care when they see a patient for preemployment or insurance examinations or on other occasions when the request comes from someone other than the patient, as when a school athletic department requests assessment of a potential athlete.

Medical Assistant Rights

The medical assistant has the right to be free from sex discrimination. This may involve a man or woman being refused employment because the job is usually filled by someone of the opposite sex. It can involve promotions, paying less for the same work, or being treated as inferior in any way.

Title VII of the Civil Rights Act of 1964 defines sexual harassment as "Unwelcome sexual advances, requests for sexual favors, and other verbal or physical conduct of a sexual nature when submission or rejection of this conduct explicitly or implicitly affects an individual's employment, unreasonably interferes with an individual's work performance or creates an intimidating, hostile or offensive work environment." Sexual harassment can occur in a variety of circumstances. It may include but is not limited to:

- The victim as well as the harasser may be a woman or a man. The victim does not have to be of the opposite sex.
- The harasser can be the victim's supervisor, an agent of the employer, a supervisor in another area, a coworker, or a nonemployee.
- The victim does not have to be the person harassed but could be anyone affected by the offensive conduct.
- Unlawful sexual harassment may occur without economic injury to or discharge of the victim.
- The victim has a responsibility to establish that the harasser's conduct is unwelcome.

It is in the victim's best interest to directly inform the harasser that the conduct is unwelcome and must stop.

FORM A-1

LETTER OF WITHDRAWAL FROM CASE

Dear Mr. _____:

I find it necessary to inform you that I am withdrawing from further professional attendance upon you for the reason that you have persisted in refusing to follow my medical advice and treatment. Since your condition requires medical attention, I suggest that you place yourself under the care of another physician without delay. If you so desire, I shall be available to attend you for a reasonable time after you have received this letter, but in no event for more than five days.

This should give you ample time to select a physician of your choice from the many competent practitioners in this city. With your approval, I will make available to this physician your case history and information regarding the diagnosis and treatment which you have received from me.

Very truly yours,

_____, M.D.

FIGURE 3-7 Letter of withdrawal from case. (Courtesy American Medical Association)

Each instance reported to authorities is handled on a case-by-case basis and involves a thorough investigation.

Negligence ....

Torts is the branch of private law that deals with **breach** of legal duty. Torts **encompass** such wrongs as invasion of privacy, personal injury, malpractice, and slander or libel. The tort of negligence is a primary cause of malpractice suits.

Physicians are expected to be as well trained and to exercise the same degree of skill with the same degree of judgment as other physicians in similar circumstances. These **criteria** are used in determining the standard of care. In lawsuits involving specialists, the standard of care is that practiced nationally rather than that in a given community.

In a case of negligence the patient must establish that he or she was examined by the physician, that the physician did something another physician under similar circumstances would not have done, and that the negligence injured the patient. Testimony of a physician as an expert medical witness is almost always necessary in a case of negligence. In some cases the testimony of an expert witness is not required. In these instances the **doctrine** is **res ipsa loquitur,** or *the thing speaks for itself.* These cases involve such situations as a sponge or instrument left in the patient during surgery, an injury done to the bladder while performing a hysterectomy, and an infection caused by the use of unsterilized instruments. This doctrine has different interpretations in different states.

Physicians are responsible for the actions of their employees. This liability is expressed in the doctrine of **respondeat superior** (*let the master answer*). This is the law of agency, and you are an agent for the physician. Any individual entering the profession of medical assisting is considered to be accepting a position as a health care professional. If you violate the standard of care, you create the basis for a medical malpractice lawsuit. The physician is responsible for the acts of the medical assistant in the care of patients, and it is reasonable to expect the care to be as professional as the care given by the physician. A medical assistant is not licensed to practice medicine and cannot decide for a patient what care should be given.

After a Roche Laboratories medicolegal seminar, the Los Angeles County Medical Society sent the following directive to its doctors:

> When you ask your office assistant to instruct or refill a prescription, you are placing both the assistant and yourself in jeopardy. The physician's aide who directs a pharmacist to fill or refill a prescription becomes guilty of practice of medicine without a license. A physician who directs his assistant to do this places his license in jeopardy by assisting an unlicensed person to practice medicine. The

conclusion of this directive is that when you want a pharmacist to fill or refill a prescription, let him or her hear the doctor's own telephone voice, or better, have written orders on a regular prescription blank.

Negligence is not doing something that a reasonable person would do in a given situation. Malpractice is a professional's negligence. Under ordinary circumstances, a medical assistant performing the administrative duties of a receptionist or secretary would be considered a person who could be charged with negligence. A medical assistant performing clinical procedures such as drawing blood or administering injections would be considered a professional and charged with malpractice.

Medical assistants who have had special training are expected to perform at a higher standard of care than those with no special knowledge or training.

The medical assistant is not always covered by the physician's insurance, but insurance is available for the protection of medical assistants.

Good Samaritan Act

The Good Samaritan Act originated in California in 1959 to protect the physician who gives emergency care from liability for any civil damages. The physician could help in an emergency without fear of being charged with neglect or abandonment for follow-up care. Now all states have Good Samaritan statutes. The statute requires that the emergency care be given to the best ability of the person providing the care. In some states, the statute includes coverage for any health professional or citizen with first aid skills. The Good Samaritan law does not cover physicians if they receive compensation for the emergency care.

An implied agreement is considered to be a legal contract in a medical office. The medical assistant should never make a promise of a cure. You should be certain the patient understands the instructions you give come directly from the physician or from written instruction sheets. When you hand a patient a written instruction sheet you need to be certain the patient can read the instructions. Illiterate people are often reluctant to let anyone know that they cannot follow the directions for use of medications or preparation for a diagnostic test. One indicator of illiteracy might be the patient who becomes a "pest" by asking over and over for office staff to explain the instructions given by the physician. This patient might also ask you to explain a printed instruction sheet as a means of getting you to read it aloud.

The importance of doing everything possible to avoid a medical malpractice suit cannot be overemphasized. Simply being accused has a severe effect on the physician and his or her family, as well as on the community at large. A physician can be ethical, honest, and **compe-**

tent, and still be sued for medical malpractice by a single patient who for some reason did not realize the expected result of treatment. The great increase in malpractice cases has caused physicians to order more tests and X rays than are really necessary because they need to protect themselves from the possibility of missing a diagnosis and therefore being sued by the patient. The medical assistant is an extremely important person in the practice of preventive medicine in the medical office. When a friendly, harmonious interpersonal relationship is found in the office, the patient is much less likely to feel angry about anything associated with the care received. The well-trained medical assistant will understand the basic skills in good human relations and will then avoid confrontations that could lead to lawsuits against the office.

The following is the beginning of a chapter regarding medical office staff written by Melvin Belli, an internationally known attorney:

> A woman once came to me with a complaint that she'd been incorrectly treated by a "dumb doctor."
>
> "How do you know he's dumb?" I asked her.
>
> "Because everybody who works for him is dumb."
>
> It's common for patients to relate a doctor to his or her staff. Therefore, quite often, patient dissatisfaction with an office assistant will put the doctor on a malpractice spot.
>
> (Reproduced with permission from Melvin M. Belli, Sr., and John Carlova. *For Your Malpractice Defense*, Oradell, New Jersey: Medical Economics Company, Inc., 1986.)

The patient who suffers nerve damage as the result of a medical assistant giving an improperly administered injection may sue both medical assistant and physician under this doctrine. You should always inform the physician immediately of any mistakes you have made in the care of a patient so that corrective measures may be taken. You should never attempt to perform a procedure for which you have not been trained. Finally, you should be sure you understand your job responsibilities as outlined in a written procedures manual, which should be periodically updated.

You must be especially careful what you say about a patient within hearing of anyone but the physician or other office personnel. Statements regarding patients may be considered defamation of character and a breach of confidentiality. If you should make public the fact that a patient has a venereal disease, for example, this could be damaging to the patient.

You play an important role in preventing negligence by scheduling appointments for careful follow-up, knowing how and where to reach the physician at all times during the day, and making sure that the telephone is adequately covered at all times. The patient who feels well cared for will not be anxious to sue the physician. The patient who can never reach the physician for advice or who has difficulty obtaining an appointment will be much more apt to sue on the grounds of negligence.

The medical assistant should investigate use of an arbitration agreement procedure by contacting your local or state medical society. Not all states have an arbitration statute at the present time but it is well worth investigating as a possible way to settle legal problems without going to court.

Because the incidence of malpractice suits has increased, the medical assistant may need to be involved in preparing materials for court. This may include the professional training and experience of the physician as well as the patient medical record.

The attorneys may agree to taking the testimony of the physician by deposition. A deposition is oral testimony and may be taken in the attorney's office, or the physician's office in the presence of a court reporter.

A medical assistant may also receive a subpoena duces tecum to appear in court with patient records. This occurs when the physician is not available at the time needed in court.

Statutes of Limitations

A statute of limitations is a law that designates a specific limit of time during which a claim may be filed in malpractice suits or in the collection of bills. Each state is obligated to protect individuals by establishing the statutes that regulate the time period. It is important to research the current law by contacting your state medical association.

Medical Records ....

The medical office staff must understand the importance of maintaining accurate, up-to-date records on all patients. You must have complete records to give adequate care to patients. Your records may be used in research into certain illnesses or forms of treatment, and your records must be complete for protection in case of a lawsuit. A patient record that would meet this criterion would include (1) personal information such as full name, address, occupation, marital status, and insurance carrier; (2) patient's personal and family medical history; (3) all details of physical examinations, laboratory and X-ray findings, diagnoses, and treatments; and (4) consent forms for procedures done and authorization forms for release of medical information. Procrastination cannot be tolerated in handling medical records. As legal documents, they are subject to critical inspection at any time.

You should always take a medical history in a private room or ask the patient to complete the information. Make entries on the patient medical record only as requested by the physician. All entries should be factual. All results of findings on a patient should be recorded even if they are normal or negative. Errors on a medical record must be corrected by drawing a single line through incorrect material and adding your initials, the date, and the reason for the change. All prescription refills should be noted along with missed appointments, the reason for the missed appointment, and follow-up. Requests for medical information should be noted along with the information given. Any failure to follow the treatment or advice of the physician should be noted. All notations should be in blue or black ink, as pencil is too easily erased. Standard abbreviations should be used. Upon the death of a patient, a copy of the death certificate should be filed in case of subsequent requests for information. A quality medical record indicates quality medical care.

Medical records are considered the property of the physician who treats the patient. No record should be shown to a patient without the knowledge of the physician, as there may be some reason the patient should not see all of the record.

Each office should have a written policy regarding releasing information from a medical record. This policy must take into consideration local or state statutes. In some states, the legislature has given the patient, his or her physician, or authorized agent the right to examine or copy the medical record. The requirement of confidentiality regarding the medical record is no longer recognized when the patient initiates a malpractice claim against a physician.

Physicians cannot agree on whether patients should be allowed to review their own records. The physician must be careful of personal opinion notes placed in the chart if there is a possibility the patient will be reading it. The following are two examples of patients reading medical records that were not recorded for their viewing:

> A female patient was being professionally treated by a young physician when the doctor was suddenly called away from his office and left her medical record open on his desk. The patient read the first sentence: "This woman is a crock." Needless to say, she became very distraught and angry. (From "Personal Comments in Medical Records May Cause Trouble," *Medical World News*, Jan. 12, 1976, 128.)
>
> While waiting to see a physician, a patient had been given her own record. Curious, she took out the notes and read them only to find that the doctor had written on the heading of the page, "Beware, hysterical and manipulative, determined to be unwell." She left immediately. (From "Case Conference: Fain Would I Change That Note," *Journal of Medical Ethics*, 4 [1978] 207–209.)

Any review of the chart by the patient should be done when the physician is present to interpret medical terms or abbreviations. Some physicians give patients a copy of their medical records and believe this reduces any anxiety regarding their health.

The following are six basic principles for preventing unauthorized disclosure of information:

1. When in doubt, err by not disclosing rather than by disclosing. There are exceptions to this principle but a mistaken refusal to disclose confidential data is, at least, reversible.

2. Remember that the owner of the privilege to keep information confidential is the patient, not the doctor. If the patient is willing to release the data, the physician may not ethically decide to withhold it even 'for the patient's own good.'

3. Apply the concept of confidentiality equally to all patients despite the physician's assessment of their goals, mores and lifestyles. A physician cannot ethically inform an insurer of suspicions that a patient is trying to defraud an insurer.

4. Be familiar with the federal, state and local law plus ordinances, rules, regulations and administrative decrees of various agencies such as public health departments.

5. When required to divulge a confidence, discuss the situation with the patient. When obligations to society conflict with those of the patient, the physician should discuss the conflict with the patient. When legal guidelines are absent or vague, the criteria for decision are the immediacy and degree of danger to either the patient or society.

6. Get written authorization from the patient before divulging information. To meet standard situations such as requests from third parties, have the patient sign a blanket authorization in advance to release pertinent data to specific third parties.

(Reprinted with permission from Leif C. Beck, "Patient Information: When—and When Not—to Divulge," *Patient Care*, April 15, 1972.)

The AMA has several forms for authorization for disclosure. It is a good policy to refuse to answer a telephone question as to whether an individual is a patient. A person coming to the office for information regarding a patient should produce an authorization to disclose information before any is given. It is important to check the specific details authorized to be released and to ask for identification of the individual or organization requesting the information. The signed authorization should be placed in the patient chart with a copy of the information released. According to Myrtle Flight, "when the information requested is disclosed, it must be accompanied by a note forbidding redisclosure" (*Law, Liability, and Ethics for Medical Office Personnel*, 134).

The complete, unaltered medical record is a legal document and is the best defense for a physician who is charged with malpractice. The first step a lawyer will take in a malpractice case against a physician is to obtain a copy of the patient's records and have them examined by an independent physician. The following office procedures have caused problems in malpractice suits:

1. Procrastination in filing lab test results
2. Incomplete medical records
3. Illegible records

4. Unexplained altered medical records
5. Faking or forging a document or signature
6. Loss of records

There are acceptable methods of making changes in medical records. A single line should be drawn through an incorrect entry. An initial of the person making the correction should be written in the margin along with the date the error was discovered. The corrections should appear in the record in chronological order.

The contents of a medical record have been enumerated. In addition to having complete, up-to-date records you must be aware of the need for keeping these records even after care has ceased or the patient has expired. Records should be kept as long as the statute of limitations is in effect on a case history. A few states stipulate the length of time records must be kept. You have a responsibility to see that necessary records are kept for any narcotics used in the office. You also may be responsible for keeping accurate financial records.

Complete Chapter 3, Unit 2 in the workbook to help you meet the objectives at the beginning of this unit and therefore achieve competency of this subject matter.

REFERENCES

American Association of Medical Assistants. "Law for the Medical Office—1984."

Flight, Myrtle. *Law, Liability, and Ethics for Medical Office Personnel*. Albany: Delmar, 1988.

Hasty, Frederick E., III. "Your Most Dangerous Malpractice Gamble." *Medical Economics for Surgeons*. August 20, 1984.

Horsley, Jack E. "Who Can Sue You For Not Rendering Care?" *Medical Economics*. August 20, 1984.

Isele, William. "Legal and Ethical Concerns of the Medical Assistant." *The Professional Medical Assistant*. July–August 1977.

Kinn, Mary E., and Derge, Eleanor. *The Medical Assistant: Administrative and Clinical*, 6th ed. Philadelphia: W. B. Saunders, 1988.

Lewis, Marti, and Warden, Carol. *Law and Ethics in the Medical Office*. Philadelphia: F. A. Davis, 1983.

Monahan, James S. "How Your Office Staff Can Get You Sued." *Medical Economics*. August 22, 1983.

Physician's Guide to Ohio Law. Ohio State Medical Association, Columbus, 1987.

The Professional Medical Assistant. "Ethics, a Roundtable Discussion." September–October, 1979.

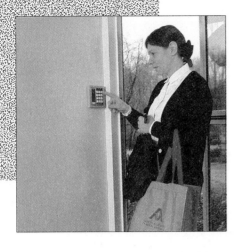

C H A P T E R   4

Safety and Security in the Medical Office

UNIT 1
Equip Office for Emergency

UNIT 2
Office Safety

UNIT 3
Documenting Emergency Situations

The medical office must be run as a business whether it is a solo practice or a large number of physicians operating as a corporation. Every business is responsible for the safety of those who enter the premises. The medical assistant is part of the team responsible for recognizing any safety hazards, helping to eliminate them, and warning patients of any dangers.

U N I T   1

Equip Office for Emergency

OBJECTIVES

Upon completion of the unit, the student will meet the following terminal performance objectives by verifying knowledge of the facts and principles presented through oral and written communication at a level deemed competent.

1. Define a medical emergency.
2. List the appropriate drugs, supplies, and equipment for an emergency tray.
3. Know what telephone numbers should be posted near each telephone.
4. Know the procedures for handling narcotic drugs in the office.
5. Know which emergencies require special evaluation procedures.
6. Identify special needs of a laboratory for safety of personnel.
7. Spell and define, using the glossary at the back of the text, all the words to know in this unit.

WORDS TO KNOW

activated	grillwork
antihistamine	hyperventilation
diabetic	hypoglycemic
emetic	sharps
evacuation	snap locks
eyewash	

A medical emergency is any situation in which an individual suddenly becomes ill or has an injury or circumstances calling for decided action.

As part of your preparation for an emergency, you and your employer should list the supplies and equipment necessary to handle an emergency that would come under your care. Then set aside a place in your office where these items will always be ready for use. All employees in the office should know where the items are and how they are to be used.

The easiest way to be prepared for an emergency is to purchase a prepared emergency kit, which is available through most medical supply houses, Figure 4–1, page 42. If your physician feels this is not necessary, you must assemble your own. You should have a supply of sterile dressings, bandage material, and adhesive tape; easily activated hot and cold packs; disposable syringe and needle units with adrenaline, narcotics, and antihistamines. Adrenaline (epinephrine) is available in cartridge

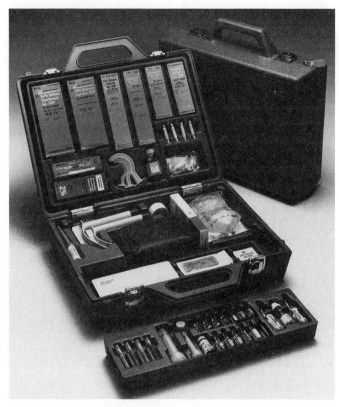

FIGURE 4–1 Prepared emergency kit (Courtesy of Banyan International Corporation)

units ready for use. Other supplies include ipecac, an effective emetic; tubes of glucose for use in diabetic patients suffering from a severe hypoglycemic reaction; and an oxygen tank with a mask. Other items your physician might include would be alcohol wipes, aromatic spirits of ammonia, blood pressure cuff, stethoscope, bandage scissors, airways of different sizes, penlight, paper and pencil, and a small bag for hyperventilation.

Every employee should be certified in first aid and cardiopulmonary resuscitation and this certification must be current. The office should have written guidelines outlining the scope of care to be given by medical assistants and the location in the office where this care should be given. A list of all the necessary telephone numbers for police, fire, ambulance, hospitals, and poison control centers should be near each telephone.

Anything recognized as a possible office hazard should be remedied. All employees need to follow safety procedures in the proper disposal of drugs. Any unwanted samples should be donated to a clinic where they can be used. Dated samples should be checked and any that have been kept beyond the expiration date should be properly discarded. Potentially dangerous equipment, such as syringes and needles, must be disposed of in sharps containers. Several protective safety adapters are available to reduce the risk of patient-to-staff contamination by accidental needle sticks. Contaminated dressings

need to be placed in special disposable containers. Always keep narcotics in a locked cupboard in an area not usually seen by patients.

Your office should have a well-planned procedure and route for evacuation in the event a fire should occur in the office building. All office personnel should know the location of fire extinguishers and how to use them, Figure 4–2. All personnel should know the location of the nearest fire escape. Battery-powered lights should be available to use in the event of a power failure.

All office personnel should know the procedure to use during a tornado or severe storm. The safest area of the building should be identified. Your local disaster service can assist you in identifying the safest location.

The laboratory should have an emergency eyewash station. Every office laboratory and operating room should be equipped with disposable latex gloves, protective glasses, and masks for the protection of staff and patients.

The medical assistant should take the precaution of washing hands before and after dealing with each patient. When it is necessary to clean up any examination area after any patient, wear latex gloves and use a solution of 20% chlorine and water.

The increased incidence of robbery and rape makes it extremely important that snap locks be used on doors between the office and reception area. Police have advised that any opening between the reception area and office should be covered with a grillwork, which would prevent entry by undesirable individuals. Private entry doors to the office should not be left unlocked. If you must enter or leave the office after dark, the outside area should be well lighted and security people should be available if necessary.

Complete Chapter 4, Unit 1 in the workbook to help you meet the objectives at the beginning of this unit and therefore achieve competency of this subject matter.

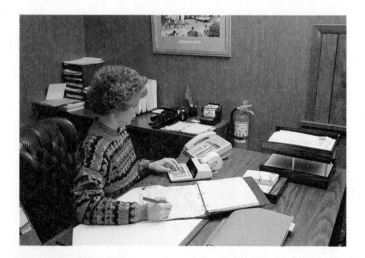

FIGURE 4–2 Know the location of fire extinguishers and how to use them. (Courtesy of American LaFrance)

U N I T 2

Office Safety

WORDS TO KNOW ....

attenuated	ergonomics
automation	inoculating loops
carpal tunnel syndrome	keying
concealed	procurement
contaminated	volatile

Computers should be situated so that glare is not present on the screen. Employees using computers or word processors should rest the eyes by looking away from the screen at regular intervals of one to three minutes at least every hour. A vertical document holder, which may be either free standing or attached to a flexible equipment arm, eases eyestrain and improves posture, Figure 4–3.

Ergonomics is the science that deals with people's performance and well-being in relation to their job tasks, their equipment, and their environment. Ergonomics in an office is valuable for maintaining the health and safety of employees and for improving performance. The increased automation of the office with the use of computers has made it necessary to consider health issues of employees.

It is important for chairs to fit the employee who must sit for long periods. The height and back need to be adjustable. It is important to relax periodically by standing and moving about. Variety in the work will be helpful. Plan work so that you might balance keying with filing, talking on the telephone, or preparing documents. This variety helps to keep you mentally alert and also requires physical movements away from the computer. The use of a footrest, Figure 4–4, page 44, or wrist supports may also aid in avoiding posture problems. An armrest on your chair can help to keep your wrists as straight as possible. If you do not have armrests on your chair, a wrist support should be used, Figure 4–5, page 44. The wrist support needs to be the same thickness as the keyboard and needs to extend the length of the keyboard. A good wrist support should have rounded edges, be padded, and be about two inches wide. The problem of carpal tunnel syndrome can be prevented with proper wrist position while you are keying. The fingers should be lower than the wrist.

Never leave a file drawer open at floor level when you are away from the file cabinet. There is danger of tripping over such an obstacle. In a vertical file cabinet if you pull out more than one drawer at a time you may cause the cabinet to tip forward and cause injury. Cupboard doors left open are a hazard.

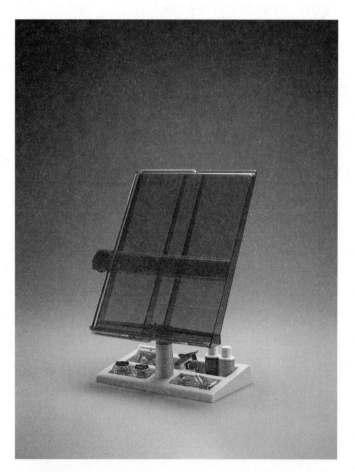

FIGURE 4–3 Vertical document holder (Courtesy of Eldon-Rubbermaid Office Products)

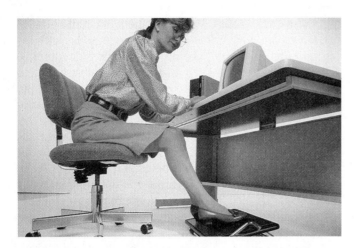

FIGURE 4–4 Using a footrest may help in avoiding posture problems. (Courtesy of Magnuson Group, Inc.)

Be sure to unplug appliances such as coffee makers and sterilizers at the end of the day because they are a fire hazard if allowed to boil dry.

Laboratory Area

If chemicals are kept in the office for laboratory work, care must be taken to store them properly. Some chemicals become volatile when kept beyond the expiration date, so these dates need to be monitored carefully.

Gloves should always be worn when handling contaminated instruments or when processing patient specimens. The Centers for Disease Control in Atlanta has outlined universal precautions to be followed concerning laboratory workers. These precautions will be discussed in connection with the clinical procedures in this text.

Every office should have a general safety procedure book that employees must be familiar with through an employee training program. This book should include guidelines for handling of hazardous medical wastes.

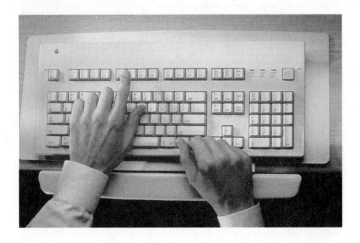

FIGURE 4–5 Wrist support (Courtesy of Details, a subsidiary of Steelcase, Inc.)

The U.S. Occupational Safety and Health Administration (OSHA) was established to help the employer provide a safe working environment for the employees. Hazardous medical wastes include blood products, body fluids, tissue cultures, live and attenuated vaccines, sharps, table paper with body fluids, gloves, speculums, cotton swabs, and inoculating loops.

Reception Room

The medical assistant should conduct a visual check of the reception area daily to be sure the furniture is clean and in good repair. All electrical cords should be checked routinely for frayed wires and should be removed immediately if defective. Children's toys or books should be off the floor when not in use. All toys should be washable and made of safe materials. It is common practice to display a "no smoking" sign in the office. Smoking is a health hazard and fire can result from careless smoking.

Examination Rooms

The examination table should be cleaned carefully after each patient. Any dropped objects or spills should be cleaned up immediately to prevent slipping or falling, Figure 4–6. Small children will pick up any loose object and put it in their mouth. Extremely ill patients or children should not be left alone on an examination table, where they could fall. All equipment cords should be concealed where people will be moving about. No prescription blanks should be left where they can be forged and used illegally for drug procurement.

Complete Chapter 4, Unit 2 in the workbook to help you meet the objectives at the beginning of this unit and therefore achieve competency of this subject matter.

U N I T 3

Documenting Emergency Situations

OBJECTIVES

Upon completion of this unit, the student will meet the following terminal performance objectives by verifying knowledge of the facts and principles presented through oral and written communications at a level deemed competent.

1. Describe the two general kinds of emergencies that may be encountered in a medical office.
2. List examples of accidents that may take place in the office.

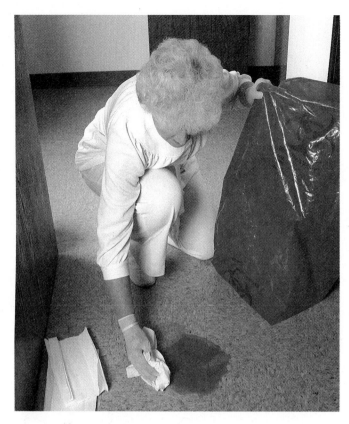

FIGURE 4–6 Always pick up dropped objects or clean up spills immediately to prevent accidents.

3. List examples of accidents that may take place outside of the office.
4. Describe illnesses that may be emergency situations.
5. Prepare a sample accident report form.
6. Describe where accident reports should be kept.
7. Spell and define, using the glossary at the back of the text, all the words to know in this unit.

WORDS TO KNOW ....

anaphylactic shock
asphyxiation
disposition

epilepsy
hypothermia
illicit

Every office should have guidelines in the office procedure manual regarding methods to handle each type of emergency that might occur in the office. All office personnel should understand their individual roles in handling emergencies in the office. The patient could be involved in an accident in or out of the office. The patient could be suffering from diabetic coma, anaphylactic shock, heart attack, or an illicit drug reaction.

Emergencies that might require cardiopulmonary resuscitation are airway obstructions, smoke inhalation, brain injury, chest wall injury, drug or medication reaction, electrocution, drowning, cardiac arrest, trauma, respiratory arrest, hypothermia, allergies, electric shock, asphyxiation, stroke, and epilepsy.

A decision must be made as to who is responsible for recording detailed information in the patient's medical record. The information necessary to be recorded should include:

■ Date and time of accident or emergency
■ Full name of injured party
■ Notation as to whether this individual is a patient, visitor, or office staff member
■ Address of injured party with telephone number
■ Location in office where incident occurred
■ Detailed description of incident
■ Names of staff involved in any way
■ Names, addresses, and telephone numbers of witnesses other than staff
■ Action taken; medications given; physician examined; patient referred to hospital, other medical office, or home
■ Signature of person preparing report with time and date

The above information should be on a printed form approved by the physician and liability insurance company.

When the report of an accident or illness is completed, the office needs to have established guidelines for disposition of the form. It may be advisable to have legal input as to whether to place the form in the patient's medical record or file it in a special incident file.

Complete Chapter 4, Unit 3 in the workbook to help you meet the objectives at the beginning of this unit and therefore achieve competency of this subject matter.

REFERENCES

Cody, John P. Cardiopulmonary Resuscitation. The ABCs of Basic Life Support. *The Professional Medical Assistant.* July-August, 1990.
Jett, Ernestine. Enforcement of Safety and Security in the Medical Office. *The Professional Medical Assistant.* November-December, 1986.
Joyce, Marilyn and Wallersteiner, Ulrika. *Ergonomics. Humanizing the Automated Office.* Cincinnati: South Western Publishing, 1989.
Keir, A. Lucille. Safety in the Medical Office. *The Professional Medical Assistant.* September-October, 1986.

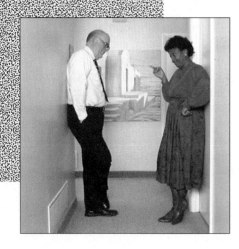

CHAPTER 5

Interpersonal Communications

One of the most important skills a medical assistant can possess is the art of communicating effectively with others. Both clinical and administrative duties require a constant exchange of written, oral, and nonverbal information.

You must be able to convey messages to many different people and receive vital information in the same manner. You will have daily contact with patients, colleagues, and other professionals, by phone, face to face, or by letter. Telephone and written communications and office mail will be discussed later in this text. This chapter deals with both verbal and nonverbal messages. Understanding how one gives and receives these is vital in the exchange of communication.

Stress management and stress and related illnesses will be covered in this chapter, as will a basic overview of behavioral adjustments that interfere with the communication process. Basic coping skills that can be applied in all aspects of living are also provided. These topics are included in the hope that you will benefit from having this information and so that you may be of greater assistance to others who need support in times of personal conflict.

In dealing with patients and their families, learning to listen and to offer advice in a calm, professional manner will help to reduce unnecessary stress for all concerned. Times of sadness and pain can be extremely difficult for those closely involved. You can be instrumental in providing comfort and compassion to those in need.

Since the medical office is usually a very active place, with many people coming and going, asking questions and making payments or appointments, intraoffice communication can become ragged and ineffective. A harmonious team effort makes for an efficient as well as a pleasant work environment. If an atmosphere of accord and cooperation exists among the staff, patients will sense this during their visits. If an uneasy situation exists, with friction evident, this may add to a patient's apprehensions and anxieties. Working together for the single purpose of providing quality health care to patients in a relaxed and friendly manner will help ease the daily pressures for the members of the medical office team and contribute greatly to their collective effectiveness.

U N I T   1

Verbal and Nonverbal Messages

OBJECTIVES ....

Upon completion of the unit the student will meet the following terminal performance objectives by verifying knowledge of the facts and principles presented through oral and written communication at a level deemed competent.

1. Describe the basic pattern of communication.
2. Give examples of nonverbal communication.
3. Explain how verbal and nonverbal communication can sometimes be misinterpreted.
4. Describe ways that tone and speed of speech can affect the message.
5. Discuss the importance of dress in nonverbal communication.
6. Define *perception* and state its importance in communication.
7. Spell and define, using the glossary at the back of the text, all the words to know in this unit.

WORDS TO KNOW ....

articulate	empirically	perception
conceptualize	incongruous	scrupulously
contradict	intangible	
distort	intuition	

To become effective in the art of communication, it may help to conceptualize the communication process, Figure 5–1. The message originates with the sender. The encoded message takes form based upon the sender's reference points (or frames of reference), and off it goes. The message is picked up by the intended receiver, who immediately begins to decode it based on his or her reference points (or frames of reference). In responding (or providing feedback) the whole process is reversed: the original receiver becomes the sender, and the original sender becomes the receiver. In receiving this feedback, the original sender (now the receiver) can assess and evaluate how well the original message was received and interpreted and make any necessary adjustments or clarification.

The whole process seems simple enough, and generally it works well. However, many things can happen to affect the quality of the message or even distort it. You must be aware of these potential problems.

Foremost is the issue of reference points. For example, the spoken messages may include terminology familiar to you but unknown to the patient. Therefore, though the message will be heard, it may not be understood. Talking to patients on a level that they can easily understand is a skill requiring quick judgment. You will have to adapt to a vast number of different personalities in conveying information.

Some patients may be hearing- or sight-impaired, developmentally disabled, or non-English speaking, and will therefore require extra understanding. If a patient is in some way handicapped, a family member or friend usually accompanies the person, thereby helping with your task of transmitting necessary information.

Other factors may interfere, such as interruptions or simply the way you feel. These factors must be recognized and dealt with if effective communication is to occur.

The spoken word must be delivered in an articulate, clear manner if the intended message is to be received. Correct pronunciation and proper grammar help to convey the meaning. You must also be aware of the rate of the spoken word. Patients need to be spoken to in an unrushed manner so that the information has a chance to register and questions can be asked. Speaking in a pleasant tone of voice is necessary to keep the listener's interest in what you are saying.

Common courtesy is an art which seems to have been lost to some degree. In a professional setting it is essential to be scrupulously polite. *Please, Thank you,*

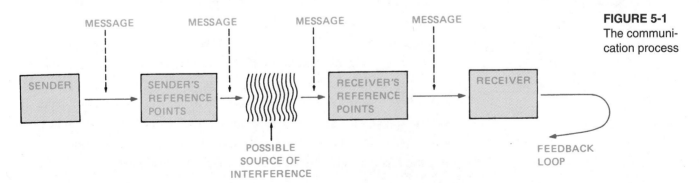

FIGURE 5-1
The communication process

Excuse me, and *May I help you?* should be words in frequent use. In this way the entire health care staff will show respect for others and a sense of caring.

Perception

Perception in the context of communication may be considered as being aware of one's own feelings and the feelings of others. The feelings you have about other people's moods and the way they act are perceptual, nonspoken communication between you. Intuition is another term for perception in this sense. While they cannot be measured empirically, these feelings may be strong indeed. Therefore, they must be recognized and reckoned with.

Being perceptive is a skill acquired with experience and practice. Keeping your eyes and ears open to the needs of others and what is going on will help you develop it. Developing the ability to perceive your own needs is a part of perception that will enhance your effectiveness. Planning and thinking ahead will help you develop in this area.

Body Language

The image you project is of utmost importance. Your overall appearance sends out messages to anyone who looks at you. Appropriate dress, uniform, or businesslike attire should be worn. Your professional appearance sends a nonverbal message that you have authority and are in charge.

Proper attire may vary with the medical specialty. For instance, many pediatric practices prefer medical assistants to dress in normal street clothes so as to make young patients feel more at ease. Children sometimes associate a white uniform with an unpleasant hospital visit. Psychiatry and psychology medical office assistants may also be more inclined to wear businesslike dress, for clinical duties are few, if any, and a uniform may not be necessary. However, casual wear is considered unprofessional, and jeans, sandals, and excessive jewelry are out of the question during working hours. Looking like a professional will not only encourage the respect of others for your profession, but it will help you to feel an integral part of the health care team.

Personal hygiene should be impeccable, because setting a good example for others is a part of your responsibility in the care of others. Daily showering, clean attractive hair, and neatly manicured nails show others that you take pride in yourself and give them a model to pattern themselves after, Figure 5–2.

Another part of your appearance, something intangible but very real, is your attitude. Your attitude shows *everyone* who sees you or speaks to you (by telephone or in person) how you feel about your work, others, and yourself. You display your attitude in the way you get along with others and interact with them. The importance of a positive attitude cannot be overemphasized. The many

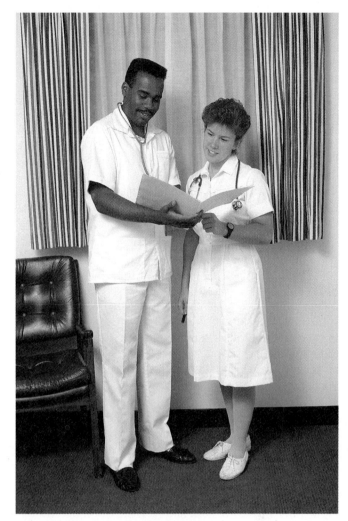

FIGURE 5-2 Pride in appearance

hassles and conflicts that can, and do, arise with patients and colleagues during everyday activity in the busy medical office can be handled much more effectively if you possess and project a positive attitude. Constant complaining only makes situations worse and breeds contempt. Having a good outlook on life carries over into every area and promotes well-being. Pleasant, agreeable working conditions increase productivity and efficiency besides giving one a sense of satisfaction on the job.

Facial Expression

Part of perception is being aware of how others think you feel, or see you. You create this impression partly by your facial expression. It is possible to contradict a verbal message by an inappropriate or incongruous facial expression. The most common example of a positive, happy facial expression is a smile, Figure 5–3, page 49. This nonverbal signal conveys a positive attitude. Frowning and looking glum only add to other people's troubles. It is especially important to be pleasant and friendly to those seeking medical attention, because their worries concerning their condition are already on their minds. Adding your troubles to theirs is highly inappropriate. A positive attitude and a receptive awareness will show in your facial expression.

Eye contact shows that you are interested in giving and receiving messages of mutual concern and interest. It has been said that the eyes are the windows of the soul. Looking into another's eyes while engaging in conversation permits an open, honest transmission of thoughts and ideas. Looking away while people are talking to you makes them feel that what they are saying is not important. Interest and attention soon disappear and the intent of your message may be distorted or lost.

Gestures

Still another way of transmitting nonverbal messages is by gesturing. Gestures are body movements that enhance what is being said. You may know people who seemingly could not talk if they had to sit on their hands. Try to follow their example. Using hand and body gestures to accentuate a point can help the receiver understand your meaning.

A handshake is a sign of friendship. Another meaningful body movement is a hug to convey feelings of warmth and affection. A comforting touch helps patients feel that you care and gives them a sense of security and acceptance. Studies have shown that patients who have been touched, by a hand on the shoulder or a hand held, respond significantly better in treatment than those not touched. Patting someone on the back and saying "Good for you" is a positive reinforcer. You might do that in praise of a patient who followed the prescribed treatment of the physician and lost 10 pounds and who needs positive recognition of these achievements to encourage continued compliance. In reinforcing a patient, you should display a positive attitude, facial expression, gestures, and eye contact—all the communication skills so far mentioned. In addition, your tone of voice should be happy and sincere. Patients who believe you are pleased with their progress are more willing to strive to follow future treatment because of the resulting positive feelings.

Another powerful nonverbal communication tool is silence. This method can indeed be most frustrating to the person for whom it is directed. In dealing with patients who exhibit this nonverbal way of communicating, it is best if the inexperienced medical assistant ask for help from a supervisor, a physician, or another staff member who has skill in dealing with this type of situation. Patients who exhibit behavior such as this may have serious underlying problems.

Complete Chapter 5, Unit 1 in the workbook to meet the objectives at the beginning of this unit and therefore achieve competency of this subject matter.

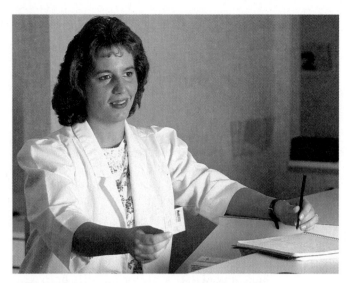

FIGURE 5–3 A smile conveys a positive attitude.

UNIT 2
Managing Stress

OBJECTIVES ....

Upon completion of the unit the student will meet the following terminal performance objectives by verifying knowledge of the facts and principles presented through oral and written communication at a level deemed competent.

1. Describe the phenomenon of stress and differentiate between "good" stress and "bad" stress.
2. List and describe stress-related illnesses.
3. List positive methods for dealing with stress.
4. Describe type A and type B personalities.
5. List the four basic human physical needs.
6. List the four basic human developmental needs.
7. Describe steps you can take to eliminate unnecessary stress.
8. List mental health resources for referral of patients.
9. Spell and define, using the glossary at the back of the text, all the words to know in this unit.

WORDS TO KNOW ....

absolute	implement	psychosomatic
absurdity	leisure	receptors
conflict	nurture	rejuvenate
discretion	perspective	respite
exemplify	prioritize	
impending	psychosis	

As you become familiar with patients' symptoms and their diagnoses, it will be evident that a great many illnesses may be ultimately stress-related. Some persons are more stress-prone than others, operating at such a hectic pace and with such compulsiveness or perfectionism that they create many stressful situations for themselves. In general, these persons are referred to as type A personalities. There is a type B personality as well, exemplified by a tendency to operate at a slower pace and not to worry as much. These typings are neither absolute nor evaluative; that is, one is not better than the other, and most people probably demonstrate characteristics of both types at different times and in different situations. For the most part, though, we lean toward one type or the other in our general actions. Although both type A and type B personalities inevitably face stressful situations, the type As probably face them more frequently than the type Bs. Hence, type A personalities should pay particular attention to recognizing stress and learning to deal with its effects.

Basic human survival needs are really few. Physical needs include protection, food, water, and oxygen. Developmental needs are physical, emotional, intellectual, and spiritual nurturing. Often materialistic values override real needs to the point of absurdity. The quality of personal relationships and meaningful endeavors determine the quality of life more than material things.

A certain amount of stress is necessary to provide motivation. This is "good" stress. The degree of stress that is necessary or helpful varies with the individual. Goals must be set realistically and kept in perspective. Reaching goals produces a sense of pride in accomplishment, and these positive feelings reinforce continued personal growth and development. Failure tends to produce feelings of worthlessness and even despair. These negative feelings, if not properly vented, can cause many psychosomatic problems. For example, they may lead to aggressive behavior, which is itself stress-producing to the one who displays it as well as to others. Feelings of hostility toward others may lead to difficulty in coping with pressures from change in employment or unemployment, family or personal conflicts, and many other problems, usually known only to the individual.

Difficulty in planning the use of time can produce stress. The feeling of being inefficient and unproductive can lead to a vicious cycle of defeat and despair. This negative attitude may encourage dependence on drugs or alcohol to find some pleasure in life and respite from feelings of worthlessness. Exaggeration? No. People vary in their coping skills for dealing with stress. Those who have no one to encourage or support them in their lives may have a particularly hard time.

Office Stress

The hectic pace of a medical office practice creates pressure. On some days there may be little time to exchange even a complete sentence with a coworker. Therefore, lunch and rest breaks are essential to your well-being. Time away from the pressures of patient care can give a whole new outlook on a problem. Some offices schedule time for the lunch period between morning and afternoon patients and block the time routinely in the appointment book. This is a good practice. You return to work refreshed and are more productive as a result. Most medical practices have a heavy schedule and working overtime is a frequent reality. Many find that trading evenings with another employee is a good practice. Since patients do not get sick by appointment, schedules will never run perfectly. Flexibility must be acquired early. A great number of problems stem from the high-pressure nature of the job itself. Realizing this will be of great help in learning to cope well with whatever situation presents itself.

However, there may be times when you are tired or have a cold or a headache or are worried about a personal problem that things will start to go awry and it seems that everything follows suit. This is the time when every patient who calls has a major health problem or a mistake with their bill or insurance claim.

Taking one thing at a time and completing it before starting something else can ease many tensions. Everyone must learn to help out on days when life itself seems to be a chore. Exchanging common courtesies and being considerate of each other's feelings can also reduce stressful situations. Just knowing that someone cares is what patients need sometimes. You should give this consideration to colleagues as well.

Since you can be the target of patients', and sometimes coworkers', pent-up feelings from time to time, it is clear that your own feelings will need expression, too. Everyone needs to get rid of negative feelings. The bad as well as the good times must be shared; it is human nature to do so. This may lead to feeling over-burdened at times, but these emotions must be directed into proper channels. Realizing the difference between the things we can and cannot control is important.

Stress and Related Illness

Stress in itself is a most useful reaction for it is a signal for one to respond to a stimulus. There is both good and bad stress. Good stress is known as *eustress* such as special events we look forward to and plan for, or even deadlines to meet (when planned). Those things ultimately beneficial and rewarding to us are motivating and energizing. The stress is temporary and useful to us.

All of us are constantly processing various stimuli that aid us in our daily communications and activities. The difficulty in regard to stress occurs when the stressor is chronic (constant) and causes us to be troubled. Because no short-cut or fast relief can resolve the stressor or situation causing the stress, it becomes *distress* or bad stress. The effects of this chronic stress stay with the affected person, so that a potentially dangerous physical and mental state ensues.

Stress manifests itself in individuals in many ways. The most commonly recognized stress-related illnesses are asthma, headaches (migraines), gastritis, heart disease, insomnia, mental (emotional) illness, and peptic ulcers.

The effect of stress is that the nerve receptors send nerve impulses to the brain, where the sympathetic function of the autonomic nervous system reacts by sending a message of impending danger to the adrenal glands. These glands pour adrenaline into the circulatory system, as do special nerve cells, to give the body extra strength to deal with the impending threat or danger. The heart beats faster, respirations are increased, and digestion slows down to allow the circulation of adrenaline. As the problem is resolved or removed, the body begins to reorganize impulses. The parasympathetic function sends impulses to slow the previously supercharged body functions back to normal levels. The sympathetic and parasympathetic functions work to create a balance of nerve impulses to regulate the activities of the body.

If one is living under constant stress, the heart and circulatory system, the lungs, and intestinal tract are constantly being literally turned on and off, leaving insufficient time for normal body functioning. The human body, given too much to deal with too often, eventually breaks down and needs repair, as does an automobile run too hard and too long without proper maintenance.

The body reacts to stress by showing various symptoms. Constipation or diarrhea, frequent colds and flu, indigestion, and migraine headaches are a few of the common physical complaints of patients who overtax themselves. Those who seek medical attention for these types of complaints are usually referred to a counseling service, where the cause of the stress may be discovered and eliminated. Once this is accomplished the symptoms usually disappear.

There are, of course, patients whose symptoms have developed over a long period of time and whose physical problems have progressed into a major illness. These patients need counseling as well as medical supervision and treatment.

Since physicians have become so specialized, there is usually little or no time for counseling during a routine office visit. The general practitioner used to know the whole family and was often the counselor of all members. Some family and general practice physicians still do domestic counseling in a limited manner. You will notice if a patient who has always been pleasant and smiling during previous office visits suddenly demonstrates a change in mood. This patient may begin to complain of headaches or other aches and pains without apparent cause. After the physician's examination and lab reports have been reviewed, if no major cause has been found, the physician may suggest that the patient seek counseling.

In almost every community large or small hospitals, health centers, and clinics offer mental health services. The county medical society will be helpful in referring patients to a physician, psychologist, or psychiatrist if listings are not available in the local phone directory.

Inquiries about mental health services should be treated with discretion. Mental illness can be a difficult and delicate problem to deal with, not only for the patient, but for family, close friends, and neighbors. As in all matters of medical records, confidentiality must be carefully maintained.

The family or general practitioner is usually the first professional to have contact with the patient. The referral for appropriate care of the patient will be made by the medical assistant.

Depression

Depression is treated by physicians with both counseling and medication. Some patients may respond well with counseling only, however. Where medication is given, careful supervision of patients is a must. Alerting the physician to any changes that the patient reports by phone is vital in the direction of the patient's therapy.

There are many types of depression. Depression is a predictable reaction to the death of a relative, spouse, or close friend, for example. A person may take some time to overcome this grief, the amount of time varying with the individual. Usually, after a few months, the person should begin to adjust to the loss, however. When normal functioning does not return, assistance is necessary.

Psychosomatic Illness

Psychosomatic illness is not imagined. These patients have very real symptoms. However, the symptoms are usually emotional and not organic in nature. Patients with psychosomatic illness may have deep-rooted guilt feelings, fears, frustrations, hostilities, anxieties, or phobias. The patient may not be conscious of these feelings. The stress-related illnesses described earlier are some of the common physical expressions of psychosomatic illness.

Anxiety

Anxiety is a stress-related condition in which the patient is in a constant state of worry. Those who are constantly feeling apprehension and fear have a variety of physical ailments as a result, which can lead to serious illness if not treated. Concerns over money or sexual dysfunction are common anxieties. Patients of this type usually need a combination of counseling and medication to regain a healthy outlook on life and function productively.

Psychoses

Psychosis is a more profound mental disorder characterized by impairment of normal intellectual and social functioning. These patients usually have either partially or completely withdrawn from reality. Their condition may become so severe that hospitalization is necessary. These patients have severe mood swings, sometimes experience hallucinations, and may not know who they are. Patients may be treated on an out-patient basis, but the most severe cases are hospitalized. Many persons in psychotic states can, with long-term treatment, return to normal functioning. Other psychotic states may be irreversible.

Treatment

Many public service agencies, churches, colleges, businesses, and private organizations offer educational programs in stress management. Most programs deal with methods which can be practiced by individuals in coping with their personal lives. Significant life events, such as major changes in employment or geographic location, marital status, or health create varying levels of stress. Support groups can help; meetings are held to discuss problems or situations which are too complex or difficult to figure out alone. For that matter, a close friend can be a valuable resource. Simply identifying a source of stress may relieve some of it, but some action must usually be taken to relieve most stressful situations. Finding workable solutions to problems may take a considerable amount of time and patience. Counseling can help both in defining problems and in beginning to take definitive action to implement changes. Individuals must recognize the importance of prioritizing values and standing firm in beliefs, while at the same time remaining flexible enough to cope with new and challenging situations.

Effective time management involves careful assessment of one's personal routine and deciding how and when to accomplish priorities. Then the primary goal is to eliminate activities that are not worth the time they demand. A good rule to follow is to single out one issue at a time and deal with it thoroughly and appropriately.

Activities that help you relax are a basic necessity. For some, it may be working a jigsaw puzzle, reading, or listening to music; for others, it may be taking a walk after supper, dancing, or gardening. Each person should find an enjoyable leisure activity. Something that refreshes the spirit and rejuvenates the soul is a must for sound mental and physical health. You also need to give yourself a pat on the back occasionally for doing a good job.

Following a dull pattern of work-eat-sleep-work is not enough. Personal growth and development are rewarding and essential. A hobby or interest is vital to feeling good about yourself. Many find that physical activity is the answer. Regular exercise is not only a good way to relieve tension, it keeps you in shape and stimulates more energy. A daily program of physical activity is an excellent and refreshing outlet.

Many people today participate in exercise groups through community centers, schools, work, private health clubs, or public facilities such as the YMCA/YWCA. Still others follow an individual exercise regimen. Whatever one does to stay physically fit, it will have a positive effect in reducing stress.

You may want to place exercise class announcements and other health-related tips on a bulletin board in the reception area or by the scale, or wherever patients have enough time to read and copy the information.

An excellent means of venting one's inner feelings is by associating with your peers. Talking "shop" for a while can be good therapy and can lead to friendships outside the working relationship. Membership in a professional association will provide you with many opportunities. You can make strong friendships and participate in a variety of continuing education programs for personal and professional growth. Membership is encouraged for it adds a new perspective to your career.

Because stress is perceived by each of us differently, a personal evaluation to define the cause of our individual stress is necessary for relieving or eliminating it from our lives. Developing good habits of coping can include quiet "alone" time for reflecting, meditation, daydreaming (and visualization), imaging, or other techniques that help clear the mind and renew the spirit. The old saying, "a healthy mind—a healthy body" is becoming more evident. Maintaining a daily routine of physical and mental exercises to relieve anxiety and tension is a healthy way to cope with stress. A happier healthier life results from successful stress management.

Complete Chapter 5, Unit 2 in the workbook to help you meet the objectives at the beginning of this unit and therefore achieve competency of this subject matter.

UNIT 3
Behavioral Adjustments

OBJECTIVES ....

Upon completion of the unit the student will meet the following terminal performance objectives by verifying knowledge of the facts and principles presented through oral and written communication at a level deemed competent.

1. List the commonly used defense mechanisms and give an example of each.
2. Explain what could happen to a person who habitually uses one or more of the defense mechanisms listed in this unit.
3. Discuss why it is necessary to know oneself before one can relate effectively to others.

4. List problem-solving steps and apply them to a particular problem you may have.
5. Explain the importance of one's mental and emotional status in regard to overall health.
6. Spell and define, using the glossary at the back of the text, all the words to know in this unit.

WORDS TO KNOW ···

adjustment	intellectualization	repression
analytical	malinger	stratagem
ardently	projection	sublimation
denial	rationalization	unobtrusive
displacement	regression	

We discussed in Unit 1 of this chapter how keeping a positive attitude is of primary importance in our interactions with others. Even though we strive for a good rapport with coworkers, patients, family, and friends, we must realize that we are human beings. Perfection in any relationship, even the best one, is certainly a desirable goal, but rather unrealistic. Understanding ourselves and others is essential in meaningful communications. Often in our daily transactions of conveying and receiving messages, we use certain coping skills to keep ourselves from getting hurt or to protect our image. These complex **stratagems** are called defense mechanisms.

Defense Mechanisms ·····························

These defenses are largely unconscious acts we use to help us deal with unpleasant and socially unacceptable circumstances or behaviors. They help us make an emotional **adjustment** in everyday situations. Surely we all use various defense mechanisms from time to time. However, habitual use can cause one to become somewhat out of touch with reality.

The most commonly used defense mechanisms are repression, displacement, projection, rationalization, intellectualization, sublimation, forms of withdrawal, and malingering.

Repression

The most commonly used defense mechanism is **repression,** which is the forcing of unacceptable or painful ideas, feelings and impulses into the unconscious mind without being aware of it. Certainly, we have all wished something unpleasant would happen to another person when we have experienced feelings of hostility, jealousy, or intense anger from interacting with that person. These feelings do not vanish, but are placed in our unconscious and may surface in dreams or subtle **unobtrusive** behaviors.

Repression, like all of the defense mechanisms, tends to protect us from unwanted messages about ourselves that make us feel bad.

Displacement

Displacement is the transfer of emotions about one to another. A typical example of displacement for the medical assistant might be as follows: In the course of the day, the medical assistant has many duties to perform for many others and one patient in particular becomes overly demanding and rude. The medical assistant holds back the strong feelings and deals with the situation professionally. Later in the evening at home, she feels all the pent-up anger and explodes at a family member. This is also done unconsciously, although sometimes, after the fact, we realize our actions have been displaced from the point where they originated to an innocent, unsuspecting target.

Projection

In **projection,** one might blame another unconsciously for one's own inadequacies. An extreme form of projection can lead to hostile, even aggressive behavior if one perceives another to be the cause of the painful feelings. An obese patient may blame a medical assistant for his/her gaining of a few pounds saying that the scales were set up or read incorrectly.

Rationalization

With **rationalization,** one justifies behavior with socially acceptable reasons and tends to ignore the real reasons underlying the behavior. This self-discipline unconscious act is relatively harmless. Habitual use of this defense mechanism, as well as all the others discussed in this unit, can become nonproductive or even destructive because they distort reality. A typical rationalization might be, "I dieted very strictly all day; therefore, it's okay to eat a couple of candy bars later in the evening after supper."

Intellectualization

Intellectualization is still another means of denying socially unacceptable feelings or strong feelings that cannot be easily expressed. With this mechanism, one uses reasoning to avoid confronting emotional conflicts and stressful situations. One might discuss all the facts and provide endless information about how to begin caring for an elderly relative, elaborating on special diets and home health care to avoid dealing with the true feelings of sadness over a relative's illness.

Sublimation

Sublimation is used unconsciously to express socially unacceptable instinctive drives or impulses in approved and acceptable ways. An example of sublimation might be a 30-year-old father and frustrated athlete forcing his child to excel in a sport.

Temporary Withdrawal

Temporary withdrawal is a defense mechanism in that it is a retreat from facing a painful or difficult situation. This avoidance of something that is unpleasant is another way of protecting ourselves from disagreeable feelings. Watching TV excessively or reading to avoid dealing with an issue are common types of withdrawal.

Putting off issues only makes the situation worse. It produces anxiety and makes the problem more difficult to face the longer the withdrawal goes on.

Malingering

Another common defense mechanism is malingering. One who malingers deliberately pretends to be sick to avoid dealing with situations that are unpleasant or that cause anxiety. A malingering individual might stay home sick on a day when he or she was to give a presentation, when in fact, that person is as healthy as always, enjoying the time at home.

Denial

Denial seems to be a commonly used defense mechanism. It is the refusal to admit or acknowledge something so the person does not have to deal with a problem or situation. When one is not accepting of the phases of life that may produce anxiety, as an emotional defense one sometimes uses denial. It is usually seen only in psychosis in adults who have reacted to a traumatic situation of extreme stress.

When one who has been given the diagnosis of a terminal illness does not accept the reality of it and believes that a recovery is certain, that person is going through the denial stage.

Regression

Regression is behaving in ways that are typically characteristic of an earlier developmental level. This usually happens in times of high stress.

A college student consoles herself during final exam week with eating hot fudge sundaes as she did as a child with her mother whenever problems at school piled up.

Indeed, we all use many, perhaps all of these defense mechanisms from time to time. Since they are mostly used without our conscious awareness, they may be relatively harmless. Again, habitual use of defense mechanisms can veil reality and interfere with facing personal issues and crises, as well as with open and honest communication with others.

Problem Solving

In our complex daily lives, we use many coping skills to deal with our difficulties. Defense mechanisms have already been discussed. Another approach to handling interpersonal problems and concerns is to develop problem-solving skills. Taking a step-by-step approach helps one look realistically and logically at a problem. This method encourages analytical thinking and confident decision making. Here is an outline of the basic steps in problem solving:

1. Determine just what the problem is and write it down.
   a. Is there a problem chain or a series of events that are contributors?
2. Gather facts and ideas to help you decide what to do about it.
3. Use analytical and creative thinking. (List your decisions and what you think their outcome will be.)
4. Prioritize your decisions and begin testing them one by one until results are satisfactory to you and others concerned.

If results are not pleasing, begin again with step one. Often, step one alone triggers an answer to a problem. Sitting down and writing out what the problem actually is can be most therapeutic. Once you begin to use this skill to think logically about major problems such as changing employment, relocating geographically, or locating a suitable day care facility, you will begin to think more logically in all matters. Making a habit of this skill will increase your peace of mind and reduce stress because you will deal with problems more efficiently and spend less time and energy worrying about what to do. This skill can be a great stride toward eliminating procrastination.

The medical assistant who concentrates on patient education may want to pass this helpful skill on to patients.

Mental and Emotional Status Influencing Behaviors ....

The medical assistant, in both administrative and clinical capacities, has many opportunities daily to observe patients' mental and emotional states. These observations have a direct influence on the medical assistants' behavior, which in turn directly influences their overall health. We must keep in mind that all medical personnel are patients too. Therefore, all of the information we learn about patients applies to us as well.

As Unit 2 points out, the stress in life can lead to ill health. A true understanding of one's self is the primary key to understanding others.

Learning about ourselves requires us to take a good hard look at who and what we really are. When assessing our "self," our individual presence may come to mind first. This presence comprises both one's physical self (our bodies) and one's self-image (how we view ourselves). Another dimension of self, as termed by psychologists, is the "self-as-process." This refers to the ongoing process inside us that deals with constant changes, or adjustments, in our lives.

Our response to others is dealt with by our social self. We have many different roles with which we identify ardently. Finally, we all have an "ideal self." This is what we picture ourselves to be, the perfect model we have of ourselves.

We are, indeed, complex beings, capable of doing just about anything we choose to. Unfortunately, many of us never come close to realizing our true potential. This may be due to never having to look at ourselves squarely. Sometimes it can be quite difficult and even unpleasant to be honest about ourselves.

A good way to begin a basic assessment of ourselves is by making a list of all the strengths we have, as well as all our weaknesses. This technique can help point out our abilities and qualities and identify areas that need to be changed.

An ideal time to reevaluate yourself and renew your goals and aspirations is annually on your birthday. Many people prefer the traditional New Year's resolution. Knowing yourself will help you become a more complete person and will help you relate to others more effectively.

Communicating Emotional States ....

In Unit 1 of this chapter, we discussed verbal and non-verbal messages. Communication is a complex process in which one must be aware of all facets for complete information exchanges to occur.

The perceptive medical assistant should be able to decide what "feeder questions" to ask a patient to determine whether the look on the patient's face matches the patient's emotional demeanor. The following are feeder questions the medical assistant may use to find out the emotional states of the patients they interview. After greeting the patient with a kind "hello," the assistant may want to ask "What seems to be the problem today?" or "What brings you here to see the doctor today?" or "Can you tell me about the problem you seem to be having?" or "Can we talk about what has been giving you concern that brings you in to see the doctor?"

For a follow-up visit, ask "Are you feeling any better since you were in to see the doctor last?" or "You don't seem to be feeling too well; do you feel any better?" or "Can you tell me how you've been doing since you were here last?"

Hearing patients' answers can provide a general idea of how they feel emotionally. Of course, one can only accomplish this by taking time to find out. That means giving the patients your undivided attention, if only for a few minutes. Unfortunately, many health care professionals lack the skills and perhaps even the concern to establish this rapport, and therefore fail to develop this skill. The medical assistant can be instrumental in pointing out

factors that can interfere with a particular treatment approach planned by the physician, Figure 5–4. Patients will likely respond to and comply with the doctor's orders far more readily if the medical assistant imparts a genuine concern for their well-being with each contact.

If a patient seems quieter than usual, for instance, the medical assistant might determine after talking to the patient (with eye contact of course) that he is preoccupied by some problem or matter that he may open up about if interest is shown and the time is taken. If the patient is not allowed to express certain feelings, he may not be attentive enough to listen to the physician's orders, which need to be followed for optimal health benefits. The medical assistant plays an important role in assisting both physician and patient in providing quality health care.

Complete Chapter 5, Unit 3 in the workbook to help you meet the objectives at the beginning of this unit and therefore achieve competency of this subject matter.

1. Travel (business or pleasure)
2. Work schedule (irregular hours)
3. Relocating/moving
4. Lifestyle/cultural influences
5. Economic concerns
6. Comprehension of physician's orders
7. Handicap/mental incompetence

FIGURE 5–4
Factors that can interfere with patient compliance in treatment plans

U N I T   4
Patients and Their Families

OBJECTIVES ....

Upon completion of the unit the student will meet the following terminal performance objectives by verifying knowledge of the facts and principles presented through oral and written communication at a level deemed competent.

1. Explain why it is important to develop rapport with patients and their families.
2. Describe means of safeguarding the patient's right to confidentiality.
3. Describe the patient's options in relation to the physician's treatment plan.
4. Describe the stages that follow diagnosis of a terminal illness.
5. Describe your role in dealing with the terminally ill patient.
6. Explain the purpose of the living will.
7. State the purpose of the Hospice movement.
8. List the services of the Hospice movement.
9. Spell and define, using the glossary at the back of the text, all the words to know in this unit.

absurd
devastate
holistic
hostility
incomprehensible

inevitable
marginal
nonchalant
terminal

The medical profession's first responsibility is to the patient. Thus you must be able to relate to people of all ages, from tiny infants to senior citizens.

The development and growth of your own personality and interests will help you do so. The ability to converse about a variety of subjects shows an interest in people and makes you interesting to be with. Conversation with patients helps to ease their anxieties and encourages a sense of friendship and trust. At times a patient needs to express pent-up feelings, and you will often be the one who provides this necessary listening service. Sincere empathy will often begin to relieve the inner fears and anxieties of a patient who is experiencing an illness for the first time.

Patients and family members may need to discuss the treatment plan the physician has already discussed with them. Often patients do not hear all of what has been said by the physician because they have been preoccupied with worry about their illness. Their questions may sometimes seem trivial, but to the patient they are real and pressing issues that need immediate attention.

Many patients have never before experienced sickness or injury. They may never have set foot in a health care facility. Having to face strange new surroundings, unfamiliar medical language, and possibly puzzling proce-

dures will add to the patient's apprehensions. The way the patient is treated in these new situations will determine how the patient, and members of the family, accept the diagnosis and prognosis of the patient's condition. Tact and good communication skills will help to promote rapport with all patients and their family members.

Right to Privacy ....

As mentioned previously, every patient has a legal right to privacy and confidentiality. Information disclosed to the health care team must be kept in the strictest confidence, and you must be ever mindful of the legal implications in handling patients' records. Information concerning patients may be given to another member of the health care team, such as a laboratory technician or referring physician, only when it pertains directly to the course of treatment. Another medical office may telephone to inquire about a patient's medical history for diagnostic purposes, to confirm symptoms, or to verify a birthdate; patients, in complying with referral appointments or scheduled tests, will have given implied consent for necessary information to be transmitted concerning their condition. In the daily routine, such procedures do not require consent forms to be signed by the patient. If this were not true, very little could be accomplished besides handling forms.

Medical information may be given to parties not concerned in the patient's treatment *only* when the patient has signed a release of information form. Medical insurance forms, for instance, have a section patients must sign to authorize the release of information to insurance companies, Figure 5–5. Only those

RELEASE AND ASSIGNMENT

Date _____

To _____
INSURANCE COMPANY

_____

Group No. _____ Certificate No. _____

I hereby authorize Dr. _____

to release to your company or its representative, any information including the diagnosis and the records of any treatment or examination rendered to me during the period of such Medical or Surgical care.

I also authorize and request your company to pay directly to the above named doctor the amount due me in my pending claim for Basic Medical, Major Medical and/or Surgical treatment or services, by reason of such treatment or services rendered to:

_____
PATIENT

_____
SIGNATURE OF INSURED

_____
WITNESS

_____
ADDRESS

FORM 3340 COLWELL CO., CHAMPAIGN, ILL.

FIGURE 5–5 Release of information form (Courtesy of Colwell Systems, Inc.)

persons specified by the patient in writing may receive information concerning the patient's condition. Usually the medical facility has a patient information release form, which is completed during the initial visit. Persons to contact in case of emergency are listed there. Inquiries should be made at this time as to who may be informed about the patient's condition. This document should be filed in the patient's chart for future reference. Those of legal age have the right to privacy in all matters of treatment, and even parents may not be given information about a patient's condition unless specific written permission accompanied by the patient's signature is secured.

In the normal course of conversation you may be told personal information that should be kept to yourself, unless doing so would be harmful to the patient. The patient will usually tell you how far the information should go, or whom to tell or not to tell. Emotional stress and other critical data should be relayed to the physician, for it may have some bearing on the condition of the patient. You must use judgment in this important area. A patient who is experiencing domestic problems, for instance, may be asking for help in telling you about them. Patients usually realize that professional persons can put them in touch with assistance and sometimes expect that it will be forthcoming if they merely suggest that help is needed. Tact is required in handling delicate matters of this nature. Patients trust the medical profession to safeguard matters discussed in the privacy of the medical office. Directly asking each patient who may receive this confidential information and having appropriate release forms signed will ensure that the patient is aware of what has been done and will also protect you from liability.

Choice of Treatment

Advising patients of the choices they have in the treatment of their illnesses is often among your responsibilities. A full explanation of the diagnosis, prognosis, and options in treating the condition are given to the patient by the physician. But, some patients have a difficult time in making up their minds and may need additional information and further discussion before deciding to accept a treatment plan, especially when it involves a major event such as elective surgery. There are life-threatening situations in which patients must make these decisions quickly. Often family members must help patients with these difficult decisions.

You play an integral part in reinforcing the physician's orders. You should become proficient in identifying those patients who still seem confused after leaving their conference with the physician. Restating what the physician has already said may be all you need to say to some patients to initiate their compliance. Some patients may have had trouble with the wording used by the physician and look

to you to interpret. It is difficult at times to make clear to patients all that is involved in the course of treatment. Great skill in perception is essential for all members of the health care team to ascertain if the approach to treatment is fully understood by the patient. This is a valuable skill which takes time and experience to master.

It is prudent to advise patients to seek a second opinion if they harbor any doubts concerning their condition. It may be that patients disbelieve the diagnosis. Having a second, or even a third, opinion will help them to accept their illness. Many insurance companies encourage patients to seek other opinions before treatment is initiated. This is wise, especially if the patient is troubled about the possible outcome.

In more routine matters patients still may have difficulty in complying with physicians' orders, as in weight reduction, exercising, or taking prescribed medicine. Patients must be given sound reasons for following the advice of the physician even though they already know that it is for their own good. The prescribed treatment plan will most likely change the patient's life-style. The patient who has just been diagnosed as hypertensive may have to cope with several life-style changes, such as losing weight, following a special diet, and giving up cigarettes. If reinforcement and encouragement are not sufficiently provided to the patient by members of the health care team, cooperation may be marginal. The risks of not following the physician's advice should be outlined in the simplest terms. Acting nonchalant or showing no interest in the patient will not be much help in prompting a patient to follow orders.

The final choice is always the patient's, to accept and follow the outlined plan of treatment or not. Knowing what is best does not always dictate compliance. Motivation is the key. Giving patients realistic suggestions can help them accept a treatment plan that may initially have seemed impossible to follow. Changing behavior will probably be resisted. The patient who experiences setbacks, who does not remember to take medication, who breaks away from the prescribed diet, and the like, will need additional encouragement to get back on track. You can be of particular value in this type of situation. You must always be reinforcing remarks made to patients concerning the intended goals of treatment. Furthermore, by being a good role model, you subtly reinforce the physician's advice. An assistant who should be, but is not, following a weight-reduction plan will give a negative impression to a patient who has just been told to do so by the physician. A patient who has been instructed by the physician in personal hygiene will be less likely to follow advice if the medical assistant could also well heed the advice.

In conversing with patients you will find that their areas of interest will prompt ideas for encouraging compliance with treatment. One good motivator is the physician's fee for services. Many patients quickly realize that they should follow the physician's advice, for it will certainly be more costly in the long run if they do not.

Terminal Illness

Dealing with patients who have been diagnosed as having a **terminal** illness will be a challenging and rewarding experience: challenging because of its difficulty and rewarding because of the knowledge that you are giving supportive care when patients and their families need it most.

Many patients have a hard time accepting the diagnosis. Their initial reaction is to deny it. Indeed, knowing that one's life is about to end is an almost **incomprehensible** fact. Patients wrestling with this new reality claim that the diagnosis is **absurd.** But ignoring the problem cannot provide solace.

As frustration mounts and anger becomes apparent, patients feel isolated, for they see others as the picture of health. Feelings of **hostility** are natural and **inevitable.** Patients in this plight may lash out at anyone with whom they come in contact. Blaming themselves and others becomes a means of dealing with their anger for a time. Questioning becomes a way of venting anger for some. "Why does this have to be?" is the most troublesome question. Following this stage of anger is a period of depression. This is the reaction to the final realization of the course of their illness. Patients in this stage are usually ready to talk about their illness, hoping someone will understand. It is a difficult subject to talk about, but you may be influential in helping them to respond and talk about their fears. Eventually the patient attempts to accept the terminal illness by bargaining, or seeking ways of "buying" more time. This sometimes gives them inner strength to stay a while longer, holding on to see someone be married, wanting to hold the new grandchild, waiting for someone to return from the service. In this stage of bargaining, patients may look for spiritual inspiration. The zest for life is strong and the fight is one not easily given up.

In the final stages of terminal disease, patients come closer to accepting the course of their disease. This is truly a sad time for patients and their families. To know that one may not see the next spring, to know that one will no longer experience the joys and pleasures of loved ones, is **devastating** to the patient. Empathy and genuine compassion may be offered to a patient who is reaching out for comfort. You will be touched deeply, and your fortitude will be challenged to the maximum in interacting with the patient and family members during this most stressful time.

Finally, patients resign themselves to impending death. An inner peace is often evident in patients in this final stage of their illness and they are willing to make plans for their final days.

Some patients prefer to spare family members the ordeal of prolonging treatment when their physicians reach the decision that death is likely to occur in the near future. The living will is a legal document that allows patients to terminate medical procedures that would sustain their lives if they became unconscious or unable to make further decisions, Figure 5–6, page 60. Also refer to Figure 3–1, page 29. This document is not recognized in all states in the United States, but is fast becoming a more acceptable way to eliminate continued life-support treatment of the terminally ill patient. With this legal form the patient and family are able to avoid an agonizingly long period in waiting for the inevitable and also keep the cost of health care to a more realistic and reasonable amount.

The patient signs this document and a copy is filed with the physician, the attorney, and the family. In assisting patients with this procedure, it would be helpful if you would remind them to make sure that all details have been worked out and that the family has been properly informed and who is responsible for honoring the document. Patients now know that they have a right to die with dignity and that they have a choice in making their last days of life more meaningful.

For many years a concerned group of individuals has recognized and commiserated with this grief-stricken group of people. These people have formed the Hospice movement to provide some health care to those with terminal illness. In recent years the Hospice movement has gained strength. Instead of the tiring and impersonal surroundings that are sometimes associated with hospital care, the Hospice movement helps the family provide care so that patients can remain in their comfortable, familiar home surroundings during the last days of their lives and be among their family members and friends more conveniently. Support and caring assistance is given to help the family learn to cope with the turbulence of the patients and their illness. Efforts are coordinated with physicians and hospital staffs when necessary to give patients the best possible care.

Patients and their families in this stage of the patient's illness may need more spiritual guidance. The counsel of a minister, priest, or rabbi, may also be found through the Hospice movement. **Holistic** care is their purpose. You should refer patients with life-threatening illness to the local Hospice movement for consultation.

Society is returning to the idea that there is a human need to share the experiences of birth and death with loved ones. These natural parts of life have been largely removed from our experience for some time

LIVING-WILL

of _____, Maker

WHEN my attending physician and one other physician decide that:

    (1) I am virtually certain to die in the near future and that I am currently unable to make or communicate my decisions regarding my medical treatment, or

    (2) I am currently unconscious and have a negligible possibility of ever regaining consciousness,

I NOW DIRECT that, under either of these conditions, all medications and medical procedures be withheld or discontinued except for those necessary to provide as complete relief from pain and other suffering as is medically possible. This comfort care should be used as generously as necessary even though it may alter my remaining life span.

THIS LIVING-WILL should be honored by my family, attorney, and physicians as the expression of my legal right to refuse treatment. I am an adult who understands and accept the consequences of its directives. To the extent that it may not be legally enforceable, those who know of its existence should regard themselves as morally bound by it.

SIGNED _____
                                      Maker

I CERTIFY that, on the date shown below, the Maker signed or acknowledged this Living-Will in my presence freely without pressure, that I believe the Maker understands and accepts the consequences of its instructions, that I am eighteen years of age or older, and that I am not related to the Maker by blood or marriage.

Signed _____ _____ _____
             witness' name   witness' address   date

Signed _____ _____ _____
             witness' name   witness' address   date

Prepared and distributed by
Association For Freedom to Die, 490 G Alden Avenue, Columbus 43201

FIGURE 5–6 Living will form (Courtesy of Association for Freedom to Die, Columbus, OH)

now. We have even become uneasy in talking about them. The need for human love in these significant times in our lives is evident in the return to the practice of entering and leaving this world at home.

Complete Chapter 5, Unit 4 in the workbook to help you meet the objectives at the beginning of this unit and therefore achieve competency of this subject matter.

UNIT 5

Office Interpersonal Relationships

OBJECTIVES

Upon completion of the unit the student will meet the following terminal performance objectives by verifying knowledge of the facts and principles presented through oral and written communication at a level deemed competent.

1. Describe relationships between the medical assistant, the employer, and coworkers.
2. List positive methods for dealing with stress.
3. Describe the reasons for staff meetings.
4. Explain methods of intraoffice communication.
5. State the purpose of an employee evaluation.
6. Discuss the obligations of the employer and the new employee in providing a smooth transition in the work place.
7. Spell and define, using the glossary at the end of the text, all the words to know in this unit.

WORDS TO KNOW

description	merit	petty
evaluation	obligation	transition
externship	perplexing	

The medical assistant employed in a medical office or clinic must learn to relate well not only to patients but to other members of the health care team as well. Dealing with the needs of patients on a day-to-day basis can sometimes become an overwhelming task. Schedules in most medical practices can easily become overbooked; sometimes it seems everyone has an emergency and must be seen by the physician today! Health care employees should be able to shift gears and handle these situations gracefully as well as efficiently. The essential ingredient in running a medical office smoothly is cooperation. When each employee contributes, a good team that works together for quality patient care results.

The field of medicine is by its nature stress-filled. Patients are troubled by an abnormal state of health and are naturally anxious and on edge. Commonly they exhibit their feelings by acting irritable and uncooperative at times. They not only expect but demand patience and understanding from medical personnel.

Staff Arrangements

Picture the ideal medical office where patients and medical staff are going about the business at hand in a pleasant, efficient manner. Everyone gets along well with everyone else, patients are smiling and friendly, and every interchange is courteous. The schedule is kept down to the minute, all the filing is caught up, the phone rings only when there is nothing else pressing at the moment, referral reports are all back, and everything runs like clockwork. This picture is unreal. This ideal situation is what every medical practice hopes to achieve. But to bring this model practice into existence would require the perfection of all persons involved. This is, of course, impossible. Nevertheless, each member of the staff has a unique set of values, principles, and standards and each must respect the others to ensure compatible relationships.

The number of employees varies in the many types of medical practices. Some physicians in private practice employ only one medical assistant to perform both administrative and clinical duties. This is a tremendous responsibility and requires a highly motivated and mature personality. Medical assistants must realize that sometimes long hours and limited benefits may be the result. A good rapport with the employer is necessary to accomplish the objectives of daily patient care. Usually a good friendship develops between physician and medical assistant over a period of time, and working together is an enjoyable learning experience for both. Interest in each patient is easy to cultivate since individual contact is made at each office visit. You may get to know patients even better than the physician because of frequent phone conversation. You will soon become the physician's right hand by supplying important patient information obtained in this manner.

Communication lines must remain open with this one-to-one relationship, as in all employer-employee relationships. If misunderstandings occur, they must be rectified as soon as possible. More complex problems can mushroom if incidental misunderstandings are not cleared up. Solutions to these problems must be worked out together. You will have to be assertive in decisions concerning administrative, clinical, and personal employment matters. Being on one's own as a medical assistant in a private practice has its rewards as well as its disadvantages.

Many physicians in private or group practice find it necessary to employ several medical assistants. Although this can be an enjoyable experience for all members of the staff, a great deal of cooperation and respect for one another is necessary for a harmonious relationship among the staff members to be maintained. Specific job **descriptions** encourage each employee to remain in a particular area and promote efficiency. Overstepping boundaries may cause friction and misunderstandings. At the same time all staff members must be willing to pitch in where help is needed. Again, a positive attitude is needed to create a pleasant work environment.

The physician usually delegates responsibility for office management to one of the employees, most often the one with greatest seniority, qualifications, or both. This frees the physician to attend to patients and also relieves the physician of personnel management. This is a major area of concern, especially in large clinics with many employees, and, as a rule, is an area physicians are not trained to handle. Many of these supervisory or personnel management positions are filled by registered nurses, but they also have little or no specific training in medical office management. Their training centers primarily around the hospital model and direct patient care. Since a trained medical assistant can, in most states, perform most of the procedures that a nurse can, under the supervision of a physician, resentment may arise. You must come to grips with this reality before accepting a position where it may be a source of irritation and discontent.

Many physicians and office managers appreciate the versatility of the medical assistant, respect their initiative and industriousness, and employ them with pride and satisfaction. However, each medical practice has its own unique office policy regarding employees. There are still those physicians who would rather take charge of their own office business affairs.

Working closely with others can have both positive and negative effects. In a large office practice or clinic, when there are many employees, a certain amount of give and take must prevail. Completing assigned tasks is expected so that the work is shared equitably. Petty differences should be settled with tact. Sharing enlightening experiences and significant events with other employees is a natural inclination. This is fine if it does not interfere with the patient care. A certain amount of self-discipline and self-control are necessary in a professional setting. Remaining aware of the situation at hand will help you perceive what is appropriate.

Intraoffice Communication

Many physicians hold regular staff meetings that all employees are expected to attend. They are usually held in the medical office either before or after patients have been seen and are announced far enough in advance so that arrangements can be made to attend. At these meetings decisions concerning office policy changes are reached and problems are discussed. This is a time for new ideas to be expressed and exchanged. It also allows all members of the staff to get to know each other.

Some situations between employees may be impossible to iron out. These are usually personality conflicts, and the usual course of action if the situation does not improve is termination of one of the employees, usually the one who is more troublesome or less valuable to the practice. This kind of perplexing problem may be discussed during a staff meeting. Personnel managers are often aware of these problems before they are reported, and they are usually handled privately.

Employers sometimes use office meeting time for in-service programs, such as training in cardiopulmonary resuscitation. Some employers encourage holiday celebrations on occasion to promote better working relationships.

An intraoffice memo is a means of communicating important information to members of the staff, especially between regularly scheduled staff meetings. Each employee is instructed to read the memo and initial it, indicating that the information has been received, and then pass it on to another employee. This helps ensure that all employees are informed. Word of mouth is not a sure way to relay an important announcement for it may get distorted en route.

Some offices and clinics use a bulletin board as a means of intraoffice communication. Notices of educational programs, seminars, or meetings are posted for all members of the staff to read, in an area such as the staff room or eating area. Meetings of the American Association of Medical Assistants should be posted there.

Career Entry

According to recent statistics, there is an increasing need for qualified medical assistants across the nation. Employers in the health care field are recognizing the benefits of employing medical assistants who have had specific training in this most versatile field. This, of course, eliminates the need for extensive and expensive additional training on the job. Externship plans are very successful in cooperative programs that provide soon-to-graduate medical assistant students. These students are usually hired at a part-time rate, and the supervisor agrees to allow the instructor to periodically visit the facility and observe the student's performance. (Many programs do not allow the students to be paid.) Other training programs require only that students observe for a certain number of hours to fulfill the program's standards. In either case, the trend is most welcomed after the past practice of hiring assistants without any training in the field, who sought either full-time or part-time employment in the physicians' offices or clinics.

The transition from student to medical assistant, at any age, poses certain adjustment considerations to all concerned in the health care setting. Employers have an obligation to assist the new employee in feeling accepted in the profession and to give helpful advice with patience. The new employee is obligated to strive to perform skills with both proficiency and efficiency. An effort to get along with others is required of each member of the health care team. A smooth transition by the new member of the team is possible if each employee recognizes the individual worth of each person and the value of each position in fulfilling the health care needs of the patients they serve.

Employee Evaluation

In most employment situations, an evaluation of work performance is made on an annual basis. This is filed in your record. The initial employment review is usually held after a probationary period of 90 days. In this meeting, you and your employer will discuss your job performance. Most evaluation forms are basically the same, Figure 5–7. They outline the most important qualities and abilities needed for the job and include a section for strengths and weaknesses to be listed. Qualities and abilities are assessed on a point system. High scores will be worthy of praise and recognition, usually in the form of a merit raise. Employers are always aware of an employee's behavior. Little goes unnoticed when you share a daily routine. Your attitude shows at all times. Even though the word *attitude* may not be a part of the evaluation, the other categories cover it comprehensively.

Initiative is an important factor. Demonstrating resourcefulness will help you advance in your career. Following office policy is also important. Being on time and being dependable on the job are always pleasing to employers. Absences and tardiness are difficult to tolerate from employees who make it a habit. Another area of extreme importance to employers is the quality and quantity of your work. Performing assigned tasks in a reasonable amount of time, without needing to be reminded, is a valuable trait.

The employee evaluation need not be a threat to the conscientious medical assistant. It is a time when questions about advancement and salary may be openly discussed. If you have lived up to the standards of the job, your performance should receive a favorable review.

FIGURE 5–7
Employee evaluation form

```
EMPLOYEE EVALUATION
_____

Employee's name        Position/Title         Date of Review
_____

Department             Supervisor             Date Employed
_____

Type of Review: ____ Probationary ____ Six Month ____ Annual ____*Other

*Explain_____

Date of Last Evaluation _____  Previous Rating _____
_____

Total days absent _____  Total of tardies _____  Total times left early ___
_____

Place  Appropriate Number for each of the following on the line to the right.

                   0  1  2  3  4  5  6  7  8  9  10  11  12  13  14  15
Quantity of Work:  inferior / careless/ does / average/ above / exceptional
Volume and                            just            average
   Consistency                        enough                            ___

Quality of Work: very poor/ fair / good/ acceptable/ excellent/ superior
Accuracy and
   Neatness                                                            ___

Initiative:      lacking/ needs pushing/ adequate/ excellent/ superior
Motivation                                                             ___

Judgement:       poor/ unreliable/ limited/ plans well/ reliable/ superior
Planning work,
Make decisions                                                         ___

Adaptability:    poor/ slow / satisfactory/ good/ excellent/ superior
   Adjusts to
   change                                                              ___

Cooperation:     uncooperative/ difficult / cooperative/ excellent/superior
Getting along
   with others                                                         ___

Speed:           slow/ moderate/ average/ above average/ superior
   Rate of
   work                                                                ___

Job Knowledge:   very little/ limited/ adequate/ average/ good/superior
                 (almost none)                                         ___
_____
                                                     Total             ___

Since last evaluation employee has:        Recommended for pay increas

____ Improved  ____ No change  ____ Regressed    ____ Yes    ____ No

Overall impression of this employee:

____ Unsatisfactory ____ Poor ____ Fair ____Good ____ Excellent ____Exceptional

Comments of strengths/weaknesses:    Supervisor's signature
```

Some employers find that annual evaluations motivate employees and keep communication lines open. Others choose not to have official evaluations, but wish employees to discuss whatever is on their mind at any time. For some office personnel this works quite well. For the private practice physician with a single medical assistant this is usually the case.

Complete Chapter 5, Unit 5 in the workbook to help you meet the objectives at the beginning of this unit and therefore achieve competency of this subject matter.

MEDICAL-LEGAL ETHICAL HIGHLIGHTS

Throughout this chapter you should be mindful of all medical-legal/ethical implications. Listed below are a few important reminders.

1. Be constantly aware of how you project yourself, verbal and nonverbal messages.
2. Develop and maintain good personal health habits to be alert on the job.
3. Respect the rights of all individuals.
4. Attend all in-service and staff meetings.
5. Follow office policy where employed.

Ms. Right

attends the monthly staff meeting where office policy is reviewed. She is considerate of all coworkers and patients by addressing them with their appropriate titles courteously in a pleasant tone of voice. Her body language exhibits professionalism as her appearance is consistently fresh, neat, and clean without excessive use of makeup, perfume, or jewelry. Patients sense her sincerity because she makes eye contact while speaking to them and she listens carefully when spoken to. She never talks about patients where other patients may overhear her.

Employment outlook: Continuous

Ms. Wrong

rudely calls patients by their first names regardless of their age or status. She does so while alternating cracking her gum, blowing bubbles, sneezing, and coughing. She missed the staff meeting because she was sick, again. Her appearance is untidy, her uniform and "jogging" shoes are obviously dirty. She complains to patients that she's the one who should be seeing the doctor and ignores the patients' questions. She pays no attention to reminders regarding office policy. She talks and laughs about patients where other patients can hear her.

Employment outlook: Termination

REFERENCES

Bates, Richard C. *The Fine Art of Understanding Patients*, 2d ed. Oradell, NJ: Medical Economics, 1972.

Calhoun, James F., and Acocella, Joan Ross, *Psychology of Adjustment and Human Relationships*, 2d ed. New York: Random House, 1983.

Kinn, Mary E., and Derge, Eleanor. *The Medical Assistant: Administrative and Clinical*, 6th ed. Philadelphia: W. B. Saunders, 1988.

Kubler-Ross, Elizabeth. *On Death and Dying*. New York: MacMillan, 1969.

Milliken, Mary Elizabeth. *Understanding Human Behavior*, 5th ed. Albany: Delmar, 1993.

Physician's Desk Reference. Oradell, NJ: Medical Economics, updated annually.

Purtilo, Ruth. *Health Professional/Patient Interaction*. 2d ed. Philadelphia: W. B. Saunders, 1978.

Riker, Audrey Palm, and Riker, Charles. *Me: Understanding Myself and Others*, rev. ed. Peoria, IL: Bennett, 1982.

Sehnert, Keith W., M.D. *Stress/Unstress*. Augsburg Publishing House, 1981.

Thompson, Ella M. *Textbook of Basic Nursing*. Philadelphia: J. B. Lippincott, 1973.

U.S. Department of Health and Human Services. *Saying No*. 1981. Alcohol, Drug Abuse, and Mental Health Administration, 5600 Fishers Lane, Rockville, MD 20857.

Wright, H. Norman. *How to Have a Creative Crisis*, Berkley ed. New York: Berkley Publishing Group, 1987.

The Administrative Assistant

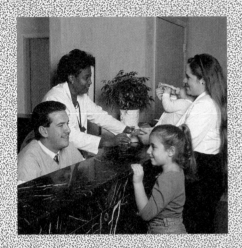

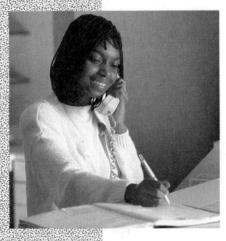

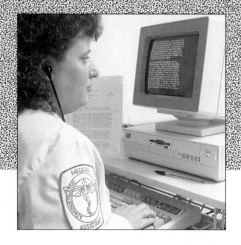

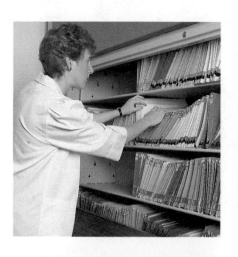

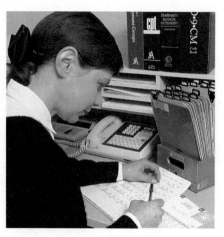

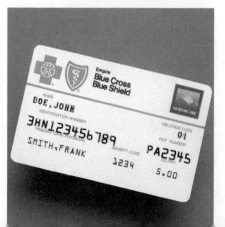

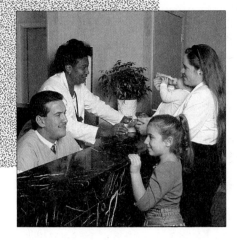

C H A P T E R　6

Reception

One of the most vital of the medical assistant's responsibilities is the role of receptionist. The receptionist's appearance and tone of voice in answering the telephone reflect directly on the physician-employer. Because of this, the assistant must always be professional, courteous, and friendly. The importance of appearance extends to the waiting room atmosphere, as this also reflects on the physician's practice. The office assistant must also have sufficient knowledge of medical terminology to deal efficiently with the unending variety of phone calls received daily.

U N I T　1

Planning the Day

OBJECTIVES

Upon completion of the unit, the student will meet the following terminal performance objectives by verifying knowledge of the facts and principles presented through oral and written communication at a level deemed competent, and will demonstrate the specific behaviors as identified in the terminal performance objectives of the procedures, observing safety precautions in accordance with health care standards.

1. Prepare a checklist for opening the office.
2. Prepare a checklist for closing the office.
3. Describe the importance of time management.
4. List information points that might be included in a practice information brochure.
5. List skills necessary for the medical assistant to use in maintaining patient satisfaction with the office.
6. Spell and define, using the glossary at the back of the text, all the words to know in this unit.

WORDS TO KNOW

brochure　　　　　　　　　　monitor
confidentiality

Preparing for Patients

The receptionist should always arrive 15 to 20 minutes before the scheduled time for opening the office. This time is needed for a visual check of office readiness.

You will need to **monitor** the temperature and cleanliness of all rooms; check to see that all supplies are in place and ready for use; and call the answering service for any telephone messages. In addition, the charts of returning patients should be prepared. Any correspondence or laboratory reports since their previous visit should be added to their charts and the date of visit should be written or stamped on the progress notes sheet.

Closing the Office

At the close of the day, the charts should be filed in locked cabinets. Money received from patients should be deposited at the bank or locked in the office safe. Check to be sure doors are securely locked when you leave.

P R O C E D U R E

Open the Office

TERMINAL PERFORMANCE OBJECTIVE: In a simulated situation the student will role play each of the skills identified in this procedure, taking into account the assignment and time schedule for completion of the procedures. The instructor will evaluate the procedure.

1. Unlock the reception room door.
2. Adjust heat or air conditioning for the comfort of the patients.
3. Check for safety hazards in the office. **Key Point: Check for frayed electric wires, damaged furniture, objects on the carpet which might cause patients to fall.**
4. Check magazines for condition and current date. **Key Point: Be sure magazines are current. Torn or damaged magazines should be removed from the waiting room.**

5. Check the telephone answering device or call the answering service for any messages.
6. Pull the charts of patients to be seen. **Key Points: Write or stamp with today's date. Check the patient's previous visit to see if any studies were ordered. If so, be certain that results are filed in the chart before the patient is seen.**
7. Check examining rooms to be sure they are clean and stocked with supplies. **Key Point: This is often done in the evening before leaving, but on occasion the physician does see a patient after office hours and may not have put things away.**
8. If it is the policy of the office, prepare a list of the patients to be seen and the times of their appointments and place this list on the physician's desk so that he/she can follow the schedule for the day without checking the appointment book.

P R O C E D U R E

Close the Office

TERMINAL PERFORMANCE OBJECTIVE: In a simulated situation, having been given an office environment problem, the student will identify all steps to be taken covering all applicable criteria identified within the procedure. The instructor will evaluate the response.

1. Check to see that records are complete and filed in locked cabinets.
2. Place any money received in safe if not to be deposited.
3. Check to see that all electrical appliances are turned off. **Key Point: Many offices ask that you unplug electri-**

cal appliances.
4. Check that rooms are all cleaned and supplied for the next day.
5. Straighten waiting room if time allows.
6. Pull charts for the next day if time allows.
7. Activate answering device on phone or call answering service with information about when you will be back in the office.
8. Turn off lights.
9. Securely lock doors. **Key Point: Activate alarm system if necessary.**

Organizing Your Time ....

To have a successful career as a medical assistant, you need to organize your time. When you know what is expected of you and what must be done, make a work schedule for yourself and try to follow it as closely as possible. You might have interruptions during the day that prevent you from following your schedule entirely, but it will serve as a reminder so that nothing will remain undone. This checklist could be used for several in an office or for an individual responsible for all the work. A sample schedule might look like this:

1. Call the physician's answering service.
2. Check all the rooms for appearance.
3. Fill sterilizer if necessary and connect all electrical appliances to be used.
4. Sort and open the mail.
5. Place a list of the appointments for the day on the physician's desk.
6. Pull medical histories out of the file for all patients expected. Stamp current date on progress sheet under last entry.
7. Prepare trays and setups for the day's appointments.
8. Type yesterday's dictation.

9. Transfer the patients' charges and payments to the patients' ledger cards. Set up pegboard for the day if that is the system used.
10. Check the supplies and order what is needed.
11. Check the physician's bag if one is used.
12. Do yesterday's filing.
13. Prepare bank deposit.

Practice Information Brochure ....

Each office should have an attractive **brochure** used to welcome new patients and to furnish information regarding your office. This is an excellent timesaver for office staff and should include:

1. The name of the office practice
2. Name or names of physicians and their specialty
3. Address of office
4. Map of office location
5. A description of specialty service offered
6. Procedure for making appointments, the best hours to call if not an emergency, hours the office is open
7. Any special instructions for first appointments
8. Any special rule regarding canceling of appointments
9. Instructions for emergency situations
10. Instructions regarding telephone calls, who may answer questions, when the physician returns calls
11. Comments regarding charges, billing, and insurance
12. Your policy regarding referrals and consultations
13. A statement regarding **confidentiality** of records
14. A statement regarding availability of qualified staff, educational materials, and any other special services offered (such as transportation to office)

Timesavers in the office include preprinted forms and use of inked rubber stamps.

Patient Relations ....

The receptionist has the first opportunity to ensure good patient relations for the office. Studies have shown that a patient gains the first impression of the office in the first 4 minutes in the office. The receptionist must be attentive by immediately welcoming patients with a smile, a pleasant tone of voice, and eye contact. Always attempt to call the patient by his or her full name. Be sure to explain any delays. Listen with undivided attention for verbal messages and note any observed nonverbal messages. The medical assistant must always be well-groomed and professional. It is a sign of professionalism to be polite and courteous. Look for opportunities to show that you care about the patients and their problems.

Complete Chapter 6, Unit 1 in the workbook to help you meet the objectives at the beginning of this unit and therefore achieve competency of this subject matter.

U N I T   2

The Reception Room Atmosphere

OBJECTIVES ....

Upon completion of the unit, the student will meet the following terminal performance objectives by verifying

---

P R O C E D U R E

Obtain Preliminary Patient Information

TERMINAL PERFORMANCE OBJECTIVE: In a simulated situation, having been assigned a patient, the student will clearly communicate instructions and will then follow up by completing the steps designated in the procedure within acceptable time limits. Consideration must be given the confidential needs of the patient and the details necessary for a completed medical record. The instructor will observe and evaluate the procedure.

1. Take new patient to private room to ask preliminary questions.
2. Ask new patient to complete a data sheet.
   Key Points:
   a. **Give the patient a clipboard to write on.**
   b. **Offer assistance.**

c. **Ask the patient to return the form when it is completed.**
d. **Any medical history is a** potential **legal document. Check to be sure the form is completed accurately and legibly.**
3. Prepare a patient folder by typing the patient's name on a label and attaching it to the tab of the folder.
4. Transfer information from the data sheet to the chart sheet.
5. Insert the chart and data sheets in the folder.
6. Prepare charge slip.
7. Place the folder in the area reserved for charts of patients to be seen. **Key Point: If you have received any referral material on a new patient be sure to place it with the chart you have prepared.**

knowledge of the facts and principles presented through oral and written communication at a level deemed competent, and will demonstrate the specific behaviors as identified in the terminal performance objectives of the procedures, observing safety precautions in accordance with health care standards.

1. Describe methods of providing for patient comfort in a reception room.
2. Describe techniques of monitoring interpersonal relationships in a reception room.
3. Obtain preliminary information on new patients.
4. Prepare a new patient chart.
5. Prepare a charge slip for each patient.
6. Spell and define, using the glossary at the back of the text, all the words to know in this unit.

WORDS TO KNOW ....

adequate   potential
alleged   preliminary
compliance   rapport
inappropriate   reluctant
interpersonal   tactfully
obstetrical

Physical Surroundings ....

It is the receptionist's responsibility to make the reception room (waiting room) a pleasant and comfortable place to be. The work day should begin with a special check to see that there is proper lighting, a comfortable temperature, and safe, adequate seating. A variety of current reading materials appropriate for all ages, both male and female, should be attractively arranged. When magazines become outdated they should be removed. The receptionist should monitor the subscription expiration dates to see that magazines are reordered when needed. Reading material of a medical nature is probably inappropriate in the waiting room because it may upset the patients.

Many physicians have developed brochures to give to new patients to serve as an orientation to the office. It is helpful to have the brochure available in the waiting room for patients to use as they wish.

You should make a daily visual check of the furniture to be sure it is clean and in good repair. Any wood furniture should be checked for splinters or rough places. Springs may wear out and protrude through cushions causing injury to an unsuspecting patient. Electric cords should routinely be checked for frayed wires and should be removed immediately for repair or discarded if found defective. An electric shock could seriously injure a patient. The carpet should be in good repair and there should never be throw rugs that can cause patients to trip or slip. A wastebasket should be provided.

If there are children's toys or books they should be off the floor when not being used. All toys for children should be washable and should be of a safe material with no sharp edges and no part small enough for a child to

swallow. The toys should be cleaned regularly so that children will not be infected by contaminated toys.

It is common practice to display a "No Smoking" sign in the office. If smoking is permitted, you not only allow smoke contamination and irritation to nonsmoking patients, but you invite the danger of matches being dropped in a wastebasket or into furniture, where a fire could start. Furniture and carpeting can be damaged by a dropped match or cigarette even if no fire results. If you allow smoking, a cigar smoker might light up and offend almost everyone. The best way to handle this situation is to take the patient to the next available examining room. If the patient leaves the cigar in an ash tray in the waiting room, be sure to dispose of it by flushing it down the commode. Any type of smoking can cause a patient with asthma or other respiratory conditions to have serious breathing problems.

Care should be taken to make the reception area accident proof. An injury in the office can result in a patient's demanding that the physician pay for the alleged pain and suffering. If anyone should be injured in the waiting room, no matter how slightly, the medical assistant must be sure the individual is examined by the physician.

The reception desk should be placed so that the medical assistant can have a clear view of the waiting room, but it should not be in the waiting room. It is generally advisable to have a window, which can be closed for privacy when you are engaged in telephone conversation or interviewing a patient.

Police officials now inform us that if your business office is accessible to the general public through the waiting room, the office entrance window should be covered with a grille to prevent individuals from entering the office to take drugs or to rob the cash drawer.

Social Climate ....

As patients begin to arrive for their scheduled appointments the assistant should greet each one by name, in a friendly, courteous, and cheerful manner. Of course, the medical assistant should be neat and well groomed. Building a good rapport is the key to patient compliance and continuation in the physician's practice. Remember to ask former patients if there has been any change of address, telephone number, marital status, or place of employment when they report to the reception desk.

You must be alert to monitor interpersonal relationships in the waiting room. Be alert to discussions of religion or politics as they can lead to angry differences of opinion. The best way to break up such a discussion is to place the patients in individual examination rooms where they will see the physician.

Patients who are very ill should not be left in the waiting room but placed in an examination room where they can be made more comfortable. No small child or very ill patient should ever be left alone on an examination table because of the danger of a fall.

Children who accompany patients, or those to be seen as patients, should be given books or easy-to-clean toys to keep them entertained while they wait. If they appear to be annoying patients, you may have to tactfully provide additional distractions in the form of reserved books or toys. This is especially true when the parent seems not to notice the situation.

Unexpected delays should be explained to patients on their arrival. If possible, an estimate of the length of time involved should be given. Patients can be given the option of waiting or rescheduling their appointments.

New Patients

A patient's initial visit is very important. Greet the patient promptly and courteously. Make an extra effort to make the patient feel comfortable and at ease.

The receptionist must be responsible for the completion of a new patient information form for each new patient seen in the office. If the medical assistant is not going to complete the form for the patient in a private area in the office, a clipboard and pen should be furnished to the patient so the individual can complete the preliminary information. You must be sure to give clear instructions and always offer help if needed. Patients who cannot read may be reluctant to admit their problem. Be sure the insurance information is complete. Many offices routinely make a copy of both sides of insurance cards to be sure of the necessary billing information. Be sure the form is signed by the responsible party. Figure 6–1, page 72, is an example of a new patient information form.

Charge Slips

Most medical offices have a slip that lists most, if not all, of the procedures performed in the office. This charge slip has space for the name of the patient and is attached to each patient's chart. Some large clinics even have charge-a-plates which they use to stamp the patient's name and account number on the charge slip. When the physician has completed the treatment, he or she gives the patient the slip indicating the services provided, and the patient gives the slip to the receptionist.

In an office where computers are used, you will find a variety of forms. Every office will design a form to fit its specialty, the number of physicians practicing in the office, and the type of computer program being used.

Figure 6–2, page 73, is an example of a computer form used in a medical clinic with a laboratory, X-ray, and physical therapy departments. The form should be preprinted with the name and address of the patient. If it is not attached to the chart, the receptionist may hand it to the patient to give to the physician. The physician completes the form with services provided the patient. The form is then returned to the front office desk by the patient before leaving the office.

Figure 6–3, page 74, is an example of a medical clinic form where obstetrical care and office surgery are offered.

Complete Chapter 6, Unit 2 in the workbook to help you meet the objectives at the beginning of this unit and therefore achieve competency of this subject matter.

MEDICAL-LEGAL ETHICAL HIGHLIGHTS

Throughout this chapter you should be mindful of all medical-legal/ethical implications. Listed below are a few important reminders.

1. Eliminate safety hazards: post warnings of dangers.
2. Clearly post exit signs.
3. Display fire, tornado, earthquake, and other emergency instructions for public safety.

Mr. Right

checks the reception area daily before patients arrive, making sure furnishings are in the proper place to eliminate any hazards. He knows hazards in the reception room could lead to a lawsuit if a patient is injured. He periodically inspects all exit sign lights and emergency instructions to ensure their visibility to patients for their safety. He is efficient in getting charts out for the day's schedule before patients arrive.

Promotion outlook: Excellent

Ms. Wrong

ignores her duty of checking for hazards in the reception area and takes no interest in patient safety. She has a habit of leaving boxes from deliveries in the hall or near exits for long periods because she tends to work slowly. She places emergency instructions on the wall behind the coat rack. She looks for charts as patients arrive.

Promotion outlook: None

PATIENT INFORMATION

DATE:

PATIENT'S NAME		MARITAL STATUS	DATE OF BIRTH	SOCIAL SECURITY NO.
		S	M	W	DIV	SEP		

STREET ADDRESS	☐ PERMANENT	☐ TEMPORARY	CITY AND STATE		ZIP CODE	HOME PHONE NO.

PATIENT'S EMPLOYER	OCCUPATION (INDICATE IF STUDENT)	HOW LONG EMPLOYED?	BUSINESS PHONE NO.

EMPLOYER'S STREET ADDRESS	CITY AND STATE	ZIP CODE

IN CASE OF EMERGENCY CONTACT:	DRIVERS LIC. NO.

SPOUSE'S NAME

SPOUSE'S EMPLOYER	OCCUPATION (INDICATE IF STUDENT)	HOW LONG EMPLOYED?	BUSINESS PHONE NO.

EMPLOYER'S STREET ADDRESS	CITY AND STATE	ZIP CODE

WHO REFERRED YOU TO THIS PRACTICE?

IF THE PATIENT IS A MINOR OR STUDENT

MOTHER'S NAME	STREET ADDRESS, CITY STATE AND ZIP CODE		HOME PHONE NO.
MOTHER'S EMPLOYER	OCCUPATION	HOW LONG EMPLOYED?	BUSINESS PHONE NO.
EMPLOYER'S STREET ADDRESS	CITY AND STATE		ZIP CODE
FATHER'S NAME	STREET ADDRESS, CITY, STATE AND ZIP CODE		HOME PHONE NO.
FATHER'S EMPLOYER	OCCUPATION	HOW LONG EMPLOYED?	BUSINESS PHONE NO.
EMPLOYER'S STREET ADDRESS	CITY AND STATE		ZIP CODE

INSURANCE INFORMATION

PERSON RESPONSIBLE FOR PAYMENT, IF NOT ABOVE	STREET ADDRESS, CITY, STATE AND ZIP CODE		HOME PHONE NO.
☐ COMPANY NAME & ADDRESS	NAME OF POLICYHOLDER	CERTIFICATE NO.	GROUP NO.
☐ COMPANY NAME & ADDRESS	NAME OF POLICYHOLDER	POLICY NO.	
☐ COMPANY NAME & ADDRESS	NAME OF POLICYHOLDER	POLICY NO.	
☐ MEDICARE	MEDICARE NO.	☐ MEDICAID	PROGRAM NO.	COUNTY NO.	ACCOUNT NO.

In order to control our cost of billing, we request that office visits be paid at the time service is rendered. We would rather control our billing costs than be forced to raise our fees.

AUTHORIZATION: I hereby authorize the physician indicated above to furnish information to insurance carriers concerning this illness/accident, and I hereby irrevocably assign to the doctor all payments for medical services rendered. I understand that I am financially responsible for all charges whether or not covered by insurance.

_____
Responsible Party Signature

FIGURE 6-1 New patient information record

PATIENT INFORMATION

PATIENT'S LAST NAME	FIRST	INITIAL	BIRTHDATE		SEX ☐ MALE ☐ FEMALE	TODAY'S DATE
ADDRESS	CITY	STATE	ZIP	RELATIONSHIP TO SUBSCRIBER		INJURY DATE
SUBSCRIBER OR POLICYHOLDER				INSURANCE CARRIER:		
ADDRESS	CITY	STATE	ZIP	INS. I.D.	COVERAGE CODE	GROUP

ASSIGNMENT AND RELEASE: I HEREBY AUTHORIZE MY INSURANCE BENEFITS TO BE PAID DIRECTLY TO THE UNDERSIGNED PHYSICIAN. I AM FINANCIALLY RESPONSIBLE FOR NON-COVERED SERVICES. I ALSO AUTHORIZE THE PHYSICIAN TO RELEASE ANY INFORMATION REQUIRED.

OTHER HEALTH COVERAGE ☐ YES ☐ NO   IDENTIFY

DISABILITY RELATED TO:
☐ ACCIDENT ☐ INDUSTRIAL ☐ ILLNESS ☐ OTHER

SIGNED (PATIENT, OR PARENT, IF MINOR) _____ Date _____

DATE SYMPTOMS APPEARED, INCEPTION OF PREGNANCY, OR ACCIDENT OCCURRED:

✔	DESCRIPTION	CPT/MD	FEE	✔	DESCRIPTION	CPT/MD	FEE	✔	DESCRIPTION	CPT/MD	FEE
	OFFICE VISITS	NEW PT			LABORATORY (Cont'd.)				PROCEDURES		
	Moderate Complex	99203			Wet Mount	87210			EKG	93000	93005
	Moderate/High Comp.	99204			Pap Smear	88150			Resp. Function Test	94010	
	High Complexity	99205			Handling	99000			Ear Lavage	69210	
	OFFICE VISITS	EST. PT			Hemoccult Stool	82270			Injection Inter. Jt.*	20605	
	Minimal	99211			Glucose	82948			Injection Major Jt.*	20610	
	Self Limited Comp.	99212			INJECTIONS				Anoscopy	46600	
	Low/Moderate Comp.	99213			Vitamin B12/B Complex	J3420			Sigmoidoscopy	45355	
	Moderate Complex	99214			ACTH	J0140			I & D*	10060	
	High Complexity	99215			Depo-Estradiol	J1000			Electrocautery*	17200	
	CONSULTATIONS	OFFICE			Depo Testosterone	J1070			Thromb Hemor.*	46320	
	Moderate Complexity	99243			Imferon	J1760			Inj. Tendon*	20550	
	Mod. to High Comp.	99244			Tetanus Toxoid	J3180					
	HOME	EST. PT			Influenza Vaccine - Flu	90724			MISCELLANEOUS		
	Moderate Complexity	99352			Pneumococcal Vaccine	90732			Drugs, Supplies, Materials	99070	
	ER				TB Tine Test	86585			Special Reports	99080	
	Moderate Severity	99283			Aminophyllin	J0280			Services After Hrs.	99050	
	High Severity	99284			Terbutaline Sulf.	J3105			Services 10pm - 8am	99052	
	LABORATORY				Demerol HCL	J0990			Services Sun. & Holidays	99054	
	Urinalysis - Complete	81000			Compazine	J0780			Counseling	99403	
	Hemoglobin	85018			Injection Therapeutic	90782					
	Culture, Strep/Monilia	87081			Estrone Susp.	J1410					

DIAGNOSIS:

☐ Allergic Rhinitis 477.9	☐ Chronic Fatigue Synd. 300.5	☐ Hemorrhoids 455.6	☐ Peripheral Vascular Dis. 443.9
☐ Anemia 280.9	☐ COPD 496	☐ Hiatal Hernia 553.3	☐ Pharyngitis 462.0
☐ Angina Pectoris 413	☐ Costochondritis 733.99	☐ Hiatal Hernia c̄ Reflux .. 530.1	☐ Pneumonia, Bacterial .. 482.9
☐ Anxiety 300.00	☐ CVA 431	☐ HVD 402.10	☐ Pneumonia, Viral 480.9
☐ Aortic Stenosis 424.1	☐ Cystitis 595.9	☐ Hyperlipidemia 272.4	☐ Prostatitis, Chronic/Acute . 601
☐ ASCVD 429.2	☐ Deg. Disc. Disease, CX .. 722.4	☐ Hypoestrogenism 256.3	☐ Rectal Bleeding 569.3
☐ ASHD 414.9	☐ Deg. Disc. Dis., Lumbar ... 722.52	☐ Hypothyroidism 244.9	☐ Renal Failure, Chronic .. 585
☐ Asthma 493.9	☐ Depression, Endogenous . 296.2	☐ Impacted Cerumen 380.4	☐ Rheumatoid Arthritis 714.0
☐ Atrial Fibrillation 427.31	☐ Dermatitis 692.9	☐ Influenza, Viral 487.1	☐ Sinusitis 461.9
☐ Bigeminy 427.89	☐ Diabetes Mellitus, Adult .. 250.0	☐ Irritable Bowel Syndrome . 564.1	☐ Supraventr. Tachycardia . 427.0
☐ BPH 600	☐ Diarrhea 558.9	☐ Laryngitis 464.0	☐ T.I.A. 435.9
☐ Bronchitis, Acute 466.1	☐ Diverticulitis 562.11	☐ Menopausal Syndrome .. 627.2	☐ Tachycardia 426.89
☐ Bronchitis, Chronic 491.9	☐ Esophagitis 530.1	☐ Mitral Insufficiency 396.2	☐ Tendinitis 726.90
☐ Bursitis 726	☐ Fibrocystic Breast Disease . 610.11	☐ Moniliasis 112	☐ Tc sillitis 463
☐ Cardiomyopathy 425.4	☐ Fissure In Ano 565.0	☐ Myocardial Infarction 410.9	☐ Ulcer Duodenal 532.9
☐ Carotid Artery Disease . 433.1	☐ Gastroenteritis 558.9	☐ Neuritis 729.2	☐ Ulcer Gastric 531.9
☐ Cerebral Vascular Disease . 437.9	☐ Gout 274.9	☐ Osteoarthritis 715.9	☐ URI 465.9
☐ CHF 428.0	☐ HCVD 429.2	☐ Osteoporosis 733.0	☐ UTI 599.0
☐ Cholecystitis 575.1	☐ Headache, Vascular 784.0	☐ Otitis Media 382.9	☐ Vaginitis 616.10
	☐ Headache, Migraine 346.9	☐ Parkinsonism 332	☐ Vertigo 780.4

DIAGNOSIS: (IF NOT CHECKED ABOVE)

REF. DR. & #

DOCTOR'S SIGNATURE / DATE	NO SERVICES PURCHASED	SERVICE PERFORMED	ACCEPT ASSIGNMENT	TODAY'S FEE	

INSTRUCTIONS TO PATIENT FOR FILING INSURANCE CLAIMS

1. MAIL THIS FORM DIRECTLY TO YOUR INSURANCE COMPANY. ATTACH YOUR OWN INSURANCE COMPANY'S FORM.

PLEASE REMEMBER THAT PAYMENT IS YOUR OBLIGATION, REGARDLESS OF INSURANCE OR OTHER THIRD PARTY INVOLVEMENT.

OFFICE ☐   YES ☐   AMT. REC'D. TODAY

E.R. ☐

HOME ☐   NO ☐   TOTAL DUE

INSUR-A-BILL ® BIBBERO SYSTEMS, INC. • PETALUMA, CA • © 7/89 (T-7) # 153-158   (REV. 2/92)

FIGURE 6-2 Charge form for medical clinic (Courtesy Bibbero Systems, Inc., Petaluma, CA 94954)

Patient First Name	Patient Last Name	DATE OF ONSET FOR ILLNESS OR ACCIDENT
Responsible Party Last Name	Patient Last Name (If Different)	Date / /

CHANGE OF: ☐ NAME ☐ ADDRESS ☐ PHONE ☐ INSURANCE ☐ EMPLOYER

DIAGNOSIS:	CODE	DIAGNOSIS:	CODE	DIAGNOSIS:	CODE	DIAGNOSIS:	CODE	DIAGNOSIS:	CODE
___ Abdominal Pain	789.0	___ Chest Pain	786.50	___ Enteritis	008.0	___ Impetigo	684	___ Pneumonia	486
___ Abrasion	959.9	___ CHF	428.0	___ Esophagitis	530.1	___ Insomnia	780.51	___ Post Menopaus. Atr. Vag.	627.3
___ Abscess	682.9	___ Cholecystitis	575.1	___ Fatigue	780.7	___ Irritable Bowel Synd.	564.1	___ Pregnancy	V22
___ Acne	706.1	___ Cirrhosis	571.5	___ Flu Syndrome	487.1	___ Keratosis	701.1	___ Prostatis Hypertrophy	600
___ Alcoholism	303.9	___ Colitis	558.9	___ FUO	780.6	___ Labyrinthitis	386.3	___ Prostatitis	601.9
___ Allergic Reaction	995.3	___ Concussion	850.9	___ Furuncle	680.9	___ Laceration	882.0	___ Pyelonphritis	590.10
___ Allergic Rhinitis	477.9	___ Conjunctivitis	372.3	___ Gastritis	535.5	___ Laryngitis	464.0	___ Radiculitis	729.2
___ Amenorrhea	626.0	___ Constipation	564.9	___ Gastroenteritis	558.9	___ Low Back Pain	847.9	___ Renal Failure	586
___ Anemia	281.9	___ Costochondritis	733.6	___ GI Bleeding	578.9	___ Lumbar Disc Dis.	847.2	___ Rheum. Arthritis	714.0
___ Angina Pectoris	413.9	___ Contusion	924.9	___ Gingivitis	523.1	___ Lumbar Strain	846.7	___ Sebaceous Cyst	706.2
___ Anxiety State	300.00	___ COPD	496	___ Gout Unspecified	274.9	___ Menopausal Syndr.	672.2	___ Seborrhea	690
___ Appendicitis	541.	___ Corneal Abrasion	918.1	___ Headache, Migraine	346.9	___ Menorrhagia	626.2	___ Seizure Disorder	345.1
___ Arrhythmia	427.9	___ Cough	786.2	___ Headache, Tension	307.81	___ Mult. Contusions	924.0	___ Sinusitis	473.9
___ ASHD	414.0	___ CVA	431	___ Hematuria	599.7	___ Myocard. Inf	429.1	___ Sprain	848.9
___ Asthma	493.9	___ Cystitis	595.9	___ Hemorrhoids	455.6	___ Myositis	729.1	___ Suture Removal	V58.3
___ Atrial Fibrillation	427.31	___ Dementia	331.0	___ Hernia Hiatal	553.3	___ Nephrosclerosis	403.9	___ Tendonitis	726.90
___ Back Pain	724.2	___ Depression	296.2	___ Hernia Ventral	553.20	___ Nose Bleed	784.7	___ Thrombophleb	451.9
___ Breast Fibrocystic Dis.	610.1	___ Derangement Knee	717.9	___ Hernia, Inguinal	550.9	___ Obesity	278	___ Tonsilitis	463
___ Breast Tumor	239.3	___ Dermatitis	692.5	___ Herpes Simplex	054.9	___ Osteoarthritis	715.9	___ Urethritis	597.80
___ Bronchitis Nos.	493.9	___ Diabetes Mellitus	250.00	___ Herpes Zoster	053.9	___ Otitis Externa	380.12	___ URI	460
___ Bursitis	727.3	___ Diarrhea	558.9	___ Hypercholesteremia	272.0	___ Otitis Media	382.9	___ Vaginitis No.s	616.1
___ CAD	746.85	___ Diverticulitis	562.11	___ Hyperlipidemia	272.4	___ Ovarian Cyst	620.2	___ Vaginitis Trich	131.01
___ Cellulitis		___ Duodenal Ulcer	532.1	___ Hypertension	401.9	___ Pancreatitis	577	___ Vaginitis Candida	112.1
___ Cerv. Disc. Disease	722.9	___ Dysfunct. Uterus Bld.	626.8	___ Hyperventilation	786.01	___ Paronychia, Finger	681.02	___ Vertigo	780.4
___ Cervical Strain Syndr.	723.8	___ Dysmenorrhes	625.3	___ Hypoestrogenism	256.3	___ Paronychia, Toe	681.11	___ Warts, Viral	078.1
___ Cervicitis Chronic	616.0	___ Electrolyte Imb.	276.9	___ Hypothyroidism	244.9	___ Pharyngitis	462		
___ CHD	414.9	___ Endometriosis	617.9	___ Impacted Cerumen	380.4	___ PID	614.9		

DIAGNOSIS: (IF NOT CHECKED ABOVE)

✔ DESCRIPTION	CODE/MD	DX	FEE	✔ DESCRIPTION	CODE/MD	DX	FEE	✔ DESCRIPTION	CODE/MD	DX	FEE
OFFICE VISIT - ESTABLISHED PATIENT				**LABORATORY**				**DIAGNOSTIC PROCEDURES (Cont'd)**			
Minimal Exam	99211			Venipuncture-DR.	36410			Spirometry	94010YB		
Limited Exam	99212			Venipuncture	36415			Holter Recording	93224YB		
Intermediate Exam	99213			Handling	99000			Sigmoidoscopy	45330		
Extended Exam	99214			Throat Culture	87060			High Sigmoidoscopy	45360		
Comprehensive Exam	99215			Monilia Culture	87086			Sigmoidoscopy w/ Biopsy	45331		
				Urinalysis	81000						
OFFICE VISIT - NEW PATIENT				Urine Culture	87086						
Limited Exam	99202							**PHYSICAL THERAPY**			
Intermediate Exam	99203			**PROCEDURES**				Hydrocollator	97010		
Extended Exam	99204			Arthrocentesis Small Joint	20600			Ultrasound	97128		
Comprehensive Exam	99205			Arthrocentesis Interm. Joint	20605			PT Unlisted	97039		
Accident Work-up	90020			Arthrocentesis Major Joint	20610						
				Trigger Point Injection	20550			**SUPPLIES**			
INJECTIONS				Cryosurgery Cervix	57511			Surgical Tray A4550	99070		
B12 J3420	90782			Face Cryosurgery	17000			Sterile Kit	84550		
Cortisone J0810	90782			Not Face, 1st	17100						
Flu	90724			Not Face, 2nd	17101			**MISCELLANEOUS**			
Pneumovax	90732			Not Face 3 or More, Each	17102			Special Reports	99080		
Tetanus Toxoid	90703			Ear Lavage	69210			Emergency O.V.	99058		
DPT	90701							Review X-Ray Report	76140-26		
Polio	90712										
MMR	90707										
HIB	90729										
Estrogen J0970	90782			**DIAGNOSTIC PROCEDURES**							
Lidocaine J2000	90782			Audiometry	92552						
Skin Test (TB, Cocci, Histo)	86585			ECG	93000YB						
Therapeutic Inj.	90782			ECG (Medicare)	93005						
Drug:	Dose:										
Antibiotic Inj.	90788										
Drug:	Dose:										

REC'D. BY:	TOTAL FEE	
☐ CASH		
☐ CK. # _____		
☐ CO-PAY	AMT. REC'D.	
☐ MC/VISA		

Authorization/Responsibility Agreement

I hereby authorize any insurance company to pay the proceeds of any benefits due me directly to: JAY RICHARD HODES, M.D. A copy of this can be considered as an original for insurance purposes.

Signed: _____ Date: _____

I hereby agree to pay my account as services are provided. If for any reason there is a balance owing on my account, I agree to pay promptly upon receipt of the monthly statement.

Signed: _____ Date: _____

I acknowledge and understand that I am responsible for all of the charges for all of the services rendered to me or any member of my family.

Although I have requested the doctor to bill my insurance company on my behalf, I clearly understand that it is still my responsibility to make sure the bill is paid in a reasonable time. If for any reason any portion of my bill is not paid by my insurance. I further agree to make arrangements for prompt payment of the bill.

Signed: _____ Date: _____

NEXT APPOINTMENT

MON	TUES	WED	THUR	FRI	SAT
2 WKS		1 M		2 M	
3 M		6 M		12 M	

DOCTOR'S SIGNATURE & DATE

FIGURE 6-3   Charge form for medical clinic (Courtesy Bibbero Systems, Inc., Petaluma, CA 94954)

REFERENCES

Frederick, Portia and Kinn, Mary E., and Derge, Eleanor. *The Medical Assistant: Administrative and Clinical*, 6th ed. Philadelphia: W. B. Saunders, 1988.

Simmers, Louise. *Diversified Health Occupations*, 3rd ed. Albany: Delmar, 1993.

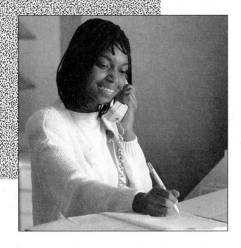

CHAPTER 7

Oral and Written Communications

The office assistant must have sufficient knowledge of medical terminology to deal efficiently with the unending variety of telephone calls received daily. A pleasant voice and good listening skills are essential. The medical assistant needs to have legible handwriting for recording appointments and messages. Typing skills are necessary if appointments are to be made on a computer. The student who enjoys typing has an opportunity to develop this skill as an administrative medical assistant. You will have an opportunity to demonstrate your knowledge of anatomy, medical terminology, spelling, grammar, and punctuation as you complete progress notes on charts. You will use these skills also in the completion of correspondence. You may have the responsibility of processing incoming and outgoing mail. Written communication skills must be as flawless as possible. A number of people may view the letters or forms you send out and each will receive a mental picture of you and your office—good if the work is neat and correct, and definitely questionable if it is inaccurate or messy.

UNIT 1

Telephone Communications

OBJECTIVES ....

Upon completion of the unit, the student will meet the following terminal performance objectives by verifying knowledge of the facts and principles presented through oral and written communication at a level deemed competent, and will demonstrate the specific behaviors as identified in the terminal performance objectives of the procedures, observing safety precautions in accordance with health care standards.

1. Organize desk space for efficient use of the telephone.
2. Demonstrate a professional method of holding and answering the phone.
3. Describe methods of screening incoming calls.
4. Locate information in a telephone directory.
5. Demonstrate a procedure for referring a patient to another health facility.
6. Spell and define, using the glossary at the back of the text, all the words to know in this unit.

WORDS TO KNOW ....

colleague	etiquette	prompts
confirmed	expressed	rely
empathy	personality	screening
enunciating	pertinent	verification

Telephone Messages ....

A telephone message pad and pen or pencil should be placed by each office telephone. You cannot **rely** on memory in a busy office where there are constant interruptions. Individual offices have a variety of methods for recording telephone messages. You may use a preprinted duplicate message pad; the top sheet is removed and the carbon remains as a permanent record of calls received. The office may use a secretarial notebook that is dated each day; calls are recorded and checked off when returned. You need to develop a follow-up method to be sure calls have been returned. The call pad or messages should not be filed until the requests have been responded to. Some offices have a stamp made up to indicate in the patient chart a telephone communication and a brief note with the date the patient was contacted. It is not advisable to have loose slips of paper in the file as they are too easily lost. If it is desired to keep these in the chart, they should be filed shingle fashion on a sheet of bond paper with the latest call on top. The slips should be fastened with a piece of transparent tape horizontally across the top of the slip. A vertical piece of tape along the side allows curling of the edges of the slip, resulting in a messy record that is difficult to read.

Adhesive telephone message forms are helpful in establishing effective control of patient calls. One of these forms comes in single looseleaf style with a stub which remains in a binder for future reference. Another style has a duplicate copy which remains in a spiral binder and provides a master reference for future review. When a call is received from a patient, the message form is completed. After completing the form, tear it at the perforation and attach the form to the patient's chart by removing the adhesive protection strips at each end on the back of the form. If a patient call requires a return call from the physician, the form is stuck to the front of the patient's chart and given to the physician. When the physician completes the call and records the message, the form is simply removed from the front of the chart and restuck on the inside of the chart for future reference, Figure 7–1. Another telephone message form is a log sheet and message slip with carbon. The benefits of this system are that you do not have to rewrite the message in the patient's chart, use a telephone stamp, or be concerned about loose slips of paper falling out of the chart. The carbon copy is a permanent record of calls for reference. Examples of telephone message forms are shown in Figure 7–1 and 7–2.

The important items of a telephone message are:

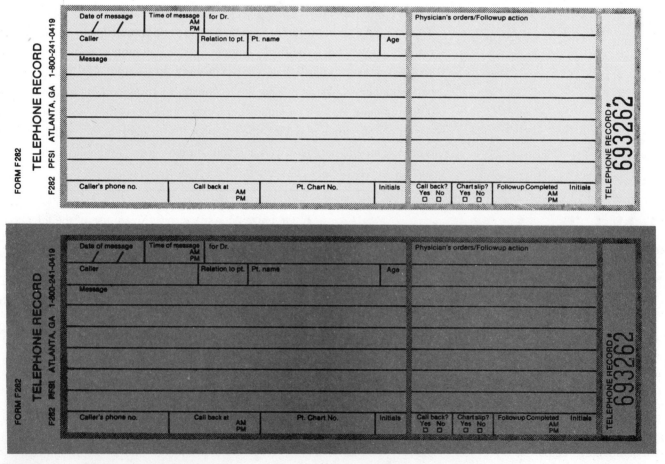

FIGURE 7–1   Telephone message form with adhesive strip backing on each end and carbon copy to stay in record book (Courtesy of Professional Filing Systems, Inc.)

- Caller's name, spelled correctly
- Brief note indicating the nature of the call
- Action required
- Date, time of call, initials of person receiving call
- Phone number of caller. Include the area code if this is a long distance call.

A telephone should always be answered promptly. If you are speaking with a patient in the office, excuse yourself and answer the telephone. You can never be sure when an emergency situation may be presenting itself. Hold the receiver 2 to 3 inches in front of your mouth and clearly identify your office, yourself, and say, "May I help you?" This prompts the individual on the phone to state his or her name and the reason for the call.

TELEPHONE MESSAGE LOG

Date_____ Time Of Call _____
Caller_____ Patient _____
Address _____ Age_____
Complaint_____

Medication Taken_____ How Long Sick _____
Cough_____ Productive_____ Temp_____
Vomiting_____ Diarrhea_____
Pain_____ Location _____
Bleeding_____ How Long _____ From _____ How Much _____
Nurse Return Call_____ Doctor Return Call_____ Phone No._____
Appointment Made and
Response or/Prescription given _____

PHONE MESSAGE

FOR ....

M ....

OF ....

TELEPHONE NO ....

☐ Telephoned   ☐ Please Return Call
☐ Will Call Again   ☐ Came In
☐ Returned Your Call   ☐ Important
☐ See Me   ☐ Wants To See You

MESSAGE..

....

....

....

....

....

....

DATE .... TIME .... BY ....

FIGURE 7–2 Telephone message forms (Courtesy Coldwell Systems)

When you are finished with the conversation, it is best to allow the caller to hang up first. If you hang up first you might miss something the patient wanted to add. It is not considered professional to say "Bye-Bye" when you finish the call. You should say "Goodbye."

When you have more than one telephone line coming in to the office, never answer the second line with "Hold the line, please," and then go back to your first call. You need to place the first call on hold and find out who is on the second line. Then you can determine whether or not it is an emergency and if it is not, ask the second caller to hold for you to finish the first call. Make all calls as brief as possible. You should keep any personal calls to a minimum.

Your voice is an important part of your personality at any time, but over the telephone, your voice is you. Callers form a picture of you as they listen to your voice. Does your telephone personality reveal a confident, courteous, friendly, and efficient medical assistant? It is equally easy to be heard as uncertain, irritated, abrupt, or inefficient.

The most common causes of poor communication are speaking too fast, too slowly, or too softly, and enunciating poorly. The phone is the heart of the office and should not be taken lightly. Since the phone call is often the first contact a patient has with the office, your manner of speaking and empathy are critical to your success as a receptionist, Figure 7–3.

Common Types of Phone Calls ....

The process of screening calls requires that you be aware of the most frequent types of phone calls that will be received in the medical office. They are:

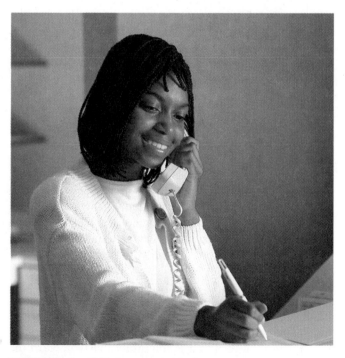

FIGURE 7–3 Telephone conversation

- Patients who are calling for appointments, prescriptions, or the results of tests
- Emergency calls
- Other physicians, hospitals, or laboratories
- Personal calls and general business calls

The American Medical Association has a workbook and cassette titled *Handling Patients' Telephone Calls Effectively*, which is used in the Department of Practice Management as a guideline for workshops on this important aspect of the management of a medical office.

Appointments, Prescriptions, and Test Results

Patients who phone for appointments should be given a choice of two appointment times. Usually one of the times will be satisfactory and this will eliminate the patient asking for multiple dates and times that are not available. Do not say "When would you like to come in?" It is better to say "Do you prefer mornings or afternoons?" Do not say "Are you a patient here?" It is better to say "When did we last see you?" Do not say "What is the problem?" It is better to say "Can you tell me what the problem is so that we can schedule you properly?" The appointment should be confirmed by reading the scheduled time back to the patient after it has been recorded in the appointment book.

You will find that patients will frequently ask to speak with the physician. Never say "The doctor is busy," as this may give the impression that the doctor does not want to be bothered by the caller. Be aware of the statements you make in reporting why the physician cannot speak on the telephone. The cliche, "The doctor is tied up right now," might suggest someone tied with a rope, bound to a chair. It would be much better to state "the doctor is with a patient now. May I take a message and we will return the call?" The caller will usually respect the right of others to have the full attention of the physician and will not expect to interrupt the doctor except for an emergency.

Transferring Telephone Calls

If it is necessary to transfer a call to the physician or someone in another part of the office, it is not professional to raise your voice to call another person to the telephone. If a patient is calling for information, be sure to pull the patient chart and hand it to the physician so that the needed information will be at hand. If the physician is with another patient when you relay the message that a call needs to be answered, it is best to hand the physician a note to protect the confidentiality of the caller.

Prescriptions

Each office will have its own rules for giving information to patients regarding tests or for calling pharmacies for prescription refills. It is important that you learn the rules for the office you work in and follow them without

exception. The general rule is that a medical assistant does not give out information or call in a prescription without the expressed direction of the physician.

Write messages requesting prescriptions or test results in legible handwriting. If a patient requests a prescription refill, you need to know the name and phone number of the pharmacy as well as the name of the medication, strength, and prescription number. You also should record a telephone number where the patient can be reached in case the physician needs to talk with the patient before prescribing the medication. The physician may need to examine the patient first and you would need to call and schedule an appointment.

Emergency Calls

Emergency calls should be put through to the physician immediately. Calls in this category would relate to:

- Severe chest pain
- Abdominal pain
- Shortness of breath
- Severe injury
- Possible poisoning

After you find out the symptoms, you must ask how long they have been present. You should have a series of questions in mind which will be triggered by the caller's statements. Your office protocol should provide you with a checklist of questions to be asked. These questions can be a part of the specially designed message pads for your office. Callers are often so upset they forget important information. You must remain calm and get the name of the caller, the address, and telephone number.

Caller: "I need to see the doctor right away."
Medical Assistant: "What symptoms are you having?"
Caller: "I am having a lot of pain."
Assistant: "Where is the pain? How long have you had it? Have you had pain like this in the past?"

You should be able to determine the urgency from the responses to the questions. The patient may need to be seen right away in the office or even need to be referred to a hospital emergency room. If the caller is alone you may need to call an emergency team or paramedics to go to the patient. Be sure in that case that the patient or someone near will be able to admit the squad when they arrive.

You should know what procedures are to be followed in handling an emergency when the physician is available and in the absence of the physician. The procedures should be written in the office procedure manual and should be near the telephones at all times. This procedure sheet should list the complaints your physician considers to be emergencies. These might include bleeding from injury, bleeding during pregnancy, vomiting blood, severe chest pains, difficulty breathing, unconsciousness, fractures, seizures, sudden loss of feeling in any part of the body, a child swallowing poison, or an eye injury. In each case, the procedure manual should give you guidelines to follow. The guidelines should include whether the patient should be seen in the office or be referred to a hospital. There should be a listing of the physicians to refer special problems to when your employer is not available. The referral should give a choice of two or three physicians for the patient to choose from.

Emergency numbers should be near the telephone so that you can make immediate referrals if the physician is away from the office. The list should have the telephone numbers for ambulance, fire, police, local hospital emergency rooms, and the poison control center. Never put an emergency call on hold before you determine the nature of the emergency.

Never give advice over the phone or in the office without the express instruction in each instance from the physician. You may know what the physician is going to say but you must hear it from the physician and then with permission relay it to the patient.

Professional Calls

When a physician telephones to speak to your employer, politely ask the caller for his or her name and inform the physician. Professional **etiquette** dictates that a physician will not keep a **colleague** waiting unless the physician is involved with an emergency or a surgical procedure.

Any calls that come into your office for the purpose of giving X ray or laboratory results need to be recorded accurately. Always record the name of the person making the report. It is best to read back everything you have written down to be sure it is correct and complete before allowing the caller to leave the line.

The physician should review and initial all reports the day they arrive at the office. Pull the patient chart and attach the report. Never file a report that the physician has not seen and initialed. The patient or referring physician may need to be notified of the results by your physician employer. After this is completed, the report will be ready to file.

Some physicians also dictate reports, which you will be required to transcribe and mail. Always be sure to make a copy of any correspondence mailed out so you have a copy to file in the patient chart. This is always filed with the most recent correspondence on top when the folder is opened.

When a patient calls for test results, you should never give them without receiving the physician's instructions on what to report. You would never give information to other people about a patient without the written permission of the patient and the approval of the physician.

Business and Personal Calls

Your employer should let you know how to handle calls from family members, business associates, and salespeople. Calls from attorneys requesting information on a patient must be handled with great caution. Attorneys know the patient must give written permission to divulge information to anyone regarding their health, yet attorneys will call and ask for information. Pull the patient chart and look for authorization listing the name of the attorney and the signature of the patient. If you find it, you may answer questions about the patient. If you do not find authorization listing the name of the attorney, you must tell the caller to send an authorization signed by the patient and then you will be able to release information. It is advisable to return a call from an attorney even if you have authorization so you can be sure whom you are talking to. Anyone can call and claim to be a patient's attorney. Unless you know the caller, you cannot be sure you are talking to the correct individual.

Only information that has been authorized by the patient in writing, with the patient's signature, may be given to another party. Otherwise, the patient record is considered confidential information.

Angry Calls

You may receive calls from patients regarding their statement or their insurance. If you are very careful in your accounting and billing, these should be infrequent calls. If you do receive a call from a patient who is angry, be sure you listen attentively, then tell the patient "please hold so I can get your record." If you have made an error, be sure you admit it, apologize, and offer to send a revised statement. Never raise your voice or allow yourself to blame someone else for a mistake you have made. Sometimes it is best to say you will check the records and call back. Always keep your word and follow up with the promised action. Patients will soon learn to trust you if you gain a reputation for careful follow-up of promises. Frequently patients need to know if insurance has paid the bill or how much was paid by insurance. You can quickly check the record and answer the questions.

Reports from Patients

When the physician routinely tells patients, "Call me and let me know how you are getting along," you can expect to receive calls to report how the patient is feeling or to report reactions to medications. These reports should be carefully recorded and given to the physician. You need to indicate whether or not the physician is expected to respond to the call.

Physician Visits Outside the Office

When a patient calls and requests a house call, be sure you check with your physician employer before you schedule one. If your employer makes house calls, you should have a city map or county map to help locate any new patient scheduled.

Many physicians visit patients in nursing homes on a regular basis. You need to establish a method of recording these visits and hospital calls. The physician should have a list of calls to be made each day along with a checklist of needed follow-up and charges for services.

Answer the Office Phone

TERMINAL PERFORMANCE OBJECTIVE: In a simulated situation, with a telephone, paper, and pen or pencil, the student will answer the telephone by the third ring, identifying the office and self. The voice must be clear, distinct, and at a moderate rate, expressing consideration for the needs and safety of the patient according to accepted medical standards.

1. Answer the phone promptly and pleasantly. **Key Point: Answer by the third ring.**
2. Identify office by name (Dr. Brown's office).
3. Identify yourself by name (_____ speaking). **Key Point: Your employer will tell you how to identify the office and yourself.**
4. Ask the caller if you can be of assistance (May I help you?).
5. Listen to the name of the caller and the reason for the call. **Key Points:**
   a. **Be sure to obtain correct spelling of name. If in doubt, ask for spelling.**
   b. **Never ask an emergency call to wait.**
   c. **If you put callers on hold, let them know so they won't think you have hung up on them. Return to the line every 2 minutes to let them know they are not forgotten.**
   d. **Always wait for a response. They may not be able to hold or may wish to call back or to call again later. Always give an option.**
   e. **When you place a call on hold, go back and complete the call that was interrupted.**
   f. **Never leave an angry patient. If necessary get another person to take over or answer other lines.**
6. If a patient is calling to talk with the physician and your employer is busy, say, "I'm sorry, but the doctor is with a patient now. May I be of assistance?" If you cannot help, say, "May I have your telephone number so that your call may be returned?" **Key Point: Sometimes callers will allow you to help when they find the physician is unable to come to the phone.**
7. Write down the response requested by the caller.
8. Close the conversation politely (Thank you for calling). **Key Point: Say "Goodbye," never "Bye-bye." Use patients' names in thanking them.**
9. Make sure the conversation is completed before replacing the receiver. **Key Point: Allow caller to hang up first.**

Long Distance Calls

You may need to place long distance calls. If you are calling an area outside of your time zone, you should consult the telephone directory for the map of time zones so you can establish the appropriate time to call. Be sure you know the code number needed to dial for your long distance service, in addition to the telephone numbers of the persons you need to call. A record book should be kept on all long distance calls made.

Call Monitoring

When your employer asks you to monitor a call, listen quietly and take notes of the conversation. It is important to make certain the caller agrees to your listening and taking notes. It is illegal for you to do this without the consent of the caller.

Refusal to Identify

Your office may have a specific method of handling individuals who call and refuse to identify themselves. A good general rule is to suggest that the individual write a letter to the physician and mark it *personal*, in which case the physician will receive it unopened. Most physicians do not wish to talk to unidentified callers during busy office hours.

Finding Phone Numbers ....

You can save a great deal of time by keeping an up-to-date index of your most frequently called numbers by the telephone. In addition, when you need to use the telephone directory, it is helpful to know how it is organized.

The introductory section usually contains:

- Emergency numbers
- Community service numbers
- General telephone information
- Directory assistance information
- Rates for telephone calls
- Out-of-city area codes and time zones
- Money-saving tips on use of the telephone
- Directions for making international calls

You will find an alphabetic listing of individuals in the white pages. There may be separate listing of business and professional organizations in a second section of the white pages. An index of city, county, state, and U.S. government offices may be found in a separate section of pages. Local zip code numbers by street address are usually in the introduction or a separate section of the telephone book. The yellow pages (or classified directory) list the name, address, and phone number of every business subscriber, grouped under product and

PROCEDURE

Receive, Evaluate and Record a Phone Message

TERMINAL PERFORMANCE OBJECTIVE: In simulated situations, with a telephone, paper, and pen or pencil, the student will answer the telephone by the third ring, identifying the office and self. The voice must be clear, distinct, and at a moderate rate, expressing consideration for the needs and safety of the patient according to accepted medical standards for each situation presented.

1. Answer phone promptly and pleasantly. **Key Point: Speak distinctly and use good grammar.**
2. Identify the office and yourself.
3. Screen calls. Write the caller's name on the message sheet. **Key Points:**
   a. **The patient may often be satisfied by scheduling an appointment.**
   b. **When the patient requests a refill on a prescription, write down the name and phone number of the pharmacy to be called, the medication being requested, and prescription number. Record the phone number of the patient in case the physician does not wish to allow a refill and needs to see the patient first.**
   c. **On patient requests regarding test results, you will need to show the patient record to the physician and receive instructions regarding information to be given to the patient.**
   d. **If a patient requests that you give information to an employer, attorney, or insurance company, inform the patient that the request must be written and signed and in the file before such information can be released.**
   e. **If the physician must return a call, be sure the pertinent information (number to be called, reason for call, and whether or not the call is urgent) is written on the message pad.**
   g. **If a business person is calling, record name, company, and company's phone number along with reason for the call.**
   h. **If it is a personal call from another physician, notify your employer immediately.**

   i. **If it is a personal call from a member of your employer's family, you will have instructions about how to handle it (usually put through immediately).**
   j. **If it is a personal call of a general nature, write the person's name and phone number and where he or she may be reached by phone.**

EMERGENCY CALLS

   a. **By calmly asking pertinent questions, you may be able to recognize whether a patient is simply upset or whether a real emergency exists.**
   b. **The physician or office manager in each office should train staff in the questions to ask and procedures to be followed when the physician is in or out of the office.**
   c. **If specific training is not given, the medical assistant should request instructions before an emergency arises.**
   d. **In general, the questions would be:**
      What are the symptoms?
      How long have you had them?
      What have you done for the symptoms?
      Have you ever had similar symptoms?
      Where are you?
      Could you get someone to bring you to the office or an emergency facility?
4. Write the time and date of the phone call.
5. Sign your initials.
6. Write the complete message as stated by caller.
7. Note the response requested by caller (action to be taken).
8. Read the information you have recorded to the caller for **verification**.
9. Close the conversation politely.
10 Make sure conversation is completed before replacing the receiver. **Key Point: Allow the caller to hang up first.**
11. Pull patient chart and attach message.

service headings. The classified directory also contains an index that can help you determine the headings under which a specific type of product or service may be listed.

Answering Device and Service ....

Your office may have an answering device which you will set to answer the telephone when you are not in the office. This machine will tell the patient how to contact

the physician or how to leave a message. It will usually be your responsibility to play back any messages received when you return to the office.

The telephone in the medical office must be answered any time a patient calls during day or night every day of the year. Many physicians prefer not to have calls come to their home and therefore subscribe to a telephone answering service. Some answering services are owned and operated by the local medical society and some are

PROCEDURE

Arrange Referrals by Phone

TERMINAL PERFORMANCE OBJECTIVE: In a simulated situation requiring patient referral reason, and using patient information, phone, paper and pen or pencil, and a phone directory, the student will accurately dial number, provide patient information, record referral data covering all criteria identified in procedure. The instructor will evaluate the procedure.

1. Receive name of patient, reason for referral, and other instructions from physician.
2. Place call to the referred physician or laboratory.
   Key Points:
   a. **Give name, address, and telephone number of the patient.**
   b. **State reason for referral.**

   c. **Indicate whether you will be sending a letter with information (be sure you have a signed release from the patient if doing this).**
   d. **Record the appointment time and place.**
3. Give the patient the name, address, and phone number of the doctor or laboratory to be visited with the date and time of the appointment and general directions on how to reach the place of appointment.
4. Give the patient instructions for any special tests to be completed. **Key Point: This should be a pretyped instruction sheet.**
5. Write the date and time of the appointment and the name of the physician or laboratory on the patient's chart along with a note of any instructions given to the patient.

---

privately owned. The answering service will have an arrangement to contact the physician in the event of an emergency. The contact can be made by telephone or through use of a "pager" carried by the physician. If the "pager" is activated, the physician knows to call the answering service for the message. Some answering services are connected with the phone in the physician's office and home. This service will answer the phone if it is not answered in the office or home after a predetermined number of rings.

The answering service is to be contacted the first thing in the morning for calls not picked up by the physician during the night, at noon if no one is going to be in the office, and at night to let the service know the destination of the physician.

Telephone answering services bill per call after a predetermined number of calls has been reached (example: 500 per month). For this reason, it is important to call the answering service as soon as you reach the office in the morning.

The rules for handling the physician's telephone can be summarized as follows:

1. Answer the telephone as promptly as possible.
2. Keep a pad and pencil next to the telephone at all times.
3. Verify the caller's name and correct spelling. If an adult calls about a child, make sure you have the correct last name. Do not assume the child's last name is the same as the caller's name.
4. Determine the reason for the call.
5. Handle as many telephone calls as you possibly can without disturbing the physician.

6. If the physician prefers to speak to patients, call physician to the telephone after saying who is calling. Take out the patient's chart and give it to the physician.
7. Whenever possible, if you cannot handle the call alone, take a message for the physician, so it can be read at leisure. The physician will tell you what to do or call the patient back when time allows.
8. Make a memorandum for the physician of every telephone call. Use printed telephone memorandum pads that show date of call, time of call, name of caller, telephone number, and message.
9. Always know where to reach the physician. If the message is urgent and the physician is not in the office, telephone at once and relay the message.
10. If the physician cannot be reached, have the message by your phone. When your employer checks in, you may relay the message.
11. Learn how much medical information the physician wishes you to give over the telephone. Patients frequently call the office because they have forgotten the physician's instructions about treatments or medications. If these instructions are clearly stated in the chart, it may be possible for the assistant to repeat them to the patient.
12. When answering a second line, determine if it is an emergency or another physician before placing tne caller on hold and returning to finish the first call.
13. End all telephone conversations on a friendly note. In general, let the caller be the first one to hang up or say "good bye."
14. *Never* promise a cure over the telephone or in person. Never say "I am sure the physician can help you."

PROCEDURE

Record Telephone Message on Recording Device

TERMINAL PERFORMANCE OBJECTIVE: In a simulated situation with a telephone recorder or tape recorder, paper, and pen or pencil, the student will compose, record and verify message according to the accepted medical standards specified in the procedure.

1. Write out the message you wish to record.
2. Activate the recorder.
3. Read the message you wish to record. **Key Point: Speak naturally but be aware of your speed and clarity.**
4. Play the message back so you can evaluate how well you have done.

Key Points:
a. **Did you identify the office?**
b. **Did you ask the caller to leave a message and if so did you give clear instructions as to how to do this?**
c. **If you give information did you include everything necessary?**
d. **Was your voice clearly understood?**

5. Set the machine to play the recording when you are unable to answer or are unavailable to answer the phone.

PROCEDURE

Obtain and Record Messages from Answering Service

TERMINAL PERFORMANCE OBJECTIVES: In a simulated situation with a telephone, paper, and pen or pencil, the student will call the answering service, record messages, and verify information according to accepted medical standards specified in this procedure. The instructor will observe the procedure.

1. Dial the answering service number and ask for all messages.
2. Accurately record the messages given. **Key Point: Use a separate form for each message.**
3. Read back the messages to be sure you have made no mistakes in recording the information.

Complete Chapter 7, Unit 1 in the workbook to help you meet the objectives at the beginning of this unit and therefore achieve competency of this subject matter.

U N I T   2

Schedule Appointments

OBJECTIVES ....

Upon completion of this unit, the student will meet the following terminal performance objectives by verifying knowledge of the facts and principles presented through oral and written communication at a level deemed competent, and will demonstrate the specific behaviors as identified in the terminal performance objectives of the procedures, observing safety precautions in accordance with health care standards.

1. Describe modified patient wave scheduling.
2. Describe cluster patient schedules.
3. Describe establishing a matrix.
4. List ways an office can establish the most desirable method for scheduling.
5. List the most important points in determining appointment scheduling when the patient calls the office.
6. Define the two types of listening.
7. State rules for handling a cancelled appointment.
8. Describe the best way to schedule a patient who is always late.
9. List goals of the patients in making appointments.
10. List goals of the physician in making an appointment schedule.
11. List goals of the medical assistant in making an appointment schedule.
12. List the common appointment abbreviations and what they mean.
13. Define the term *detail person*.
14. List advantages of a computer scheduling system.
15. Discuss advantages of open office hours.
16. State information needed in a procedure manual that is helpful in making appointments outside of the office.
17. Describe the procedure for making a follow-up appointment.
18. Spell and define, using the glossary at the back of the text, all the words to know in this unit.

Structuring ••••••••••••••••••••••••••

Office hours may be scheduled, with appointments at specific times, or left as an open, **unstructured** block of time.

If patients are to be seen at specific times, the most suitable method for scheduling appointments must be determined. Several supply houses produce books that can be used to schedule an entire year, each day printed with hours ranging from 8 A.M. to 5 P.M. or later, Figure 7–4. Some offices use individual appointment sheets for each month and may be able to schedule only a month or 6 weeks at a time. Many offices are now using a computer, which can be adapted for unstructured time frames. The computer is particularly useful when several physicians are working in the same office because it eliminates the need for several appointment books.

Some changes in scheduling that have helped offices improve efficiency are modified wave-and-cluster scheduling. In modified wave, three patients might be scheduled for 9 A.M., two at 9:15, and one at 9:20, with a catch-up period at the end of the hour. The patients are seen in order of arrival. This would be a possibility if the average time needed for these patients is only 10 minutes. Obviously, you would not schedule more patients than the physician could see in an hour as you consider the average time used for each.

Some offices find it helpful to cluster patient schedules according to needs: diabetics, hypertensives, well babies, obese patients, or new patients. In using this type of scheduling, you do not need to shift mental gears so often. You can offer more comprehensive patient educational programs. The physician may have video programs that the medical assistant can set up for review by these patients.

Establishing a matrix on the appointment schedule consists of blocking off any time the physician will be out of the office and unable to see patients. Some offices prefer to highlight the appointment schedule book for medical meetings, surgeries, and vacations, Figure 7–5. This prevents scheduling patients during these periods.

Patients frequently become angry at having to wait a long time to be seen. This usually results from improper scheduling. It may be helpful to do a survey to determine the actual time required to see different types of patients. An average time for each type can then be determined so that you can estimate more effectively and be more accurate in scheduling.

A conference with other office personnel and the physician may make it possible for you to establish a time to be set aside for returning calls. A method for working in urgent cases during the day can also be determined.

The key to successful operation of any office is the extent to which employees are willing to share ideas and information regarding what needs to be accomplished. If the office manager discovers that employees do not participate in this sharing of honest communication, it is best to discuss this problem and try to improve the communication. The development of a team feeling should allow all employees to be honest, consistent, loyal, considerate, and by all means to avoid gossip. A professional image is reflected through attitude, abilities, appearance, and ethics.

The physician generally expects the medical assistant scheduling appointments to schedule patients in time slots that are realistic for the presenting complaints. A guideline for scheduling some typical patient visits follows:

annual physical exam   30 minutes
dressing change   15 minutes

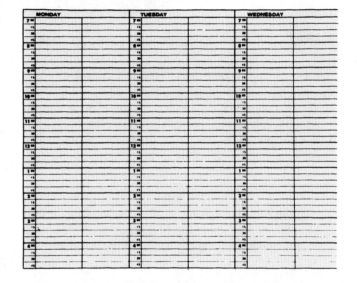

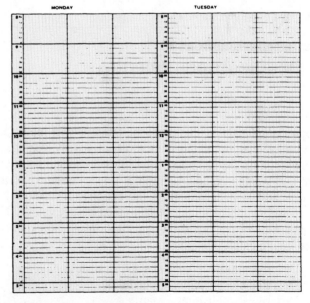

FIGURE 7–4 Examples of appointment schedules

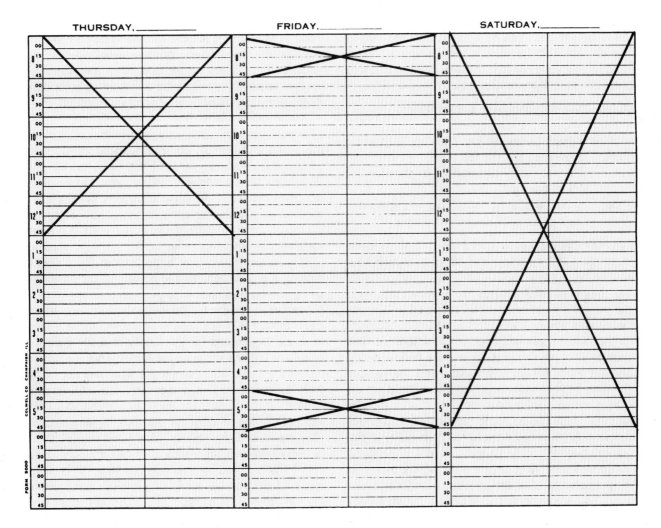

FIGURE 7–5 Appointment schedule with matrix established

surgery follow-up	15 minutes
cast removal	15 minutes
gynecological exam/pap smear	30 minutes
prenatal exam	15 minutes
postnatal exam	15 minutes
general follow-up exam	15 minutes
new patient exam	60 minutes
minor office surgery	30 minutes
routine office call	15 minutes

It is also your job to help the physician keep on schedule by realizing there must be free time on the schedule for emergencies to be worked in. This is individualized to suit the practice. In the winter there are more cases of colds, influenza, and pneumonia, so a general practitioner needs more time kept unscheduled to work in these patients. When the ground is covered with ice, a medical assistant working for an orthopedist knows more fractures are likely to occur and need immediate attention, so more time is left for emergencies. If the time is not taken up with patients, the physician almost always has telephone calls to make or medical dictation to catch up with.

The physician and the office staff should work together to find a system that meets the needs of the patients and the specialty office staff. Such organization requires effort on the part of the physicians and the office staff. If the physicians do not keep the office well-informed as to when they will be in the office, it is extremely important to try to get a better understanding of how you should schedule patients.

When an office has difficulty in scheduling patients so that they do not have long waiting times, steps should be taken to correct that problem. Management experts suggest an evaluation of old appointment sheets for a 12- to 15-week period. When you determine the number of work-ins, cancellations, and no shows you will get an idea of the number of work-in spaces you need each day. You need to establish a listing of most often seen cases, most done procedures, and the length of time needed for these appointments. You can then determine time slots needed for short, medium, long, and extra-long appointments.

When a patient calls for an appointment, it is important to determine whether the patient is new or has been in the office previously. If the patient is new, it is important to get the name correctly spelled. Don't be afraid to confirm spelling (Smith can be spelled Smithe, Smyth and Smythe). Ask for the reason for the appointment. You should have a series of questions in mind which will be triggered by the caller's statements.

> *Caller:* "My daughter has a temperature."
> *Assistant:* "What is the temperature?"
> *Caller:* "I don't know, she just feels hot."
> *Assistant:* "How long has she felt hot?"
> *Caller:* "I'm not sure, I just noticed it when I picked her up."
> *Assistant:* "What other symptoms have you noticed? Crying? Cough? Excessive sleeping?"

The answers you receive will help you determine when to suggest the appointment should be and how long it should be.

Decide, based on instructions from your employer, where the patient should be seen. Be prepared to hear "If I knew what was wrong I wouldn't need to see the doctor." You then must find out symptoms to determine first of all whether your physician is the one the patient needs to see. If you work for an orthopedist and the patient thinks she may be pregnant, the orthopedist could not do much to help but an obstetrician could. In this case, your employer may want you to name physicians who could help the patient or you may want to refer the caller to the local medical bureau. Some patients do not understand the terminology associated with specialists and you should be prepared to offer the assistance they need (see Chapter 2). You are expected to schedule patients your physician employer can treat effectively.

You will learn with practice and experience the importance of careful listening to what the patient says. There are two kinds of listening: automatic and concentrated. In *automatic listening*, you are hearing but not registering what you hear because you are thinking about something else. This may cause you to have to ask the caller to repeat what was said. When a caller must repeat statements, it creates a concern as to your ability to respond adequately to the patient's concerns. On the other hand, *concentrated listening* requires that your total interest be centered on what is said. Concentrated listening allows you to detect tones of voice that could be important to relay to the physician. Some examples of these would be excitement, anger, impatience, and depression.

You need to be aware of the needs of the patient when you schedule appointments because you have to estimate the amount of time needed and you must make the best use of your office facilities and equipment. If you have one room for minor surgical procedures you only schedule one patient at a time for surgical procedures. It is advisable if there are several physicians in an office to have a special schedule book for such procedures as electrocardiograms, sigmoidoscopies, and minor surgical procedures so that appointments are coordinated.

It is important for you to know the kinds of instructions to be given to patients who are to have special examinations. If you have a patient who needs special preparation, you should give or send printed instructions so that the patient will be ready for the examination on the day of the appointment. You will find some helpful information on diagnostic examinations in Chapters 16 through 18.

Some offices also send an information pamphlet to new patients along with a confirmation of the appointment. This important communication should cover all of the information you find yourself telling patients: directions for finding your office, your office hours, the hospital where your physician has privileges, your method of scheduling appointments, how refills of prescriptions are taken care of, and your payment and insurance procedures.

If you are making an appointment for a continuing patient, it is still important to be sure of the spelling of the name so you will be able to pull the patient's chart for the physician to review for previous illnesses and treatments. Even though it is not legally advisable, some offices may have all the records for the family in a file with the husband's or father's name on the folder. This is a difficult situation for a new office employee who may not be familiar with the names of family members. It is still important to determine the reason for the visit so you will know the amount of time to allow for the visit. Be sure to determine who the caller is by saying "May I ask who is calling?" It is fairly common for a patient to call and say "I need an appointment." You have to find out who "I" is. Try not to insult a lady who has a cold or a low-pitched voice by saying "What is your name, sir?", and don't insult a gentleman with a high tenor voice by calling him "Ma'am."

A cancelled appointment should be crossed out in the appointment book with a single line and the time given to another patient. It should also be noted in the patient's chart, and the physician should be made aware of it. This procedure provides legal protection if a lawsuit is filed against the physician for failure to provide needed care for the patient. For example, if a patient is being treated for a wound that requires follow-up for a dressing change, the patient may cancel and the wound area could become infected. The patient may then decide to sue the physician for poor care. The record of the canceled appointment would be important in proving that the patient had failed to follow instructions. Some offices find it useful to have a stamp that can be used to record in the patient chart the fact that an appointment was canceled. You would need to add only the date and any reason for cancellation.

Every office should include appointment scheduling information in the office procedure manual. The appointment book is an important document and should be as legible as possible. It should be kept for 3 years. Management advisors state no liquid paper or erasures should be used in this book.

You must work at keeping the physician on schedule throughout the day. If you have a patient who always comes late for an appointment, try scheduling that person last. If the patient does not come on time, he will find you have gone home. If the physician is taking more than the scheduled amount of time with a patient and you have reason to believe they are just visiting, you might work out a plan with your employer whereby you knock on the door and take the physician out of the patient's hearing range, then point out how many patients are waiting to be seen.

The first step in analyzing any scheduling problem in the office is to establish the goals of the appointment schedule. The goals of the patient, the physician, and the medical assistant need to be considered. In general, the *goals of the patients* are:

1. A minimum wait for an appointment
2. A minimum wait in the office
3. Maximum time with the physician

The general *goals of the physicians* are:

1. Cost-effective use of time
2. To spend needed time with the patients
3. Uninterrupted time
4. Time for referrals, emergencies, and so on

The general *goals of the medical assistant* are:

1. A smooth-running office
2. To close the office on time
3. A lunch hour
4. Everything the patient and physician want

Studies have shown that while a 10-hour day is 25 percent longer than an 8-hour day, the increase in productivity only rises 6 percent because of the increased likelihood of making errors.

Surveys have shown that patients usually do not mind as much as a half-hour wait, but tend to become angry after half an hour.

When the physician and office staff have made a decision regarding the best scheduling method for the office, any professional stationery company will help you print appointment schedules to meet your needs.

You might prefer to write appointments in pencil so that changes can be done neatly, but they should be traced over in ink at the end of the day. Your appointment schedule is a legal record. One abbreviation commonly used in the appointment book for cancelled appointments is CC (called and cancelled). The abbreviation for a patient who did not keep an appointment is NS (no show).

In recording an appointment, it is important to block off the time correctly depending on the length of the appointment. Most books allow for 15-minute time intervals. When the patient needs only 15 minutes, you would record the name, phone number, and reason for the visit on one line. The patient who requires 30 minutes would require two units of time. The patient who will have a comprehensive physical examination may need an hour, so you would block four units of time, Figure 7–6.

Each office has abbreviations that are used in the appointment schedule. Everyone in the office needs to know what these abbreviations are, and they should be used consistently. Some of these might be:

1. NP—new patient
2. CPE or CPX—complete physical examination
3. FU—Follow-up examination
4. NS—no show
5. RS—reschedule
6. Can—cancel
7. Ref—referral
8. RE√—re-check
9. PT—physical therapy
10. Cons—consultation
11. Inj—injection
12. ECG—electrocardiogram
13. Sig—sigmoidoscopy
14. Surg—surgery
15. Lab study abbreviations are also commonly used

In addition to emergency situations that may disrupt the schedule, you must be prepared to handle other common disruptions. Salespeople from pharmaceutical companies make regular visits to see physicians. The common name is *detail person*, and they may leave literature concerning new medications or samples of medications your employer uses to treat patients. Some physicians require that the detail persons make appointments: others will see them for a few minutes whenever they come. Sales representatives from insurance companies or specialty supply firms may also call to see the physician. When other physicians come to see your employer, they are usually taken immediately into the office to see your employer.

When your physician is ill or late, you need to cancel or reschedule patients as quickly as you can. This is eas-

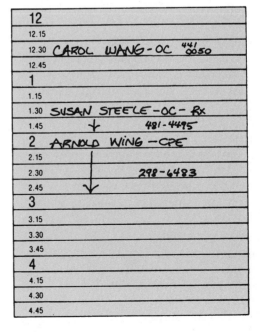

FIGURE 7–6
Scheduling appointments according to the purpose of the visit

ier to do if you have recorded the telephone numbers as the appointments are made.

A patient who has an appointment and brings along another family member to be seen can also complicate the schedule. When a patient arrives with no appointment, you need to tell the patient the physician has a full schedule and would prefer that the patient have an appointment. You need to explain that the physician would then be able to spend as much time as needed to care for the patient. Your employer might want you to ask him or her before turning away a walk-in patient.

You might have patients who only need an injection or a lab study performed, with no need to be charged for an office visit. These patients are usually recorded in the appointment book with an indication "injection only" or "lab only." When you call these patients from the waiting room, try to indicate "The nurse can see you now," or "I can give your injection now," or "We are ready to do your lab studies." This indicates to patients who may have been waiting longer to see the physician that later arrivals are not being taken in to see the physician ahead of them.

It may not be considered cost effective to purchase a computer for scheduling of appointments. If the office has installed a computer system for managing accounts receivable, it would be important to research the possibility of using the system for scheduling also. When you use computerized appointment scheduling, you totally replace the paper appointment book. You should certainly have an accounts receivable system well established before converting to appointment scheduling. This feature should not be added if you have a single terminal, but can be effective if you have several terminals. You also must consider how you would handle "downtime," when, for whatever reason, the computer is not functional. This is a reality you need to plan for before it takes place so the office will run as smoothly as possible through the downtime.

A computerized appointment system locates automatically the next available time; gives you a record of all appointments already made; allows you to locate a specific date and time; and prints copies of the daily schedule. These printed copies should be filed with the accounting records of the day as a legal document that you could be called on to produce in the event of an IRS audit of the office practice. Some computer systems can be used to print charge slips for the patients as they are seen. It is not recommended to try to add an appointment scheduling procedure to the computer until you have a smooth operation under the handwritten system.

The main points to remember in making appointments are:

1. Have the name exactly right.
2. Make the appointment for the next hour available.
3. Be sure the date and time are clearly understood.
4. Allow enough time for each appointment.
5. Check to see that no one else is scheduled at the same time for the same service.
6. Try to remember the time of day each patient prefers for an appointment.
7. When scheduling a series of appointments for the same patient, try to use the same day and time to make it easier for the patient to remember.
8. Offer a choice: "Would you like to come today at 3:00 or tomorrow at 9:00?"
9. If you have to refuse a request for an appointment at a certain time, explain why this is necessary and try to find another time that is convenient for the patient.
10. Enter the appointment in your appointment book or computer.
11. Complete an appointment card and hand it to the patient.
12. Try to allow extra time for emergencies each day.

The office should have a policy for allowing time for emergencies in the morning and in the afternoon. Sometimes this time is used as a telephone hour when calls can be returned. It is really a buffer zone to be used for whatever arises during the day to disrupt the schedule. If this method is used in the office, it should be marked off on the schedule before any appointments are entered.

Some offices elect to have patients arrive any time within specified hours, sign in with the receptionist, and be seen in order of arrival. The greatest disadvantage of this "open hours" system is that you cannot have patient's charts pulled and prepared in advance. In addition, patients frequently end up with a long wait.

As you would not want the appointment book to be seen by all who come to the office, it is also not advisable to have the sign-in sheet where it can be seen. Therefore, it is best to record the patients' names yourself as they arrive.

Appointments Outside Medical Office ....

When a patient develops a condition or requires an examination that your office cannot take care of, your employer will refer the patient to an appropriate colleague or facility. The office should have a page in the office procedures manual listing the names, addresses, and phone numbers of physicians your employer wishes to refer patients to in the different specialty areas. You should give at least two names. You should have the name, address, and phone number of facilities you might refer patients to, such as laboratories, X ray facilities, and community clinics.

When a patient is to be admitted to the hospital, it is important to know what admission information the hospital will require. Be prepared when you call to give the necessary information regarding the patient.

Hospitals have established guidelines for admitting patients. The purpose of these guidelines is to cut the cost of hospital care. If the care needed by the patient can be given in an outpatient facility, this must be the method used. Many insurance companies and the government sponsored programs require a preadmission evaluation of the need for hospitalization of a patient. To determine the need for admission, a criterion statement would need to be composed by the admitting physician using specific terminology as to severity of the illness and an assessment of need. Definitions that may be given for these terms are:

acute onset—symptoms occurred within last 6 hours

sudden onset—symptoms occurred within last 24 hours

recent onset—symptoms occurred within past week

recently or newly discovered—symptoms not present on previous examination

In some cases, in addition to terms describing the severity of the illness, the vital signs (temperature, pulse, respiration, and blood pressure), laboratory workup, any functional impairment, the physical findings, the need for monitoring, the medications needed, and the procedures, along with criteria for discharge, must be considered as part of the determination for need of admission.

In scheduling an admission, you may be asked to identify the attending physician for the admission, the service admitting under (i.e., whether medical, surgical, obstetrical, and so on), the admission date requested, and the type of reservation. The type of reservation might be: In-patient; admitting day surgery (ADS); ambulatory surgery (ASU), or patients who walk in, have surgery and go home; or outpatient. Some hospitals furnish nearby hotel rooms for chemotherapy patients or other patients who need daily treatment for several hours but do not need to be admitted to a hospital room. Other information needed would be:

1. Full name of the patient (include maiden name of married female patient)
2. Age and date of birth
3. Sex of patient
4. Marital status
5. Social security number
6. Address (including zip code)
7. Telephone number (home)
8. Primary insurance guarantor and Social Security number of this individual
9. Employer of guarantor and work telephone number
10. Hospital insurance coverage along with verification if prior authorization granted
11. Name and address of referring physician
12. The physician needs to furnish the diagnosis and plan of care needs for the utilization committee review.
13. If surgery is to be scheduled, you need to give the date of surgery, expected length of procedure in hours, name of procedure, type of anesthesia, units of blood needed, and whether X rays will be taken.
14. When preadmission testing is to be carried out, you need to know the date, time, and names of tests, X rays, ECG, etc. If a generally required test is not ordered, you need to explain why it was not ordered.

The following conditions will generally justify inpatient hospital care for an otherwise outpatient procedure if the severity of the illness or intensity of service needed warrant it:

1. Severe myocardial insufficiency (with or without angina)
2. Chronic congestive heart failure

P R O C E D U R E

Schedule Appointments

TERMINAL PERFORMANCE OBJECTIVE: In a simulated situation with an appointment book and pen the student will greet the patient in a clear, distinct voice, expressing consideration for the needs of the patient according to accepted medical standards. The student must consider the emergency needs of the office and the schedule of the physician. The instructor will observe and evaluate this procedure.

1. Determine appropriate appointment book or daily record method.
2. Mark off the hours when the physician will be unable to see patients. **Key Point: This would include lunch hour and time when the physician is attending meetings, making hospital rounds, or taking a vacation.**
3. Attempt to give patients two choices of times when they need an appointment.
   Key Points:
   a. If the patient's name is recorded in pencil during the day, be sure the name is retraced in black or blue ink at the end of the day.
   b. Record the telephone number of the patient so that you can easily call if the need arises.
4. As patients are preparing to leave the office, be sure to ask if they need another appointment.
5. Write their names on the appointment schedule.
6. Complete an appointment card and give it to the patient. **Key Point: Always record the scheduled appointment before making out the appointment card.**
7. Avoid overscheduling. It is important to have time for urgent patients to be worked in during the day.
8. Allow time for the physician to return patient calls during the day. The patient chart should be put with the phone messages to be returned. **Key Point: the physician should tell you how he or she wants this situation handled.**

3. Chronic obstructive lung disease
4. Bronchial asthma
5. Diabetes
6. Thyroid disease
7. Hypertension

Guidelines are generally established with a detailed listing by ICDA–9–CM codes (International Classification of Diseases, 9th revision, Clinical Modification) for elective outpatient procedures, for elective procedures that might require a preoperative length of stay, and for those procedures to be done on admission day.

Follow-up Appointments ....

It is the medical assistant's responsibility to assist patients with their payments and any necessary follow-up or referral appointments after the physician has seen them.

The need for a follow-up appointment may be marked by the physician on the charge slip, or the patient may be told to inform you of this need. The patient should be given the choice of two appointment times, and only after the entry is made in the appointment book should an appointment card be prepared and given to the patient. This practice will prevent the possibility of forgetting to enter the patient's name in the book.

Physicians who treat patients who need regular follow-up but do not make appointments for 6 months or a year in advance may choose to send a recall notice. This notice could be a preprinted card sent to the patient as a reminder to call or write for an appointment. An example would be a reminder for an annual Pap test. Some offices find it helpful to send a reminder notice of appointments that were made far in advance. You might even ask the patient to address such a card at the time the appointment is made. The patient is handed an appointment card which he or she may lose, and at the same time addresses a card with the appointment time marked on it. You place this in a file under the date when it should be mailed. This practice might be helpful for the forgetful geriatric patient, the overworked housewife, or the busy executive who may forget to put the appointment in the date book along with business appointments.

Complete Chapter 7, Unit 2 in the workbook to help you meet the objectives at the beginning of this unit and therefore achieve competency of this subject matter.

U N I T   3

Compose and Type Letters

OBJECTIVES ....

Upon completion of this unit, the student will meet the following terminal performance objectives by verifying knowledge of the facts and principles presented through oral and written communication at a level deemed competent, and will demonstrate the specific behaviors as identified in the terminal performance objectives of the procedures, observing safety precautions in accordance with health care standards.

1. List the types of letters medical assistants may need to compose.
2. Name some uses of form letters.
3. Demonstrate knowledge of grammar, spelling, punctuation, and sentence structure in composing original letters.
4. Produce a mailable letter by use of a dictating machine.
5. Demonstrate knowledge of business letter styles.
6. Correct typewritten copy.
7. Name "danger zones" needed to focus on when proofreading.
8. Use standard proofreading marks.
9. Correctly fold letters and address envelopes.
10. Describe the use of numbers in the ZIP + 4 postal code.
11. Spell and define, using the glossary at the back of the text, all the words to know in this unit.

WORDS TO KNOW ....

context	galley proofs	sector
contractions	mailable	thesaurus
critique	modifies	watermark
denote	postscript	
ellipses	redundant	

Composing Letters ....

The medical assistant should be able to compose effective business letters for the signature of the physician or for his or her own signature. The assistant who can perform these skills well can quickly advance to a position as executive secretary.

The physician may wish to review the mail and give notes and suggestions to assist in answering mail, such as:

- Appointment for new patient or cancellation of appointment
- Acknowledgment of an announcement
- Return-to-work or school certifications
- Transmission of laboratory study results
- Collection letters
- Letter of congratulations

The medical assistant will find it extremely helpful to prepare and use form letters for collecting accounts. This is especially easy to do now with a word processor or computer. The series of letters can be stored on a floppy disk and when the need arises to send a first, second, or third notice on a past-due account, you can bring up the desired format. You then insert the date, name, address, amount due, and salutation, and print the letter. You can

P R O C E D U R E

Compose and Type Business Correspondence

TERMINAL PERFORMANCE OBJECTIVE: Given a situation requiring a letter answer, the student will compose and perfect the letter, following steps in the procedure. The instructor will proofread the final copy.

1. If you are to answer a letter, first read it carefully and underline facts to be covered.
2. Make a note of any additional facts to be covered.
3. Make a note of reaction, if any, you expect from recipient.
4. Write or type rough draft of your letter.
   Key Points:
   a. Use simple, easy-to-understand words in sentences that are short and interesting, with one idea to a sentence.
   b. Avoid the use of *I* and *we*.
5. Reread the rough draft to check grammar, spelling, and punctuation.
   Key Points:
   a. Eliminate any redundant phrases.

   b. Be sure to use a dictionary, a thesaurus, a reference for grammar and punctuation, and a style manual when in doubt. (Every office should have such references available.) A list of general spelling rules is given in Figure 7–7.
   c. Ask a coworker of your employer to read and critique your letter. Accept criticism gracefully.
6. Type final copy.
   Key Points:
   a. Final copy must be well placed on the page and free of obvious corrections or errors.
   b. Office employees using letterhead stationery should always identify themselves by position and provide a courtesy title, which is enclosed in parentheses.
   Examples:
   (Ms.) Mary Jones
   Office Manager
   (Mr.) John Smith, Medical Assistant

Rule 1. Write *ie* when the sound is *ee*, as in:

achieve	piece
field	shield
grief	yield

EXCEPT after c, as in:
conceive
deceive
perceive
receive
EXCEPTIONS:
leisure
neither
seize
weird

Rule 2. Write *ei* when the sound is not long *e*, especially when the sound is long *a*, as in:

freight	veil
height	vein
sleigh	weigh

EXCEPTIONS:
friend
mischief

Rule 3. The prefixes *mis, il, in, im* and *dis* do not change the spelling of the root word:
mis + spell = misspell
il + legal = illegal
il + literate = illiterate

in + audible = inaudible
im + mature = immature
dis + appear = disappear

Rule 4. Only one word in English ends in *sede*: supersede.
Only three words end in *ceed*: exceed, proceed, and succeed.
All other words of similar sound end in *cede*, as in:
concede
recede
precede

Rule 5. The suffixes *ly* and *ness* do not change the spelling of the root word:
sudden + ness = suddenness
final + ly = finally
truthful + ly = truthfully
lean + ness = leanness
EXCEPTIONS: Words ending in y preceded by a consonant change y to i before any suffix not beginning with *i*:
kindly + ness = kindliness
happy + ly = happily
happy + ness = happiness
Words ending in y preceded by a vowel also follow this rule.

FIGURE 7–7   Spelling reference rules

Rule 6. Drop the *e* from the end of a word before adding the suffixes *al, ed, ing,* and *able*:

    complete—completed—completing
    care—caring
    fine—final
    love—lovable
    observe—observable
    EXCEPTIONS: Words ending in *ce* and *ge* usually keep the silent *e* when the suffix begins with *a* or *o* in order to preserve the soft sound of the final consonant:
    notice + able = noticeable
    change + able = changeable

Rule 7. Keep the final *e* before a suffix beginning with a consonant:

    large + ly = largely
    care + ful = careful
    care + less = careless
    state + ment = statement
    EXCEPTIONS:
    argue + ment = argument
    true + ly = truly

Rule 8. With words of one syllable ending in a single consonant preceded by a single vowel, double the consonant before adding *ing, ed,* or *er*:

    sit + ing = sitting
    hop + ed = hopped
    dip + er = dipper
    run + ing = running
    swim + ing = swimming

Rule 9. If a one-syllable word ends in a single consonant not preceded by a single vowel, do not double the consonant before adding *ing, ed,* or *er*:

    reap + ed = reaped
    heat + ing = heating

Rule 10. To make a word ending in *y* plural, check the letter before the *y*. If it is a vowel, just add *s*:

    birthday—birthdays

    day—days
    ray—rays
    toy—toys
If it is any other letter, change the *y* to *i* and add *es*:
    city—cities   lady—ladies
    study—studies   guppy—guppies
    fly—flies

Rule 11. Most nouns (names of people, places, things, ideas) become plural by adding *s*:

    boy—boys
    dog—dogs
    desk—desks
    window—windows

Rule 12. The plural of nouns ending in *s, x, z, ch,* or *sh* is formed by adding *es*.

    wax—waxes
    dish—dishes
    waltz—waltzes

Rule 13. The plural of most nouns ending in *f* is formed by adding *s*. The plural of some nouns ending in *fo* or *fe* is formed by changing the *f* to *v* and adding *s* or *es*:

    gulf—gulfs
    belief—beliefs
    knife—knives
    life—lives
    half—halves
    loaf—loaves
    thief—thieves
    wolf—wolves

Rule 14. The plural of nouns ending in *o* preceded by a vowel is formed by adding *s*. The plural of nouns ending in *o* preceded by a consonant is formed by adding *es*.

    patio—patios
    ratio—ratios
    tornado— tornadoes
    hero—heroes
    EXCEPTIONS:
    Eskimo—Eskimos
    silo—silos

FIGURE 7–7 (continued)   Spelling reference rules

generate personalized letters very quickly. If you do not have a word processor or computer, you can compose your series of collection letters and have them copied. You need to allow a blank space within the letter to fill in the amount due. When you use the form, carefully line up your margins and type in the date, name, address, salutation, and amount due. Then sign and send the letter.

You can also make good use of form letters to recall patients for follow-up therapy, Pap tests, eye examinations, and the like. You may want to compose forms to use for back-to-work permits, back-go-school permits, or back-to-athletic activities permits. This type of form is available from companies who furnish medical forms if you do not wish to make up your own. You may want to compose a form to be used for procedures done in the office, for release of information, or for giving instructions to patients. The use of form letters or information sheets depends on the type of practice and the desires of the physician.

1. Keep a list of your own misspelled words to use as a reference when you proofread.

2. Use the following steps to correct your errors:
  a. Make a mental picture of the word correctly spelled.
  b. Pronounce the word correctly several times.
  c. Write the word, dividing it into syllables and inserting accent marks.
  d. Write or type the word several times.
3. Learn to use the dictionary if in doubt.
4. Learn to proofread carefully.

When you proofread a rough draft you may use informal markings, but there are standard markings you should be familiar with. Many physicians write for publication and the publisher will send galley proofs that must be checked, corrected, and returned. Ask a coworker to read the original copy while you check copy

from the printer for typographical errors and omissions. It is important to follow the instructions of the editor on the proper method of indicating corrections. The most common proofreader's marks are shown in Figure 7–8.

Typing Letters

You are usually responsible for making appointments for patients referred by other physicians, although some employers may prefer that you consult with them before doing so. The referring physician will often send a letter asking that such an appointment be made, Figure 7–9, page 97. You then enter the appointment in the book, being sure to allow time for your letter to reach the patient. You compose a short letter giving the reason for

PROOFREADER'S MARKS

Mark	Meaning	Mark	Meaning
∧	Insert	⌐	Move left
ℰ	Delete	⌐	Move right
#	Insert space	⌐	Move up
⌒	Close up space	⊔	Move down
ℰ	Delete and close up	⌐⌐	Center
#	Close up, but leave normal space	⌃	Insert comma
eq.#	Equal space between words	⌄	Insert apostrophe
‖	Align type vertically	:|	Insert colon
=	Align type horizontally	⊙	Insert period
sp	Spell out (Wd) or (5)	?|	Insert question mark
TR	Transpose letters words or	⌄ ⌄	Insert quotation marks
BF	Boldface type	⌃	Insert semicolon
ROM	Roman type	=	Insert hyphen
ITAL	Italic type	⊥/M	Insert em dash
CAP	Capital letter	⊥/N	Insert en dash
LC	Lower case letter	⌃2	Subscript
SC	Small caps	2⌄	Superscript
STET	Let it stand	¶	Paragraph indent
WF	Wrong font	no ¶	No indent; run in
		⌐	Break; start new line

FIGURE 7–8 Proofreader's marks

the appointment and the time and asking the patient to notify you if unable to keep the appointment. As a courtesy, you would send a copy of the letter to the referring physician. When the patient has been seen, your employer will send a letter to the referring physician listing the findings and the diagnosis along with suggested treatment.

There are definite standards for a mailable letter. The typewriter type must be clean, the ribbon well inked, and there should be no smudges on the paper. The placement of the letter on the page should be attractive, with the right margin fairly even and generous margins on all sides, Figure 7–10, page 98. Punctuation and spacing should follow acceptable business practice. The typing should show no errors, strikeovers, or words incorrectly divided at the end of a line. Be certain that the content of the letter is accurate as dictated and that you have used the dictionary for any questions regarding spelling. It is a fairly simple matter to change the meaning of a sentence with the use of poor grammar and spelling errors.

Proofreading

The task of proofreading is a skill which you must develop if you are to compose letters or copy of any kind for office use. If you use a word processor or computer with a dictionary built in, you can still have words that are spelled correctly but are out of context.

There are danger zones on which you should first focus. The danger zones are words ending in *s*, apostrophes, combinations of punctuation, periods and commas, double letters in words, capital letters, two-letter words, hyphens, numbers (those below ten should be spelled out), and dashes.

If you must do your own proofreading be aware of your weaknesses. Focus on them so you can conquer them. If spelling is your problem, you should have a dictionary readily available to check words. If it is possible, have someone else check the work for errors that you feel you might miss.

It is not recommended to proofread on a screen. This cannot replace proofing the printed copy, and reading the printed copy will not overtire your eyes. It is helpful to read lines from right to left to catch misspelled words.

Parts of Speech. To proofread for grammar you must remember the eight parts of speech and how they are identified.

1. A noun is the name of anything. It may be a person, a place, an object, an occurrence, a quality, a measure, or a state. Examples of words that may be used as nouns are *assistant, laboratory, instruments, office, empathy, manners, kindness,* and *attention.*
   Examples:
   The *assistant* draws *blood* and takes it to the *laboratory.*
   The *assistant* shows *kindness, empathy,* and *attentiveness* to all *patients* in the *office.*

2. A pronoun is a word that is used as a noun substitute. The most often used pronouns are *I, me, she,*
her, you, he, him, who, which, that, one, all, some, everyone, it, their, they, any* and *nobody.*

3. A verb is a word (or word group) that expresses action or state of being. Every sentence must have a verb. Examples of words which may be action verbs are *do, write, speak, hesitate, educate, perform, assist, obtain,* and *attend.* Examples of verbs that may express state of being are *am, are, is, will be, have been, feel, seem,* and *appear.*

4. An adjective is a word that describes, limits, or restricts a noun or pronoun.
   Examples:
   The *conscientious* medical assistant reports for work on time.
   She is an *energetic, efficient,* and *dedicated* employee.

5. An adverb is a word that modifies a verb form, an adjective, or another adverb. The most common ending for adverbs is *ly.* Adverbs should be used to answer questions such as: How? When? Where? How often? To what degree? It is incorrect to say "I did real good on the terminology test." You should say, "I did very well on the terminology test."
   Examples:
   Sometimes the assistant reports *early* at the office and stays *late.*
   Usually when a patient *angrily* confronts an assistant, she should answer *calmly* and *quietly* after the patient has finished talking.

6. A preposition shows the relationship of an object to some other word in the sentence. Prepositions *must* have an object. If a pronoun is the object of a preposition, it must be in the objective case.
   Examples:
   Medical supplies arrived *for* the doctor, the nurse and *me.*
   Between you and *me* that physician's handwriting is most difficult to read.
   Some common prepositions include: *with, without, for, against, above, below, on, under, through, between, by, during, among, concerning, in, from, to,* and *of.*

7. Conjunctions are connectives that join words, phrases, and clauses. Examples are *and, but, or, nor, for, yet, because, if,* and *since.*

8. An interjection is a word used to express strong feeling or emotion. Examples are *ouch, hurray, well,* and *oh.* These words are usually followed by an exclamation point or a comma. Examples of sentences containing all eight parts of speech:
   Yes! A busy medical practice like theirs always employs efficient and energetic medical assistants.
   Well, a conscientious medical assistant like you will sit confidently for the certification examination and pass it!
   Oh, that emergency patient canceled after he had rested and settled down.

```
                    Kerry  Peoples,  M.D.
                    101  Fitness  Lane
                    Anywhere,    U.S.A.  00000




October 7, 19--




Robert Jones, M.D.
5000 North High Street
Columbus, Ohio 43200

Dear Dr. Jones:

I am referring Mary Ellen Lewis to your office for evaluation
of severe headaches of approximately six months duration.  She
was treated initially at a pain clinic in Cleveland.  Mary Ellen
will be calling your office for an appointment.  I am sure you
will find her to be a most cooperative patient.

I would appreciate a report of your diagnosis and recommended
course of treatment.

Sincerely,



Kerry Peoples, M.D.

lk
```

FIGURE 7–9   Sample referral letter

Sentence Structure. When writing letters, write in complete thoughts. A **simple sentence** consists of only one complete thought, that is, one independent clause with a subject and a verb.

Examples:
Physicians examine patients.
Physicians prescribe medication.
The receptionist scheduled appointments.

A **compound sentence** contains two or more independent clauses.

Examples:
The physician dictates letters and the medical assistant transcribes them.
Administrative medical assistants perform clerical duties and clinical medical assistants perform nursing skills.
Laboratory technicians analyze specimens and medical assistants assist with physical examinations.

A **complex sentence** contains one independent clause and one or more dependent clauses. A dependent clause cannot stand alone as a sentence.

Examples:
The doctor, who is off on Thursdays, sees allergy patients in the morning. (an adjective clause)

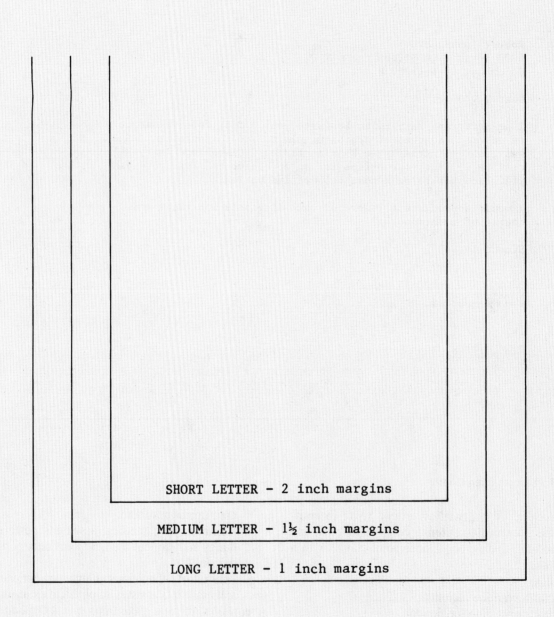

KERRY PEOPLES, M.D.
101 FITNESS LANE
ANYWHERE, U.S.A. 00000

SHORT LETTER – 2 inch margins

MEDIUM LETTER – 1½ inch margins

LONG LETTER – 1 inch margins

FIGURE 7–10 Spacing of letter

Patients are sometimes quite apprehensive when they come to the office for diagnostic examination. (an adverb clause)

Physicians require that patients receive proper instructions for diagnostic procedures. (noun clause) A compound–complex sentence contains two or more independent clauses plus one or more dependent clauses.

Example:

Medical assistants should seek continuing education because medical technology is constantly changing, and the medical assistant must keep current with new procedures.

Punctuation.   A comma or period should appear in front of an ending quotation mark (,” .”). There are four general rules for the use of a comma:

1. Use between main clauses connected by *and, but, so, for, or, nor,* and *yet*. If main clauses are short, no comma is needed.
2. Use following long introductory phrases or clauses that may begin with words such as *after, whenever, if, until, since,* and *once*.
3. Use to separate items in a series.
4. Use to set off nonrestrictive modifiers. A nonrestrictive phrase or clause is a nonessential phrase or clause. It just adds descriptive or explanatory detail. A restrictive modifier restricts or limits the noun it modifies.

Example:

The medical assistant, being dedicated to her profession, helps the doctor in countless ways.

The medical assistant, who is a part of the medical team, needs to be especially careful in attending to details.

Apostrophes need your attention. An apostrophe is used in contractions to signify that one or more letters have been left out. Be sure if you use *it’s* that you mean *it is*. *Who’s*, meaning *who is*, should not be confused with *whose*, and *there’s*, meaning *there is*, is not to be confused with *theirs*.

An apostrophe is also used to signify possession in a noun.

Example:

The medical assistant’s pen, pencil, and note pad are always beside the office telephone.

The assistant’s stethoscope hangs in the examination room.

Carefully check all hyphens at the end of a line to be sure the word is divided correctly. Check your dictionary if you are in doubt.

Two forms of ellipses may be used—three and four dots. The three-dot ellipsis is used with spaces on either end, and between the dots, to signify an omission of words.

Example:

“They come in two varieties—the three-dot variety . . . and the four-dot variety.”

The four-dot ellipsis signifies an omission of words and the end of a sentence with no space between the last letter and the first dot.

Example:

“The four-dot. . . .”

Capitalization.   Capitalize names of persons and places, the first word in a sentence, names of holidays, principal words in titles of major works, and any product or title that might be trademarked. Many medical terms begin with a capital letter because they are names of the physicians who named them. Medications are usually trademarked. Again, use your dictionary when in doubt.

Be especially careful to check every word in a heading or title for correct spelling. Use your medical dictionary or a good general dictionary. Always have these reference books in the office.

Numbers.   The use of numbers must be consistent. If you follow a specific reference style book (e.g., *The Chicago Manual of Style, CBE Style Manual, AMA Manual of Style*), you should follow its instructions for using numerals or spelling out the numbers. Also, follow the rules your employer wishes to be used for your office.

Letter Style

The letter should be consistent in following a full block or modified block style, Figures 7–11, page 100, 7–12, page 101, and 7–13, page 102. Your employer may have a preference so be sure you know what is preferred. In full block style, the dateline, address, salutation, body of letter, complimentary close, typed signature, and initials of typist are flush with the left margin. This is a popular style as no tab stops are needed. The most popular style is the modified block with the dateline, complimentary close, and typed signature beginning a bit right of center. This style is compatible with most letterheads. The dateline sets the style. If you place the date at the right, you must follow with modified block style, lining up the complimentary close and typed signature with the date. The least popular of the three styles customarily used in the medical office is the modified block with indented paragraphs.

The medical secretary will often be responsible for ordering typing supplies. The stationery letterhead is usually the choice of the physician. Letterhead stationery and matching envelopes are usually 16-, 20-, or 24-pound weight. The larger the number, the heavier the paper. It is usually ordered by the ream, which consists of 500 sheets of paper. Continuation pages are plain bond and should match the weight of the letterhead.

A watermark appears on bond paper and should read across the paper in the same direction as the typing. You can determine the correct watermark side by holding the paper to the light. If you type on the wrong side of erasable paper you will lose the erasable quality.

Be certain to make a copy of every business letter or report to be sent from the office. Copies of correspondence regarding patients need to be filed in the patient chart. Correspondence in answer to business letters need

Kerry Peoples, M.D.
101 Fitness Lane
Anywhere, U.S.A. 00000

August 15, 19—   **(DATELINE)**

Robert Jones, M.D.
5000 North High Street   **(INSIDE ADDRESS)**
Columbus, Ohio 43200

RE: Krista Smith   **(REFERENCE)**

Dear Dr. Jones: **(SALUTATION)**

I am referring Krista Smith to your office for an eye examination. She is complaining of some difficulty with reading. She will be entering school soon and
wants to be sure she can maintain the high level of academic achievement she has
enjoyed in the past.

She will call your office for an appointment. I would appreciate a report of your
findings.

Sincerely yours,   **(COMPLIMENTARY CLOSE)**

                                                  (SIGNATURE OF SENDER)

Kerry Peoples, M. D.   **(SIGNATURE TYPED)**

lk   **(REFERENCE INITIALS)**

(ENCLOSURE IF ANY)

FIGURE 7–11 Sample full block letter

Kerry Peoples, M.D.
101 Fitness Lane
Anywhere, U.S.A. 00000

August 15, 19—   **(DATELINE)**

Robert Jones, M.D.
5000 North High Street   **(INSIDE ADDRESS)**
Columbus, Ohio 43200

RE: Krista Smith   **(REFERENCE)**

Dear Dr. Jones: **(SALUTATION)**

I am referring Krista Smith to your office for an eye examination. She is complaining of some difficulty with reading. She will be entering school soon and wants to be sure she can maintain the high level of academic achievement she has enjoyed in the past.

She will call your office for an appointment. I would appreciate a report of your findings.

(COMPLIMENTARY CLOSE)   Sincerely yours,

                                     (SIGNATURE OF SENDER)

(SIGNATURE TYPED)
(TITLE IF NEEDED)   Kerry Peoples, M. D.
lk   **(REFERENCE INITIALS)**

(ENCLOSURE IF ANY)

FIGURE 7–12   Sample modified block letter

Kerry Peoples, M.D.
101 Fitness Lane
Anywhere, U.S.A. 00000

August 15, 19—   **(DATELINE)**

Robert Jones, M.D.
5000 North High Street   **(INSIDE ADDRESS)**
Columbus, Ohio 43200

RE: Krista Smith   **(REFERENCE)**

Dear Dr. Jones: **(SALUTATION)**

I am referring Krista Smith to your office for an eye examination. She is
complaining of some difficulty with reading. She will be entering school soon and
wants to be sure she can maintain the high level of academic achievement she has
enjoyed in the past.

She will call your office for an appointment. I would appreciate a report of
your findings.

(COMPLIMENTARY CLOSE)   Sincerely yours,

                                        (SIGNATURE OF SENDER)

(SIGNATURE TYPED)
(TITLE IF NEEDED)   Kerry Peoples, M. D.
lk   **(REFERENCE INITIALS)**

(ENCLOSURE IF ANY)

FIGURE 7–13   Modified block letter with indented paragraphs

to be copied and filed in the appropriate files. If your office prefers to use carbon paper for copies of correspondence, be sure carbon copies are carefully corrected whenever corrections are made on the original copy.

Addressing Envelopes ....

The United States Postal Service (USPS) uses optical character readers (OCRs) and bar code sorters (BCSs) to read the addresses on envelopes you mail. The BCS equipment is capable of sorting over 30,000 pieces of mail per hour but only if envelopes are properly addressed.

The bar code is a series of little lines you often see at the bottom of letters from utility companies, banks, retailers, and other businesses, Figure 7–16, page 104.

Each piece of mail passes by the computer's scanner for a quick read of the delivery address. Then, it flies past the OCR's printer, which sprays on a bar code representing the zip code or ZIP + 4 code for the address. Next, the mail piece zooms to one of the OCR's sorting channels reserved for the proper delivery area. From there, the bar coded mail is fed to BCSs for the final separations. The BCS processes mail just as fast and in much the same way as the OCR reads addresses, except its scanner recognizes only one thing—the bar code. As the bar code on your mail piece shoots past the BCS lens, it is quickly read and sent to the appropriate channel for delivery.

Addresses should be typewritten or machine printed to be processed on automated equipment. Script or Executive type should not be used. The USPS prefers that the entire address be printed in upper case letters and, except for the hyphen in the ZIP + 4 code, all punctuation should be omitted. Lines of the address should be formatted with a uniform left margin, Figure 7–17, page 107.

For domestic mail, the post office (city), state, and zip code or ZIP + 4 should appear in that order on the bottom line of the address. However, if all three elements will not fit on that line, the zip code or ZIP + 4 may be placed on the line immediately below the post office and state, aligned with the left edge of the address block. The standard two-letter state abbreviations should also be used, Figure 7–18, page 108. The ZIP + 4 codes should always be printed as five digits, a hyphen, and four digits. The hyphen should be treated as any other character as far as spacing and stroke width are concerned.

The line immediately above the post office (city), state, and zip code line is designated the *delivery address line*. The street address, post office box number, rural route number and box number, or highway contract number and box number should appear on this line. Mail addressed to multiunit buildings should include the apartment number, suite, room, or other unit designation immediately after the street address of the building, on the same line. When the length of the delivery address is such that it prevents the placement of the unit number or other designation on the same line, the number or designator should be placed on the

line immediately above the delivery address line. When use of the building name in the address is necessary, it should also be placed on the line above the delivery address line, Figure 7–19, page 108.

The name of the intended recipient (business or individual) should appear on the line above the delivery address line. This should be either the third or fourth line from the bottom, depending on possible overflow from the delivery address line, whether or not dual addresses are used, and so on. The line above the name of recipient line is an optional line for additional address information. When needed, it should be used to direct mail to the attention of a specific person when a business name has been placed on the name of recipient line or to provide other information that will facilitate delivery (i.e., the name of a department within a company).

Mail addressed to foreign countries should include the country name printed in capital letters (no abbreviations) as the only information on the bottom line. For example:

MR THOMAS CLARK
117 RUSSELL DRIVE
LONDON WIP6HQ
ENGLAND

Mail addressed to Canada may use either of the following formats when the postal delivery zone number is included in the address:

MRS HELEN SAUNDERS   MRS HELEN SAUNDERS
1010 CLEAR STREET   1010 CLEAR STREET
OTTAWA ON K1AOB1   OTTAWA ON CANADA
CANADA   K1AOB1

The post office will furnish additional information on mailing to foreign countries if assistance is needed.

Address Block Location

The shaded area in Figure 7–20, page 108, illustrates the area on the face of the mail piece where address information should be located to be read by the OCRs. The OCRs and BCSs register mail pieces on the bottom edge; therefore, all vertical measurements are relative to the bottom edge.

Where possible, the entire address (exclusive of the optical lines above the name of recipient line) should be contained in an imaginary rectangle which extends from 5/8 inch to 2 3/4 inches from the bottom of the mail piece, with 1-inch margins on each side. At a minimum, all characters of the last line of the address block—the post office (city), state and zip code or ZIP + 4—should be located within an imaginary rectangle which extends from 5/8 inch to 2 1/4 inches from the bottom of the mail piece with 1-inch margins on each side.

Care must be taken to make the lines straight, as slanted lines cannot be read by the OCR process. The only abbreviations permitted in the name of the city are those found in the "Abbreviations" section of the

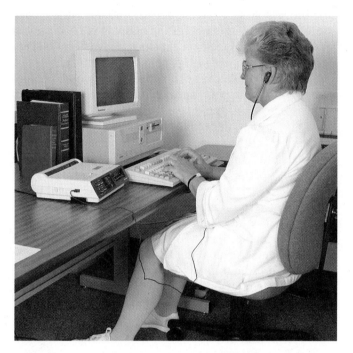

FIGURE 7–14 Transcribing medical dictation

The last two numbers denote a delivery segment, which might be one floor of an office building, one side of a street, specific departments in a firm, or a group of post office boxes. If your office has a large volume of mail, use of ZIP + 4 offers a discount in postal rate. The USPS will offer assistance in converting to ZIP + 4, but the confidential nature of medical office records means that patient interests would best be served by converting your own records. The customer service representative at the post office can answer your questions on the use of the *ZIP + 4 National/State Directory*, which is on computer tape.

Completing Mailing

When you are satisfied that your letter and envelope are complete, place the flap of the envelope over the top of the letter and secure it with a paper clip. If enclosures are indicated, be sure these are included. It is a good idea to have a signature folder to place finished mail in.

When the mail has been signed, fold it and place it in the envelope. A standard-size letter should be folded by

```
(Down one inch from top of page)

RE: Mary Ellen Lewis              2              October 7, 19--
(name of patient)           (page number)              (date)


RE: Mary Ellen Lewis
Page 2
October 7, 19--
```

FIGURE 7–15 Horizontal and vertical heading for second page

National Zip Code Directory. The OCR cannot read a non-standard abbreviation.

Special notations for the post office such as *Special Delivery* or *Certified Mail* should be typed in all capitals two lines below the postage. Be sure you are above the address zone. Special notations for the recipient such as *Personal* or *Confidential* should be typed in all capitals aligned with and 2 lines below the return address.

The zip code is critical to the rapid delivery of mail. The first number of the zip code stands for a region of the United States, from 0 for the East coast to 9 for the West coast and Hawaii. The next two numbers stand for the major post office in the region, and the final two stand for local delivery post offices. The newer ZIP + 4 coding will make even better use of automated processing in that the first two new numbers denote a delivery sector, which may be several blocks, a group of streets, several office buildings, or other small geographic area.

|ₗₗₗₗₗ|ₗₗₗ||ₗₗₗ|ₗₗ|ₗₗ|ₗₗₗ|||ₗₗₗₗₗ||ₗ|ₗ|ₗ||ₗₗₗₗ||ₗₗ|

FIGURE 7–16 Example of bar code (Courtesy of United States Postal Service)

bringing the lower third of the letter up and making a crease, then folding the top third of the letter down to about half an inch from the creased edge and making a second crease. The second crease goes into the envelope first. To fold a standard-size letter for a 6 3/4 envelope, bring the bottom edge to within half an inch of the top edge and crease. Fold from the right side about one third the width of the sheet and crease. Fold from the left edge to within half an inch of the second crease. Insert the left-edge crease into the envelope first.

If you have a large number of envelopes to seal you can speed up the process by placing eight or ten envelopes address side down with flaps open in fan fashion. Use a damp sponge to wet all the flaps at once and then starting with the lower letter turn down each flap

Type Business Letter from Dictating Machine

TERMINAL PERFORMANCE OBJECTIVE: Given typewriter, transcriber, dictation tapes, typing paper, and correction tape the medical assistant will complete mailable copy following designated format as the procedure requires in a time specified by the instructor, Figure 7–14, page 104. The instructor will proofread the final copy. The instructor will also designate the number of times the student is allowed to re-do the copy to achieve mailable copy.

1. The date should be no less than three lines below the letterhead. It may be lower in a short letter.
   Key Points:
   a. **The date must be in keeping with the style of letter (block or modified block).**
   b. **It should be the day the letter was dictated.**
   c. **Spell out the month in full.**
      Example: August 28, 19__ for traditional style
      28 August, 19__ for military style
      (number before month)
2. The inside address is flush with left margin on about the fifth line below the date (may be moved down in shorter letter or up in longer letter).
   Key Points:
   a. **The name should be copied exactly from letterhead or as printed in phone book or medical society directory.**
   b. **A courtesy title (Mr., Mrs., Miss, or Ms.) is used before a name.**
   c. **Use title Mr. if you do not know whether man or woman.**
   d. **Do not use Dr. before name of a physician with M.D. following name.**
      Example:
      William Smith, M.D. (correct)
      Dr. William Smith, M.D. (incorrect)
   e. **If street address and box number are given, use box number.**
   f. **Abbreviations such as NE, SW, SE, and NW may be used after street names, but North, South, East, and West preceding names and Road, Street, Avenue, and Boulevard are not abbreviated.**
   g. **Apartment and Suite are typed on same line as street address and separated by a comma. Apartment may be abbreviated if the line is unusually long.**
   h. **The name of the city is spelled out and separated from the state name by a comma.**

i. **The state name may be spelled out or abbreviated and is separated from the zip code by one space and no punctuation. The state abbreviations are not used without zip codes.**

3. Double space after the last line of the address and type the salutation followed by a colon. **Key Point: In writing to a firm, *Dear Sir or Madam* or *Gentlemen* is correct.**
4. A reference line is used often in medical correspondence and should be two spaces below the salutation. It may be flush with left margin or centered.
   Key Points:
   a. **This is often placed incorrectly because the dictator commonly dictates it before the salutation. Type RE followed by a colon.**
   b. **When using modified block style, you may place the reference line between the last line of the address and the salutation, lined up with the date. When it is not placed in this position it must appear after the salutation.**
5. Double space below the salutation or the reference line if one is used and begin the body of the letter.
   Key Points:
   a. **Always double space between paragraphs.**
   b. **The first line of each paragraph is flush with the left margin in block style and in modified block.**
   c. **Tabulated copy is indented 5 spaces from each margin.**
   d. **If necessary to continue to a second page, do so at the end of a paragraph if possible. If not, type at least 2 lines of a paragraph on the first page.**
   e. **Type no farther than 1 inch from the bottom of the page.**
   f. **Do not divide the last word on a page.**
   g. **Proofread pages before removing them from the typewriter and make any necessary corrections.**
6. Line up the complimentary close with the date a double space below the last line in the body of the letter.
   Key Points:
   a. **Only the first word of the complimentary close is capitalized.**
   b. **The complimentary close is followed by a comma.**
   c. **The formality of the letter determines the complimentary close. An informal complimentary close is *Cordially* or *Sincerely*; a more formal complimentary close is *Very truly yours*.**
7. The signature should be typed exactly as it appears on the letterhead, 4 spaces below the complimentary close

CONTINUED

and lined up with it. **Key Point: An official title may follow the name on the same line, preceded by a comma, or be directly below the name with no comma necessary.**

8. Reference initials identify the typist and are placed flush with the left margin on the second line below the typed signature in lowercase letters.
   Key Points:
   a. **If the dictator will not be signing the letter, then both the dictator's and typist's initials are used.**
   b. **If the typist has an unusual combination of initials, use the initials that would be least confusing or humorous.**
   c. **The typist does not place reference initials on a letter he or she signs.**

9. If the dictator is enclosing any items, *Enclosure* or *Enc.* is typed 1 or 2 lines below the reference initials. **Key Point: If more than one enclosure, number and identify them.**

10. If carbon copies are to be sent to others, type *cc* 1 or 2 spaces below reference initials or last notation made.
    Key Points:
    a. **If more than one carbon copy is to be sent, the individuals should be listed alphabetically or by rank.**
    b. **Never type *cc* without a name following it.**
    c. **If a copy is to be sent without the letter recipient knowing, it is called a *blind copy*. The notation *bcc* is made on the file copy and the copy mailed but no notation is made on the letter itself.**

11. A *postscript* is typed a double space below the last notation and is introduced by the abbreviation *P.S.*

12. The second page of a letter should have a heading typed starting on the seventh line of the page.
    Key Points:
    a. **The heading should include name of patient, page number, and date, in horizontal or vertical form, Figure 7–15, page 104. When the letter does not concern a patient, the name of the correspondent is listed in place of the patient's name.**
    b. **The letter should be continued on the third line after the heading.**
    c. **The page should contain at least 2 lines of a paragraph.**

 P R O C E D U R E

Make Corrections on Typewritten Copy

TERMINAL PERFORMANCE OBJECTIVE: Given typewriter, copy needing correction, and correction supplies, the medical assistant will demonstrate the ability to align letters and make neat acceptable corrections using various methods described in the procedure. The instructor will proofread the corrected copy.

Useful materials for making corrections:

- Eraser
- Soft brush
- Correction paper in white or colors to match the paper you use
- Correction fluid in white or colors
- Correction tape to be used only if you are making a master copy to be copied

1. If you are fortunate and have a correcting ribbon on your typewriter, use it to make corrections.
2. If you use erasable paper, a pencil eraser will do a neat job. Use a brush to clear off eraser crumbs.
   Key Points:
   a. **If using a Selectric typewriter, move the element so crumbs do not fall on it.**
   b. **Erase only the error, being careful not to erase any surrounding letters.**
   c. **Place a guard between carbon paper and carbon copy while erasing. Be sure to remove it before you resume typing.**
3. If you use correction paper, choose color to match paper you are typing on. Insert over error and type error. Remove paper and type in correction.
4. Correction fluid should be used only for very small errors as it is quite noticeable.
5. If paper has been removed from the typewriter before an error is found, learn how to realign the line of typing for a correction to blend in.
   Key Points:
   a. **Study the relationship of letters on the page to lines on the paper guide so that you can realign the paper.**
   b. **Insert a piece of scratch paper in typewriter and clean keys you plan to use by striking several times on stencil setting. Reinsert letter and, with ribbon still on stencil, strike letters to be inserted. If alignment is good, put ribbon back on print and type in correction.**

```
Nonaddress Data Line . . . . . . . . . . . . . . . . . . . . . . . . XXXXXXXXXXXXXX
Information/Attention Line . . . . . . . . . . . . . . . . . . MR. STANLEY DOE
Recipient Line . . . . . . . . . . . . . . . . . . . . . . . . . . . . . LAST NATIONAL BANK
Delivery Address Line . . . . . . . . . . . . . . . . . . . . . . PO BOX 345
Last Line . . . . . . . . . . . . . . . . . . . . . . . . . . . . . . . . NEW YORK NY 10163-0345
```

MR JAMES F JONES
4417 BROOKS ST NE
WASHINGTON DC 20019-4649   **EXAMPLE OF INDIVIDUAL ADDRESS**

LAW DEPARTMENT
US POSTAL SERVICE
475 LENFANT PLAZA SW RM 6627
WASHINGTON DC 20260-1120   **EXAMPLE OF ATTENTION LINE**

ACME INSURANCE CO
CAREW TOWERS
320 E MAIN ST RM 1121
MEMPHIS TN 38166-1121   **EXAMPLE OF BUILDING ADDRESS**

H E BOWN
RR 3 BOX 9
CANTON OH 44730-2521   **EXAMPLE OF RURAL ROUTE ADDRESS**

B G LIGHT CO
MC 2 BOX 293A
DULUTH MN 55811-9702   **EXAMPLE OF HIGHWAY CONTRACT ADDRESS**

MISS JANICE SMITH
PO BOX 34
DULUTH MN 55803-0034   **EXAMPLE OF POST OFFICE BOX ADDRESS**

CRPS 03672
MR S ONEILL PRES
SEAN ONEILL INC
4321 MAPLE ST
OAKTON MD 12345-6789   **EXAMPLE OF NONADDRESS DATA**

FIGURE 7–17 Examples of addresses (Courtesy of United States Postal Service)

and seal. Be sure that the sponge is not too wet as it will wet the envelopes and may spread glue so that letters stick together before you can seal them.

Complete Chapter 7, Unit 3 in the workbook to help you meet the objectives at the beginning of this unit and therefore achieve competency of this subject matter.

ALABAMA	AL	IDAHO	ID	MONTANA	MT	RHODE ISLAND	RI
ALASKA	AK	ILLINOIS	IL	NEBRASKA	NE	SOUTH CAROLINA	SC
ARIZONA	AZ	INDIANA	IN	NEVADA	NV	SOUTH DAKOTA	SD
ARKANSAS	AR	IOWA	IA	NEW HAMPSHIRE	NH	TENNESSEE	TN
CALIFORNIA	CA	KANSAS	KS	NEW JERSEY	NJ	TEXAS	TX
CANAL ZONE	CZ	KENTUCKY	KY	NEW MEXICO	NM	UTAH	UT
COLORADO	CO	LOUISIANA	LA	NEW YORK	NY	VERMONT	VT
CONNECTICUT	CT	MAINE	ME	NORTH CAROLINA	NC	VIRGINIA	VA
DELAWARE	DE	MARYLAND	MD	NORTH DAKOTA	ND	VIRGIN ISLANDS	VI
DISTRICT OF COLUMBIA	DC	MASSACHUSETTS	MA	OHIO	OH	WASHINGTON	WA
FLORIDA	FL	MICHIGAN	MI	OKLAHOMA	OK	WEST VIRGINIA	WV
GEORGIA	GA	MINNESOTA	MN	OREGON	OR	WISCONSIN	WI
GUAM	GU	MISSISSIPPI	MS	PENNSYLVANIA	PA	WYOMING	WY
HAWAII	HI	MISSOURI	MO	PUERTO RICO	PR		

FIGURE 7–18 Two-letter state abbreviations

Annex	ANX	Knolls	KNLS	Road	RD
Apartment	APT	Lake	LK	Room	RM
Association	ASSN	Lakes	LKS	Route	RT
Attention	ATTN	Lane	LN	Rural	R
Avenue	AVE	Manager	MGR	Rural Route	RR
Boulevard	BLVD	Meadows	MDWS	Secretary	SECY
Canyon	CYN	North	N	Shore	SHR
Causeway	CSWY	Northeast	NE	South	S
Circle	CIR	Northwest	NW	Southeast	SE
Court	CT	Palms	PLMS	Southwest	SW
Department	DEPT	Park	PK	Square	SQ
East	E	Parkway	PKY	Station	STA
Expressway	EXPY	Pike	PIKE	Street	ST
Freeway	FWY	Place	PL	Terrace	TER
Heights	HTS	Plaza	PLZ	Treasurer	TREAS
Highway	HWY	Post Office	PO	Turnpike	TPKE
Hospital	HOSP	President	PRES	Union	UN
Institute	INST	Ridge	RDG	Vice President	VP
Junction	JCT	River	RIV	View	VW

FIGURE 7–19 Examples of USPS approved address abbreviations (Courtesy of United States Postal Service)

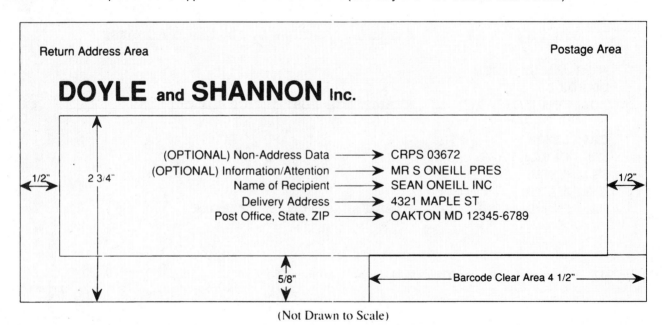

FIGURE 7–20 Example of address block location (Courtesy of United States Postal Service)

UNIT 4

Office Mail

OBJECTIVES

Upon completion of the unit the student will meet the following terminal performance objectives by verifying knowledge of the facts and principles presented through oral and written communication at a level deemed competent, and will demonstrate the specific behaviors as identified in the terminal performance objectives of the procedures, observing safety precautions in accordance with health care standards.

1. Categorize, open, and annotate incoming mail.
2. Describe how vacation mail might be handled.
3. Identify postal services that may be required by an office.
4. List points to remember in processing metered mail.
5. List three methods for classifying mail.
6. List examples of first class mail.
7. List examples of second class mail.
8. List examples of third class mail.
9. List examples of fourth class mail.
10. Describe express mail service.
11. Describe use of certificate of mailing.
12. Describe use of certified mail.
13. Describe purpose for use of registered mail.
14. Spell and define, using the glossary at the back of the text, all the words to know in this unit.

WORDS TO KNOW

annotating	dedicated
categories	integrity
confirmation	judgment
consecutively	

Incoming Mail

The amount of mail coming into the physician's office depends on the number of physicians. There are many categories of mail to be sorted and distributed. In smaller offices the task is manageable but in large clinics it may be necessary to have a mail clerk who is responsible for sorting and delivering the mail within the clinic.

The first class mail may consist of:

Special delivery mail

Mailgrams

Special messenger mail

Correspondence from patients

Payments from patients

Payments from insurance companies

Insurance forms to be completed

General correspondence
    a. referral letters or reports from physicians

    b. laboratory reports
    c. hospital reports
    d. professional organization mail
    e. miscellaneous mail

Other classes of mail:

Professional journals

Magazines

Newspapers

Advertisements

Promotional literature and samples from pharmaceutical companies

The office procedure manual should give instructions regarding the handling of mail. If no procedure manual is available, the office manager or the physician should be consulted. Following are some generally accepted procedures.

Sorting Mail

Incoming mail should first be sorted. Any mail marked *personal* should be placed on the physician's desk unopened. Special delivery mail, mailgrams, or special messenger mail should be opened immediately. (The mailgram is a postal service offered jointly by the USPS and Western Union. Mailgrams are transmitted over Western Union's communication network to printers located in over 140 post offices, then placed in special envelopes carrying the postal service emblem and delivered the next day by regular carrier. First class mail may be sorted into mail from patients, from physicians, from insurance companies, and miscellaneous. Magazines, professional journals, and newspapers should be separated from drug samples and advertisements.

Opening Mail

You will need a letter opener, paper clips, a stapler, and a date stamp. The medical assistant who is dedicated to efficiency will stack all envelopes so that they are facing in the same direction. A quick tap on the desk will shake contents away from the flap side of the envelope. You are then ready to cut all letters along the flap edge before emptying them. Be careful to remove all contents from each envelope. As the mail is removed be sure the contents contain the same name and return address shown on the envelope. Some offices want you to keep the envelope with the mail received, and certainly you should if it is needed to help identify the contents. Otherwise you may discard the envelopes.

Date-stamp the correspondence and attach any enclosures. If an enclosure is indicated on the letter but is missing, it is necessary to write "none" after the "Encl." notation and circle it to indicate need for follow-up.

Processing Incoming Mail

You should exercise judgment in determining which mail can be handled without the aid of the physician.

Such mail would include checks for deposit. If cash is received in the mail, you should always seek a witness as to the amount of money and have that person sign a receipt along with you to be sent to the patient. This helps avoid the possibility of the patient saying that more was sent than was actually found in the envelope, which can happen quite innocently with elderly patients who have a poor memory. The medical assistant needs to have flawless integrity and this simple procedure can help demonstrate that integrity.

The mail will contain copies of hospital summaries and operative notes if you work for a surgeon. These can be filed in the patient chart if your employer was the attending physician. Any other hospital reports, laboratory reports, or special examination reports you receive should be seen by the physician and initialed before they are filed. Any requests regarding patients or other office matters should be placed in a designated area for the physician to see and dispose of each day.

The medical assistant can perform a valuable, time-saving service for the physician by annotating the incoming mail, or identifying important points to be noticed. If any correspondence or a patient chart is needed in answering mail, it should be pulled and placed with the mail to be answered.

Notifications of meetings, miscellaneous correspondence, and professional journals are placed under the stack of mail to be answered. Some physicians want to see all supply catalogs and pharmaceutical company descriptions of products. In other offices, many of these items are disposed of immediately, especially if they concern items the office has no use for. Items of this nature that may be needed for future reference should be placed in a designated file.

Drug samples that your office may use should be placed in a designated area for future use. Samples you will not use should never be placed in the trash where they could cause harm to individuals using them ignorantly. Often charity clinics or organizations within the community can make good, safe use of unwanted samples, and you should have a box for this purpose.

Vacation Mail

When the physician is away from the office for professional meetings or for vacation, it is the duty of the medical assistant to carefully read all mail and decide how each piece of mail will be handled. You should discuss what to do with urgent mail before the physician leaves. The physician may want you to call, or in some cases, to copy the mail and forward it. Never send the original copy. If the physician will be away for a long time, you may need to mail urgent mail more than once. If so, be sure to number the envelopes consecutively and keep track of what you send so that you can be sure all the urgent mail is received. You may also wish to send brief notes explaining the reason for the delay in answering

mail. If the office will be closed completely, be sure to go to the post office and complete a form to have mail held or forwarded to another address. Never send this form by mail as it may be delayed. The USPS cannot take verbal orders for this purpose. Allowing mail to pile up in the mail slot invites theft.

Sending Mail

The cost of sending mail is an expense that must be examined and understood to be sure you obtain the most for your money. Your local post office can furnish you with current information. Postage rates, categories, and regulations are changeable, so you must be alert to keep current.

Mail may be either stamped or metered. Stamps may be purchased at a post office or obtained through the mail by using a specially printed envelope available through the post office. If you have a large volume of mail, it is preferable to use a postage meter. This machine can be leased from several authorized dealers, but the license to use it must be obtained from the USPS. A medical office can obtain a license by submitting an application to the post office where the metered mail will be deposited.

Postage meters contain a sealed unit that houses the printing die and two recording counters. One counter adds up all postage printed by the meter. The other counter subtracts and shows the balance of postage remaining in the meter. When you purchase an amount of postage, the post office will open the meter with a key, set the counter for the amount of postage purchased, and relock the meter. When the prepaid amount runs out, the meter will lock automatically. The postage meter prints prepaid postage either directly on the mail or on adhesive strips that are then affixed to the mail. The metered mail imprint, or metered stamp, serves as postage payment, postmark, and cancellation mark. All classes of mail may be metered, any amount of postage may be metered, and any quantity of mail may be metered. Metered mail, when bundled, can provide faster service than stamped mail because it is already postmarked and will bypass postal cancellation equipment.

To expedite the processing of metered mail, remember to: (1) change the date on the meter daily, (2) apply the correct amount of postage by weighing the mail before affixing postage, (3) check the imprint to be sure it is clear and readable, and (4) use fluorescent ink in the meter, Figure 7–21.

Mail is classified according to type, weight, and destination. First class mail includes handwritten and typewritten messages, payments from patients or insurance companies, laboratory reports, and any other business mail which weighs up to 11 ounces. (Postage is figured by the ounce.) All first class mail over 11 ounces is considered priority mail. The cost of priority mail is determined by the weight and zone of destination. The maximum weight for priority mail is 70 pounds. If you

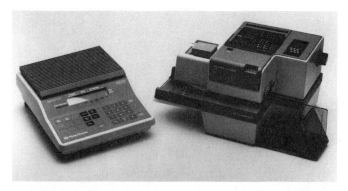

FIGURE 7–21 Postage meter machine (Courtesy Pitney Bowes)

need to send first class mail that is larger than the usual number 10 business envelope, the envelope should have a green diamond border which signals the post office that the letter is to go first class.

The office should have a mail scale so that you can determine the amount of postage necessary for your mail. The second ounce does not cost as much as the first.

Second class mail includes newspapers and other periodicals issued regularly at least four times a year. You are not likely to use this classification unless you work for a medical society that mails its own journal.

Third class mail includes circulars, printed booklets, catalogs, newsletters, and merchandise weighing up to but not including 16 ounces, which is not required to be mailed at first class rates or as priority mail. Anything 16 ounces or more must be mailed fourth class or priority mail.

Fourth class mail is commonly known as parcel post. The classification also includes bound printed matter, books, 16 mm or narrower films, sound recordings, and manuscripts. Fourth class postage is computed by weight and the zone of destination.

In combination mailing, a first class letter is sent with a parcel, either by placing the letter in an envelope and attaching it to the outside of the package or by enclosing it within the parcel, in which case you write *letter enclosed* just below the postage. This method is used frequently in the field of medicine for sending X rays with an accompanying report. Separate postage is paid for the two items.

Express mail service is a reliable, speedy delivery service available in most major metropolitan areas for anything mailable up to 70 pounds and 108 inches in combined length and girth. You are given a receipt when the letter or package is mailed and the addressee is required to sign a confirmation of delivery. Each express shipment is insured against loss or damage at no additional charge. Postage varies according to weight and the type of express mail service chosen. A form with a large *A* or *B* on it will be attached to express mail to designate it as post office-to-post office or post office-to-addressee. *A* designates post office-to-post office service: mail which is deposited by 5:00 P.M. at an express post office will be shipped to the destination post office for customer pickup the next day as early as 10:00 A.M. *B* designates post office-to-addressee service: mail which is deposited

by 5 P.M. at a designated post office will be delivered to the addressee no later than 3:00 P.M. the next day (weekends and holidays included). A full refund of postage will be made if shipments are delivered later than the service standard called for. You apply at the originating post office for the refund. Express mail envelopes and labels are available at the post office as well as a network directory of all destinations that can be served.

Special delivery may be purchased for all classes of mail to provide prompt delivery at the destination post office. Smaller post offices and rural routes do not offer this service, so it is best to check before mailing a letter to such an address. Do not send special delivery to a box number because it is considered delivered when it is put in the box.

A certificate of mailing provides evidence of mailing. The postal clerk will date and initial the slip you prepare to show that a piece of mail was dispatched from that post office on a particular date. The service is inexpensive and is often used to prove that an income tax form was mailed by the deadline. Certified mail provides an opportunity to restrict delivery to addressee only and to request a signed return receipt for an additional fee. This method of mailing should always be used for letters requesting that the patient find another physician. This is sometimes necessary if the patient will not follow the instructions of the physician for treatment or follow-up, and you must have proof that the patient received the notification. The signed return receipt needs to be filed in the patient chart as your proof that the patient received the letter.

Registered mail is the best method to use if sending valuable articles. Paying the extra fee for this service guarantees extra security in the form of locked mail bags and signed releases for each step through which the mail passes. The full value of the mailing must be declared, and it can be insured up to $10,000. Only first class and priority mail can be registered.

You can insure any class of mail against loss or damage. You can also request a return receipt and restrict the delivery.

If you have deposited mail and find you want it back, you can do this by written application at the local post office. You will need an envelope addressed exactly as the one you wish returned. If the post office finds that the letter has left the local post office, the postmaster will telephone or telegraph the destination post office at your expense to have the letter returned to you.

When a letter is returned to you after an attempt has been made to deliver it, you must prepare a new envelope and put on new postage before remailing the letter. This sometimes happens if you have made an error such as transposing numbers in an address. If you have returned mail because the patient has moved and left no forwarding address, you can try contacting the employer for a new address or talking with the individual who referred the patient.

Complete Chapter 7, Unit 4 in the workbook to help you meet the objectives at the beginning of this unit and therefore achieve competency of this subject matter.

Throughout this chapter you should be mindful of all medical-legal/ethical implications. Listed below are a few important reminders.

1. Use only blue or black ink for documenting messages.
2. Draw a single line through an error then initial, date, and state error.
3. Keep office policy handbook updated on a routine basis.
4. Cover telephones adequately at all times.
5. Chart reasons for all missed appointments.
6. Establish and maintain good rapport with patients.
7. Never give information over the telephone to anyone concerning a patient unless written authorization from that patient is on file.

Mr. Right. . .

uses black ink when documenting information about patients. If an error is made, he draws a single line through it, initials and dates it, and then briefly states the error. He is polite in speaking to patients over the telephone and never leaves telephones unattended. When a patient misses an appointment, he records the reason on the chart. He never gives information to anyone on the telephone (or otherwise) unless written permission is obtained from the patient. When it comes time to revise the office policy handbook, he offers helpful suggestions. He is efficient in office correspondence and in scheduling appointments.

Advancement potential: Excellent

Miss Wrong. . .

never worries about what color she uses in recording patient information. She frequently uses "white out," or erases errors on the patients' records, schedule book, and other documents. She is short and rude with patients over the telephone when she does answer it. She has been known to put callers on hold for long periods or even hang up on them. She is careless about taking messages and forgets to write them down. When a caller requests information about a patient she tells the caller she'll get it if she can find it. She pays no attention to the office policy handbook because she thinks it is silly. She makes appointments when she remembers and is negligent in correspondence.

Advancement potential: None

REFERENCES

Fordney, Marilyn, and Diehl, Marcy. *Medical Transcription Guide: Do's and Don'ts*. Philadelphia: W. B. Saunders, 1990.

Frew, Mary, and Frew, David. *Comprehensive Medical Assistant: Administrative and Clinical Procedures*, 2nd ed. Philadelphia: F. A. Davis, 1988.

Kinn, Mary, and Derge, Eleanor. *The Medical Assistant: Administrative and Clinical*, 6th ed. Philadelphia: W. B. Saunders, 1988.

United States Postal Service. "Postal Addressing Standards," Publication 28, May 1990.

———. "A Guide to Business Mail Preparation," Publication 25, August 1988.

———. "Address Information Systems," Publication 40, May 1990.

———. "Addressing for Success," Notice 221, April 1990.

———. "ZIP + 4 Code Procedures," Notice 189, March 1990.

———. "Two-Letter State and Possession Abbreviations" and "Abbreviations for Street Designations," Publication 28, May 1990.

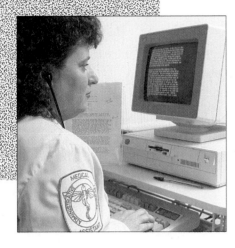

C H A P T E R   8

Office Equipment

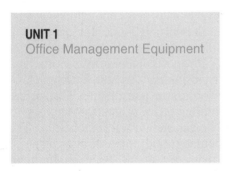

The medical assistant may be responsible for the operation of a variety of business equipment in performing administrative duties. The typewriter is a familiar business machine and a skilled medical transcriptionist has many opportunities for employment. Many offices are turning to computer systems in order to cope with the increased amount of paper work. The medical assistant will need to know the basic computer terminology and the functions that a computer can perform in an office. You will learn the uses of many other business machines in this chapter.

U N I T   1

Office Management Equipment

OBJECTIVES ••

Upon completion of the unit the student will meet the following terminal performance objectives by verifying knowledge of the facts and principles presented through oral and written communication at a level deemed competent, and will demonstrate the specific behaviors as identified in the terminal performance objectives of the procedures, observing safety precautions in accordance with health care standards.

1. Demonstrate use of a calculator, with emphasis on accuracy.
2. Describe use of a copier in the office.
3. List steps necessary to use a check writer.
4. Discuss advantages of a FAX machine in the office.
5. Cite at least five office functions that may be completed with the use of a FAX machine.
6. Describe the nine general rules to follow in the operation of a FAX machine.
7. Explain two uses for a microfilm and microfilm reader-printer.
8. Identify the helpful hints that may make the use of dictation-transcription equipment successful.
9. State the advantages of computer use in the medical office.
10. Define the computer terminology described in this unit.
11. Describe advantages of out-of-house computer services.
12. List specific functions a computer system can perform in the billing, insurance, and collection functions in the office.
13. Describe the types of printers used with computers.
14. Name three general main functions computers should perform for an office.
15. Describe use of a word processor.
16. Spell and define, using the glossary at the back of the text, all the words to know in this unit.

WORDS TO KNOW ••

acronym	documentary	thermally
adequate	microfiche	transmitted
ascertain	polling	
delete	scan	

Many pieces of equipment will improve the efficiency of the office. The typewriter and postage meter have been discussed.

Adding Machine

An adding machine or calculator will aid in preparing statements for patients, billing for insurance, receipts of checks and cash, and bank deposits. Of course, the machine is only as accurate as the person who operates it. Figures must always be double-checked. If you do not have a tape on your machine, do the calculation a second time to see if your answer is the same, Figure 8–1.

Copy Machine

The office copy machine is extremely important to office efficiency. Use of the machine to copy correspondence has been discussed. In addition, a copy of all forms prepared in the office should be kept in the patient chart. Some offices use a copy machine for monthly billing: the accounting record is copied, folded, inserted in an envelope, and mailed. It is also easy to keep a supply of patient information forms and patient release forms on hand when you have a good copy machine, Figure 8–2.

Check Writer

A check writer imprints a check so that the figures and name of payee cannot be altered. The figures and name are set on the machine, a lever is pulled, and the check is imprinted. It is essential that you double-check your figures to be sure they are correct before you imprint the check. If it is imprinted incorrectly, you must void the check and write a new one. The check should then be signed by the physician, or other designated person, Figure 8–3.

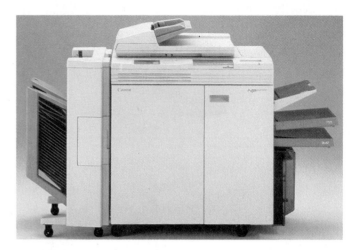

FIGURE 8–2 Copy machine

FAX Machines

Facsimile (FAX) machines, Figure 8–4, page 115, are used by hospitals, physicians offices, and clinics to send and receive information over telephone lines, regarding patients. The machine makes it possible to send and receive letters, medical reports, laboratory reports, and insurance claims. Physicians may use the FAX machine to send prescription orders to pharmacies. The office may also use it for ordering office or medical supplies.

A FAX machine is connected to a telephone line. The machine scans a document and converts the image to electronic impulses that are transmitted over the telephone lines. The receiving FAX machine converts the impulse back to an identical copy of the original, and a printed copy is created. FAX machines may print on thermally treated paper or plain paper. The thermally treated paper fades when exposed to sunlight; therefore, you would usually photocopy an important document onto bond paper.

The FAX machine is available with many special features. Certainly a concern in the medical office is the trans-

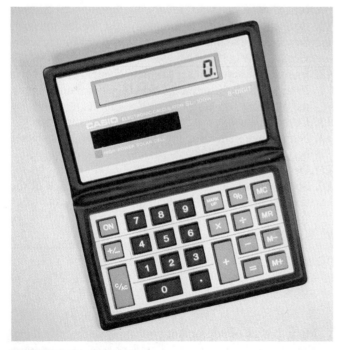

FIGURE 8–1 Calculator

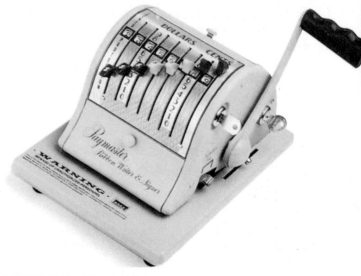

FIGURE 8–3 Check writer

Total Charges on Calculator

TERMINAL PERFORMANCE OBJECTIVE: Given completed ledger cards and calculator, the student will calculate all charges and report with 100% accuracy. The student must follow all steps in the procedure and complete it within a time period specified by the instructor. The instructor will observe each step.

1. Pull patient ledger card. **Key Point: If a patient is seen only in consultation and has not been a patient previously, there may be no ledger card.**
2. Turn on calculator.
3. Clear machine to be sure you are not adding on to something already there.
   Key Points:
   a. **Ideally you should have a calculator with a digital display plus a printer which will deliver a hard copy.**
   b. **The digital display window or printed tape gives visual evidence that the machine is cleared.**
4. Enter figures from ledger card.
5. Enter fee for report, if charged.
6. Enter any fee for X rays or special examination, etc., not listed on ledger card.
7. Total fees.
8. Double-check tape or refigure on digital display to be sure you get the same answer twice.
9. Add consultation and report fees to ledger card and make a copy to send with the report. **Key Point: In some cases two copies of the bill may be required. If there is no ledger card, type a copy of the bill on a statement and make needed copies.**

mission of confidential material. It is possible to have a secret code that will lock out unauthorized polling. The machine may also store multiple documents in memory and have automatic dialing with redialing when a busy signal is detected. The paper is automatically cut to the length of each page of the received message. If the recording paper runs out, the message is stored in memory and will be automatically printed out when new paper is loaded. A battery safeguards the document memory in case of power failure. The machine may be equipped with a white line skip function that automatically skips over horizontal blank spaces on a document. This feature allows a standard document to be transmitted in as little as 12 seconds.

You will need to learn the procedures for operating the FAX machine you will be required to use. General rules which would be important to the use of any machine are:

1. Always remove paper clips and staples from material to be scanned so you will not damage the FAX machine.
2. Make a test copy if the document has color. Dark colors may block copy and can slow transmission.
3. Do not use correction tape or fluid on documents to be transmitted.
4. Do consider typing words for numbers to avoid problems with interpretation.
5. If the material you are sending is confidential, you should call recipients before sending the information to alert them to be watching for the material.
6. The first page of any transmission is called the FAX page. It includes the date, name of recipient, recipient's address and FAX number, and the number of pages being sent (includes FAX page). Also the name and FAX number of the sender will be included. Any other special information required for routing instructions may be added.
7. Be familiar with the error messages the FAX machine may indicate and how to correct these problems. The machine may be equipped with built-in service diagnostic codes that can be automatically transmitted over the telephone lines to a service provider. Most service calls can be resolved by telephone and this, of course, reduces costly equipment downtime and labor costs.
8. You may need to resend a message if noise or interference on the telephone line interfered with a clear transmission.
9. Be sure the transmission is completed before you leave. A copy of your FAX document will be produced by the machine. It will indicate the message was sent, identifying the data and time of transmission. Remove the originals and the copy from the machine.

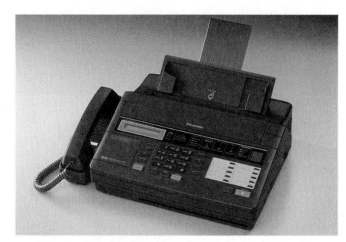

FIGURE 8–4 FAX machine (Courtesy of Panasonic Communications & Systems Co.)

PROCEDURE

Operate Copy Machine

TERMINAL PERFORMANCE OBJECTIVE: Given material to be copied and a copy machine, the student will demonstrate the ability to make decisions as to machine settings and operate the copy machine following procedures listed. The instructor will observe the student in completing the steps in this procedure.

1. Assemble material to be copied.
2. Determine number of copies needed.
   Key Points:
   a. **You usually make one file copy of every letter you send. If copies are to be sent, you need additional copies.**
   b. **Two copies are needed of most medical legal reports.**
   c. **If you are making copies of instruction sheets for patients, copy enough for a month's use at one time.**
3. Turn on copy machine.

4. Check settings to see that they are appropriate for what you want to copy.
   Key Points:
   a. **Set for legal- or letter-size paper.**
   b. **Regular copy/lighter/darker may be adjusted on some machines.**
   c. **Set for number of copies.**
5. Check to see that paper supply is adequate. **Key Point: Some machines will jam if paper supply becomes too low.**
6. Feed copy in or lift cover and place material face down on glass.
7. Replace cover and push print.
8. Remove copy and original. **Key Point: Some offices leave the machine on all the time because it requires a warm-up period before it can be used. If this is not your office policy, turn the machine off when finished.**

Microfiche

The medical assistant needs to be familiar with the microfilming process, Figure 8–5. Microfilming is a method of preserving documentary material by reducing it to minute film images. Microfilming of office records can provide the necessary record security while using a minimum of storage space. The machine is easy to operate. The microfilmed documents may be read at any time with the use of a microfilm reader. In seconds, the reader–printer can provide a hard copy of microfiche material printed on plain bond paper.

You may find that some patients will present an insurance card that needs to be read with the help of a microfilm reader-printer, Figure 8–6.

Dictation-Transcription Machine

The most common units to be used in the physician's office are the desktop machines, Figure 8–7. Several kinds of

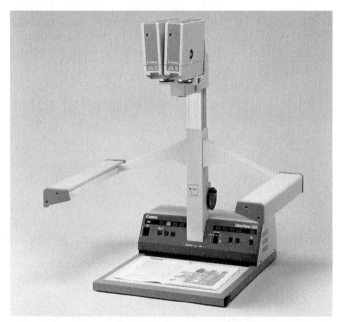

FIGURE 8–5 Microfilm machine (Courtesy of Canon, Inc.)

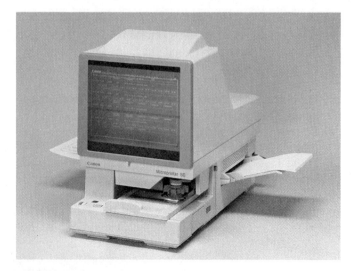

FIGURE 8–6 Microfilm reader-printer machine (Courtesy of Canon, Inc.)

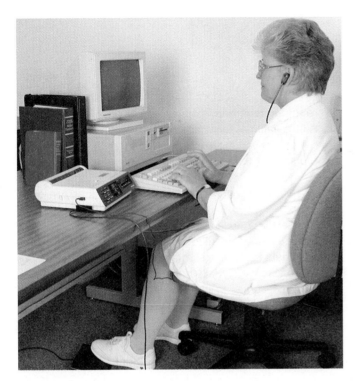

FIGURE 8–7 Dictation-transcription machine

units are available: a unit for dictation only, a unit for transcription only, or a combination unit that can be used for both purposes. Many physicians use a portable dictating machine, which can be operated by battery or electricity. The physician may use this machine in the office, in the car, at home, or while attending meetings. The medical assistant can help the physician use the equipment more efficiently by discussing any problems encountered while transcribing. This can be done tactfully because you are doing it to improve your efficiency and productivity as an employee. When the machine is in the office, the transcriptionist should check to be sure the equipment is ready for use. Be

sure the battery is replaced as needed and that transcribed tapes are erased and ready for reuse. Tell the physician when the dictation is good. Sometimes a list of helpful hints to improve dictation and reduce the chance of error can be used to help both the physician and the transcriptionist. The list might include the following:

1. Check machine to be sure it is recording.
2. Indicate date and what is being dictated (chart note, letter, research paper, report, and so on).
3. Recognize that you are talking to a person through the machine.
4. Dictate the name of the patient and the name of the person or firm who will be the recipient of the message.
5. Dictate the street address, city, state, and zip code to which correspondence is to be sent and the number of copies needed.
6. Dictate punctuation such as "period," "comma," or "paragraph."
7. Encourage the physician to refrain from eating, drinking, or listening to loud music or television while the dictation is being done.
8. Speak in a normal clear voice.
9. End with an appropriate message to indicate the dictation is completed.

The transcription machine has a foot control that starts the machine. When the pedal is released the machine stops. It also has a backup pedal that allows you to relisten to the transcription if you need to hear it again before you transcribe. You will learn to press the pedal, listen, then begin typing the sentences with a minimum of time. With practice and speed, you may be able to type and listen almost simultaneously. The machine has controls for automatic rewind and fast forward. The speed control can be adjusted to either slow or speed up the voice message. The speed control should generally be adjusted for the normal voice quality for the physician making the dictation.

P R O C E D U R E

Operate Check Writer

TERMINAL PERFORMANCE OBJECTIVE: Given necessary equipment and supplies, the student will prepare a check for a specified amount and then imprint it with the check writer with 100% accuracy. The instructor will observe each step of the procedure.

1. Determine to whom check is to be written and amount of the check.
2. Type date, name of payee, and amount of check on check.
3. Set figures to desired amount by adjusting number levers on check writer. **Key Point: Double-check to be sure check writer is set correctly.**
4. Insert check in check writer.
5. Press down on lever to imprint dollar amount and perforate payee name in one operation. **Key Point: No change can be made in name or amount after they are imprinted.**
6. Remove check and have it signed by the physician or designated person.

Operate Transcriber

TERMINAL PERFORMANCE OBJECTIVE: Given a transcriber, a dictated tape, headset with earphones, foot control, typewriter and paper, or a computer, the student will operate the transcriber with 100 percent accuracy. While transcribing recorded messages, the student will follow all steps in the procedure and complete the transcription within a time period specified by the instructor. The instructor will observe each step.

1. Turn on the transcriber.
2. Verify that headset with earphones and the foot control are attached to the unit.
3. Select tape. **Key Point: Type rush reports or oldest dictation first.**
4. Adjust headset with earphones. **Key Point: Earphones should not be shared as a safeguard from spreading ear infections.**
5. Insert tape. Press play tab or the pedal to listen for the beginning of the dictation. **Key Point: Sometimes you need to rewind the tape to find the beginning.**
6. Listen for physician's instructions. **Key Point: The material to be typed will guide you in selecting the appropriate paper to be put in the typewriter or printer. It may be a chart note, a report, or a letter requiring letterhead paper.**
7. Adjust volume, tone, and speed controls for clearest communication reception. **Key Point: A speed that is too slow or too fast will distort the sound.**
8. Set typewriter or computer margins and tabulator stops.
9. Insert paper in typewriter or bring up blank screen on computer and type recorded information.
10. Alternately press and release foot pedal to listen and transcribe the recorded message. **Key Point: If you are unable to understand a word or words for any reason, leave a blank, note the place on the tape and ask someone else to listen. Consult a dictionary, if the word is unfamiliar. If necessary, ask the dictating physician for assistance so you can complete the work.**
11. Save the dictation on the tape, in case questions should arise, or until the physician reads and approves the report or signs the letter.
12. Erase tape, following report approval or signature of physician on letter, so it can be used again.
13. Turn off the machine, place accessory items in proper storage space.

Because you cannot always judge the length of the message when you begin to listen, it may be advisable to run the tape to determine its content before typing if you are using a standard typewriter. You may also need to make an initial rough draft copy, setting your margins, headings, and tabs later according to content involved.

Computer

In a text titled *Computer Fundamentals for an Information Age*, authors Shelly and Cashman define a computer as follows:

> A computer is an electronic device, operating under the control of instructions stored in its own memory unit, which can accept and store data, perform arithmetic and logical operations on that data without human intervention, and produce output from the processing.

Physicians are becoming more aware of the advantages to be gained by using computers in the office. Large clinics often have direct-line insurance reporting by computer: the necessary information is programmed into the clinic computer and travels directly to the insurance company computers. This eliminates paper work, and the speed of processing claims is enhanced considerably.

Computer Terms

- **backup**—duplicate of data files made to protect information. Records should be backed up daily. Some experts recommend twice daily.
- **batch**—an accumulation of data to be processed.
- **boot**—to start up a computer.
- **bug**—an error in a program.
- **catalog**—a list of files on the storage media.
- **characters per second**—term used to measure printer output.
- **CPU**—central processing unit, or the brain of the system. The memory is made up of **bits**. A bit is a single **BI**nary digi**T**. *Binary* refers to a situation in which there are only two choices: for example, yes/no, on/off, pass/fail. Digit refers to a single number. A bit is either 0 or 1. A **byte** is the fundamental group of bits that a computer will treat as a word. A byte consists of 8 bits. A 16-bit processor is twice as fast as an 8-bit processor. One **K** is equal to 1,024 bytes. A 64-K computer can handle 65,536 bytes. The greater the number of bytes, the greater the memory.
- **cursor**—a marker on the screen that shows where the next letter, number, or symbol will be placed (may be an underline dash or a blinking rectangle or square).
- **daisy wheel printer**—a printer that uses a changeable

printwheel, named for its shape.

- **data**—information that can be processed or produced by a computer.
- **debugging**—finding errors and correcting them in computer programs.
- **disk**—a magnetic storage device made of rigid material (hard disk) or flexible plastic (floppy disk).
- **disk drive**—the device used to get information on and off a disk.
- **DOS**—(**D**isk **O**perating **S**ystem) a program that tells the computer how to use the disk drive.
- **dot matrix printer**—printer that uses dots to form letters and numbers.
- **downtime**—a period of lost work time during which a computer is not operating or is malfunctioning because of machine failure.
- **electronic mail**—the transmission of letters, messages, or memos from one computer to another over telephone lines.
- **external memory**—recording on floppy disks.
- **file**—a single, stored unit of information that is given a file name so it can be accessed.
- **file maintenance**—adding, changing, or deleting information from data contained in file.
- **floppy disk**—a thin magnetic storage device made of flexible plastic.
- **font**—a family or assortment of characters of a given size or style.
- **GIGO**—**G**arbage **in** **g**arbage **o**ut. The standard explanation when the computer output does not make sense. If you get nonsense out of a computer, you must have put nonsense in.
- **hard copy**—the readable paper copy or printout of information.
- **hardware**—the electronic, magnetic, and electromechanical equipment of a computer system (keyboard, disk drive, monitor, and printer).
- **initialize**—to prepare a diskette to receive data. This is sometimes referred to as *formatting* the disk.
- **input**—data processed from peripheral equipment into the machine via the keyboard or the floppy disk for internal storage.
- **interface**—the hardware and software that enable individual computers and components to interact.
- **K**—computer shorthand for 1,024 bytes; a term used to measure computer memory capacity.
- **keyboard**—an input device resembling a typewriter keyboard that converts keystrokes into electrical signals which are displayed on the screen as words or symbols.
- **kilobyte**—one thousand bytes.
- **main memory**—the internal memory of the computer.
- **memory**—data held in storage.
- **menu**—a display of available machine functions for selection by the operator.
- **microcomputer**—a self-contained computer system that uses a microprocessor as the central processing

unit. Often called a desktop or personal computer. Has limited capacity for internal memory.

- **microprocessor**—a single chip where the computer computes.
- **minicomputer**—a computer significantly smaller in size, capacity, and software capability than its larger mainframe counterparts.
- **modem**—**MO**dulator/**DEM**odulator. A peripheral device that enables a computer to communicate with other computers or terminals over normal telephone lines.
- **monitor**—visual display unit with a screen called a cathode-ray tube (CRT).
- **mouse**—a hand-held computer input device, separate from a keyboard, used to control cursor position on a VDT (video display terminal), sometimes called a joystick.
- **output**—what the computer produces after recorded information is processed, revised, and printed out.
- **peripheral**—anything you plug into a computer; for example, a printer, a disk drive, CRT terminal, or printer.
- **printer**—a device that produces hard copy. It may be dot matrix, letter quality, or laser.
- **program**—a set of instructions written in computer language and designed to tell a computer how to complete every operation.
- **prompting**—messages issued to a user requesting information necessary to continue processing.
- **RAM**—acronym for **R**andom **A**ccess **M**emory. This is temporary, or programmable memory. You can put new information into RAM. When you turn off the computer, the memory is gone.
- **ROM**—acronym for **R**ead **O**nly **M**emory. This is permanent memory. You cannot put new information into ROM. It has been determined by the computer manufacturer.
- **scrolling**—moving cursor up, down, right, or left through information on a computer display to view information otherwise excluded.
- **security code**—a code the operator must enter in before procedure may be completed. Used to prevent unauthorized access to data in system.
- **software**—computer programs necessary to direct the hardware of a computer system to perform specific tasks.
- **terminal**—a device used to communicate with a computer, usually a keyboard. Terminals depend on the main (host) computer for their abilities. An office may have several terminals and a host computer physically removed from any of them.
- **write-protect**—process or code that prevents overwriting of data or programs on a disk.

Input into a computer is by means of a keyboard very much like that on a typewriter. There are added keys to give you expanded capability. You do not need to be an expert on computer technology or programming to make good use of a computer. Any computer, like a typewriter, will occasionally need to be serviced and when this happens you call a repair person.

In learning about computers you will find references to *hardware* and *software*. The hardware consists of the keyboard, the disk drive, the monitor, and the display screen. The software consists of the instructions that enable a computer to perform its tasks. These are usually stored on a disk, commonly called a floppy disk, Figure 8–8. This floppy disk looks very much like a small phonograph record enclosed in a protective jacket. Figure 8–9 provides guidelines for the care of floppy disks.

You will also find the use of the hard disk important in the medical office. A hard disk consists of oxide-coated metal platters that are sealed inside a housing to ensure dust-free operation. They store much more information than floppy disks, and you have faster access to the information. The disks may be 8, $5\frac{1}{4}$, $3\frac{1}{2}$, $3\frac{1}{4}$, or $2\frac{1}{2}$ inches in diameter.

The information stored on a disk is called a *file*. It is necessary to assign a code to information to be saved on a file so that it may be *called up* from the storage disk by using the code. Computer manufacturers usually provide basic software programs that are compatible with the hardware. Many companies design special programs of software for use with specific computers. A computer would be useless without the software instructions for using input data.

Computer Printers ....

To produce hard copy, you must have a printer. Printers may be equipped with a single-sheet feeder or a tractor feeder that automatically advances the paper. Three types of printers are appropriate for a medical office: dot matrix, letter quality, or laser. The dot matrix, Figure 8–10 produces print made up of pin-head dots and can

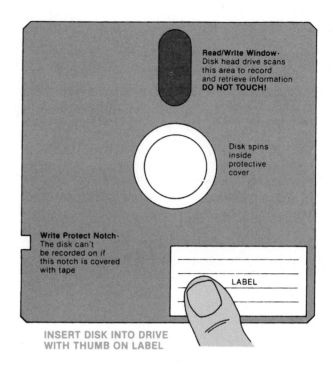

Rules for Handling Floppy Disks

DO · Handle the disk by its jacket and label.
Store disks upright in their envelopes.
Store disks away from direct sunlight, moisture, or extremes of heat or cold.

DO NOT · Spill soda, coffee, or any liquids on disk.
Set disks on top of monitors or television sets.
Get disks near magnets or electrical devices.
(especially telephones, motors and televisions)

FIGURE 8–9 Care and feeding of floppy disk

produce "near letter quality" printing. Depending on the type of printer you have, you may set "draft mode," and the printer will print more than twice as fast as it will on letter quality. For example, one popular model prints 180 characters per second in draft mode and 60 characters per second in letter quality. The print wheel in most cases will be bidirectional (prints from left to right and right to left) as this offers more speed. The letter-quality printers may have many print styles (fonts) built in, and more can be loaded into the printer. Laser printers are more expensive than the other varieties but may print as few as six pages per minute. The print quality is comparable to typesetting.

Use of Computer Software ....

Computer software capabilities are virtually limitless. Software companies are continually designing programs that make it possible to direct a computer to produce different prescribed information. It takes anywhere from 12 to 24 months to research, write, and test a comprehensive software system. When the project is begun, the newest technology is used. By the time the project is completed

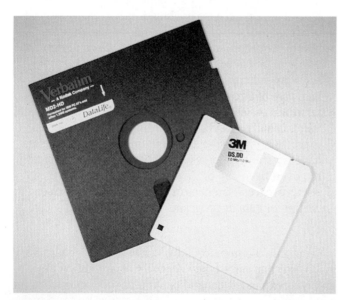

FIGURE 8–8 Floppy disk

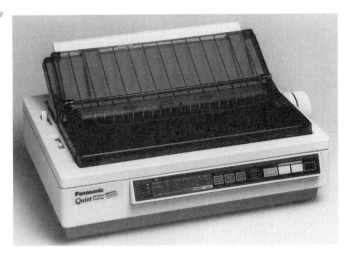

FIGURE 8–10 Dot matrix printer (Courtesy of Panasonic Communications & Systems Co.)

and fully tested, the newest technology is now 2 years or more outdated. It is important to keep this in mind if you are in a position to recommend use of software.

Medical management software is available from many different companies. An example is the MEDWARE program available from Computer Solutions. The software programs make it possible to keep patient information with no limit to the number of patients except the capacity of the computer memory. It provides information needed from billing such as primary and secondary insurance. It is easy to look up patient treatment or payment history, print patient mailing labels, phone listings, or set up a recall/reminder system.

The number of procedure and diagnosis codes that may be entered is limitless, Figure 8–11. The codes may be looked up by number or by description. New codes may be added, changed, or deleted at any time, Figure 8–12, page 122.

The computer program allows all posting charges and payments to be completed. The input screen is modeled from the standard insurance form (HCFA-1500), Figure 8–13, page 122. The program allows the medical assistant to input the necessary information and then push one key to print a completed insurance form. The information in the computer may be automatically looked up at any time.

Reports can be prepared with a minimum of effort when data are regularly put into the computer. Accounts receivable may be printed by date or aging, or alphabetically. Accounts receivable may be broken down between insurance company and patient. A detailed summary of income between two given dates may be easily prepared. The report of charges between any two dates may be accessed in detail or summary. A day sheet can be easily prepared. Physicians may find a need for a statistical report of diagnosis and procedure code usage, which can be retrieved from the stored data.

The computer gives immediate access to the names and addresses of the most commonly used insurance companies. It also allows immediate access to the names and provides numbers of referring physicians, Figure 8–14, page 123. The system can accommodate offices where multiple physicians are practicing. Figure 8–14 also shows the other programs you have entered with the request for the password to enter those programs.

```
WILDER DAN V                    ‖BC    BC / BS OF FLA ‖ BELL  BELLSOUTH DED.  ‖A

 1   271.1  ┌─────────────── Select Diagnosis ──────────── 8,297 ──┐ letter and then
 2   794.31 │                                                       │   bring up the
 3    53.5  │ dia                                          ◄-type   │ al listing of
 4          │                                                       │ codes.
 ═════════  │ DIABETES  INSIPIDUS                           253.5   │ ═══════════════
   FROM     │ DIABETES  MELLITUS                           250.    │ NSURANC   PATIENT
11/19/91 1‖ │ DIABETES  MELLITUS OF MOTHER, WITH DELIVE    648.01  │   0.00     75.00
11/26/91 1‖ │ DIABETES  MELLITUS WITHOUT MENTION OF COM    250.0   │   0.00     33.00
           │ DIABETES  WITH HYPEROSMOLAR COMA             250.2   │
           │ DIABETES  WITH KETOACIDOSIS                  250.1   │
           │ DIABETES  WITH NEUROLOGICAL MANIFESTATION    250.6   │
           │ DIABETES  WITH OPHTHALMIC MANIFESTATIONS     250.5   │
           │ DIABETES  WITH OTHER COMA                    250.3   │
           │ DIABETES  WITH OTHER SPECIFIED MANIFESTAT    250.8   │
           │ DIABETES  WITH PERIPHERAL CIRCULATORY DIS    250.7   │
           │ DIABETES  WITH RENAL MANIFESTATIONS          250.4   │
           │                                                       │
           │ ENTER TO SELECT    [INS] TO ADD [F10] TO CHANGE       │
 HOLD FOR  │ [DEL] TO DELETE                [F6] VIEW BY NUMBER    │   0.00|   108.00
           └───────────────────────────────────────────────────────┘ .00

  [INS]      [DEL]    [F10]   [F3]     [F4]      [F5]       [F6]      [F7]     [F8]*    [F9]
 Next Proc  Delete   Done   Walkout  HCFA 1500 Payment   Transfer    Hold    Recall  Path/Lab
```

FIGURE 8–11 Diagnosis and procedure codes may be quickly called up alphabetically or numerically. (Courtesy of Computer Solutions, New Smyrna, FL)

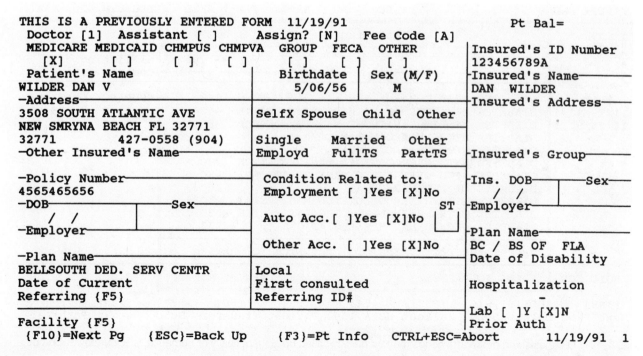

```
WILDER DAN V                    ‖BC    BC / BS OF  FLA ‖ BELL  BELLSOUTH DED.  ‖A
┌──────────────────────────────────────────────────────────────────┐
1  271 │         Procedures in Alphabetical Order           1,035 │ then
2  794 │                                                           │ the
3  253 │                                      ◄─Type to locate     │ of
4      │                                            A        B      │
───────│ 3 LEAD ECG MONITOR  (PROF, COMP)     93040    0.00     0.00│────────
 FROM  │ A & P ┌──────────────Record will be Added──────────┐  0.00│ PATIENT
11/19/ │ A-S ( │ PROC#                                       │  0.00│  75.00
       │ ABDOM │ DESCRIPT                                    │  0.00│
 2/26/ │ ABDOM │ MEDICAL?   (Y or N)    Press {F1} for more info  0.00│  0.00
       │ ABO G │                                             │  0.00│
       │ ACE B │ FEES:  A    0.00   (usually MEDICARE)       │  0.00│
       │ ACETO │        B    0.00   (usually private patient)│  0.00│  Dr 1
       │ ACID  │        C    0.00   (usually PPO, HMO, etc.) │  0.00│
       │ ACID  │        D    0.00                            │  0.00│
       │ ACNE  │        E    0.00                            │  0.00│
       │ ACTH  │                                             │  0.00│
───────│ ENTE  │ TYPE OF SERVICE CODE FOR THIS PROCEDURE   1 │──────
       │       └─────────────────────────────────────────────┘
 HOLD  │   [DEL] TO DELETE        F6 TO VIEW IN NUMERICAL ORDER   │ 108.00
       └──────────────────────────────────────────────────────────┘
  [INS]    [DEL]    [F10]    [F3]     [F4]      [F5]      [F6]     [F7]    [F8]*   [F9]
Next Proc Delete   Done   Walkout HCFA 1500  Payment  Transfer  Hold   Recall Path/Lab
```

FIGURE 8–12   New codes may be added at any time. (Courtesy of Computer Solutions, New Smyrna, FL)

Figure 8–15 shows one of many functions of main menus. Each selection on the screen will take you to one of the modules where the work of the program is accomplished.

Figure 8–16 shows an example of a main menu, which lists all the major functions of your program. Each selection on the screen will take you to one of the modules where the work of the program is done.

Figure 8–17, page 124 shows the new patient entry screen. This screen provides for the entry of account information for each patient or family group. All the data needed to properly bill the account are included. Note the ability to enter aged balance information for each account. This means that you can begin your computerized system with all accounts properly aged.

Figure 8–18, page 124 is an example of the new

```
THIS IS A PREVIOUSLY ENTERED FORM  11/19/91                  Pt Bal=
  Doctor [1] Assistant [ ]      Assign? [N]  Fee Code [A]
  MEDICARE MEDICAID CHMPUS CHMPVA  GROUP  FECA  OTHER      Insured's ID Number
   [X]     [ ]      [ ]    [ ]     [ ]    [ ]    [ ]       123456789A
  Patient's Name                Birthdate   Sex (M/F)      ┌Insured's Name─────
  WILDER DAN V                   5/06/56      M            DAN  WILDER
 ─Address─                                                 ┌Insured's Address──
  3508 SOUTH ATLANTIC AVE      ┌SelfX Spouse  Child  Other
  NEW SMRYNA BEACH FL 32771    │
  32771        427-0558 (904)  ├Single    Married    Other
 ─Other Insured's Name─        │Employd   FullTS    PartTS  ┌Insured's Group───

 ─Policy Number─               ├Condition Related to:      ┌Ins. DOB──┬──Sex──
  4565465656                   │Employment [ ]Yes [X]No      / /
 ─DOB─              ┌─Sex─     │                      ST   ├Employer─────────
    / /             │          │Auto Acc.[ ]Yes [X]No  ┌─┐
 ─Employer─                    │                       │ │ ├Plan Name─────────
                               │Other Acc. [ ]Yes [X]No       BC / BS OF  FLA
 ─Plan Name─                                                  Date of Disability
  BELLSOUTH DED. SERV CENTR    │Local
  Date of Current              │First consulted              Hospitalization
  Referring {F5}               │Referring ID#                -
                                                            Lab [ ]Y [X]N
 Facility {F5}                                              Prior Auth
   {F10}=Next Pg   {ESC}=Back Up   {F3}=Pt Info  CTRL+ESC=Abort   11/19/91  1
```

FIGURE 8–13   Screen modeled on the HCFA-1500 layout (Courtesy of Computer Solutions, New Smyrna, FL)

```
              Last              First          MI Sex | FEE  ASSIGN? DOC ASSIST
      Name WILDER                                                    1
   Address 3508 SOUTH AT  ┌─────────────────────────────────────────┐
      City NEW SMRYNA BE  │        Select Referring Physician         │ 32771
    Home # 427-0558 (904  │                                           │
[F5] Refr THOMAS          │         ◄─Begin typing last name          │
   Status: Single  Marr   │                                           │  T. Student
MCARE MCAID CHUS CHVA     │  THOMAS JOLLY          64452              │  [N] "Y" or "N"
  [X]  [ ]  [ ]  [ ]      │  THOMAS VALERIE G      04821              │
                          │  THOMAS CHRISTOPHE     TH155008           │     BELL [F6]
            PRIMARY       │  TORKELSON ANDREW      086429024         │
   CO. BC / BS OF  FLA    │  TOUB FRANK            07227              │ RV CENTR
STREET P O BOX 1798       │  TRELOAR H.S.B.        64175              │
  CITY JACKSONVILLE       │  WAHBA WAHBA           79793              │
 STATE FL         ZIP     │  WALKER JOHN           22583              │ 35283
  ID # 123456789A         │  WARSETT DUANE         30676              │
 GROUP                    │  WEINTRAUB             1465210            │
X-SELF  -SPOUSE   -CHI    │  WEISS RICHARD         47117              │
                          │  WELSH RUSSELL         64099              │
                          │                                           │
INSURED DAN  WILDER       │  [ENTER] TO SELECT       [INS] TO ADD     │
 STREET                   │  [F10] TO CHANGE                          ]
   City                   └───────────────────────────────────────────┘ f applic) [ ]
  Phone                                                                  / /
    DOB    /  /  Sex        [TAB]   [ESC]   [F8]   [F9]   [F10]   [F1]
 Emplyer                   JUMP  BACK UP RECALL  label   DONE    HELP
```

FIGURE 8–14 Information screen with look-up windows for insurance company addresses and referring physicians (Courtesy of Computer Solutions, New Smyrna, FL)

patient insurance entry screen. Any information required to properly submit claims to the proper carrier is included on this screen. Each account can have as many as ninety-nine different insurance plans, if needed. One of the data entries is the insurance form to be used when billing the plan.

Figure 8–19, page 124, illustrates the daily transactions entry screen. This is where all charge entries are done, as well as the entries for payments made at the time of service. Up to five entries may be made on each screen, and the screen will repeat until you indicate that you are through. In other words, the number of charges per visit is unlimited. If the charges being entered are for

an insurance account, special items such as the dates of disability or hospitalization, or indicators for emergency or accident can be entered in the suffix field. During charge entry, a running total of the account is displayed at all times. When you have finished making entries for the patient, the account updates immediately. There is no cumbersome batch entry, and you can always count on an accurate and up-to-date account balance. When you have finished your entries for each patient, you will be given the option of printing an insurance claim form, a patient statement, or both.

Figure 8–20, page 124, is an example of a reports menu of all the reports and billing options available to you. Most of the reports options are available either on

```
┌──────────────────────────────────────────────────────┐
│ Function - Password Selection        Screen ID # 3-3   │
│ Message -                                              │
│ ────────────────────────────────────────────────────  │
│                                                        │
│ Enter Master Password _____  < - Required │
│ Use Master Password for all ___                        │
│ Enter System Password _____  < - Required │
│ Enter Update Password _____  < - Optional │
│ Enter Utility Password _____  < - Optional │
│ Enter Reports Password _____  < - Optional │
│ Enter Install Password _____  < - Optional │
│ Enter Daily Password _____  < - Optional │
│ Enter New Patient Password _____  < - Optional │
│ Enter Post Password _____  < - Optional │
│ Enter Recall Password _____  < - Optional │
│ Enter Pull Password _____  < - Optional │
│                                                        │
│                                                        │
│ E - Edit, S - Save, R - Remove Passwords ___           │
└──────────────────────────────────────────────────────┘
```

FIGURE 8–15 Sign-on screen (Courtesy of Artificial Intelligence, Inc., Renton, WA)

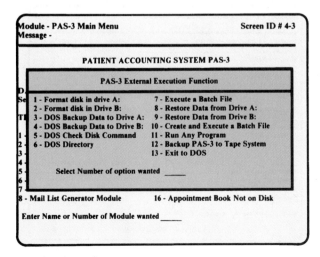

FIGURE 8–16 Main menu (Courtesy of Artificial Intelligence, Inc., Renton, WA)

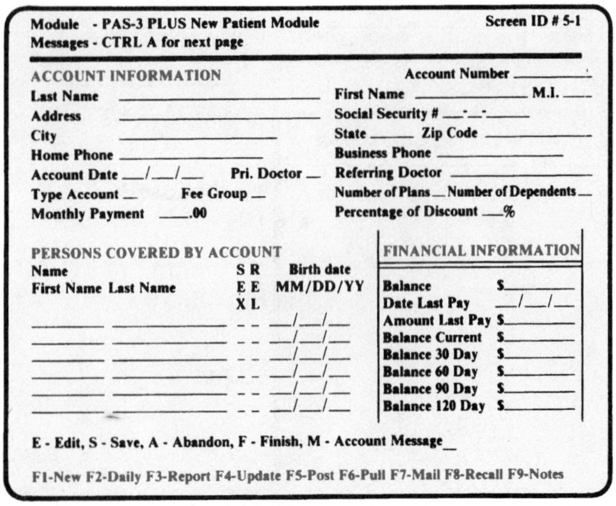

FIGURE 8–17 New patient entry screen (Courtesy of Artificial Intelligence, Inc., Renton, WA)

FIGURE 8–19 Daily transactions entry screen (Courtesy of Artificial Intelligence, Inc., Renton, WA)

the screen or printed out on paper. Many of the reports can be printed either for the practice as a whole or for each provider within the practice. The billing and insurance billing functions accessed from this menu are the lifelines of the medical practice. Prompt billing of patients means faster payment, and efficient, accurate submission of claims means a higher payment ratio. The patient encounter system, which is also accessed from this menu, tracks your charge slips and helps to eliminate the problem of lost charges.

Figure 8–21 is an example of a medical style daily transactions report.

Figure 8–22 is an example of an update menu. This module provides a way for all account information to be updated or corrected. Any data pertaining to the account can be changed, if necessary. In addition to the main account update screen, there are screens where updates can be made to dependent, activity, and insurance data. The update module can be password-protected to prevent unauthorized person-

nel from making changes to the accounts. Your account records are always safe from tampering.

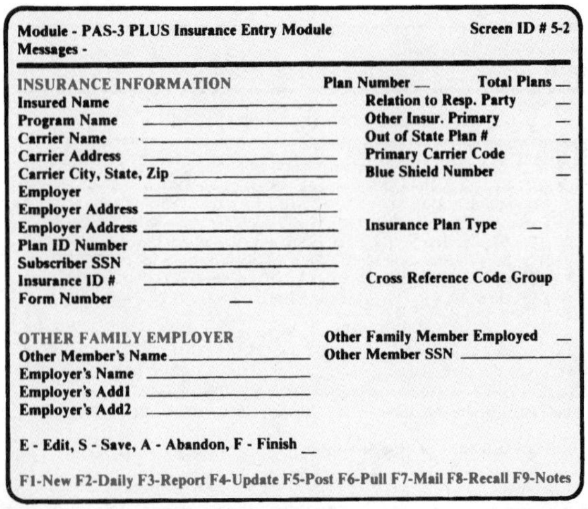

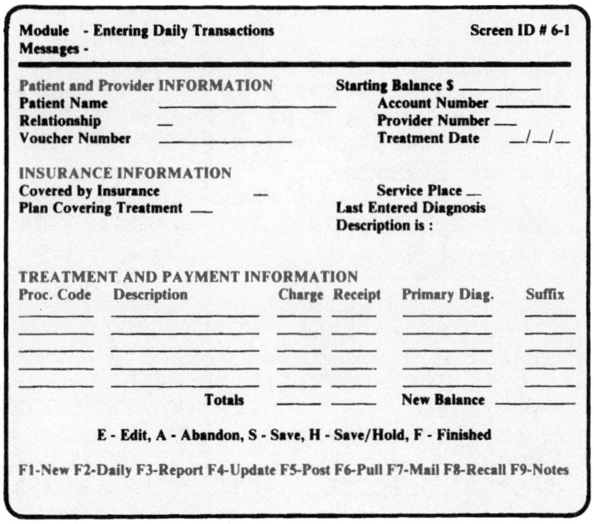

Figure 8–23 is an example of a utility menu screen. This screen gives you access to all the functions that let you set up and maintain the custom files to be used by the system, establish the format for your custom forms, and do the maintenance work to keep your system running efficiently. Among the files set up in utility code are the procedure codes, diagnosis codes, provider, insurance company, hospital, and referring doctor. Once these files are established, the data in them is a keystroke away when the system is in use. The custom forms generator gives you the advantage of being able to use any patient billing form and charge slip you may wish, and of submitting claims on almost any insurance form. The formats for up to ninety-nine insurance forms can be stored in the system at one time. The maintenance functions allow you to purge old activity data, unlock files, reclaim

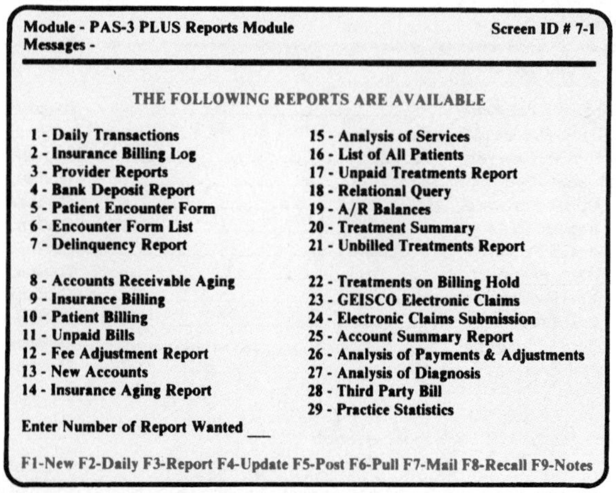

FIGURE 8–18 New patient insurance entry screen (Courtesy of Artificial Intelligence, Inc., Renton, WA)

FIGURE 8–20 Reports menu (Courtesy of Artificial Intelligence, Inc., Renton, WA)

Mode of operation - Daily data only

Page 1

DATE	ACCNT #	ACCOUNT NAME	PAT NAME/ PMT. SOURCE	DOCTOR	PROC	DIAG	VOUCHER	CHARGES	RECEIPTS	TODAYS BALANCE	BILLED P	I	INS
03/08/90	2	Brown	Rachael	1	82996	V22.2	2	$18.00	$0.00	$134.00	N	N	Y
03/08/90	4	Gonzales	Joseph	1	93000	785.1	1	$36.00	$0.00	$36.00	N	N	Y
03/08/90	6	O'Brien	Janet	1	85022	285.9	3	$23.00	$23.00	$75.00	N	N	N
03/08/90	9	Williams	Ryan	1	90071	780.7	7	$44.00	$0.00	$144.00	N	N	Y
03/08/90	1	Takamoto	Credit Adj.	1	M02		5	-$18.00	$0.00	$78.00	N	N	Y
03/08/90	10	Young	David	2	73090	848.9	6	$54.00	$54.00	$0.00	N	N	N
03/08/90	15	Anderson	Nancy	1	86300	075	4	$18.00	$0.00	$62.00	N	N	Y
03/08/90	12	Lightfoot	James	2	92551	389.9	8	$36.00	$0.00	$36.00	N	N	Y
03/08/90	11	Roberts	Debit Adj.	1	M01		9	$0.00	-$25.00	$75.00	N	N	N
03/08/90	13	Paulson	Jon	2	95000	477.9	10	$44.00	$0.00	$144.00	N	N	Y
03/08/90	14	Bond	PAYMENT	1	M91		11	$0.00	$75.00	$200.00	N	N	Y

TOTALS $255.00 $127.00

Total interest included in Charges $0.00
Total Debit Adjustments - $25.00
Total credit Adjustments - $18.00
Mode of operation - Daily data only

FIGURE 8–21 Daily transactions report (Courtesy of Artificial Intelligence, Inc., Renton, WA)

back-up files, reconstruct the internal hashtables, and sort files.

Figure 8–24, page 126, is a new accounts report listing all new accounts for any given month. The name of the referring doctor is indicated by a number.

These illustrations of computer screens are only a sampling of the many office procedures possible with computers. It is important to note that many of the software manufacturers make programs which are compatible with more than one brand of computer. Many of the software systems run on IBM® computers. MAI Systems Corporation has developed its own computer and the software for

medical offices, Figure 8–25. Healthcare Communications™ makes software exclusively for Macintosh™ SE.

Some believe that in the future it will be common practice to use a hand-held scanner (like those used in department stores) to scan the bar code on the patient charge slip and thus automatically enter the code number of the procedure or illness and the charge for service. This would eliminate the possibility of error in typing the figures into the computer.

The computer should be useful for inventory control of office supplies, to personalize form letter mailings for collections, to reschedule annual checkups, and to gather research data. The computer is expected to decrease in size as it is constantly improved.

Some physicians find the computer essential if they are engaged in research and need to quickly identify all patients with a specific diagnosis. It is also valuable in

---

Function - PAS-3 PLUS Update Module   Screen ID # 8-1
Message -

NAME or ACCOUNT NUMBER of Patient _____
Name - _____   Account # ____
_____
Phone _____   Type Account ____
Additional Persons Covered by this Account
_____
Is this the Proper Account (Y/N) ____

Function - PAS-3 PLUS Account Update   Screen ID # 8-2
Messages -

Account of _____   Account Number _____

Name _____   Type _____
Address _____   Day Phone ( ) _____
City _____ State __ Zip ____   Night Phone ( ) _____
Referred by _____   SSN ___-__-____
Date of Birth __/__/__   Sex __   Primary Doctor No. __
Last Bill   Last Pay   Pay Amount   # Plans   # Dep Fee Group
__/__/__   __/__/__ $_____
Discount % __   Monthly Payment $ __
Dependents

FINANCIAL INFORMATION

Name	Last Name	Sex	Rel	D.O.B.

Balance Current $_____
Balance 30 Days $_____
Balance 60 Days $_____
Balance 90 Days $_____
Balance 120 Days $_____

Total Balance $_____

E - Edit   S - Save   F - Finished   D - Dependents   U - User Screen
A - Activity   I - Insurance   R - Recalls   N - Next Record   O - Options

F1-New F2-Daily F3-Report F4-Update F5-Post F6-Pull F7-Mail F8-Recall F9-Notes

FIGURE 8–22 Update menu (Courtesy of Artificial Intelligence, Inc., Renton, WA)

Module - PAS-3 PLUS Utility Module   Screen ID # 11-1
Message -

THE FOLLOWING OPTIONS ARE AVAILABLE

1 - Procedure Codes
2 - Diagnosis Codes
3 - Copy all Files to Backup Disk
4 - Delete Patient Record
5 - Reconstruct Hash/Key Tables
6 - Selective Activity Purge
7 - Move Record to Inactive Disk
8 - Change Billing Forms Format
9 - Set Up Practice Data Files
10 - File Checker
11 - Reclaim Backup Files
12 - Sort Procedure/Diag/Key Code File
13 - Split the Disk

14 - Enable Rebill Insurance/Patient
15 - Create and Add Records to Files
16 - Provider Files
17 - Unlock All Files
18 - Insurance Company File
19 - Hospital/Facility Files
20 - Referring Doctors File
21 - Encounter Form Setup
22 - Dunning Messages Establish
23 - Change Insurance Forms Format
24 - Relationship Cross Reference
25 - Format User Defined Data Screen
26 - Format Third Party Billing Forms

Warning Do not Run Utility options while another terminal is using files.

Enter number of option wanted ____

F1-New F2-Daily F3-Report F4-Update F5-Post F6-Pull F7-Mail F8-Recall F9-Notes

FIGURE 8–23 Utility menu (Courtesy of Artificial Intelligence, Inc., Renton, WA)

```
Function - New Accounts Report                    Screen ID # 7-17
Message -

Month that you want new account for 12
Do you want a printout (Y/N)

        Function - New Accounts Report                    Screen ID # 7-17
        Message -

        Month that you want new account for 12

F1-

        F1-New  F2-Daily  F3-Report  F4-Update  F5-Post  F6-Pull  F7-Mail  F8-Recall  F9-Notes
```

FIGURE 8–24 New accounts report (Courtesy of Artificial Intelligence, Inc., Renton, WA)

the quick identification of patients taking a particular drug if the manufacturer should issue a warning about side effects. You may be involved in the use of a computer for patient education. This is similar to the television programs used by some offices. The medical assistant may load the programs into the computer, discuss with patients what they will see, and ascertain whether patients have further concerns after they complete the viewing. Information programs have been developed for diabetes, cancer, pregnancy, health hazards of smoking, and many other conditions.

The use of a computer as a word processor is probably the most exciting advantage for the medical secretary. The qualifications for a word processing operator are similar to those of a medical assistant in some ways. You need to be organized, be able to follow directions, and to work well under pressure. You need to be able to type accurately and be skilled in the written communica-

tion skills of grammar, spelling, punctuation, and sentence structure. The medical assistant must have an adequate knowledge of medical terminology and use this knowledge with 100 percent accuracy. It is possible to have a medical dictionary program stored in the computer, which can be very helpful. This will not take the place of having a working knowledge of anatomy and medical terminology, however.

Most word processing software has a standard built-in dictionary that helps with spelling. Misspelled words are highlighted when the spell-check is activated. You still must read carefully to be sure you typed the correct words for the message you wish to convey. You must be accurate in your proofreading.

Continuous letterheads and new continuous envelopes make your work much faster. There is no need for a typewriter to address envelopes.

You have learned in this unit that using computers in medical offices can be extremely important in helping to complete your work. You should use any opportunity you have to practice with the computer. You should learn the vocabulary and how to read and understand an instruction manual. You need to practice on a typewriter if a computer is not available so that you will have accurate keyboarding skills.

Important Steps in Selecting a Computer System

The medical assistant employed in the office planning to consider automation with computers will be able to look forward to the experience if there is an opportunity to take part in the planning.

It is important to research the kinds of software available, the kinds of computers the software can be used

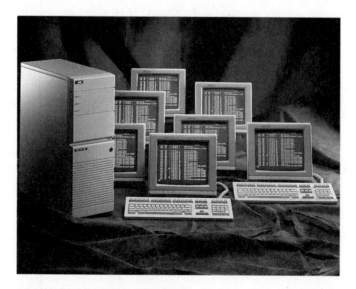

FIGURE 8–25a and b Record tracking in a multi-user PC environment using the MAI GP™ Series 50. (Courtesy of MAI Systems Corporation, Tustin, CA)

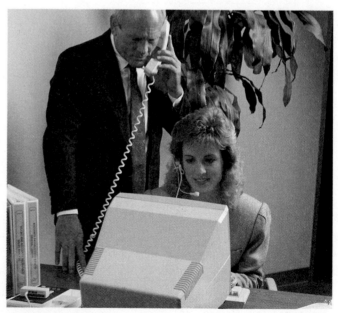

with, the costs, how long the supplier has been in business, and the kinds of support offered after installation.

A good source for this information is *The Computer Talk Directory of Medical Computer Systems*, which is published semiannually by:

Computer Talk Associates, Inc.
485 Norristown Road, Suite 112
Blue Bell, PA 19422
(215) 825-7686

There are hidden costs to consider. The office will need to provide necessary electrical outlets at the areas where the computer terminals and printers will be located. The office will need desk space for both computers and printers. A maintenance contract should be available for both software and hardware. Investigate the costs or availability of insurance to cover theft, natural disasters such as a tornado, and internal disasters such as fire or flood damage. Determine the availability and cost of a consultant to supervise the training of the office staff.

It is always important to obtain cost estimates from at least three companies. The companies should also refer you to current users to help you determine the reliability of the software and hardware. Find out if the software company can furnish new formats when needed. Very often the specialist is neglected in preparing software programs.

When the physicians decide what they want to accomplish with the system and the costs have been obtained, a decision must be made as to whether the return will justify the cost.

If the determination is made that the cost is justified, the first task is to select software that will meet the needs of the office. The hardware is then selected to be compatible with the software. The computer system should meet the needs of the office in accounting and office management, and should furnish a data base for research. Arrangements must be made to back up every program on the office computer daily, and off site on a regular basis, so that an emergency in the office would not wipe out all the work put into setting up the system. If several people will be working with the computers, it is important the system be multiuser and multitasking.

Electronic Claims Submission

Client Support

Under this system, the central computer calls each practice every night (five nights a week) and records the data entered in that office computer on magnetic tape at the central computer site. These data are permanently stored and retained for a full calendar year. Year-to-year records can be supplied on magnetic tape or an optical laser disk. If for any reason data stored on the hard disk in the office computer are lost, the information can be restored from this central data base. The information is loaded into a new hard disk drive; then that disk drive is

shipped by a courier directly to the practice, where it is exchanged for the existing unit. Each day's data are accumulated on a reel of magnetic tape for all practices. This tape is then used to update the practice's main files and produce the monthly statements and reports.

Processing is performed once a month on a preset billing day. The statements are laser-printed on standard letterhead stationery, custom designed to the practice's specification. Statements are zip sorted and mailed with a postmark that shows only zip code number and not city or state of origin. Statements are mailed in a double window envelope with the practice's own return address printed in the upper window. The top half of the statement, which identifies the patient, has the practice return address printed on the reverse side. This address is removed and inserted in a window envelope with the patient's check and returned to the practice, thus identifying the patient who paid the money.

Word Processors

The word processor, Figure 8–26, is an electronic typewriter with the added features of fast daisy wheel printing, spelling checks, and spelling corrections. They also have insertable disk drive units for line or screen display models, which allow you to store text on a microfloppy disk for later use. They also allow an auto cut sheet feeder and tractor feeder to be added.

Word processors offer functions such as automatic correction, adding words and deleting words, centering, right margin alignment, decimal tabs, and column layout. You might be able to make tables or activate automatic indent. Word processors offer special features such as automatic word or single letter underline, boldface type, subscripts, and superscripts. Because you can visualize the copy on the screen and move words, lines, or

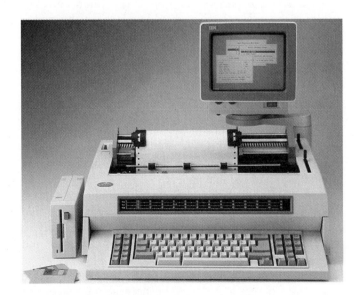

FIGURE 8–26 Word processor (Courtesy of International Business Machines Corporation)

paragraphs with the use of special key functions, there is no excuse for printing anything but perfect copy.

When you have perfected your copy you print it. You may compose standard letters for return appointments, collection letters, instructions for patients for special examinations, and special diets and store these on floppy disks. Then when you need a particular document you insert the disk, find the one you want on the list which appears on the screen, indicate this to the computer, and it is immediately there for you to see. You may personalize it for individual patients and have it printed out. The printer in the medical office should be letter quality rather than dot matrix. In some cases typewriters have cable connections to the computer so that they are the printer. The more rapid printers designed for use with computers print not only from left to right but from right to left as they come back across the page. Letter-quality printers of ink-jet or laser technology, Figure 8–27, produce near-professional typographical appearance. Postscript styles will allow infusion of many graphic applications to customize office correspondence, patient information sheets, reports, and professional papers.

You will find that larger offices and clinics have much more in the equipment line to improve the speed and efficiency of the operation. Smaller offices are likely to use less special equipment primarily due to costs and operating personnel.

All computer systems and word processors have instruction books which will be helpful references for both beginners and experienced operators. Most distributors of computers offer training for office personnel as an introduction to the use of the equipment.

Complete Chapter 8 in the workbook to help you meet the objectives at the beginning of this chapter and therefore achieve competency of this subject matter.

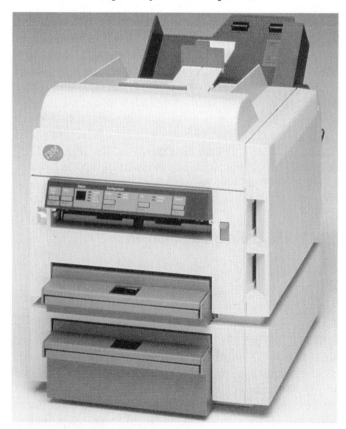

FIGURE 8–27 Laser printer (Courtesy of International Business Machines Corporation)

Operate Office Computer

TERMINAL PERFORMANCE OBJECTIVE: Given a program on a floppy disk, the student will demonstrate the ability to activate the computer, monitor and printer; load the disk; select the program; type in assigned information; proofread and make corrections as necessary; run the program and turn off the computer. The instructor will proofread the finished copy for expected 100% accuracy.

The following procedure is written specifically for the Apple IIE computer because it is one of those commonly used in schools. There are many different disk drives on IBM machines from single disk to double disk and combinations with hard drive, so it will be necessary to consult your manual for operating instructions on those machines.

1. Turn on the machine using switch on back lower left corner of central processing unit (as you face the unit).
   Key Points:
   a. **A green light turns on just to the left of the space bar when power is on.**
   b. **Check power plug attachment if no response.**
2. Turn on monitor with switch on front top right corner. **Key Point: A light tells you the monitor is activated.**
3. Turn the disk drive off by finding the CONTROL key on the left of the keyboard and the RESET key on the right side of the keyboard, pressing both keys in a 1-2 motion, and releasing them simultaneously. **Key Point: You will know the disk drive is on as a red light is activated when the computer is turned on.**
4. Select program disk to be used.
5. Activate disk drive by locating the CONTROL key, the OPEN APPLE key (to the left of the space bar), and the RESET key. Press the keys in 1-2-3 motion as listed and let go simultaneously.
   Key Points:
   a. **This activates the disk drive to "boot the disk" and will feed information from the disk into the computer memory.**
   b. **If you are going to store information on a new disk it must be initialized first. Check your computer instruction book for this procedure.**
6. Insert disk into drive slot and pull down front cover.
   Key Points:
   a. **Remove disk from sleeve or protective jacket by grasping label. DO NOT TOUCH any other portion of the disk.**
   b. **Always store disks in protective covers in upright position away from direct sunlight, moisture, or extremes of heat and cold.**
   c. **Be careful to keep food and drink away from disks as these could cause permanent damage.**
   d. **Do not set disk on top of monitors, television sets, or near magnets or electrical devices such as telephones or motors as this may erase the disk.**
7. Select program from menu.
8. Type in assigned information.
9. Proofread information and correct any errors.
10. Insert printer paper into printer.
11. Activate printer until hard copy is printed out.
12. Turn off printer, monitor, and central processing unit.
13. Remove disk and store in protective cover.

REFERENCES

American Medical Association. *The Physicians' Current Procedural Terminology.*

Diehl, Marcia, and Fordney, Marilyn. *Medical Typing and Transcribing Techniques and Procedures.* Philadelphia: W. B. Saunders, 1984.

Fordney, Marilyn. *Insurance Handbook for the Medical Office.* Philadelphia: W. B. Saunders, 1982.

Frew, Mary, and Frew, David. *Comprehensive Medical Assisting, Administrative and Clinical Procedures,* 2nd ed. Philadelphia: F. A. Davis, 1988.

Kaabes, Elaine. *Medical Secretary's Guide.* West Nyack, NY: Parker, 1972.

Kinn, Mary E., and Derge, Eleanor. *The Medical Assistant: Administrative and Clinical,* 6th ed. Philadelphia: W. B. Saunders, 1988.

McClung, Christina; Guerrieri, John; and McClung, Kenneth, Jr. *Microcomputers for Medical Professionals.* New York: Wiley, 1984.

Seraydarian, Patricia. *Metroplex Clinic: A Medical Typing Simulation.* Boston: Houghton-Mifflin, 1980.

_____. *Word Processing Applications for Electronic Typewriters.* Boston: Houghton-Mifflin, 1980.

Shelly, Gary B. and Cashman, Thomas J. *Computer Fundamentals in an Information Age.* Anaheim, CA: Anaheim Publishing Company, Incorporated, 1984.

United States Department of Health and Human Services. *International Classification of Diseases.* 1992.

Vocabulary for Data Processing, Telecommunications, and Office Systems. IBM, 1981.

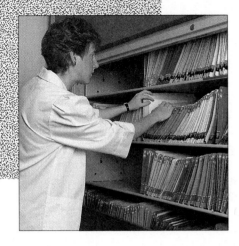

C H A P T E R   9

Records Management

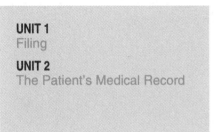

UNIT 1
Filing

UNIT 2
The Patient's Medical Record

Medical records consist of a history, physical examination and treatment notes that allow the physician to provide necessary care for patients. The records must be accurate, complete, and filed so that they may be quickly found when needed.

The confidentiality of the records is maintained by careful management as they are used. Filing is essential to a well-run medical office and needs to be current at all times.

U N I T   1

Filing

OBJECTIVES

Upon completion of the unit the student will meet the following terminal performance objectives by verifying knowledge of the facts and principles presented through oral and written communication at a level deemed competent, and will demonstrate the specific behaviors as identified in the terminal performance objectives of the procedures, observing safety precautions in accordance with health care standards.

1. Apply the rules of indexing for records management.
2. Explain basic filing methods.
3. List the steps used in filing.
4. Describe methods of removing and replacing patient files.
5. List the storage media used for "paperless" filing systems.
6. Spell and define, using the glossary at the back of the text, all the words to know in this unit.

WORDS TO KNOW

accumulated
caption
data
expedite
illuminating
purge

sequence
subsequent
supplemented
systematically
unproductive

Importance of Filing

Assembling and filing the patient's medical record are necessary to good patient care. Records must be filed accurately and systematically. Carelessly filed records produce chaos in the office. Reports lost or filed in the wrong chart or hidden in stacks of unfiled material result in many hours of unproductive time spent searching for them. An efficient office requires accurate filing done daily. Not only does this maintain efficiency, it also reduces the chance of accidental loss of correspondence and reports.

Filing Steps

Folders or cards are easily filed alphabetically or numerically, but the procedure for filing reports and letters requires several steps.

The first step is to inspect each report or piece of correspondence to see if it is released for filing. After the physician looks at a report, a call or dictation of a letter may be required to give results to the patient or to the referring physician. The physician will place a check mark or initials on the form (usually in the upper righthand corner) indicating that the report has been seen, Figure 9–1.

The second step is indexing. This requires that you make a decision as to the name, subject, or other caption under which you will file the material. Materials for patients should be filed under the patient name. Research papers can be filed under illness, procedure, treatment, medication, or author. A cross-reference may be helpful in finding things later, Figure 9–2. For example, a research paper might be filed under the title, *Diabetes*, and a cross-reference to the article placed under the author's name, *Allen, John*.

Coding is the third step, and is done by marking the index caption on the papers to be filed. If the name, subject, or a number appears on the paper, you can underline or circle it, preferably with a colored pencil. (Your employer may have a preference as to the color to be used for the coding process.) If the name, subject, or other caption does not appear on the material to be filed, write the caption in the upper right-hand corner, Figure 9–3.

The fourth step is to sort the material. A desk sorter may be used to put papers in alphabetical order after they have been coded. This speeds up the process of filing, Figure 9–4, page 134.

The final step is storing. You must first locate the file drawer or shelf with the appropriate caption. Then find the folder in which the reports will be stored. Lift the folder and place it on a flat surface before adding any material. This procedure makes it easier for you to make sure the caption on the folder agrees with the caption on the paper to be filed. Place the papers with the heading to the left and the most recent material on top. Some offices attach laboratory reports to the folder in a "shingle" fashion, Figure 9–5, page 135. The first is attached at the bottom of the page and each subsequent report partially overlaps the previous ones.

✓

Patient: Carol Sue Lamp

City hospital
Troy, Ohio

ROENTGEN FINDINGS

Examination of the pelvis. AP supine including the upper thirds of the femora bilaterally visualizes advanced degenerative arthritis of the right hip with narrowing almost to obliteration of the hip joint space and with degenerative changes and cystic formation affecting the articulating surfaces of the head of the femur as well as the acetabulum. The remaining pelvis and left hip appears essentially normal.

Impression: Advanced degenerative arthritis right hip, otherwise normal pelvis and left hip.

FIGURE 9–1 Record released for filing

PATIENT JANKOWSKI, EMILY LOUISE

CROSS REFERENCE

PEDEN-JANKOWSKI, EMILY LOUISE

PATIENT PENDEN-JANKOWSKI, EMILY LOUISE

CROSS REFERENCE

JANKOWSKI, EMILY LOUISE

FIGURE 9–2 Cross-reference

Filing Units

Every office that requires you to file paper records will have storage units for this purpose. Files come in many different styles, shapes, and sizes. There are vertical or lateral file cabinets, card index files, open shelf files, tub files, various types of movable or automated files, and special-purpose file units, such as those used to store computer printouts. It is reasonable for employers to expect you to understand how to use these storage units, Figures 9–6 and 9–7, page 136.

Safety is an important consideration when you work with file cabinets. When you leave a file drawer open at floor level where someone can fall over it, you are setting up an accident scene. If you pull out more than one file drawer at a time in a vertical file cabinet, it can tip over and injure you. Be careful when pulling a file drawer out to reach material in the back because some drawers do not have a stop to prevent the entire drawer from falling out.

Filing Supplies

Filing supplies include guides, OUTguides or OUTfolders, folders, vertical pockets, and labels, Figures 9–8 and 9–9, page 136. A properly organized filing system will have many dividers or guides that identify sections

Patient: Marsha Leonard

Tri-County Hospital
Miami, Ohio

ROENTGEN FINDINGS

Films of 8/31 __. Review of the PA and lateral chest film of 8/31__ shows the traches to be shifted slightly to the left by a soft tissue mass in the right thoracic inlet in the superior mediastinal area. This probably represents tumor and is again seen on the lateral view lying in the anterior portion of the thoracic inlet on the right. Heart is otherwise normal. Lungs are otherwise clear.

FIGURE 9–3 Coding

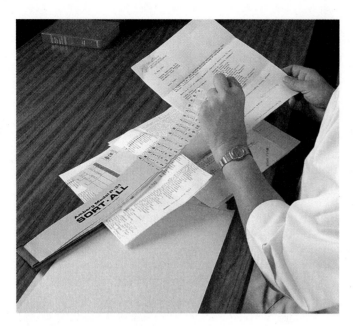

FIGURE 9–4 Desk sorter

within the file. The guides should be constructed of heavy material to stand up under continual wear. They reduce the area to be searched and allow you to locate a folder more quickly. Some authorities recommend a guide for every eight or ten folders, but this would occupy a great deal of space. The number of guides used is a matter of personal preference and will be determined by each office.

An OUTguide or folder is used to temporarily replace a folder that has been removed. It is thick and may be of a distinctive size and color for easier detection. The use of OUTguides makes refiling much easier and also alerts the medical assistant to missing files. The OUTguide may also have lines for recording information, such as where the missing folder may be located, or have a plastic pocket for inserting an information card. In a large office, with several physicians and employees, it is essential to know who has the folder when it is out of the file. Occasionally, a record may be sent to another physician or treatment facility and it is extremely important that this information be recorded. The OUTfolder is also useful in providing a place to file material until the original folder is returned.

A color coding system may be used to expedite both filing and finding of folders. Ordinary manila folders may be coded with colored strips or dots along the edge of the folder. The coding may be used to identify portions of the alphabet or patients of different physicians within an office. Color coding is also useful in identifying different types of insured patients. Everyone should have a key to the color coding through use of a procedure manual or posted chart.

Paperless Files

With computers outputting volumes of information at unbelievable speeds and the cost of office space steadily increasing, many offices have installed "paperless" filing systems. These systems record information for storage on such media as magnetic tape reels, cartridges, or cassettes; magnetic disks; and/or microforms. The use of such media has dramatically reduced the need for storage space. It is estimated that microforms (microfilm and microfiche) use less than 2 percent of the storage space required for traditional paper files. (Microfiche is a rectangular sheet of clear film containing rows of tiny negatives. Each negative represents a separate page of a document or report. See Chapter 8).

Storage units used to house such paperless media are either card files, drawers, open shelves, or racks. Shelves or drawers are used to store boxed rolls of microfilm. Card files are used for microfiche and aperture cards. (Aperture cards are one tiny negative mounted on a data processing card.) These types of records require an illuminating and magnifying viewing device to read the stored information.

If you are hired to work with a paperless filing system, you will be taught how to use the special filing equipment on the job. You will learn about the camera used to produce reduced images on film and the viewers used to read the blown-up film images. You will be using word processors and duplicating equipment to handle data and printers to produce hard copy from film images. There will be automatic storage and retrieval units to master.

Filing Systems

Most filing systems are based directly or indirectly on an alphabetic arrangement. In alphabetic filing, the names of persons, firms, or organizations are arranged as in the telephone directory. This is the simplest and most commonly used method of filing. In numeric filing, the material is arranged in numerical order in the main file. The main file is supplemented by an alphabetically arranged card index. The number under which a given item is to be filed can be determined by referring to the alphabetical card index file.

A subject file is based on an outline or classification of the subject matter to which the material refers. In a physician's office, it is customary to maintain files or reference materials accumulated by subject matter.

In geographic filing, material is arranged alphabetically by political or geographic subdivisions such as country, state, city, and even street, and each subdivision is alphabetized.

Chronological filing refers to filing according to date.

LABORATORY REPORTS

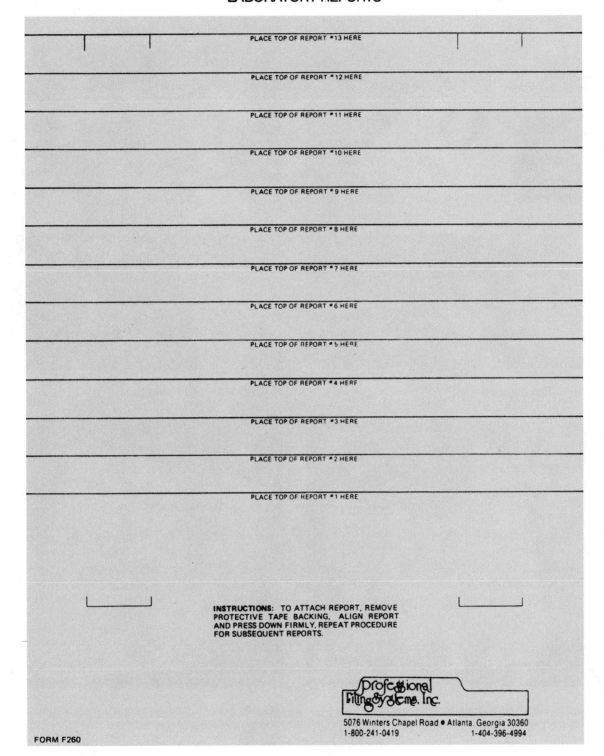

PLACE TOP OF REPORT #13 HERE

PLACE TOP OF REPORT #12 HERE

PLACE TOP OF REPORT #11 HERE

PLACE TOP OF REPORT #10 HERE

PLACE TOP OF REPORT #9 HERE

PLACE TOP OF REPORT #8 HERE

PLACE TOP OF REPORT #7 HERE

PLACE TOP OF REPORT #6 HERE

PLACE TOP OF REPORT #5 HERE

PLACE TOP OF REPORT #4 HERE

PLACE TOP OF REPORT #3 HERE

PLACE TOP OF REPORT #2 HERE

PLACE TOP OF REPORT #1 HERE

INSTRUCTIONS: TO ATTACH REPORT, REMOVE PROTECTIVE TAPE BACKING, ALIGN REPORT AND PRESS DOWN FIRMLY, REPEAT PROCEDURE FOR SUBSEQUENT REPORTS.

Professional Filing Systems, Inc.

5076 Winters Chapel Road • Atlanta, Georgia 30360
1-800-241-0419   1-404-396-4994

FORM F260

LABORATORY REPORTS

FIGURE 9–5   Report form for filing laboratory reports shingle fashion (Courtesy Professional Filing Systems, Inc.)

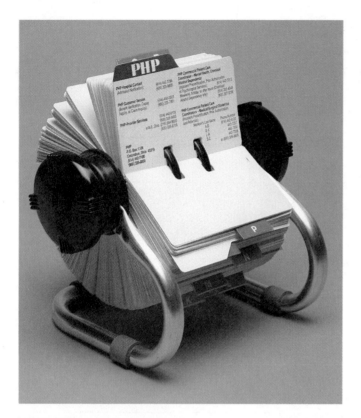

FIGURE 9–6   File storage units

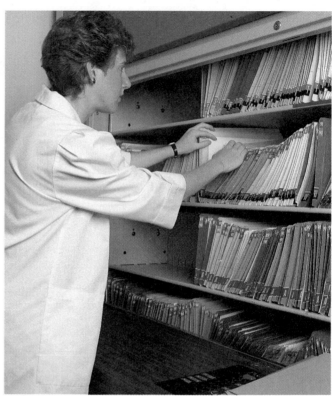

FIGURE 9–7   File storage units

FIGURE 9–8   Outguides (Courtesy of Professional Innovations, Inc.)

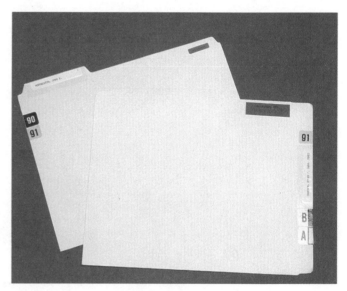

FIGURE 9–9   Top cut and end cut folders (Courtesy of Professional Innovations, Inc.)

How to File Alphabetically ....

The most common method of filing is alphabetical. The rules for filing material alphabetically must be learned. They are as follows.

Rule 1. In filing the names of persons, the surname or last name is considered first, the first name or initial second, and the middle name or initial third.

Example: John E. Brown is filed as Brown, John E.

Rule 2. Names are filed alphabetically in an A to Z sequence from the first to the last letter, considering each letter in the name separately and each unit separately. The following names are listed in correct filing order:

Allard, Wm.
Allen, E. S.
Allen, Edna

Allen, Wm. A.
Allen, William C.
Allens, M. R.

a. When the surnames of two persons are spelled differently, the first and middle names or initials need not be considered. See the first two names in the preceding list. The order of these two names is determined by the fourth letter in the surname.

b. When a shorter surname is identical with the first part of a longer surname, the shorter name is listed first. The rule is sometimes stated as "nothing before something." See the fifth and sixth names in the preceding list.

c. When the surnames are alike, the order in filing is determined by the first names or initials. When the surname and first names or initials are alike, the filing order is determined by the middle names or initials. See the fourth and fifth names in the preceding list.

d. An initial is listed before a name beginning with the same letter. See the second and third names in the preceding list. This again is the example of "nothing before something."

e. An abbreviated first or middle name is treated as if it were spelled out in full. See the fourth and fifth names in the preceding list.

Rule 3. A prefix (also called a surname particle), such as Mc, Mac, De, Le, and von, is considered as part of the surname.
Examples:
> MacAdams, Bruce
> McAdams, Helen
> VonBergen, T. R.

Rule 4. In filing the name of a married woman, her legal name is used. The title Mrs. is disregarded in filing, but is placed in parentheses after the name.
Example: Mrs. R. A. (Betty A.) Smith is filed as Smith, Betty A. (Mrs. R. A.).

Rule 5. Most firm names are filed as they are written. The apostrophe is disregarded in filing.
Examples:
> Herb's Auto Service
> Walters Printing Company

Rule 6. Firm names that include the full name of an individual are filed with the name of the individual transposed.
Example: Edward Wenger Company is filed as Wenger, Edward Company.

Rule 7. When the article *the* is part of a title, it is placed in parentheses and disregarded in filing.
Examples: Sam the Barber is filed as Sam (the) Barber; The Family Steak House is filed as Family Steak House (The).

Rule 8. *And, for, of,* etc. are disregarded in filing but are not omitted.

Example: Adams & Smith Pharmacy is filed as Adams (&) Smith Pharmacy.

Rule 9. Abbreviations such as *Co., Inc.,* or *Ltd.,* in a firm name are indexed as though spelled out.
Example: Frank Smith Co. is filed as Smith, Frank Company.

Rule 10. Hyphenated surnames and hyphenated firm names are indexed as one unit.
Examples: Dunning-Lathrop & Assoc. Inc. is filed as Dunning-Lathrop (&) Associates, Incorporated; Lester Smith-Mayes is filed as Smith-Mayes, Lester.

Rule 11. Numbers are usually filed as though spelled out.
Example: 5th Avenue Store is filed as Fifth Avenue Store.

Rule 12. Professional or honorary titles are not considered in filing but should be written in parentheses at the end of the name for identification purposes.
Examples: Dr. Anne Lewis is filed as Lewis, Anne (Dr.); President John Kennedy is filed as Kennedy, John (President); Prof. William S. Smith is filed as Smith, William S. (Prof.).

a. Titles are filed as written when they are part of a firm name. Foreign or religious titles followed by one name are also filed as they are written.
Examples:
> Dr. Scholl's Foot Powder
> Prince Phillip

Rule 13. Terms of seniority, such as *Junior, Senior, Second,* or *Third,* are not considered in filing. If two names are otherwise identical, the address is used to make the filing decision in the order: state, city, street.
Examples:
> Willard Keir, Sr.
> Willard Keir, Jr.
> *Filed as:*
> Keir, Willard, Sr. (Cleveland, Ohio)
> Keir, Willard, Jr. (Columbus, Ohio)

Rule 14. File the names of federal, state, or local government departments first by political division and then by name of department.
Example: Drug Enforcement Administration, Cincinnati, Ohio is filed as Cincinnati, City, Drug Enforcement Administration, Cincinnati, Ohio.

How to File Numerically

The second filing method used, especially in very large clinics, is the numerical system. This system provides the most patient privacy, as all that is visible on the folder is the patient number. As mentioned before, a cross-index or cross-reference is required in the form of an alphabetical card file, and a number is assigned to each patient. You first locate the alphabetical card to determine the patient's number and then locate the numbered file.

P R O C E D U R E

File Folders or Cards Alphabetically

TERMINAL PERFORMANCE OBJECTIVE: In a simulated situation, given folders and cards to be filed alphabetically, the student will observe office safety and with 100% accuracy, store the items within acceptable time limits. The instructor will observe and evaluate the procedure.

1. Use the rules for filing material alphabetically.
2. Locate the appropriate storage unit.

3. If you are filing new material, scan the guides for the area nearest to the letters you are dealing with.
4. Be sure to insert the new file between two other folders and not within another folder where it could be lost.
5. If you are filing material previously in the file, scan for the OUTguide. Remove the OUTguide when you return the folder. Check to be sure it was marking the space for the file you just returned and not another.

Most offices use the same number of digits for each number assigned, and the numbers are always filed in order from smallest to largest. If the zero (0) falls before another number, it is disregarded when filing. A system using six digits would begin 000001, 000002, 000003, etc.

Some systems use the same terminal digit or digits to designate shelves or drawers. The patients are assigned numbers, which are separated into twos or threes. The numbers are then read from the right hand group of numbers to the left hand group. After the last two or three digits are sorted together in numerical order, you next consider the middle digits and sort them in order. Finally, you consider the first group of digits and sort them in order.

For example, the numbers of charts in one series might end in 25 and another series might end in 35. Charts labeled 10-07-25 and 02-17-25 would then be filed separately from charts labeled 08-17-35 and 12-25-35. The order of the charts numbered above would be:

02-17-25
10-07-25
08-17-35
12-25-35

How to File by Subject ....

In the medical office it is necessary to have files for business information. You must file financial records, copies of inventory, copies of orders, and records of supplies and equipment received. You should have a file for tax records, insurance policies, and canceled checks. The subject headings of the above would be relatively easy to determine, but it is more difficult to determine where to file some general correspondence or reprints of medical research publications.

Very often reprints are filed with a cross-index, one file for the subject and one for the author with a listing of reprint subjects available. The miscellaneous folder is an important subject file. When you have one letter on a subject it should go into the miscellaneous file indexed by subject or names. The material in each subject file is filed in chronological order with the most recent entry on top. When five papers are assembled in the miscellaneous file on one subject or person, a separate folder should be prepared and the material removed from the miscellaneous file.

P R O C E D U R E

File Folders Numerically

TERMINAL PERFORMANCE OBJECTIVE: In a simulated situation, given folders to be filed numerically, the student will observe office safety, and with 100% accuracy, store the folders within acceptable time limits. The instructor will observe and evaluate the procedure.

1. Locate the appropriate storage unit.

2. Match the first two or three numbers with those already in the file. **Key Point: If using terminal digits, match last two numbers.**
3. Match remaining numbers with those in the file. **Key Point: If you have assigned a number to a new patient it should probably be at the very end of the file.**

PROCEDURE

Pull File Folder From Numerical File

TERMINAL PERFORMANCE OBJECTIVE: In a simulated situation, given the names of patients, the student will observe office safety, and with 100% accuracy, record numbers of patients, locate files, and prepare an OUTguide within acceptable time limits. The instructor will observe and evaluate this procedure.

1. Find the name of the patient in the alphabetical card file.

2. Write down the number assigned to that patient.
3. Locate the corresponding section of the numerical file.
4. Scan the files for the number.
5. Fill in an OUTguide with the number and name of the patient you are removing from the file; initial with your name and the date.
6. Pull the folder and insert the OUTguide in its place.

How to Use a Chronological File ·················

This file is commonly called a "tickler file" and is used as a follow-up method for a particular date. The file may be an expanding file, a card file, or even a portion of a file drawer. It consists of dividers with the names of all the months and dividers numbered from one to thirty-one for the days of the month. Some offices have patients fill out a card to be sent as a reminder to return for examination, testing, or injections. The patient addresses the card and the office retains it in the tickler file to be mailed by you at the appropriate time. You place the month card in the front of the file each month and check each day to see if anything needs to be done. The patients who would benefit are those who need regular or long-range follow-up for Pap tests, tests for follow-up of cancer therapy, or any long-range follow-up care. This file can be used to remind you to order supplies or to renew subscriptions, send tax information, or any task you need to be reminded about.

Periodically you will find it necessary to purge inactive files to storage to make room for the current files. File boxes may be used for this purpose, but they do need to be easily available in the event the patient returns. Transferring records of deceased patients should be delayed until you are sure there will be no more requests for forms to be completed. At that time, the files are closed.

You are far too busy in an office to spend time trying to locate a misplaced file or misplaced material regarding a patient. You need to be extremely careful when filing to be sure you are placing material in the correct folder. You should remove the folder and place the material to be filed in the folder with the top of the material toward the top of the folder when it is opened. The material is placed in chronological order with the latest date on top. File laboratory reports according to your office policy, usually in shingle fashion from bottom to top of the page with the latest on top.

All office records should be in closed files when not in use. Professional liability insurance policies, life insurance policies, canceled checks, wills, licenses, deeds, stocks, and bonds should be kept in a safe or at least in a fireproof file. Receipts for business equipment and any warranties should also be kept in fireproof storage until you no longer have the equipment.

Complete Chapter 9, Unit 1, in the workbook to help you meet the objectives at the beginning of this unit and therefore achieve competency of this subject matter.

UNIT 2

The Patient's Medical Record

OBJECTIVES ···

Upon completion of the unit the student will meet the following terminal performance objectives by verifying knowledge of the facts and principles presented through oral and written communication at a level deemed competent, and will demonstrate the specific behaviors as identified in the terminal performance objectives of the procedures, observing safety precautions in accordance with health care standards.

1. Describe the importance of the medical record as a legal document.
2. List examples of subjective information.
3. List examples of objective information.
4. Describe methods of recording progress notes.
5. Describe the correct procedure for making corrections of progress notes.
6. List the differences between a conventional record and the Problem Oriented Medical Record.
7. Spell and define, using the glossary at the back of the text, all the words to know in this unit.

WORDS TO KNOW ··

charting
procrastinators

progress notes

The patient history is the most important record kept in the medical office. The dates of any injuries, dates of treatment, and all notes regarding the condition of the patient must be accurate in every detail. In a lawsuit resulting from an injury, the patient chart information could win or lose the case.

Each office has its own method of charting patient visits. Some physicians ask the medical assistant to record the findings of a physical examination as it is being completed. Some physicians take the time to write all physical findings and progress notes for each visit. Many physicians prefer to dictate progress notes; then it becomes the duty of the medical assistant to type them.

The complete medical record has several important purposes:

1. It serves as a basis for planning patient care and for continuity in evaluating the patient's condition and treatment. The combination of the personal and family history with the findings of the physician must be combined with the results of laboratory studies, X rays, and any indicated special tests. The review of all of these facts together help the physician determine the diagnosis and course of treatment. This would not be possible without a well-documented, accurate record. The patient history or family history may alert the physician to certain conditions such as a family history of diabetes or exposure to hazardous substances.

2. The medical record furnishes documentary evidence of the course of the patient's medical evaluation, treatment, and change in condition. The charting of progress notes is extremely important and should give an indication of the patient comments, physician's evaluation, prescribed treatment, and need for further follow-up.

3. The record furnishes evidence of communication between the physician and any other health professional contributing to the patient's care. The chart should include a record of reports from other physicians asked to evaluate the patient with special laboratory, X-ray, or diagnostic procedures.

4. It affords protection of the legal interests of the patient and the physician. The complete accurate record would be necessary if the patient wishes the physician to testify in an injury case. The complete accurate record is also necessary if the patient sues the physician for malpractice. The patient must always sign an authorization form before any information may be released. An authorization must indicate who is to be allowed to receive the information.

5. The medical record helps to establish a data base for

use in continuing education and research. The accurate record of patients is a useful resource for research concerning response to medications or procedures in every phase of medical treatment.

The information in the medical record is classified as subjective or objective. The subjective information is supplied by the patient. The objective information is supplied by the physician. The *subjective information* includes the routine information about the patient, past personal and medical history, family history, and chief complaint. The *objective information* supplied by the physician should include examination, results of any laboratory studies, special procedures, X rays, the diagnosis, treatment prescribed, and progress notes.

The progress notes should be arranged in chronological order with the most recent date on top. If several notes are recorded on a page, the last on the page should be the most recent. The chart should be carefully dated for each visit. As discussed in the chapter on medical-legal considerations (see Chapter 3), each no-show, cancellation, telephone call, or prescription needs to be recorded as a progress note in the record of the patient, along with the date each took place, and initialed by the individual making the entry.

Some examples of progress notes might be:

12/14/91 Patient returns 10 days postop left 2d metatarsal osteotomy, some symptoms of pain on walking, area well healed, sutures removed. Continue boot, limited activity and return in 3 weeks. (Initials)

1/6/92 Patient returns, some slight complaint of pain with increased activity. Able to wear flat leather walking shoe. AP and lateral X rays reveal healing, advised activity to tolerance. Return necessary only if symptoms remain after 2 weeks. (Initials)

2/8/92 Patient called and reported feeling fine. (Initials)

2/9/92 Patient canceled appointment. (Initials)

2/15/92 Prescription for Aldomet renewed at ABC Pharmacy. (Initials)

2/15/92 Patient did not keep appointment. Note to referring physician notifying him of this. (Initials)

Dating, Correcting, and Maintaining the Chart

It is extremely important that the date be recorded on the page for progress notes each time the patient is seen. The date may be written in ink or stamped. Every time a patient is given a prescription over the phone or is given a report or advice should also be recorded with the date. Failure of a patient to keep an appointment should always be recorded by the date stamp on the chart. When it is necessary to start a new page, the patient's name and the date should always be written at the top of the new page. If office staff other than the physician are making notes on the chart, these should be initialed by the person making the notation.

In making a correction on progress notes, a handwritten entry should have a single line drawn through it and the correction written above or following it. An indication of correction should be made in the margin and should bear the initials of the person making the correction. Typing should be corrected at the time by use of correcting ribbon or whiteout. An error found at a later time is corrected in the same manner as in a handwritten record, but there should be no need to do this if typed material is carefully proofread in the typewriter.

Each medical field has its own specialized terms. You should make a correctly spelled list of these terms so you won't have to continually refer to a dictionary. These may be anatomical terms, surgical terms, appliances, medications, or simply English vocabulary the physician uses frequently. You will also find that the physician frequently uses abbreviations in hand-written notes or even in dictation, and a knowledge of these is also useful.

The medical assistant should check the charts each day to see whether notes have been dictated or written. Some physicians find it useful to keep a chart each day that reflects patients seen and has a check-off block for progress notes, referring physician if any, report dictated, and charges for service rendered. The physician can then see at a glance if all necessary work is completed on each patient.

Example:

DATE	PATIENT NAME		
10/1/93	Jane Doe		
Progress Notes	Referring M.D.	Letter Dictated	Charges
X	John Smith	X	25.00

Many fine physicians are procrastinators when it comes to completing paper work in the office. It is the duty of the medical assistant to see that it gets done even if this requires daily reminders.

The Problem Oriented Medical Record ....

In the early 1970s Lawrence L. Weed, M.D., a professor of medicine at the University of Vermont's College of Medicine, originated a system of record keeping for patients that he named the Problem Oriented Medical Record (POMR). In the traditional medical record, the progress notes are recorded according to the source they come from—the physician, laboratory, or physician's assistant—with no special attempt to record a relationship between them. The POMR record begins with the standard data base, which includes patient profile, chief complaint, review of systems, physical examination, and laboratory reports. The patient chart is then further built up by adding a numbered and titled page for each problem the patient has that requires management. Each problem is then followed with the SOAP approach for all progress notes:

S—Subjective impressions
O—Objective clinical evidence
A—Assessment or diagnosis
P—Plans for further studies, treatment, or management

This process makes the chart easier to review and helps in follow-up of all problems the patient may have, Figure 9–10.

Complete Chapter 9, Unit 2 in the workbook to help you meet the objectives at the beginning of this unit and therefore achieve competency of this subject matter.

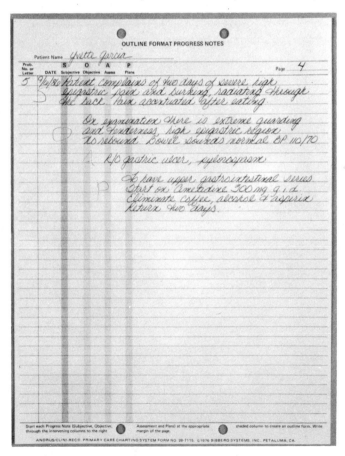

FIGURE 9–10 Example of POMR progress note page (Courtesy of Bibbero Systems, Inc., Petaluma, CA)

Throughout this chapter you should be mindful of all medical-legal/ethical implications. Listed below are a few important reminders.

1. Keep patient records according to your state statute of limitations.
2. File timely, accurately, and systematically to prevent loss of records.
3. Secure important documents in a safe or fireproof storage.
4. Obtain and file patient authorization for release of information.

Miss Right. . .

keeps the filing caught up by organizing her work so that she can file a few items between other duties. She purges files and stores them safely according to the state statute to prevent loss of important records. All important documents are placed in a fireproof storage box as they are received. She always obtains and files the proper authorization to release information about a patient. She checks the patient's chart for this signed form before giving information to anyone whether in person or by phone request.

Employment outlook: Continuous

Ms. Wrong. . .

doesn't like to file, so she lets it pile up and does it only after several reminders by her supervisor. She leaves important documents wherever she puts them and isn't concerned about their safe-keeping. She sometimes obtains the signature of patients for release of information when she remembers it. If she can't find the proper authorization form in a patient's chart, she gives out information without prior consent so the party won't call back about it.

Employment outlook: Termination

REFERENCES

Bonewit, Kathy. *Clinical Procedures for Medical Assistants.* Philadelphia: W. B. Saunders, 1990.

Kinn, Mary and Derge, Eleanor. *The Medical Assistant: Administrative and Clinical,* 6th Ed. Philadelphia: W. B. Saunders, 1988.

Simmers, Louise. *Diversified Health Occupations.* 3rd Ed. Albany: Delmar, 1993.

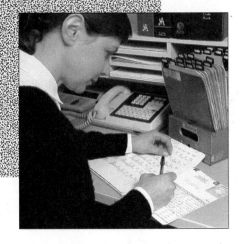

Collecting Fees

The medical assistant must be concerned with the collection of fees from patients, as there are many expenses to be covered in the practice of medicine. The medical assistant needs to know the local clinics where limited income patients can be referred for care at a reduced fee. The medical assistant can help patients plan a payment schedule for a costly surgical procedure, therapy, or for the birth of a baby. It is important to determine who is responsible for the payment for the services of the physician. If it is not the patient, it may be an employer, an insurance company, or a school.

U N I T 1

Medical Care Expenses

OBJECTIVES ....

Upon completion of this unit, the student will meet the following terminal performance objectives by verifying knowledge of the facts and principles presented through oral and written communication at a level deemed competent, and will demonstrate the specific behaviors as identified in the terminal performance objectives, observing all aseptic and safety precautions in accordance with health care standards.

1. Name the factors in determining fees for patient care.
2. List the types of patients who pay no fees or reduced fees.
3. Discuss the pitfalls of reducing fees.
4. List the information that should be obtained about every new patient.

5. Spell and define, using the glossary at the back of the text, all the words to know in this unit.

WORDS TO KNOW ....

complexity	nominal	subsequent
indigent	pitfalls	verify

Physicians traditionally are reluctant to discuss fees with patients. It is fairly common for the medical assistant to be the one who must answer these questions. When a patient is unhappy about medical costs, it is important to listen and try to explain why the charges are as stated. The physician should always be told when a patient is unhappy with the cost of treatment. It may be necessary for the physician to talk with the patient about the concern regarding cost of care.

Physicians must set their fees based on their professional financial profile and the fees appropriate for similar specialists in the community.

In considering the fee for services to the patient the physician must consider the time spent with the patient, the complexity of the diagnosis, and the treatment. In addition, the cost of maintaining an office and staff must be considered. The physician can obtain usual and customary fee schedules from the local medical society or a medical practice management firm.

In some instances now, you will find that insurance companies and government agencies will establish a fee profile for the physician based on the charges averaged over a period of time. This is one of the reasons it is so critical to learn to code patient visits accurately. When such a profile is established, it represents the highest payment the insurance company or government agency will make for the services listed in the profile.

No Fee or Reduced Fee

Although most physicians accept patients of all socioeconomic levels, the medical assistant should be aware of various pitfalls of reducing fees. Indigent patients receive the same care as paying patients and the same records are kept. The charge will be recorded as *n/c* (no charge) on the financial records for the day. Most physicians find it necessary to limit the number of indigent patients they accept, for obvious reasons. Therefore, you may be faced with the task of telling a patient who wishes to be seen, and who indicates indigent status, that your office cannot accept new patients. You should know the names, addresses, and eligibility requirements of local clinics operated by social service agencies for such referrals. These clinics provide services from qualified physicians as well as other health care at no cost or a nominal cost.

When your employer has treated a patient and the patient encounters difficulty in paying the bill, it is important to check for possible insurance coverage and the possibility of local or state public assistance. Physicians may simply write off an account they feel cannot be collected. They may also decide to reduce the fee. In that case, it should be done in writing with a date setting the time limit within which the account is to be paid. The words *without prejudice* should be part of the written agreement. This precaution will allow the physician to collect the total bill if the reduced amount is not paid. Two copies of the written statement should be made, and should be witnessed as they are signed. The original should be kept in the office and the copy given to the patient. You should continue to bill for the total amount with the understanding that when the reduced amount is paid the remainder will be written off. A fee should not generally be reduced for a patient who has died, because the family may see this as an indication that the physician was at fault. It is also not considered good practice to reduce a fee because of a poor result or to avoid sending the bill to a collection agency.

Physicians traditionally treat one another and the immediate family of close physician friends without charge or accept any insurance payment as payment in full, writing off any difference. This is considered a professional courtesy. Physicians may also treat members of the clergy and allied health professionals employed in their own offices or offices of close associates without charge or at a discount. If any of these individuals insist on paying or offer insurance to cover the charges, payment should be accepted.

MEDICAL INSURANCE RECORD

Name of Subscriber ______ LAST FIRST MIDDLE
Address ______
City ______ State ______ Zip ______
Date of Birth ______ Social Security Number ______
Phone No. (Home) ______ Phone No. (Work) ______
Employer ______
Address ______ STREET CITY STATE ZIP

INSURANCE INFORMATION

Insurance Company ______
Policy Number ______ Group Number ______ Union Local ______
If Group Insurance, Name of Policy Holder (i.e., employer, union) ______
Insured's I.D. or Medicare No. (include any letters) ______
Effective Date of Insurance ______
Coverage ______
Exclusions or Exceptions ______
Claim Form Supplied ☐Yes ☐No Standard Form Acceptable ☐Yes ☐No

INSURED DEPENDENTS' NAMES

Spouse ______ NAME RELATIONSHIP TO SUBSCRIBER BIRTHDATE
Others ______ NAME RELATIONSHIP TO SUBSCRIBER BIRTHDATE
______ NAME RELATIONSHIP TO SUBSCRIBER BIRTHDATE
______ NAME RELATIONSHIP TO SUBSCRIBER BIRTHDATE

ADDITIONAL COVERAGE

Does Patient Have Other Health Insurance? ☐Yes ☐No
If Yes, Name of Policy Holder ______
Plan Name and Address ______
______ Policy or Medical Assistance Number ______

Please complete reverse side

Form 9126 Colwell Co., Champaign, Illinois

FIGURE 10–1 Personal data sheet (Courtesy of Colwell Systems)

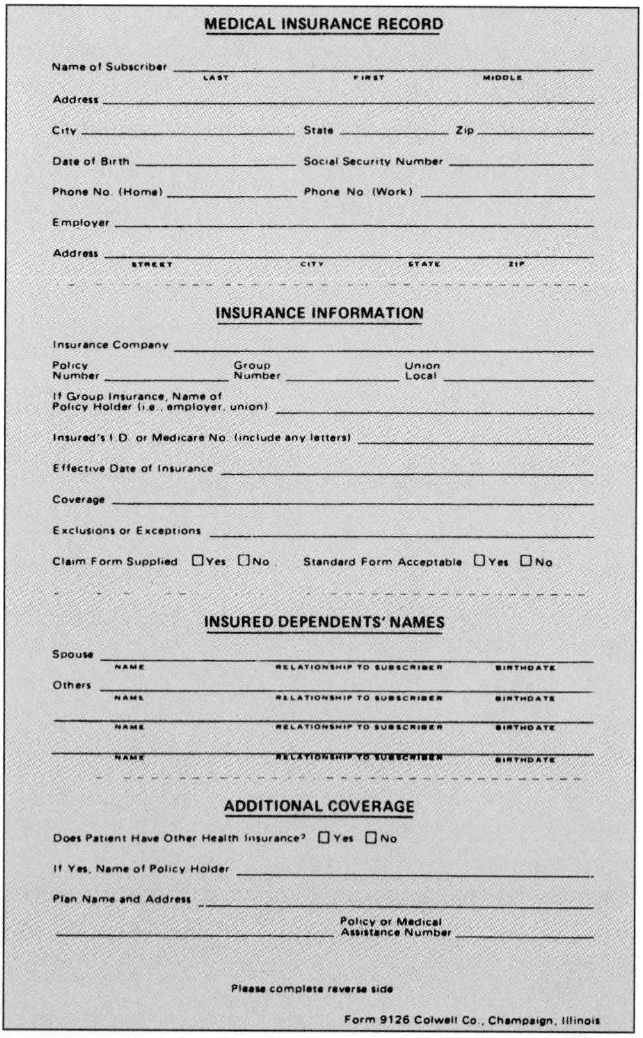

Personal Data Sheet

A personal data sheet should be completed the first time patients are seen in the office, Figure 10–1. On subsequent visits you should routinely verify the address, place of employment, and insurance information. You may type the form while interviewing the patient in private, or the patient may complete the form. The following information should always be obtained.

Kerry Peoples, M.D.
101 Fitness Lane
Anywhere, U.S.A. 00000

DATE ____________________

NAME OF PATIENT ____________________

I ____________________ agree to pay for the
(name of responsible party)
examination and treatment of ____________________
(name of patient)
on ____________________
(dates of treatment)

WITNESS ____________________

DATE ____________________

FIGURE 10–2 Third party liability statement

BEST CLINIC ASSOCIATION
PHILLIP H. BEST, M.D.
DEAN E. McLAUGHLIN, M.D.
P.O. BOX 136
LOVINGTON, ILLINOIS 61937

RECORDS RELEASE Date ____________________

To ____________________

I hereby authorize you to release to ____________________

any information including the diagnosis and records of any treatment or examination rendered to me during the period from ____________ to ____________

____________________ SIGNATURE

____________________ WITNESS ____________________ ADDRESS

FIGURE 10–3 Records release form (Courtesy of Colwell Systems)

- Patient's full name correctly spelled.
- Date of birth. This is useful if you have two people with the same or similar names.
- Social Security number. This is used as the identification number with insurance carriers in many cases.
- Marital status.
- Current address and length of time at that address. A person who moves frequently may lack stability in payment of bills.
- Telephone number at home and at work.
- Name and relationship of person legally responsible for charges. Under normal circumstances parents are considered responsible for the charges of their children. However, if a third party is involved, an oral agreement is not binding and the individual who will pay the bill needs to sign a simple statement before care is given. This statement may be a form you have prepared or it may be a handwritten statement, Figure 10–2.
- Patient's occupation, with name and address of employer. If a patient has a spouse, you should also obtain spouse's occupation and name and address of employer.
- Name of person referring patient. This information can be valuable if the patient later moves without leaving a forwarding address.
- Health insurance information. Ask to see the patient's identification card or cards, if they are covered by more than one plan. You need to make a copy of both sides of the card(s) on your copy machine to be sure you have all the information. Some states require a consent for release of information separate from the printed one on insurance forms. If this is the case in your state, be sure that this form also is completed at the time of the first visit, Figure 10–3. Be sure you have complete information on all insurance carried.

Complete Chapter 10, Unit 1 in the workbook to help you meet the objectives at the beginning of this unit and therefore achieve competency of this subject matter.

UNIT 2

Credit Arrangements

OBJECTIVES

Upon completion of this unit, the student will meet the following terminal performance objectives by verifying knowledge of the facts and principles presented through oral and written communication at a level deemed competent.

1. List circumstances when you may need to discuss payment planning with a patient.
2. Describe credit arrangements used to finance medical care.
3. Describe the reason for accepting credit cards as payment for services rendered.
4. Spell and define, using the glossary at the back of the text, all the words to know in this unit.

WORDS TO KNOW ....

solicit   substantial

Payment Planning ....

The medical assistant can be a great help to patients who are going to have a baby, surgery, or extensive therapy by helping plan for payment. When the patient knows in advance that there will be costly medical expenses, the medical assistant should review the patient's health insurance coverage. Some physicians use a cost estimate sheet to give the patient an idea of the cost for surgery or long-term treatment, Figure 10–4. The estimate may include the approximate cost of the anesthetist, any consultants, and hospital charges.

If it appears that the patient will need to pay a substantial sum out-of-pocket, the medical assistant should discuss the manner in which payments will be made. If the patient does not have current resources to pay the full amount in one payment, the medical assistant should offer the option of a fixed sum as a down payment and regular payments of a fixed amount on specified dates. The Truth in Lending Act, which is enforced by the Federal Trade Commission, specifies that when there is an agreement between the physician and a patient to accept payment in more than four installments, the physician is required to provide disclosure of finance charges. Most

FIGURE 10–4
Estimate sheet

```
                    SURGICAL COST ESTIMATE

NAME OF PATIENT_____DATE_____

Procedure_____

_____

       Your surgery is scheduled at_____Hospital

on_____.  You should report to the Admitting Office between  the
hours of _____(a.m.)(p.m.) and (a.m.) (p.m.).

     Although medical and hospital expenses are often covered by insurance,
knowing in advance what expenses to expect and how to plan for them is beneficial
to the patient.  This estimate is prepared to assist you in budgeting, if necessary,
to cover your surgical costs.

                         PROFESSIONAL FEES

     When you have major surgery, the surgical team includes the operating
surgeon, the assistant surgeon and the anesthetist.  Each has an important
part in your care, and each will render a separate statement for services.
While each physician will set his/her own fee, it is usually possible to make
an estimate in advance of the approximate range of fees.  Assuming an uncomplicated
course for your surgery, the charges are estimated as follows:

          Operating Surgeon        $_____ to $_____

          Assistant Surgeon        $_____ to $_____

          Anesthetist              $_____ to $_____

The assistant surgeon and anesthetist usually base their fees on the length
of the operating time; consequently, if a surgical procedure requires more
time, the charges may be correspondingly increased.

     The estimated duration of your hospital stay is _____ days at $_____
a day for a (semi-private) (private) room.  During your hospital stay there will
be charged for laboratory tests, medications as required, and other services.
It is impossible to estimate in advance what these charges will be, they will
be itemized on your hospital bill.  If you have health insurance, please take
the appropriate forms and I.D. information with you on the day you are admitted
to the hospital.

            PLEASE KEEP IN MIND THIS IS ONLY AN ESTIMATE
```

medical offices do not charge for financing but this makes no difference; the form still must be completed, Figure 10–5. The patient must sign this form in your presence and the disclosure statement must be kept on file for 2 years. If the physician makes no specific arrangement for more than four payments and bills each month for the full amount, rather than installment amounts, there is no need for the signed statement.

Credit Card Usage

Patients are currently using many methods of financing medical care. The AMA Code of Ethics includes several guidelines for physician participation in credit card programs. Physicians may not increase their charges for services to patients who wish to use credit cards; they may not encourage patients to use credit cards or use the credit card as a way to solicit patients; physicians may offer credit card payment as a convenience for patients but cannot advertise this fact outside the office.

The advantage of credit card use for paying for medical services is the monies are generally available to the physician within 24 hours of depositing. Also, it removes the responsibility from the physician for collection. This service does not come without cost to the physician. Generally, a fee of 1% to 3% is assessed, based on the volume of credit cards used. Many physicians feel this is to their advantage because the office time is not used for collection of any delinquent accounts.

Some banks have set up financing programs in which the bank sends the money directly to the physician after deducting a handling charge. It is important for the physician to be sure that any outside financing arranged for patients is managed in a professional manner and that no unreasonable pressure tactics are used. In larger cities the physician may want to check credit references before extending credit for a large surgical fee. Some large medical societies have Bureaus of Medical Economics that perform a collection service and also provide credit information.

If you should receive a request from a credit bureau, you can say when a patient's account was opened, the current balance, and the largest amount of the account at any time. You will be in violation of the law if you make any statements regarding paying habits of the patient or the character of the patient.

Complete Chapter 10, Unit 2 in the workbook to help you meet the objectives at the beginning of this unit and therefore achieve competency of this subject matter.

UNIT 3
Bookkeeping Procedures

OBJECTIVES

Upon completion of this unit, the student will meet the following terminal performance objectives by verifying knowledge of the facts and principles presented through oral and written communication at a level deemed competent, and will demonstrate the specific behaviors as identified in the terminal performance objectives of the procedures.

1. Transfer charges from charge slip to daily log.
2. Post charges from daily log to patient ledger card.
3. Type itemized statement.
4. Describe exceptions to usual billing procedures.
5. Describe the advantages of one-write bookkeeping system.
6. Spell and define, using the glossary at the back of the text, all the words to know in this unit.

WORDS TO KNOW

assets	equities	petition
bankruptcy	journalizing	posted
bookkeeper	ledgers	proprietorship
chemotherapy	liabilities	trial balance

FIGURE 10–5 Federal truth in lending form (Courtesy of Colwell Systems)

LEONARD S. TAYLOR, D.D.S.
2100 WEST PARK AVENUE
CHAMPAIGN, ILLINOIS 61820

TELEPHONE 351-5400

FEDERAL TRUTH IN LENDING STATEMENT
For professional services rendered

Patient _____

Address _____

_____

Parent _____

1. Cash Price (fee for service) $ _____
2. Cash Down Payment $ _____
3. Unpaid Balance of Cash Price $ _____
4. Amount Financed $ _____
5. FINANCE CHARGE $ _____
6. Finance Charge Expressed As
   Annual Percentage Rate   _____
7. Total of Payments (4 plus 5) $ _____
8. Deferred Payment Price (1 plus 5) $ _____

"Total payment due" (7 above) is payable to _____
at above office address in _____ monthly installments of $ _____
The first installment is payable on _____ 19 ____, and each subsequent payment is due on the same day of each consecutive month until paid in full.

_____   _____
Date   Signature of Patient; Parent if Patient is a Minor

FORM 9402 COLWELL SYSTEMS INC CHAMPAIGN ILLINOIS

Bookkeeping Terms ....

Some of the basic terminology used in recording office business transactions includes:

- *Daily journal* or day sheet. All patient charges and receipts are recorded here each day.
- *Account.* Record for each patient, which will show charges, payments, and balance due.
- *Accounts receivable.* All of the outstanding accounts (amounts due).
- *Posting.* Transfer of information from one record to another.
- *Debit.* A charge, added to existing balance.
- *Credit.* A payment, subtracted from existing balance.
- *Balance.* Difference between debit and credit.
- *Adjustment.* Professional courtesy discounts, write-offs, or amounts not paid by insurance. If no adjustment column is included, discounts are listed in red in the debit column.
- *Debit balance.* Shows that the patient paid an amount less than the total due.
- *Credit balance.* Shows that the patient paid more than was due or is paying in advance. A credit balance is written in red ink, circled, or noted in parentheses.

Daily Log

The medical assistant should record the charges for each patient on the daily log sheet, Figure 10–6. They should be itemized and a total only put in the charge column. Payments should be placed in the credit (paid) column. The daily log sheet will reflect the names of all patients treated in the office each day as well as any payments received in the mail or from patients who come to the office just to pay the bill. Unassigned columns on the daily log may be used to distribute charges or receipts among partners or to distribute charges by departments, such as laboratory, X ray, physical therapy, or medication in such cases as **chemotherapy.**

Ledger Cards

The medical assistant who must transfer the charges from the day sheet to the patient account card should do this when there will be a minimum of interruptions. The variety of ledger cards available makes it possible to increase efficiency by using the one which best suits your needs, Figure 10–7, page 150. It is a good policy to place a small check mark on the day sheet after each entry has been **posted** to the account card. Then if you are interrupted you will know where to begin again in your posting job.

Statements

Statements must be accurate in every detail, from the name of the patient to the figures for charges and payments, Figure 10–8, page 150. If your office uses monthly billing, send the bills on the last day of the month. Your patients are more likely to pay if statements are received on a regular basis. If you have a large number of statements to send, cycle billing should be used. With this system, you divide your account cards into groups to correspond to the number of times you will be billing. You then maintain the same cycle each month so that patients learn when to expect your statement. You might send A through F on the tenth of each month, G through M on the twentieth, and N through Z at the end of the month.

Medical assistants are generally more concerned with bookkeeping as an entry level employee. A **bookkeeper** is one who records information. You may be required to keep a record of accounts receivable and payable. The office accountant will inform you of any records you need to provide to prepare summary reports of financial information, which are as important in the practice of medicine as in any well-run business. The accountant will analyze the figures and prepare reports that not only tell the present status of accounts receivable and payable, but compare current reports with other years or periods of time. A breakdown of the most cost-efficient procedures and least cost-efficient procedures may be revealed in such a summary. The accountant may be the person designated to prepare payroll checks and pay the quarterly amounts due to government agencies for taxes withheld.

The medical assistant who is going to do bookkeeping must be accurate in every detail. There is no "almost right" in bookkeeping. The work is 100% correct or it is incorrect and must be corrected. The bookkeeper must enjoy detail work and must make clear, legible figures using a fine point black ink pen. Care must be taken to record figures in correct columns as debit or credit and always in straight columns. Care must also be taken to place the decimal point correctly and always double-check figures on a calculator or adding machine. An adding machine tape is helpful in that you can double-check figures easily. Employees have been fired from their jobs because of carelessness with figures in simple math. You should practice adding and subtracting numbers without the use of paper or pen or computer. The bookkeeper who can independently compute answers quickly and accurately is considered an asset to any office.

Single and Double Entry Bookkeeping ....

If complete records are to be maintained in the medical office, it is necessary to carefully record all transactions that affect the accounting elements. The accounting elements are expressed in one of two equations:

$$\text{assets} = \text{liabilities} + \text{proprietorship}$$
or
$$\text{assets} = \text{liabilities} + \text{owner's equity}$$

When any two of these elements are known, it is always possible to calculate the third element. **Assets** are anything that has value and is owned by a business.

HOUR	NAME	SERVICE RENDERED	√	CHARGE		PAID	
1							
2							
3							
4							
5							
6							
7							
8							
9							
10							
11							
12							
13							
14							
15							
16							
17							
18							
19							
20							
21							
22							
23							
24							
25							
26							
27							
28							
29							
30							
31							
32							
33							
34							
35							
36							
37							
38							
39							
40							
41							
42							
43							
44		TOTALS					

FORM 7241 COLWELL CO., CHAMPAIGN, ILL.

FIGURE 10–6 Daily log sheet (Courtesy of Colwell Systems)

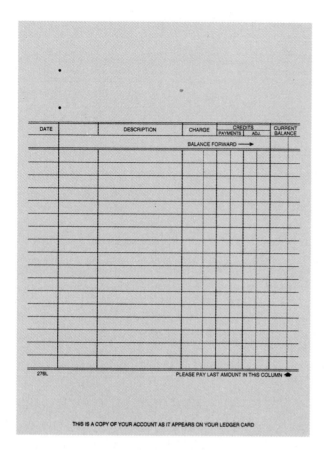

FIGURE 10–7 Ledger card (Courtesy of Professional Innovations, Inc.)

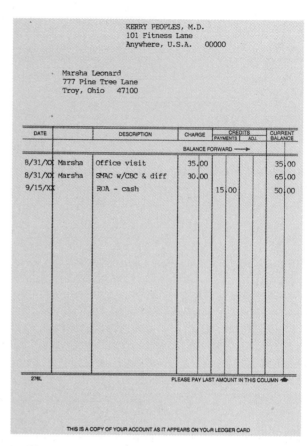

FIGURE 10–8 Itemized statement (Courtesy of Professional Innovations, Inc.)

Common examples of assets would be office furniture, equipment, building, land on which the building stands, supplies, money, and accounts receivable. The simplest definition of equities is that they are the claims that various parties have against the assets. The owner's equity, therefore, equals the amount of assets remaining after liabilities have been subtracted. These values are always recorded by dollar value. An accountant must analyze every financial transaction affecting a business to determine the effect of the transaction on either the assets or the equities or in some cases both. The equation must always balance in dollar amounts after every transaction. It might help you to understand this equation if you start with a simple "dollar value of assets = dollar value of equities." You then need to realize that normally there are both creditor's equities and owner's equities. The commonly accepted accounting term for creditor's equities is *liabilities*. This takes you back to "assets = liabilities + owner's equity." Examples of liabilities are the obligations to pay for supplies, equipment, salaries, rent or mortgage, loans, and taxes. The proprietorship is the amount by which assets exceed liabilities. In double entry bookkeeping, every transaction must be recorded on each side of the accounting equation and the two sides must always balance.

The left side of a ledger account is the debit side and the right side is the credit side. This might be more easily understood by the following example of the equation:

	Name of Business or Equity
	Liabilities and Owner's
Assets	Equity
debit for additions	credited for additions
credit for subtractions	debited for subtractions

A group of patient accounts are known as ledgers. A general ledger contains the records of all the asset and equity accounts. A medical assistant would need special training to carry out all of the details needed, and an accountant is usually paid to perform these services for the medical office. The use of computer programs for accounting have made it much easier for everyone to accomplish more complex accounting procedures.

In single entry bookkeeping, the medical assistant prepares the daily log or journal and posts charges and payments to the patient ledger card. The entries on the daily log are called journalizing. The journalized entries should be entered in chronological order. The single entry bookkeeping system allows you to record increases or decreases in assets without the balancing information regarding the increases and decreases in equity. The total amount of checks and cash should be recorded on a cash control sheet. This may be a daily record sheet or a record showing an entire month with a line used each day to show income in cash and checks, any deposits made, and any amounts not deposited and therefore carried over to the next day, Figure 10–9.

You can see when a balance is carried forward it is important to record it under "previous balance" for the next day, where it will be added to "total received" to calculate "total on hand." This kind of record is also helpful in double-checking your bank deposit slip. The cash and checks should be equal to the amount shown on your cash control record.

An accounts receivable record should be kept daily. This record represents the total owed the physician for services rendered. This total should be the same as the total of balances on all the active patient ledger records. The process of running such a total is called a trial balance. The accounts receivable balance is carried forward from month to month and added to the daily charges. The payments made by patients and any adjustments are subtracted to determine true accounts receivable each day.

The accounts payable procedures involve keeping a careful record of invoices for supplies and equipment. Always check orders received against the invoice listing to be certain the entire order was received. Be careful to check any statements or invoices before paying the amount due. If an accountant is writing the checks for the office, the medical assistant may be responsible for preparing a folder of invoices to be paid. When the medical assistant is responsible for paying bills and payroll, there is an added responsibility of keeping accurate checkbook records.

The normal disbursements in an office with one physician could include payment of rent or mortgage, utilities, salaries, office supplies, office equipment, insurance, and personal expenses of the physician. In a partnership or an incorporated clinic setting with many physicians, it is customary for the physicians to be paid a salary, which eliminates any personal expenses paid by the office account.

Exceptions to Usual Procedures

There are a number of exceptions to the usual billing procedures. Many companies make arrangements for annual physical examinations to be completed by community physicians. In these cases, the statements are sent to the employer rather than the patient. Some physicians complete physical examinations for individuals applying for insurance coverage. In this case the bill is sent to the insurance company. Physicians who specialize in sports medicine and examine athletes may be paid by the school or team referring the patient.

When it is necessary to collect a bill owed by a deceased patient, the statement is sent to the estate of the deceased in care of any known next of kin at the patient's last known address. You do not address the statement to a relative unless you have a signed agreement that that person will be responsible for the bills. You may need to contact the Probate Court to obtain the name of the administrator of the estate if the patient died in a nursing home and had no known next of kin.

When your office receives an official notice that a patient has filed for bankruptcy you send no more statements and can make no attempt to collect the account. The patient who has filed a wage earner's bankruptcy will pay a fixed amount to the court to be divided among the creditors. Your office may receive only a dollar at a time. Accept this and credit the account. You will be notified of a creditors' meeting in a straight petition for bankruptcy, but it is usually best just to be sure they have a copy of the statement and wait to see if you will receive any money. Sometimes the patient wishes to continue seeing the physician and will make payments on the account independently on a cash basis.

The physician may examine a patient in consultation in a legal claim, and in this case the person or agency requesting the consultation is responsible for the charges. The statement is sent with the consultation report. Other examples of third party billing are auto accidents, Workers' compensation, and Medicaid.

CASH CONTROL							**January 19__**
Day	Total Received	Total Cash	Total Checks	Previous Balance	Total on Hand	Deposit	Balance Carried Forward
5	7,650.00	250.00	7,400.00	——	7,650.00	7,650.00	——
6	500.00	——	500.00	——	500.00	——	500.00
7	5,950.00	550.00	5,400.00	500.00	6,450.00	6,450.00	——

FIGURE 10–9 Cash control record

Prepare Patient Ledger Card

TERMINAL PERFORMANCE OBJECTIVE: In a simulated medical office situation and provided with all necessary equipment and supplies, the student will prepare a patient ledger card following the steps in the procedure. The instructor will observe each step.

1. Type name of patient, last name first.
2. Type complete address with zip code. **Key Point: On a ledger card to be photocopied the name and address are completed in the same manner as an** address on an envelope since the copy of the card is folded and mailed in a window envelope.
3. Type name and address of person responsible for charges if different from patient.
4. Type telephone number of patient.
5. Type name of insurance company.
6. Type referring individual.
7. If this is a continuation of a previous card, carry forward any balance due.

Record Charges and Credits

TERMINAL PERFORMANCE OBJECTIVE: In a simulated medical office situation, and provided with all necessary equipment and supplies, the student will record charges and credits following the steps of the procedure. The instructor will observe each step.

1. Pull ledger card for patient.
   Key Points:
   a. **If you can record charges near your ledger file it will be efficient to do one at a time. Tilt up the card behind as a marker.**
   b. **If you must post away from your ledger file pull all the cards you need at one time; then return all to file.**
2. Post all charges and credits for a patient and check off on day sheet before you go on to the next patient.
   Key Points:
   a. **Use small, neat figures.**
   b. **Note the dividing line between dollars and cents. In some cases this is a darker line.**
   c. **Never use dollar signs on account cards.**
3. Charges are posted in the debit column. **Key Point: If a balance is shown on the card add the new debit to get a new balance.**
4. Payments are posted in the credit column and are subtracted from the balance due. **Key Point: If the credit is greater than the balance due, the difference is a credit balance and is shown in red.**
5. The balance column should always reflect the current status of the account.

Some offices send copies of charge slips to an outside billing service. In this case you need to be sure all charges and payments are sent so that the statements will be accurate and complete. The disadvantage of this system is that you do not have records in your office of current balances for your patients.

Pegboard System

Many offices use the one-write pegboard system mentioned earlier for their accounting records. The base or board has pegs, which you should place up and to the left. This log holds all of your daily entries; it becomes a listing of patients seen, as well as a complete financial record of charges made and payments received. You position a shingle of receipt/charge slips on top of the daily log, with the notches fitted over the pegs. Working downward from the top of the daily log, the shingle must be placed so that the charge/receipt slip nearest the top of the pegboard has its posting line directly over the first available line on the daily log. At the beginning of each day this will be at the top of the daily log. These forms are prenumbered in the lower right corner; be sure to use them in numeric sequence to preserve the strong audit trail designed into the system. The receipt/charge slip serves several functions. It is the charge slip for current fees; a receipt for any payment received either by check or cash; a statement of account showing previous balance, today's charges, today's payments, and the new balance; it also shows the next appointment if there is one. When this is completed you are ready for your first patient of the day, Figure 10–10.

PROCEDURE

Type Itemized Statement

TERMINAL PERFORMANCE OBJECTIVE: In a simulated medical office situation, and provided with all necessary equipment and supplies, the student will type itemized statements with 100% accuracy following the steps in the procedure. The instructor will observe each step.

1. Stack ledger cards beside typewriter.
2. Assemble statement forms and window envelopes.
3. Stamp ledger card on line below last entry with date stamp.
4. Type name and complete address in area that will show in window envelope.
5. If there is a balance from previous month, list that first under services.

6. Type each service charge and payment for the current month.
7. The last line should show current balance due.
8. Fold and place in envelope with the address showing through window in envelope.

   Key Points:
   a. **You may want to stuff all the envelopes after you have typed all the statements.**
   b. **Be careful to place only one statement in each envelope.**

9. Fan out several envelopes with flaps exposed.
10. Dampen a sponge and wipe over all flaps at once.

    Key Point: Be careful not to overwet.

11. Fold down flaps and seal.

When you check in a patient, pull the appropriate ledger card from your file tray. If the patient is new to your practice, prepare a ledger card. Post to the first available charge/receipt slip the existing balance (if zero, write—0—), and the patient's name. What you are writing on the charge/receipt slip is being written simultaneously on the daily log sheet. You then detach the charge slip portion at the perforation and forward it to the doctor with the patient's clinical record. The doctor will check the services received by the patient and give the slip to the patient to return to the receptionist. This gives the patient an opportunity to review the services and to ask any questions about the charge. The medical assistant will then position the ledger card so that the posting line of the receipt slip is directly over the first available line on the ledger card and post the receipt number, date, and professional services rendered, using the codes preprinted on the form. The total charges are figured from the charge slip and entered in the charge space on the receipt slip. This is the time to ask for payment. If there is no charge the entry is written *n/c*.

Post any payment received in the paid space on the receipt slip. If no payment, record as —0—. Post the new balance in the appropriate space and again, if zero, write —0—. In one writing you have created for the patient a combination receipt and statement. With the same one-write system, you have recorded the financial data you need on both the patient's ledger card and the daily log sheet. You are now ready to detach the receipt slip from the shingle at the perforation and remove it from the pegboard.

Arrange a new appointment, if necessary, and record the date and time in the appropriate spot on the receipt slip. Also be sure to record the appointment in the appointment book before handing the receipt to the

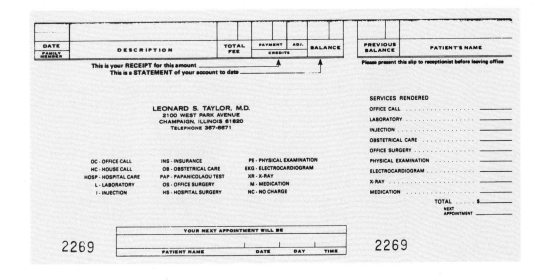

FIGURE 10–10
Pegboard charge slip, receipt, and appointment slip (Courtesy of Colwell Systems)

patient. Never write in the appointment space while the receipt is still attached to the shingle.

The last step is to return the patient ledger card to its proper position in the file tray.

If payment is made other than when service is rendered, the receipt slip is used if the payment is made in person. If the payment is received in the mail, it is written directly on the ledger card and through it to the daily log sheet. The new balance is then posted on the ledger card after it is removed from the daily log sheet.

At the close of the day, remove remaining charge/receipt slips from the pegboard and verify that all receipt numbers are listed on the daily log. You will usually have several blank lines at the bottom of the sheet; on the last line write "End of (date)." Use a new log sheet each day. Add each column and post totals in spaces provided. Save your tapes and double-check the figures. It is a simple matter to have an up-to-date account of accounts receivable at all times with this system. The total owed to the physician by all patients is increased by the day's charges and reduced by the day's receipts. The total of the receipts should be the amount of the bank deposit each day.

To protect the employees of the office against a possible bank error, the daily cash summary and the bank deposit slip should be initialed by at least two persons.

Complete Chapter 10, Unit 3 in the workbook to help you meet the objectives at the beginning of this unit and therefore achieve competency of this subject matter.

UNIT 4
Computer Billing

OBJECTIVES ....

Upon completion of this unit, the student will meet the following terminal performance objectives by verifying knowledge of the facts and principles presented through oral and written communication at a level deemed competent, and will demonstrate the specific behaviors as identified in the terminal performance objectives, observing all aseptic and safety precautions in accordance with health care standards.

1. Describe the advantages of computerized billing.
2. Describe different ways to locate an account in a computer system.
3. Describe an account history.
4. List reasons why billing statements would/should be withheld.

WORDS TO KNOW ....

account history   alpha search

Billing is the most common use for a microcomputer in the medical office. Many different computer systems are available and it is important to determine the needs of the office first. When this is accomplished, it is possible to make a decision as to which system would best meet the needs of the office. Unfortunately, not all systems will do all you want them to, so it is important to make a wise choice at the outset.

The computer terminology for a patient ledger is account history. This is simply a record of the information that should be obtained for every new patient. You need to know the name and address of the person responsible for payment of the account, all data regarding insurance, and all necessary information regarding family members under the same insurance. Generally, account histories follow the same organized plan you used for ledger records of patients. You may have a choice in determining how you will find an account entered in the computer system. When the system will accept a number only, you must maintain a cross-reference file of an alphabetical listing of patients along with their account numbers. The easiest and fastest method is called an alpha search. You type in the first few letters of the name and the screen will automatically list all names of patients starting with those letters. You select the name you wish to make an entry for and type in the appropriate entry. The account history automatically shows the balance of the account and the number of days the account has been due. The entire account activity is available to see on the screen or to make a printout for the patient. Your system should allow you to remove inactive accounts from the computer just as you remove inactive ledger cards. When a physician's office converts to a computerized system, it is important to choose the Current Procedural Terminology (CPT) codes commonly used in the practice. They are then programmed into the computer along with the descriptions of the codes and the fees to be charged for each. The International Classification of Diseases (ICD) diagnostic codes must be programmed into the computer for insurance claims use. The computer can be coded to indicate the source of the payment: insurance, cash, or check. Adjustment codes can be used for returned checks, courtesy discounts, and any cancelled account balances.

Some computers can be programmed to create charge slips (see Chapter 6, Unit 2). When the patient hands a computer-generated or hand-written charge slip to the receptionist, the charge and payments may be entered on the patient account history. A courtesy discount can also be recorded as an adjustment. In some offices, the receptionist would check to be sure the services rendered were indicated on the charge slips and then send them to the business office for processing in the computer. All charge slips must be accounted for each day. The computer can create a statement or receipt to be handed to the patient before leaving the office.

Computers can be programmed to lead you through the entry of every transaction by means of questions flashed on the screen or statements telling you what to do next. A medical assistant should be an accurate typist to operate a computer efficiently. If an error is posted on a transaction, there are ways to delete the transaction and start over again with a correct entry.

The computer insurance claims can greatly improve cash flow as a claim can be completed in a matter of seconds for every patient visit. This is a great advantage for patients who pay cash and need to be reimbursed as soon as possible. When the physician accepts the insurance payment, the computer can be programmed to print "patient signature on file" in the signature portion of the claim, so that there is no need to have the patient sign the form. Where there is no such system, the form must be signed by the patient or sent to the patient for signature in the hope that it will be forwarded to the insurance company.

The computer can speed up monthly billing and can be programmed to withhold statements on accounts for which you do not need or wish to send statements. Examples would be welfare patients, Workers' Compensation, or families of patients who have recently died. The computer statement is considered to be an efficient collection method for the office because it not only shows an itemized account of all transactions, but the age of the account can also be listed. The statement should show the portion of the amount due that is current, over 30 days, over 60 days, and over 90 days, Figure 10–11.

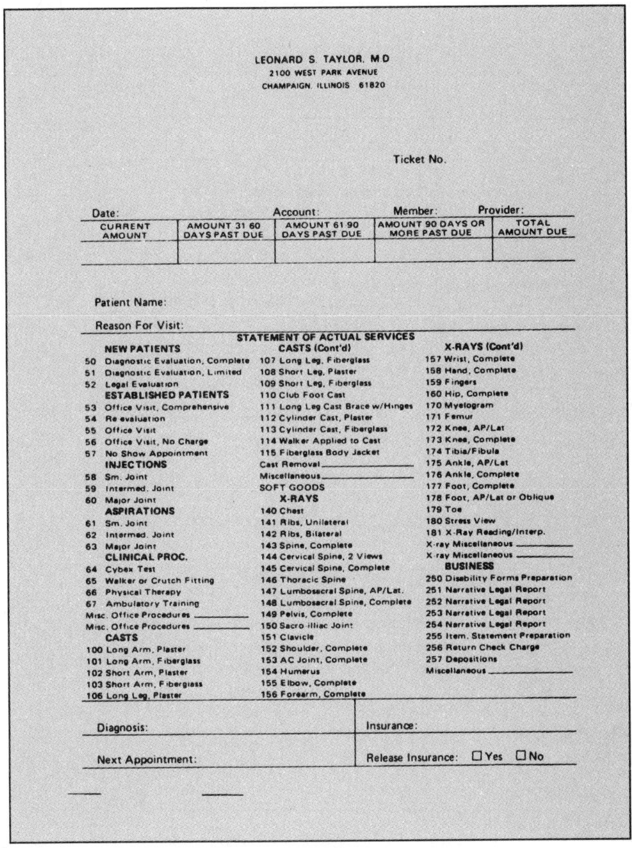

LEONARD S. TAYLOR, M.D.
2100 WEST PARK AVENUE
CHAMPAIGN, ILLINOIS 61820

Ticket No.

Date: Account: Member: Provider:

CURRENT AMOUNT	AMOUNT 31 60 DAYS PAST DUE	AMOUNT 61 90 DAYS PAST DUE	AMOUNT 90 DAYS OR MORE PAST DUE	TOTAL AMOUNT DUE

Patient Name:

Reason For Visit:

STATEMENT OF ACTUAL SERVICES

NEW PATIENTS	**CASTS (Cont'd)**	**X-RAYS (Cont'd)**
50 Diagnostic Evaluation, Complete	107 Long Leg, Fiberglass	157 Wrist, Complete
51 Diagnostic Evaluation, Limited	108 Short Leg, Plaster	158 Hand, Complete
52 Legal Evaluation	109 Short Leg, Fiberglass	159 Fingers
ESTABLISHED PATIENTS	110 Club Foot Cast	160 Hip, Complete
53 Office Visit, Comprehensive	111 Long Leg Cast Brace w/Hinges	170 Myelogram
54 Re evaluation	112 Cylinder Cast, Plaster	171 Femur
55 Office Visit	113 Cylinder Cast, Fiberglass	172 Knee, AP/Lat
56 Office Visit, No Charge	114 Walker Applied to Cast	173 Knee, Complete
57 No Show Appointment	115 Fiberglass Body Jacket	174 Tibia/Fibula
INJECTIONS	Cast Removal ______	175 Ankle, AP/Lat
58 Sm. Joint	Miscellaneous ______	176 Ankle, Complete
59 Intermed. Joint	SOFT GOODS	177 Foot, Complete
60 Major Joint	**X-RAYS**	178 Foot, AP/Lat or Oblique
ASPIRATIONS	140 Chest	179 Toe
61 Sm. Joint	141 Ribs, Unilateral	180 Stress View
62 Intermed. Joint	142 Ribs, Bilateral	181 X-Ray Reading/Interp.
63 Major Joint	143 Spine, Complete	X-ray Miscellaneous ______
CLINICAL PROC.	144 Cervical Spine, 2 Views	X-ray Miscellaneous ______
64 Cybex Test	145 Cervical Spine, Complete	**BUSINESS**
65 Walker or Crutch Fitting	146 Thoracic Spine	250 Disability Forms Preparation
66 Physical Therapy	147 Lumbosacral Spine, AP/Lat.	251 Narrative Legal Report
67 Ambulatory Training	148 Lumbosacral Spine, Complete	252 Narrative Legal Report
Misc. Office Procedures ______	149 Pelvis, Complete	253 Narrative Legal Report
Misc. Office Procedures ______	150 Sacro-illiac Joint	254 Narrative Legal Report
CASTS	151 Clavicle	255 Item. Statement Preparation
100 Long Arm, Plaster	152 Shoulder, Complete	256 Return Check Charge
101 Long Arm, Fiberglass	153 AC Joint, Complete	257 Depositions
102 Short Arm, Plaster	154 Humerus	Miscellaneous ______
103 Short Arm, Fiberglass	155 Elbow, Complete	
106 Long Leg, Plaster	156 Forearm, Complete	

Diagnosis: Insurance:

Next Appointment: Release Insurance: ☐ Yes ☐ No

FIGURE 10–11 Superbill (Courtesy of Colwell Systems, Inc.)

The computer can furnish you with a daily journal report. This report can be a record of cash control also, as a listing of checks and cash can be shown separately. All computer systems should be set up to record deleted transactions as a printed safeguard against anyone being tempted to steal money by entering a transaction and then deleting it.

The computer can be used to print out monthly summaries of charges, payments, and accounts receivable. Year-to-date reports can be easily produced. You may print out a record of all outstanding accounts with an analysis of account age.

The computer can provide a detailed list of patients seen by each physician in a large clinic and the services rendered. It can be used to determine the number of patients seen with a specific diagnosis or for a particular procedure for research summaries.

The medical assistant may be able to program the computer to print out a list of hospital and nursing home patients to be seen. Such a list improves the accuracy in recording all out-of-office patient charges.

When you have a computer system with many of the printout possibilities detailed here, you will find the business management of the office much more efficient. You will find you can complete all of these procedures in a fraction of the time required to do them by more conventional methods.

Complete Chapter 10, Unit 4 in the workbook to help you meet the objectives at the beginning of this unit and therefore achieve competency of this subject matter.

UNIT 5

Collecting Overdue Payments

OBJECTIVES

Upon completion of this unit, the student will meet the terminal performance objectives by verifying knowledge of the facts presented through oral and written communication at a level deemed competent, and will demonstrate the specific behaviors as identified in the pupil performance objectives of the procedure.

1. Define "aging of accounts."
2. Demonstrate use of the telephone for collection of accounts.
3. Compose collection letters suitable for a variety of situations.
4. Define the statute of limitations.
5. Spell and define, using the glossary at the back of the text, all the words to know in this unit.

WORDS TO KNOW

antagonize
convey
expended
harassment
reputable
specified
termination

Computers can help in analyzing accounts receivable for accounts past due. This process is known as *aging of accounts*. It is basically a means of dividing accounts into categories according to the amount of time since the first billing date. Accounts are considered current if within 30 days of the billing date. Some medical assistants place a colored metal tag on accounts 60 days past due to indicate that a reminder was placed on the statement. At 90 days the tag color is changed and a letter is sent requesting prompt attention. Some offices use the numbers 1, 2, and 3 after the stamped date on the ledger card to indicate that past due notices were attached to the statement. The notices can be in the form of pressure-sensitive colored stickers that are progressively more severe in wording and in colors which are sure to attract attention, Figure 10–12. The first one might be a mild yellow, the second an orange, and the third and final one a red. No account should be referred to a collection agency unless the physician has given approval for this to be done. However, federal law requires that when you have stated you will turn the account over for collection you must follow through and do so if the bill is not paid. You cannot make idle threats.

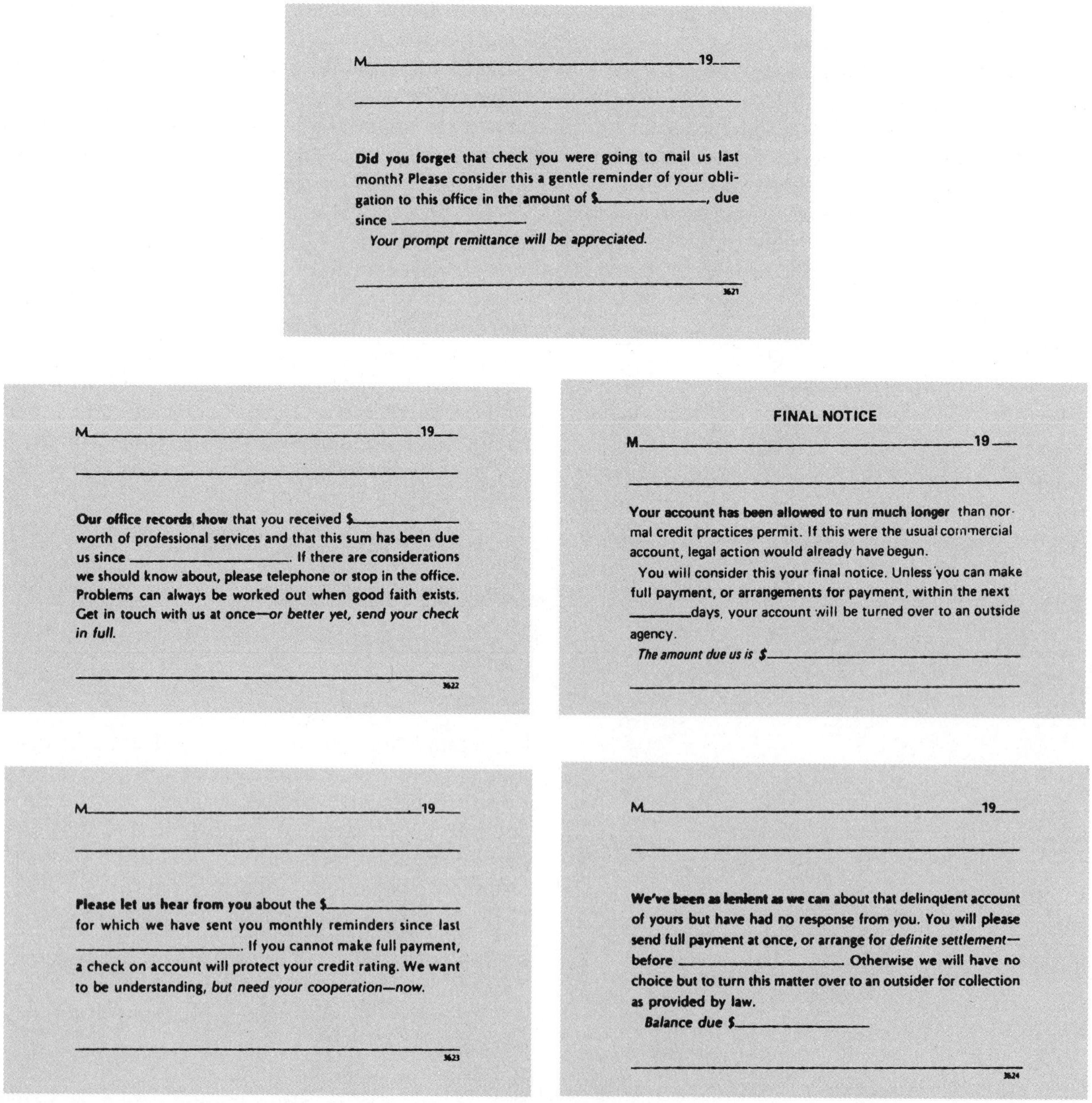
M____________ 19__

Did you forget that check you were going to mail us last month? Please consider this a gentle reminder of your obligation to this office in the amount of $________, due since ________

Your prompt remittance will be appreciated.

3621

M____________ 19__

Our office records show that you received $________ worth of professional services and that this sum has been due us since ________. If there are considerations we should know about, please telephone or stop in the office. Problems can always be worked out when good faith exists. Get in touch with us at once—*or better yet, send your check in full.*

3622

FINAL NOTICE

M____________ 19__

Your account has been allowed to run much longer than normal credit practices permit. If this were the usual commercial account, legal action would already have begun.

You will consider this your final notice. Unless you can make full payment, or arrangements for payment, within the next ______days, your account will be turned over to an outside agency.

*The amount due us is $*________

M____________ 19__

Please let us hear from you about the $________ for which we have sent you monthly reminders since last ________. If you cannot make full payment, a check on account will protect your credit rating. We want to be understanding, *but need your cooperation—now.*

3623

M____________ 19__

We've been as lenient as we can about that delinquent account of yours but have had no response from you. You will please send full payment at once, or arrange for *definite settlement*—before ________ Otherwise we will have no choice but to turn this matter over to an outsider for collection as provided by law.

*Balance due $*________

3624

FIGURE 10–12 Collection cards (Courtesy of Colwell Systems)

A personal telephone call will often result in payment of overdue accounts. If you make collection calls, never do so without the consent of your employer, and confine your calling to your normal office hours. If you make calls early in the morning or late at night you can be held liable for harassment. Confine your calls to a place in the office where you will not be overheard by other patients. It is generally not a good policy to call a patient at work. If the patient has no home phone it may be necessary to call at work but you should simply ask the patient to return your call at a time when he or she can discuss the problem with you. Remember that you will violate the confidentiality of patient-physician relationships if you talk to anyone other than the patient or the individual responsible for the charges. When the telephone is answered, use the full name of the patient in asking, "May I speak to Jane Ann Jones, please?" Always ask if it is convenient to talk at this time; if it is not try to set a definite time when you may call, or ask the patient to call you at a specified time. If the phone is answered by someone other than the patient, identify yourself by name only. When the patient is on the phone, come directly to the point by saying that you are calling regarding the past due account. Approach the task with a positive attitude. Say that you are sure non-payment of the bill is an oversight and, if not, that you want to help them make arrangements for payment. Make every attempt to establish a date when the bill will be paid, and make a notation on the ledger card indicating when that will be. Be sure you have a reminder file to help you follow up on promises to pay. If the patient indicates dissatisfaction with the results of medical care be sure that you convey this information to the physician.

Some physicians feel that collection cards or stickers are a sufficient reminder, but others prefer the use of collection letters. Consult the office procedure manual or your employer regarding preferences for follow-up on the collection of accounts. You may want to compose a series of standardized letters that you can personalize as needed, Figure 10–13. When composing collection letters, avoid words that tend to antagonize, such as *forgot*, *neglected*, *overlooked*, and *failure*. Decide whether you are going to use a series of three, four, or five letters. The last letter in the series will usually inform the patient that you must resort to a collection agency if you do not receive payment by a *specified* date. Use your knowledge of the patient to decide what type of letter to use. You would use a stronger sounding first letter for someone with a poor payment record. For a patient who has an excellent payment record your first letter would be a gentle reminder. Every effort must be expended to collect as many accounts as possible

Since your last office visit in May we haven't received any word of how you are feeling or any payments on your account.

If arrangements can't be made to pay the full amount of $_____ by June 12, please let us know so that the office can help you make arrangements for your payments.

We have had a balance of $_____ on our books since September, and have heard no word from you about your account in the past month.

If you have any questions in regard to your statement, feel free to contact the office so that we may discuss them with you. If not, we would appreciate the full amount by May 16th.

You have always paid promptly on your account in the past, so you must have accidently overlooked the statements we've sent. If that is the case, please accept this as a friendly note to remind you of your account due in the amount of $_____ .

Our office has mailed three statements for the services you received in June. Unless special credit arrangements are made, bills are payable at the time of the visit.

Please send your full payment by September 22th or get in touch with us to answer any questions you may have.

We can no longer carry your account on our books. The balance of $_____ must be paid within 10 days.

Our collection agency receives all delinquent accounts on the 25th of each month.

FIGURE 10–13 Collection letters

without resorting to a collection agency, which charges a percentage of everything collected. Most offices avoid collection agencies if at all possible.

An example of a form letter that can be used to obtain an answer in writing of reasons for nonpayment of an account is shown in Figure 10–14. If you can get this kind of letter signed by the patients, you not only know the reasons for nonpayment, but you have a signed paper acknowledging the amounts they owe the physician. If you know the reason for nonpayment, it is easier to help work out a solution for payment. If the payment is not made within the prescribed period used by your office, the fact that you have a signed statement from the patient acknowledging the amount owed is helpful in a collection situation. The patient cannot deny the debt.

Each state has laws (called *statutes of limitations*) which establish the number of years during which legal collection procedures may be filed against a patient. If a patient is being treated for a chronic illness, there is no termination of the illness or treatment unless the patient dies or changes physicians. The last date of debit or credit on the patient account card is the starting date for that particular debt. If the last date was June 1990, a 2-year statute could be collected through June 1992. In written contracts the statute of limitations starts from the date due. Some states have a shorter time limit on the statute of limitations on single entry (single charge) accounts.

When statements you have mailed are returned marked *moved, no forwarding address*, you have to consider the possibility that the patient is a *skip* (collection agency slang), or has moved to avoid payment of bills. The first step is to check your records to make sure you mailed to the correct name, address, and zip code. If these are all correct, place a telephone call to see if perhaps the old phone number was transferred to a new address. You may call referring individuals to try to obtain a new address for the patient, although you must not indicate your reason for needing the new address other than that you need to verify it. You may call the patient's employer for information regarding address change, identifying yourself by name only and asking that the patient return your call. You may find the patient simply forgot to inform the post office of an address change. You may also find the patient has left his or her place of employment, in which case you should check with your employer about referring the account for collection. The longer you wait, the less chance you have to collect.

Your employer should have arrangements with a reputable collection agency. The office reputation can be severely damaged if the agency you work with uses unethical collection methods. When your employer has made the decision to refer an account for collection, send the collection agency the full name of the patient, name of spouse or person responsible for the bill, last known address, full amount of debt, date of last entry on ledger card, occupation of debtor, and business address. Send no further statements, and refer any calls regarding the account to the collection agency. If you should receive any information regarding the account or any payments, you should forward it to the collection agency.

Complete Chapter 10, Unit 5 in the workbook to help you meet the objectives at the beginning of this unit and therefore achieve competency of this subject matter.

P R O C E D U R E

Compose Collection Letter

TERMINAL PERFORMANCE OBJECTIVE: In a simulated medical office situation, and provided with all necessary equipment and supplies, the student will compose and type appropriate collection letters for assigned accounts to be collected following the procedure. The instructor will observe each step.

1. Identify patients to whom an initial collection letter should be sent. **Key Point: If you categorize your collection accounts you will be more efficient. Complete all #1 letters before proceeding to all #2 letters, etc.**

2. Compose a rough draft with the first paragraph indicating *why* you are writing.

3. The second paragraph should indicate what response or reaction you expect.

4. Reread the rough draft to be sure you have written clearly, correctly spelled words, and correctly punctuated sentences.

5. Type the letter.
   Key Points:
   a. **Follow standard letter form (block or modified block).**
   b. **Proofread the letter.**
   c. **Sign the letter with your name unless the physician wishes to sign. Remember to type your position below your name and your title (Mr., Mrs., Miss, or Ms.) before your name.**
   d. **Do not use identification initials if you sign the letter.**

6. Type the envelope.

7. Fold the letter, seal, and mail.

Kerry Peoples, M.D.
101 Fitness Lane
Anywhere, U.S.A. 00000

(Date)

(Patient name)
(Patient address)

Dear

Normally, at this time, because your account in the amount of _____ is long past due, this account would be placed with our collection agency. However, we prefer to hear from you regarding your preference in this matter.

( ) I would prefer to settle this account. Payment in full is enclosed.

( ) I would like to make regular weekly/monthly payments of $_____ until this account is paid in full. My first payment is enclosed.

( ) I would prefer that you assign this account to a collection agency for enforcement of collection. (Failure to return this letter will result in this action.)

( ) I don't believe I owe this amount for the following reason(s):

signed _____

Please indicate your preference above and return this letter.

Sincerely,

Kerry Peoples, M.D.

FIGURE 10–14 Collection letter requesting statement from patient of reason(s) for nonpayment of account

MEDICAL-LEGAL/
ETHICAL HIGHLIGHTS

Throughout this chapter you should be mindful of all medical-legal/ethical implications. Listed below are a few important reminders.

1. Keep financial records accurate and complete.
2. Respect the privacy and confidentiality of patients' records.
3. Obtain and file written authorization for release of information.
4. Obtain a written contract if a third party is responsible for payment of medical treatment.

Mrs. Right. . .

organizes her work so that she can devote quality time in posting financial transactions on records. She is mindful in keeping this information confidential, respecting the privacy of patients. She makes sure that a signed authorization is obtained and filed when a third party payment contract is made for payment of services.

Promotion outlook: Excellent

Mr. Wrong. . .

is careless when posting charges on records because he does this between other duties. He delays posting charges and payments because he doesn't like to do this kind of work. He makes errors and doesn't recheck his work. He is also negligent in obtaining proper authorization forms signed by patients regarding third party contract for payments. He confronts patients in hallways or in the waiting area in front of others concerning their accounts. He is known for discussing payments and other confidential information with other patients.

Promotion outlook: Poor

REFERENCES

American Medical Association. "The Business Side of Medical Practice."

Frew, Mary Ann, and Frew, David R. *Comprehensive Medical Assisting: Administrative and Clinical Procedures,* 2nd Ed. Philadelphia: F. A. Davis Company, 1988.

Kinn, Mary E., and Derge, Eleanor. *The Medical Assistant: Administrative and Clinical,* 6th Ed. Philadelphia: W. B. Saunders Company, 1988.

Simmers, Louise. *Diversified Health Occupations,* 3rd Ed. Albany: Delmar Publishers, 1993.

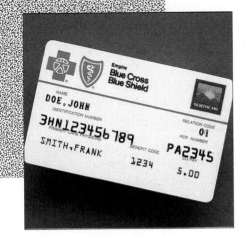

CHAPTER 11

Health Insurance

UNIT 1
Health Insurance Terms

UNIT 2
Health Care Plans

UNIT 3
Coding Systems

T he medical assistant needs to be aware of insurance terms and the types of insurance that patients may have. Medical insurance is the type which is the most important. A large portion of the income in the office is paid from some form of medical insurance.

U N I T 1

Health Insurance Terms

OBJECTIVES

Upon completion of this unit, the student will meet the following terminal performance objectives by verifying knowledge of the facts and principles presented through oral and written communication at a level deemed competent.

1. Distinguish between the two major classes of health insurance.
2. Define the insurance terms described in this unit.
3. Spell and define, using the glossary at the back of the text, all the words to know in this unit.

WORDS TO KNOW

catastrophic	primary
comprehensive	secondary
inclined	stipulations
premium	

Most patients have some form of health and accident insurance coverage, because they realize that a serious illness or injury can be **catastrophic** to family or individual finances. Insurance seldom pays all medical costs, however.

Many insurance policies include a "nonduplication of benefits" or "coordination of benefits" clause. If both husband and wife carry insurance coverage that overlaps, the insured's coverage is considered **primary** and the spouse's is **secondary**. The charges are filed first with the primary carrier; after payment is received the explanation of benefits and completed claim form is then submitted to the secondary carrier for consideration. When the couple has children covered by both policies, the Birthday Rule applies—whichever parent's birthday falls first in the calendar year that parent's insurance is the primary coverage. For example, if the father's birthday is in June and the mother's is in March, then the mother's policy would be the primary insurer and the father's the secondary one.

The two major types of health insurance are individual and group. Any individual may buy individual health insurance by paying the required premium. Group health insurance generally costs less and is more **comprehensive.** The group may be employees of a single employer or a number of employers, a union, or any other. Complete coverage may or may not be paid by the employer. The employee may have to pay a premium for other family members to be covered.

When patients come to the office they often seem to have little comprehension of the kind of coverage they have. They may bring a policy to show you that they have insurance, but you may discover that the policy is life insurance and have to explain to them that it will not pay for medical expenses. On the other hand, auto insurance or home owners' insurance may pay for an injury received in the auto or the home.

Each office must develop a method for dealing with insurance forms. This will vary with your employer's practice. A physician with a surgical practice is likely to make the medical assistant fully responsible for processing the claims. A general practice physician is usually more **inclined** to ask patients to pay when examined and then provide a superbill to be used by the patient in filing insurance papers. In this case the medical assistant should be able to offer information helpful to the patient in processing the forms.

The following terminology is common to health insurance policies.

■ *Assignment of benefits.* Specification of who is to receive payment, the patient or the physician. Most physicians prefer the patient to request that payment be sent directly to the physician. If the insurance is sent directly to the patient, the check is often used for purposes other than the physician's charges. The Blue Shield Advance Plan guarantees that payment will go to the physician if the physician signs a contract stating he will accept the payment allowed as payment in full. If the physician does not sign the contract, the payment is sent to the patient.

■ *Capitation.* The health care provider is paid a fixed amount for each person served regardless of services provided.

■ *Claim.* A request for payment under an insurance contract.

■ *Coding.* Transference of words into numbers to facilitate the use of computers in claim processing.

■ *Coordination of benefits.* Procedures used by insurers to avoid duplicate payment on claims when the patient has more than one policy. One insurance company will become the primary payer and no more than 100% of costs are covered.

■ *Copayment* or *coinsurance.* A type of insurance in which the insured must pay a specified portion toward the charge for professional services rendered.

■ *Deductible.* A predetermined amount that the insured must pay each year before the insurance company will pay for an illness or injury. The amounts vary and are stated in the policy. For example, if the deductible is $100, then after the insured has paid the first $100 of the covered benefits in a calendar year, the insurance

company will begin to pay, in many cases 80% of the charges from that point.

■ *Diagnostic related groups (DRGs).* A system developed by Yale University to group together major diagnostic categories, organized by body systems from which the 470 DRGs are drawn. DRGs require physicians to follow strict guidelines for hospital admission and the number of days that will be paid for under each DRG.

■ *Effective date.* The date when the insurance goes into effect. In some cases the policy specifies a waiting period during which no benefits will be paid. This may be true in the case of a pregnancy if the policy was not in effect for 9 months prior to delivery.

■ *Fee schedule.* A list of approved professional services for which the insurance company will pay and the maximum fee it will pay for each service.

■ *Group insurance.* Insurance offered by an employer to all employees.

■ *Health maintenance organization (HMO).* A prepaid group practice that can be sponsored and operated by the government, medical schools, clinics, foundations, hospitals, employers, labor unions, community or consumer groups, insurance companies, the "Blue" plans, hospital-medical plans, or the Veterans' Administration. Public Law 93-222 was the HMO Act of 1973. It was an amendment to the Social Security laws providing for comprehensive health care at a fixed periodic payment.

■ *Independent practice association (IPA).* A group of individuals who prepay a fee for treatment by a group of physicians who continue to practice independently in their own offices. The physicians treat nonmembers as well as members. The fee for nonmenbers is billed directly to the patients. The fee for members is billed to the IPA.

■ *Individual insurance.* Insurance purchased by an individual for self and any eligible dependents.

■ *Loss-of-income benefits.* Payments made to an insured person to help replace income lost through inability to work because of an insured disability.

■ *OR procedure.* Operating room procedure.

■ *Out-of-area.* An HMO member is generally covered for emergency services out of his or her geographic area, but other coverage might not always be provided.

■ *PAT.* Preadmission testing.

■ *Patient status.* Insurance companies frequently have **stipulations** that services be provided on an *inpatient* or *outpatient* basis. There are also requirements for *prior authorization* from the insurance company for certain services or procedures to be performed.

■ *Precertification.* Prior authorization must be obtained before patient is admitted to the hospital.

■ *Preexisting condition.* A condition that existed before the insured's policy was issued. Some policies do not cover preexisting conditions, whereas others provide compensation after a prescribed waiting period.

- *Preferred provider organizations (PPOs).* This plan offers different insurance coverage depending on whether the patient receives services from a contracting physician. The benefits are higher if the physician provider is a member of the PPO.
- *Premium.* Monies paid for an insurance contract.
- *Release of medical information form.* A form that must be signed by the patient before information may be given to an insurance company.
- *Service area.* The geographic area served by an HMO.
- *Third party payer.* An insurance carrier who is not the doctor or patient who intervenes to pay the hospital or medical bills per contract with one of the first two parties.
- *Usual and customary fee.* The usual fee is the charge physicians make to their private patients. The customary fee is one within the range of usual fees charged by physicians in a given geographic and socioeconomic area who have similar training and experience. Some insurance plans do not publish a fee schedule but agree to pay all or a percentage of the usual and customary fee.
- *Utilization review.* A review carried out by allied health professionals at predetermined times to assess the necessity of the particular patient to remain in an acute care facility.

Complete Chapter 11, Unit 1 in the workbook to help you meet the objectives at the beginning of this unit and therefore achieve competency of this subject matter.

U N I T   2

Health Care Plans

OBJECTIVES

Upon completion of this unit, the student will meet the following terminal performance objectives by verifying knowledge of the facts and principles presented through oral and written communication at a level deemed competent.

1. Describe important health care plans.
2. Describe the important government health insurance plans.
3. Spell and define, using the glossary at the back of the text, all the words to know in this unit.

WORDS TO KNOW

annuity	per capita	supplement
connotations	periodic	unique
illegible	statutory	

Private Health Care Plans

The Blues

Blue Cross and Blue Shield health insurance plans are generally well known. Physicians helped originate them, and physicians and medical societies have control over premiums paid and benefits received. The Blue Shield plans are generally better known in the medical office since they are used to pay for the services of the physician. Blue Cross was originally set up to pay for hospital expenses but now covers outpatient services.

The Blue Shield plans are **unique** in employing a large staff of provider/professional relations representatives. These representatives make personal calls on physicians' offices and conduct seminars for medical assistants. You should learn who your representative is because this person will be able to keep you informed of any procedural changes and answer questions on the completion of forms.

Most Blue Shield plans are not-for-profit voluntary associations allowing subscribers to pay in advance for health care expenses. A person becomes a subscriber (not a policy holder) by paying regular dues. Blue Cross and Blue Shield may also assist federal and state governments in administering other health care plans. Blue Shield issues membership identification cards that indicate type of coverage and provides a guide that can be used to help interpret the kinds of coverage indicated on the identification card.

When a Blue Shield patient has an out-of-area plan, it is important to check the card for the reciprocity code. This is a double-end red arrow symbol with an "N" followed by three digits. The insurance for patients with this card can be billed to the local Blue Shield plan. In the absence of the symbol, the bill must be sent to the subscriber's Blue Cross or Blue Shield plan listed on the back of the ID card, Figure 11–1.

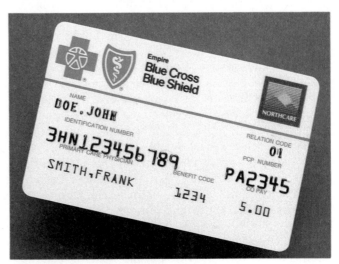

FIGURE 11–1 Blue Shield identification card (Courtesy of Empire Blue Cross/Blue Shield)

If you have a large number of patients who live outside of your area, or if you have difficulty obtaining the addresses of insurance companies, you may want to obtain a health insurance directory or check with your local hospital to see their directory. *The Nationwide Hospital Insurance Billing Directory* can be obtained from:

Francis B. Kelly & Associates
123 Veteran Avenue
Los Angeles, California 90024
1-800-328-4144

This association also publishes the *Casualty Insurance Claims Directory*, which also may be a useful reference for the office.

Commercial Health Insurance

A large segment of the population is covered by commercial health insurance policies. These private, commercial insurance companies control the price of premiums paid and specify the benefits they will pay for.

Prepaid group practice plans, which are extremely popular, began in 1929 in California. In addition, there are two different types of foundations for medical care operations: a comprehensive type that designs and sponsors prepaid health programs or sets minimum benefits of coverage, and a claims review type that provides for peer review to evaluate the quality and efficiency of services rendered to the patient in cases where an insurance claim exceeds local guidelines for the fee and/or service.

These plans are referred to as health maintenance organizations (HMOs), which is a plan set up to provide comprehensive health care services at fixed periodic fees. The medical assistant needs to understand the differences in their structures; there are three basic types. Physicians may form an independent group and contract with a health care plan to provide medical treatment to the members. The physicians are paid a salary by their independent group rather than by the health plan administrators. The second type is a plan in which the health plan pays the physicians' salaries. The third is the individual practice association (IPA), in which the physician is paid fees for services from premiums paid to the organization, which sells the health plan to patients.

The law states that an employer of 25 or more persons may offer employees the services of an HMO clinic as an alternative to commercial health insurance or Blue Cross and Blue Shield. To qualify as an HMO, an organization must present proof of its ability to provide comprehensive health care. To retain eligibility, the HMO must submit **periodic** performance reports to the Department of Health and Human Services. If your employer is engaged in treating patients who are enrolled in HMOs, the accuracy and completeness of their medical records will help the HMO to determine status. Eligible individuals are those who have voluntarily enrolled in the plan from a specific geographic area,

or who are covered by an employer who has paid an established amount per person. The federal government reimburses HMOs on a **per capita** basis, depending on the size of enrollment.

Many state and local medical associations sponsor foundations for medical care (FMCs). The comprehensive FMC may qualify as an HMO by assuming a portion of the underwriting risk for a definite population and providing health care for a fixed yearly sum on each patient. A claims-review type of FMC provides for a peer review evaluation of services that are more costly than the average established for a given community. There is an incentive reimbursement for participating physicians in that they receive an income in proportion to the number of services provided. The patient is not billed for benefit services but may be billed for nonbenefit items and deductible coinsurance. Medicare and Medicaid beneficiaries may join an HMO in which case the bill is sent to the group rather than to Medicaid (MediCal). Since regular reports of ability to provide comprehensive health care must be furnished to the offices of the Department of Health and Human Services, the office must maintain complete, accurate records to continue to qualify.

Managed Care Delivery Systems ....

Preferred provider organizations (PPOs) are structured more traditionally and operate on the assumption that members will select preferred providers for most of their care. The PPO negotiates rates with hospitals and physicians on the basis that these providers will have an increase in the number of patients in return for moderate discounts. Since utilization control is necessary for successful operation in a PPO, this may be accomplished by provisions for coinsurance, deductibles, second opinion policies, and hospital admission review.

PPOs offer more flexibility to patients who are subscribers. If the patient selects a participating physician, the highest level of benefits is available. The patient understands that a lower level of benefits is available for services from a nonparticipating physician. Some states require that the higher level of benefits should be paid if the referral is made by a participating physician to a nonparticipating physician.

There are many HMOs and PPOs. There are also many different managed care delivery systems throughout the country, but HMOs are subject to both federal regulations and state laws. PPOs must adhere to state laws.

Government Health Plans ....

Workers' Compensation

Employees in the United States have the benefit of being covered by Workers' Compensation laws. For many years the name of the coverage was known as Workman's Compensation but it was changed to avoid **connotations** of sex bias. Every state has these laws to cover employees who are injured while working or become ill as a result of their work. In addition to state statutes there are federal statutes covering federal employees injured on the job—United States Longshoremen's and Harbor Workers Compensation; Federal Coal Mine Health and Safety Compensation; and special benefits for workers in the District of Columbia. The state compensation laws cover those workers not protected by federal statutes. The employer pays the premium for Workers' Compensation insurance, with the premium based on the risk involved in performance of the job.

Physicians who treat patients under Workers' Compensation plans are usually required to register with the state Workers' Compensation Board on an annual basis. The code assigned to each physician will limit care to a particular medical specialty.

There are four principal types of state benefits: (1) the patient may have medical treatment in or out of a hospital; (2) if there is determined to be a temporary disability, the patient may receive weekly cash benefits in addition to medical care; (3) when a percentage of permanent disability is found, the patient is given weekly or monthly benefits and in some cases a lump sum settlement; (4) payments are made to dependents of employees who are fatally injured. Benefits also include comprehensive vocational rehabilitation for severely disabled employees.

In most states the report of an industrial injury is initiated by the employer and sent to the physician who reports to the insurance company responsible for paying the claims, Figure 11–2, pages 166–167. A few states have their own state fund for Workers' Compensation, and in these states the forms must be forwarded to the state office responsible. Time requirements for filing a claim vary. When the physician receives the form, it is considered authorization for treatment.

A patient who has an industrial injury should have a separate file set up for that injury and a separate account card. If the patient record is required in a court case for settlement of the claim, there is no chance of violating the patient's confidence if other records are a separate file. The patient is never billed in these cases unless treatment was given without authorization or was considered excessive by the Workers' Compensation Commission, in which case the patient may be billed for the portion denied by the commission.

The medical assistant must keep current files of procedures to be followed and forms to be used as these are frequently changed. The public affairs section or office services section of your state Workers' Compensation carrier will furnish any needed information.

Patients who have a continuing partial or permanent disability must usually be reevaluated at intervals and the physician must then promptly furnish a supplemental report. The description of injuries must be exact in the written report, and in case of fracture or amputation the anatomy diagram found on the reverse side of some of the forms must be clearly marked, Figure 11–3, page 168.

The medical assistant can help ensure prompt payment by paying close attention to all necessary details in the preparation of forms. An accurate claim number must appear on all forms and the bills. The complete name of the patient, date of service, and nature of health care treatments must be on the bill. The payee number and payee name and address must be on the form and the form must be signed by the physician. One common reason for delay in payment of claims is that they are **illegible.** The forms should be typed, and to save time a rubber stamp with the name of the physician, full address, and payee number should be used on each form. The fee totals must be carefully checked for accuracy. If billing includes laboratory work or X rays, the interpretations must be attached to the bill. Any surgery billing should include a copy of the operative report. A bill may be disallowed if it is not filed within the **statutory** time limit. If your records can prove your original billing was filed within the statutory time limit, that information should be submitted for reconsideration of the claim. You should always retain a copy of your billing and be careful to avoid duplicate billing. If computerized billing is used, a code number should identify each patient.

Medicaid

Title 19 of the Medicare Act of 1965 provides for Medicaid agreements with states for low-income families, the elderly, the blind, families with dependent children, and in some states other specified individuals. The states establish eligibility requirements and these are constantly being reviewed. Eligible citizens are issued monthly cards or coupons to identify their Medicaid status. As a general rule, prior authorization is needed to provide medical treatment except in an emergency. There are usually time limits for submission of claims. Again, the medical assistant must be aware of current rules for submitting claims. You should always check carefully to see if the card is current so that your office can be reimbursed for services. One of the important functions of the medical assistant is to assure the patient that the physician gives the same quality care to all patients regardless of their financial status.

Medicare

Medicare is a program of health insurance under Social Security for people over the age of 65 who are eligible and who have filed. The disabled or those insured under the Social Security retirement system are eligible as well as kidney dialysis or replacement patients. The patient should show you the red-white-and-blue membership card indicating coverage, Figure 11–4, page 169.

APPLICATION for payments of Medical Benefits Only

Claim Number (B.W.C. use only)

- This form is to be used in injury cases where only medical expenses are involved. (Seven calendar days of disability or less.)
- No compensation for lost time will be paid on this application
- Incomplete and/or improper completion of this form will result in a delay in processing
- Mail completed application to: Bureau of Workers' Compensation Claims Section 246 North High Street, Columbus, Ohio 43215

PART I *(Items 1 through 18 are to be completed by the Employee) Please Print or Type*

		Do Not Use This Column
Employee's Name **John Steele**	Social Security Number **410-20-9821**	Claim No.
Home Address (Number & Street) **410 N. Tony Road** / Apartment No.	Telephone No. & Area Code **(614)431-4495**	Claimant Name
City, State, Zip Code **Columbus, Ohio 43294** / County **Franklin**	Sex ☒ Male ☐ Female	Filing Date
Marital Status **Married** / Birth Date **10/6/48** / Age **40**	Number of Dependents **2**	Last Date Worked
Employer's Name **Moon Battery Company**	Employer's Telephone No. **(614)899-7776**	Return to Work Date
Employer's Address **79 S. 4th Street**	County **Franklin**	Date of Death
City, State, Zip Code **Columbus, Ohio 43205**	Length of time on job which injury occurred **7 years**	Full Weekly Wage **000000**
Your Occupation (Job Title) **Plant Superintendent**		Average Weekly Wage **000000**

PERSONAL / EMPLOYER / ACCIDENT/INJURY INFORMATION / CERTIFICATION

Date & Time of Accident **11/4/88 8:30 A.M.** / Date & Time Reported to Employer **11/4 9.00 A.M.** / Last Date Worked **11/4/88**	Date Returned to Work **11/9/88**
Accident Location (Street, Number, City, State, Zip Code) **Battery department 79 S. 4th. 43205**	Was Accident actually on Employer's premises? ☒ Yes ☐ No

Witnesses' Name(s), Address(es) and Phone No(s). (Attach additional sheet if needed)
John Wang, 2349 E. Remington Rd., 43295 441-0050

Hospital—if any (Name, Address, City, State, Zip Code)

Attending Physician (Name, Address, City, State, Zip Code, Phone No.)
I. M. Healthy, M.D., 350 E. Broad Street, Columbus, Ohio 43209 (614)463-1234

Describe Accident: In detail describe the events which resulted in the injury. What happened? How did it happen? If you were lifting an object, state approximate size, weight, and distance lifted. (Attach additional sheet if needed)

walking through battery department, slipped and fell on wet floor, pain in left knee, turned left ankle.

Do Not Use This Column (right):
- Clt. Coun/Acc. Loc.
- Clt. Sx/Mar.St./Age
- Dependents
- Occ./Job Time
- Acc. Time
- Claimant Rep.
- Nature of Injury
- Part of Body
- Source of Injury
- Exposure Type
- Wages/Sick W./Org. -9-
- Received BWC

Give exact nature of injuries (amputation, laceration, fracture, etc.) and exact parts of body affected (first joint of left index finger, right lower leg, lower right side of back, etc.) (Attach additional sheet if needed)

Nature of Injury	Part of Body	Nature of Injury	Part of Body
1. contusion	left knee	4.	
2. sprain	left ankle	5.	
3.		6.	

B.W.C. Use Only

	Yes	No
Have you ever filed a previous application for this injury?	☐ Yes	☒ No
Did you receive your wages during this disability?	☒ Yes	☐ No
Have you filed any other claims with the Bureau or Industrial Commission?	☐ Yes	☒ No

(If yes, give claim number(s) and parts of body injured)

READ CAREFULLY BEFORE SIGNING

I hereby apply for recognition of my claim under the Ohio Workers' Compensation Act for injuries which I did not purposely self-inflict and request payment as provided under the Act for medical expenses as allowable on this form.

By signing this application I expressly waive all provisions of law which forbid any person, persons, or medical facility who heretofore did or who hereafter may medically attend, treat or examine me or who may have information of any kind which may be used to render a decision in my claim from disclosing such knowledge or information to the Bureau of Workers' Compensation, or Industrial Commission.

To expedite this claim, if it is allowed, I waive any notices to which I may be entitled for hearings. Direct payment to the provider of any medical services is authorized.

Claimant's Signature *John Steele*   Date **11/4/88**

Date Coded / Coded By / Manual No. / Risk No.

BWC-1106 (Rev. 12/83)
C3

FIGURE 11–2 First report form for Workers' Compensation for payment of medical fee only (Courtesy of Ohio Bureau of Workers' Compensation)

Part A Medicare is for hospital coverage, and any person who is receiving monthly Social Security is automatically enrolled. The deductible amount has increased each year. Many patients now feel it is necessary to carry a supplemental insurance plan to pay that deductible amount. One such plan by Blue Cross is called *Medi-Fill*. The term *Medigap* is also used to describe this supplemental insurance program.

Part B of Medicare is for payment of medical expenses outside the hospital, including office visits and the services of a physician in or out of the hospital. The premiums are automatically deducted for those who wish the coverage

PART II *(Items 19 through 24 must be completed by the Employer)*

19 Name of Employer (Must be exactly as shown on Certificate) Moon Battery Company		Area Code-Telephone Number (614)899-7776
20 Business Address (Number, Street, City, State, Zip Code) 79 S. 4th Street, Columbus, Ohio 43205		Federal I.D. or Social Security Number 00-000000
21 Nature of Business (farming, coal mining, etc.) Battery manufacturing	Was claimant... ☐ Owner of Business ☐ Partner ☒ Member of Firm	B.W.C. Use Only
22 Type of Organization (Partnership, Corporation, etc.)-If Public Employer, indicate type of jurisdiction (School Board, City, Township) Company		
23 The earnings of the injured employee for services rendered at the time of injury were being reported on the payroll reports of ... ▶	Risk No. 456789 Manual No. 8410	

READ CAREFULLY BEFORE SIGNING (This section must be completed)

By signing below I hereby certify that I have authority to execute this Employer's Report and the answers in this Employer's Report are correct to the best of my information and belief.

(Employer Note: If neither box below is checked, the Bureau will assume that the employer signed to the "Full Certification" as enumerated in the 1st paragraph below and the Bureau will process this claim accordingly.)

CHECK WHICHEVER APPLIES

Full Certification ☒ This employer further certifies that the facts set forth in this application are correct and the claim, for Medical Expenses Only, is valid. The Employer hereby waives notice of receipt from the Bureau of Workers' Compensation of this claim application and order approving its payment, as provided in O.R.C. 4123.512-513, in order that Medical Expenses be promptly paid.

24 Rejection of Claim ☐ The Employer rejects the validity of this claim for the following reasons: _____

Signature *John Doe*	Date 11/5/88	Name & Title John Doe, President Moon Battery Company Department

PART III *The attending Physician should complete items 25 through 31 and return this form to the employer within two (2) weeks of the date of the first treatment. If further treatment is needed use form C-19 for future billings. (If space on this form is inadequate you may attach additional sheet.)*

25 Give coded diagnosis (written description and appropriate numeric code using ICD-9-CM Manual, 9th Edition International Classification of Diseases.

924.11 Contusion left knee
845.01 Sprain left ankle

26 Give Names and Addresses of parties rendering services ordered by you (Hospital, X-ray, Ambulance, etc.)
I.M.Healthy, M.D. 350 E. Broad Street, Columbus, Ohio 43209

27 Is further treatment or medication indicated? ☐ Yes ☒ No If yes, give brief prognosis

28 ITEMIZED FEE BILL (first fee bill for no more than 2 weeks treatment)

Date	Place	Service Description	Amount
11/4/88	office	x-ray examination left knee	30.00
		x-ray examination left ankle	30.00
		examination left knee and ankle	50.00

29 If any part of this bill has been paid, indicate amount .... $

And by whom paid ▶ Name _____
(Name, Address, Zip Code)   Address _____

TOTAL CHARGES $ 110.

30 | Payee Number
34776-01 | Billing Code or Date
11/10/88 | Federal I.D. Number
11-000000 | B.W.C. Use Only |

Physician's Name, Address, City, State, Zip Code-Phone Number (Please Print, Stamp or Type)
I. M. Healthy, M.D., 350 E. Broad St., Columbus, OH 43209

31 I hereby certify that the information on this report is true and correct to the best of my knowledge and belief.

Physician's Signature *I. M. Healthy* Must Be in Physician's own handwriting   Date *11/10/88*

PART IV – EMERGENCY SERVICE ONLY *The hospital providing emergency service should complete items 32 through 36 and return form to employer upon release of patient.*

32 | Date of Service | Service Performed |

33 Check appropriate service furnished ☐ Production of x-ray plate ☐ X-ray interpretation .... Give brief x-ray interpretation

34 If any part of this bill has been paid indicate amount .... $
And by whom paid ▶ Name _____
(Name, Address, Zip Code)   Address _____

TOTAL CHARGES $

35 | Payee Number | Billing Code or Date | Federal I.D. Number | B.W.C. Use Only |

36 Hospital Name, Address, City, State, Zip and Phone Number (Please Print, Stamp or Type)

by _____   Signature of Hospital Billing Officer   Date _____

FIGURE 11–2 (continued)
First report form for Workers' Compensation for payment of medical fee only (Courtesy of Ohio Bureau of Workers' Compensation)

and are on Social Security, railroad retirement, or civil service annuity. Other individuals who are eligible pay premiums directly to the Social Security Administration.

Remember that Medicare B is the coverage that will pay for visits to the physician's office. If you are to assume responsibility for completing the forms, be sure to enter the Medicare identification card number in your records for the patient. The number is the Social Security number followed by a letter. A husband and wife will have separate cards.

Many physicians ask the patient to pay when examined and collect from Medicare for the allowed amount.

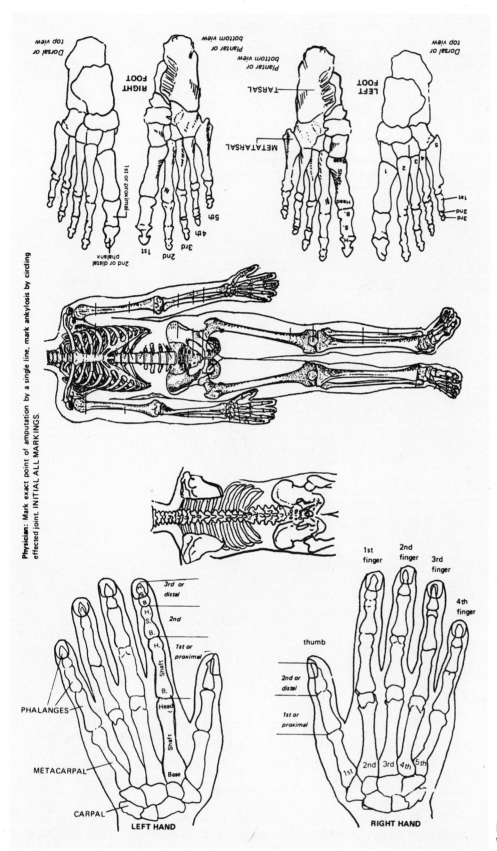

FIGURE 11–3 Anatomy chart for Workers' Compensation

After the deductible amount is met Medicare will pay 80% of the covered costs. The Omnibus Budget Reconciliation Act (OBRA) of 1989 requires that all physi- cians and suppliers submit Medicare claims for their patients since September 1990. Physicians and suppli- ers are not responsible for filing the Medicare claim if the service is not covered by Medicare or for other health insurance claims. Claims must be filed within a year of the time the service is received by the patient. In some cases the Medicare insurance carrier will automatically send the amount not covered on to the private insurance carrier, which will pay the deductible and the 20% not covered with no need to fill out additional forms.

Physicians who treat Medicare patients have the option to decline an assignment. If the physician wishes to receive the check, assignment always must be checked "yes" and Medicare will pay 80% of the approved amount after the deductible for the year has been met. Medicare will reject the claim if the physician has agreed to accept assignment and the form has not been filled out completely to reflect this fact.

Physician payment reform (PPR) is another part of OBRA passed by Congress, which will make sweeping changes in the payment of physician services by Medicare Part B.

- The PPR payment will be based on a fee schedule, which will be formed using a resource-based relative value system.
- Medicare volume performance standards (MVPS) have been established to track annual increases in Medicare Part B benefit payments for physician services and levels for future years.
- Various financial protections for the beneficiary have been developed.
- Payment and medical policies used by Medicare carriers will be more standardized.

Although all physicians are paid on a fee schedule basis, which began in January 1992, the fee schedule amounts for some services are subject to a 5-year transition policy to avoid extreme changes in the Medicare payment amount.

You must know and understand the current law because the physician who accepts assignment must accept the lower payment. If you have a computer billing system with a program to write off a certain percentage on Medicare claims, you will need to adjust your program each time a new law readjusts the reimbursement percentage.

The patient pays the 20% of charges that Medicare does not cover. It is important for you to have a record of any other insurance coverage the patient has to cover the deductible and the 20% coinsurance. If you have a patient on Medicare who is unable to pay the 20% coinsurance, the patient may be eligible for Medicaid. In this case, Medicare is the primary insurer and the balance would be billed to Medicaid. You would need to see both cards to establish that this is the case. The medical assistant should make a copy of the cards to keep on file.

Current Medicare requirements specify that nonparticipating physicians must notify all patients, in writing, of the surgeon's estimated charge, the estimated Medicare

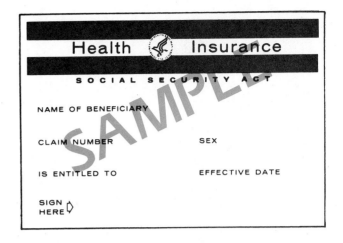

FIGURE 11–4 Medicare identification card (Courtesy of Social Security Administration)

allowable charge, and the difference between the two in advance of elective operations that involve charges over $500. Preprinted forms will help you comply with this requirement, Figure 11–5, page 170.

Claims received after May 1, 1992 must be submitted on the original HCFA–1500 claim form. Copies will not be accepted and will be returned for both assigned and nonassigned claims. You will need to check with the insurance carrier who pays the Medicare claims to find out the approved printers of the HCFA–1500 claim form.

The Health Care Financing Administration (HCFA) has designated the HCFA–1500 as the uniform health claims processing form, Figure 11–6, pages 171–172, and requires all Medicare contractors to use it. The special bar code at the top of the form allows the claims processor to assign a unique identification number to the claim during microfilming.

Medical assistants who submit Medicare insurance claims with the stamped statement "patient's signature on file" must be prepared to make these files available in the event the files are audited by the insurance carrier. The only time a signature is not needed is when a patient has services performed without being physically present in the office. An example of this would be the laboratory where a specimen collected in the physician's office was analyzed. In this case, the insurance form should state "Patient not physically present for services." Signatures of welfare patients are not required if the state agency maintains records of the signatures. It was suggested by Nationwide Mutual Insurance Company in a *Medicare Newsletter* that the office have a form prepared for the signature of Medicare patients. This could be signed once and kept on file and it would not be necessary to obtain the signature of the patient on every form. The form should list the name and Medicare claim number of the patient along with the following statement:

I request that payment of authorized Medicare benefits be made either to me or on my behalf to Dr._____ for

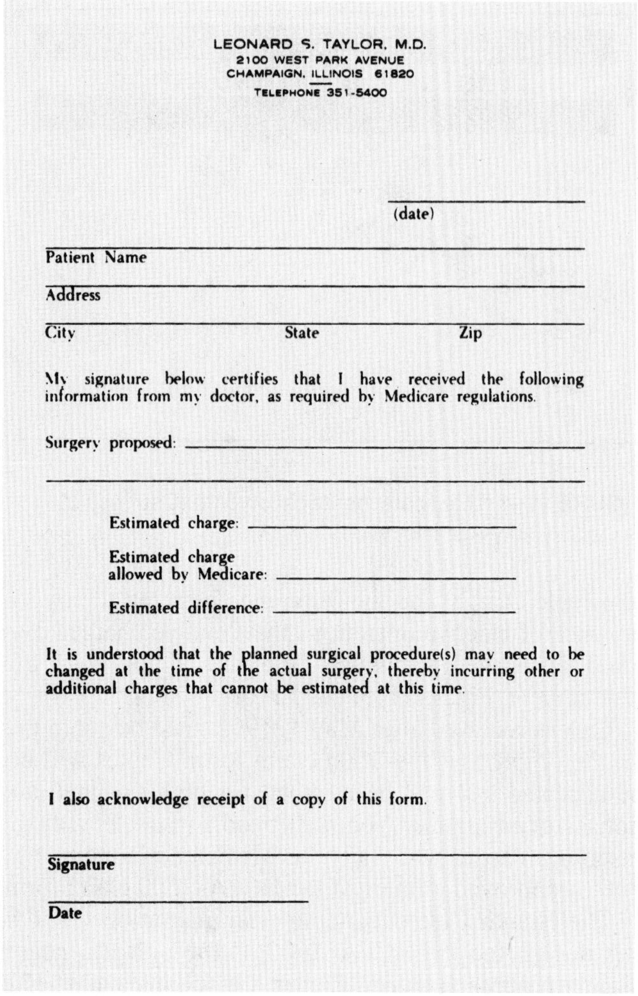

LEONARD S. TAYLOR, M.D.
2100 WEST PARK AVENUE
CHAMPAIGN, ILLINOIS 61820
TELEPHONE 351-5400

_____
(date)

Patient Name _____

Address _____

City _____ State _____ Zip _____

My signature below certifies that I have received the following
information from my doctor, as required by Medicare regulations.

Surgery proposed: _____

_____

Estimated charge: _____

Estimated charge
allowed by Medicare: _____

Estimated difference: _____

It is understood that the planned surgical procedure(s) may need to be
changed at the time of the actual surgery, thereby incurring other or
additional charges that cannot be estimated at this time.

I also acknowledge receipt of a copy of this form.

Signature _____

_____
Date

FIGURE 11–5 Form for estimate of surgery charges for Medicare patient (Courtesy of Colwell Systems, Inc.)

any service furnished me by that physician. I authorize release to the Health Care Financing Administration and its agents any medical information about me needed to determine these benefits or benefits payable for related services.

The form should be signed by the patient and dated.

The HCFA has developed codes for Medicare that allow for uniformity throughout the country. The three levels of codes range as follows:

1. CPT codes established and updated by the American Medical Association. These are five digit numeric codes ranging from 00000 to 99999 for physicians' services, such as examinations, surgeries, radiology, and pathology. Most Medicare B coverage is covered by CPT codes.
2. HCPCS codes are established and updated by HCFA. These alpha-numeric codes range from A0000 to V9999 and are used for physician and non-physician services not listed in the CPT.
3. W0000 to Z9999 are reserved for local assignment.

These codes are not present in CPT and are not common to all carriers.

Other codes which may be necessary to complete insurance forms are the Unique Physician's Identifying Number (UPIN), which is one letter and five digits. The UPIN of the referring physician must be included for any consultations and for physical therapy. The physician's identifying number (PIN), which is two letters and seven digits, must be filled in at Block 33 on the current form HCFA–1500.

In processing Medicare insurance forms, you must use ICDA codes for diagnosis, CPT codes for treatment, and HCPCS codes for any supplies or appliances used. Coding is discussed in more detail in Unit 3.

CHAMPUS

As part of the United States Department of Defense, the Civilian Health and Medical Program of the Uniformed Services (CHAMPUS) was established to aid dependents of active service personnel, retired service personnel and their dependents, and dependents of service personnel who died on active duty, with a supplement for medical care in military or Public Health Service facilities. The word *dependents* refers to spouses and dependent children only; this program does not cover active duty military personnel. All members of CHAMPUS over the age of 10 are issued an identification card. A patient who lives within 40 miles of a uniformed services hospital will need a *nonavailability statement* to be cared for in a civilian or physician's office. This simply means that the necessary services are not available at the service hospital or that for medical reasons it would be better to continue care under the civilian physician who has been treating the patient. Authorization is not necessary if the patient lives more than 40 miles from a military medical facility that could furnish the necessary care.

The Civilian Health and Medical Program of the Veterans' Administration (CHAMPVA) was established in 1973 for the spouses and dependent children of veterans who have total, permanent, service-connected disabilities. This service is also available for the surviving spouses and dependent children of veterans who have died as a result of service-connected disabilities. The local VA hospital determines eligibility and then issues identification cards. The insured members can then choose their own private physicians. There are deductibles and cost-sharing requirements your office needs to be aware of.

If your office needs additional information on military benefit programs, you can contact your local health benefits advisor (HBA) at the nearest military hospital or clinic or the office of CHAMPUS, Aurora, CO 80045-6900. The CHAMPUS phone number is (303) 361-3907; the phone number for CHAMPVA is (303) 782-3804.

APPROVED OMB-0938-0008

CARRIER →

HEALTH INSURANCE CLAIM FORM

| | PICA | | | | | | PICA | |

1. MEDICARE	MEDICAID	CHAMPUS	CHAMPVA	GROUP HEALTH PLAN (SSN or ID)	FECA BLK LUNG (SSN)	OTHER	1a. INSURED'S I.D. NUMBER	(FOR PROGRAM IN ITEM 1)
(Medicare #)	(Medicaid #)	(Sponsor's SSN)	(VA File #)			(ID)		

2. PATIENT'S NAME (Last Name, First Name, Middle Initial)

3. PATIENT'S BIRTH DATE
MM | DD | YY   SEX
M   F

4. INSURED'S NAME (Last Name, First Name, Middle Initial)

5. PATIENT'S ADDRESS (No., Street)

6. PATIENT RELATIONSHIP TO INSURED
Self   Spouse   Child   Other

7. INSURED'S ADDRESS (No., Street)

CITY   STATE

8. PATIENT STATUS
Single   Married   Other

Employed   Full-Time Student   Part-Time Student

CITY   STATE

ZIP CODE   TELEPHONE (Include Area Code)
(   )

ZIP CODE   TELEPHONE (INCLUDE AREA CODE)
(   )

9. OTHER INSURED'S NAME (Last Name, First Name, Middle Initial)

10. IS PATIENT'S CONDITION RELATED TO:

11. INSURED'S POLICY GROUP OR FECA NUMBER

a. OTHER INSURED'S POLICY OR GROUP NUMBER

a. EMPLOYMENT? (CURRENT OR PREVIOUS)
YES   NO

a. INSURED'S DATE OF BIRTH
MM | DD | YY   SEX
M   F

b. OTHER INSURED'S DATE OF BIRTH
MM | DD | YY   SEX
M   F

b. AUTO ACCIDENT?   PLACE (State)
YES   NO

b. EMPLOYER'S NAME OR SCHOOL NAME

c. EMPLOYER'S NAME OR SCHOOL NAME

c. OTHER ACCIDENT?
YES   NO

c. INSURANCE PLAN NAME OR PROGRAM NAME

d. INSURANCE PLAN NAME OR PROGRAM NAME

10d. RESERVED FOR LOCAL USE

d. IS THERE ANOTHER HEALTH BENEFIT PLAN?
YES   NO   If yes, return to and complete item 9 a-d.

PATIENT AND INSURED INFORMATION →

READ BACK OF FORM BEFORE COMPLETING & SIGNING THIS FORM.
12. PATIENT'S OR AUTHORIZED PERSON'S SIGNATURE I authorize the release of any medical or other information necessary to process this claim. I also request payment of government benefits either to myself or to the party who accepts assignment below.

SIGNED _____ DATE _____

13. INSURED'S OR AUTHORIZED PERSON'S SIGNATURE I authorize payment of medical benefits to the undersigned physician or supplier for services described below.

SIGNED _____

| 14. DATE OF CURRENT: ILLNESS (First symptom) OR INJURY (Accident) OR PREGNANCY(LMP) MM | DD | YY | 15. IF PATIENT HAS HAD SAME OR SIMILAR ILLNESS. GIVE FIRST DATE MM | DD | YY | 16. DATES PATIENT UNABLE TO WORK IN CURRENT OCCUPATION MM | DD | YY FROM TO MM | DD | YY |

17. NAME OF REFERRING PHYSICIAN OR OTHER SOURCE

17a. I.D. NUMBER OF REFERRING PHYSICIAN

18. HOSPITALIZATION DATES RELATED TO CURRENT SERVICES
MM | DD | YY   MM | DD | YY
FROM   TO

19. RESERVED FOR LOCAL USE

20. OUTSIDE LAB? $ CHARGES
YES   NO

21. DIAGNOSIS OR NATURE OF ILLNESS OR INJURY. (RELATE ITEMS 1,2,3 OR 4 TO ITEM 24E BY LINE)

1. |___.___| 3. |___.___|

2. |___.___| 4. |___.___|

22. MEDICAID RESUBMISSION CODE   ORIGINAL REF. NO.

23. PRIOR AUTHORIZATION NUMBER

24. A DATE(S) OF SERVICE From To MM DD YY MM DD YY	B Place of Service	C Type of Service	D PROCEDURES, SERVICES, OR SUPPLIES (Explain Unusual Circumstances) CPT/HCPCS	MODIFIER	E DIAGNOSIS CODE	F $ CHARGES	G DAYS OR UNITS	H EPSDT Family Plan	I EMG	J COB	K RESERVED FOR LOCAL USE
1											
2											
3											
4											
5											
6											

| 25. FEDERAL TAX I.D. NUMBER   SSN EIN | 26. PATIENT'S ACCOUNT NO. | 27. ACCEPT ASSIGNMENT? (For govt. claims, see back) YES   NO | 28. TOTAL CHARGE $ | 29. AMOUNT PAID $ | 30. BALANCE DUE $ |

31. SIGNATURE OF PHYSICIAN OR SUPPLIER INCLUDING DEGREES OR CREDENTIALS (I certify that the statements on the reverse apply to this bill and are made a part thereof.)

SIGNED _____ DATE _____

32. NAME AND ADDRESS OF FACILITY WHERE SERVICES WERE RENDERED (If other than home or office)

33. PHYSICIAN'S, SUPPLIER'S BILLING NAME, ADDRESS, ZIP CODE & PHONE #

PIN#   GRP#

PHYSICIAN OR SUPPLIER INFORMATION →

(APPROVED BY AMA COUNCIL ON MEDICAL SERVICE 8/88)

PLEASE PRINT OR TYPE

FORM HCFA-1500 (U2) (12-90)
FORM OWCP-1500   FORM RRB-1500

FIGURE 11-6a   Health insurance claim form (Courtesy of Colwell Systems, Inc.)

BECAUSE THIS FORM IS USED BY VARIOUS GOVERNMENT AND PRIVATE HEALTH PROGRAMS, SEE SEPARATE INSTRUCTIONS ISSUED BY APPLICABLE PROGRAMS.

NOTICE: Any person who knowingly files a statement of claim containing any misrepresentation or any false, incomplete or misleading information may be guilty of a criminal act punishable under law and may be subject to civil penalties.

REFERS TO GOVERNMENT PROGRAMS ONLY

MEDICARE AND CHAMPUS PAYMENTS: A patient's signature requests that payment be made and authorizes release of any information necessary to process the claim and certifies that the information provided in Blocks 1 through 12 is true, accurate and complete. In the case of a Medicare claim, the patient's signature authorizes any entity to release to Medicare medical and nonmedical information, including employment status, and whether the person has employer group health insurance, liability, no-fault, worker's compensation or other insurance which is responsible to pay for the services for which the Medicare claim is made. See 42 CFR 411.24(a). If item 9 is completed, the patient's signature authorizes release of the information to the health plan or agency shown. In Medicare assigned or CHAMPUS participation cases, the physician agrees to accept the charge determination of the Medicare carrier or CHAMPUS fiscal intermediary as the full charge, and the patient is responsible only for the deductible, coinsurance and noncovered services. Coinsurance and the deductible are based upon the charge determination of the Medicare carrier or CHAMPUS fiscal intermediary if this is less than the charge submitted. CHAMPUS is not a health insurance program but makes payment for health benefits provided through certain affiliations with the Uniformed Services. Information on the patient's sponsor should be provided in those items captioned in "Insured"; i.e., items 1a, 4, 6, 7, 9, and 11.

BLACK LUNG AND FECA CLAIMS

The provider agrees to accept the amount paid by the Government as payment in full. See Black Lung and FECA instructions regarding required procedure and diagnosis coding systems.

SIGNATURE OF PHYSICIAN OR SUPPLIER (MEDICARE, CHAMPUS, FECA AND BLACK LUNG)

I certify that the services shown on this form were medically indicated and necessary for the health of the patient and were personally furnished by me or were furnished incident to my professional service by my employee under my immediate personal supervision, except as otherwise expressly permitted by Medicare or CHAMPUS regulations.

For services to be considered as "incident" to a physician's professional service, 1) they must be rendered under the physician's immediate personal supervision by his/her employee, 2) they must be an integral, although incidental part of a covered physician's service, 3) they must be of kinds commonly furnished in physician's offices, and 4) the services of nonphysicians must be included on the physician's bills.

For CHAMPUS claims, I further certify that I (or any employee) who rendered services am not an active duty member of the Uniformed Services or a civilian employee of the United States Government or a contract employee of the United States Government, either civilian or military (refer to 5 USC 5536). For Black-Lung claims, I further certify that the services performed were for a Black Lung-related disorder.

No Part B Medicare benefits may be paid unless this form is received as required by existing law and regulations (42 CFR 424.32).

NOTICE: Any one who misrepresents or falsifies essential information to receive payment from Federal funds requested by this form may upon conviction be subject to fine and imprisonment under applicable Federal laws.

NOTICE TO PATIENT ABOUT THE COLLECTION AND USE OF MEDICARE, CHAMPUS, FECA, AND BLACK LUNG INFORMATION
(PRIVACY ACT STATEMENT)

We are authorized by HCFA, CHAMPUS and OWCP to ask you for information needed in the administration of the Medicare, CHAMPUS, FECA, and Black Lung programs. Authority to collect information is in section 205(a), 1862, 1872 and 1874 of the Social Security Act as amended, 42 CFR 411.24(a) and 424.5(a) (6), and 44 USC 3101;41 CFR 101 et seq and 10 USC 1079 and 1086; 5 USC 8101 et seq; and 30 USC 901 et seq; 38 USC 613; E.O. 9397.

The information we obtain to complete claims under these programs is used to identify you and to determine your eligibility. It is also used to decide if the services and supplies you received are covered by these programs and to insure that proper payment is made.

The information may also be given to other providers of services, carriers, intermediaries, medical review boards, health plans, and other organizations or Federal agencies, for the effective administration of Federal provisions that require other third parties payers to pay primary to Federal program, and as otherwise necessary to administer these programs. For example, it may be necessary to disclose information about the benefits you have used to a hospital or doctor. Additional disclosures are made through routine uses for information contained in systems of records.

FOR MEDICARE CLAIMS: See the notice modifying system No. 09-70-0501, titled, 'Carrier Medicare Claims Record,' published in the <u>Federal Register</u>, Vol. 55 No. 177, page 37549, Wed. Sept. 12, 1990, or as updated and republished.

FOR OWCP CLAIMS: Department of Labor, Privacy Act of 1974, "Republication of Notice of Systems of Records." <u>Federal Register</u> Vol. 55 No. 40, Wed Feb. 28, 1990, See ESA-5, ESA-6, ESA-12, ESA-13, ESA-30, or as updated and republished.

FOR CHAMPUS CLAIMS: <u>PRINCIPLE PURPOSE(S):</u> To evaluate eligibility for medical care provided by civilian sources and to issue payment upon establishment of eligibility and determination that the services/supplies received are authorized by law.

<u>ROUTINE USE(S):</u> Information from claims and related documents may be given to the Dept. of Veterans Affairs, the Dept. of Health and Human Services and/or the Dept. of Transportation consistent with their statutory administrative responsibilities under CHAMPUS/CHAMPVA; to the Dept. of Justice for representation of the Secretary of Defense in civil actions; to the Internal Revenue Service, private collection agencies, and consumer reporting agencies in connection with recoupment claims; and to Congressional Offices in response to inquiries made at the request of the person to whom a record pertains. Appropriate disclosures may be made to other federal, state, local, foreign government agencies, private business entities, and individual providers of care, on matters relating to entitlement, claims adjudication, fraud, program abuse, utilization review, quality assurance, peer review, program integrity, third-party liability, coordination of benefits, and civil and criminal litigation related to the operation of CHAMPUS.

<u>DISCLOSURES:</u> Voluntary; however, failure to provide information will result in delay in payment or may result in denial of claim. With the one exception discussed below, there are no penalties under these programs for refusing to supply information. However, failure to furnish information regarding the medical services rendered or the amount charged would prevent payment of claims under these programs. Failure to furnish any other information, such as name or claim number, would delay payment of the claim. Failure to provide medical information under FECA could be deemed an obstruction.

It is mandatory that you tell us if you know that another party is responsible for paying for your treatment. Section 1128B of the Social Security Act and 31 USC 3801-3812 provide penalties for withholding this information.

You should be aware that P.L. 100-503, the "Computer Matching and Privacy Protection Act of 1988", permits the government to verify information by way of computer matches.

MEDICAID PAYMENTS (PROVIDER CERTIFICATION)

I hereby agree to keep such records as are necessary to disclose fully the extent of services provided to individuals under the State's Title XIX plan and to furnish information regarding any payments claimed for providing such services as the State Agency or Dept. of Health and Humans Services may request.

I further agree to accept, as payment in full, the amount paid by the Medicaid program for those claims submitted for payment under that program, with the exception of authorized deductible, coinsurance, co-payment or similar cost-sharing charge.

SIGNATURE OF PHYSICIAN (OR SUPPLIER): I certify that the services listed above were medically indicated and necessary to the health of this patient and were personally furnished by me or my employee under my personal direction.

NOTICE: This is to certify that the foregoing information is true, accurate and complete. I understand that payment and satisfaction of this claim will be from Federal and State funds, and that any false claims, statements, or documents, or concealment of a material fact, may be prosecuted under applicable Federal or State laws.

Public reporting burden for this collection of information is estimated to average 15 minutes per response, including time for reviewing instructions, searching existing date sources, gathering and maintaining data needed, and completing and reviewing the collection of information. Send comments regarding this burden estimate or any other aspect of this collection of information, including suggestions for reducing the burden, to HCFA, Office of Financial Management, P.O. Box 26684, Baltimore, MD 21207; and to the Office of Management and Budget, Paperwork Reduction Project (OMB-0938-0008), Washington, D.C. 20503.

FIGURE 11–6b   Health insurance claim form (Courtesy of Colwell Systems, Inc.)

Easter Seal/Crippled Children

All states operate Crippled Children's Services with federal support under Title V of the Social Security Act. The intent of this service is to locate crippled children under 21 or those who have potentially crippling conditions to see that appropriate health care is furnished. Part or all of this treatment may be paid for if the family's resources are not adequate. Some Crippled Children's Services are being changed to Easter Seal rehabilitation centers because of the stigma attached to the words *crippled children*. Some Easter Seal rehabilitation centers are now operated as private nonprofit organizations.

Complete Chapter 11, Unit 2 in the workbook to help you meet the objectives at the beginning of this unit and therefore achieve competency of this subject matter.

UNIT 3
Coding Systems

OBJECTIVES ....

Upon completion of this unit, the student will meet the following terminal performance objectives by verifying knowledge of the facts and principles presented through oral and written communication at a level deemed competent, and will demonstrate the specific behaviors as identified in the pupil performance objectives of the procedures.

1. Describe coding systems for professional services.
2. Describe the advantages of the standard health insurance claim form.
3. List the common errors causing claim payment delays.
4. Define the purpose of coding.
5. Describe the method of following up claims when payment has not been received within 30 days.
6. Spell and define, using the glossary at the back of the text, all the words to know in this unit.

WORDS TO KNOW ....

complexity   nomenclature

The medical assistant must use great care in the completion of claim forms so that the insurance company can understand the complexity of surgical procedures or medical care given to the patient. The companies that process insurance claims are using computers and optical scanning equipment in processing payment of claims. This processing is improved by the use of numerical designations in place of the usual medical terminology to describe diseases, injuries, surgery, and procedures. Sometimes it is necessary to put several code numbers rather than a single overall diagnosis to justify a charge. The most important diagnosis must be listed first. Secondary diagnoses and procedures follow in order of importance.

The purpose of coding is to unify data for reporting, compiling, and comparing of health care information for statistical evaluation, clinical use, and reimbursement.

Coding is transforming verbal and/or written descriptions of diseases, injuries, and procedures into numerical designations to meet internal and external demands for medical information. Coding must be performed accurately and precisely if meaningful profiles are to be established. The use of vague terminology places you at a considerable risk in the development of future "fee profiles."

To become a proficient coder, two things are necessary: a working knowledge of medical terminology and an understanding of ICD-9 characteristics, terminology, and conventions.

The general coding rules are:

1. Code correctly and completely any diagnosis or procedure that affects the care, influences the health status, or is a reason for treatment on that visit.
2. Code the minimum number of diagnoses that fully describe the patient's care received on that visit. For example, the diagnosis must reflect the patient's need for treatment, X rays, diagnostic procedures, or medications.
3. Code each problem to the highest level of specification (3rd, 4th, 5th digit) available in the classification.
4. Codes must be sequenced correctly so that it is possible to understand the chronology of events, for example, reason for visit and patient care.

The following are the four basic steps to obtain the correct code for a diagnostic statement:

1. Analyze the medical terminology (identify the main term in a physician's statement).
2. Locate the main terms in the Alphabetic Index (Volume 2 of ICD book).
3. Assign a tentative code using the Alphabetic Index.
4. Check the code against the Tabular List (Volume 1 of ICD book) to verify that it is the accurate code for the described disorder according to the classification.

In the following statements, the key words are italicized:

1. Acute *arthropathy* associated with infection (rheumatic *fever*).
2. *Migraine* versus acute frontal *sinusitis*.
3. *Fibrocystic* disease of breast.
4. *Irritable* colon.
5. Urinary tract *infection* due to E. coli.

Some of the specialty academies are now printing special notebooks listing ICD diagnostic codes and the CPT codes which would commonly accompany each diagnosis. The following list might be a sample of the ICD diagnostic codes to be used by a medical clinic.

789.0	Abdominal pain
530.0	Achalasia esophagus
253.0	Acromegaly
255.4	Addison's disease
791.0	Albuminuria
303.90	Alcoholism, chronic
626.0	Amenorrhea
565.0	Anal fissure
280.9	Anemia, hypochromic iron def.
281.0	Anemia, pernicious
285.9	Anemia, unspecified
441.9	Aneurysm, aortic
413.9	Angina pectoris
783.0	Anorexia
300.0	Anxiety reaction and state
424.1	Aortic endocarditis stenosis
540.9	Appendicitis, acute
447.1	Arterial insufficiency
719.4	Arthralgia
716.9	Arthritis, acute
274.0	Arthritis, gouty
715.9	Arthritis, osteo.
714.0	Arthritis, rheumatoid
721.90	Arthritis, spine
789.5	Ascites
493.9	Asthma
518.0	Atelectasis
427.31	Arterial auricular fibril.
426.10	A V heart block
791.9	Azotemia
724.5	Back pain
351.0	Bell's palsy
533.40	Bleeding ulcer
560.9	Bowel obstruction
494	Bronchiectasis
466.0	Bronchitis, acute
491	Bronchitis, chronic
485	Bronchopneumonia
727.1	Bunion
726.10	Bursitis, shoulder

174.9	CA breast
153.9	CA colon
189.0	CA kidney
162.9	CA lung
183.0	CA ovary
185	CA prostate
154.0	CA rectosigmoid junction
154.1	CA rectum
151.9	CA stomach
592.9	Calculi, urinary system
429.3	Cardiomegaly
366.9	Cataract
682.9	Cellulitis
343.9	Cerebral palsy
437.9	Cerebral vasc. insufficiency
380.4	Cerumen in ears
622.7	Cervical polyp
723.8	Cervical root syndrome
722.4	Cervical spine disc disease
847.0	Cervical strain
616.0	Cervicitis
786.5	Chest pain
575.1	Cholecystitis
574.20	Cholelithiasis
310.9	Chronic brain syndrome
786.2	Chronic cough
582.9	Chronic glomerulonephritis
496	Chronic obstructive pul. dis.
571.5	Cirrhosis, liver and portal
443.9	Claudication
556	Colitis, ulcerative
460	Common head cold
310.2	Concussion syndrome
428.0	Congestive heart failure
372.30	Conjunctivitis
564.0	Constipation
780.3	Convulsion
414.0	Coronary artery disease
416.9	Cor. pulmonale
255.0	Cushing's syndrome
436	CVA
595.0	Cystitis, acute
618.0	Cystocele, female
389.9	Deafness
311	Depression

300.4	Depressive reaction
618.1	Descensus uteri
250	Diabetes mellitus
250.0	Diabetes mellitus w/o comp.
250.60	Diabetes neuropathy
558.9	Diarrhea
562.10	Diverticulitis
995.2	Drug intoxication
304.90	Drug dependence, unspecified
532.90	Duodenal ulcer
532.40	Duodenal ulcer with hemorrhage
535.6	Duodenitis
625.3	Dysmenorrhea
787.2	Dysphagia
692.9	Eczema
782.3	Edema
492.8	Emphysema
323.9	Encephalitis
421.0	Endocarditis, bacterial
555.9	Enteritis, regional
604.9	Epididymitis
345.1	Epilepsy, convulsive
622.0	Erosion of cervix
787.3	Eructation
530.1	Esophageal reflux, esophagitis
530.5	Esophagospasm
376.30	Exophthalmos
780.2	Fainting
780.7	Fatigue, weakness
560.39	Fecal impaction
780.6	Fever, und. origin
610.1	Fibrocystic disease, breast
729.0	Fibrositis
005.9	Food poisoning
117.9	Fungus infection
680.9	Furuncle
727.43	Ganglion
531.90	Gastric ulcer
535.0	Gastritis
558.9	Gastroenteritis
056.9	German measles
277.4	Gilbert's disease
240.0	Goiter, simple nontoxic
242.30	Goiter, toxic nodular
274.9	Gout

611.1	Gynecomastia
477.9	Hay fever
854.00	Head injury
307.81	Headache, tension
784	Headache, vascular
346.9	Headache, migraine
785.2	Heart murmur, benign
342.9	Hemiplegia
372.72	Hemorrhage, subconjunctival
455	Hemorrhoids
572.2	Hepatic coma
573.3	Hepatitis
571.40	Hepatitis, chronic
070.1	Hepatitis, infectious
789.1	Hepatomegaly
053.9	Herpes zoster
553.3	Hiatus hernia
201.90	Hodgkin's disease
603.9	Hydrocele
591	Hydronephrosis
272.0	Hypercholesterolemia
272.4	Hyperlipemia
401	Hypertension
401.1	Hypertension, benign
242.90	Hyperthyroidism
786.01	Hyperventilation
251.2	Hypoglycemia
276.8	Hypokalemia
253.2	Hypopituitarism
244.9	Hypothyroidism
300.1	Hysteria
684	Impetigo
075	Infectious mononucleosis
487.1	Influenza
550.90	Inguinal hernia
780.52	Insomnia
745.5	Interatrial defect
564.1	Irritable colon
414	Ischemic heart, chronic
782.4	Jaundice
701.1	Keratosis
737.10	Kyphosis
386.3	Labyrinthitis
464.0	Laryngitis
426.3	Left bundle branch block

208.9	Leukemia	427.2	Paroxysmal tachycardia
204.1	Leukemia, chronic lymphatic	614.9	Pelvic inflammatory disease
702	Leukoplakia	533.90	Peptic ulcer
214.9	Lipoma, unsuspected site	523.4	Periodontitis
737.20	Lordosis	443.9	Peripheral vascular disease
724.5	Low back pain	462	Pharyngitis
722.52	Lumbar disc disease	696.3	Pityriasis rosea
847.2	Lumbar strain	511.9	Pleural effusion
710.0	Lupus, disseminated	511.0	Pleurisy
695.4	Lupus erythematosus	485	Pneumonia, bronchial
289.3	Lymphadenitis	512.8	Pneumothorx, spontaneous
457.2	Lymphangitis	753.1	Polycystic kidney
200.10	Lymphosarcoma	238.4	Polycythemia vera
579.9	Malabsorption syndrome	211.3	Polyp, colon, unspecified
578.1	Melena, blood in stool	788.4	Polyuria
386.00	Meniere's disease	627.1	Postmenopausal bleeding
627.2	Menopause	459.1	Postphlebitis syndrome
626.2	Menorrhagia	427.60	Premature beats
424.0	Mitral insufficiency	625.4	Premenstrual tension
394.0	Mitral stenosis	569.49	Proctitis
625.2	Mittelschmerz	600	Prostatic hypertrophy, benign
924.8	Multiple contusions	601.9	Prostatitis
340	Multiple sclerosis	698.0	Pruritis ani
072.9	Mumps	696.1	Psoriasis
848.9	Muscle strain	306.9	Psycho. disease, unspecified
358.0	Myasthenia gravis	415.1	Pulmonary embolism
323.9	Myelitis	515	Pulmonary fibrosis
410.9	Myocardial infarction, acute	427.69	PVC
412	Myocardial infarction, old	590.80	Pyelonephritis
429.0	Myocarditis	537.81	Pylorospasm
729.1	Myositis	729.2	Radiculitis
347	Narcolepsy	443.0	Raynaud's disease
787.0	Nausea, vomiting	569.3	Rectal bleeding
580.9	Nephritis, acute	465.9	Respiratory infection, acute
582.9	Nephritis, chronic	390	Rheumatic fever, acute
698.3	Neurodermatitis	398.90	Rheumatic heart disease
278	Obesity	714.0	Rheumatoid arthritis
459.9	Occlusive vascular disease	477.9	Rhinitis, allergic vasomotor
604.90	Orchitis	807.01	Rib fracture, single
715.0	Osteoarthosis	722.2	Ruptured intervertebral disc
733.00	Osteoporosis	295.6	Schizophrenia, chronic
380.10	Otitis externa	737.30	Scoliosis
382.9	Otitis media, acute	706.3	Seborrhea
577.0	Pancreatitis, acute	780.3	Seizure disorder
332.0	Parkinsonism	797	Senility

290.0	Senile dementia
786.09	Shortness of breath
461.9	Sinusitis, acute
462	Sore throat
720.0	Spondylitis, rheumatoid
536.8	Stomach pain
528.0	Stomatitis
378.9	Strabismus
034.0	Strep throat
625.6	Stress incontinence, female
788.3	Stress incontinence, male
692.71	Sunburn
780.2	Syncope
785.0	Tachycardia
451	Thrombophlebitis
241.0	Thyroid nodule
245.9	Thyroiditis
733.6	Tietze's syndrome
388.30	Tinnitus
463	Tonsillitis
333.1	Tremor, essential
350.1	Trigeminal neuralgia
011.9	Tuberculosis
597.80	Urethritis
599.0	Urinary tract infection
708.9	Urticaria
623.5	Vaginal discharge
627.3	Vaginitis, atrophic
616.1	Vaginitis and vulvovaginitis
131.01	Vaginitis, trichomonas
454.9	Varicose veins
780.4	Vertigo
078.1	Warts, plantar
426.7	Wolff-Parkinson-White syndrome

Coding Manuals

You should use standard nomenclature code books. The AMA publishes *The Physicians' Current Procedural Terminology* (CPT). The United States Department of Health and Human Services publishes the *International Classification of Diseases* (ICD).

Any medical assistant who is going to work with patient accounts or insurance needs to be very familiar with the CPT book, which is prepared and published annually by the AMA. This book lists the descriptive terms and identifying codes for reporting medical services and procedures performed by physicians. The AMA also has prepared codes on computer tapes for those offices using computers for billing and processing insurance.

Medicine is changing constantly with research and development of new therapy and procedures. For this reason the AMA constantly reviews the terminology and regularly drops obsolete codes to replace them with new up-to-date terminology and codes. The CPT codes are updated annually.

The introduction in the CPT code book gives excellent instructions on the use of CPT terminology and coding. The book is divided into specialty sections, but a specialist may use codes from any section to give an adequate description of a treatment or procedure rendered by a qualified physician. In reading the introduction, you will find guidelines are presented at the beginning of each section to define items that are necessary to interpret and report the procedure and services to be found in the section. In some instances a specific procedure or service may need to be slightly altered and the instructions and appendix explains the use of modifiers. Some examples of when these would be used are if unusual events occurred, if a service was performed by more than one physician, or if a procedure had both professional and technical components. Other examples are listed.

If you cannot find a code listed for a procedure or service your employer has performed, a provision has been made for the use of specific code numbers for reporting unlisted procedures. In these instances a description of the service must also be provided.

It is important to have a new code book each year to check the codes you are using often to be sure they have not been changed. A special appendix in the book provides a complete list of the codes deleted, revised, and added to the book, and also for the computer tape revision.

The introduction also defines and lists examples of the terms and phrases common to the practice of medicine. Coding for office visits, or *E*valuation and *M*anagement services, has recognized levels of service and is divided into categories or subcategories of E/M services; there are three to five levels of E/M services for reporting purposes. Levels of E/M services are not interchangeable among different categories or subcategories.

The levels of service include examination, evaluation, treatment, conferences with or concerning patients, preventive pediatric and adult supervision, and similar medical services. The levels of E/M service include the wide variation of skill, time, effort, responsibility, and medical knowledge required for the diagnosis and treatment of illness or injury and promotion of optimal health.

Seven components are recognized; six are used in defining the levels of E/M services. The components are:

- History
- Examination
- Medical decision-making
- Counseling

- Coordination of care
- Nature of presenting problem
- Time

The first three are considered key components in selecting the level of E/M services. The next three are contributing factors in a majority of encounters. The time factor is included to help the physician select the most appropriate level of E/M service.

The introduction also describes the magnetic computer tapes available—either the full procedure tape listing the complete text of the CPT manual or the Short Description Tape including narrative in nonmedical language.

At the end of the book are the appendix and the index. At the end of the index is a page listing instructions for the use of the CPT index. The index has six general categories: 1) procedure or service; 2) organ; 3) condition; 4) synonyms; 5) eponyms; and 6) abbreviations. Examples of each category are given to add to the understanding of each category.

The CPT code book also includes the order form for the standard insurance form provided through the AMA, see Figure 11–6.

The medical assistant who is routinely responsible for billing and preparation of insurance forms should take every opportunity to attend workshops or seminars to help you understand the use of the codes and the completion of insurance forms. In processing claims, it is absolutely necessary to code every individual procedure and service so the patient will receive full benefit. Even if the physician requests payment from the patient first and reimbursement from the insurance company is to go to the patient, the patient is more likely to pay promptly if the reimbursement is timely.

When a patient has surgery or a fracture, there is usually a flat fee for the procedure. The follow-up office visits are at no charge. Insurance companies and Medicare may average all charges to make up a fee profile that establishes the top amount to be paid to a physician for services rendered. If you use inaccurate codes, you could be lowering the rate the physician will be paid and may even keep yourself from receiving an increase in salary.

When a new patient receives an injection on the first visit, you may use a special code. When patients are seen for emergencies, use the emergency code in addition to the codes for office services. An additional charge may be made for materials and supplies, such as a sterile tray, by adding the CPT code. A professional component code may be added when the physician reads and evaluates X rays taken elsewhere.

You will need to refer to the current CPT book for the coding of services as these numbers are based on several components and may be changed with the annual CPT upgrade. Proper coding of services is a must for optimal reimbursement.

As examples of the extent to which the physician and office staff must evaluate the patient visit in order to determine the CPT codes, the following codes are offered for the new patient:

99201—Office or other outpatient visit for the evaluation and management of a new patient, which requires these three key components:
A problem focused history;
A problem focused examination;
Straightforward medical decision making.

99202—Same statement as 99201, with these components:
An expanded problem focused history;
An expanded problem focused examination;
Straightforward medical decision making.

99203—Same statement as 99201, with these components:
A detailed history;
A detailed examination;
Medical decision making of low complexity.

99204—Same statement as 99201, with these components:
A comprehensive history;
A comprehensive examination;
Medical decision making of moderate complexity.

99205—Same statement as 99201, with these components:
A comprehensive history;
A comprehensive examination;
Medical decision making of high complexity.

The following code determinations would need to be considered for the established patient:

99211—Office or other outpatient visit for the evaluation and management of established patient, that may not require the presence of a physician. Usually the presenting problem(s) are minimal.

Typically 5 minutes are spent performing or supervising these services.

99212—Office or other outpatient visit for the evaluation and management of established patient, which requires at least two of these three components:
A problem focused history;
A problem focused examination;
Straightforward medical decision making.

Physicians typically spend 10 minutes face to face with the patient and/or family.

99213—Same statement as 99212, with these components:
An expanded problem focused history;
An expanded problem focused examination;
Medical decision making of low complexity.

Physicians typically spend 15 minutes face to face with the patient and/or family.

99214—Same statement as 99212, with these components:
A detailed history;
A detailed examination;
Medical decision making of moderate complexity.

Physicians typically spend 25 minutes face to face with the patient and/or family.

99215—Same statement as 99212, with these components:

A comprehensive history;

A comprehensive examination;

Medical decision making of high complexity.

Physicians typically spend 40 minutes face to face with the patient and/or family.

The following are examples of operative reports and a breakdown of the codes for processing insurance forms:

PREOPERATIVE DIAGNOSIS: 40+ week intrauterine pregnancy. Fetal distress. Perineal condylomata.
POSTOPERATIVE DIAGNOSIS: Same.
OPERATION: Primary low transverse cervical cesarean.
PROCEDURE: The patient was taken to the OR after adequate epidural anesthesia. The abdomen was prepped with Betadine solution and draped in a sterile manner. A Pfannenstiel incision was made through a previous scar and carried through subcutaneous fat, and the fascia of the rectus muscle, the latter being separated from each other in the midline. Peritoneum was opened without complications and the bladder flap was taken down by sharp and blunt dissection. Transverse incision was made in the uterus which was enlarged digitally. A normal appearing male infant, Apgars 8 and 9, was then delivered. The cord was doubly clamped and cut and the infant given to Dr. _____ and Dr. _____, who were both in attendance. The placenta was delivered spontaneously after cord blood was collected. The uterus was cleaned of clots and remaining placental fragments. The uterus was then closed using two lengths of 1-Chromic; the first being interlocking stitch and the second being imbricating suture. After being satisfied that hemostatis was achieved, the bladder flap was closed with 2/0 Chromic catgut. Inspection revealed normal fallopian tubes and ovaries bilaterally without evidence of endometriosis or pelvic adhesions. Both round ligaments were S/P round ligament shortening and had ruptured through. The abdomen was then closed using continuous 0-Chromic for peritoneum, two lengths of continuous 1-Vicryl for fascia, interrupted 3/0 Dexon for subcuticular skin closure, and Dexon for subcutaneous skin closure.

At this point, the patient was placed in the stirrups and a right perineal condyloma was excised using a 15 blade and using 4/0 Vicryl for subcuticular skin closure. This incision was Steri-stripped for hemostatis.

The patient and the infant tolerated the procedure well, and the patient was taken to the RR in stable condition.
EBL: 1,000 ccs.
Final sponge and needle counts noted to be correct at termination of the procedure.

PREOPERATIVE DIAGNOSIS: Chronic mastoiditis.
POSTOPERATIVE DIAGNOSIS: Same.
OPERATION: Mastoidectomy.
INDICATIONS: This man had a mastoidectomy years ago, and has had chronic drainage since despite intensive medical therapy. He is admitted for revision mastoidectomy.

PROCEDURE: Under general anesthesia, a postauricular incision was made. A Koerner's flap developed, and the mastoid exposed in this way. Any overhang was removed with a drill and granulation tissue found present in the cavity. The cavity was cleaned out. There was a drill exposure high medially and somewhat posterior and the facial nerve was exposed in its horizontal dimension as it passed over the oval window. No ossicles were present except possibly a remnant of incus. The facial ridge was taken down. *A pedicle of temporalis muscle fascia and soft tissue was developed inferiorly based and swung into the cavity to obliterate.* The Koerner's flap was then positioned back in the ear, and the canal packed. The posterior incision was closed with interrupted chromic gut and the usual head wrap applied. Patient went to RR in good condition.

The italicized area above helps to identify code to be used. The CPT code for this would be 69604—revision mastoidectomy, resulting in tympanoplasty.

OPERATION: Under general anesthesia, the Crowe-Davis scope was used to expose the lingual tonsillar area and the lingual tonsils were removed with the scissors with sharp dissection. Bleeding controlled with Bovie cautery unit, and the patient tolerated the procedure well. He went to the RR in good condition.

The code would be 42870—excision lingual tonsil (separate procedure).

PREOPERATIVE DIAGNOSIS: Dysphagia, etiology uncertain.
POSTOPERATIVE DIAGNOSIS: Normal tracheoesophageal function and anatomy.
OPERATION: Laryngoscopy; bronchoscopy; esophagoscopy.
PROCEDURE: Under general anesthesia, this patient, who has been choking quite violently at times, was scoped. Laryngoscopy, bronchoscopy, and esophagoscopy all were done. No abnormalities were found of the anatomy with any of these procedures. They all went well. The patient was taken to the recovery room in good condition.

The code would be 31515—laryngoscopy direct; for aspiration.

PREOPERATIVE DIAGNOSIS: Serious otitis media.
POSTOPERATIVE DIAGNOSIS: Same.
OPERATION: Bilateral Tube Insertion.
PROCEDURE: A myringotomy was performed through the anterior middle portion of the ear drum. Fluid was removed from the middle ear space and a small Teflon tube was inserted without difficulty through the incision. The tube was an Arrow tube.

The code would be 69437—tympanostomy (requiring insertion of ventilating tube bilateral).

PREOPERATIVE DIAGNOSIS: Bilateral nasal polyps with polyps in the right antrum.

POSTOPERATIVE DIAGNOSIS: Same.

OPERATIONS: Bilateral nasal polypectomy; partial ethmoidectomy; right Caldwell Lac with removal of polyps from the antrum.

PROCEDURE: Under anesthesia, the nose was inspected and polyps found projecting from the middle meatus. The polyp forceps and small cup forceps were used to grasp the polyps and remove them along with some of the ethmoid sinus. This was done on both sides of the nose. Incision was made in the canine fossa on the right side and carried by blunt and sharp dissection of the face of the maxillary sinus. The sinus was opened with a chisel and polypoid tissue present in the sinus was removed with the polyp forceps. The procedure was then terminated and the patient went to the RR after closing the incision with interrupted chromic gut.

The codes would be 30116—excision, nasal polyps, extensive, bilateral; 31200—ethmoidectomy; 31033—radical, bilateral (Caldwell-Lac) with removal antrochoanal polyps.

PREOPERATIVE DIAGNOSIS: Cyst, right vocal cord.
POSTOPERATIVE DIAGNOSIS: Same.
OPERATION: Microlaryngoscopy with removal cyst right vocal cord with stripping of the left vocal cord.
PROCEDURE: Under general anesthesia, with the patient in position, a self-retaining laryngoscope was placed in the larynx, visualized the right vocal cord, which had a cyst on its anterior third. Cyst was removed with a small micro right biting cup forceps and the right vocal cord stripped. The left cord was somewhat roughened and slightly swollen, compatible with her history of heavy smoking, and the left vocal cord was stripped although the commissure was spared. The entire larynx, hypopharynx, and oral pharynx were viewed with the laryngoscope and the procedure terminated. Patient left for the RR in good condition.

The code would be 31541—laryngoscopy, direct, operative, with excision of tumor and/or stripping of vocal cords with operating microscope.

PREOPERATIVE DIAGNOSIS: Perforated tympanic membrane.
POSTOPERATIVE DIAGNOSIS: Same.
OPERATION: Tympanoplasty.
PROCEDURE: Under general anesthesia, a postauricular incision was made, Koerner's flap was developed, and the ear canal and drum exposed. The posterior perforation occupied the posterior inferior third of the ear drum and went back to the annulus. A tympanomeatal flap was developed, and the parts of the drum that were retracted to the promontory elevated. A secondary membrane portion was adherent to *the inferiormost edge of the stapes, and it was elevated and removed.* A fascial graft of temporalis fascia, which was pressed and dried, and the tympanomeatal flap replaced in its normal position. The graft was held in place with Gelfoam. The incision was closed with interrupted chromic gut, and the usual head wrap

applied. The patient went to recovery room in good condition.

The code would be 69632—tympanoplasty with ossicular chain reconstruction.

Processing Claims

The AMA has worked for many years on improvement of a standard claim form that can be used for both group and individual insurance claims, see Figure 11–7. This claim form should be used whenever possible. When a patient brings in a claim form from a private insurance company, be sure the patient has completed the patient's portion of the form and that it is signed. This form can then be attached to the standard claim form. The advantage of the standard form is that you can fill it in more quickly because of its familiarity.

Many medical software packages for computers include programs that simplify completion of standard insurance claim forms. The programs prompt the medical assistant to provide the necessary information and the computer responds by printing the information in the appropriate spaces on the form.

When a patient applies for insurance coverage and lists prior medical care from your employer you will usually receive a request for information regarding the patient. There are agencies that will do the abstracting of your records for the insurance company, coming into the office with a signed authorization from the patient. Your employer will decide whether to let an outside agency abstract the records. If so, it saves you time; if not, you will need to read the record and fill in the required information on the request form.

In a recent survey of insurance companies, the following common errors were listed as causes of claim payment delays:

1. The patient's—not the policyholder's—Social Security number is used as the certificate number. The claim would be rejected for lack of membership.
2. The "Coordination of Benefits" section is not completed, thereby suspending the claim for additional information.
3. Use of incorrect ICD-9 (International Classification of Diseases) codes.
4. Use of an incorrect or deleted CPT code could result in a decreased payment or a rejection.
5. Use of incorrect provider identification number could result in misdirection of payment.
6. Superbills attached to a claim form are sometimes illegible. Always attach additional information to back of claim, upper left-hand corner.
7. Member does not respond to our request for clarification of insurances covering injury or illness when another party might have responsibility.
8. Lack of operative report if procedure is unusual, complicated, or fee is unusual.

FIGURE 11–7 AMA-approved insurance form (Courtesy of Colwell Systems, Inc.)

Completing the Claim Form

TERMINAL PERFORMANCE OBJECTIVE: Given the patient chart, ledger, universal claim form, and typewriter, the student will complete the claim form with 100% accuracy within the time limit prescribed by the instructor. The instructor will evaluate the completed form.

1. Check for a photocopy of the patient's insurance card. (You need to know which block to check at the top of the form.)

2. Check the chart to see if the patient signature is on file for release of information and assignment of benefits. (If not on file, the patient must sign the form. It is best to have it signed before the form is completed. If the completed form is forwarded to the patient to be signed and sent to the insurance company, it is best to send a stamped and addressed envelope so there will not be a delay in forwarding the form to the insurance company.)

3. Using Figure 11–6 as a guide, complete the following entries:
   (Be certain the name used on the form is the same as that on the identification card.)
   2. Name of patient
   3. Birth date and check box for male or female
      (Use six digits to write birthdate, i.e., 02/17/21)
   1a. Insured's ID number
   4. Insured's name
   5. Patient's full address and telephone number
   6. Patient's relationship to insured
   7. Insured's full address and telephone number
   8. Patient's status
   9. Other insured's name
   9a. Other insured's policy or group number
   9b. Other insured's birthdate and box for male or female
   9c. Employer's name or school name
   9d. Insurance plan name or program name
      (Fill in "none" or N/A, for not applicable, so there is no doubt you have observed this section.)
   10. Check the appropriate box regarding employment and accident. (Do not leave all these boxes blank.)

   11. Insured's policy number
   11a. Insured's birthdate and box for male or female
   11b. Employer or school name
   11c. Insurance plan name or program name
   11d. Is there another health benefit plan?
   12–13. May stamp "signature on file" if you have the record to prove it.
   14. Date illness began
   15. Date patient was first treated for illness
   16. Complete with dates or state N/A
   17–17a. Complete with name and ID number or state N/A
   18. Complete with dates or state N/A
   19. Leave blank
   20. Mark appropriate box
   21. Fill in separate line for each diagnosis
   22. Complete if applicable
   23. Complete if applicable
   24. Complete A through G with appropriate codes
      (List each service separately with the most important listed first in case of surgery.)
   25. The physician's Social Security number or practice tax identification number and mark appropriate box
   26. Patient's account number if applicable
   27. Check one box
      (Must be marked "yes" for assignment)
   28–30. Total charged; amount paid; any balance due (Form will be rejected if not completed.)
   31. Physician's signature (Medicare will accept stamped signature.)
   32. Name and address of facility where services were rendered, if other than office
   33. Physician's name, address, and telephone number and specific identification numbers for Medicare or other group plan if applicable (Another good place to use a stamp)

   Be sure you obtain current directions for completion of the HCFA-1500 form for Medicare; any medical office that sends in a form that has been completed without explicitly following directions will find the form is rejected.

9. Incorrect spelling of patient's name.
10. Inconsistent use of patient's name will suspend claim processing; for example, middle name is used as first, nicknames are used instead of correct first name (Bill instead of William).
11. An incorrect patient birthdate is reported.

12. Use of an incorrect place of service code will suspend a claim.

Following up Delinquent Claims ....

Once a claim has been submitted to the insurance carrier for payment, processing should be completed within 30 days. If you have not received a payment or denial within 30 days you will need to follow up your claim with the carrier. Most carriers provide toll-free telephone numbers on their claim forms. When calling the carrier with an inquiry have the patient's name, identification number, and group name or number available. Once they have identified the subscriber they will request the date(s) of service and the total amount submitted. The carrier will then give you the status of the claim. If the claim is in process, ask how soon you can expect payment. If the claim is pending for further information from the patient, contact the patient and ask if he or she received the request and if the response was returned to the carrier. If the claim was not received, ask if you could submit a copy of the claim previously submitted and verify the mailing address. Also ask if you could direct the claim to a specific person in case further follow-up is necessary. If the carrier says the claim has been paid, ask when the payment was made and to whom it was directed. If payment was made to the patient, you will need to send the patient a statement.

Complete Chapter 11, Unit 3 in the workbook to help you meet the objectives at the beginning of this unit and therefore achieve competency of this subject matter.

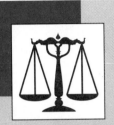

MEDICAL-LEGAL/ ETHICAL HIGHLIGHTS

Throughout this chapter you should be mindful of all medical-legal/ethical implications. Listed below are a few important reminders.

1. Obtain and file written authorization for release of information.
2. Obtain written contract if third party is responsible for payment of medical treatment.
3. Maintain careful records in handling patient claim forms.
4. Respect patients' privacy and confidentiality.

Ms. Right. . .

keeps proper authorization forms and other important documents filed in patients' charts as they are received. She checks for signatures as necessary on claim forms and never releases any information to anyone unless she first checks for the appropriate forms. She keeps abreast of any changes in claims processing or coding procedures to ensure a proper and efficient payment schedule. She makes sure that a copy of each claim form is made and placed in the patient's chart before sending it to be processed. She respects patients' privacy.

Advancement potential: Excellent

Miss Wrong. . .

obtains and files proper authorization forms with signatures when she remembers it. She is careless in her filing of claim forms and other important information. She neglects to read about changes in claims processing or coding procedures and therefore payment is held up until corrections are made. She never makes copies of forms before sending to be processed. She has a habit of discussing patient information with other patients and friends, as well as in public.

Advancement potential: None

REFERENCES

American Medical Association. *The Physicians' Current Procedural Terminology,* updated annually.

Fordney, Marilyn. *Insurance Handbook for the Medical Office.* Philadelphia: W. B. Saunders, 1989.

Nationwide Mutual Insurance Company. *Medicare Newsletter,* Columbus, OH: June, 1990.

Nationwide Mutual Insurance Company. *Medicare Newsletter,* 1991 HCPCS Update. Columbus, OH: February, 1991.

United States Department of Health & Human Services. *International Classification of Diseases,* 1992.

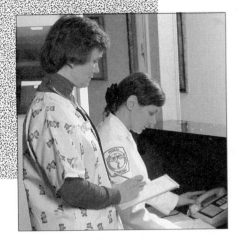

CHAPTER 1 2

Medical Office Management

Many different methods are used to affect the overall management of the medical office. A one- or two-physician office that employs only a few people could assign someone to deal with all the office management duties. However, most physicians find that a professional accounting firm or professional management company is best suited for the preparation of tax forms and financial statements and maintenance of salary records. Medical assistants with adequate office experience and management abilities are often selected to be the office manager. However, large group practices, clinics, and physician corporations with several physicians and many employees may choose an individual with a business background or degree to be the office manager or elect to use a professional management service, in addition to an accountant.

It would be impossible to include specific management instruction in this text to cover all variables because individual physician preference results in a wide array of possibilities. Therefore, this chapter discusses the general administrative duties and responsibilities of the medical assistant and also includes information regarding the role of an office manager. Regardless of who is serving as manager, you must be aware of the records the accountants will need. You will probably be responsible for maintaining certain financial and tax records.

The physician places great confidence in a manager to handle efficiently and accurately the business affairs of the office. The following units outline the skills and duties related to the fiscal and physical operation of a medical office and include such things as:

- Processing received payments for banking
- Preparing checks for office expenses
- Maintaining office accounting records
- Maintaining employer records
- Maintaining office equipment
- Obtaining essential reference materials
- Attending office management update seminars

U N I T   1

The Language of Banking

OBJECTIVES

Upon completion of this unit, the student will meet the following terminal performance objectives by verifying knowledge of the facts and principles presented through oral and written communication at a level deemed competent.

1. Differentiate between savings and checking accounts.
2. Explain the significance of the ABA and MICR codes.
3. Define the banking terms listed in this unit.
4. Differentiate between cashier's, certified, limited, postdated, stale, traveler's, and voucher checks.
5. Explain the difference between overdraft and overdrawn.
6. Discuss the "stop payment" process.
7. Spell and define, using the glossary at the back of the text, all the words to know in this unit.

WORDS TO KNOW

agent	endorsement	payee
certified	insufficient	power of attorney
currency	issue	warrant
deposit	negotiable	withdrawal

This unit presents the most common banking terms with their definitions to help you understand financial transactions. The medical assistant must have a good working knowledge of banking and basic accounting procedures. These skills are not only important in the physician's office but also in the management of your own personal finances.

Banking Terms

- *ABA number.* A code number found in the right upper corner of a printed check. It may be above the check number on a business check or below the check number on a personal check. This number was originated by the American Bankers Association. The purpose is to have a method of identifying the area where the bank on which the check is written is located, and to identify the bank within the area. It may be written as a fraction: $\frac{51-44}{119}$ on a business check, or 25-2/440 on a personal check.
- *Agent.* An agent is a person authorized to act for another person. You are the agent for your employer in the office. Bank officials are agents for the bank.

- *Bankbook.* In the case of a savings account it is called a savings passbook and contains a record of deposits, withdrawals, and interest earned, with the dates of all the transactions. This book must be presented with each deposit or withdrawal. At regular intervals, usually quarterly, interest earnings are credited to an account. These earnings should be entered in the passbook by the bank. Some banks indicate the passbook should be presented for interest entry at least once in a 3-year period.
- *Bank statement.* A record of a checking account sent to the customer, usually on a monthly basis, showing the beginning balance, all deposits made, all checks drawn, all bank charges, and the closing balance. The customer's canceled checks are returned with the statement.
- *Cashier's check.* The purchaser pays the bank the full amount of the check. The bank then writes a check on its own account payable to the party specified. This type of check "guarantees" to the recipient that the full amount of money indicated on the check will be paid on processing.
- *Certified check.* The bank stamps the customer's own check *certified* and then holds the certified amount in reserve in the customer's account until the check is cashed. This is a guaranteed check and so is always acceptable when a personal check is not.
- *Check register.* Also referred to as a check stub. It is a record showing the check number, person to whom check is paid, amount of check, date, and balance, and is kept by the person writing the check, as a record of the transaction.
- *Checking account.* A bank account against which checks may be written. The bank will issue the checks and deposit slips.
- *Currency.* Paper money issued by the government.
- *Deposit.* An amount of money (cash and/or checks) placed in a bank account.
- *Deposit record.* A record of a deposit that is given to the customer at the time of the deposit. It is important to keep the deposit record as proof of the deposit in case the bank fails to list the deposit on the bank statement.
- *Deposit slip.* An itemized list of cash and checks deposited in a checking account. It is important to keep a copy of all deposit slips.
- *Electronic fund transfer systems.* Methods of crediting or debiting accounts by computer without checks or deposit slips.
- *Endorsement.* The payee's signature on the back of a check. It is a transfer of title on the check to the bank in exchange for the amount of money on the face of the check.
- *Endorser.* The payee on a check. If the name is spelled incorrectly on the face of the check, it should be endorsed in the same way and then endorsed correctly.
- *Insufficient funds.* A bank term used to indicate that the writer of the check did not have enough money in his or her account to cover the check. An office usu–

ally has a policy regarding returned checks, which normally involves contacting the patient immediately, asking the person to pick up the check and bring a cash payment. These checks are sometimes described as *bounced,* and the account is called *overdrawn.*

■ *Limited check.* A check that will be marked void if written over a certain amount. These checks are often used for payroll or for insurance payments. A check may also list a time limit during which it must be cashed. It must be cashed within the time limit or you will find it is not **negotiable.**

■ *Maker.* The individual who signs a check or the corporation that pays it.

■ *MICR.* Magnetic Ink Character Recognition. This technique consists of characters and numbers printed in magnetic ink at the bottom left side of checks and deposit slips, Figures 12–1 and 12–2, page 188. This information is specific to each checking account and is imprinted on each check and deposit slip by the company printing the checks. The first series of numbers is the routing information that identifies the bank and area. The second series identifies the account numbers. The last series corresponds to the check number. When the bank processes the check, additional magnetic ink numbers are printed across the bottom identifying the amount of the check. These characters and numbers can be read by high-speed machinery, which greatly enhances the book-keeping procedures in the bank by simplifying the sorting of checks and the printing of individual monthly statements.

■ *Money order.* Negotiable instrument often used by individuals who do not have checking accounts or to meet the requirement for purchasing an item or service. Money orders may be purchased for a fee from banks, credit unions, post offices, and many other money order service locations.

■ *Note.* Legal evidence of a debt. A promissory note is a written promise to pay. A collateral note is a written promise to pay with the additional requirement that the maker of the note must list marketable securities that may be sold by the creditor if the maker does not pay the note within the time limit promised.

■ *One-write check writing.* System that makes it possible to make a record on a check register as you write a check. This is excellent for payroll because you can record deductions for the employee and office records in one writing.

■ *Overdraft checking accounts.* Accounts that allow checks to be written for a larger amount than is currently in the account. The overdraft is covered by the bank in the form of a loan for which interest is charged.

■ *Payee.* The person to whom a check is written. The name of the payee is listed on the check after the words *Pay to the order of.*

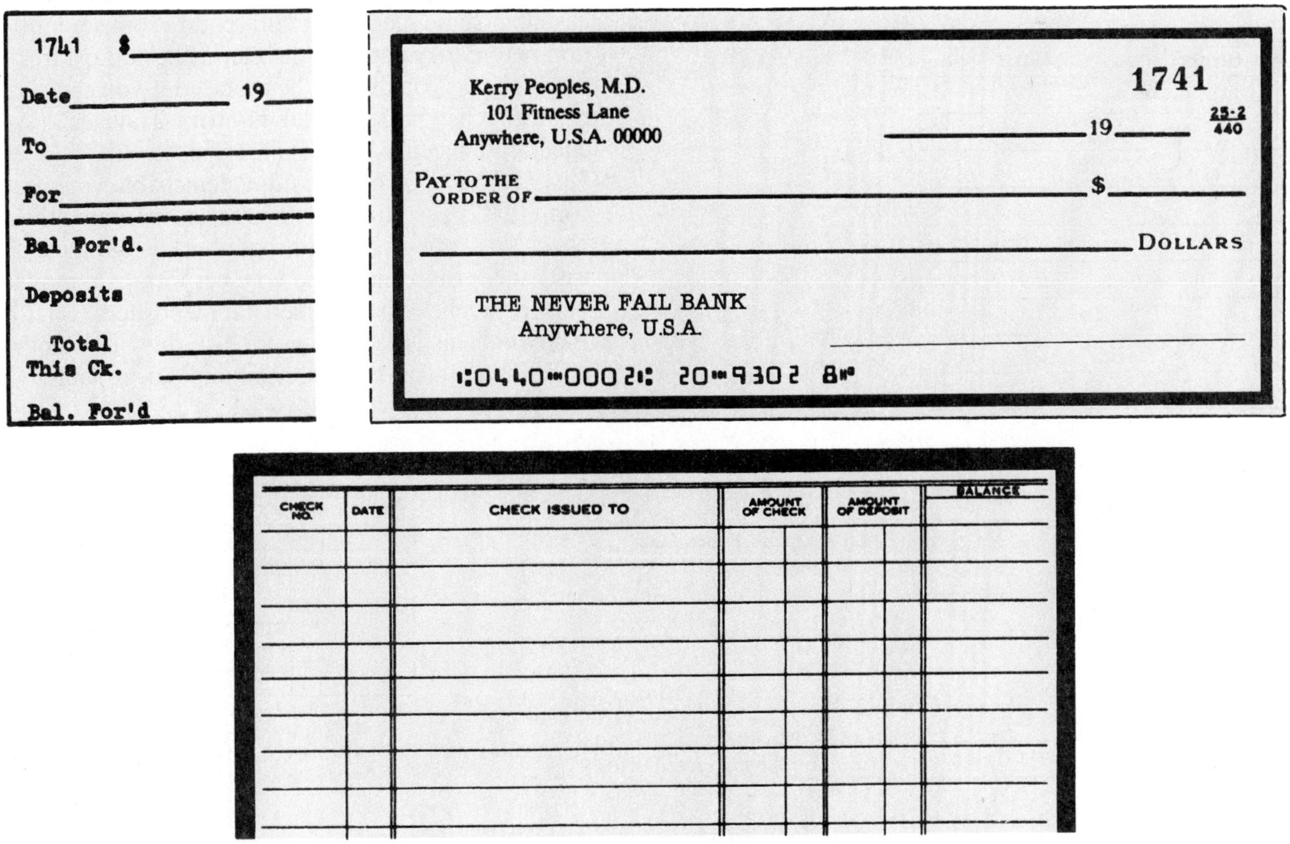

FIGURE 12–1 Check, check stub, and check register

- *Payer.* The person who signs the check.
- *Postdated check.* A check made out with a future date. You may have patients who wish to pay while they are in the office but will not have the money in their account until next pay day, which is the date they will put on the check. Never deposit these checks until the date for which they are made out. This practice is illegal in some states; be sure you know the law in your state.
- *Power of Attorney.* A legal procedure that authorizes one person to act as an agent for another. This is often necessary when patients are not physically or mentally capable of taking care of their own financial affairs.
- *Savings account.* A bank account upon which the depositor earns interest. The amounts deposited may be recorded in a passbook. (Note that many banks now also give interest on checking accounts if a minimum balance is maintained.)
- *Service charge.* Fees charged by the bank on a monthly basis for services rendered. If a specified minimum balance is maintained in the account the bank may not charge because they have the use of that money. Some banks charge for every transaction, whether putting money in or writing checks.
- *Special checking account.* Many different names and definitions apply, depending on the area of the country. It may be an account on which interest is paid if an established minimum balance is maintained in the account; an account for senior citizens for which no handling charges are made; or a fee for checks only. Banks are continually offering new plans to attract depositors.
- *Stale check.* A check presented too long after it was written to be honored by the bank. Some checks specify that they must be cashed within 90 days and if presented after that date the bank will not honor payment. A period of 6 months is generally considered enough time for a check to be presented for payment.
- *Stop payment.* A method by which the maker of a check may stop payment. The bank charges a sizable fee for this service. Some banks will accept a stop order by phone if it is promptly followed by completion of a form, which the bank furnishes. The payer must furnish the number of the check, date issued, name of payee, amount of the check, and the reason for stopping payment. The bank will then refuse to honor the check. A stop payment order is used when a check is lost or if there is a disagreement regarding a product or service received.
- *Teller.* The bank employee who is the main contact between the customer and the bank.
- *Traveler's check.* A special check used by individuals who are traveling and do not wish to carry a large amount of cash. Personal checks are usually not accepted outside of the area of the bank upon which they are drawn. Therefore, in exchange for cash, banks will issue traveler's checks. These must be signed individually at the time of purchase and again when they are used. They are usually considered the same as cash, but some merchants still require some identification before they accept a traveler's check. Lost traveler's checks can usually be replaced if you can produce a list of their serial numbers. Traveler's checks are listed as checks on a deposit slip.
- *Voucher check.* A check with a detachable voucher form that is used to show the reason for which the check was drawn. This kind of check is often used by insurance companies. The voucher form is removed before the check is endorsed and deposited.
- *Warrant.* This is evidence of a debt due but is not negotiable. It can be converted into a negotiable

CHECKS LIST SINGLY	DOLLARS	CENTS
1		
2		
3		
4		
5		
6		
7		
8		
9		
10		
11		
12		
13		
14		
15		
16		
17		
18		
19		
TOTAL		

ENTER TOTAL ON THE FRONT OF THIS TICKET

Kerry Peoples, M.D.
101 Fitness lane
Anywhere, U.S.A. 00000

DATE____________________19____

CASH	CURRENCY		
	COIN		
LIST CHECKS SINGLY			
TOTAL FROM OTHER SIDE			
TOTAL			
LESS CASH RECEIVED			
NET DEPOSIT			

USE OTHER SIDE FOR ADDITIONAL LISTING

BE SURE EACH ITEM IS PROPERLY ENDORSED

The Never Fail Bank
Anywhere, U.S.A.

⑆044000024⑆ 028941108 6⑈

CHECKS AND OTHER ITEMS ARE RECEIVED FOR DEPOSIT SUBJECT TO THE PROVISIONS OF THE UNIFORM COMMERCIAL CODE OR ANY APPLICABLE COLLECTION AGREEMENT

FIGURE 12–2
Deposit slip

instrument or cash. An insurance adjustor may issue a warrant as evidence that a claim should be paid. The warrant authorizes the insurance company to issue a check to settle the claim.

- *Withdrawal.* Removal of funds from a depositor's account. This may be done by means of a passbook, a withdrawal slip, a check, or electronic fund transfer.

Complete Chapter 12, Unit 1 in the workbook to help you meet the objectives at the beginning of this unit and therefore achieve competency of this subject matter.

UNIT 2

Currency, Checks, and Petty Cash

OBJECTIVES

Upon completion of this unit, the student will meet the following terminal performance objectives by verifying knowledge of the facts and principles presented through oral and written communication at a level deemed competent, and will demonstrate the specific behaviors as identified in the terminal performance objectives of the procedures.

1. Write a check.
2. Discuss precautions with checks received from patients.
3. Explain blank and restrictive endorsement.
4. Prepare a bank deposit.
5. Discuss special concerns with mail deposits.
6. Reconcile office records with bank statements.
7. Discuss establishing and maintaining a petty cash fund.
8. Spell and define, using the glossary at the back of the text, all the words to know in this unit.

WORDS TO KNOW

authorization	register	void
depleted	third party	voucher
reconcile	transaction	

Writing Checks

The medical assistant may often be required to write checks to pay for equipment, supplies, or wages. These are then given to the physician for signature before being mailed or otherwise distributed, see Figure 12–1. Some physicians will give check signature power to an office manager to eliminate the need for their personal signature. A signature authorization card obtained from the bank must be completed to allow someone other than the recorded owner of the account to execute checks. Some offices, as a means of monitoring expenditures and preventing employee embezzlement, require two signatures

on a check or have a policy that the individual writing the check (e.g., bookkeeper) must have another authorized person (often the office manager) sign the check. This also provides an opportunity to question expenditures and maintain a sense of cash flow.

One area of expenditure that must be carefully monitored is payment of invoices for office equipment and supplies. When a statement is received from a supplier, it is essential to know that everything on the invoice and the amount or number of each item(s) has, in fact, been received. The shipment must be compared to packing slips or invoices at the time they are received and notification of any discrepancy made to the supplier. Frequently, partial shipments are sent and some items are on back order. Payment of the total amount of the invoice would represent payment for goods not received. Some difficulty may also arise in trying to obtain materials not sent once you have paid in full for the shipment. The provider assumes everything was shipped as stated on the invoice because no questions were raised when the shipment was received.

If a mistake is made in writing a check, it is necessary to write "VOID" across the check and stub and rewrite the check.

Checks Received from Patients

The medical assistant should take certain precautions when accepting checks from patients:

- Be sure the check has the correct date, amount, and signature, and that no corrections have been made.
- Do not accept a third party check unless the check is from an insurance company. A third party check is generally one made out to the patient by someone unknown to you. Since you do not know how creditworthy the check writer is or have any personal information about the individual, it is unwise to accept a check that person has written.
- You might have patients who want to write a check for more than the amount due so they can have some cash in hand. This is generally not a good policy, and it would be advisable to refuse such a check. When you accept the check as payment and give out an additional amount in office cash, you risk the check not being honored by the bank. Your office will lose not only the amount owed by the patient, but also will lose the cash given out.
- Do not accept a check marked "payment in full" unless it does pay the account in full including charges incurred on the day the check is written. If there is still a balance, you will be unable to collect if you accept and deposit such a check. The statement "payment in full" should be written on the back of a check where it is to be endorsed. When you receive a check, you should stamp it with the deposit endorsement to protect against theft. If you do this, you will be sure to see any statement written on the check and

Write a Check

TERMINAL PERFORMANCE OBJECTIVE: In a simulated medical office situation and provided with all necessary equipment and supplies the student will prepare a check following the steps of the procedure with 100% accuracy. The instructor will observe all steps.

1. Fill out check register or stub with the check number, date, name of person or business to receive check, and amount of check. Also enter balance from previous stub.
   Key Points:
   a. **Always complete register before writing check.**
   b. **Use only black or blue ink.**
   c. **The stub may have the check number preprinted.**
   d. **If a deposit has been made, add to previous balance.**
   e. **Subtract amount of check and enter new balance.**
2. Enter date on check. **Key Point: May be typewritten or entered in black or blue ink.**
3. Enter name of payee on check.
4. Enter in figures the amount of the check. **Key Point: Keep figures close to the dollar sign so other figures cannot be inserted to change the amount of the check.**
5. Write out the amount of the check in words beginning as far to the left as possible.
   Key Points:
   a. **After writing the amount, fill in remaining space with a line to prevent insertion of words that would increase the amount.**
   b. **All amounts are written in terms of dollars and fractions of dollars. A check for $10 is written "Ten and no hundredths." A check for $12.65 is written "Twelve and sixty-five hundredths."**
   c. **When writing a check for less than a dollar, write the word Only and then the amount. ("Only ninety-five hundredths.")**
6. The check should be signed with the same signature used on the authorization card to open the checking account.

you can be sure the payment is indeed in full before accepting the check.

■ Do not accept a postal money order with more than one endorsement because two are the limit honored.

Endorsement

An endorsement is a signature or a signature plus other information on the back of a check. The endorsement of a check transfers all rights in the check to another party. Endorsements should always be made in ink and may be made with a pen or rubber stamp. The end of the check to be endorsed can be identified by holding the check on the right end as you look at it, turning it over, and endorsing the opposite or left end. All checks received in the office, whether in person or through the mail, should be protected by endorsement at the time received.

The two kinds of endorsement commonly used are blank endorsement and restrictive endorsement. A *blank endorsement* is a signature only. It should not be used until the check is to be cashed, because if the check is stolen with such an endorsement, someone else could endorse the check below your name and cash the check. A *restrictive endorsement* is used to endorse checks when they are received. It is a stamp or written information that states, "PAY TO THE ORDER OF (name of bank where check is to be deposited)" followed by the name of the physician. If such a check is stolen it could not be used in any way.

If the name of the payee is misspelled, it should be endorsed the same way followed by the correct signature directly below.

Effective September 1, 1988, new federal regulations required all endorsements to be within $1\frac{1}{2}$ inch of the "trailing edge" of all checks. Checks on which the endorsement extends beyond the $1\frac{1}{2}$ inch area may be refused by the financial institutions for improper endorsement. To avoid processing delays, be sure to endorse all checks as described, Figure 12–3.

Making Deposits

The medical assistant is also expected to deposit cash and checks received in the office. This may be a daily task or it may be as infrequent as once a week for a physician with a limited practice. Deposit slips are imprinted with the account number in magnetic ink character recognition numbers, which match those on the checks. These numbers make it possible for checks and

BACK

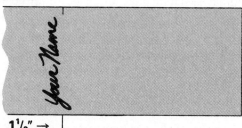

1½" →

FIGURE 12–3 Proper placement of signature for endorsement

P R O C E D U R E

Prepare a Deposit Slip

TERMINAL PERFORMANCE OBJECTIVE: In a simulated medical office situation and provided with all necessary equipment and supplies, the student will prepare a bank deposit slip, at 100% accuracy, following the steps in the procedure. The instructor will observe each step.

1. Separate money to be deposited by check or currency.
2. Currency is usually listed first.
   Key Points:
   a. **All bills should be sorted so that the bills of each denomination are together, facing in the same direction, and with portrait side up.**
   b. **Place in stack with largest bills on top and smallest on the bottom.**
   c. **Total currency and record on deposit slip.**
3. If a large number of coins are included they should be placed in wrappers. Record the total on the slip.
4. List checks by number, name of maker, and amount.

Key Points:
a. **The check number is sufficient if you have an office copy on which you list the names also.**
b. **Money orders are listed as money order and name or MO and name.**
c. **Be sure checks are stamped with endorsement. This should be done as they are received to prevent cashing if stolen. Use no more than $1\frac{1}{2}$ inch to endorse the checks.**
d. **If the endorsement is not stamped, write *For deposit only* and sign name of payee.**
5. Total all amounts.
6. Make a copy for your office files.
7. Enter deposit total in checkbook.
8. Deposit at bank. **Key Point: Be sure you receive a record of deposit either personally or by mail if you make a night deposit. This record is necessary to prove a deposit was made if the bank fails to give credit for it on the monthly statement.**

---

deposit slips to be sorted and recorded by computer. Banks will accept a list of deposited items on something other than the bank-provided deposit slip as long as the bank deposit slip is attached, see Figure 12–2, page 188.

Deposit by Mail

Checks may be deposited by mail. You should avoid sending cash or currency by mail, but if you must, then send it by registered mail. The deposit slip and money are prepared as for any deposit. The checks should be endorsed by restrictive endorsement only. If no stamp is available, the hand-written notation "for deposit only to the account of (name of your employer)" will suffice. You should request a receipt, as this record is necessary to prove a deposit was made. It is extremely important that you have an accurate record of all checks deposited with the check number, whom the check is from, and the amount of check so that you can follow up if the mail is lost. If this should happen, it will be necessary to notify all payees to stop payment and issue you new checks.

Reconciling Bank Statements

An important part of banking is the reconciliation each month of the bank statement with the office records. You need to be sure that you and the bank agree as to the amount of money in the account. You will receive a statement that shows all banking transactions concerning the account along with the checks which the bank

has received and processed. Most statements contain a section that allows you to list outstanding checks and do other calculations to reconcile the amounts, Figure 12–4.

Petty Cash and Other Accounts

Since it is not reasonable to write checks for small office transactions, most physicians have a petty cash fund. The physician will determine the amount of the fund and for what it will be used. The fund is established by writing a check payable to Cash or Petty Cash. The check is then

RECONCILING THE BANK STATEMENT

Bank Statement Balance $_____

   Less Outstanding Checks

  # _____ $ _____
  # _____ $ _____
  # _____ $ _____
  # _____ $ _____
  # _____ $ _____
  # _____ $ _____
  # _____ $ _____

   Total _____ $ _____
   Plus deposits not shown $ _____

CORRECTED BANK STATEMENT $ _____

   Checkbook balance $ _____
   Less bank charges $ _____

CORRECTED CHECKBOOK BALANCE $ _____

FIGURE 12–4 Reconciliation form

P R O C E D U R E

Reconcile a Bank Statement

TERMINAL PERFORMANCE OBJECTIVE: In a simulated medical office situation and provided with all necessary equipment and supplies, the student will prepare at 100% accuracy a bank reconciliation form following the steps in the procedure. The instructor will observe each step.

1. Compare the opening balance on the new statement with the closing balance on the previous statement. **Key Point: If they do not agree, contact the bank.**
2. List the bank balance in the appropriate space on the reconciliation worksheet.
3. Compare the check entries on the statement with the returned checks. **Key Point: The bank may have your checks in numerical order; if not, you should place them in order.**
4. Determine if you have any outstanding checks. **Key Points:**
   a. **An outstanding check is one you have written that does not appear on your bank statement and has not been returned by the bank.**
   b. **Put a red check mark on each check stub or check register entry that appears on your**

statement.
   c. **Any stub or entry not marked indicates an outstanding check, which you list on your worksheet in the column provided.**
   d. **Total the outstanding checks.**
5. Subtract from your checkbook balance items such as automatic payments or service charges that appear on the statement but not in the checkbook. **Key Point: These items are indicated by a code such as *AP* for automatic payment or *SC* for service charge.**
6. Add to your checkbook any interest payments indicated on your statement. **Key Point: Some banks pay interest if a specified minimum amount is maintained in the account.**
7. Add to the bank statement balance any deposits not shown on the bank statement (*e.g.,* deposited since statement prepared).
8. The balance in your checkbook and the bank statement should agree. **Key Point: If they do not agree, subtract the lesser figure from the greater for a possible clue to the error and recheck all figures.**

---

cashed and the money kept in a locked cash box. (All patient payments should be kept in a separate money box.) The money is often used for postage due letters, inexpensive office supplies, and small charitable donations.

A voucher form should be completed each time payment is made from this fund. When the amount in the fund is nearly depleted, another check is written for the difference between the original fund and the amount remaining. The vouchers are kept in a file to verify the use of the petty cash fund. Figure 12–5 shows a petty cash fund ledger form to monitor expenditures.

Complete Chapter 12, Unit 2 in the workbook to help you meet the objectives at the beginning of this unit and therefore achieve competency of this subject matter.

U N I T 3

Salary, Benefits, and Tax Records

OBJECTIVES

Upon completion of this unit, the student will meet the following terminal performance objectives by verifying knowledge of the facts and principles presented through oral and written communication at a level deemed competent.

1. Explain the W-4, W-2, and I-9 forms.
2. Differentiate between hourly wage and a salary.

DATE	DESCRIPTION	VOUCHER NUMBER	TOTAL AMOUNT	OFFICE EXPENSE	DONA-TIONS	MISC.	BALANCE
10/1	Fund established						25.00
10/5	Postage due	1	.40	.40			24.60
10/8	Parking fee	2	1.60			1.60	23.00
10/10	Coffee	3	2.98				20.02

FIGURE 12–5 Petty cash form

3. Identify the information required for payroll records.
4. List the four factors that affect the amount of federal tax withheld.
5. Differentiate between gross and net salary.
6. Discuss salary benefits, identifying six examples.
7. Spell and define, using the glossary at the back of the text, all the words to know in this unit.

WORDS TO KNOW

accountant
benefits
deductions
disability
exemption
gross

longevity
net
profit sharing
unemployment
vested

Employee Requirements and Records

All employees in a physician's office must have a Social Security number. This is a nine-digit number which is obtained from the Social Security Administration. Forms to apply for a Social Security number can be obtained from local Social Security office, Internal Revenue office, and post offices. Each employee must also complete an Employee's Withholding Exemption Certificate (W-4 form) indicating the number of exemptions claimed, Figure 12–6, pages 194 and 195. Any employee who fails to complete a W-4 form will have withholding figured on the basis of being single with no exemptions. A new W-4 form must be completed if there is a change in marital status or a change in the number of exemptions.

Recent federal legislation requires employees to complete an Employment Eligibility Verification Form I-9, Figure 12–7, page 196. The form is issued by the Department of Justice, Immigration and Naturalization Service. Its purpose is to ensure all persons employed are either United States citizens, lawfully admitted aliens, or aliens authorized to work in the United States. By law, this form must be completed before an individual can be officially hired. Accountants will not permit salary to be paid to individuals who do not have a form I-9 on file.

In addition to these federal requirements, forms must also be processed for state and local tax records. Local government tax is paid to the city where employment occurs regardless of where the employee lives.

Medical Office Requirements and Records

The physician's office must have a federal tax reporting number, which is obtained from the Internal Revenue Service. In states that require employer reports, a state employer number must also be obtained.

When payroll checks are prepared, a record must be kept showing Social Security, federal taxes, any state and city taxes, and insurance amounts deducted from earnings. Employees may be paid an hourly wage or a salary (a fixed amount paid on a regular basis for a prescribed period of time). The Federal Fair Labor Standards Act regulates the minimum wage and requires that overtime be paid to wage earners at a minimum rate of $1\frac{1}{2}$ times the regular rate for hours over and above 40 hours per week. It is necessary to keep records of hours worked, total pay, and all deductions withheld.

Several office supply houses furnish forms for payroll record keeping. There should be a page for each employee's payroll record. The heading should give the name, address, telephone, Social Security number, and date of employment. In columns there should be a record of date of check, hours worked (regular and overtime), gross salary, and individual deductions (including federal income tax, Social Security tax, and any state and local taxes). There might also be deductions for insurances or uniforms. The final column should show the amount of net pay, that is, the actual amount of the paycheck after deductions. When an accountant or management firm is employed to prepare payroll, office records must be given to them by a designated date(s) each month in order that payroll can be prepared and records maintained.

The amount of federal tax withheld is based on the amount earned, marital status, number of exemptions claimed, and the length of the pay period. The Internal Revenue Service will provide the charts used to figure deductions for federal income tax and Society Security tax. State and local taxes are usually a percentage of gross earnings. The net pay (pay actually given to the employee) is the gross earnings minus taxes and other deductions. The physician must provide the employee with a statement of gross pay and deductions along with the check each pay period. The tax deductions withheld must be sent on a quarterly basis to the federal, state, and local government offices along with the reporting forms provided by the tax offices. The local, state, and federal governments supply the guidelines necessary to complete these reports.

A W-2 form, which is a summary of all earnings for the year and all deductions withheld for federal, state, and local taxes, must be provided to each employee by January 31st of each year. The Social Security Administration must receive a report of W-2 forms each year. The physician who has several employees may also need to submit reports to the state and federal government for unemployment taxes. This tax is not deducted from the employee's earnings for federal tax but may be deducted in some cases for state unemployment tax.

Benefits

Full-time employed medical assistants and other medical office employees can expect benefits in addition to their

19**92** Form W-4

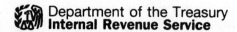
Department of the Treasury
Internal Revenue Service

Purpose. Complete Form W-4 so that your employer can withhold the correct amount of Federal income tax from your pay.

Exemption From Withholding. Read line 7 of the certificate below to see if you can claim exempt status. *If exempt, complete line 7; but do not complete lines 5 and 6.* No Federal income tax will be withheld from your pay. Your exemption is good for one year only. It expires February 15, 1993.

Basic Instructions. Employees who are not exempt should complete the Personal Allowances Worksheet. Additional worksheets are provided on page 2 for employees to adjust their withholding allowances based on itemized deductions, adjustments to income, or two-earner/two-job situations. Complete all worksheets that apply to your situation. The worksheets will help you figure

the number of withholding allowances you are entitled to claim. However, you may claim fewer allowances than this.

Head of Household. Generally, you may claim head of household filing status on your tax return only if you are unmarried and pay more than 50% of the costs of keeping up a home for yourself and your dependent(s) or other qualifying individuals.

Nonwage Income. If you have a large amount of nonwage income, such as interest or dividends, you should consider making estimated tax payments using Form 1040-ES. Otherwise, you may find that you owe additional tax at the end of the year.

Two-Earner/Two-Jobs. If you have a working spouse or more than one job, figure the total number of allowances you are entitled to claim on all jobs using worksheets from only one Form

W-4. This total should be divided among all jobs. Your withholding will usually be most accurate when all allowances are claimed on the W-4 filed for the highest paying job and zero allowances are claimed for the others.

Advance Earned Income Credit. If you are eligible for this credit, you can receive it added to your paycheck throughout the year. For details, get Form W-5 from your employer.

Check Your Withholding. After your W-4 takes effect, you can use **Pub. 919,** Is My Withholding Correct for 1992?, to see how the dollar amount you are having withheld compares to your estimated total annual tax. Call 1-800-829-3676 to order this publication. Check your local telephone directory for the IRS assistance number if you need further help.

Personal Allowances Worksheet   For 1992, the value of your personal exemption(s) is reduced if your income is over $105,250 ($157,900 if married filing jointly, $131,550 if head of household, or $78,950 if married filing separately). Get Pub. 919 for details.

A   Enter "1" for **yourself** if no one else can claim you as a dependent . . . . **A** _____

B   Enter "1" if: { • You are single and have only one job; or
                        • You are married, have only one job, and your spouse does not work; or
                        • Your wages from a second job or your spouse's wages (or the total of both) are $1,000 or less. } . . **B** _____

C   Enter "1" for your **spouse.** But, you may choose to enter -0- if you are married and have either a working spouse or more than one job (this may help you avoid having too little tax withheld) . . . . **C** _____

D   Enter number of **dependents** (other than your spouse or yourself) whom you will claim on your tax return . . . . **D** _____

E   Enter "1" if you will file as **head of household** on your tax return (see conditions under "Head of Household," above) . **E** _____

F   Enter "1" if you have at least $1,500 of **child or dependent care expenses** for which you plan to claim a credit . . **F** _____

G   Add lines A through F and enter total here. **Note:** *This amount may be different from the number of exemptions you claim on your return* ▶ **G** _____

For accuracy, do all worksheets that apply.   { • If you plan to **itemize or claim adjustments to income** and want to reduce your withholding, see the Deductions and Adjustments Worksheet on page 2.
• If you are **single** and have **more than one job** and your combined earnings from all jobs exceed $29,000 OR if you are **married** and have a **working spouse or more than one job,** and the combined earnings from all jobs exceed $50,000, see the Two-Earner/Two-Job Worksheet on page 2 if you want to avoid having too little tax withheld.
• If **neither** of the above situations applies, **stop here** and enter the number from line G on line 5 of Form W-4 below. }

------------------ **Cut here and give the certificate to your employer. Keep the top portion for your records.** ------------------

Form **W-4**	**Employee's Withholding Allowance Certificate**	OMB No. 1545-0010
Department of the Treasury Internal Revenue Service	▶ **For Privacy Act and Paperwork Reduction Act Notice, see reverse.**	19**92**

1 Type or print your first name and middle initial	Last name	**2** Your social security number

Home address (number and street or rural route)	**3** ☐ Single ☐ Married ☐ Married, but withhold at higher Single rate. **Note:** *If married, but legally separated, or spouse is a nonresident alien, check the Single box.*
City or town, state, and ZIP code	**4** If your last name differs from that on your social security card, check here and call 1-800-772-1213 for more information ▶ ☐

5   Total number of allowances you are claiming (from line G above or from the Worksheets on back if they apply) . . | **5** |

6   Additional amount, if any, you want deducted from each paycheck . . . . | **6** $ |

7   I claim exemption from withholding and I certify that I meet **ALL** of the following conditions for exemption:

• Last year I had a right to a refund of **ALL** Federal income tax withheld because I had **NO** tax liability; **AND**
• This year I expect a refund of **ALL** Federal income tax withheld because I expect to have **NO** tax liability; **AND**
• This year if my income exceeds $600 and includes nonwage income, another person cannot claim me as a dependent.

If you meet all of the above conditions, enter the year effective and "EXEMPT" here . . . ▶ | **7** 19 |

8   Are you a full-time student? (**Note:** *Full-time students are not automatically exempt.*) . . . . | **8** ☐ Yes ☐ No |

Under penalties of perjury, I certify that I am entitled to the number of withholding allowances claimed on this certificate or entitled to claim exempt status.

Employee's signature ▶ _____   Date ▶ _____ , 19 ____

9 Employer's name and address (Employer: Complete 9 and 11 only if sending to the IRS)	**10** Office code (optional)	**11** Employer identification number

Cat. No. 10220Q

FIGURE 12–6a   Form W-4: Employee's Withholding Allowance Certificate and worksheet

Deductions and Adjustments Worksheet

Note: *Use this worksheet only if you plan to itemize deductions or claim adjustments to income on your 1992 tax return.*

1   Enter an estimate of your 1992 itemized deductions. These include: qualifying home mortgage interest, charitable contributions, state and local taxes (but not sales taxes), medical expenses in excess of 7.5% of your income, and miscellaneous deductions. (For 1992, you may have to reduce your itemized deductions if your income is over $105,250 ($52,625 if married filing separately). Get Pub. 919 for details.)   **1** $ _____

2   Enter: { $6,000 if married filing jointly or qualifying widow(er)
              $5,250 if head of household
              $3,600 if single
              $3,000 if married filing separately }   . . .   **2** $ _____

3   **Subtract** line 2 from line 1. If line 2 is greater than line 1, enter -0-   . . . . .   **3** $ _____

4   Enter an estimate of your 1992 adjustments to income. These include alimony paid and deductible IRA contributions   **4** $ _____

5   **Add** lines 3 and 4 and enter the total   . . . .   **5** $ _____

6   Enter an estimate of your 1992 nonwage income (such as dividends or interest income)   . . . . .   **6** $ _____

7   **Subtract** line 6 from line 5. Enter the result, but not less than -0-   . . . .   **7** $ _____

8   **Divide** the amount on line 7 by $2,500 and enter the result here. Drop any fraction   . . . . .   **8** _____

9   Enter the number from Personal Allowances Worksheet, line G, on page 1   . . . .   **9** _____

10 **Add** lines 8 and 9 and enter the total here. If you plan to use the Two-Earner/Two-Job Worksheet, also enter the total on line 1, below. Otherwise, **stop here** and enter this total on Form W-4, line 5, on page 1   . . . .   **10** _____

Two-Earner/Two-Job Worksheet

Note: *Use this worksheet only if the instructions for line G on page 1 direct you here.*

1   Enter the number from line G on page 1 (or from line 10 above if you used the Deductions and Adjustments Worksheet)   **1** _____

2   Find the number in **Table 1** below that applies to the **LOWEST** paying job and enter it here   . . . .   **2** _____

3   If line 1 is **GREATER THAN OR EQUAL TO** line 2, subtract line 2 from line 1. Enter the result here (if zero, enter -0-) and on Form W-4, line 5, on page 1. **DO NOT** use the rest of this worksheet   . . .   **3** _____

Note: *If line 1 is **LESS THAN** line 2, enter -0- on Form W-4, line 5, on page 1. Complete lines 4–9 to calculate the additional dollar withholding necessary to avoid a year-end tax bill.*

4   Enter the number from line 2 of this worksheet   . . . .   **4** _____

5   Enter the number from line 1 of this worksheet   . . . .   **5** _____

6   **Subtract** line 5 from line 4   . . . .   **6** _____

7   Find the amount in **Table 2** below that applies to the **HIGHEST** paying job and enter it here   . . . . .   **7** $ _____

8   **Multiply** line 7 by line 6 and enter the result here. This is the additional annual withholding amount needed   **8** $ _____

9   Divide line 8 by the number of pay periods remaining in 1992. (For example, divide by 26 if you are paid every other week and you complete this form in December of 1991.) Enter the result here and on Form W-4, line 6, page 1. This is the additional amount to be withheld from each paycheck   . . . . . .   **9** $ _____

Table 1: Two-Earner/Two-Job Worksheet

Married Filing Jointly		All Others	
If wages from **LOWEST** paying job are—	Enter on line 2 above	If wages from **LOWEST** paying job are—	Enter on line 2 above
0 - $4,000	0	0 - $6,000	0
4,001 - 8,000	1	6,001 - 10,000	1
8,001 - 13,000	2	10,001 - 14,000	2
13,001 - 18,000	3	14,001 - 18,000	3
18,001 - 22,000	4	18,001 - 22,000	4
22,001 - 26,000	5	22,001 - 45,000	5
26,001 - 30,000	6	45,001 and over	6
30,001 - 35,000	7		
35,001 - 40,000	8		
40,001 - 60,000	9		
60,001 - 80,000	10		
80,001 and over	11		

Table 2: Two-Earner/Two-Job Worksheet

Married Filing Jointly		All Others	
If wages from **HIGHEST** paying job are—	Enter on line 7 above	If wages from **HIGHEST** paying job are—	Enter on line 7 above
0 - $50,000 . . .	$340	0 - $27,000	$340
50,001 - 100,000 . . .	640	27,001 - 58,000	640
100,001 and over . . .	710	58,001 and over	710

Privacy Act and Paperwork Reduction Act Notice.—We ask for the information on this form to carry out the Internal Revenue laws of the United States. The Internal Revenue Code requires this information under sections 3402(f)(2)(A) and 6109 and their regulations. Failure to provide a completed form will result in your being treated as a single person who claims no withholding allowances. Routine uses of this information include giving it to the Department of Justice for civil and criminal litigation and to cities, states, and the District of Columbia for use in administering their tax laws.

The time needed to complete this form will vary depending on individual circumstances. The estimated average time is: **Recordkeeping** 46 min., **Learning about the law or the form** 10 min., **Preparing the form** 70 min. If you have comments concerning the accuracy of these time estimates or suggestions for making this form more simple, we would be happy to hear from you. You can write to both the **Internal Revenue Service,** Washington, DC 20224, Attention: IRS Reports Clearance Officer, T:FP; and the **Office of Management and Budget,** Paperwork Reduction Project (1545-0010), Washington, DC 20503. **DO NOT** send the tax form to either of these offices. Instead, give it to your employer.

*U.S. Government Printing Office: 1991 — 285-081

FIGURE 12–6b   Form W-4: Employee's Withholding Allowance Certificate and worksheet

EMPLOYMENT ELIGIBILITY VERIFICATION (Form I-9)

1 **EMPLOYEE INFORMATION AND VERIFICATION:** (To be completed and signed by employee.)

Name: (Print or Type) Last	First	Middle	Birth Name
Address: Street Name and Number	City	State	ZIP Code
Date of Birth (Month/Day/Year)		Social Security Number	

I attest, under penalty of perjury, that I am (check a box):

☐ 1. A citizen or national of the United States.

☐ 2. An alien lawfully admitted for permanent residence (Alien Number A _____) .

☐ 3. An alien authorized by the Immigration and Naturalization Service to work in the United States (Alien Number A _____ .
or Admission Number _____ , expiration of employment authorization, if any _____) .

I attest, under penalty of perjury, the documents that I have presented as evidence of identity and employment eligibility are genuine and relate to me. I am aware that federal law provides for imprisonment and/or fine for any false statements or use of false documents in connection with this certificate.

Signature	Date (Month/Day/Year)

PREPARER TRANSLATOR CERTIFICATION (To be completed if prepared by person other than the employee). I attest, under penalty of perjury, that the above was prepared by me at the request of the named individual and is based on all information of which I have any knowledge.

Signature	Name (Print or Type)		
Address (Street Name and Number)	City	State	Zip Code

2 **EMPLOYER REVIEW AND VERIFICATION:** (To be completed and signed by employer.)

Instructions:

Examine one document from List A and check the appropriate box, **_OR_** examine one document from List B **_and_** one from List C and check the appropriate boxes. Provide the **_Document Identification Number_** and **_Expiration Date_** for the document checked.

List A Documents that Establish Identity and Employment Eligibility	List B Documents that Establish Identity	**and**	List C Documents that Establish Employment Eligibility
☐ 1. United States Passport ☐ 2. Certificate of United States Citizenship ☐ 3. Certificate of Naturalization ☐ 4. Unexpired foreign passport with attached Employment Authorization ☐ 5. Alien Registration Card with photograph	☐ 1. A State-issued driver's license or a State-issued I.D. card with a photograph, or information, including name, sex, date of birth, height, weight, and color of eyes. (Specify State)_____) ☐ 2. U.S. Military Card ☐ 3. Other (Specify document and issuing authority) _____		☐ 1. Original Social Security Number Card (other than a card stating it is not valid for employment) ☐ 2. A birth certificate issued by State, county, or municipal authority bearing a seal or other certification ☐ 3. Unexpired INS Employment Authorization Specify form # _____
Document Identification #_____ **_Expiration Date (if any)_** _____	**_Document Identification_** #_____ **_Expiration Date (if any)_** _____		**_Document Identification_** #_____ **_Expiration Date (if any)_** _____

CERTIFICATION: I attest, under penalty of perjury, that I have examined the documents presented by the above individual, that they appear to be genuine and to relate to the individual named, and that the individual, to the best of my knowledge, is eligible to work in the United States.

Signature	Name (Print or Type)	Title
Employer Name	Address	Date

Form I-9 (05/07/87)
OMB No. 1115-0136

U.S. Department of Justice
Immigration and Naturalization Service

FIGURE 12–7 Form I-9: Employment Eligibility Verification

salary. These are sometimes known as "fringe benefits." Benefits will vary according to the situation of the employee and the generosity of the physician(s). The following are examples of benefits that may be offered.

- Vacation. Usually a minimum of 2 weeks with pay after completing a year of full-time employment; will increase with longevity.
- Holidays. A minimum of six paid holidays per year—New Year's, Memorial Day, July 4th, Labor Day, Thanksgiving, and Christmas.
- Health insurance. Available; may require some copayment and may not be provided if employee is covered by insurance with spouse's employment.
- Disability insurance. Will cover a percentage of the salary if the employee is unable to work because of a disabling condition.
- Life insurance. Usually for a set amount such as equal to a year's salary.
- Profit sharing. A form of pension plan to employees who meet certain requirements such as: at least 21 years old, work a minimum of 1000 hours in a year, employed for at least a year to establish eligibility. Each plan will have its own requirements. An amount equal to a certain percentage of the employee's salary is deposited annually into the plan by the employer. This amount accumulates interest and grows tax free until it is withdrawn. The employee is normally responsible for the taxes due. There is usually a period of time, 5 years for example, before an employee becomes vested in the plan. This means the person must be employed at least 5 years before being eligible to receive the money in the account should employment be terminated. This type of benefit can add up to a nice sum. As an example, a person earns $10 per hour, $20,800 per year. If 10% of the salary ($2080) is placed into the plan for 10 years, it would be valued at $20,800 plus the interest earned. Even if there were no increase in salary and therefore no increase in annual contributions, with an interest rate of only 5%, the amount would be approximately $23,000 at the end of 10 years—a very impressive fringe benefit.

Another benefit, which is often overlooked, is the medical care you may receive as an employee. Depending on the type of practice in which you work, you may realize a considerable amount of complimentary health care. It is also of benefit to be a physician's employee when you need referral to another physician or medical specialist.

Medical practices that offer a good benefit package in addition to a competitive salary usually have a much more stable staff. This, in turn, results in reduced expense and maintenance of a high level of productivity because training time for new employees is not needed.

Complete Chapter 12, Unit 3 in the workbook to help you meet the objectives at the beginning of this unit and therefore achieve competency of this subject matter.

U N I T 4
General Management Duties

OBJECTIVES ....

Upon completion of this unit, the student will meet the following terminal performance objectives by verifying knowledge of the facts and principles presented through oral and written communication at a level deemed competent.

1. Discuss refunds to patients.
2. Explain why no-shows are a concern.
3. Discuss a method to ensure inventory supplies.
4. Identify office equipment requiring frequent attention.
5. Describe a manager's responsibility to the employees.
6. Describe a manager's responsibility to the physicians.
7. List general facility responsibilities.
8. Spell and define, using the glossary at the back of the text, all the words to know in this unit.

WORDS TO KNOW ....

calibration	fiscal	management
delegation	inventory	negligent
expenditure	maintenance	reimbursement
extensive		

Many duties performed in a medical office can be categorized under the broad classification of general management duties. These are activities that coordinate and maintain the functions within an office. This unit identifies a wide range of miscellaneous duties to acquaint you with those "behind the scenes" activities needed to efficiently operate a successful medical practice.

Daily and Monthly Account Records ....

Medical offices use a variety of bookkeeping and accounting systems. Regardless of the system used, some method will be needed to maintain a sense for fiscal status. It is essential to identify expenditures and income totals to ensure the practice is earning sufficient income to meet office expenses, taxes, insurance premiums and benefits payments and to provide an income for the physician. In addition, it is necessary to build assets for equipment purchases, investments, and perhaps hiring additional employees when needed.

In a medical practice, a percentage of patients may be negligent in paying for services. This can represent a sizeable amount of lost income and if it is allowed to continue or increase in percentage, it can present a serious problem and must be dealt with by the manager. Because of this fact, many physicians now require payment when services are delivered. In long-term care situations, such as with obstetrical patients, a standard fee to cover the anticipated form of delivery is established and the patient makes periodic payments prior to the delivery.

It is necessary to keep a record of accounts receivable. You can do this with a record page that allows you to begin the month with the amount carried over from the preceding month. Then each day you list charges and receipts and increase or decrease your total accounts receivable balance depending on whether your receipts or charges were greater. A trial balance, or total of all outstanding accounts, should be calculated each month. The total should agree with the accounts receivable balance.

The accounts payable records include all invoices for purchases, the checkbook, and the disbursement journal. All expenditures must be carefully entered in the disbursement journal. Office expenses must be separated from the physician's personal expenses. Office expenses are tax deductible but not all personal expenses are.

In an office where a computer is used for accounting transactions, you will receive instructions before being expected to perform the work. Every system has special features not found in other systems.

Many offices send their billing and invoices to a computerized accounting service through a telephone-linked terminal. Still other offices prepare all accounting records in a batch and take them to an accounting service computer center to be processed.

When a personal accountant is employed, the records will be maintained and a report provided to the medical practice each month, which indicates the expenditures, balances, and accounts receivable.

Another related area that a manager may need to address is missed appointments. If a patient does not show, no payment is received for that scheduled time of the day. In addition, another patient who needed to schedule an appointment was either scheduled at another time or referred if necessary. As an example, say there is one no-show for an average charge of $32. If this occurs 3 days in a week for 48 weeks during a year, $4608 income is lost. A policy of calling to remind patients may be established or a fee assessed for additional missed appointments after the patient has been notified in writing.

Office Policy Manual

The office manager would be responsible for developing and maintaining the policy and procedure manual for the office. There should be regular staff meetings to allow input from employees and exchange of ideas. This can help greatly in maintaining office harmony. To have a successful meeting, it is necessary to have an agenda or order of business so that you will be organized and know in advance what topics will be covered. If you are making decisions that will affect office operation, you should be sure a written record in the form of minutes is kept so that you will have a reference for any necessary changes

in the policy and procedure manual. The office manager should be familiar with basic parliamentary procedures.

Patient Refunds

Managers usually assume the responsibility of verifying overpayment to a patient's account before approving reimbursement to the patient. This situation occurs when both the patient and the insurance company pay the physician or an error in the amount due is made.

Equipment Maintenance and Supply Inventory

The manager or the medical assistant is expected to keep track of equipment maintenance and maintain an inventory of clinical and administrative supplies. An office that has been in operation for several years will have an established list of companies that supply its needs. You should not change to another company without consulting the physician. You should be alert to the best quality for the best price, however. You will be a valuable member of the health care team if you are able to control costs without sacrificing the quality of the products and supplies you use. New medical assistants will usually have to prove their capability to handle routine office affairs before being entrusted with maintaining an inventory.

The best method for organizing office supplies is to prepare a separate inventory card for each item used. These should be reviewed and updated in a systematic manner. Some high usage items may require a daily update, whereas a weekly update is sufficient for others. The inventory card should indicate the supplier's name, address, phone number, and the cost of the item. A file should be maintained of the maintenance contracts on equipment along with the names and phone numbers of service personnel to be called.

Good housekeeping rules must be followed in storage of supplies. The storage areas should be clean and dry. All medications should be stored in a cool, dark area to avoid deterioration. Narcotics should always be in a locked cabinet. Some laboratory supplies must be refrigerated. Supplies should be stored near the area where they will be used.

It is not possible to give quality care to patients with faulty office equipment. You must be aware of daily, weekly, or monthly maintenance that must be carried out to keep equipment in good working order. Always go through a troubleshooting checklist to see if you can correct a problem before requesting outside help. Maintenance personnel charge for plugging in a machine just as they do for repair service.

Autoclaves require regular cleaning to work effectively in sterilization procedures. Typewriters should be covered when not in use. The calibration of aneroid sphygmomanometers should be checked periodically. The mercury level of mercury manometers should be checked to ensure an accurate blood pressure reading (see Chapter 15, Unit 2).

Electrocardiograph machines must be maintained. Light sources on sigmoidoscopy, otoscope, and ophthalmoscope should be checked and replaced when necessary. There should always be a supply of batteries and light bulbs to be used in maintenance of equipment.

A part of office maintenance that cannot be overlooked is linen supplies. Some offices use gowns, towels, pillow cases, and sheets, which must be sent to a laundry. If disposable items are used, there must be an adequate supply at all times.

Payroll Records

All employees are expected to work the assigned number of hours per day, week and month. Any time off must be reconciled on the payroll records and the salary adjusted according to office policy.

Responsibility for Decision-Making

In large practices, clinics, and corporations, it is advisable to divide the decision-making responsibilities among the physicians according to their area of interest or expertise. When decisions need to be made, the manager has to confer with only that physician or two instead of the total partnership. An example of division of responsibility is:

- Employment/personnel concerns
- Purchasing and office facility concerns
- Lab and radiology
- Fees, investments, and other financial matters

Decisions made by designated physicians are then usually discussed at the general meeting.

Responsibilities to Employees

The manager in large practices often has the following responsibilities related to the support staff employees.

- Interview, hire, and terminate employees in concert with physicians if desired.
- Supervise or personally train employees. This applies to new personnel as well as updating current staff.
- Conduct staff meetings to inform, discuss, and exchange information.
- Make out work schedules.
- Arrange vacations and coverage if needed. Work in the position if necessary.
- Conduct performance evaluations, establishing probationary periods as deemed necessary.
- Consult physicians concerning salary increases and benefit changes.

Responsibility for the Facility

The physical structure of the office must be observed and maintained. The manager assumes responsibility for:

- Maintenance of office services such as cleaning and laundry
- Subscriptions to magazines and health-related literature
- Monitoring and paying utilities
- Suggesting improvements: repairs, decorating, organization of rooms

Responsibilities to Physicians

Physicians also need to be kept informed and aware of conditions affecting the practice. The manager has a great deal of obligation to the physicians. Some areas the manager must consider are:

- Assist in creating or updating business policies to increase efficiency
- Attend meetings pertaining to office management such as those sponsored by the medical association and other professional organizations
- Update physicians on Medicare, health plans, and insurance company policy changes, fee schedules, and reimbursement rates (for example, changes in ICD or CPT codes or descriptors or the reduction in Medicare coverage affecting reimbursement when accepting consignment). Approximately 85% of a physician's income is from third party payers, either directly or indirectly. It is critical that physicians learn to code their services correctly to obtain the full amount allowed for their care.
- Order CPT and ICD books annually. Review for deleted numbers.
- Hold physician meetings to discuss practice concerns.

Tax Records

In addition to those already mentioned, the 1099 forms issued by third party payers, which indicate the total amount paid directly to the physician during the year, must be saved and given to the accountant for inclusion with the tax forms.

Manager's Rewards

The role of office manager can be as limited or **extensive** as the physician(s) feel comfortable in the **delegation** of authority. A trusted employee who performs well in the role of office manager becomes a tremendous asset to the practice. This role in large medical offices carries a great amount of authority and responsibility, but the rewards are worthwhile both financially and personally. It is a challenge you should look forward to accepting should the opportunity arise.

Complete Chapter 12, Unit 4 in the workbook to help you meet the objectives at the beginning of this unit and therefore achieve competency of this subject matter.

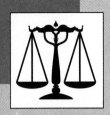

MEDICAL-LEGAL/ ETHICAL HIGHLIGHTS

Throughout this chapter you should be mindful of all medical-legal/ethical implications. Listed below are a few important reminders.

1. Keep accurate and complete records.
2. Secure important papers and documents in safe or fireproof storage.
3. Keep records private and confidential.
4. Stay abreast of current changes in tax laws and interest rates.

Ms. Right. . .
        is organized and efficient in completing information on patients' records. She is mindful in storing important documents in a fireproof storage for safekeeping. She respects the privacy of patients and never leaves charts or records out where other patients can read them. When bulletins are received, she carefully reads them and notes important changes in tax laws and interest rates.

Employment outlook: Continuous

Mrs. Wrong. . .
        is careless in leaving charts and other important documents out in full view of other patients. She leaves charts and other information out wherever she pleases and has a difficult time finding things. She ignores bulletins concerning tax laws and interest rates because she doesn't like to read. She is negligent in recording important information on patients' charts because she is so disorganized.

Employment outlook: Termination

REFERENCES

American Medical Association. "The Business Side of Medical Practice."

Diehl, Marcia, and Fordney, Marilyn. *Medical Typing and Transcribing Techniques and Procedures.* Philadelphia: W.B. Saunders, 1984.

Douglas, Lloyd V., James T. Blanford, and Ruth I. Anderson. *Teaching Business Subjects,* 3d Ed. Englewood Cliffs, NJ: Prentice Hall, 1973.

Erlich, Ann, M.A. *The Role of Computers in Medical Practice Management.* Champaign, IL: Colwell Systems, Inc., 1981.

Frew, Mary, and Frew, David. *Comprehensive Medical Assisting: Administrative and Clinical Procedures,* 2nd Ed. Philadelphia: F.A. Davis, 1988.

King, Colleen, RN. Office Manager, Northwest Family Physicians. Interview, October 1991.

Kinn, Mary E. and Derge, Eleanor. *The Medical Assistant: Administrative and Clinical,* 6th Ed. Philadelphia: W. B. Saunders, 1988.

Simmers, Louise. *Diversified Health Occupations,* 3d Ed. Albany: Delmar, 1993.

Structure and Function of the Body Systems

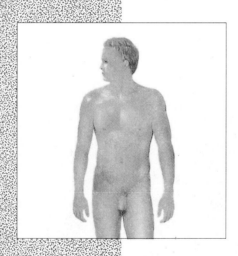

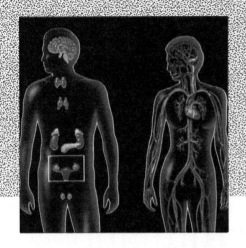

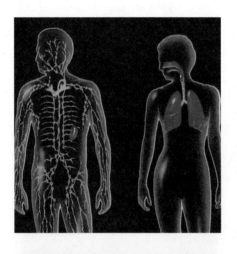

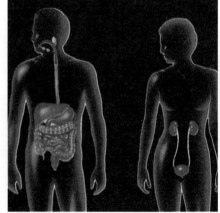

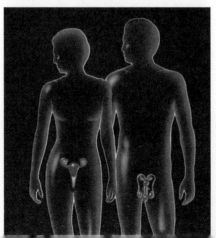

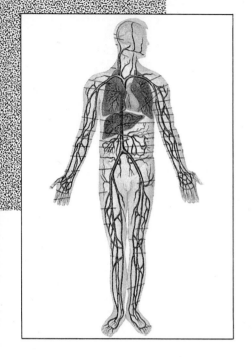

CHAPTER 13

Anatomy and Physiology of the Human Body

The human body is a fantastic combination of parts that function in an organized manner, far more efficiently and effectively than any machine ever developed. This chapter describes the body's fundamental structure, the body systems, and discusses how the parts work together.

The diseases and disorders affecting the human body are a result of impairment, deterioration, or malfunction of one or more of its component parts. Within this chapter, the anatomy of each body system will be presented as well as how that system physiologically functions within itself and with the other body systems. Following the presentation of each system will be a discussion of characteristic pathophysiological conditions and disorders, many of which result from the body's inability to adapt or defend itself. A basic discussion of the critical role of the immune system in maintaining a healthy state will help you to correlate your knowledge of the body's complex interrelationships. With this understanding you will be able to see how the patient's concerns and complaints, the physician's examination, and the clinical findings fit together to indicate the diagnosis and the plan of treatment the physician prescribes.

U N I T   1

Anatomical Descriptors and Fundamental Body Structure

OBJECTIVES ....

Upon completion of this unit, the student will meet the following terminal performance objectives by verifying knowledge of the facts and principles presented through oral and written communication at a level deemed competent.

1. Describe the anatomical position.
2. Apply the appropriate terminology to points of reference on the human body.
3. Locate the four body cavities.
4. Name the major organ(s) located within each body cavity.
5. Identify the regions of the abdomen.
6. Describe the basic characteristics of the cell.
7. Describe the six ways molecules pass through cell membranes.
8. Describe the four main types of body tissues.
9. Name the 10 systems of the body.
10. Spell and define, using the glossary at the back of the text, all the words to know in this unit.

WORDS TO KNOW ....

abdominal	elements
abdominopelvic	endocytosis
anatomical	endoplasmic reticulum
anatomy	epigastric
anterior	epithelial
biochemistry	exocytosis
buccal	extremities
cardiac	filtration
caudal	frontal
cavities	gene
cell membrane	Golgi apparatus
centrioles	gross anatomy
chromosomes	histology
connective	histotechnologist
coronal	homeostasis
cranial	horizontal
cytology	hypertonic
cytoplasm	hypochondriac
cytotechnologist	hypogastric
dehydration	hypotonic
diaphragm	iliac
diffusion	inferior
distal	inguinal
dorsal	involuntary
edema	isotonic

Keloid	pathophysiology
lateral	pelvic
lumbar	phagocytosis
lysosomes	physiology
medial	pinocytosis
membrane	posterior
microscopic anatomy	proximal
midline	pubic
mitochondria	quadrant
mitosis	retroperitoneal
muscle	ribosome
myelin	sagittal
nasal	skeletal
nerve	smooth
neurilemma	spinal
neuron	striated
normal saline	superior
nucleolus	system
nucleus	thoracic
orbital	tissue
organ	transverse
organelles	umbilical
osmosis	ventral
osseous	voluntary

Anatomy and Physiology Defined ....

Two terms are used in discussing the study of the human body: anatomy, which is the study of the physical structure of the body and its organs; and physiology, which is the science of the function of cells, tissues, and organs of the body. In other words, anatomy describes the framework and physical characteristics while physiology explains how everything works together to support life.

Anatomy can be subdivided into various areas of study. For instance, the term gross anatomy refers to the study of those features that can be observed with the naked eye by inspection and dissection. As an example, the pathologist, when examining a tissue specimen, will describe its gross anatomical surface appearance and then proceed with the dissection and its description.

An area of study known as microscopic anatomy deals with features that can be observed only with the use of a microscope. Referring again to the pathologist, a fragment of a specimen can be properly prepared on a slide and observed with a microscope to complete the description of the specimen's characteristics and formulate an opinion as to its identity or state of condition.

There are two related areas of microscopic anatomy, cytology, the study of cell life and formation and histology, the study of the microscopic structure of tissue. Pathologists are assisted by laboratory specialists known as cytotechnologists and histotechnologists who precisely prepare materials for microscopic examination and diagnosis.

Physiology is the study of the interrelationships of all the functioning structures of the body. When everything is in harmony and all biological indicators are within acceptable limits, the individual is referred to as being in a "steady state" or "normal." When the normal physiology is disrupted to the point of instability and begins to deteriorate, pathophysiological mechanisms are likely to occur and may result in the development of a disease condition. Pathophysiology is the study of mechanisms by which disease occurs, the responses of the body to the disease process, and the effects of both on normal function.

Pathophysiology attempts to bring together the clinical signs and symptoms present with the knowledge of the effects of the disease processes on the body, from the cellular level to the total human being. Often close observation of the clinical signs of a disease state has led to the discovery of physiological functions previously unknown. This is currently apparent in the great effort to understand the immune system to find a way to effectively control and eventually eliminate AIDS and cancer.

Fortunately, the healthy body has an enormous capacity to protect itself by compensating, defending, and adapting to the pathophysiological effects of disease. However, when this fails, appropriate medical intervention can often correct or at least control the disease process.

Language of Medicine ....

The members of the health care team must be able to accurately communicate information, findings, and instructions among themselves. Much of the language of medicine is precise and is specific to the field of health care. For instance, it is necessary to not only know about the human body but also to be able to physically as well as verbally locate body structures or describe the site of a patient's complaint or injury. The following fundamental descriptive terminology will be essential to the understanding of body references.

Anatomical Directional Terms ....

Certain directional terms are universally used in describing anatomical structures. A body is said to be in anatomical position when standing erect, with arms down at the sides, and the palms of the hands facing forward, Figure 13–1. This means that when the person is facing you, his right side is on your left, as if you were looking in a mirror. When reference is made to a body structure or a specific area, it is in relationship to this anatomical position. The same is true when you are studying illustrations in this textbook or labeling a drawing in the workbook.

Dividing the body vertically down the front will result in a right and left half. This imaginary line is known as the median or sagittal plane. The right and left designations always refer to right and left in anatomical position. Anything located toward the midline is said to be

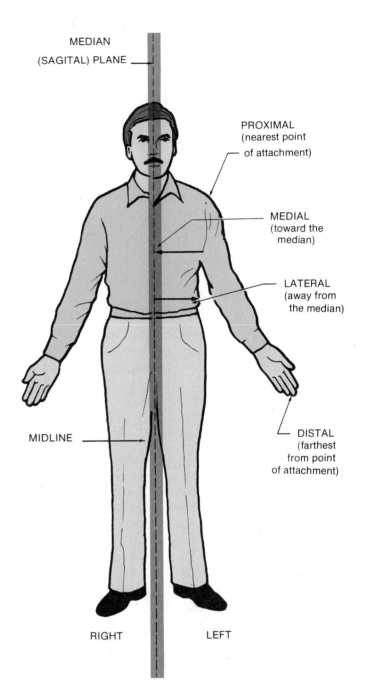

FIGURE 13–1 Anatomical position with directional references

medial, while anything away from the midline is said to be lateral.

Two other terms are used to describe the relationship of the extremities or ends of the body, such as the arms and legs, to the trunk of the body. Proximal indicates nearness to the point of attachment, while distal indicates distance away from the point of attachment. These terms are also applicable when describing parts of the arms, legs, fingers, or toes. For example, the thumb and great toe have proximal and distal sections while the other fingers and toes have proximal, middle, and distal sections.

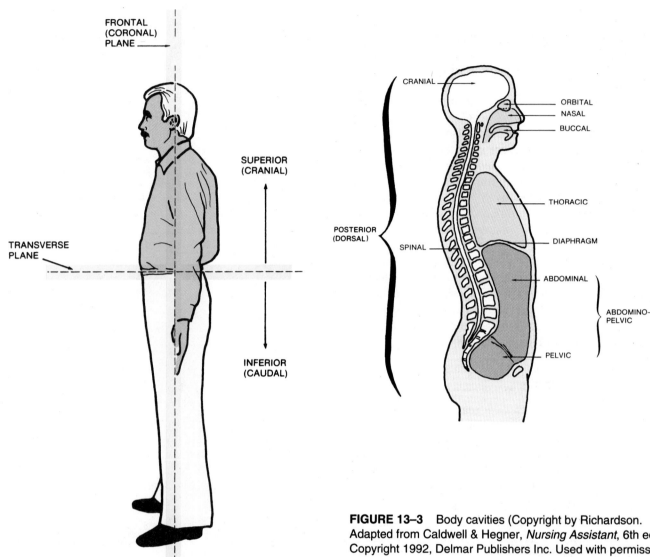

FRONTAL
(CORONAL)
PLANE

SUPERIOR
(CRANIAL)

TRANSVERSE
PLANE

INFERIOR
(CAUDAL)

ANTERIOR (VENTRAL) ◄─────► POSTERIOR (DORSAL)

CRANIAL

ORBITAL
NASAL
BUCCAL

POSTERIOR
(DORSAL)

SPINAL

THORACIC

DIAPHRAGM

ABDOMINAL

ANTE
(VENT

ABDOMINO—
PELVIC

PELVIC

FIGURE 13–3 Body cavities (Copyright by Richardson. Adapted from Caldwell & Hegner, *Nursing Assistant*, 6th ed. Copyright 1992, Delmar Publishers Inc. Used with permission.)

FIGURE 13–2 Anatomical directional references

If you draw a line vertically through the side of the body, from the top of the head, to the feet, you will make a front and back section, Figure 13–2. This line is known as the frontal or coronal plane. The front is known as the anterior or ventral section; the back is called the posterior or dorsal section.

Finally, drawing an imaginary line horizontally (across) the body creates a transverse plane. The portion of the body above the line is known as superior or cranial. The portion below the line is called inferior or caudal. It is not necessary that the body be divided into equal parts. The terms superior and inferior refer to any relation-

ship of structures above or below a "line" and depends on where it is drawn. For example, with a transverse line at the waist, the chest is superior to the abdomen but if at the neck, the chest is inferior to the head. All anatomical directional terms are appropriate only when describing the relationship of one structure to another.

These planes or sections can also be applied to internal structures as well as to the body as a whole. *Incisions* (cuts) made on the body surface or into organs are often made along a plane. The surgeon's description of the operation will identify the location of the incisions made using referencing planes. A tissue specimen cut along the transverse plane is known as a *cross section*.

Body Cavities and Organs ....

The body is divided into two main cavities, an anterior or ventral cavity and a posterior or dorsal cavity, Figure 13–3. A dome-shaped muscle known as the diaphragm divides the anterior cavity into an upper **thoracic** cavity and a lower **abdominopelvic** cavity. The thoracic cavity (chest) has a wall of ribs that protects its vital organs—the heart, lungs, and the great blood vessels, Figure 13–4.

The diaphragm alternately contracts and relaxes to move the lungs, causing breathing to occur.

The abdominopelvic cavity has two parts, an upper **abdominal** portion and a lower **pelvic** portion. The abdominal portion extends from the diaphragm to the top edge of the pelvic girdle (bones). The organs found in the abdomen are the stomach, small intestines, most of the large intestine, the liver, spleen, pancreas, and gallbladder. The kidneys are located in the dorsal abdominal area but are behind the peritoneal **membrane** that lines the cavity and so are technically outside the abdominal cavity. This space is referred to as **retroperitoneal,** behind the peritoneum. The pelvic cavity is surrounded by the pelvic girdle, which provides protection for the urinary bladder, the last portion of the large intestine, and the internal reproductive organs.

The cranial cavity is totally encased by the bones of the skull, which provides protection for the brain. The cranial cavity is joined at its base by the **spinal** cavity, which extends through the center of the column of vertebrae (bones). This bony structure contains the spinal cord and protects it from injury.

There are three other small cavities, the **orbital** for the eyes, the **nasal** for the structures of the nose, and the **buccal** or mouth.

Abdominal Regions

The abdomen is such a large area of the body that it is necessary to divide it into regions for purposes of identification or reference. There are two recognized methods of division. One creates **quadrants** known as the right and left upper quadrants (RUQ and LUQ) and the right and left lower quadrants (RLQ and LLQ), Figure 13–5.

A more exacting division results in nine regions identifiable by location and an anatomical reference point. The three central areas are called **epigastric** (over the stomach), **umbilical** (around the umbilicus), and **hypogastric** (below the stomach; also called **pubic**). The six side areas are called the right and left **hypochondriac** (below the cartilage, referring to the ribs), the right and left **lumbar** (loin or side region; also called lateral); and the right and left **iliac** (referring to the ileum portion of the pelvic bone; also known as the **inguinal,** meaning groin, region), Figure 13–6, page 208.

The Cell

To understand the structure of the body, you must first learn about its basic building block, the cell. This fascinating wonder is a living, working, microscopic image

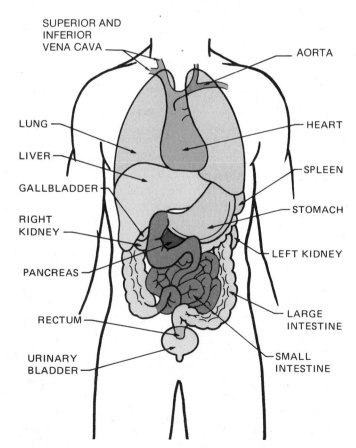

FIGURE 13–4   Thoracic and abdominal organs

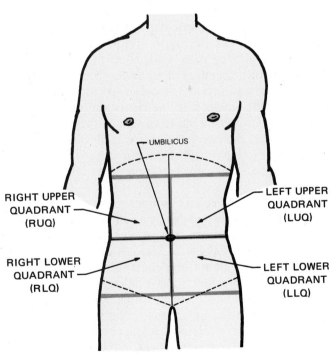

FIGURE 13–5   The four abdominal quadrants (Adapted from Caldwell & Hegner, *Nursing Assistant*, 6th ed. Copyright 1992, Delmar Publishers Inc.)

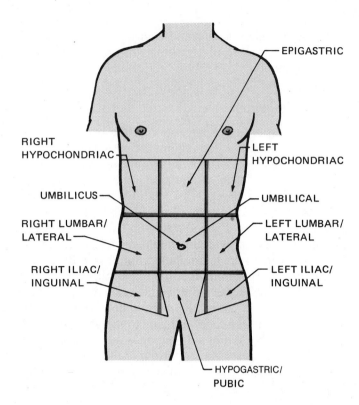

FIGURE 13–6 Nine regions of the abdomen (Adapted from Caldwell & Hegner, *Nursing Assistant*, 6th ed. Copyright 1992, Delmar Publishers Inc.)

of the body. It requires food and oxygen to survive, performs specific functions, produces heat and energy, gives off waste products, and can reproduce itself.

Cells vary greatly in size and shape due to their various activities. The body contains about 75 trillion cells. Whenever cells of a particular type are destroyed, the remaining cells of that type divide until they have replaced the missing cells. Cells come in different varieties to perform specific duties. Some secrete materials, some receive and transmit impulses, or some enable us to move. Still others carry nutrients and oxygen, clot blood, or destroy bacteria. Even though they are microscopic in size, their proper function is absolutely essential to life. No man-made apparatus can match the cell for the number of chemical reactions that occur in such a small space.

A conventional cell is composed of a fluid called **cytoplasm** and is surrounded by a cell membrane, Figure 13–7. The **cell membrane** separates the cell from the surrounding environment. It consists of protein and fat molecules. The membrane controls what enters and leaves the cell; therefore, it plays an important role in the health and welfare of the cell, which will be seen later. Enclosed within the membrane is the sticky semifluid material known as cytoplasm. It is a combination of protein, lipids (fat), carbohydrates, minerals, salts, and water (over 70%). Chemical reactions such as respiration and protein synthesis occur in the cytoplasm.

Within the cytoplasm of the cell are many minute bodies called **organelles** that perform amazing tasks.

The organelles are the **nucleus, mitochondria, ribosomes, centriole, endoplasmic reticulum, Golgi apparatus,** and **lysosomes.** Scientists still do not understand how some functions are carried out so when describing them they may use the word "magical." They do know some organelles physically separate the chemical reactions occurring in the cytoplasm because many reactions are not compatible. Organelles also control the time when reactions take place, such as producing or processing a molecule in one organelle then later using the molecule in another reaction.

The *nucleus* is a dense mass within the cytoplasm. It is surrounded by its own nuclear membrane. Materials pass in and out of the nucleus from the cytoplasm through pores in the membrane. The membrane is continuous with the endoplasmic reticulum, which often has ribosomes attached. The nucleus is the control center of the cell. It regulates the chemical reactions and controls the process of **mitosis** (cell division) for reproduction. Within the nucleus are the structures called **chromosomes.** Each member of a species has a specific number of chromosomes. Human beings have 46 individual or 23 pairs of chromosomes that store the hereditary material passed on from one generation to another. Twenty-two pairs of chromosomes are autosome (same in number and kind) and one pair are sex chromosomes, either both X if female, or an X and a Y, if male. Chromosomes have molecules known as deoxyribonucleic acid (DNA), which contain the genes and carry the genetic coding necessary for the exact duplication of the cell.

The DNA structure varies from one cell to another in that the sequence of the base pairs of the DNA molecule are arranged differently. The sequence is what determines heredity factors. A gene is the specific sequence of about 1000 base pairs. Approximately 100,000 genes compose the DNA molecule of one chromosome. Since humans have 46 chromosomes, we therefore have about 4 1/2 million genes in each cell. This helps explain why there is so much variety in the human race.

The nucleus itself will have at least one **nucleolus.** In a nucleolus, portions of ribonucleic acid (RNA) are assembled with proteins to make subunits of the ribosomes, which then pass through the nuclear pores of the nuclear membrane into the cytoplasm, to become a complete two-part ribosome to synthesize protein. Ribosomes are found circulating in the cytoplasm or attached to the endoplasmic reticulum.

Centrioles are the two cylinder-shaped organelles near the nucleus. During mitosis, the centrioles separate and form spindle fibers that attach to the chromosomes to ensure their equal distribution to the two new daughter cells.

Endoplasmic reticulum crisscrosses the cytoplasm in a network fashion. When attached to the nuclear membrane, it serves as a passageway for the transportation of materials in and out of the nucleus. If grouped

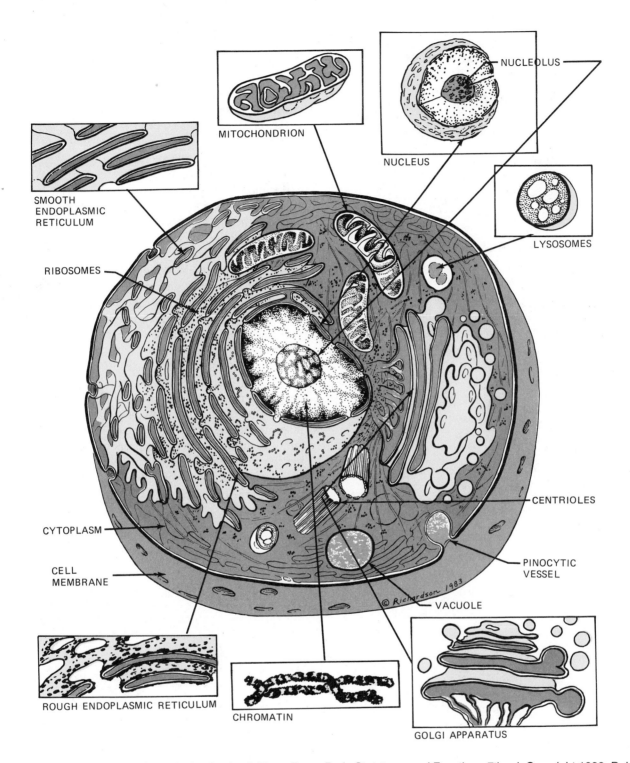

FIGURE 13–7 Fine structure of a typical animal cell (From Fong, *Body Structures and Functions*, 7th ed. Copyright 1989, Delmar Publishers Inc.)

together, they can store large amounts of protein. The difference between rough and smooth endoplasmic reticulum is the presence of *ribosomes* on the membrane. Ribosomes give the membrane a coarse and rough appearance.

Mitochondria are round or rod-shaped organelles that supply the cell's energy. There may be from one to over a thousand in each cell depending on how much energy

that type of cell requires. Mitochondria have a double-membraned structure with the inner membrane folding into ridges. Chemicals known as enzymes are located in the ridges. The cell is capable of respiration because the enzymes break down nutrient molecules to provide carbon dioxide and water.

The *Golgi apparatus* is a stack of membrane layers, which are believed to synthesize carbohydrates and com-

TABLE 13–1
Summary Table of Cell Organelles

Organelle	Function
Cell membrane	Regulates transport of substances into and out of the cell.
Cytoplasm	Provides an organized watery environment in which life functions take place by the activities of the organelles contained in the cytoplasm.
Nucleus	Serves as the "brain" for the control of the cell's metabolic activities and cell division.
Nuclear membrane	Regulates transport of substances into and out of the nucleus.
Nucleoplasm	A clear, semifluid medium that fills the spaces around the chromatin and the nucleoli.
Nucleolus	Functions as a reservoir for RNA.
Ribosomes	Serve as sites for protein synthesis.
Endoplasmic reticulum	Provides passages through which transport of substances occurs in cytoplasm.
Mitochondria	Serve as sites of cellular respiration and energy production.
Golgi apparatus	Manufactures carbohydrates and packages secretions for discharge from the cell.
Lysosomes	Serve as centers of cellular digestion
Pinocytic vesicles	Transport of large particles into a cell.
Centrosome and centrioles	Contains two centrioles that are functional during animal cell division.

(From Fong, *Body Structures and Functions*, 7th ed. Copyright 1989, Delmar Publishers Inc.)

bine them with molecules of proteins. The organelle appears to store and prepare secretions to excrete from the cell. Therefore, the cells of the gastric, salivary, and pancreatic glands have large numbers of Golgi apparatus.

Lysosomes are round or oval structures. They have a strong digestive enzyme that consumes protein molecules such as those found in old worn cells, bacteria, or foreign matter. This is a very important function of the body's natural immune system.

Pinocytic vesicles are pocket-like formations in the cell's membrane. These structures permit large molecules like protein and fat, which cannot pass through the pores of the cell membrane, to enter with the extracellular fluid into the vesicle. Then the "pocket" closes forming a vacuole (bubble) in the cytoplasm. This process is called endocytosis. When liquid droplets, instead of protein or fat molecules, are enclosed, the process is known as pinocytosis, which means "cell drinking." A related term, exocytosis, refers to a similar process whereby substances are moved from the cell to the outside. On entering the cytoplasm, most vesicles fuse with lysosomes and their contents are digested. Special white blood cells known as phagocytes rely on endocytosis to destroy harmful bacteria in the body. As you learn more about your body, you will begin to appreciate what a magnificent piece of "equipment" it is and how important it is that you care for it properly. You have the physical and mental power to have great impact on your health and even your very life.

Table 13–1 summarizes the organelles and their role in the function of the cell.

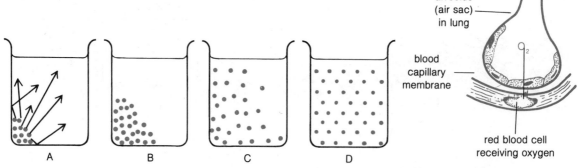

Diffusion:

(A) A small lump of sugar is placed into a beaker of water, its molecules dissolve and begin to diffuse outward. (B&C) The sugar molecules continue to diffuse through the water from an area of greater concentration to an area of lesser concentration. (D) Over a long period of time, the sugar molecules are evenly distributed throughout the water, reaching a state of equilibrium.

Example of diffusion in the human body: Oxygen diffuses from an alveolus in a lung where it is in greater concentration, across the blood capillary membrane, into a red blood cell where it is in lesser concentration.

FIGURE 13–8 The process of diffusion (From Fong, *Body Structures and Functions*, 7th ed. Copyright 1989, Delmar Publishers Inc.)

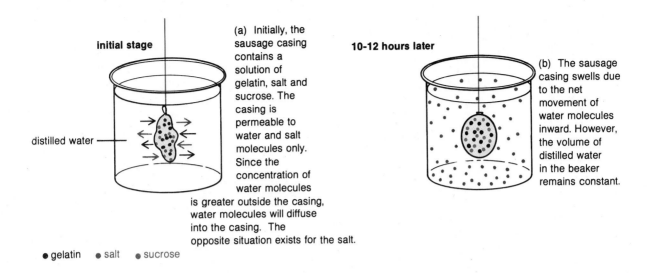

initial stage

(a) Initially, the sausage casing contains a solution of gelatin, salt and sucrose. The casing is permeable to water and salt molecules only. Since the concentration of water molecules is greater outside the casing, water molecules will diffuse into the casing. The opposite situation exists for the salt.

distilled water

10-12 hours later

(b) The sausage casing swells due to the net movement of water molecules inward. However, the volume of distilled water in the beaker remains constant.

● gelatin   ● salt   ● sucrose

FIGURE 13–9   Osmosis: the diffusion of water through a selective permeable membrane is illustrated. (A sausage casing is an example of a selective permeable membrane.) (From Fong, *Body Structures and Functions*, 7th ed. Copyright 1989, Delmar Publishers Inc.)

Passing Molecules Through Cell Membranes ·····················

As stated before, the cell membrane controls materials entering and leaving the cell. This is necessary for the cell to acquire substances from its environment to be processed for its use, or for secretion, or for excretion of the waste materials. There are six processes by which materials pass through a cell membrane; diffusion, osmosis, filtration, active transport, phagocytosis and pinocytosis.

Diffusion is a process whereby gas, liquid, or solid molecules distribute themselves evenly through a medium. When the medium is a fluid and the molecules are solid, they are called solutes, Figure 13–8. When solutes and water pass across a membrane to distribute themselves, they will move from an area of higher concentration to an area of lesser concentration. Diffusion plays a vital role in the body. For example, higher concentrations of oxygen in the alveolus (air sac) of the lung cross the membrane into the lesser concentrated area of the red blood cell in the capillary, Figure 13–8. The blood cell, now with a high concentration of oxygen, circulates in the blood to a body cell with lower oxygen concentration and exchanges its oxygen for the cell's higher concentration of waste products. And so the body's cells "breathe" in a process called *internal respiration*.

Osmosis is a process of diffusion of water or another solvent through a selected permeable membrane, one through which some solutes can pass but others cannot, Figure 13–9. In the illustration, the membrane will only allow the salt and water to pass through; therefore, the

hypertonic solution   **hypotonic solution**   **isotonic solution**

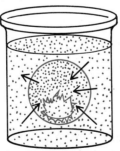
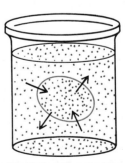

Hypertonic solution (seawater)
a red blood cell will shrink and wrinkle up because water molecules are moving out of the cell.

● water molecules

Hypotonic solution (freshwater)
a red blood cell will swell and burst because water molecules are moving into the cell.

Isotonic solution (human blood serum)
a red blood cell remains unchanged, because the movement of water molecules into and out of the cell are the same.

FIGURE 13–10   Movement of water molecules in solutions of different osmolalities. (From Fong, *Body Structures and Functions*, 7th ed. Copyright 1989, Delmar Publishers Inc.)

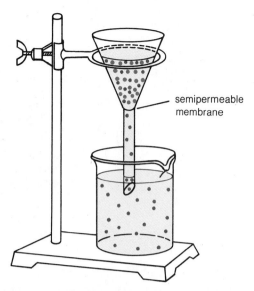

semipermeable
membrane

Filtration: Small molecules are filtered through the semi-permeable membrane, while the large molecules remain in the funnel.

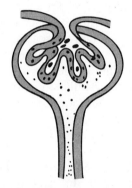

Example of filtration in the human body: Glomerulus of kidney, large particles like red blood cells and proteins remain in the blood, and small molecules like urea and water are excreted as a metabolic excretory product—urine.

FIGURE 13–11 Filtration: a passive transport process (From Fong, *Body Structures and Functions*, 7th ed. Copyright 1989, Delmar Publishers Inc.)

salt leaves the greater concentrated area within the membrane to go to the lesser concentrated water. At the same time, the water leaves its higher concentrated area to enter the lesser concentrated area within the membrane. When the water molecules are equal on both sides, the diffusion will stop. The pressure of the water molecules inside the membrane is then said to be at *equilibrium,* a state known as the *osmotic pressure.*

The osmotic characteristics of solutions are classified by their effect on red blood cells, Figure 13–10, page 211. If the solution is of the same osmotic pressure as blood serum it is known as an isotonic solution. A 0.9% salt (NaCl) solution has the same salt concentration as that of the red blood cell and is called normal saline. If the osmolality is lower, the solution is hypotonic and the blood cell will swell with water and burst. In a

hypertonic solution, the cell will release its water and shrink.

Filtration is the movement of solutes and water across a semipermeable membrane as a result of a force such as gravity or blood pressure. The particles move from a higher to a lower area of pressure. The size of the pores of some membranes allow only small molecules to leave. This process occurs in the kidneys where small molecules of water and waste products are filtered from the blood in the capillaries while the large protein molecules and red blood cells are retained, Figure 13–11.

Active transport refers to molecules moving across a membrane from an area of low concentration to an area of higher concentration due to the presence of ATP (adenosinetriphosphate), a high-energy compound from the cell membrane. It appears as a "carrier" molecule, temporarily binding with another molecule on the outer edge of the membrane. The carrier crosses the membrane and releases its "passenger" into the cytoplasm. The carrier then receives more energy from the membrane and returns to the outer surface to transport another molecule. The carrier can also reverse the process and carry molecules from the inside to the outside.

Phagocytosis is known as "cell eating." White blood cells become phagocytes and engulf bacteria, cell fragments, or damaged cells, Figure 13–12. The white cell forms a vacuole by enfolding its membrane and enclosing the particle. When it is completely enclosed, digestive enzymes enter from the cytoplasm and destroy the trapped material. This process is extremely important to the body's ability to maintain a healthy state.

Pinocytosis, as discussed earlier, is called "cell drinking" and involves the engulfing of large molecules of liquid material. Once inside the cytoplasm, the fluid is digested by the cell.

Another area of great importance to the welfare of the human body is its chemistry. When chemical reactions within the body are studied, it is referred to as biochemistry. The basic building blocks of all matter are called elements, substances in their simplest form. There are 92 natural and at least 13 man-made elements. Of these, about 20 are in all living things. Four of these 20 elements make up 97% of all living matter. They are carbon, oxygen, hydrogen, and nitrogen. The remaining 16 elements are sodium, chloride, magnesium, phosphorus, sulfur, calcium, potassium, iron, copper, manganese, zinc, boron, tin, vanadium, cobalt, and molybdenum. Because the last four occur in the body in such minute amounts, they are known as *trace elements.*

Many elements combine together in specific amounts to form new substances known as *compounds.* Some common compounds are water (hydrogen and oxygen), carbon dioxide (carbon and oxygen), salt (sodium and chloride), hydrochloric acid (hydrogen and chlorine), and sodium bicarbonate (sodium, hydrogen, carbon, and oxygen). Compounds can be classified in one of three groups: acids, bases, or salts. An acid compound will

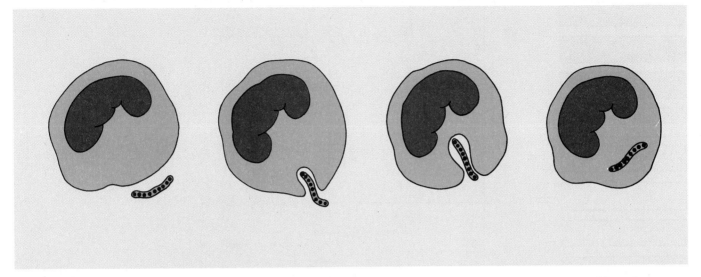

FIGURE 13–12 Phagocytosis of bacteria by a white blood cell. Phagocytosis can occur in the blood stream or white cells may squeeze through capillary walls and destroy bacteria in the tissues.

have positively charged ions of hydrogen and negatively charged ions of some other element. They have a sour taste such as found in some citrus fruits (limes and lemons). However, an unknown substance should not be tasted to determine its acidity, but rather tested by the special dyes contained in litmus paper. If acid is present, blue litmus paper will turn red.

A base compound is also called an alkali. A base substance will have negatively charged hydroxide ions and positively charged ions of a metal. Bases have a bitter taste and will turn red litmus paper blue. Table 13–2 lists

some common acids and bases and identifies where they are found.

When an acid and a base are combined, they form a salt and water. A common example is sodium chloride (table salt), which is the result of combining hydrochloric acid with sodium hydroxide. When the water evaporates, the salt remains.

Frequently the determination of acidity or alkalinity of a body fluid or solution is desired. This measurement is referred to as the *p*H. A *p*H value of 7.0 on the *p*H scale indicates the solution has the same amount of hydrogen ions as hydroxide ions and therefore is neutral. An example of a neutral solution is water. A *p*H value between 0 and 6.9 indicates an acidic solution. The lower the number the stronger the acid or hydrogen ion concentration. A *p*H value of 7.1 to 14.0 indicates the solution is basic or alkaline. The higher the number is above 7.0 the stronger the base or hydroxide ion concentration. The *p*H values of some common acids, bases, and human body fluids and their effect on a *p*H testing strip are shown in Figure 13–13, page 214.

TABLE 13–2
Names, Location, or Use of Some Common Acids and Bases

Name of Acid	Where Found or Used
Acetic acid	Found in vinegar
Boric acid	Weak eyewash
Carbonic acid	Found in carbonated beverages
Hydrochloric acid	Found in stomach
Nitric acid	Industrial oxidizing acid
Sulfuric acid	Found in batteries and industrial mineral acid

Name of Base	Where Found or Used
Ammonium hydroxide	Household liquid cleaners
Magnesium hydroxide	Milk or magnesia
Potassium hydroxide	Caustic potash
Sodium hydroxide	Lye

(Adapted from Fong, *Body Structure and Functions,* 7th ed. Copyright 1989, Delmar Publishers, Inc.)

Cellular Division

The division of cells is known as mitosis and is controlled by the nucleus of the cell, Figure 13–14(a), page 215. When a cell is preparing to divide, the two pairs of centrioles, just outside the nucleus, move to opposite sides of the cell (b). Threadlike substances trail behind them, forming a spindle. The nucleus then duplicates exactly its chromatine material (c). As division begins, the nuclear membrane breaks up and the pairs of chromosomes attach to the spindles (d) and are pulled to the center of the cell (e). As the spindles enlarge, the centrioles are pushed farther apart (f) until the chromosomes break in half (g). The spindles then dissolve and a

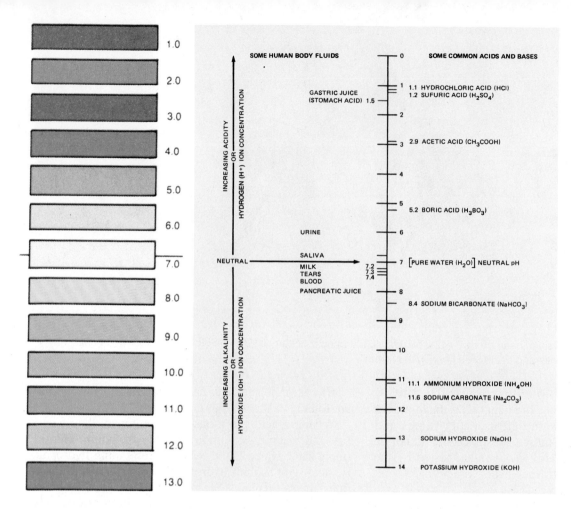

FIGURE 13–13   pH Values of some common acids, bases, and human body fluids and the color changes that can occur to a pH strip when tested. (From Fong, *Body Structures and Functions*, 7th ed. Copyright 1989, Delmar Publishers Inc.)

nuclear membrane develops around each new set of chromosomes (h). For unknown reasons, the cell then pinches itself in two, thereby making two new cells (i) called daughter cells. Mitosis results in the formation of two daughter nuclei with the exact same genes as the mother cell nucleus. The purpose of cell division is to provide exact duplication of cells for growth and repair of the body. In the unit on immunity, you will discover what happens when an antigen (foreign matter) interferes with this process.

All cells do not reproduce at the same rate. The blood-forming cells of the bone marrow, the cells of the skin, and the cells of the intestinal lining reproduce continuously. Muscle cells only reproduce every few years; however, muscle tissue formed of voluntary muscle cells may be enlarged with exercise. This is apparent from the great increase in muscle size produced by body builders who use weight and repetitions of routines to achieve muscle definition and enlargement. Cells of the nerve tissue, or neurons, do not increase in number after birth, and some cannot be regenerated if damaged or destroyed.

There are many kinds of cells with different shapes and sizes. The characteristics shown in Figure 13–7 are common to most cells. However, cells like those in the blood (red, white, and platelets) and the nerve cells are very different and perform specialized functions. With this specialization, some of the other cell functions may be lost, such as the ability of some nerve cells to reproduce. Specialization also results in an interdependence among cells to enable them to carry out their activities. One type of cell that is very different is the sex cell (gamete), which is responsible for reproduction. During a process known as meiosis, the ovum from the female and the spermatozoon from the male each reduce their respective 46 chromosomes to 23, one half the normal amount. When fertilization occurs, the two cells combine to form a single cell called a zygote, which will then have the full set of 46 chromosomes, 23 from each parent. The zygote will subsequently, by mitosis, divide again and again until the new being is fully developed. This cellular activity will be more fully discussed in the section on the reproductive system.

Homeostasis

The body has many control systems, some of which operate within the cell. It is important that the fluid within the cell (*intracellular fluid*) maintain the proper chemical balance for the cell to maintain life. The fluid surrounding the cells (*extracellular fluid*) mixes with the fluid of the blood to supply the cell with food and other substances. When the internal environment is functioning properly and all the organs and tissues of the body are performing their appropriate tasks, a condition of **homeostasis** exists. This is a stable condition of the internal environment. This condition continues until one or more of the control systems loses the ability to maintain it. When this occurs, all cells of the body suffer. A moderate dysfunction causes illness; a severe dysfunction leads to death.

Genetic Cellular Change ....

Several disorders result from improper sex cell division at the time of fertilization or from the inheritance of an altered gene or genes. These are collectively called genetic disorders. Some result in structural defects such as cleft lip, cleft palate, club foot, spinal bifida, and congenital heart disease.

A condition resulting from the absence or alteration of a protein enzyme is known as phenylketonuria (PKU). Before birth the mother's blood supplies the missing chemical compounds, but at birth the baby is unable to handle some metabolic products, thereby impairing brain development, causing profound retardation, seizures, and stunted growth. Checking newborns with a heel stick blood test permits early diagnosis and dietary treatment to prevent the consequences of the disorder from developing.

A genetic disorder known as galactosemia occurs when a byproduct of lactose (milk sugar) cannot be metabolized. It is caused by the mutation of a single gene. About 1 in 100,000 newborns have this condition.

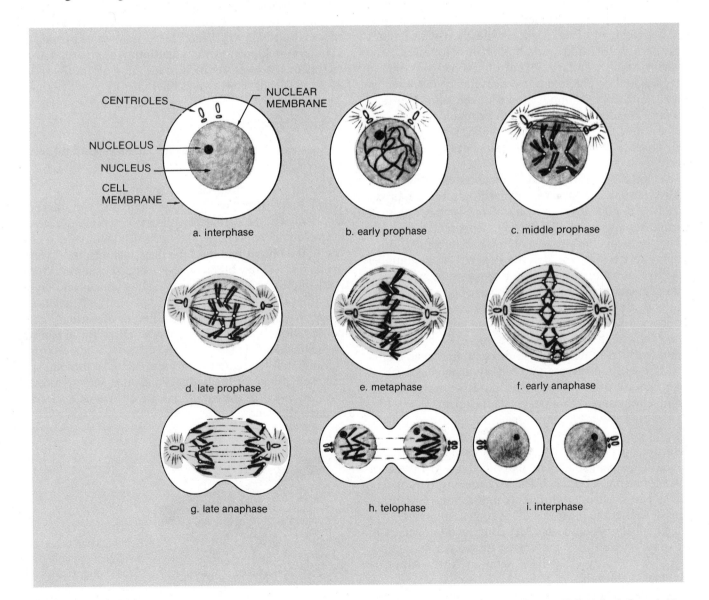

FIGURE 13–14   Stages of mitosis in animal cells (Adapted from Schraer & Stolze, *Biology: The Study of Life*, 2d ed. Copyright 1987 Allyn and Bacon, Inc.)

Early symptoms include malnutrition, diarrhea, and severe vomiting. Often the eyes, liver, and brain become damaged. Children who are not treated will die. If the abnormality is detected early enough, infants can be fed a diet including milk substitutes and grow up to be symptom free as long as they avoid galactose.

Some disorders are known as sex-linked because they are carried by the X or Y chromosome, which differentiates males and females. Probably the best known is hemophilia, a bleeding disorder caused by a lack of protein. The disorder is carried by the female but occurs only in males. This condition is now treatable by administration of factor VIII, a human blood clotting factor.

Another sex chromosome abnormality is called Turner's syndrome. About 1 in 5000 newborn females will have the disorder. Affected individuals have only 45 chromosomes; because of a failure of the sex cells to divide correctly in meiosis, only one sex chromosome is present in their cells. Turner's syndrome causes a short stature, webbing of the neck, a wide chest with broadly spaced nipples, and poor breast development. The ovaries and secondary sexual characteristics fail to develop, making the female sterile. Often it is not recognized until lack of menses and developing genitalia become apparent. Treatment with estrogen (female hormone) after age 13 to 15, to prevent stopping growth, will produce a menstrual cycle but will not reverse the sterility.

A similar condition affecting males is called Klinefelter's syndrome and affects, in varying degrees, approximately 1 in 600. It is the result of one or more extra X chromosomes. It usually becomes apparent at puberty when the penis and testicles fail to mature fully, often leading to sterility. The severity depends on the number of extra chromosomes. Other symptoms are breast enlargement, mental retardation, sparse body hair, abnormal body build (long legs with short obese trunk), tall, a tendency toward alcoholism, and often personality disorders. Treatment with testosterone, the male hormone, if begun early may help reverse the feminine characteristics, but will not reverse the sterility or mental retardation. Psychotherapy is indicated when sexual dysfunction causes emotional maladjustment.

A well-known chromosomal abnormality resulting from improper cell division is Down's syndrome. In this disorder, the number 21 chromosome is in triplicate rather than a pair, so that the individual has 47 instead of 46 chromosomes per cell. The *syndrome* (group of features) causes structural defects consisting of slanting eyes, a fold at the inner eye, large tongue, pug nose, and microcephaly (small head). Mental retardation occurs in all cases as well as some degree of growth restriction. About 1 in every 1000 live births in North America develops the disorder.

Amniocentesis, a diagnostic test, is indicated when prenatal interviews indicate the possibility of a genetic problem. A small amount of amniotic fluid, which surrounds the fetus, is removed from the pregnant uterus. Skin cells from the fetus are in the fluid and can be grown in a culture for examination. The test can relieve anxiety or permit early pregnancy termination if findings indicate cause for concern.

Tissues

As previously stated, not all cells are alike. They may be transparent as in the eye, or transmit electrical impulses or nutrients. Some have long thin fibers, and others produce secretions. When cells of the same type group together for a common purpose, they form a **tissue.** Tissues are from 60 to 99% water. The essential substances needed by the body are either dissolved or suspended in the tissue fluids. Therefore, water is indispensable to cell life, and lack of it causes death more rapidly than lack of any other substance, except oxygen.

Two common medical terms describe the opposites of tissue fluid balance. When there is too little fluid, the condition is known as **dehydration.** An abnormal accumulation of excess fluid, causing puffiness of the affected tissues, is known as **edema.**

Tissue Classifications

Tissues can be classified into four main types: **epithelial, connective,** nerve, and muscle.

Epithelial. Epithelial tissues form the body's glands, cover the surface of the body, and line the cavities. Epithelium is the main tissue of the skin, which serves as a protective covering for the body. Epithelium also covers all the organs and lines the intestinal, respiratory, and urinary tract, the blood vessels, and the uterus. Some epithelial tissues secrete fluids such as mucus and digestive juices. Others selectively absorb nutrients, chemical elements, and water. The epithelium of the urinary bladder is uniquely arranged in folds to allow for expansion as the bladder fills.

Epithelial tissues in glands specialize to provide specific secretions for the body. Glands that secrete directly into the blood in the capillaries are known as *endocrine* or ductless glands.

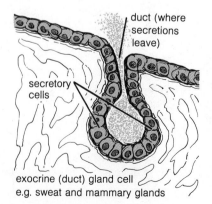

FIGURE 13–15
Epithelial cell tissue of an exocrine gland. (From Fong, *Body Structures and Functions*, 7th ed. Copyright 1989, Delmar Publishers Inc.)

Glands that produce secretions through ducts within the body are classified as *exocrine,* Figure 13–15. Two glands, the liver and pancreas, produce both endocrine and exocrine secretions.

Connective. Connective tissue forms the supporting structure of the body, connecting other tissues together to form the organs and body parts. There are several categories of connective tissue but they can also be simply divided into soft or hard tissues. A soft type is adipose or fat tissue, which stores the body's reserve of food, fills in between tissue fibers, insulates against heat and cold, and pads the body structures, Figure 13–16. Another form of soft connective tissue is stretchable and forms the subcutaneous layer of the skin. A soft but dense connective tissue in the form of tendons, ligaments, and organ capsules serves to support and protect organs and lend elasticity to the walls of arteries, Figure 13–17.

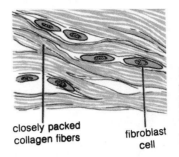

FIGURE 13–17 Dense fibrous connective tissue in ligaments and tendons (From Fong, *Body Structures and Functions,* 7th ed. Copyright 1989, Delmar Publishers Inc.)

closely packed collagen fibers

fibroblast cell

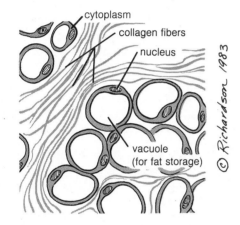

cytoplasm

collagen fibers

nucleus

© Richardson 1983

vacuole (for fat storage)

FIGURE 13–16 Adipose tissue throughout the body (From Fong, *Body Structures and Functions,* 7th ed. Copyright 1989, Delmar Publishers Inc.)

Blood and lymphatic vessels, lymph, the blood, and blood cells are all considered to be connective tissues. Cells in the blood carry nutrients and oxygen to the cells and pick up metabolic wastes for elimination. Lymph fluid consists of water, glucose, fats, and salt and is present in the spaces between the cells of the tissues as well as within the lymph vessels. Soft connective tissue plays a major role in the repair of damaged body tissue. The repair process involves new blood vessel formation and the growth of new connective tissue known as scar tissue. Excessive blood vessel development in the early stages results in a condition called "proud flesh." In instances of surgery or suturing (sewing) of a clean wound, the need for tissue regrowth and therefore the resulting scar is reduced because the cut edges are brought together closely by the surgical process. An excessive growth of scar tissue is called a **Keloid.**

Hard connective tissue can be found in the cartilage and bones of the body. Cartilage is located between the bones of the spine (where it acts as a shock absorber and allows for flexibility) and in the ear, nose and voice box (to provide shaping). Bone tissue is actually cartilage with the addition of calcium salts. This addition takes place gradually from birth until the tissue becomes hardened, Figure 13–18.

Bone tissue, which is also called **osseous** tissue, is not a lifeless material. Within most bone is a medullary cavity filled with yellow marrow, which is composed of fat, connective tissue, and blood vessels. Some long bones contain cavities filled with red marrow, which manufactures red blood cells. Because bone is a living tissue with a blood supply and nerves, it can easily repair itself when it is damaged.

Nerve. Nerve tissue is found throughout the body. It serves as the body's communication network. The basic structural unit of the tissue is the neuron, which consists of a nerve cell body and fibers that resemble tree branches, Figure 13–19, page 218. The dendrites bring impulses to the cell body; the axon conducts impulses away. Neurons range from a fraction of an inch up to 3 feet in length.

There are three types of nerve cells or neurons. A *sensory neuron* in the skin or sense organs picks up a stimulus and sends it toward the spinal cord and brain. An *interneuron,* or *connecting neuron,* carries the impulse to another neuron. A *motor neuron* receives an impulse and sends a message, which causes a reaction.

Clusters of neurons form the nerve tissue. Nerves throughout the body join together to form the spinal cord, which in turn transmits electrical impulses to and from the brain. Nerves outside the brain and spinal cord are called *peripheral nerves.* The fibers of these nerves are covered with a fatty insulating material called a **myelin** sheath, which is then covered with a thin membrane called **neurilemma.** If a sheathed nerve fiber is damaged

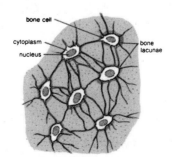

bone cell

cytoplasm

nucleus

bone lacunae

FIGURE 13–18 Hard connective tissue found in bone (From Fong, *Body Structures and Functions,* 7th ed. Copyright 1989, Delmar Publishers Inc.)

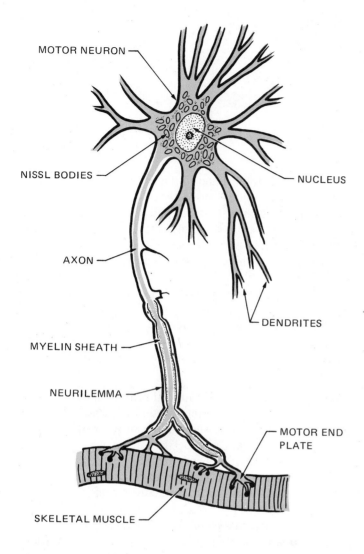

or cut, it can be surgically repaired and a new fiber may form within the sheath, but nerve tissue recovers very slowly, if at all. Unfortunately, fibers of the brain, spinal cord, optic (eye), and auditory (ear) nerves lack sheaths and cannot be repaired by surgery when damaged or cut.

Muscle. Muscle tissue is designed to contract on stimulation. Tissue that can be controlled at will with impulses from the brain is called **voluntary** muscle tissue. This type is found connected to the bones of the body, and is called **skeletal** or **striated** muscle, Figure 13–20(a). It gives us the ability to move our bodies.

Involuntary muscle action occurs without control or conscious awareness. There are two types of involuntary muscle tissue. One type, called **smooth** muscle tissue, is found within the walls of all the organs of the body except the heart. This type of tissue moves food and waste material through the digestive tract and changes the size of the iris of the eye and the diameter of arteries, Figure 13–20(b). The other type of involuntary muscle tissue, called **cardiac** muscle tissue, is found only in the heart. Cardiac muscle fibers are joined in a continuous network and must contract together in a forceful, rhythmic action to pump blood throughout the body, Figure 13–20(c).

Organs ....

The **organs** of the body are made of two or more types of tissue that work together to perform a specific body function. For example, the stomach is constructed with walls of smooth muscle tissue to "churn" the food; it is lined with one type of epithelial tissue, which secretes gastric juices, and covered with another type, which protects the organ; connective tissue fills the spaces between the other tissue fibers; nerve tissue controls the rate at which material is emptied from the stomach. (The roles of the organs will be discussed in more detail in the remaining units of this chapter.)

FIGURE 13–19   A motor neuron (From *The Wonderful Human Machine*, copyright 1979, American Medical Association)

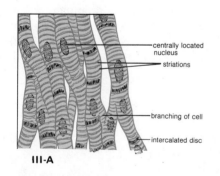

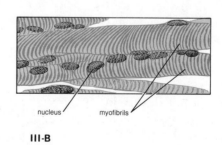

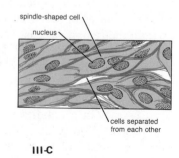

FIGURE 13–20

(a) Cardiac muscle tissue of the heart.

(b) Skeletal muscle tissue (straited voluntary) attaches to bone.

(c) Smooth muscle tissue in walls of organs and blood vessels.

(From Fong, *Body Structures and Functions*, 7th ed. Copyright 1989, Delmar Publishers Inc.)

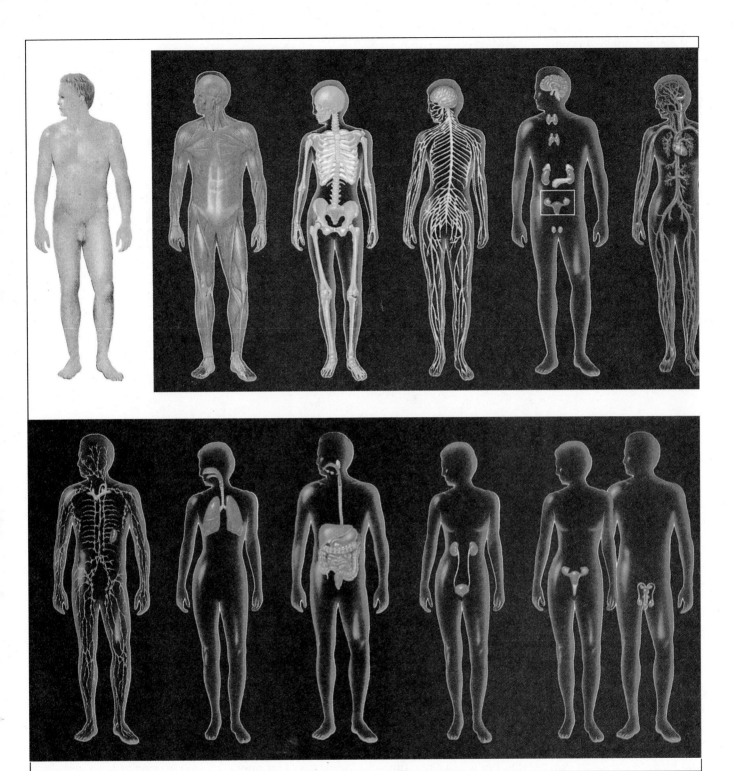

FIGURE 13–21   The body systems (From Starr & Taggart, *Biology, The Unity and Diversity of Life*, 5th ed. Copyright 1989, Wadsworth Publishing Co.)

Systems

Organs of the body that perform similar functions are organized into a body system. Using the stomach again as an example, it joins with the mouth, throat, esophagus, and small and large intestines to make up the alimentary tract of the digestive system. The alimentary tract combines with the teeth, tongue, salivary glands, liver, pancreas, and gallbladder to form the total digestive system. The other systems of the body, which will be discussed individually, are the integumentary, skeletal, muscular, respiratory, circulatory, urinary, nervous, endocrine, and reproductive systems.

One additional "system" will also be discussed later in this chapter. The immune system is not normally considered, at least at the present time, as being a "system." However, the body's health and well-being so directly depend on an intact and effective immune response, that it requires you have a basic knowledge of its role in disease response. As scientists begin to better understand how it functions and what can be done to correct a malfunction, perhaps we can solve the mysteries of cancer and AIDS, as well as many other immunologically based disorders. The basics of the complex subject of immunology are discussed in Unit 9.

Even a body system cannot function alone. All systems must combine their individual contributions for the health and well-being of the total human body. Figure 13–21, page 219 illustrates the body systems and briefly describes their functions.

Note: Figure 13–21 includes the lymphatic system. This system is usually considered as part of the circulatory system.

Complete Chapter 13, Unit 1 in the workbook to help you meet the objectives at the beginning of this unit and therefore achieve competency of this subject matter.

U N I T 2

The Nervous System

OBJECTIVES

Upon completion of this unit, the student will meet the following terminal performance objectives by verifying knowledge of the facts and principles presented through oral and written communication at a level deemed competent.

1. Name the two main divisions of the nervous system.
2. Identify the two types of peripheral nerves and explain the function of the spinal nerves.
3. Describe simple and complex reflex actions.
4. Describe a synapse and the effects of various substances on its action.
5. Describe the purpose of the automatic nervous system and explain the action of its two divisions.
6. Identify the main parts of the brain and their functions.
7. Name the coverings of the brain and spinal cord and describe their purpose.
8. Describe the function of cerebrospinal fluid.
9. Name common diagnostic tests used to identify neurological disorders and possible reasons for their use.
10. List the functions of the hypothalamus.
11. Describe 21 diseases or disorders of the nervous system.
12. Spell and define, using the glossary at the back of the text, all the words to know in this unit.

WORDS TO KNOW

action potential	medulla oblongata
angiography	meninges
arachnoid	midbrain
arteriography	migraine
auditory	motor
autonomic	myelography
axon	occipital
brain scan	olfactory
central	optic
cerebellum	parasympathetic
cerebrospinal fluid	parietal
cerebrum	peripheral
computerized axial tomography (CAT)	pia mater
	plexuses
cranium	pneumoencephalograph
dendrite	pons
dura mater	sciatica
electroencephalography (EEG)	sensory
	spina bifida
electromyography	subarachnoid
frontal	subdural
ganglion	sympathetic
hypothalamus	synapse
interneurons	syndrome
longitudinal fissure	temporal
lumbar puncture	thalamus
magnetic resonance imaging (MRI)	thorax
	ventricle

The nervous system is the communication network that organizes and coordinates all the body's functions. It is a complex and somewhat difficult system to understand, and in most texts is not usually discussed early in the study of the body systems. However, in this text, it is being presented first. It is believed that this will help you to more easily understand the involvement of the nervous system's regulatory action in the functioning of the other body systems, as they are discussed.

You might think of the system as being something like your telephone system. You can make local, in-state, national, and international calls. You can easily call next door but the further away the more number messages and the more "routing" of signals needed to complete your call. The phone picks up your voice (stimulus), converts it to impulses, and sends it along a charged line to a bundle of lines and on to phone company switching equipment. Every so often, the impulse is "boosted" to maintain your "voice." It may even be given a special treatment and sent through space and bounced off a satellite, but the message is forwarded to its destination. Your nervous system operates in a similar but much more complicated manner. The system has two main divisions: the **central** nervous system (CNS), which consists of the brain and the spinal cord, and the **peripheral** nervous system, which includes all the nerves that connect the CNS to every organ and area of the body. The autonomic nervous system is a specialized part of the peripheral system and controls internal organs and other self-regulating body functions.

Like in all systems, the basic functioning unit is the cell; in this system the unit is a nerve cell or neuron. As described in Unit 1, there are three types of neurons in nerve tissue; sensory, connecting and motor. They receive stimuli or impulses, transmit impulses to other neurons, and deliver response actions to the muscles and glands. Connecting neurons are also called *associative* or *internuncial neurons.* Figure 13–22 illustrates the three types of neurons.

All nerve cells have a nucleus, cytoplasm, and a cell membrane. Scattered throughout the cytoplasm are little microscopic granular "dots" called Nissl bodies, see Figure 13–19. They may represent a store of nervous energy. The cell body has processes that are extensions of cytoplasm called dendrites and axons. A neuron may have many dendrites but only one axon. These extensions are also called *fibers.* Around the long thin axons of peripheral nerves are the Schwann cells. They form a tight protective covering called the myelin sheath and also play a part in the transmission of messages. The myelin is then surrounded by the neurilemma, an elastic sheath covering.

A nerve is composed of bundles of nerve fibers bound together by connective tissue. If a nerve is composed of fibers going from the sense organs to the spinal cord or brain, it is a *sensory* or *afferent nerve.* If it is carrying impulses from the brain or spinal cord to a muscle, organ, or gland it is known as a *motor* or *efferent nerve.* Some nerves have both kinds of fibers and are known as *mixed nerves.*

Membrane Excitability

Nerves carry impulses by creating electric charges in a process known as membrane excitability. Neurons have a membrane that separates the cytoplasm inside from the extracellular fluids outside the cell, thereby creating two chemically different areas. Each area has differing amounts of potassium and sodium ions and some other charged substances, with the inside being the more negatively charged. When a neuron is stimulated, ions move across the membrane creating a current, which if large enough, will briefly change the inside of the neuron to be more positive than the outside area. This state is known as action potential. Neurons and other cells that produce action potentials are said to have membrane excitability.

To understand how impulses are carried along nerves or throughout a muscle when it contracts, we need to learn a little more about membrane excitability. Ions cross a membrane through channels, some of which are open and allow ions to "leak" (diffuse) continuously. Other channels are called "gated" and open only during

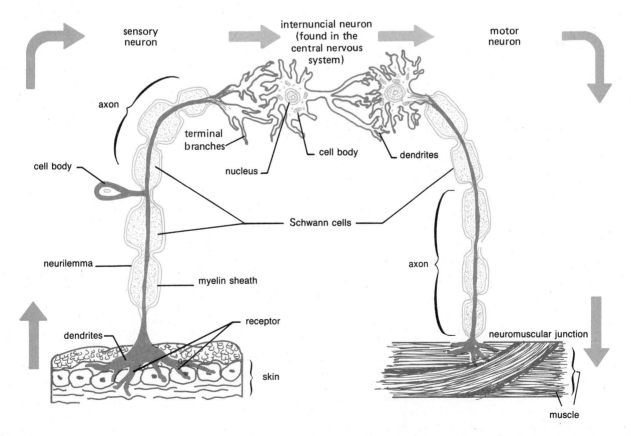

FIGURE 13–22 Types of neurons (From Fong, *Body Structures and Functions*, 7th ed. Copyright 1989, Delmar Publishers Inc.)

action potential. Another membrane opening is called a sodium-potassium pump which, by active transport, maintains the flow of ions from higher to lower concentrations levels across the membrane and restores the cytoplasm and extracellular fluid to their original value, after an action potential occurs. This action is in response to the fact there is an imbalance between the cytoplasm and the extracellular fluid. When diffusion takes place, particles move from an area of greater concentration to an area of lesser concentration.

The following simplified description explains how this whole process works.

1. A neuron membrane is "at rest." There are large amounts of potassium (K+) ions inside the cells but not very many sodium (NA+) ions. The reverse is true outside the cell in the extracellular fluid. Most of the open channels are for potassium to pass through, so it leaks out of the cell.

2. As the K+ ions leave, the inside becomes relatively more negative until some K+ ions are attracted back in and the electrical force balances the diffusion force and movement stops. The inside is still more negative and the amount of energy between the two differently charged areas is ready to work (carry an impulse). This state is called *resting membrane potential,* Figure 13–23(a). The membrane is now polarized. The sodium ions are not able to move "in" since their channels are closed during the resting state; however, if a few leak in, the membrane pump sends an equal number out.

3. Now suppose a sensory neuron receptor is stimulated by something, a sound for instance. This will cause a

change in the membrane potential. The stimulus energy is converted to an electrical signal and if it is strong enough, it will depolarize a portion of the membrane and allow the gated sodium ion channels to open initiating an action potential, Figure 13–23(b).

4. The sodium ions move through the gated channels into the cytoplasm and the inside becomes more positive until the membrane potential is reversed and the gates close to sodium ions.

5. Next the potassium gates open and large amounts of potassium leave the cytoplasm resulting in the repolarization of the membrane, Figure 13–23(c). After repolarization, the sodium-potassium pump restores the initial concentrations of sodium and potassium ions inside and outside the neuron.

This whole process occurs in a few milliseconds. When this action occurs in one part of the cell membrane, it spreads to adjacent membrane regions, continuing away from the original site of stimulation, sending "messages" over the nerve. This cycle is completed millions of times a minute throughout the body, day after day, year after year.

But what happens when the impulse reaches the end of the neuron? You will recall that impulses travel across a neuron from the dendrites to the cell body and then to the axon. Here there is a minute space between the dendrites of the next neuron called a **synapse,** which the impulse must "jump" chemically. This space is technically called a *synaptic cleft.* Impulses from the sending cell release "transmitter substances" into the cleft, Figure 13–24. These substances are signaling molecules that can cause a rapid change in the membrane potential of the receiving cell. These chemicals can either speed up or slow down the transmission. Normally nerve impulses travel about 200 miles per hour. The intake of alcohol, for instance, seems to aid the chemical that causes impulses to be blocked and our reactions are therefore slowed down. Other chemicals, such as stimulant drugs and wartime nerve gases, cause the release of a chemical that allows the transmission of impulses to speed up, even to the point of causing a flood of impulses to the brain resulting in the possible breakdown of the body's ability to function.

A disease condition called tetanus results from the effects of the bacteria *Clostridium tetani* on the nervous and muscular systems. Bacteria invade the body through a puncture wound from a contaminated object or an animal bite. The tissues deep in the puncture do not receive oxygen, so they die off and the bacteria multiply. A substance is released by the bacteria, which is toxic to the motor neurons that innervate the muscles. A neuron normally stimulates muscle tissue through balanced chemical messages, which alternately contract and relax the muscle tissue. This balance is essential to our ability to maintain erect stature and movement. However, with the release of the neurotoxin from the bacteria, excitation is

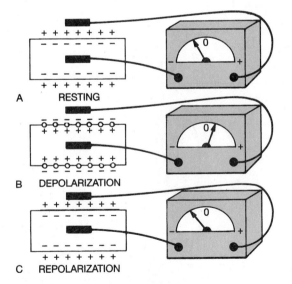

FIGURE 13–23 Sequence of events in membrane potential and relative positive and negative states
(a). Normal resting potential—(negative inside/positive outside)
(b). Depolarization—(positive inside/negative outside)
(c). Repolarization—(negative inside/positive outside)

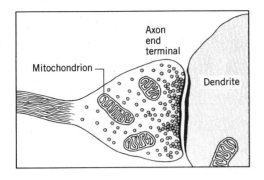

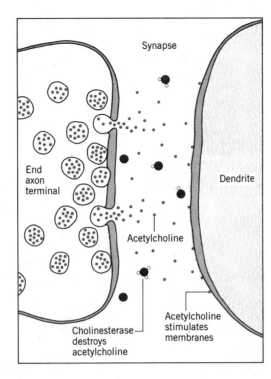

FIGURE 13–24
Transmission of a nerve impulse across a synapse is chemical. Acetylcholine and cholinesterase are often the chemical mediators. (From Burke, *Human Anatomy and Physiology in Health and Disease*, 3d ed. Copyright 1992, Delmar Publishers Inc.)

unbalanced and the inhibitory synapses of the motor neurons of the brain and spinal cord are affected, thereby allowing excessive contraction of the muscles. (Without the control of the "inhibitor" the message goes on full permission to contract.) The muscles cannot relax and there is a prolonged, spastic paralysis of the muscles, which can result in death.

With this one example, it is apparent how the function of the nervous system affects the total welfare of the body. It is now important to learn how the nerves are organized in the communication network.

Peripheral Nervous System and Spinal Cord ....

The peripheral nervous system includes 12 pairs of cranial nerves that connect the brain directly to the sense organs (eye, ear, tongue, nose, and skin), the heart, lungs, and other internal organs. Some cranial nerves, like the optic from the eye, have only sensory fibers, whereas others, like those to the heart and lungs, are mixed nerves containing both sensory and motor fibers. The peripheral system also includes 31 pairs of spinal nerves. The spinal nerves are both motor, to provide a function or movement, and sensory, to perceive stimuli; therefore they are also mixed nerves.

All spinal nerves enter and leave the spinal cord, which is located within the canal created by an opening in each of the bones (vertebrae) of the spinal column. A cross section of the cord would reveal a rounded white mass of myelinated nerve fibers with a notched area on the anterior surface, Figure 13–25. The white matter is mainly axons of **interneurons.** Some axons are grouped together into major sensory nerves going to a specific section of the brain. Others are grouped into major motor nerves going to their muscle or organ destination. Still others connect with each other up, down, and within the gray matter to provide control over activities that occur within the cord itself. In the center of the white area is a gray area in the shape of an H, which is the nerve cell bodies and their fibers without the myelin covering. The gray matter is involved mainly with reflex connections in the spinal cord that deal with the reflexes involved in such things as walking or blinking.

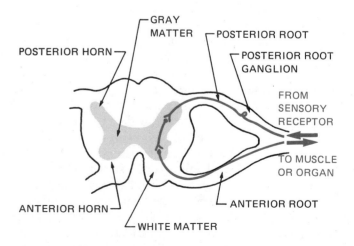

FIGURE 13–25   Cross section of the spinal cord

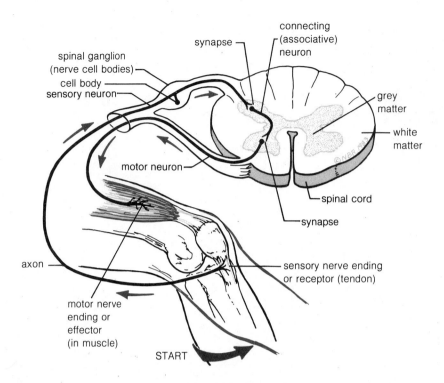

spinal ganglion
(nerve cell bodies)

cell body
sensory neuron

synapse

connecting
(associative)
neuron

grey
matter

white
matter

motor neuron

spinal cord

synapse

axon

sensory nerve ending
or receptor (tendon)

motor nerve
ending or
effector
(in muscle)

START

FIGURE 13–26   Reflex action. In this example, tapping the patellar tendon of the knee results in extension of the leg, producing the knee jerk reflex. (From Fong, *Body Structures and Functions*, 7th ed. Copyright 1989, Delmar Publishers Inc.)

A spinal nerve splits into two roots as it enters the cord. The rear root carrying sensory fibers to the cord enters at the rear horn of the H. The bulge on the rear root contains the sensory nerve cell bodies and is called a **ganglion.** The front root of the nerve leaves at the anterior horn of the H carrying motor nerve fibers which have their cell bodies inside the gray matter of the cord. Neurons within the cord itself connect sensory to motor nerves.

Sensory neurons transmit messages from millions of special receptor cells to the spinal cord and on to the brain for interpretation and decisions. If a reaction is needed, impulses from the CNS are transmitted to the appropriate muscle or organ over the motor neurons. Connecting interneurons route impulses throughout the body, permitting any nerve to communicate with any other nerve.

In very simple reflex actions where no interpretation or decision is required, the nerve impulse travels only to the spinal cord and back. The knee jerk test often used by physicians illustrates such a simple reflex and provides an evaluation of the nervous system. When the knee is hanging completely relaxed, the leg should kick up sharply when the tendon below the kneecap is lightly tapped, Figure 13–26. If there is no response, a nervous system disease or disorder can be suspected.

In more complicated reflex actions, such as a hand coming into contact with something hot, the sensory impulse is relayed through nerve cells to the spinal cord and up to the brain, Figure 13–27. There the impulse is interpreted and the motor neurons carry the message back down the spinal cord and out the appropriate nerves. The eyes see the object, the hand will jerk away, and the voice may speak out.

Autonomic Nervous System

The autonomic nervous system is part of the peripheral nervous system. These nerves are involuntary and unconsciously regulate functions such as breathing, heartbeat, and digestion. The system consists of nerves, ganglia, and **plexuses** (networks of nerves). There are two divisions of the autonomic system. The **sympathetic** division accelerates activity in the smooth, involuntary muscles of the body's organs, and the **parasympathetic** division reverses the action and slows down activity. For example, the sympathetic nerves constrict blood vessels and speed up the heartbeat; the parasympathetic nerves dilate the blood vessels and slow down the heartbeat. These activities continuously balance each other to maintain homeostasis in the body. However, this on or off mechanism does not apply to all organs, because some do not have a dual nerve supply. Also, nerves in both divisions can have excitatory or inhibitory effects. At any given time, the actual effect depends on the net outcome of the two opposing signals.

The *sympathetic nervous system* begins at the base of the brain and runs down both sides of the spinal column in two tracts. These consist of nerve fibers and ganglia. The sympathetic nerves extend to all the vital internal organs, the blood vessels, the iris of the eye, and even to the sweat glands, Figure 13–28, page 226.

The *parasympathetic system* has two important nerves, the vagus and the pelvic nerve. The vagus extends from the medulla oblongata of the brain and branches to the neck, chest, and upper abdominal organs. The pelvic nerve exits the spinal cord around the hip

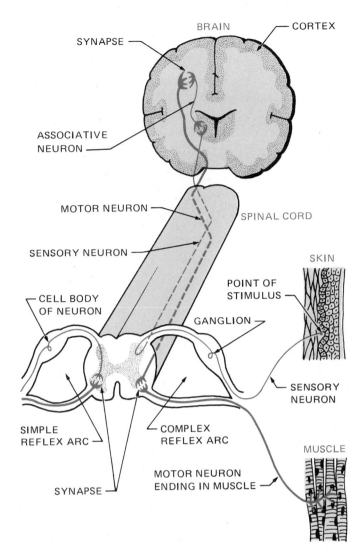

The figure labels (clockwise): BRAIN, CORTEX, SYNAPSE, ASSOCIATIVE NEURON, MOTOR NEURON, SPINAL CORD, SENSORY NEURON, SKIN, POINT OF STIMULUS, CELL BODY OF NEURON, GANGLION, SENSORY NEURON, SIMPLE REFLEX ARC, COMPLEX REFLEX ARC, MUSCLE, SYNAPSE, MOTOR NEURON ENDING IN MUSCLE

FIGURE 13–27 Complex reflex action (From *The Wonderful Human Machine*, copyright 1979, American Medical Association)

area and branches into the lower abdominal and pelvic organs. Both systems are strongly affected by emotions such as fear, anger, and stress.

The action of the autonomic system is extremely important to our ability to react in an emergency. It is frequently called our "flight-fright mechanism," because it accelerates our body functions to permit escaping or otherwise dealing with danger.

Central Nervous System ....

The Brain

The brain is a large mass of nerve tissue with about 100 billion neurons. It is protected and supported by surrounding membranes known as meninges, Figure 13–29, page 227. It is further protected by the cranium (skull). The brain surface has extensive deep furrows and folds and is divided into two hemispheres by a longitudinal

fissure. The hemispheres are connected internally with nerve fibers and share information. The cerebral surface is covered with ridges and furrows known as *fissures,* if they are deep, or *sulci* if they are shallow. The elevated ridges between the sulci are called *convolutions.*

The brain is divided into five parts. The largest is the cerebrum, which controls sensory and motor activities. The cerebrum is further divided into lobes, Figure 13–30, page 227. The frontal lobe behind the forehead seems to be related to emotions, personality, moral traits, and intellectual functions. The frontal lobe is also the motor area for active voluntary muscle movements as well as two areas that control speech. The occipital lobe is the far back portion of the cerebrum. This area is associated with vision. The impulses of color and light received by the eyes are transmitted by the optic nerve fibers to the occipital lobe for interpretation. Between the frontal and occipital lobes is the parietal lobe. The motor area governing speech lies at its junction with the frontal lobe. It is the parietal lobe that receives impulses from receptors in the hands, feet, and tongue, among others, and sends impulses that cause movement in all these parts in response. This area also receives nerve impulses from sensory receptors for pain, touch, heat, and cold. A small temporal lobe lies on the side of the cerebrum. The auditory nerve association area is here, which provides us with the sense of hearing. The olfactory area, which provides our sense of smell, is within a small projection under the temporal lobe. It is connected by nerve fibers to receptors in the nasal cavity.

Beneath the cerebrum lies the part of the brain known as the cerebellum. This section is responsible for smooth muscle movement, muscle tone, and coordination of sensory impulses with muscular activity, particularly for equilibrium, walking, and dancing. If the cerebellum is damaged, many activities requiring coordination of muscles cannot be performed.

The medulla oblongata is the part of the brain that adjoins the spinal cord. The medulla influences, through the autonomic nervous system, the function of the heart and lungs, stomach secretions, and the size of the openings in blood vessels.

Just above the medulla is the pons. This part of the brain also helps to regulate breathing. It is the reflex center for chewing, tasting, and secreting saliva. A small part called the midbrain is superior to the pons. This area is the control center for some of the reflex movements of the eyes, such as blinking and changing the size of the pupil. It also conducts impulses between the brain parts above and below it.

In an area between the cerebrum and the midbrain are two major structures, the thalamus and the hypothalamus. The thalamus acts as a relay station for impulses going to and from the brain as well as those from the cerebellum and other parts of the brain. The hypothalamus lies below the thalamus and is connected to the pituitary gland, midbrain, and thalamus by a bundle of nerve

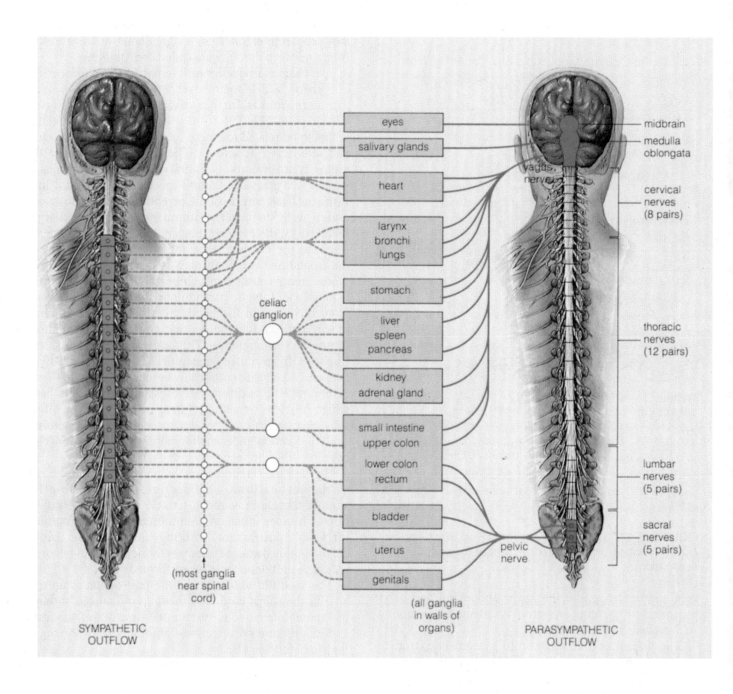

FIGURE 13–28 Autonomic nervous system. Shown here are the main sympathetic and parasympathetic pathways leading out from the central nervous system to some major organs. As the lists of examples suggest, in some cases the sympathetic and parasympathetic nerves operate antagonistically in their effects on the organ. Keep in mind that both systems have paired nerves leading out from the brain and spinal cord. (From Starr & Taggart, *Biology, The Unity and Diversity of Life*, 5th ed. Copyright 1989, Wadsworth Publishing Co.)

fibers. The hypothalamus performs many vital functions such as:

1. Autonomic nervous control
2. Controling blood pressure by regulating the heart beat and blood vessel constriction and dilation

3. Maintaining body temperature
4. Stimulating the production of an antidiuretic hormone to conserve water in the body and to cause thirst to maintain normal water balance
5. Assisting in the regulation of appetite

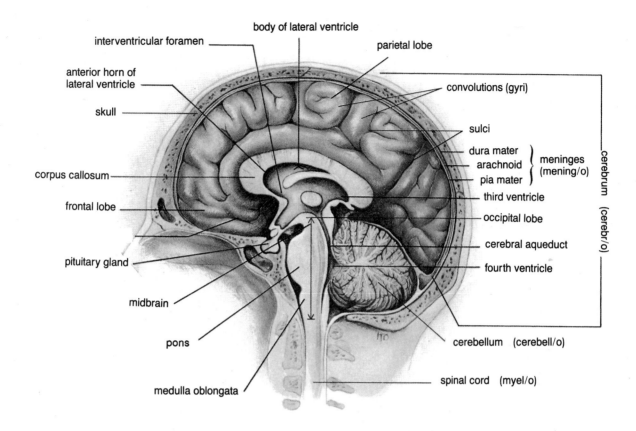

FIGURE 13–29 Cross section of brain (Adapted from Smith, *Medical Terminology, A Programmed Text*, 6th ed. Copyright 1991, Delmar Publishers Inc.)

6. Increasing secretions and motility in the intestinal tract
7. Playing a role in emotions such as fear and pleasure
8. Helping maintain wakefulness when it is necessary

The midbrain, pons, and the medulla make up the brain stem. Doctors learned long ago that nerve fibers from the right side of the body cross over in the brain stem to the left side of the brain. The body's left side is

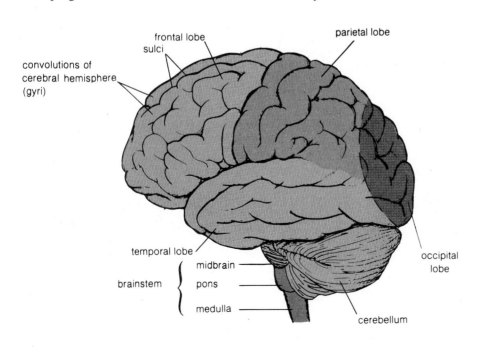

FIGURE 13–30 The parts of the brain (From Fong, *Body Structures and Functions*, 7th ed. Copyright 1989, Delmar Publishers Inc.)

LATERAL VIEW

likewise controlled by the right side of the brain. Therefore, when a person is paralyzed on the right side, it may be that there is damage to the left side of the brain.

Meninges

Because of their common origin, the brain and the spinal cord are covered with the same meninges (membranes), Figure 13–31. Three membrane layers make up the meninges. The innermost layer is called the pia mater, a delicate, tight-fitting covering containing blood vessels to nourish the nerve tissue. The middle layer, the arachnoid, is a delicate, lacelike membrane. The outer layer, called dura mater, is a tough, fibrous tissue which protects the CNS from being damaged from contact with the bony surfaces of the skull and spine. The space between the dura mater and the arachnoid is called the subdural space. The subarachnoid space is between the arachnoid and the pia mater.

Cavities of the Brain and Spinal Cord

Within the brain are several hollow areas called ventricles. They extend into the lobes of the cerebrum and into contact with the other sections of the brain by means of small passageways. The central canal of the spinal cord is directly associated with the most inferior ventricle. There are also connections from the ventricles into the subarachnoid space of the meninges.

Cerebrospinal Fluid

The hollow cavities within the brain and spinal cord are filled with a liquid called cerebrospinal fluid (CSF). This fluid acts as a watery cushion or shock absorber to provide additional protection for the delicate tissues of the CNS. The fluid transports nutrients, primarily proteins and carbohydrates, to the brain and spinal cord. CSF is formed continuously within the ventricles of the brain at the rate of 450 ml (15 oz) per day. Only 150 ml are present at any one time in a normal adult. The fluid circulates within the cavities of the brain and spinal cord and the subarachnoid space, being reabsorbed into the blood vessels in special structures called *arachnoidal villi.*

Diagnostic Tests ....

Diagnosis of neurological disorders and diseases may require the use of specific tests. Some of the more common tests and a few possible findings are as follows:

■ Arteriography—(cerebral angiography)—A catheter (small tube) is inserted into an artery and threaded up to the carotid artery in the neck. A dye is injected through the catheter to show the cerebral blood vessels when X rays are taken. This test can detect an aneurysm, hemorrhage, evidence of a cerebrovascular accident, and arteriosclerosis.

■ Brain scan—Radioisotopes are injected into the blood and then measured by a special scanner to

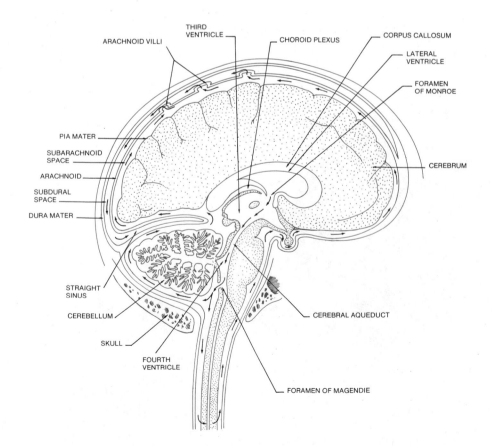

FIGURE 13–31 A diagrammatic representation of the meninges and the circulation of cerebral spinal fluid from its formation in the choroid plexus until its return to the blood in the cranial venous sinus. (Adapted from Burke, *Human Anatomy and Physiology in Health and Disease,* 3d ed. Copyright 1992, Delmar Publishers Inc.)

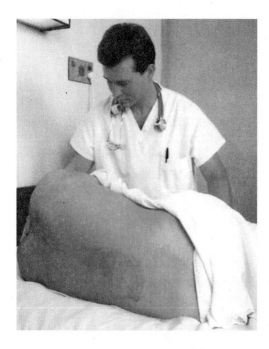

FIGURE 13–32

(a) Positioning of patient.

tumors, bleeding, a blood clot, decrease in brain size, and brain edema.

■ **Electroencephalography (EEG)**—A brain wave test to detect abnormal electrical impulses which could be caused by a tumor, epilepsy, retardation, or psychological disorder. New technology has developed an ambulatory EEG monitor that helps diagnose neurological conditions including fainting "spells" and seizures, by permitting continuous monitoring.

■ **Electromyography**—Needles are inserted into selected skeletal muscles. When the patient contracts the muscles, the nerve impulses are recorded and the conduction time is measured to detect neuromuscular disorders or nerve damage.

■ **Lumbar puncture**—A spinal needle is inserted into the subarachnoid space between the vertebrae of the lower back, and CSF is removed for examination, Figure 13–32. The procedure is indicated when infection is suspected, when there is hemorrhage from injury, or when the fluid pressure must be measured. When measurement is desired, a calibrated glass tube is attached to the needle and the level of the fluid is observed and recorded.

detect abnormal masses or blood vessel lesions within the brain. Used less frequently due to development of magnetic resonance imaging.

■ **Computerized axial tomography (CAT)** scan—A series of X rays of layers of the brain to construct a three-dimensional picture. Useful for identifying

■ **Magnetic resonance imaging (MRI)**—Uses magnetic waves to give results similar to a CAT scan but has much better quality. It is very useful for detecting

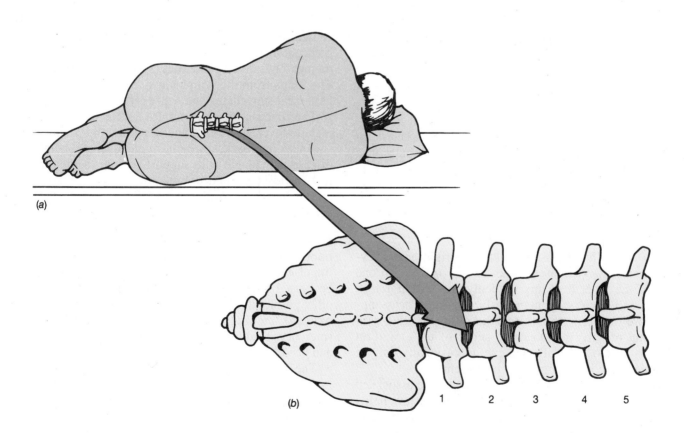

(a)

(b)   1   2   3   4   5

FIGURE 13–32   (b) Site of lumbar puncture

problems with the spine and the brain.

- Myelography—A lumbar puncture is performed, removing CSF and instilling a dye to outline the structures on X ray. This will show irregularities or compression of the spinal cord. If air is instilled following removal of CSF to visualize cerebral cavities, the procedure is called a **pneumoencephalograph.** Used less frequently due to new technology.
- Skull X ray—To identify fractures and dense areas which indicate a tumor or increased pressure within the skull.

Diseases and Disorders ....

Amyotrophic Lateral Sclerosis (ALS; Lou Gehrig's disease). ALS is a common motor neuron disease causing degeneration of the upper motor nerves in the medulla oblongata and the lower nerves in the spinal cord. It results in atrophy (wasting away) of the muscles. The onset occurs between the ages of 40 and 70 and is usually fatal within 3 to 10 years due to aspiration pneumonia or respiratory failure. The rate of incidence is 2 to 7 people for every 100,000. It affects men four times as frequently as women. About 10% of the cases are from an inherited autosomal trait. Other causes are from vitamin E deficiency, which damages cell membranes; metabolic interference in the production of nucleic acid by the nerves; an autoimmune disorder; and the effects of a nutritional deficiency of the motor neurons.

Factors that often precipitate the development of ALS are trauma, acute viral infections, and physical exhaustion. The symptoms are muscular atrophy and weakness, especially of the hands and forearms, plus problems with speech, chewing, and swallowing. If the brain stem is involved, respirations will be affected, as well as occasional choking and excessive drooling. Mental deterioration does not usually occur; therefore, the patient is acutely aware of the progressive physical deterioration, so depression due to the consequences of the disease, may happen. No effective treatment is available, only methods to control symptoms and provide emotional and physical support.

Bell's Palsy. This disease of unknown origin of the seventh cranial nerve causes weakness or *paralysis* on one side of the face. It occurs suddenly and within 1 to 8 weeks will usually spontaneously subside. The symptoms are drooping mouth (on the affected side) with drooling of saliva, a distorted sense of taste, and an inability to close the affected eye. Occasionally pain in the area of the jaw's angle may be present.

Treatment with steroids aids in reducing the associated edema. Moist heat applied to the face and jaw helps relieve any pain, but care must be taken to avoid burning the skin. It may be advisable to protect the eye with an eye patch while outdoors or if exposed to dust or pollutants.

Cerebral Palsy. This disorder is associated with birth and involves both nerves and muscles. It is the most common crippler of children. Cerebral palsy appears in about 15,000 live births per year, 25% of which are either small or premature, weighing less than 5 1/2 pounds. There are three forms of cerebral palsy: spastic, athetoid, and ataxic. About 70% of those affected have the spastic type. Characteristics of this form are hyperactive tendon reflexes, rapid alteration between muscular contraction and relaxation, contracture tendency (permanent muscle shortening), and underdevelopment of the affected extremities. Approximately 40% of the children affected are also mentally retarded, 25% have seizures, and 80% have speech impairment.

Cerebral palsy is probably caused by conditions that resulted in a lack of oxygen to the brain, hemorrhage, or brain damage. Prenatal conditions include rubella (German measles), toxemia, maternal diabetes, and malnutrition. At the time of birth such difficulties as forceps delivery, breech presentation, premature placental separation, premature birth, and either a too rapid or too prolonged labor are considered causative factors.

There is no cure for cerebral palsy, only supportive treatment including physical, occupational, and speech therapy; psychological assistance; braces or splints; perhaps orthopedic surgery for severe contractures; muscle relaxors; and, when indicated, barbiturates and anticonvulsants to control seizures.

Encephalitis. This severe brain inflammation, usually caused by a virus-bearing mosquito or tick, can also be contracted from viruses that cause polio, herpes, or mumps or following measles, rubella, or a vaccination. The fluids from the lymphatic system infiltrate the brain tissue, causing edema and nerve cell destruction.

The disease onset is sudden and acute. Symptoms include fever, headache, and vomiting and progress to a stiff neck and back, drowsiness, and eventual coma. The disease is treatable with supportive drug therapy to control restlessness and convulsions, reduce edema, and relieve headache. Antiviral agents are ineffective except against herpes virus encephalitis.

Epilepsy. This seizure disorder affects 1% to 2% of the population. It is associated with abnormal electrical impulses from the neurons of the brain. It is believed to be caused by either abnormal brain chemistry or several other possibilities including birth trauma, anoxia (lack of oxygen), meningitis, encephalitis, ingestion of toxins (mercury, lead, carbon monoxide), brain tumor, PKU, and head injury.

The disorder is characterized by either petit or grand mal seizures. Petit mal seizures are of short duration and mild. Grand mal seizures may last up to 5 minutes, with convulsions, loss of control of bodily functions, and unconsciousness.

Diagnosis is made upon evidence of seizure characteristics, a positive EEG, and various X-ray procedures. Treatment consists of drug therapy to control the seizures, and psychological support.

Headache. Headaches are commonly classified as vascular, muscle contraction (tension), or traction–inflammatory. Both muscle contraction and traction–inflammatory types cause dull, persistent aching and a feeling of a tight band around the head, with tender spots on the head or neck. Most chronic headaches result from tension that may be caused by emotional stress, fatigue, or environmental conditions. Other causes include inflammation of the sinuses, diseased teeth, and muscle spasms of the neck and shoulder.

Vasodilators, such as nitrates, alcohol, and histamine, expand arteries causing pressure against the brain's nerve endings and are often the causative factors. Many people are affected by anything aged or fermented such as cured or processed meats and wine, especially red wine. Other foods or additives cause headaches by the vasoconstricting action of amines in such things as MSG, chocolate, and aspartame. A condition known as hypoglycemia (low blood sugar) can result in vasodilation and headaches but can be easily avoided by eating three meals a day, preferably five smaller ones.

A migraine headache is characterized by prodromal (beginning) symptoms, which may include fatigue, visual disturbances, such as zig-zag lines and bright lights; sensory symptoms such as tingling of the face and lips; and sometimes motor symptoms like staggering. Migraines frequently occur in people with compulsive personalities and within families. They usually happen on weekends and holidays. A migraine headache is a severe throbbing pain caused by initial constriction then dilation of the blood vessels in the brain. Frequently, it is accompanied by sensitivity to light, nausea, and vomiting. The headache can occur suddenly and last from a few hours to a few days. It cannot be prevented but medication can reduce frequency and intensity. Ergotomine, especially with caffeine, seems to be fairly effective, if taken early; it is available in suppository form if vomiting prevents oral administration. There is no cure for migraine headaches, only control. Drugs known as beta blockers and tricyclic antidepressants appear to be very effective in prevention.

It seems to be best to lie quietly in bed in a darkened room until the symptoms subside. Limited relief may be obtained from regular analgesics and some people feel an ice bag to the head and a wet cloth over the eyes and forehead are beneficial. Usually, it is just a matter of waiting out the episode.

When headaches are frequent, unusual, such as causing awakening in the middle of the night, persistent or become increasingly more intense, medical attention should be sought. It may be important to rule out the presence of pathology such as an aneurysm, abscess, intercranial bleeding or tumor.

Herpes Zoster (shingles). This is an acute inflammation of the dorsal root ganglion by a herpes virus that also causes chickenpox. It is characterized by fluid-filled vesicle lesions on the skin and severe pain from the affected nerves. The onset is characterized by fever and discomfort followed by severe deep pain, itching, and abnormal skin sensations. The vesicles erupt in about 2 weeks, spreading around the thorax or vertically on the extremities. The episode may last from 1 to 4 weeks.

Treatment consists of medication, sometimes even narcotics, to relieve the pain and itching, plus a systemic antibiotic if infection develops.

Hydrocephalus. This excessive accumulation of CSF within the ventricles of the brain, occurring most frequently in newborns, may result from overproduction of CSF, obstruction of the flow of CSF or a lack of absorption. The increased fluid compresses the brain tissue resulting in brain damage. Hydrocephalus is characterized by an abnormally enlarged head; distended scalp veins; fragile, shiny scalp skin; a high-pitched, shrill cry; irritability; and vomiting.

Surgery is the only treatment for hydrocephalus. A shunt (passageway) is inserted into a ventricle in the brain to drain off excess fluid into either the peritoneal cavity or the atrium (upper chamber) of the heart for absorption by the body.

Meningitis. This inflammation of the meninges of the brain and spinal cord is due usually to a bacterial infection from the ears, sinuses, or lungs (pneumonia), or a brain abscess. Mortality is 70% to 100% if left untreated.

Meningitis is characterized by a high fever, chills, headache, vomiting, and specifically by positive Brudzinski's and Kernig's signs, Figure 13–33, page 232. Brudzinski's sign is demonstrated by the flexing of the hips and knees when the head and neck of a dorsal recumbent person are raised and pulled forward. Kernig's sign is demonstrated by pain and resistance when the knee is straightened after flexing at the thigh and knee.

Diagnosis of meningitis is confirmed by a lumbar puncture that shows elevated pressure, cloudiness from the excess white cells, and identification of the causative organism after culturing. Treatment consists of antibiotics, medication to reduce cerebral edema, pain relievers for headache, and an anticonvulsant. Isolation may be indicated in certain instances.

Multiple Sclerosis (MS). This disease, causing the demyelination of the white matter of the brain and spinal cord, results in double or blurred vision and sensations of tingling and numbness. Onset occurs between the ages of 20 and 40. MS is usually characterized by a series of attacks and periods of remission. Its symptoms are tremor, muscular weakness, paralysis, urinary frequency, incontinence, and emotional swings. Symptoms and extent of remission depend on the body's ability to remyelinate and restore synaptic function.

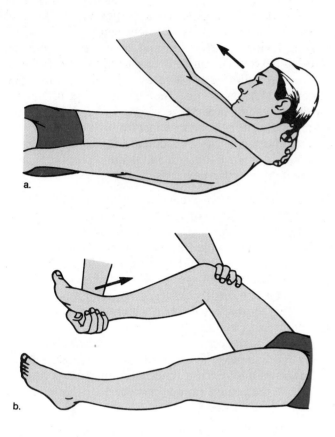

FIGURE 13–33 Two telltale signs of meningitis: (a). Brudzinski's sign (b). Kernig's sign

The cause of MS is unknown. Theories suggest the cause could be a slow-acting virus, an allergic reaction to an infectious agent, trauma, lack of oxygen, or nutritional deficits, in addition to others. Treatment consists of ACTH (adrenocorticotropic hormone) and steroids to relieve symptoms and hasten remission. Drugs for the emotional swings, urinary problems, and muscular spasticity are used as required. Bed rest to prevent fatigue is important during acute phases.

Neuralgia. Severe cutting pain along the course of a nerve may be due to inflammation, pressure on the nerve, toxins, or a change in the root ganglia. The term is used to describe general nerve pain.

Neuron and Spinal Cord Damage. This results in a loss of sensation and voluntary motion due to destruction of the neurons.

Hemiplegia is paralysis on one side of the body because of damage to the opposite side of the brain. Trauma, a tumor, or cerebrovascular accident (CVA) are the usual causative factors. Hemiplegia is characterized by unilateral paralysis of the tongue, face, arm, and leg, causing muscular contractures. Often the patient has difficulty comprehending written or verbal communication and is unable to perceive sensory stimuli on the affected side.

Paraplegia is a motor or sensory loss in the lower extremities due to spinal cord injury from trauma, most frequently from automobile, motorcycle, or sports-related accidents. Incomplete spinal cord injury is evident when ability to flex toes, control bodily functions, and feel perianal sensations is present. With complete spinal cord injury, there is a total lack of sensation and muscular control for at least 24 hours, and return of functions is unlikely. Accurate assessment of the extent of paralysis cannot be made until a year after the injury.

Quadriplegia is paralysis of the arms, legs, and body below the level of the injury to the spinal cord. It usually occurs from injury sustained in an automobile or a sporting accident and is often in the area of the fifth to seventh cervical vertebrae. Spinal cord injuries above the fifth vertebrae dramatically affect body systems such as the respiratory and the circulatory in addition to body paralysis. A complete physical and neurological examination is necessary to assess remaining motor function and determine if the cord injury is complete or partial. The condition occurs most frequently among young men. Athletic activities such as diving, gymnastics, and trampoline usage are often the cause of spinal cord injury.

Parkinson's Disease. This condition is characterized by severe muscle rigidity, a peculiar gait, drooling, and a progressive tremor. The body becomes bent forward, with head bowed. The steps become faster and faster with increasing forward body inclination, which often results in falling.

There is no known cure for the disease, although a drug called Levodopa relieves most of the symptoms until the necessarily increased dosage begins to cause serious side effects. In selected patients a surgical procedure can either freeze, electrically coagulate, or radioactively destroy a small area of the brain to prevent the involuntary motions.

Reye's Syndrome. This acute childhood illness causes fatty infiltration of the liver and increased intracranial pressure (ICP). Further damage from fat infiltration occurs in the kidneys and possibly the muscle of the heart. The syndrome (group of symptoms) affects children from infancy to adolescence, occurring equally in males and females, but affects whites more than blacks. Reye's syndrome almost always follows within 1 to 3 days of an acute viral infection such as influenza, upper respiratory infection, or chickenpox.

The syndrome prognosis depends on the degree of CNS depression from ICP. At one time, mortality was 90%; now with early treatment and ICP monitoring, the rate has been reduced to 20%. Death usually results from cerebral swelling, respiratory arrest, or coma.

The symptoms occur in stages of severity beginning with vomiting, lethargy, and liver dysfunction, then progression to hyperventilation, delirium, hyperactive reflexes, and coma. The condition worsens as symptoms of rigidity, deepening coma, large fixed pupils, seizures, and eventual respiratory arrest occurs.

Sciatica. Inflammation and severe pain of the **sciatic** nerve causes sharp, piercing pain in the back of the thigh extending down the inside of the leg. Primary causes may be exposure to wet and cold, impingement on the nerve by the spinous processes (bony projections of the vertebrae), or uneven length of the legs, causing improper vertebral alignment. Treatment consists of bed rest, heat, medication for pain, and sometimes the use of traction.

Spinal Cord Defects (Spina bifida, meningocele, myelomeningocele). These spinal cord defects result from failure of tissues to properly close during the first 3 months of pregnancy. They occur most frequently in the lumbosacral area. **Spina bifida** occulta is the most common, characterized by the incomplete closure of one or more vertebrae, but without protrusion of the spinal cord or meninges, Figure 13–34. There is usually a depression, a tuft of hair, a port wine nevi, or a combination of these signs over the defect. In spina bifida with meningocele, the sac contains meninges and CSF. Spina bifida with myelomeningocele contains meninges, CSF, and a portion of the spinal cord or nerve roots.

The incidence is approximately 5% of live births, or about 100,000 infants per year, and is highest among persons of Welsh or Irish descent. Treatment and prognosis depend on the extent of the defect. Neurological symptoms range from minimal weakness of the feet and some bladder and bowel problems to permanent neurological dysfunction such as paralysis, inability to control the bladder and bowels, hydrocephalus, clubfoot, and sometimes mental retardation. If CSF and meninges are involved, surgical closure is required to prevent further injury. Unfortunately, the neurological conditions cannot be reversed. With hydrocephalus present, a shunt will be implanted to relieve the fluid pressure.

Subarachnoid Hemorrhage. This is a collection of blood in the subarachnoid space, usually due to the spontaneous rupture of a weakened blood vessel. The patient may complain of a sudden, severe headache and experience nausea and projectile vomiting. This may be accompanied by motor disturbances, seizures, and deviations in sensory perception, particularly in vision. Precipitating factors include hypertension, oral contraceptives, malformations of cranial blood vessels, and family history.

Subdural Hematoma. A collection of blood within the subdural space, usually resulting from injury due to a fall or accident, is a slow process in which the gradually accumulating blood causes progressive symptoms such as motor disturbances, facial weakness on the side opposite the hematoma, generalized seizures, and a decreasing level of consciousness. Surgical intervention is indicated to remove the pressure on the brain tissues caused by the hematoma when symptoms and intracranial pressure reach a significant state.

Transient Ischemic Attack (TIA). This temporary condition lasting 12 to 24 hours is characterized by symptoms such as double vision, slurred speech, dizziness, staggering gait, and falling. TIA is a warning sign of impending thrombotic CVA (stroke from a blood clot). It results from microscopic clots temporarily closing off tiny arteries in the brain and impairing blood flow. Treatment

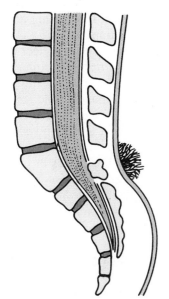

a. Spina Bifida Occulta

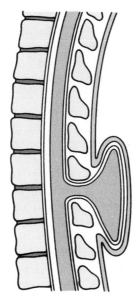

b. Meningocele

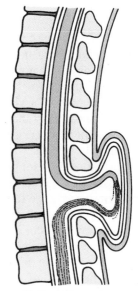

c. Myelomeningocele

FIGURE 13–34 Spinal cord defects: (a). Spina bifida occulta (b). Meningocele (c). Myelomeningocele

includes the use of aspirin and anticoagulant to reduce blood clot formation to minimize the risk of thrombosis and the resulting CVA.

Trigeminal Neuralgia (tic douloureux). This disorder of the fifth cranial nerve, on one side of the face, produces episodes of excruciating facial pain on stimulation of a trigger zone. It frequently follows exposure to heat or cold, a draft from air, smiling, or drinking hot or cold liquids. The episodes may last from 1 to 15 minutes, recurring from several times daily to a few times a year. Persons with the disorder live in fear of the next attack.

Treatment consists of oral medication and/or the injection of alcohol or phenol into the nerve branch. With frequent, severe attacks, a surgical procedure is indicated that severs the nerve, thereby relieving the pain, but also results in loss of sensation to the inner-vated area. Care must be taken afterward to protect the affected eye, avoid burns from hot food, guard against dental decay, and avoid biting the inner cheek and lip.

Complete Chapter 13, Unit 2 in the workbook to help you meet the objectives at the beginning of this unit and therefore achieve competency of this subject matter.

U N I T 3

The Senses

OBJECTIVES ....

Upon completion of this unit, the student will meet the following terminal performance objectives by verifying knowledge of the facts and principles presented through oral and written communication at a level deemed competent.

1. Name the senses of the human body identifying the corresponding organ(s) responsible for perception.
2. Identify on an anatomical illustration the structures of the eye, ear, nose, tongue, and skin.
3. Trace the path of a visual image from the cornea to the visual center of the brain.
4. Explain the effects of the lens and cornea upon the focusing of images.
5. Trace the path of sound from the entrance of the ear to the auditory center of the brain.
6. Explain the balance function of the inner ear.
7. Describe the anatomy of the olfactory organ and explain how an odor is perceived.
8. Name the taste sensations and identify the corresponding areas on the surface of the tongue.
9. Name the types of contact receptors found in the skin.
10. Describe 14 diseases or disorders of the eye, 8 of the ear, 3 of the nose, and 2 of the mouth and tongue.

11. Spell and define, using the glossary at the back of the text, all the words to know in this unit.

WORDS TO KNOW ....

accommodation	Ménière's disease
amblyopia	myopia
aqueous humor	optic disc
astigmatism	organ of Corti
auditory	otitis
cataract	otosclerosis
cerumen	papillae
choroid	polyps
cochlea	presbycusis
conjunctiva	presbyopia
cornea	pupil
enucleation	receptor
epistaxis	retina
eustachian tube	retinopathy
fovea centralis	sclera
glaucoma	semicircular canals
hyperopia	sensorineural
incus	stapes
insidious	strabismus
iris	tinnitus
lacrimal	tympanic membrane
lens	vitreous humor
malleus	

The human being is able to communicate with the surrounding environment because of a miraculous network of nerves coordinated with the organs of the five special senses, which allow us to see, hear, taste, smell, and touch. Knowledge of the environment requires the cooperation of three factors: the sense organs to perceive, intact cranial nerves to transmit, and a functioning area of the brain to interpret the received stimuli.

A stimulus is anything the body is able to detect by means of its **receptors.** Receptors are the peripheral nerve endings of sensory nerves that respond to stimuli. They are not all alike and do not respond to the same kinds of stimuli. Some respond to environmental chemical energy from ions or molecules that are dissolved in body fluids. These are chemoreceptors and are associated with the sense of taste and smell. Changes in position or pressure or the effects of acceleration create mechanical energy, which is detected by mechanoreceptors. These are associated with touch, hearing, and equilibrium. The detection of energy from light is possible due to the photoreceptors in the eyes. Thermoreceptors detect radiant energy from heat and are in the skin or connective tissues.

The stimulus, regardless of its form, is converted into energy. If the stimulus is sufficient enough to cause an action potential in the neuron, the message will travel along the sensory nerve to the brain. The reason messages are interpreted differently, such as being hot, a color, or an odor, is that certain nerves always end up in the same specific part of the brain. In other words, the sensation of heat or pain and the "seeing" of a color actually occurs in the brain, not at the point of stimulus. The ability to distinguish between hot, cold, red, or blue, for example, is the outcome of messages being received in an appropriate section of the brain, undergoing routing, being compared with stored past experiences and producing the interpretation of the stimulus.

The primary organs of the senses are familiar: the eye and the sense of sight; the ear and the sense of hearing; the tongue and the sense of taste; the nose and the sense of smell; and the skin and the sense of touch. However, these organs cannot perform their functions without the cooperation of the corresponding nerves and section of the brain.

The Eye and the Sense of Sight ....

The structure of the eyeball is frequently compared to that of a camera. The outside of the camera is made of a strong plastic or metal to protect its interior structures. To protect the eye, it is located within the bony orbital cavity of the skull. For additional protection, the outside of the eye is covered with tough, white fibrous tissue called the sclera, Figure 13–35. The sclera helps maintain the shape of the eyeball. Six extraocular or intrinsic (outside) muscles are attached to the sclera and anchored in the skull; these contract or relax as pairs to move the eyeball within its cavity. This permits rolling of the eyes in up/down, in/out, and combinations of these directions, to permit a large field of vision without moving the head, Figure 13–36, page 236. Under the sclera is another covering called the choroid, which contains the blood vessels that serve the tissues of the eye. This layer has a nonreflective pigment that makes it dark and opaque and prevents light from reflecting within the eye.

Focusing the Image

Both the eye and the camera have a lens to focus an image onto a surface for "recording." In the camera this surface is the film. In the eye it is the retina. In the camera, the distance between the film and the camera lens is adjusted to bring the picture into focus before it is recorded on the film. In the eye, the shape of the elastic lens is automatically altered by ciliary muscles of the ciliary body to focus objects onto the retina. When the ciliary body contracts, the lens becomes rounder, in a process known as accommodation for permitting near vision. With relaxation, the lens thins out to accommodate focusing on distant objects. The shape of the lens is convex on both the anterior and posterior surfaces. The shape is quite rounded in childhood, becoming more convex with age until it is nearly flat in the elderly, causing difficulty with accommodating near vision.

Controlling Light

The aperture of the camera is similar to the iris of the eye; the size of their openings is adjusted to allow varying amounts of light to enter. The iris is the colored circular muscle which surrounds the central opening called the pupil. The amount of melanin (color) and its location in the iris determines the color of the eye. When melanin is present only in the posterior area, the iris appears blue, if

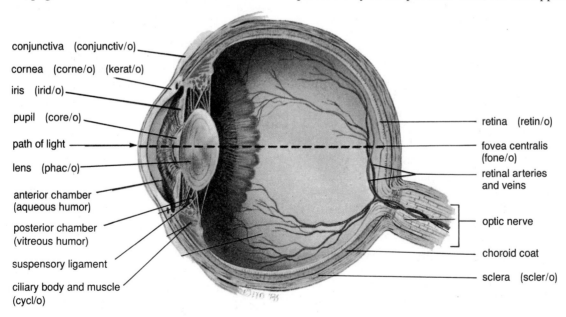

conjunctiva (conjunctiv/o)
cornea (corne/o) (kerat/o)
iris (irid/o)
pupil (core/o)
path of light
lens (phac/o)
anterior chamber (aqueous humor)
posterior chamber (vitreous humor)
suspensory ligament
ciliary body and muscle (cycl/o)

retina (retin/o)
fovea centralis (fone/o)
retinal arteries and veins
optic nerve
choroid coat
sclera (scler/o)

FIGURE 13–35   Cross section of the eye (From Fong, *Body Structures and Functions*, 7th ed. Copyright 1989, Delmar Publishers Inc.)

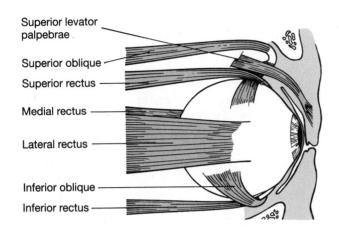

Superior levator
palpebrae

Superior oblique

Superior rectus

Medial rectus

Lateral rectus

Inferior oblique

Inferior rectus

FIGURE 13–36   Extraocular (extrinsic) muscles of the eye

it is scattered throughout, it will go from green to brown to black, depending on the amount of pigment. In the eye, the two intrinsic (inside) muscle structures of the iris regulate the amount of light that enters the eye. When the light is bright, the circular muscle fibers of the iris contract, reducing the size of the pupil, thereby permitting less light to enter. If it is dark or dimly lit, the pupil will dilate (enlarge) as the radial muscle fibers of the iris contract to pull it outward, permitting more light to enter.

The Cornea

The cornea is a transparent extension of the sclera that lies in front of the pupil. This covering has no blood vessels to interfere with vision so the tissue is nourished by lymph fluid circulating through the cellular spaces. It has both pain and touch receptors, which cause it to be extremely sensitive to any foreign body that touches its surface. If an injury to the cornea results in scarring, vision will be impaired.

The curvature of the cornea "corrects" some of the unclear image that the edge of the lens projects. If the cornea develops an abnormal shape, vision becomes blurred, and the result may be a disorder known as astigmatism.

Surface Membranes

A mucous membrane called the conjunctiva lines the inner surfaces of the eyelids and covers the anterior sclera surface of the eye. At the margin of the cornea, the conjunctiva merges with the transparent epithelium covering that protects the cornea. The conjunctiva and cornea are lubricated by tiny glands that secrete an oily substance. Further protection for the eye is provided by lacrimal glands, which secrete tears to moisten and cleanse the surface of the membrane.

Cavities and Humors

The eyeball is divided into two main areas separated by the lens and its supporting ciliary body structures. The more anterior area is subdivided into the anterior chamber, which is between the cornea and the iris, and the posterior chamber, which lies between the iris and the lens. A salty, clear fluid known as the aqueous humor fills and circulates between the chambers. It maintains the curvature of the cornea and assists in the refraction process. The eyeball behind the lens, sometimes called a vitreous chamber or vitreous body, is filled with a thick, jellylike substance called the vitreous humor. This material not only aids in refraction but also maintains the shape of the eyeball. Injury with the loss of an appreciable amount of the humor may cause damage to the eyeball, which could necessitate surgical removal of the eye by a procedure called enucleation.

The Retina

The inside layer of the eyeball is the retina, a multilayered nervous tissue. Specialized nerve cells called rods and cones transmit the stimuli focused on the retinal surface through the optic nerve to the visual center in the brain where the image is "seen." The cones, about 7 million in number, are sensitive to colors and function only in well-lighted environments. Most of them are located in a depression on the posterior surface of the retina called the fovea centralis, the area of sharpest vision. There are about 100 million rods in the more peripheral areas of the retina. The rods are very sensitive to light and permit us to see, without color, in dimly lit or nearly dark surroundings.

Optic Disc.   Two other types of nerve cells in the retina relay impulses from the rods and cones. The axons of one type form the fibers of the optic nerve. Where the optic nerves exits the retina, there are neither rods or cones so it is referred to as the optic disc or blind spot.

The Path of Light

The process of sight begins with the passage of light rays through the cornea, on through the aqueous humor, the pupil, and the lens into the vitreous humor, to focus at the back of the eyeball on the retina. Here the image is picked up by the rods and cones, transformed into nerve impulses, and transmitted over the optic nerve to the thalamus. Here some of the fibers cross over to the nerve tract of the other eye. From the thalamus, other neurons relay the impulses to the visual center in the occipital lobe of the cerebrum, where the impulses are "developed" into pictures and "seen."

Refraction Error

Each part of the eyeball refracts (deflects) the light to cause the image to focus on the retina, Figure 13–37(a). However, this does not always occur correctly. When the image is improperly refracted and focuses in front of the retina (b), the person is said to be nearsighted, or to have **myopia.** When the image focuses behind the retina (c), the person is said to be farsighted, or to have **hyperopia.** These conditions may result from abnormal curvature of the lens or cornea, or from an abnormally shaped eyeball. Note that images are inverted when they pass through the lens due to the curvature deflecting the image. Eyeglasses provide a means of refracting light to correct abnormal deflection of the image. They perform artificially what the eye's structures fail to do.

Diseases and Disorders of the Eye ....

Amblyopia (lazy eye). A condition known as amblyopia usually results from one eye turning inward, causing blurring of vision. The brain therefore suppresses the visual impulses from the inward turning eye. The condition is treated by covering the "good eye," thereby stimulating development of the "lazy eye." Amblyopia is most prevalent in children under age 5. For a good prognosis, therapy should begin before the age of 8; otherwise, eventual blindness of the affected eye may result.

Blepharitis. This inflammation is caused by the sebaceous glands producing excess secretions, which lead to greasy scales and sticky, crusted eyelids. The condition is usually associated with seborrhea of the scalp (dandruff). The itching and burning sensations cause an unconscious rubbing of the eyes resulting in red-rimmed eyelid margins. Treatment consists of frequent shampoos of the hair and daily cleansing of the eyelids with a mild shampoo to remove the scales.

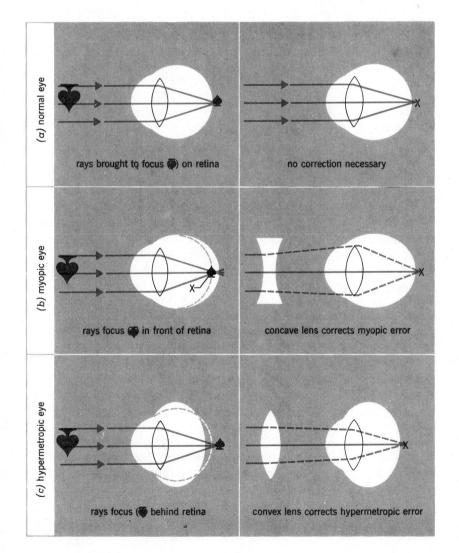

(a) normal eye

rays brought to focus on retina

no correction necessary

(b) myopic eye

rays focus in front of retina

concave lens corrects myopic error

(c) hypermetropic eye

rays focus behind retina

convex lens corrects hypermetropic error

FIGURE 13–37 The refraction of an image (a). Normal vision (b). Nearsightedness (c). Farsightedness and the type of lens required to correct the vision. (From Burke, *Human Anatomy and Physiology in Health and Disease*, 3d ed. Copyright 1992, Delmar Publishers Inc.)

Cataract. This gradually developing opacity (cloudiness) of the lens occurs most frequently in persons over 70 years of age, as part of the aging process. The probable cause of cataracts is a change in the composition of the proteins of the lens. The condition causes a painless, gradual blurring and loss of vision. The pupil turns from black to a milky white as the lens becomes visible. People with cataracts frequently complain of seeing halos around lights or being blinded at night by oncoming automobile headlights.

Cataracts are treated by surgical removal of the lens and postoperative substitution of cataract eyeglasses. Other options are possible for some patients. Contact lenses can be fitted and provide much better correction than glasses. Frequently an intraocular lens (IOL) is implanted directly behind the cornea when the cataract surgery is performed. A new "taco" style lens is inserted in a folded-over state through a very tiny incision popping open after it is implanted. Cataract surgery is now being done on an outpatient basis, with the patient detained only a few hours.

Sometime after surgery the capsule that held the lens in place, and is now behind and supporting the IOL, may become clouded, once again obstructing the path of light into the eye. This problem can be easily solved without invasive surgery, using a laser beam to make a tiny opening in the capsule, which lets in light and restores vision.

Conjunctivitis (Pinkeye). This condition results in redness, pain, swelling, and occasionally a discharge, due to inflammation of the conjunctiva. It is usually caused by an infectious organism such as bacteria (streptococcus or staphylococcus) or a virus (herpes simplex). Allergic reactions and environmental irritants can also cause the condition.

It usually begins in one eye, spreading rapidly to the other from contamination by a wash cloth or by the hands. Since it is highly contagious, other family members should not share towels, wash cloths, pillows, etc. with the infected person. The causative organism is identified by stained smears of the drainage and indicates the method of treatment. Bacterial conjunctivitis responds to antibiotics and sulfa drug therapy; the herpes viral type does not.

Corneal Abrasion. A scratch or trauma to the cornea, usually from a foreign body in the eye, is most often caused by dirt that becomes imbedded under the eyelid, small pieces of wood, metal, or paper, or an injury from a fingernail. Even if the eye waters profusely to cleanse the surface, the scratch (abrasion) remains, causing redness, tearing, and irritation. Abrasions may also occur when people fall asleep wearing hard contact lenses. Vision may be affected if the location and extent of injury are significant. Foreign bodies embedded in the cornea require removal following application of a topical anesthetic. Treatment consists of antibiotic eyedrops or oint-

ment and application of a pressure eye patch to prevent blinking. Corneal epithelium heals rapidly within 24 to 48 hours.

Corneal Ulcers. These result from bacterial, viral, or fungal infections. The first signs are pain, aggravated by blinking, and excessive tearing. Blurred vision results from the ulcerations, the corneal surface appears irregular, and exudate (pus) may be present. Instillation of an ophthalmic dye will permit confirmation of the diagnosis. A culture of the drainage to determine the causative organism will indicate appropriate medication. Broad-spectrum antibiotics are used initially to prevent corneal scarring and the resulting impairment of vision. Certain bacterially caused ulcers progress so rapidly that, without proper treatment, the cornea will perforate (be pierced with holes) and vision in the eye will be lost within 48 hours.

Diabetic Retinopathy. This form of vascular retinopathy results from juvenile or adult diabetes. Approximately 75% of patients with juvenile diabetes develop diabetic retinopathy within 20 years after the onset of diabetes. Incidence in adults with diabetes increases with the length of time a person is diabetic. About 80% of patients with diabetes of 20 to 30 years' duration develop retinopathy. The condition is a result of an interference with the blood supply to the eyes. It is the leading cause of acquired blindness in adults.

Symptoms result from an edematous retina, which causes light to scatter. Tiny capillary walls thicken and show evidence of dilation, twisting, and hemorrhage. This causes glare, blurred vision, and reduced visual acuity. If diagnosed and treated early, prognosis is good for simple forms; in extensive forms, prognosis is poor, with 50% becoming blind within 5 years. Treatment consists of sealing holes that have developed in the retina and coagulating the leaking vessels with a laser beam. If new abnormal vessels have grown onto the retina and into the vitreous body, it is possible for the retina to detach from the choroid layer, resulting in vitreous hemorrhage and blindness. With this advanced condition, open surgery will be required.

Glaucoma (Chronic). This condition of excessive intraocular pressure results in atrophy (wasting away) of the optic nerve. Glaucoma causes severe visual impairment and eventually blindness. It occurs in 20% of adults over age 40 and accounts for 15% of all blindness in the United States. It is the most easily prevented cause of blindness.

The condition results from either an overproduction of the aqueous humor produced by the epithelium of the ciliary body or the obstruction of its outflow circulating mechanisms to the canal of Schlemm for absorption into venous circulation, Figure 13–38. With chronic open-angle glaucoma, fluid cannot drain because of a blockage of the trabecular meshwork. Symptoms are insidious (gradual) and are often not recognized until late in the disease. They include mild aching, a loss of peripheral (side) vision, seeing halos around lights, and difficulty seeing at night.

In acute closed-angle glaucoma, fluid cannot drain because the iris presses against the cornea, closing off the canal of Schlemm. There is a rapid onset of symptoms and it is considered an emergency. There is pain and redness of the affected eye with a feeling of pressure. The pupil is moderately dilated and nonreactive to light. There is blurred and decreased visual acuity as well as sensitivity to light. Unless the pressure is relieved quickly, blindness will occur within 3 to 5 days. Usual treatment consists of aggressive drug therapy and a peripheral iridectomy (removal of a piece of the iris) to permit outflow of the aqueous humor.

Glaucoma is diagnosed with evidence of increased intraocular pressure as measured by a tonometer and confirmed by viewing, through an ophthalmoscope, characteristic changes in the optic disk. Initial treatment usually consists of systemic drugs to reduce the production of aqueous humor and eye drops to aid in the outflow. With inadequate response, a surgical procedure is required to create an opening for the circulation of the fluid.

Laser surgery is a quick, less expensive, and relatively painless solution to both open- and closed-angle glaucoma. In open-angle, if medication is ineffective, a laser beam is directed to open the trabecular meshwork. In closed-angle, the laser makes a tiny opening in the iris to allow the fluid to drain. A second treatment may be necessary in closed-angle glaucoma. Laser eye surgery is more effective in the early stages of the disease.

Hordeolum (Stye). This localized infection of a gland of the eyelid produces an abscess around an eyelash. The eye is red, painful, and swollen. Treatment consists of applying warm, wet compresses to relieve pain and promote drainage, and the use of eye drops or ointment to take care of the infection.

Iritis. An inflammation of the iris is often caused by an improperly healed corneal abrasion, especially if damage is from a sharp object. Iritis produces moderate to severe eye pain, photophobia, and a small nonreactive pupil due to the spasm of the iris. Prompt treatment is required to prevent complications. The pupil is dilated with mydriatics to allow the eye to rest to prevent the formation of posterior synechiae (adhesions of the iris to the lens). Corticosteroid drops are used to reduce the inflammation.

Presbyopia. This condition is characterized by inability of the lens to accommodate for near vision because of loss of elasticity. Presbyopia occurs as part of the normal aging process. The condition can be corrected by the fitting of contact lenses or eyeglasses.

Ptosis. Drooping of the upper eyelid may be a congenital condition (a condition one is born with), the result of aging, the presence of an excess fatty fold, or a neurological factor. Treatment may be required if vision is restricted or the appearance is cosmetically undesirable. A surgical procedure on the eyelid muscles will correct the disorder or a device can be attached to the eyeglass frame to elevate the eyelid.

Retinal Detachment. This disorder is characterized by the separation of the retina from the choroid layer of the eyeball. The separation may occur with aging, which causes the normal vitreous support to shrink away. This results in a small hole or tear that permits the humor to seep between the layers and cause separation. Other causative factors include severe high blood pressure, diabetes, trauma, and other systemic diseases.

Diagnosis can be made from the patient's complaints of seeing floating spots, flashes of light, and a gradual vision loss. Confirmation is possible after pupil dilation and ophthalmoscopy reveal a gray and opaque retina with indefinite margins in the affected areas. Folds, tears, and a ballooning inward of the retina may be seen. Treatment consists of limiting eye movements with a patch, bed rest, sedation, and appropriate positioning of the head. Spontaneous reattachment is rare. A coagulation laser beam can repair simple tears in the retina by "spot welding" the area with several rows of "welds," but once separation has occurred, other treatment will be necessary. Both heat and cold therapies are used to create a sterile inflammatory reaction, which causes the retina to readhere. A tight band is placed around the eye-

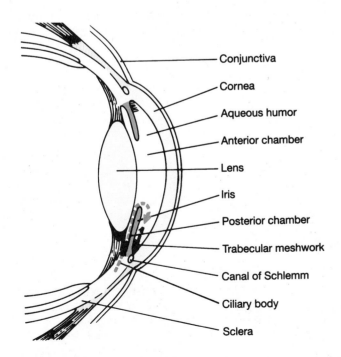

FIGURE 13–38   Normal flow of aqueous humor

- Conjunctiva
- Cornea
- Aqueous humor
- Anterior chamber
- Lens
- Iris
- Posterior chamber
- Trabecular meshwork
- Canal of Schlemm
- Ciliary body
- Sclera

ball, inside the sclera layer, which makes the choroid "indent" against the retina to maintain its closeness. Various surgical procedures to re-attach the retina to the choroid can be performed.

Strabismus. In this condition, one eye deviates, with the gaze being abnormally inward (cross-eyed), outward (walleyed), higher, or lower than that of the other eye. This condition may result from muscle imbalance or attempts to compensate for farsightedness. Strabismus is frequently associated with Down's syndrome, cerebral palsy, and mental retardation. Diagnosis is made on observation of the obvious visual symptoms and the complaint of blurred or double vision. Conservative initial treatment consists of a patch on the normal eye, corrective glasses, and specific eye exercises. Surgery to adjust the muscles that control eye placement and movement may be indicated. If strabismus develops before age 5, the deviated eye may be suppressed, resulting in amblyopia that could cause loss of vision if not treated.

The Ear and the Sense of Hearing ....

The ear is capable of receiving vibrations in the air and translating them into the sounds we recognize: the more vibrations per second, the higher the frequency, or pitch, of the sound, the stronger the vibration, the louder the sound.

The Outer Ear

Vibrations are picked up by the pinna (auricle) of the outer ear and directed down the external auditory canal to the tympanic membrane (eardrum), Figure 13–39.

The Middle Ear

The sound waves vibrate the membrane and the malleus (hammer) attached to its inner surface. The malleus in turn "strikes" the incus (anvil), which moves the stapes (stirrup). These three small bones and the space around them are called the middle ear. The middle ear communicates the vibrations to the inner ear by the stapes pushing against the fluid in the vestibule of the inner ear through the oval window.

The middle ear is connected by means of the eustachian tube to the throat. The tube is responsible for equalizing air pressure in the middle ear with the outside atmospheric pressure. Unfortunately, infections from the throat often pass through the tube into the middle ear. Rapid changes in altitude, harsh blowing of the nose, or a forceful sneeze may cause temporary air pressure inequities.

The Inner Ear

The vibrations from the middle ear continue through the coiled cochlea, which contains the organ of Corti, a collection of specialized nerve cells, Figure 13–40. These cells transmit the impulses to the auditory nerve, which passes them on to the auditory center of the temporal lobe of the cerebrum for interpretation.

The inner ear also contains three semicircular canals. These structures are responsible for maintaining equilibrium (balance). Inside the canals, hairlike nerve cell receptors are embedded in a gelatinlike material. When the head moves, the material pushes against the receptors, which transmit to the brain the change in position.

Another nerve receptor network in the semicircular canals is similarly constructed inside two small sacs. The

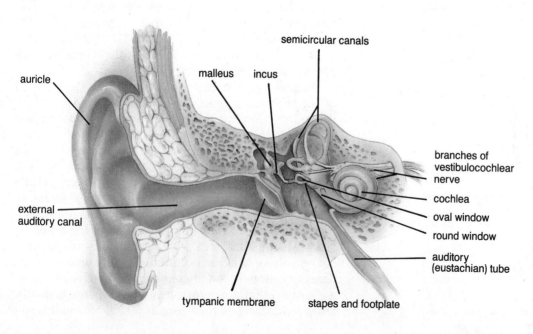

semicircular canals
malleus   incus
auricle
branches of vestibulocochlear nerve
cochlea
oval window
round window
external auditory canal
auditory (eustachian) tube
tympanic membrane   stapes and footplate

FIGURE 13–39 The ear (From Smith, *Medical Terminology, A Programmed Text*, 6th ed. Copyright 1991, Delmar Publishers Inc.)

gelatin surface here is covered with a layer of tiny lime-stone grains. When the head moves, the grains shift causing the hair cells to send out impulses.

Diseases and Disorders of the Ear ....

Auditory Canal Obstruction. The auditory canal can be obstructed by impacted **cerumen** (ear wax) or a foreign body such as a bean, pea, pebble, bead, or insect. Children often put objects into their ears. Some obstructions may cause discomfort and a degree of hearing loss. Treatment consists of a removal technique appropriate to the obstruction. Cerumen can be removed by gentle scraping with a cerumen spoon and/or irrigation by syringe or an aerated water jet (see Chapter 16). Irrigation should be stopped immediately if it causes pain. Removal of insects can be accomplished easily after killing with an instillation of 70% alcohol. Similar objects can also be removed after irrigation with alcohol if they cannot be reached with forceps. Water must be avoided if it may cause swelling of the object, such as a bean or pea.

Hearing Loss. This condition of reduced ability to perceive sound at normal levels can be either a conductive loss due to the inability to carry sound waves through the structures of the ear or a nerve loss sensorineural, due to transmission failure of the nerves within the inner ear or the auditory nerve. Loss can also be caused by a combination of lack of conduction and impulse transmission.

Conductive loss may be caused by an obstruction from a buildup of cerumen (wax), a foreign body, swelling within the auditory canal, middle ear infection, or otosclerosis.

Sudden loss of hearing without prior impairment is considered a medical emergency because prompt treatment may restore hearing. Common causes are acute infection, head trauma, brain tumor, toxic drugs, or metabolic and vascular disorders.

Hearing loss can also be noise induced and can be temporary or, over time, permanent. It follows prolonged exposure to noise in excess of 85 to 90 db (see Chapter 16). It is common among people who work in constant industrial noise, military personnel and rock musicians. This loss is preventable with the enforcement of the use of protective devices, such as ear plugs, as mandated by law in occupational exposure.

Bone and air conduction hearing loss is assessed by the Rinne and Weber tests. An audiometer can be used to give a pure tone audiometry examination to measure the threshold and degree of loudness at which sound can be perceived (see Chapter 16). A gradual loss of hearing occurs normally as part of the aging process and is known as **presbycusis.**

Ménière's Disease. The condition known as **Ménière's disease** is characterized by severe vertigo (dizziness), **tinni-**

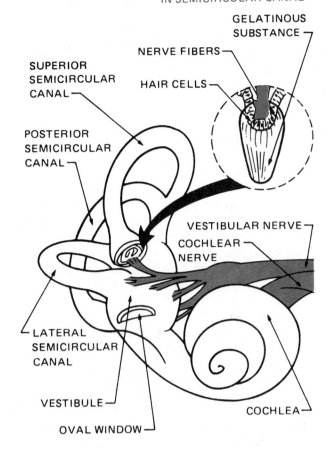

FIGURE 13–40 Enlarged view of the inner ear. (From *The Wonderful Human Machine*, copyright 1979, American Medical Association)

tus (ringing in the ears), and nerve loss, apparently from degeneration of the hair cells in the cochlea and vestibule of the inner ear. Violent attacks may last from 10 minutes to hours and cause severe nausea, vomiting, and perspiration. Often the vertigo causes loss of balance and results in the person falling. Treatment consists of drugs to reduce fluid, antihistamines, and mild sedation. If frequent severe attacks occur, surgical destruction of the cochlea may be indicated at the cost of permanent hearing loss.

Motion Sickness. This is characterized by loss of equilibrium, perspiration, headache, nausea, and vomiting brought on by irregular motion. The disorder probably results from excessive stimulation of the inner ear receptors or confusion in the brain between the visual stimulus and movement perception. Treatment consists of avoiding the causative motions, lying down, and closing the eyes. When avoidance is not possible, the head should be kept still and vision focused on distant and stationary objects. Medications to prevent vomiting are usually beneficial.

Otitis: Externa. This infection of the external auditory canal is usually caused by bacteria. Otitis causes pain and hearing loss. Otitis externa can result from contaminated swimming water (swimmer's ears); cleaning the canal with bobby pins or introducing an organism on a cotton swab; regular use of earphones or plugs which can trap moisture, creating optimal growing conditions; and scratching the ear canal with a fingernail. It is best treated with heat, pain medication, and antibiotic ear drops, following thorough cleaning.

Otitis: Media. An infection of the middle ear often associated with respiratory infections, otitis media can also result from obstruction of the eustachian tube, which causes a negative pressure to develop and "pull" serous fluid from the blood vessels into the middle ear. Otitis media is characterized by a severe, deep, and throbbing pain; fever; hearing loss; nausea and vomiting; and dizziness. The tympanic membrane may be reddened and bulge into the external canal. Excessive pressure may cause it to rupture, resulting in drainage into the canal. Recurring episodes may scar and thicken the membrane, causing a conduction hearing loss. Holes and tears from a rupture will also cause a loss of hearing.

Treatment requires antibiotics such as penicillin or erythromycin (with a sulfa drug if allergic to penicillin) in addition to pain medication. A myringotomy (incision of the tympanic membrane) is indicated if bulging and severe pain are present. Young children and infants are prone to ear infections. Anatomically, their eustachian tubes slant horizontally, which allows fluid to collect more easily and become a medium for bacterial growth. Infants who are allowed to take a bottle while lying down, especially on their backs, may get fluid into their eustachian tubes if they cough or cry. With chronic fluid collection due to obstruction, it may be necessary to insert a tiny polyethylene tube through the membrane temporarily to equalize the pressure.

Otosclerosis. The most common cause of conductive deafness is otosclerosis. The loss is slow and progressive and may be accompanied by tinnitus. It is characterized by the formation of spongy bone, which immobilizes the stapes in the oval window of the vestibule, disrupting the conduction of vibrations from the tympanic membrane to the cochlea. It appears to result from a genetic factor and often occurs among family members. Incidence in Caucasians is at least 10%, affecting twice as many females as males, usually between 15 and 30 years of age. Treatment for otosclerosis consists of surgically removing the stapes (stapedectomy) and inserting an artificial substitute, which results in partial or complete return of hearing. An appropriate type of hearing aid may be of some assistance, if a stapedectomy is not possible.

Presbycusis (Senile Deafness). This hearing loss that is an effect of aging and results from deterioration of the audi-

tory system and a loss of the hair cells in the organ of Corti. It is sensorineural in nature, normally manifesting itself through the loss of high frequency sounds. It is usually accompanied by an annoying tinnitus. The patient has difficulty understanding the spoken word and may become depressed due to inability to communicate. Presbycusis is irreversible and can be somewhat overcome with an effective and proper-fitting hearing aid.

The Nose and the Sense of Smell ....

The sense of smell is due to the olfactory organ in the top of the nasal cavity, Figure 13–41. The nerve fibers in the organ are chemoreceptors that respond to stimuli from ions or molecules dissolved in the moisture from the mucous membranes. The organ is connected by nerve fibers, which run through tiny holes in the skull bone above the nasal cavity, to the olfactory center in the brain. The nerve fibers connect with hair cells in the mucous membrane of the nose. These odor detectors can "smell" something only after it is dissolved in the mucus secretions.

Diseases and Disorders of the Nose ....

Epistaxis (Nosebleed). This usually occurs after injury, either external or internal, such as a blow to the nose, nosepicking, or foreign body insertion. Less frequent causes of epistaxis are chronic conditions such as nasal

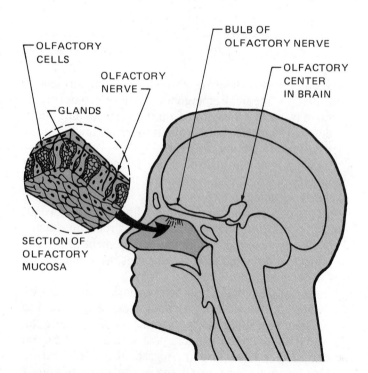

FIGURE 13–41 The sense of smell (From *The Wonderful Human Machine,* copyright 1979, American Medical Association)

or sinus infection that results in capillary congestion and bleeding, or the inhalation of irritating substances. Predisposing systemic factors include high blood pressure, anticoagulation drugs, chronic aspirin use, and blood diseases such as anemia, hemophilia, and leukemia.

Treatment varies depending on the cause, location, and severity. Even moderate bleeding is considered severe if it persists longer than 10 minutes after pressure is applied. Symptoms may include lightheadedness, a drop in blood pressure, rapid pulse, dyspnea, pallor, and other indications of shock. Initial first aid treatment may consist of: elevating the head; compression of nostrils against the septum continuously for 5 to 10 minutes; application of ice or cold compresses to nose and back of neck; preventing the swallowing of blood (to determine the amount lost); avoiding talking or blowing the nose; and observing for amount of blood loss and signs of shock.

Advanced treatment includes: for anterior bleeding, applying epinephrine-saturated cotton ball or gauze to the bleeding site and the use of external pressure, followed by cauterization by electric cautery or silver nitrate; for posterior bleeding, the insertion of a nasal pack for 48 to 72 hours may be required. Small catheters are passed through each side of the nose into the mouth. Rolled gauze packs are attached to the catheters and drawn back through the mouth and up into the posterior nasal cavity where they become lodged, making pressure against the leaking blood vessels. If necessary, anterior bleeding can be treated by packing for 24 to 48 hours. Other treatment may include supplemental vitamin K, blood transfusions, and surgical ligation (tying) of the bleeding artery.

Nasal Polyps. These benign growths, usually multiple and in both sides of the nose, often occur in large enough numbers and size to distend the nose and obstruct the airway. They are caused by prolonged mucous membrane edema associated with allergies, chronic sinusitis, rhinitis, and recurrent nasal infections. Diagnosis is made by visual observation through a nasal speculum or X rays of posterior nasal passages and the sinuses. Treatment with antihistamines, cortisone, and antibiotics if infected, will temporarily reduce the size of the **polyps.** However, surgical removal is the treatment of choice and usually necessary.

Rhinitis (Allergic). This reaction to airborne allergens causes sneezing, profuse watery discharge, itching of the eyes and nose, conjunctivitis, and tearing. Many symptoms are the result of the body's attempt to dilute or remove irritants coming into contact with its mucous membranes. Treatment consists of eliminating environmental antigens when possible, the use of antibiotics, and systemic corticosteroids. Long-term

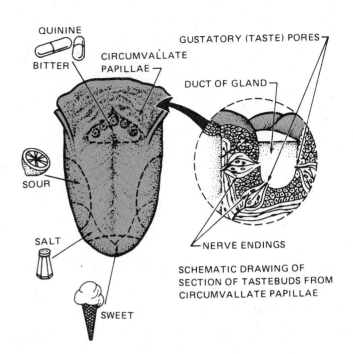

FIGURE 13–42 The sense of taste (From *The Wonderful Human Machine*, copyright 1979, American Medical Association)

management includes injections of the offending allergens to cause desensitization, the use of air conditioning, and, if severe and persistent, relocation to a safe environment.

The Tongue and the Sense of Taste

The ability to taste flavors is located in the receptors of the taste buds on the tongue. They are located at the tip, sides, and back, grouped by the taste that can be perceived, Figure 13–42. The sweet area is at the tip, the salty areas are next along the sides, followed by the sour areas and another area of salty perception. The large **papillae** (raised areas) at the back transmit the bitter sensations. Like the sense of smell, taste is possible because of the chemoreceptors that receive stimuli from ions or molecules and initiate the impulses. As with smell, taste is not possible unless the substance is moistened. This moisture is supplied by the salivary glands, in sufficient quantities to affect taste.

Diseases and Disorders of the Mouth and Tongue

Glossitis. Inflammation of the tongue caused by an organism, irritation, injury, or nutritional deficiencies is known as glossitis. Such agents as tobacco, alcohol, spicy foods, and jagged teeth may cause glossitis. The condition results in a red, swollen tongue, pain on chewing, difficult speech, and occasionally an obstructed airway. Treatment includes topical anesthetic mouthwash, systemic pain medication, good oral hygiene, and the avoidance of alcohol and hot, cold, or spicy foods.

Oral Cancer. In recent years, a significant increase in the incidence of oral cancer has been noted. There seems to be evidence that people have switched from cigarettes to smokeless forms of tobacco in an effort to alleviate the development of lung cancer. In exchange, the use of products such as chewing tobacco and snuff has caused extensive disease of the gums, tongue, and other oral structures and often results in the development of cancer within the oral cavity.

The Skin and the Sense of Touch ....

The sense of touch requires direct contact with the body through contact receptors, Figure 13–43. The sense of touch involves mechanical energy, such as pressure or traction, which activates mechanoreceptors and radiant energy, such as heat or cold, which activates thermoreceptors. The design of the receptor varies with its location on the body. Touch receptors are most concentrated in the fingertips. Pain receptors are simply bare nerve endings in the skin and other organs. Separate skin receptors perceive heat and cold. Each of the contact receptors in the skin has its own perceptive function enabling us to feel the many different sensations of pain, touch, pressure, heat, cold, traction, and tickle. This sense aids us in protecting ourselves, identifying injury, feeling pleasure, and maintaining contact with our environment. The skin is the subject of the next unit.

Complete Chapter 13, Unit 3 in the workbook to help you meet the objectives at the beginning of this unit and therefore achieve competency of this subject matter.

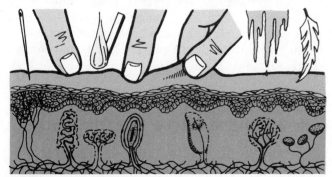

PAIN TOUCH HEAT PRESSURE TRACTION COLD TICKLE

FIGURE 13–43 The sense of touch (From *The Wonderful Human Machine*, copyright 1979, American Medical Association)

UNIT 4

Integumentary System

OBJECTIVES ....

Upon completion of this unit, the student will meet the following terminal performance objectives by verifying knowledge of the facts and principles presented through oral and written communication at a level deemed competent.

1. List the five functions of the skin.
2. Explain how the skin regulates body temperature.
3. Describe how the body cools its surface.
4. Name the three layers of skin tissue and the characteristic structures of each layer.
5. Describe the process that causes wrinkles.
6. Explain what causes a suntan to develop.
7. Identify the ABCD rules and other warning signs of melanoma and the factors that contribute to its development.
8. Explain what causes blushing, birthmarks, moles, and albinism.
9. Identify 20 diseases or disorders of the skin.
10. Spell and define, using the glossary at the back of the text, all the words to know in this unit.

WORDS TO KNOW ....

albino	macule
alopecia	melanin
carbunculosis	melanocytes
constrict	pediculosis
dermatitis	perception
dermis	pigment
dilate	psoriasis
eczema	pustule
epidermis	receptors
erythema	sebaceous
follicle	sebum
folliculitis	slough
furuncle	subcutaneous
herpes simplex	transdermal
herpes zoster	urticaria
integumentary	verrucae
inunction	vesicle
keloid	wheals
Lyme disease	whorl

The word **integumentary** refers to an external covering or skin. You may never have thought of the skin as a "body system," but according to the definition of a system in Unit 1, the skin with all its structures qualifies: it is many tissues (nerve, connective, muscle, epithelial), forming organs (sweat and oil glands), to perform a function. The skin is not usually listed as one of the body's systems, however. Most anatomists classify the skin as an organ. When listed in this category, it becomes the largest organ of the body. An average adult has about 3000 square inches of skin surface. The skin makes up about 15% of the total body weight, which would be approximately 20 pounds of a 145 pound person. The skin varies in thickness from very thin over the eyelids to quite thick on the soles of the feet.

The skin is so important to survival that the loss of even a small percentage of its vital function is a cause for concern. If about one-third of the skin of a healthy young adult is lost, death may result. Skin covers all the body's surface, preventing the tissue fluids from escaping and foreign materials in the environment from entering. At the openings to the body, such as the nose, mouth, or anus, it joins with the mucous membranes that line the openings into the respiratory and digestive systems to make a continuous internal and external covering.

Functions

The skin performs five important functions for the body: protection, perception, temperature control, absorption, and excretion. The skin protects against the invasion of bacteria by serving as a barrier. It is effective, however, only as long as it remains intact. A cut or scrape of the surface allows bacteria to enter. It also protects the delicate underlying tissues from injury by the damaging rays of the sun. Equally important, it protects the body's tissues from loss of fluid. This is of great concern when large areas of skin are lost as a result of burns, for example, which allows fluids to escape and bacteria to enter.

The skin serves as an organ of perception in cooperation with the nervous system and the sense of touch. A square inch of skin contains about 72 feet of nerves and hundreds of receptors registering pain, heat, cold, and pressure.

In that same square inch are about 15 feet of blood vessels, which provide food and oxygen, and also regulate the body's temperature. This function is of such importance to the body that the skin receives approximately one-third of the blood circulating throughout the body. When the body's temperature control center in the brain senses the body is becoming too warm, the nervous system sends messages to the surface vessels to dilate, which allows heat from the blood to escape through the skin and therefore cool the body. If heat must be retained, the vessels are ordered to constrict to reduce the loss of heat so that body temperature can be maintained at an adequate level. This important function is discussed in greater detail in Chapter 15, Unit 2, Vital Signs.

The skin also contains sweat glands, which are likewise controlled by the heat regulator in the brain. When the air temperature rises, the body produces sweat, which evaporates from its surface to provide a cooling effect and thereby reduce the amount of heat within the underlying blood vessels.

The skin is capable of absorbing some materials from its surface through the hair follicles and the glands. This function can be of use to the physician in treating certain conditions. Perhaps the two most common applications are antimotion sickness medication, which is placed on the skin's surface behind the ear, and a medicated paste strip, which is placed on the chest to treat certain heart conditions. A trend seems to be developing toward a greater amount of medications being administered through the skin. Primarily the advantages are "timed release," which spreads medication evenly over a long period of time thereby eliminating repeated dosage and the digestive system side effects from certain oral drugs. This form of drug administration is called inunction, or transdermal.

Several substances known as lipoid-soluble (e.g., vitamins A, D, and K, the sex hormones, etc.) and almost all gases (e.g., oxygen, hydrogen, and nitrogen, etc.) can pass through the skin. It is interesting to note that carbon monoxide cannot pass.

The skin's function of excretion consists primarily of eliminating water and salt plus a minute amount of other waste products. Excessive fluid loss as a result of strenuous activity or highly elevated temperature can be a matter of concern. Fluid must be replaced to maintain a proper fluid balance. The skin also combines the ultraviolet rays from sunlight with compounds normally present in the skin to produce vitamin D while screening out any harmful ultraviolet rays.

A great number of microscopic skin structures are located within an area of only one square centimeter. This is illustrated in Figure 13–44, page 246 as a small circle on the back of the hand. That this large group of anatomical structures could be located in such a small area seems inconceivable. These microscopic wonders perform an invaluable service for the body.

Structure of the Skin

The skin is composed of three layers, the epidermis on the top, the dermis in the middle, and the subcutaneous layer on the bottom, Figure 13–45, page 247. The subcutaneous layer is filled with fat globules, blood vessels, and nerves. The dermis contains blood vessels, nerves, hair follicles, and sweat and oil glands. This layer is usually referred to as the "true skin." The top of the dermis is covered with cone-shaped papillae, which create an uneven surface. The epidermis is full of ridges that fit snugly over the papillae on top of the dermis. These ridges form the whorls and patterns on the fingertips that we call fingerprints. Since no two people have exactly the same pattern of ridges, they will not have the same fingerprints, making this characteristic a suitable means of identification. Similar patterns of ridges appear on the

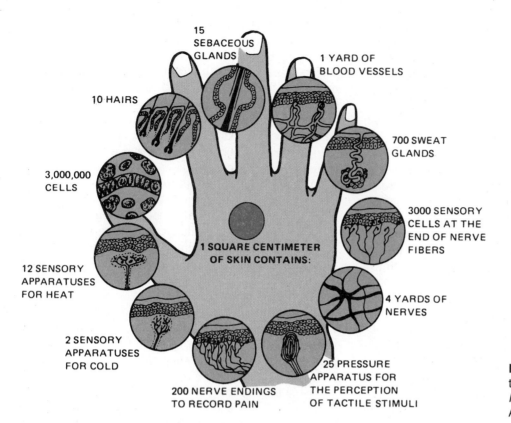

FIGURE 13–44 Structures of the skin (From *The Wonderful Human Machine*, copyright 1979, American Medical Association)

Labels in figure:
15 SEBACEOUS GLANDS
1 YARD OF BLOOD VESSELS
10 HAIRS
700 SWEAT GLANDS
3,000,000 CELLS
3000 SENSORY CELLS AT THE END OF NERVE FIBERS
12 SENSORY APPARATUSES FOR HEAT
1 SQUARE CENTIMETER OF SKIN CONTAINS:
4 YARDS OF NERVES
2 SENSORY APPARATUSES FOR COLD
200 NERVE ENDINGS TO RECORD PAIN
25 PRESSURE APPARATUS FOR THE PERCEPTION OF TACTILE STIMULI

soles of the feet and are used for identification of newborns. New cells are formed deep in the epidermis. Here rapid cell division pushes cells toward the surface of the skin to replace those that wear away, die, and flake off. The process from division to flaking off takes about 30 to 45 days. Because of the skin's ability to reproduce cells rapidly, it can repair itself quickly following cuts and abrasions.

The skin is strong, soft, flexible, and elastic in young people because of the presence of keratin in the epidermis and collagenous fibers in the dermis. Also, some dermis cells store fat. The action of the keratin and cell membranes allows skin to act as a barrier to prevent dehydration. With age, the fatty underlying tissue is absorbed and the elastic fibers decrease, leaving an excess in the outer layer which develops folds or wrinkles.

The skin has four appendages, the sweat and oil glands, hair, and the nails. The dermis contains the sweat and sebaceous (oil) glands. Sweat glands are tiny coiled tubes deep in the dermis with corkscrew tubules leading to the surface. Oil glands are located in or near hair follicles over the entire skin surface except for the palms of the hands and the soles of the feet.

A sebaceous gland contains an oily substance which helps prevent the hair and skin from becoming dry and brittle. Unfortunately, oil glands often become plugged by cell overgrowth. The gland continues to produce oil, which fills the duct and results in development of a blackhead or pimple.

Every hair has a root, which is inside a follicle (shaft) that extends deep into the dermal layer. With long hair, the root extends into the subcutaneous layer. Attached to each follicle is a small involuntary muscle. With certain emotions or sensations of coldness, the muscle contracts, causing the hair to stand erect and producing what we call "goose flesh." An inner layer of cells in the shaft of hair contains a pigment which gives the hair its color. Hair that is white has cells that contain air in place of pigment.

The hair and nails are composed of hard keratin (soft keratin is found in the epidermis). They are similar but the hard keratin is more permanent and does not slough (drop) off, which means they must be cut occasionally.

Skin Color

A brown-black pigment called melanin is produced by cells called *melanocytes,* which are present in the epidermis to protect the underlying tissues from damage by the sun. The amount of melanin affects the color of the skin as does another pigment, carotene, which is yellow. The presence of blood vessels in the dermis also contributes to the coloration of the skin. When the skin is exposed to the sun, it may become reddened due to dilation of the superficial blood vessels. The condition is known medically as erythema, but it is commonly known as sunburn. If it is not severe, the skin will acquire a brown coloration or suntan, which is produced by the melanin pigment increasing and moving to the surface to protect the underlying tissues. New melanin will replace the old in the lower cell layer. Freckles are actually small areas of melanin pigment.

Skin coloration is affected by many factors. The rich supply of blood vessels causes reddening of the skin, due to dilation, when we blush. Birthmarks may be due to coloration from a concentration of blood vessels or from patches of skin pigment. Moles are also pigmented patches. A person whose skin has little or no pigment to give it color is said to be an albino. An albino's hair also lacks pigment and will be white. Because pigment is also lacking in the coloration of the eyes, the sun and artificial light cannot be filtered out. Therefore the eyes of a person with albinism are very sensitive to light. People with this disorder must wear sunglasses or tinted lenses for comfort and to prevent eye damage.

The Skin as a Diagnostic Testing Site ....

The skin is often used to test and diagnose disorders and diseases of the body, specifically in the area of allergies. Because of its natural capacity to defend the body from foreign substances, it makes an excellent medium for testing the reaction to minute amounts of allergens. Following injection of common substances, usually on the back or inner surface of the forearm, the skin will form various-sized areas around the injection sites, reacting to those materials that initiate an allergic response. Physicians can then identify causative substances and recommend measures to reduce the problems associated with the allergic disorder. (See Chapter 18, Diagnostic Tests, X rays, and Procedures.)

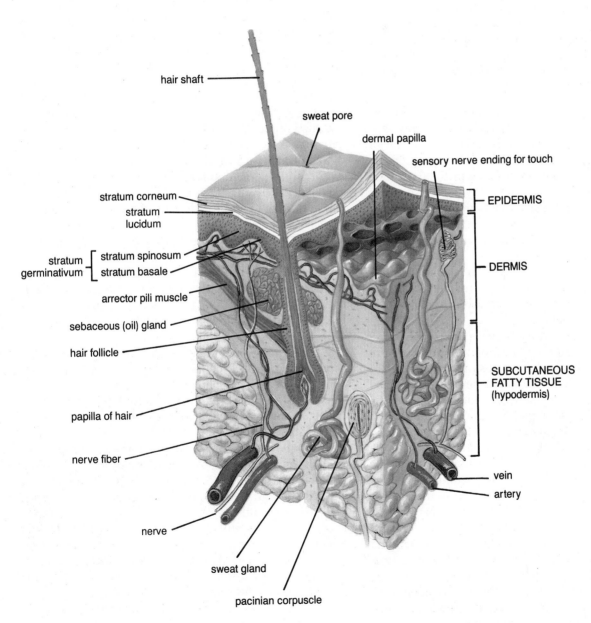

FIGURE 13–45
Cross section of skin (From Smith, *Medical Terminology, A Programmed Text*, 6th ed. Copyright 1991, Delmar Publishers Inc.)

Diseases and Disorders ....

Acne Vulgaris. This inflammatory disease of the follicles of the sebaceous glands mainly affects adolescents. The true cause is unknown. Research has determined that dietary habits appear to be less of a factor than originally thought. Present findings seem to suggest that hormonal dysfunction and an oversupply of sebum, oil from the sebaceous glands, are the probable underlying causes. It collects at the openings to the glands, hardens, and closes off the natural flow of oily secretion, causing blackheads or cysts to develop. Sometimes the area will become filled with leukocytes that cause pus to accumulate and pimples develop.

Usual treatment for severe acne includes a topical antibacterial product either alone or in combination with a topical vitamin A product. Often antibiotics applied to the skin are helpful. Antibiotics are systematically used to decrease bacterial growth. Occasionally with females who have severe disease, estrogens may be used to control the androgen (male hormone) activity, which stimulates the growth of sebaceous glands and the production of sebum.

Alopecia. This is loss of hair, usually occurring on the scalp. There are two types of alopecia. A scarring type causes irreversible hair loss and is usually the result of physical or chemical trauma or chronic tension on the hair shaft from such things as braiding or tightly rolling the hair. Certain diseases like lupus erythematosus, bacterial or viral infections, and skin tumors may also cause scarring alopecia.

The most common form of nonscarring alopecia is male-pattern baldness. It seems to be primarily due to aging and androgen levels. There is a tendency for genetic influence and it will often be displayed among male family members. Women may also exhibit the male pattern but at a lesser degree.

Other forms of nonscarring alopecia are: physiologic, which is usually temporary and occurs suddenly in infants or the mother's diffuse loss after childbirth; areata, of unknown cause but is self-limiting and occurs among both sexes from young to middle age; and trichotillomania, which is the pulling out of one's own hair and is most common among children. These people may also pull out other hair such as the eyebrows.

There is no known "cure" for male-pattern baldness; however, recent specific drug usage seems to prevent further loss and encourage some regrowth in many men. Surgical grafting of hair follicles from other parts of the scalp have proved successful. Areata alopecia usually reverses itself within 4 to 6 weeks. Trichotillomania alopecia can be controlled by a behavioral change or if necessary, psychiatric counseling.

Hair loss as a result of chemotherapy is common. Certain chemical agents destroy the cells of the hair, which result in the massive loss of hair over a 2- or 3-day period soon after the initiation of the drug. Normally, some fine hair will remain, but is very sparse. Fortunately, about 3 months after treatments end, hair will begin regrowth, sometimes a different color or texture.

Cancer. The skin may be the site of different forms of cancerous lesions such as basal cell carcinomas, squamous cell carcinomas, and malignant melanomas. Nevi (moles) are considered to be potentially malignant and require careful observation. Bleeding, itching, or a change in color, size, shape, or texture of a mole suggests a possible conversion to a malignant state.

Basal cell carcinoma is caused primarily by prolonged exposure to the sun and occurs where there are abundant sebaceous follicles, especially on the face. It is more prevalent in persons over 40, especially blond, fair-skinned males. It is the most common malignant tumor affecting Caucasians.

There are basically three types of basal cell carcinoma lesions, each with its own distinctive characteristics and usual location. They are diagnosed by appearance and surgical biopsy.

Nodulo-ulcerative lesions occur most often on the face and are small, smooth, pinkish and translucent papules. As they enlarge, the centers become depressed and the borders elevated and firm. *Superficial* basal cell carcinoma are often multiple and commonly occur on the chest and back. They are oval or irregularly shaped with sharply defined, threadlike borders that are slightly elevated. *Sclerosing* basal cell lesions occur on the head and neck. They appear yellow to white, are waxy, and do not have distinct borders.

Squamous cell carcinoma is predisposed by sunlight, presence of premalignant lesions, X-ray therapy, environmental carcinogens, and chronic skin irritation. Its incidence is highest in fair-skinned Caucasian males over the age of 60. Living in sunny climates and working in outdoor employment greatly increase the risk of development.

This form of carcinoma is commonly found on the face, ears, and back of the hands as well as other sun-damaged areas. The lesions have a tendency to metastasize with those located on unexposed skin having the greater incidence. Lesions of the lower lip and ears are exceptionally metastatic.

Malignant melanoma develops from pigment-producing cells and occurs in three forms: superficial spreading, modular malignant, and lentigo maligna melanomas. It spreads through the lymphatic and circulatory systems, metastasizing to the lymph nodes, liver, lungs and CNS. Prognosis varies with the characteristic of the lesion. Superficial tumors are curable, while deeper lesions tend to metastasize. The American Cancer Society recently released facts about the incidence of malignant melanoma. For the year 1991, 32,000 people were diagnosed; about 6500 died. This incidence translates into 1 in every 105 United States resident as compared to only

1 in every 1500 in 1935. If the trend continues, the incidence is projected to be 1 in 75 by the year 2000.

The major cause of malignant melanoma is exposure to the sun. The sun produces ultraviolet rays, mainly UVA and UVB. UVBs cause sunburn, premature aging of the skin, and skin cancers. Most sunscreens provide a degree of protection against this ray. However, recent evidence seems to suggest that the UVA rays may also be damaging the skin, perhaps aiding the cancer-forming ability of UVB.

The Cancer Society cited the primary reasons for the increase to be weekend-packed leisure time, which results in intense bursts of exposure to UVB, the loss of the ozone layer protection, UVA rays not being blocked by sunscreens, and the tendency of people to purposely lie flat in the sun for hours at a time, which allows deeper penetration of the rays. People most at risk are those who have had severe blistering sunburns during their teens or twenties.

Other contributing factors are blond or red hair, fair skin, blue eyes, and a tendency to sunburn. Persons who work or spend many hours outdoors or who live in places with intense year-round sunshine are also at risk. Arizona has the highest incidence reported. The peak of incidence occurs between 50 to 70 years of age. Incidence is slightly higher among women than men.

Dermatologists recommend avoiding sun altogether from 10:00 A.M. to 3:00 P.M. (perhaps from 8:00 A.M. to 6:00 P.M. if the ozone condition worsens), and using a sunscreen of at least 15 SPF that will block both UVA and UVB during exposure. Sunlamps, tanning pills and tanning salons should be avoided. The information and photos in Figure 13–46, page 250, show the ABCD rules and appearance signs of melanoma.

Dermatitis. The term means inflammation of the skin and can refer to any form of skin condition such as: seborrhea, eczema, contact dermatitis (from irritants), exfoliative dermatitis (large pieces of peeling skin), or stasis (from lack of blood supply). Dermatitis is often caused by allergens such as wool, detergent, cosmetics, pollen, or foods such as eggs, milk, seafood, or wheat products. Common symptoms are dry skin, redness, itching, edema, formation of lesions, and scaling. It is treated by avoiding known allergens, applying anti-inflammatory products to the skin, systemic steroids, antihistamines, and other measures specific to the type of dermatitis.

Eczema. This noncontagious skin disease is characterized by dry, red, itchy, and scaly skin. It can be acute or chronic and sometimes produces a watery discharge. Several things may initiate eczema such as diet, cosmetics, clothing, medications, soaps, occupational or environmental substances, and emotional stress.

Treatment consists primarily of removal of the causative agent where possible and the local application of ointments to alleviate the symptoms. Oral steroids are indicated to reduce inflammation and antibiotics are used if secondary infection is present.

Follicular Infections. A staphylococcal infection of the hair follicle that results in the formation of a pustule is known as folliculitis. It can be of a superficial form involving only the surface area around a single follicle or deep, involving the total hair follicle. Treatment consists of thorough cleansing of the area and the application of wet heat to promote drainage from the lesion as well as the use of topical antibiotics. If recurrent, systemic antibiotics may be indicated.

What is the Difference Between a Melanoma and an Ordinary Mole?

A normal mole is an evenly colored brown, tan, or black spot in the skin. It is either flat or raised. Its shape is round or oval and it has sharply defined borders. Moles are generally less than 6 mm in diameter (about the size of a pencil eraser). A mole may be present at birth or it may appear spontaneously, usually in the first few decades of life. Sometimes several moles appear at the same time, especially on sun-exposed areas of the skin. Once a mole has fully developed, it normally remains the same size, shape, and color for many years. Most moles eventually fade away in older persons.

Almost everyone has moles, on the average of about 25. The vast majority of moles are perfectly harmless. A sudden or continuous *change* in a mole's appearance is a sign that you should see your physician. However, a melanoma is more complicated than a mole.

Here's the simple **ABCD** rule to help you remember the important signs of melanoma:

A. **Asymmetry.** One half does not match the other half, Figure 13–46(a).

B. **Border irregularity.** The edges are ragged, notched or blurred, Figure 13–46(b).

C. **Color.** The pigmentation is not uniform. Shades of tan, brown, and black are present. Red, white and blue may add to the mottled appearance, Figure 13–46(c).

D. **Diameter greater than 6 mm.** Any sudden or continuing increase in size should be of special concern, figure 13–46(d).

Other Warning Signs of Melanoma

Change in the surface of a mole—scaliness, oozing, bleeding or the appearance of a bump or nodule; spread of pigment from the border into surrounding skin; redness or a new swelling beyond the border; change in sensation—itchiness, tenderness or pain.

(The above information reprinted, with permission, from a brochure titled *Why You Should Know About Melanoma,* distributed by the American Cancer Society and developed in cooperation with the American Academy of Dermatology.)

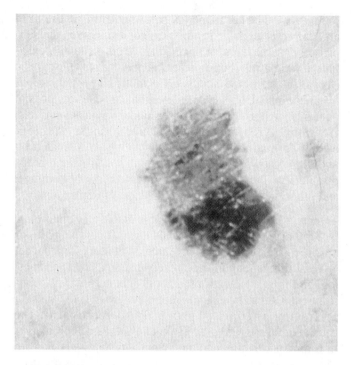

(a) Asymmetry

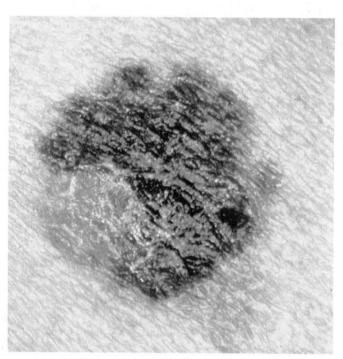

(b) Border irregularity

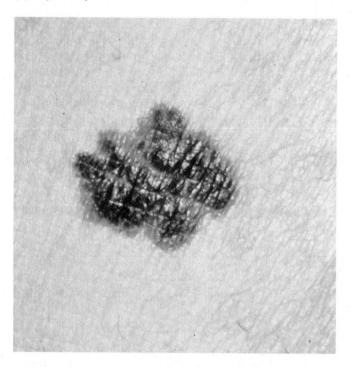

(c) Color

(d) Diameter

FIGURE 13–46   The signs of melanoma (Courtesy of the American Academy of Dermatology)

Folliculitis may lead to the development of furuncles (boils), which are hard, painful nodules that enlarge over several days until they rupture, releasing pus and dead cells through one draining point. The area remains red and swollen for a short time but the pain lessens. Furuncles may be caused by irritation, pressure, or friction of the follicular site. Treatment consists of the measures used for folliculitis with wet heat to relieve pain and

encourage "ripening" of the lesion. Often incision and drainage are required to allow complete expulsion of the material. Patients must be cautioned not to squeeze a boil because it may rupture into the surrounding tissues.

Carbunculosis follows persistent staphylococcal infection and furunculosis and is characterized by deep follicular abscesses of several follicles with multiple draining points. It is extremely painful and usually associated with fever and general malaise. Carbunculosis requires treatment with systemic antibiotics in addition to the localized heat applications and drainage. Wash cloths and towels, bed sheets, and clothing used by the infected person must not be shared with other family members to prevent spreading the bacteria. A patient with recurring furuncles should see a physician to rule out any underlying cause such as diabetes.

Herpes Simplex. This viral infection results in cold sores or blisters on the mouth or face. It is equally prevalent among males and females and occurs throughout the world. Diagnosis is made from the typical lesions that appear as vesicles with a red base that eventually ruptures making a painful ulcer. Herpes simplex has a 2- to 12-day incubation period during which tingling and itching signal the oncoming vesicle. A yellow crust develops following vesicle rupture and healing is complete after approximately 3 weeks.

Treatment consists of topical applications of tincture of benzoin at initial indication followed by various ointments to the lesion to alleviate cracking and discomfort. Some people feel that an ice cube to the lesion when it appears produces quicker healing.

Herpes Zoster. This is an acute infectious process by the virus that also causes chickenpox. In herpes zoster, also known as shingles, the dorsal root ganglia are inflamed, causing severe neuralgic pain along the area of the involved nerves. It is characterized by fever, malaise, and the eruption of vesicles in the painful area, which spread unilaterally around the back, chest, back of neck, or vertically on the extremities. (See Unit 2.)

Hirsutism. This disorder usually appears in women and children; excessive body hair develops in an adult male pattern of growth. There may be a family history of the disorder or it could be related to an endrocrine problem resulting from either pituitary dysfunction, ovarian lesions, or adrenal gland enlargement.

The most common symptom is growth of facial hair but other masculinization signs such as deepening voice, increased muscle mass, menstrual irregularity, and breast size reduction may be exhibited. Treatment consists of hair removal by shaving, depilatory creams, or waxing as well as bleaching to minimize the appearance of hair. Electrolysis will permanently destroy the hair follicles but is slow and expensive. If hormonal causes are evident, treatment may involve counteracting or controlling endocrine secretions in specific situations.

Impetigo. This contagious, superficial skin infection is usually seen in young children. Predisposing factors include anemia, malnutrition, and poor hygiene, but these are not essential to the development of the disease. The causative organism is either streptococcal or staphylococcal. If strep, a small red macule (flat area with definite edge) turns into a vesicle (raised lesion containing serous fluid), then to a pustule (lesion with purulent material), within a relatively short period of time. (The terms macule, vesicle, and pustule refer to any skin lesion that demonstrates these descriptive characteristics, not to impetigo alone.) When the lesions break, a characteristic yellow crust develops from the exudate (drainage). Other sites develop from contact with the lesions or the drainage. The staph lesion is characterized by a thin-walled vesicle, which forms a thin, clear crust from the exudate. Both forms characteristically have a clear central area and definite outer rims. The lesions appear primarily on the face, neck, and other exposed areas of the body. Contamination of others is prevented by avoiding contact through wash cloths, towels, and bed linens. Scratching of the lesions must be prohibited. Therapy includes washing the areas two to three times daily to remove the exudate, and a systemic antibiotic to prevent secondary infection.

Keloid. A scar that developed excess dense tissue as it progressed through the healing process is known as keloid.

Lyme Disease. This disease is caused by a spirochete (corkscrew bacteria) carried by the deer tick. Lyme disease was named after Old Lyme, Connecticut, where it was first identified. The deer tick is known as a three-host tick and has a 2-year life cycle. In spring, eggs are deposited and six-legged larva ticks hatch, attaching themselves to small mammals or birds to obtain their first meal of blood. The tick larva winter over, molting to a larger eight-legged nymphal stage, which attaches to dogs, squirrels, and deer. Next they molt to the adult stage in the summer and attach to a larger mammal, primarily a deer. After engorging on blood and mating, they later drop off to lay eggs. The tick can transmit the disease during any stage. Bites seem to occur most often during summer or late autumn. The ticks apparently go from these hosts to woods and field underbrush where they are picked up by people and pets.

The disease was first recognized and reported in the United States in the mid 1970s with the incidence almost doubling from 4882 cases in 1988 to 8551 cases in 1989. There were 22,570 cases reported between 1982 and 1989, with over one-third being in 1989 alone. About 80% of the cases are reported in California, Connecticut, New Jersey, New York, Pennsylvania, Rhode Island, and Wisconsin. Symptoms begin with a distinctive bullseye rash but it is not always on everyone. Usually there is a small red bump and rash at the bite site. This site can expand to an oval or round area 2 to 3 inches in diameter. The rash will fade after a few weeks, with or without treatment. Early symptoms include profound fatigue, stiff neck, flulike headache, chills, muscle aches, and fever. Later stages may produce heart and nervous system involvement with subsequent chronic arthritis beginning up to a year later.

Fortunately, treatment with antibiotics for 2 to 3 weeks is effective, especially if begun early in the disease process. The best line of treatment is defense. When hiking or camping in a wooded or brushy area, use repellents with a high concentration of Deet, applied sparingly to adult skin, but not to a child's. Use only as directed. Wear long sleeves and trousers tucked into either socks or boots to prevent tick contact with the skin. Light-colored clothing also makes it easier to spot the ticks. The most common sites are underarms, groin, or behind the knees, and on the heads of children. Pets should also be checked. The deer tick is very small, about the size of a pinhead, orange-brown with a black spot near the head. It resembles a crab. If detected on a human, it should be removed, alive if possible, and shown to a doctor or sent to proper health authorities for positive identification. When removing, grasp with forceps or tweezers at the mouth parts where attached and pull straight out. If you have to use your fingers, cover them with a tissue. Cleanse the site with antiseptic and wash clothing because ticks hide in seams and creases.

Ticks can be tested for spirochete infection. About 30% to 60% of Northeastern ticks are positive. Even if positive, you may not develop Lyme disease. If the tick is removed within 24 hours, your risk is minimal. The longer attached, the greater the chance of infection. Ticks require 18 to 48 hours to transmit the bacterium into a victim. Lyme disease is an increasingly serious public health problem, now ranked as the second most prevalent infectious disease in the United States, surpassed only by AIDS.

Pediculosis.　There are three types of **pediculosis** caused by three varieties of parasitic lice: capitis from head lice; corporis from body lice; and pubis from pubic lice, commonly called crabs. The lice feed on human blood and lay eggs known as nits on body hairs or fibers of clothing. The nits hatch and will die in 24 hours unless they feed on a host. Nits mature in 2 to 3 weeks.

Capitis is the most common form and is found primarily among children, especially girls. It is caused by poor hygiene and overcrowding. It spreads through shared combs, brushes, clothing, and hats. It is identifiable as an oval grayish, dandruff-like fleck that cannot be shaken off. Its symptoms are itching and scalp abrasions with matted, foul-smelling hair in severe cases. Nits are easily treated with gamma benzene hydrochloride (GBH) cream rubbed into the scalp at night followed by GBH shampoo the next morning. A follow-up treatment is required the next night. Nits can then be removed with a fine-tooth comb.

Pediculosis corporis lives in clothing seams except when feeding on the host. Initially small red papules appear, which itch. The resulting scratching causes rashes and wheals to develop. The usual cause is prolonged wearing of the same clothes, overcrowding, and poor hygiene. It is spread through shared clothing and linens. Treatment consists of bathing with soap and water and the use of GBH if infestation is severe. All clothing and linens must be washed or dry cleaned.

Pediculosis pubis is found attached primarily to pubic hair and is transmitted through sexual intercourse or contact with infected clothes, bedding, or towels. The lice cause itching, which results in skin irritation from scratching. Treatment consists of local applications of GBH ointment, lotion, or cream, which must remain for 24 hours or shampooing with GBH. Treatment must be repeated in a week. All clothing and linens must be washed. Sexual contacts must also be treated or reinfection will occur.

Psoriasis.　This chronic disease is characterized by itching and red papules (solid, elevated masses) covered with silvery scales. **Psoriasis** is recurrent, with alternating periods of remission or increased severity. Contributing factors are environmental (cold weather causes flare-ups), endocrine changes, pregnancy, and emotional stress.

Psoriasis cannot be cured. Scales can be softened with applications of ointments and then removed in an oatmeal bath. Ultraviolet light, either artificial or from the sun, retards cell production. Normal cells require about 2 weeks to move from their place of production to the skin surface and after another couple of weeks of wear and tear, are sloughed off. Psoriatic cells require only 4 days, which does not permit the cell to mature and results in marked proliferation of the epidermis. Steroid creams, tar preparations, and sometimes the use of coverings such as plastic gloves or plastic wrap worn overnight may help to control the disease.

A recent accidental discovery may hold promise of treatment. An experimental drug, FK 506, used to block organ transplant rejection, rapidly cleared psoriasis according to researchers at the University of Pittsburgh Medical Center. The drug suppresses a T cell in the immune system. Since psoriasis is somewhat genetically determined and researchers have identified the presence of certain antigens, it is believed it could be caused by an autoimmune deficiency.

Ringworm.　This fungus may affect the scalp (tinea capitis), the body (tinea corporis), or other areas, such as the groin, beard, or feet (tinea pedia, or athlete's foot). On the body, it is characterized by flat lesions, which are dry and scaly or moist and crusty. When they enlarge, clear central areas develop leaving an outer ring from which it gets its name. On the scalp, small papules occur causing scaly patches of baldness.

Treatment consists of systemic medication and topical applications of antifungals. Since the disease is contagious, care must be taken to prevent its spread by refraining from sharing bed linens, combs, and towels.

Scabies.　This skin infection is caused by the itch mite. The female mite burrows into the skin, laying eggs that later hatch into larvae. The larvae emerge, mate, and then reenter the skin. The condition causes an itching which becomes intense at night. The lesions are characteristically threadlike red nodules, approximately 3/8 inch long. They occur between fingers, at the inner wrist area, the elbows, in axillary folds (armpit), about the waist, on genitalia (external sex organs) of males, and on the nipples of females. The infection is spread by skin contact or sexual activity.

Treatment consists of bathing with soap and water followed by an application of pediculicide such as Kwell. It must remain on the skin for 24 hours and be repeated in 1 week to destroy the developing mites. An antipruritic (against itching) or steroid may be applied topically to help reduce the itching.

Urticaria (hives). This is a self-limiting reaction to allergens such as drugs, food, insect stings, and airborne agents. **Urticaria** often occurs during especially stressful or emotional times. The reaction produces distinct, raised **wheals** surrounded by a reddened area. They may be few in number or cover the entire body. Often they are accompanied with itching.

Urticaria is treated by eliminating or limiting the causative allergen or, when that is not possible, by gradual desensitization through interdermal injection of the allergen. Antihistamine is used to reduce itching and swelling. A barbituate may be required when the causative factor is emotional stress.

Verrucae (warts). This is a benign (noncancerous) viral infection of the skin, probably transmitted by direct or self-contact. Common **verrucae** are characterized by a rough, elevated, rounded surface, usually on the extremities, especially the hands and fingers. Plantar warts occur primarily at pressure points on the soles of the feet. Condyloma accuminatum (venereal warts) are moist, soft, pink to red warts occurring singly, but most often in large clusters, on the penis, vulva, or anus. This type of wart is transmitted by sexual contact.

Treatment of warts varies with the type, size, and location. Common types often disappear spontaneously. When removal is necessary, they can be destroyed by methods using electricity, acid, liquid nitrogen, or solid carbon dioxide. Venereal warts are treated with applications of podophyllum and tincture of benzoin.

Table 13–3 summarizes different types of skin lesions and their characteristics, which may help you to identify some common conditions.

Complete Chapter 13, Unit 4 in the workbook to help you meet the objectives at the beginning of this unit and therefore achieve competency of this subject matter.

U N I T 5
The Skeletal System

OBJECTIVES

Upon completion of this unit, the student will meet the following terminal performance objectives by verifying knowledge of the facts and principles presented through oral and written communication at a level deemed competent.

TABLE 13–3
Different types of Skin Lesions, Their Characteristics, Size, and Examples

Type of Skin Lesion	Characteristics	Size	Example(s)
Bulla (blister)	Fluid-filled area	Greater than 5 mm across	A large blister
Macule	A round, flat area usually distinguished from its surrounding skin by its change in color	Smaller than 1 cm	* Freckle * Petechia (small hemorrhage spot)
Nodule	Elevated solid area, deeper and firmer than a papule	Greater than 5 mm across	Wart
Papule	Elevated solid area	5 mm or less across	Elevated nevus (mole)
Pustule	Discrete, pus-filled raised area	Varying size	Acne
Ulcer	A deep loss of skin surface that may extend into the dermis that can bleed periodically and scar	Varies in sizes	Venous stasis ulcer
Tumor	Solid abnormal mass of cells that may extend deep through cutaneous tissue	Larger than 1-2 cm	* Benign (harmless) epidermal tumor * Basal cell carcinoma (rarely metastasizing)
Vesicle	Fluid-filled raised area	5 mm or less across	* Chickenpox * Herpes simplex
Wheal	Itchy, temporarily elevated area with an irregular shape formed as a result of localized skin edema	Varies in size	* Hives * Insect bites

(Adapted from Fong, *Body Structures and Functions*, 7th ed. Copyright 1989, Delmar Publishers Inc.)

1. Name the two divisions of the skeletal system and the bone groups in each division.
2. Describe the structure of the long bones.
3. Explain how long bones grow.
4. Identify the elements which make up bone tissue.
5. Identify the major bones of the body.
6. List the six functions of the skeletal system.
7. Name the divisions of the spinal column and the number of vertebrae in each division.
8. Describe fontanels and explain why they are essential.
9. Describe the structure of the rib cage and its primary function.
10. Identify three kinds of synovial joints and give examples of each.
11. List the parts of a synovial joint and identify the purpose of each part.
12. Name the seven types of fractures and the characteristics of each.
13. Outline the treatment of a fracture.
14. Describe the healing process of a fracture.
15. Define the term *fatty embolus,* explaining its origin and what might occur.
16. List situations predisposing to amputation.
17. Define the phantom limb sensation.
18. Discuss two diagnostic examinations.
19. Explain why the symptoms of carpal tunnel syndrome occur.
20. Name the three types of spinal curvatures, describing their physical characteristics.
21. Identify 17 diseases and disorders of the skeletal system.
22. Spell and define, using the glossary at the back of the text, all the words to know in this unit.

WORDS TO KNOW

alignment	dislocation
amputate	embolus
appendicular	epiphyses
arthritis	femur
articulation	fibula
axial	fracture
bunion	greenstick
bursa	humerus
callus	ilium
carpal	impacted
cartilage	intervertebral
cervical	ischium
clavicle	kyphosis
coccyx	laminectomy
comminuted	ligament
compound	lordosis
cranium	marrow
depressed	metacarpal
diarthrosis	metatarsal
osteoporosis	skeletal
patella	spinal fusion
periosteum	spiral
phalanges	sprain
phalanx	sternum
phantom limb	symphysis pubis
prosthesis	synovial
radius	tarsal
reduce	tibia
sacrum	traction
scapula	ulna
scoliosis	vertebrae
simple	xiphoid

The skeletal system consists of organs called bones. It may be difficult to think of bones as living, functioning organs, but they use food and oxygen and perform functions just as other organs do.

The skeleton is divided into two sections. The spinal column, skull, and rib cage make up the axial skeleton. The bones of the arms, hands, legs, feet, shoulders, and pelvis make up the appendicular skeleton, Figure 13–47.

The primary purpose of the skeletal system is to support the body. This support must be strong yet not heavy. Bone is said to be as strong as cast iron, yet it is much lighter and more flexible. The skeleton must be flexible enough to endure pressure, stress, and shock without shattering.

Bone Structure

Over 20% of the weight of bone is water. Two-thirds of the remainder are minerals and one-third, organic matter. The main minerals are calcium, phosphorus, and magnesium. The organic matter is primarily collagen, a type of protein fiber that forms the matrix (intercellular substance) of the bone.

The ends of long bones have articulating (connecting) surfaces that fit together with other bones to form joints, Figure 13–48, page 256. These ends are separated by cartilage to facilitate movement. The ends and parts of the shaft are filled with a meshlike network of spongy bone. The openings in the spongy bone are filled with red marrow. The inside of the shaft of the bone is filled with a fat or yellow marrow.

A tough membrane called periosteum covers the surface of the bone. Blood vessels and nerves pass through the periosteum and into the bone through a network of openings called Haversian canals. Some larger vessels pass directly into both the yellow and red marrow.

Number of Bones

At birth, a baby has 270 bones. As the child grows, some of the bones fuse together so that at adulthood

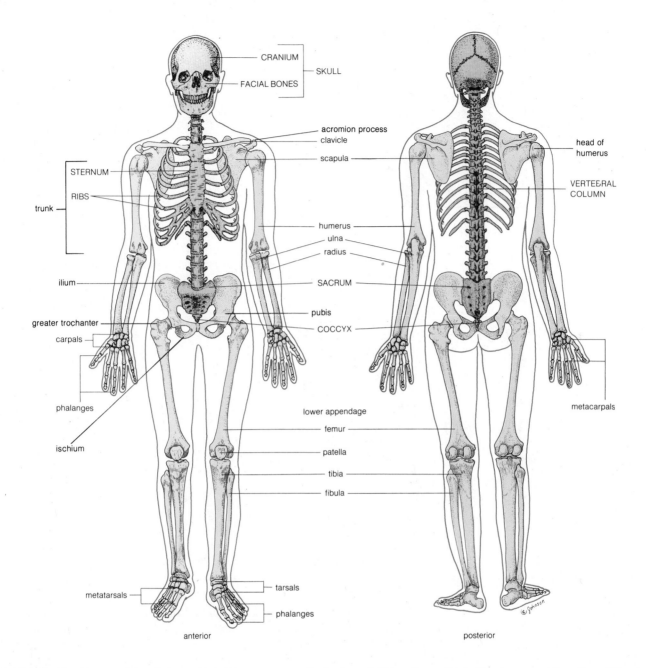

FIGURE 13–47   Bones of the skeleton (Axial in gray, appendicular in red) (From Fong, *Body Structures and Functions*, 7th ed. Copyright 1989, Delmar Publishers Inc.)

there are only 206. For example, at the lower end of the spinal column five **vertebrae** have fused to form the **sacrum** while the last four have fused into the **coccyx** (tailbone), Figure 13–49, page 257. The smallest bones in the body are the malleus, incus, and stapes of the middle ear.

Functions of the Skeleton ....

The skeleton serves at least six functions for the body. One, as previously indicated, is to support the body. The bones provide a framework for the distribution of the body's fat, muscles, and skin.

Two, the bones also serve to protect the body's vital organs. The brain and spinal cord are both located within bony cavities. The cranium also provides protection for the inner ear and parts of the eye. The heart and lungs are positioned within the rib cage. The internal reproductive organs and the urinary bladder lie within the bony pelvis.

Third, the bones are the points of attachment for skeletal muscles. When the muscles contract, they allow the joints of the skeleton to rotate, bend, or straighten, thereby providing for movement and flexibility. Fourth, the bones, along with the muscles, give shape to the body.

A fifth and vital function of bone is the formation of red blood cells. The red marrow in the spongy areas of

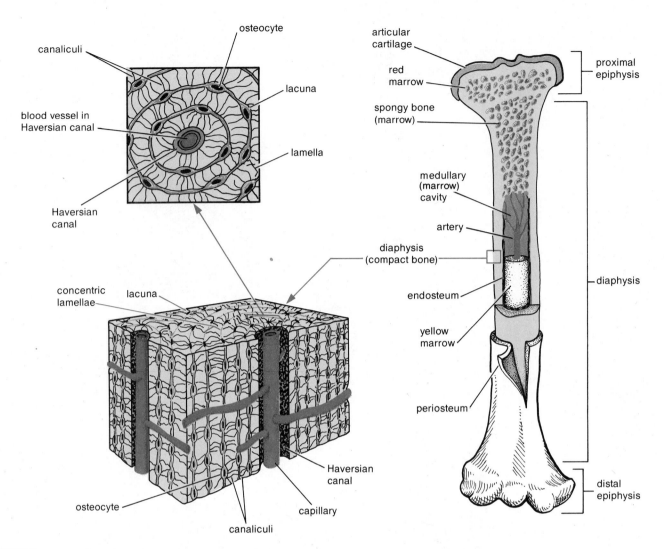

FIGURE 13–48 Structure of a long bone (From Fong, *Body Structures and Functions*, 7th ed. Copyright 1989, Delmar Publishers Inc.)

the long bones, the ribs, and the vertebrae produces millions of red blood cells a minute. This rate is necessary to replace the cells, which live only a few weeks. When the body needs more red cells than the red marrow can produce, some of the yellow marrow is converted to red.

Finally, bones store most of the body's supply of calcium. Calcium is needed by the heart to beat, by the muscles to contract, and by the blood to clot. When the calcium in the body is inadequate for all its needs, the blood takes calcium from its storage in the bone. The bone minerals are constantly being borrowed and replaced through the blood flow within the body.

Spinal Column ....

The spinal column is a stack of vertebrae that supports the head and keeps the trunk erect. As noted earlier, it provides protection for the spinal cord, which descends from the brain through its canal. The bones of the column are separated by **intervertebral** cartilage disks

between their rounded front portions, Figure 13–50. The disks permit the column to bend or twist and also absorb much of the shock received from walking, running, or jumping. The vertebrae in the column are named for the area of the body in which they are located: **cervical** (neck), thoracic (chest), lumbar (back), sacral (posterior pelvic girdle), and coccygeal (tailbone), Figure 13–51, page 258.

The spinal nerves enter and leave the spinal cord through foramen (openings) between the vertebrae. The disks maintain adequate spacing between vertebrae to prevent damage to the spinal nerves from bone-to-bone contact.

Typical vertebrae as shown in Figure 13–50 have descriptive parts, mainly the large solid part called the *body,* the winglike side projections called the *transverse processes,* a posterior projection called a *spinous process* (the part you can feel if you arch your back) and the *foramen* through which the spinal cord passes. Other processes called *articular* are where parts of two vertebrae touch.

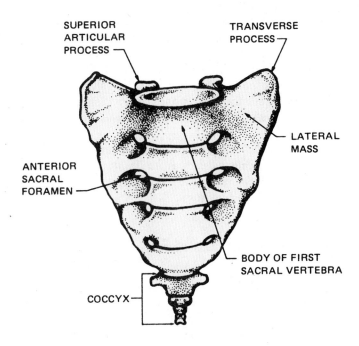

FIGURE 13–49 The sacrum and coccyx (From *The Wonderful Human Machine*, copyright 1979, American Medical Association)

The Skull ....

The skull is the bony structure of the head. It consists of a cranial and a facial portion. The cranium is actually a fusion of eight cranial bones, with the vital function of protecting the brain from injury, Figure 13–52, page 259. The main bones of the cranium are: the frontal (the forehead and upper eye sockets), two parietal bones, two temporal, and the occipital (back of the skull). The facial bones are: the mandible (lower jaw), the maxillae (upper jaw), the zygomatic (cheek bones), and the several small bones about the eyes, nose, and palate.

The cranium is not solid bone at birth. Spaces between the bones are soft incomplete bone to allow for the molding of the skull during the birth process and for enlargement of the skull as growth occurs. A large diamond-shaped anterior area where the frontal and parietal bones meet and a triangular space posteriorly where the occipital bone meets the parietals are known as *fontanels* or "soft spots," and can easily be felt. Other smaller fontanels are located along the sides of the skull. Without these areas for growth, the brain could not increase in size during late pregnancy and early infancy. The fontanels gradually close, turning the membrane and cartilage into solid bone after about 2 years. The irregular lines marking the former growth areas are called *sutures*.

The skull does not grow remarkably when compared to the rest of the body. It makes up about one-fourth of the total length of the infant's body but only one-eighth of the adult's total length.

The Rib Cage ....

Thoracic vertebrae serve as the posterior attachment points for 12 pairs of ribs, Figure 13–53, page 259. The top 10 pairs are also attached by cartilage strips to the sternum (breast bone) anteriorly. The flexibility of the cartilage attachment allows the rib cage to move when the lungs are inflated to breathe. The bottom two pairs of ribs are called floating ribs because they are attached only to the spinal column and not the sternum.

The rib cage is sometimes described in terms of true and false ribs. When this division is made, the first seven pairs of ribs are considered "true" ribs because of their posterior and direct anterior attachment. The last five

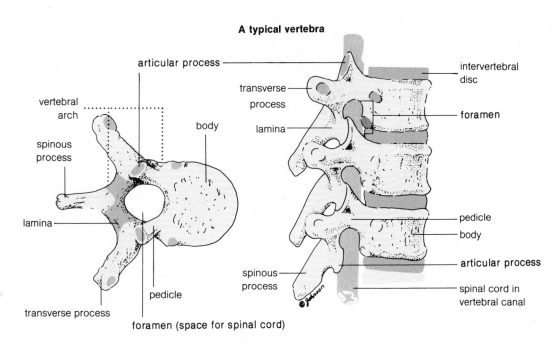

FIGURE 13–50
Vertebrae structure (From Fong, *Body Structures and Functions*, 7th ed. Copyright 1989, Delmar Publishers Inc.)

pairs are "false" ribs because they attach anteriorly to the cartilage of the rib above or have no anterior attachment.

Three other bones of the thoracic area should be mentioned. They are the clavicle (collar bone) anteriorly and the scapula (shoulder blade) posteriorly. A small bony process called the xiphoid is attached to the inferior edge of the sternum.

Long Bones

The long bones of the body are found in the extremities. To a great extent, the long bones of the lower extremities determine our height. Long bones are shaped generally like hollow cylinders to be strong with the least amount of weight. A typical long bone has a main shaft or diaphysis and ends called epiphyses. Early in life the epiphysis is mainly cartilage. Later the cartilage becomes a strip or "growth plate" which permits new tissue growth and bone length. At maturity, growth stops and the cartilage is replaced by bone.

The femur (thigh bone) is the longest bone in any species, extending from the hip joint to the knee. (Refer to Figure 13–47, page 255.) The thickness of the femur

wall depends on the size and needs of the species. For example, large animals such as the bear have a thick, heavy femur to support their weight and accommodate slow movements, whereas the deer has a very thin and light femur to permit speed. The tibia (shin bone) and fibula complete the long bones of the leg. The small bone at the knee is known as the patella.

The long bones of the upper extremities are the humerus of the arm and the radius and ulna of the forearm. The radius extends from the thumb side of the wrist to the elbow, while the ulna extends from the little finger side to the elbow joint.

Bones of the Hands and Feet

The bones of the hands and feet are similar in structure, Figure 13–54, page 260. The wrist has eight bones, known as carpals while the ankle has seven, called tarsals. In the palm area of the hand there are five metacarpals that correspond to the five metatarsals of the instep of the foot. The phalanges (fingers and toes) are further subdivided into individual sections called a phalanx. There are three phalanx sections in each finger and toe except the thumb and great toe, which have only

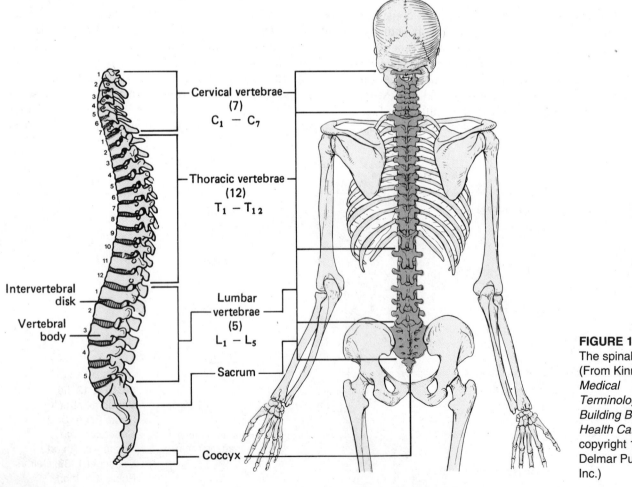

Cervical vertebrae
(7)
$C_1 - C_7$

Thoracic vertebrae
(12)
$T_1 - T_{12}$

Intervertebral disk

Vertebral body

Lumbar vertebrae
(5)
$L_1 - L_5$

Sacrum

Coccyx

FIGURE 13–51
The spinal column (From Kinn, *Medical Terminology, Building Blocks for Health Careers*, copyright 1990, Delmar Publishers Inc.)

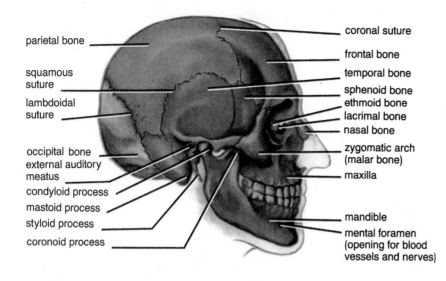

FIGURE 13–52 parietal bone

coronal suture
frontal bone
temporal bone
sphenoid bone
ethmoid bone
lacrimal bone
nasal bone
zygomatic arch
(malar bone)
maxilla

squamous
suture
lambdoidal
suture

occipital bone
external auditory
meatus
condyloid process
mastoid process
styloid process
coronoid process

mandible
mental foramen
(opening for blood
vessels and nerves)

FIGURE 13–52 The skull (From Smith, *Medical Terminology, A Programmed Text*, 6th ed. Copyright 1991, Delmar Publishers Inc.)

two. The section of a phalanx is identified as distal, medial, or proximal by its relationship to the metacarpals or metatarsals.

The Pelvic Girdle

The pelvic girdle provides the structure for the hip area. Two large bones called *os coxae* (hip bones) are joined posteriorly with the sacrum. The top blade-shaped portion is called the **ilium,** Figure 13–55, page 261. The anterior lower portion is called the pubis, with the point of attachment (right and left pubis) called the **symphysis pubis.** The posterior lower portion of the bone is called the **ischium.** The hip bone provides the recessed area where the head of the femur fits. The anatomical name for the socket is *acetabulum.*

Joints

The place where two or more bony parts join together is known as an **articulation** or joint. Strong, flexible bands of connective tissue called **ligaments** hold long bones together at joints. Ligaments can stretch and often become torn as a result of injury.

There are three main types of joints, classified primarily by their degree of movement. A movable joint such as the knee or elbow is called **diarthrosis** or **synovial** joint. A partially movable joint like where ribs attach to the spine or between the vertebrae is known as *amphiarthrosis* or *cartilaginous.* An immovable joint such as a cranial suture is called *synarthrosis* or *fibrous.*

Most of the body's joints are diarthrotic. They may have three distinct parts, articular cartilage, a **bursa** (saclike capsule), and a synovial cavity. The articulating

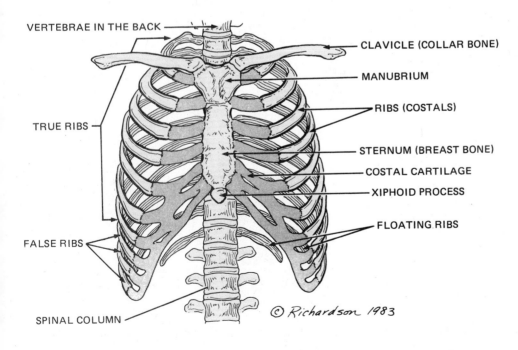

VERTEBRAE IN THE BACK
CLAVICLE (COLLAR BONE)
MANUBRIUM
RIBS (COSTALS)
TRUE RIBS
STERNUM (BREAST BONE)
COSTAL CARTILAGE
XIPHOID PROCESS
FLOATING RIBS
FALSE RIBS
SPINAL COLUMN
© Richardson 1983

FIGURE 13–53 The rib cage (Copyright by Richardson. From Fong, *Body Structures and Functions*, 7th ed. Copyright 1989, Delmar Publishers Inc. Used with permission.)

joint surfaces of bones are covered with the articular cartilage, which provides a slippery, smooth surface and enables the joint to absorb shock. An articular capsule of tough, fibrous tissue encloses the articulating surfaces and is lined with a synovial membrane, which secretes synovial fluid into the cavity, lubricating the joint and reducing friction.

The joint is surrounded with ligaments, tendons, and muscles that hold the joint together but still allow for movement. Some synovial joints have cushionlike sacs called bursa, which form from the synovial membrane and are filled with synovial fluid. These are generally located between tendons and bones. In addition, synovial membranes may also form sheaths that wrap around the tendons. Bursa and tendon sheaths cushion and lubricate tendons and help reduce friction between the tendons and the bone.

The synovial joints of the body have been copied by man to develop many useful devices, Figure 13–56, page 262. The ball and socket type of joint found in the hip or shoulder can be seen in the movement of a desk pen set. The action of the fingers, knees, and elbows is like that of a hinge. An unusual pivot type of joint appears at the wrists and elbows. When the palm of the hand is up, the radius and ulna are side by side. As the palm is turned down, the radius crosses over the ulna in a pivoting action. This type of motion is independent of the elbow's hinge action. Joints found in the wrists and ankle are formed by bones with curved surfaces, which allow for various angular movements.

Fractures

The bones of children contain a high percentage of cartilage and are much more flexible than those of an adult. Frequently the bone will crack under pressure but will not break all the way through. This type of break is known as a **greenstick fracture.**

A complete bone break in which there is no involvement with the skin surface is known as a **simple** fracture, Figure 13–57, page 263. When broken bone protrudes through the skin's surface, it is known as a **compound** fracture. This causes additional concerns because of the possibility of infection to the area. A more involved type of fracture is called **impacted,** which indicates that the broken ends are jammed into each other. A **comminuted** fracture is one with more than one fracture line and several bone fragments. A **depressed** fracture may occur

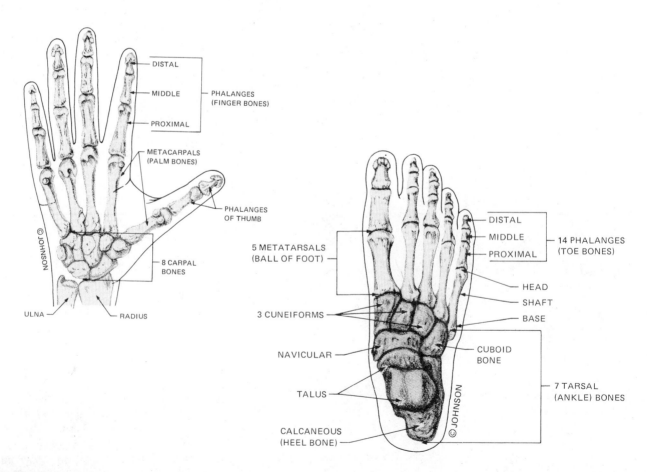

FIGURE 13–54 Bones of the hand and foot (Copyright by Johnson. From Fong, Ferris & Skelley, *Body Structures and Functions*, 7th ed. Copyright 1989, Delmar Publishers Inc. Used with permission.)

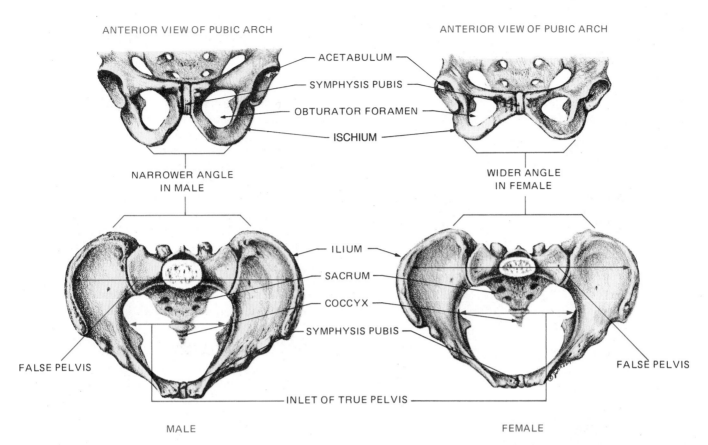

ANTERIOR VIEW OF PUBIC ARCH   ANTERIOR VIEW OF PUBIC ARCH

ACETABULUM

SYMPHYSIS PUBIS

OBTURATOR FORAMEN

ISCHIUM

NARROWER ANGLE   WIDER ANGLE
IN MALE   IN FEMALE

ILIUM

SACRUM

COCCYX

SYMPHYSIS PUBIS

FALSE PELVIS   FALSE PELVIS

INLET OF TRUE PELVIS

MALE   FEMALE

FIGURE 13–55   The pelvic girdle (Copyright by Johnson. From Fong, Ferris, & Skelley, *Body Structures and Functions*, 7th ed. Copyright 1989, Delmar Publishers Inc.)

with severe head injuries in which a broken piece of skull is driven inward. A spiral fracture may occur with a severe twisting action as in a skiing accident, causing the break to wind around the bone.

In treating fractures, immobilization of the affected part and prevention of shock are the main concerns. The extremity is splinted extending above and below the area of fracture. Elevation of the part and application of a cold pack or ice helps prevent swelling. When there is also damage to the surrounding tissues, especially to the exterior, control of bleeding may be indicated. This may require direct pressure over the wound.

When long bones are broken, they are usually pulled by the muscles attached to their surfaces into abnormal positions, often causing overlapping of their broken parts. Before the bone can be set, traction (pulling) either manually or by a system of ropes and pulleys, must be used to stretch the muscles and pull the bone pieces back into alignment. This procedure is known as reducing the fracture. Once the ends fit together properly, a splint or cast can be used to maintain the position until the bone has healed.

With involved fractures, such as compound or comminuted, an additional surgical procedure is often necessary either to repair the skin and surrounding tissues or to place all the small bone fragments in position. This procedure is called an *open reduction* because it involves

an opening into the fractured bone through the skin and overlying tissues, to achieve alignment of the bone. Sometimes the use of pins or wire is required to hold the fragments together.

Bone Healing Process

When a fracture occurs, healing begins with a sticky material, which is secreted by the blood. This material forms a bulgy deposit called a callus around the break, which holds the ends together, Figure 13–58, page 263. As time passes, the callus turns first to cartilage and then to bone. Certain bone cells build the new bone tissue while others remove the cartilage and then slowly smooth the repaired section back to approximately its original size.

A complication which may occur after a fracture of long bones is a fat embolus. An embolus is a mass of foreign material circulating within the blood vessels. This potentially fatal complication may follow the release of fat droplets from the marrow of the long bones. The trauma of the event can also cause the body to release catecholamines, which in turn activate fatty acids. The fatty acids can develop into a fatty embolus and circulate in the blood, becoming lodged in the lungs or even the brain. If the embolus causes an *infarction* (blocked blood vessel) of a large enough vessel, death can occur.

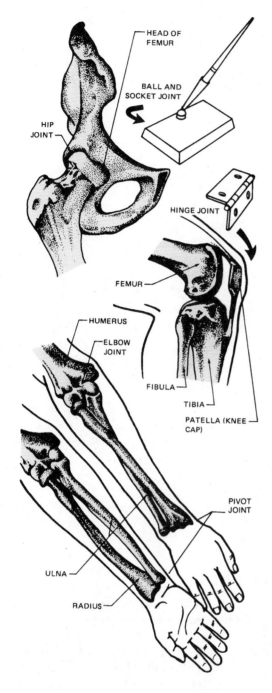

FIGURE 13–56 Types of joints (Adapted from *The Wonderful Human Machine*, Copyright 1979, American Medical Association)

Usual symptoms and signs include apprehension, sweating, fever, rapid heart rate, pallor, difficulty breathing, bluish discoloration of the skin, convulsions, and coma. If the complication occurs, it is usually within 24 to 48 hours, but may occur as late as 3 days after the fracture.

Amputation

Severe trauma, a malignant tumor, lack of circulation, or complications of other conditions, such as diabetes, may result in the need to amputate an extremity. The change in the patient's body image and function causes emotional as well as physical difficulties in coping with daily activities. Following amputation a condition often occurs known as phantom limb, the sensation that the missing extremity is still present. It is often described as an itching or tingling sensation. This may last for quite some time but will usually subside eventually. It is considered normal to experience the sensation.

When the amputated stump has healed sufficiently, a prosthesis (artificial part) may be fitted. Lower limbs are either attached directly to the remaining extremity, fastened by means of straps or belt to the waist, or hung from the shoulder. The method depends to a great extent on the amount of the remaining extremity. Upper limbs may be replaced by a "hook" device that can be opened and closed to grasp objects. A prosthesis that closely resembles a real arm and hand is often desired, even though it lacks the flexibility of the "hook."

Diagnostic Examinations

- Arthroscopy—This endoscopic procedure permits direct visual inspection of a joint, most often the knee. It is frequently used to evaluate injuries suffered by athletes. Arthroscopy is useful in detecting arthritis, torn meniscus, cysts, or loose pieces of tissue. Some surgical procedures can be performed through the scope to repair damaged joint structures, thereby eliminating open surgery.
- X ray—A frequently used test that evaluates the condition of bones in such cases as dislocations, sprains, and fractures. X ray can also be used to determine bone structure changes like those occurring in some metabolic conditions such as acromegaly (giantism), osteoporosis, or with Paget's disease.

Diseases and Disorders

Arthritis, Osteoarthritis. This common form of arthritis causes progressive deterioration of joint cartilage, most often at the hips and knees. It is accompanied by joint pain, stiffness, aching (particularly with weather changes), "grating" during joint motion, and fluid around the joint.

Osteoarthritis is best treated with aspirin, nonsteroids, intraarticular joint injections of steroids, and reducing pressure on joints through the use of a cane, crutches, a cervical collar, etc. Occasionally, disability and uncontrollable pain will require surgical intervention. This can range from scraping deteriorated bone fragments from the joint to replacing joint bone parts with prosthetic appliances (artificial joints).

Arthritis, Rheumatoid. A chronic inflammatory disease attacking joints and surrounding tissues, this is an inter-

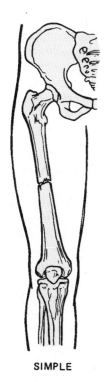
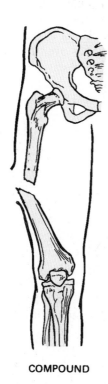
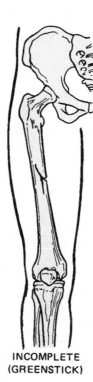
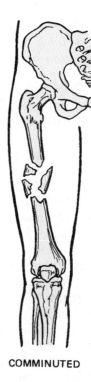

SIMPLE   COMPOUND   INCOMPLETE
                            (GREENSTICK)   COMMINUTED

FIGURE 13–57
Types of fractures
(Copyright by
Richardson. From
Fong, Ferris, &
Skelley, *Body
Structures and
Functions,* 7th ed.
Copyright 1989,
Delmar Publishers
Inc.)

mittent disease with periods of remission. It is three times more common in females than males, most often striking between the ages of 35 and 45. The cause of the condition is not thoroughly understood. The disease attacks the joint synovial membrane, causing edema and congestion. Tissue layers become granulated and thicken, eventually involving the cartilage and destroying the joint capsule and bone. Scar tissue formation, bone atrophy, and malalignment cause visible deformities, pain, and often immobility.

Bursitis.   This is a painful inflammation of the bursa. A bursa is a sac located around a joint and containing lubricating fluids that allow muscles and tendons to move freely over bony surfaces. Bursitis occurs most frequently at the hip, shoulder, or knee. It is usually associated with middle age and results from recurring trauma or stresses on a joint or from inflammatory arthritis.

Treatment consists of joint rest, often immobilization, a pain medication, and joint injection with a steroid combined with an anesthetic. It may be necessary to remove joint fluid by aspiration (withdrawal through a needle) and institute a program of physical therapy to preserve joint motion.

Carpal Tunnel Syndrome.   This condition results from the compression of the median nerve at the wrist. The carpal

tunnel is a passageway for nerves, blood vessels, and flexor tendons to the fingers and thumb. It is formed by the carpal bones and the transverse ligament. The tendon sheaths become inflamed, causing swelling, which presses the median nerve against the transverse ligament

NORMAL BONE REPAIR

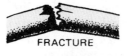

FRACTURE

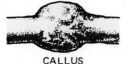

CALLUS

5 TO 6 WEEKS

4 TO 10 MONTHS

FIGURE 13–58   Normal bone repair (From *The Wonderful Human Machine,* copyright 1979, American Medical Association)

resulting in pain, tingling, numbness, and weakness of the hand. It involves only the thumb and index and middle finger. The patient will be unable to make a fist.

The condition occurs most frequently among women between the ages of 30 and 60 and is usually occupationally related. Persons most likely to develop the syndrome are those who use their hands strenuously in grasping, twisting, or turning actions such as assembly line workers and packers. Other systemic conditions that cause the carpal tunnel to swell are diabetes mellitus, pregnancy, menopause, hypothyroidism, benign tumors, and others.

Diagnosis can be made on examination that reveals decreased sensitivity of the first two fingers and the thumb on pricking with a pin, X rays showing bony abnormalities, and an electromyogram showing delayed motor nerve conduction. Patients may also have an *atrophy* (shrinking) of the muscle on the palm side of the thumb due to decreased innervation.

If the syndrome is of short duration, treatment will consist of immobilizing the hand and forearm in a splint, local injections of corticosteroids, and systemic anti-inflammatory medication. It may be necessary to seek new employment if a work-related connection is determined. If conservative treatment does not correct the problem, a surgical procedure may be indicated to section the transverse ligament and "free-up" the nerve. Usually conservative treatment is not successful and only surgery will relieve the symptoms.

Congenital Hip Dysplagia. This abnormality of the hip joint is present at birth. It is the most common hip disorder of children, affecting one or both joints. It is present in three forms: unstable, with the hip in place but easily dislocated by manipulation; incomplete dislocation, with the head of the femur on the edge of the acetabulum; and complete dislocation, with the head totally outside the hip socket. Signs of hip dysplagia include the appearance of one leg being shorter than the other or one hip being more prominent. If both hips are involved the child has a characteristic "duck waddle" or, if one hip only, a limp. Early treatment is essential to normal development. In infants, a splint device is used for 3 to 4 months to maintain proper positioning. Older babies may be placed in traction or the hips may be reduced and a cast applied for a period of 4 to 6 months.

Dislocation. Displacement of bones at a joint so that the regularly meeting surfaces are no longer in contact is a **dislocation.** This occurs most frequently at joints of the fingers, shoulder, knee, and hip. Prompt reduction (relocation) is essential to limit damage to surrounding tissues. It is extremely painful and is often accompanied with joint surface fractures. Following reduction, a splint, cast, or traction (depending on the joint involved) to immobilize the area is indicated. From 2 to 8 weeks will be needed to allow surrounding ligaments to heal completely.

Epicondylitis (Tennis Elbow). This is an inflammation of the forearm extensor tendon at its attachment to the humerus. It probably begins as a tear and is common among people who grasp things forcefully or twist the forearm. Pain occurs at the elbow and becomes intense. There is tenderness over the area where the radius articulates with the humerus.

The condition is best treated with an injection of a steroid and a local anesthetic, aspirin, an immobilizing splint, heat, and physical therapy. If the disorder is not treated, it may result in a disability.

Gout (Gouty Arthritis). This metabolic disease results in severe joint pain, especially at night. It most often affects the great toe but can involve other joints. The pain results from deposits of urates (uric acid salts), which are overproduced and/or retained by the body. Often gout is associated with another disease such as leukemia, due to cell destruction by chemotherapy. Gout may also follow drug therapy that interferes with urate excretion. Gout can be a progressive disease, initially causing severe pain and a hot, tender, inflamed joint. This attack will be followed by a symptom-free period of approximately 6 months to 2 years, when a second episode will occur. Additional attacks usually involve other joints of the feet and legs. Eventually the condition becomes chronic (ongoing), involving many joints that are persistently painful and become degenerated, deformed, and disabling.

Gout is best treated with medication to suppress uric acid formation and promote excretion of the urates. Dietary restrictions must be followed, such as avoiding alcohol, primarily beer and wine, and purine-rich foods such as liver, sardines, kidneys, and lentils.

Hallux Valgus. This is a lateral deviation of the great toe with enlargement of the first metatarsal head and a **bunion** formation. A bunion is a bursa with a callus formation. The bursa becomes inflamed, filled with fluid, and tender. The overlying skin will be red. It is common in women, most often caused by prolonged pressure on the foot from narrow, high-heeled shoes. The condition can also result from degenerative arthritis. Hallux valgus will cause bone deformity and the change will alter the person's weight-bearing pattern. Early treatment with proper shoes, and the use of padding and straightening devices as well as exercises, may correct the situation. A severe deformity and disabling pain will require surgical removal of the bunion.

Herniated Disk (Ruptured Disk). In this situation, the soft gellike material within an intervertebral disk has been forced through its outer surface. The extruded material may cause pressure on a spinal nerve exiting the spinal cord or may impinge on the spinal cord itself. A herniated disk may result from severe trauma or strain, but it is frequently related to degeneration of the intervertebral joints. It occurs most often in the lumbar or lumbosacral regions. Herniated disk usually occurs in adults, mainly men, under age 45. In elderly people with disk degeneration, herniation can occur from a minor trauma. The classic symptom is severe lower back pain, frequently radiating deep into the buttocks and down the back of the leg. It is usually unilateral (one sided). Sensory loss results from nerve compression, and the patient experiences numbness, muscle spasm, motor difficulty, and eventually weakness and atrophy of the leg muscles.

Conservative treatment consists of prolonged bed rest, often with pelvic traction, heat applications, and specific exercises. A **laminectomy** is indicated if there is neurological involvement that does not improve with conservative therapy. This procedure involves removing a portion of the lamina (flattened portion of the vertebral arch) to remove the protruding disk material. A new type of treatment, chemonucleolysis, which involves injecting an enzyme into the disk to dissolve the tissue, is being tried as an alternative to laminectomy surgery.

If pain still persists, a surgical procedure, **spinal fusion,** is performed to stabilize the adjoining vertebrae. This is accomplished by vertically "notching" the spinous process of the two or three involved vertebrae and placing a long sliver of bone taken from the ilium into the notches. When the bone heals, the joined vertebrae can no longer move independently to impinge on the nerve or spinal cord.

Kyphosis (Roundback, Humpback). This is a bowing of the back, usually at the thoracic level, due to improper vertebral alignment, Figure 13–59(a). In children and adolescents **kyphosis** is caused by growth retardation or a disturbance in epiphysis development during rapid growth periods. It occurs often in youth engaged in excessive sports activities. Adult kyphosis may result from aging and the degeneration of intervertebral disks or the collapse of vertebrae due to osteoporosis.

Kyphosis as a result of poor posture during childhood can be treated by therapeutic exercise, a firm mattress, and a Milwaukee brace to straighten the spine until spinal growth is complete. If neurological damage or disabling pain occurs in adolescents and adults (which happens rarely) a surgical procedure may be indicated, which involves posterior spinal fusion, bone grafting, and casting to straighten the severe curvature. With full skeletal maturity and debilitating curvature, a posterior spinal fusion can be accomplished with the use of a stainless steel Harrington rod mechanism to align the vertebrae.

Lordosis. This abnormal anterior convex curvature of the lumbar spine is commonly referred to as swayback, Figure 13–59(b). The body's spine normally curves in at this point; however, if it is exaggerated, it is considered to be **lordosis.** This condition can be improved, or

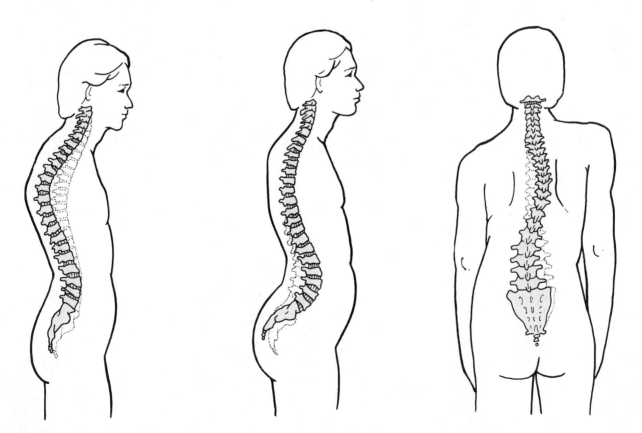

FIGURE 13–59 Abnormal curvatures of the spine. (a). Kyphosis (b). Lordosis (c). Scoliosis. (Adapted from Fong, *Body Structures and Functions*, 7th ed. Copyright 1989, Delmar Publishers Inc.)

at least prevented from progressing, by appropriate exercises, improving posture and having proper footwear.

Lumbar Myositis. This inflammation of the lumbar region muscles of the back causes low back pain. It is common and is due primarily to a straining of the back muscles. The condition is best treated with rest, mild analgesics, and muscle relaxers. When improved, a program of stretching exercises is prescribed to condition and strengthen the muscles.

Osteoporosis. A metabolic bone disorder, characterized by acceleration of the rate of bone resorption while the rate of bone formation slows down, which causes a loss of bone mass. The loss of calcium and phosphate from the bone allows it to become porous, brittle, and prone to fracture. The cause of primary **osteoporosis** may be a combination of prolonged inadequate dietary intake of calcium, faulty metabolism due to estrogen deficiency, and/or a sedentary life style. This type is also known as senile or postmenopausal osteoporosis because it affects primarily elderly, postmenopausal women. Recent statistics show the condition may affect 25 million older Americans. Secondary osteoporosis can occur following prolonged steroid therapy, bone immobilization or lack of use (with paralysis), malnutrition, alcoholism, scurvy, and hyperthyroidism. It is usually discovered following injury from bending to lift something. The individual hears a snapping sound and then feels instant pain in the lower back. The sound and pain are from the collapse of a vertebra. Other common signs are slowly developing kyphosis, loss of height, fractures of the forearm or hip from minor falls, and spontaneous vertebral fractures. The condition is treatable to prevent additional fracturing by increasing exercise, giving an estrogen supplement, and taking calcium and vitamin D to support normal bone metabolism.

Recently scientists in Philadelphia, using new biotechnology equipment, believe they have discovered the cause of postmenopausal osteoporosis. They have linked the condition to a defect on chromosome 7, leading them to think that it may be possible to develop a test that will predict who will develop osteoporosis so that preventive measures may be taken long before the symptoms would become evident.

Scoliosis. A lateral curvature of the spine, usually in the thoracic region, resulting from rotation of the spinal column. It may also be lumbar or involve both, Figure 13–59(c), page 265. The thorax usually curves to the right while the lumbar curves left. Because the body has to maintain balance, the cervical spine will also curve left, which gives the spine an "S" curve appearance.

There are two forms of **scoliosis**, functional, caused by poor posture or uneven leg lengths and structural, resulting from vertebral body deformities. Structural scoliosis can be caused by congenital defects of the vertebrae, muscular dystrophy or paralysis, or a transmitted trait that develops during the growth process. An infantile type of transmitted scoliosis occurs primarily in boys from birth to age 3 and causes left thorax and right lumbar curves. Another type known as juvenile scoliosis affects both sexes between the ages of 4 and 10. The third type, called adolescent, affects primarily girls between 10 and maturity of the skeleton, and results in varying types of curvatures. Adolescent scoliosis can be easily diagnosed. Classic symptoms are apparently uneven hemlines or unequal pants legs, one hip appearing to be higher than the other, and one shoulder appearing higher and perhaps the scapula more pronounced.

Treatment includes observation, exercises, and a brace. With curvature beyond 60 degrees, an immobilizing cast or preoperative traction system is followed by surgical correction using posterior spinal fusion and a Harrington rod for stabilization. Note the following Parent Teaching Aid for detecting scoliosis.

How to Detect Scoliosis

Parents:
To check your child for scoliosis (abnormal curvature of the spine) perform this simple test. First, have your child remove his or her shirt and stand up straight. As you look at the child's back, answer these questions:

■ Is one shoulder higher than the other, or is one shoulder blade more prominent?

■ When the child's arms hang loosely at his or her sides, does one arm swing away from the body more than the other?

■ Is one hip higher or more prominent than the other?

■ Does the child seem to tilt to one side?

Ask your child to bend forward, with arms hanging down and palms together at knee level. Can you see a hump on the back at the ribs or near the waist?

If your answer to any of these questions is "yes," your child needs careful evaluation for scoliosis. Notify your doctor.

Sprain. This complete or incomplete tear in the supporting ligaments of a joint follows a severe twisting action. **Sprains** are characterized by pain, swelling, and a black-and-blue discoloration. The ankle is the most common site. Care of sprains should follow the easy to remember R.I.C.E. method—Rest, Ice, Compression, and Elevation. Treatment consists of (1) controlling pain and swelling by elevating the joint and applying ice intermittently for the first 12 to 24 hours, (2) immobilization using an elastic wrap or, if very severe, a soft cast, and (3) the use of crutches to eliminate stress on the joint. If healing does not occur normally in 3 to 4 weeks, the torn ligaments may require surgical repair, especially if sprains reoccur.

Subluxation. This partial or incomplete dislocation of the articulating surfaces of joint bones usually results from injury or a disease process. If it results from injury, it can be painful and involve the surrounding nerves, blood vessels, ligaments, and soft tissues. Symptoms include joint deformity, impaired motion, pain, and change in length if an extremity is involved. Common sites are shoulders, elbows, wrists, knees, fingers and toes, hips, and ankles. Diagnostic X ray is usually indicated to rule out or confirm accompanying joint fracture.

Treatment consists of reduction as soon as possible to minimize swelling and muscle spasms, which make reduction difficult. The use of medication to control muscle spasm and pain and possibly a splint or cast to provide joint immobilization and support while ligaments heal depend on the joint involved.

Complete Chapter 13, Unit 5 in the workbook to help you meet the objectives at the beginning of this unit and therefore achieve competency of this subject matter.

UNIT 6

The Muscular System

OBJECTIVES ....

Upon completion of this unit, the student will meet the following terminal performance objectives by verifying knowledge of the facts and principles presented through oral and written communication at a level deemed competent.

1. Explain how muscular activity increases body heat.
2. List six functions of skeletal muscles.
3. Name and describe the three types of muscular tissue and the purpose of each.
4. Describe the purpose of a muscle team and give an example.
5. Explain what muscle tone means.
6. Describe the structure and function of a tendon and identify the body's strongest tendon.
7. Explain the terms *origin* and *insertion.*
8. Describe a muscle sheath and a bursa and the purpose of each.
9. Identify the muscles of respiration and describe how their function results in breathing.
10. Name the major skeletal muscles of the body.
11. Describe the smooth muscle action of peristalsis.
12. Explain the structure and function of a sphincter.
13. Describe four disorders or diseases of the muscular system.
14. Spell and define, using the glossary at the back of the text, all the words to know in this unit.

WORDS TO KNOW ....

abduction	latissimus dorsi
Achilles tendon	muscle team
adduction	muscle tone
anchor	musculoskeletal
aponeurosis	origin
atrophy	pectoralis major
biceps	peristalsis
contracture	quadriceps femoris
cramp	sartorius
deltoid	sheath
dystrophy	spasm
extensor	sphincter
fascia	sternocleidomastoid
flexor	strain
gastrocnemius	tendon
gluteus maximus	tendonitis
hamstring	tibialis anterior
hiccough	torticollis
insertion	trapezius
intercostal	triceps

There are approximately 600 muscle organs in the human body. Muscles are composed of muscular tissue, which is constructed of bundles of muscle fibers about the size of a human hair. The larger the muscle, the greater the number of fibers. Muscles perform their duties by alternately contracting and relaxing. All muscle activity is directed by the nervous system. Motor neuron axons innervate several muscle cells within a muscle. Signals from the brain go through the axons and cause all the cells under their control to contract at the same time. That group of cells and its motor neuron are called a *motor unit.* When only one stimulus acts on the unit causing a contraction, it is called a *twitch.* This quick, simple contraction naturally occurs occasionally as a spontaneous event in a muscle. Scientists can study these units by using an electrical stimulus, which will also activate the motor unit. A muscle contraction is a quick progression of events following a stimulus—a very brief interval before the contraction begins, then it intensifies to a peak, and decreases to relaxation. If a second stimulus is received before the first is completed, the contraction will strengthen. When repeated stimulation occurs without a relaxation time, the muscle is maintained in a state of contraction called *tetanus* (not to be confused with the disease of the same name). This occurs when we experience muscle cramps and spasms.

At all times, motor units are alternately either contracted or relaxed; there is no other state in which they exist. The units that make up the muscles are contracted in sufficient number to meet whatever need is necessary. During sleep, for instance, only a few would be contracted at a given time, yet during strenuous activity, a great number would be called on to contract, a process known as *muscle recruitment.*

Some muscles work in partnership with the bones and can be controlled voluntarily by the motor nerves of the peripheral nervous system. Other muscles function continuously without the slightest conscious concern. The autonomic nervous system directs their activities to provide the body with essential services. It is the action of these muscles that causes us to breathe and our blood to circulate.

Muscle Fuel

All body tissues must have food and oxygen to survive. The muscles receive an ample supply of both because of their importance to the body's safety and well-being. The body stores carbohydrates in its muscles in the form of a starch called *glycogen*. When muscles function, they use the stored glycogen, changing it to glucose, as their source of energy. Heat is released as this fuel is used, thereby warming the body. Strenuous exercise burns a great deal of stored glycogen and therefore often results in overheating the body.

Functions of Muscle

In addition to providing heat and the ability to move, muscles support the structures of the body and hold the body upright. The muscles along the back, shoulders, and neck hold the trunk and head erect while permitting great flexibility in movement.

The structure of the skeletal muscles protects the blood vessels and nerves that lie throughout the body. The contraction of lower leg muscles aids in the return flow of blood to the heart by squeezing the veins of the legs. Muscles also provide protective padding to shield delicate internal organs and structures from injury.

Visually, the muscles add greatly to our appearance by giving shape to the body. Body-building enthusiasts spend years developing the degree of muscle enlargement and definition they feel is desirable. Muscle fiber, and therefore the muscle, hypertrophies (grows larger) with exercise; the number of fibers does not increase, however.

Muscle Growth

Muscle tissue changes slightly with age. During infancy, muscles have little connective tissue, often being attached to the bone directly. With maturity, the connective tissue increases as do the elastic fibers. Muscles grow in relation to the structures to which they are attached. Muscles of the eye, for example, grow very little, while the large muscles of the lower extremities grow considerably.

Types of Muscle Tissue

There are three types of muscle tissue, Figure 13–60. First, there is the *skeletal* type. Skeletal muscles are attached to bones and therefore permit movement. Since

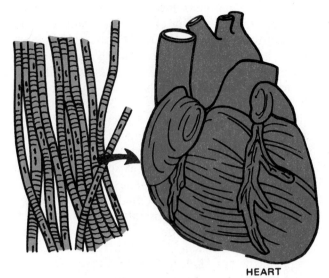

HEART

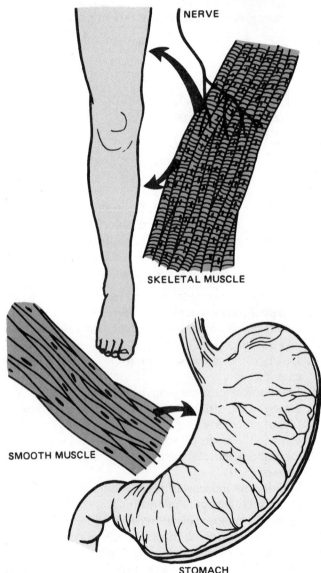

NERVE

SKELETAL MUSCLE

SMOOTH MUSCLE

STOMACH

FIGURE 13–60 Types of muscle tissue (From *The Wonderful Human Machine*, copyright 1979, American Medical Association)

we have some control over movements, this type of muscle tissue is also called voluntary. Skeletal muscle cells are long and strong, some reaching lengths up to 12 inches. These cells are held together by connective tissue to form a muscle bundle. The bundles in turn are enclosed in a tougher connective tissue **sheath** to form the muscle organs such as the **biceps** of the arm. The larger the muscle organ, the greater the number of fibers.

The second type of muscle tissue is *smooth*. Smooth muscle tissue is made of small, delicate muscle cells and is found throughout the internal organs of the body, except for the heart. Smooth muscle activity occurs continuously in such actions as breathing, moving food through the intestinal tract, changing the size of the pupil of the eye, and dilating or constricting blood vessels. These muscles function without conscious direct control, so they are also called involuntary.

The third type is *cardiac* muscle tissue. As the name implies, this type is found in the heart. These cells are joined in a continuous network without sheath separation. The membranes of adjacent cells are fused at places called *intercalated disks*. A communication system at the fused areas will not permit independent cell contraction. When one cell receives a signal to contract, all neighboring cells are stimulated and they contract together to produce the action of a heart beat. This type of muscle tissue is also involuntary, which is fortunate. It would be a full-time job to consciously contract the heart muscle 70 times a minute, 100,800 times a day.

Skeletal Muscle Action

When muscles contract they become shorter and thicker. A good example is the skeletal muscle of the upper arm, the biceps. When the biceps contract to bend the elbow, the shorter, and thicker muscle causes a bulge in the upper arm, Figure 13–61.

The skeletal muscle that bends a joint is called a **flexor,** while the action of straightening the joint is done by the **extensor** muscle. The extensor muscle that straightens the elbow is the **triceps.** The flexor and its partner, the extensor muscle, form what is known as a **muscle team** to bend and straighten joints, Figure 13–62, page 270. Muscles also contract to move extremities away from the body's center line, which is known as **abduction,** or toward the center line, which is known as **adduction,** Figure 13–63, page 270.

Muscle Tone

Most skeletal muscles are partially contracted at all times to maintain the body's erect position. It is believed that some fibers contract while others rest and that they then exchange places. This constant state of contraction is known as **muscle tone.** Physicians frequently refer tò muscle tone when examining patients. Evaluation of

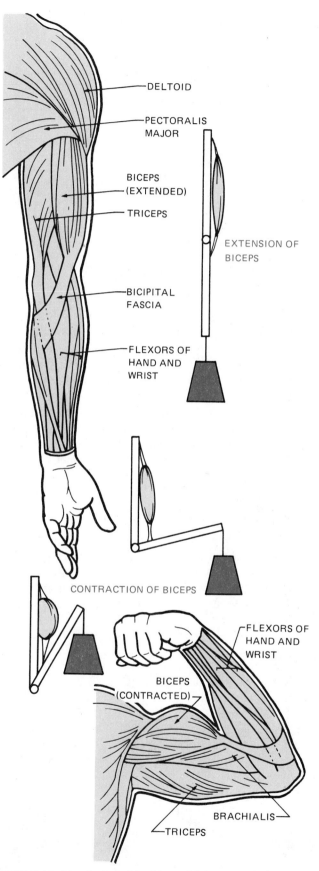

FIGURE 13–61 Action of the biceps/triceps muscle team (From *The Wonderful Human Machine*, copyright 1979, American Medical Association)

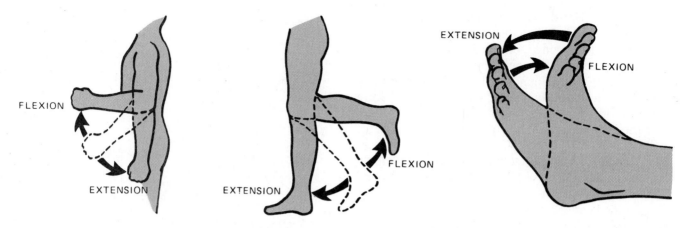

FIGURE 13–62   Flexor/extensor muscle team action

muscle tone aids in determining the status of the CNS and the motor function of the peripheral nerves.

Loss of muscle tone can occur when muscles are not used, as with severe illness, the elderly, paralysis, or temporarily when an extremity has been immobilized in a cast. With prolonged lack of use muscles will atrophy, which is a progressive wasting away of the muscle tissue. Atrophy renders a muscle useless. Another muscular condition that develops from lack of use is called contracture. Here flexor muscles become shorter and permanently bend the joints. This is a common condition with paralyzed or unconscious patients. The most common sites are the fingers, elbows, knees, and hip joints.

Muscle Attachment

Skeletal muscles are attached to bone in various ways. In some instances the connective tissue within the muscle is attached directly to the bone periosteum. Some muscular connective tissue sheaths extend to form a strong fibrous structure known as a tendon, which is attached to rough surfaces on a bone. Tendons are extremely strong and do not stretch. A tendon 1 inch thick reportedly will support 9 tons of weight. Because of this characteristic, a bone will sometimes fracture before the tendon attached to it will separate. The thickest and strongest tendon in the human body is the Achilles tendon, which attaches the gastrocnemius muscle in the calf of the leg to the heel bone.

A similar type of connective tissue is called a ligament but it does not perform the same function. A ligament is a flexible, fibrous tissue which supports organs and connects bone to bone at joints. Ligaments, unlike tendons, do stretch.

Another form of muscular attachment is by fascia, a sheetlike, tough membrane that forms sheaths to cover and protect the muscle tissue. The term aponeurosis designates either a fascia or a flat tendon type of muscle attachment.

Origin or Insertion

When skeletal muscles join bones that meet at joints, one of the bones becomes the anchor on which the muscle

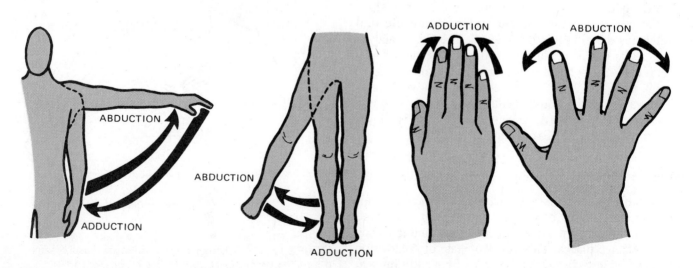

FIGURE 13–63   Abduction/adduction muscle team action

has its origin. The bone to be moved becomes the insertion end for the muscle. For example, the biceps has its origin at the shoulder and its insertion on the radius. When the biceps contracts, being firmly anchored at the shoulder, it pulls upon the insertion location on the forearm, and the arm flexes (bends).

The terms origin and insertion can also apply to muscle attachments other than at joints. Essentially, the end nearest the center of the body is described as the origin, while the distal end is referred to as the insertion. Usually the origin is relatively immobile while the insertion is into a movable structure.

Sheaths and Bursae ....

To protect the moving parts of the muscles, muscle groups are separated from each other by membranes called *sheaths* to reduce the friction from movement. Within muscle groups, individual muscles are also separated by membranes. The tendons that extend from the muscle group are also enclosed in lubricated sheaths to protect them from damage by rubbing against other tendons, bone, or cartilage.

A sheath which is shaped like a sac and has a slippery fluid lining is known as a bursa. A bursa functions as a water cushion to minimize pressure and friction over bony prominences and under tendons. The most common bursae are located at the elbow, knee, and shoulder.

Major Skeletal Muscles ....

The muscle most important in breathing divides the chest cavity from the abdominal cavity. This muscle is called the *diaphragm*, Figure 13–64. It is a dome-shaped muscle with tendons that attach it in the back to the spinal column, in the front to the tip of the sternum, and along the sides to the cartilage edge of the ribs. When the muscle contracts, it becomes shorter and therefore flatter, creating a vacuum which causes the lungs to draw in air. When the muscle relaxes, it returns to its dome shape and forces air out of the lungs. The diaphragm also plays a role in coughing, sneezing, or laughing. Spasmodic contractions of the diaphragm, followed by spasmodic closure of the space between the vocal cords, cause the common hiccough.

The orbicularis oculi and orbicularis oris are circular muscles around the eye and mouth, Figure 13–65, page 272. Their contraction enables us to squint or wink and to whistle or pucker the mouth. The sternocleidomastoid and the trapezius are the major muscles of the neck and upper back, which hold the head erect and assist with its movement, Figure 13–66, page 273. The trapezius not only supports the head but extends down the back and shoulders, giving us the ability to raise and throw back the shoulders.

The pectoralis major is the main upper chest muscle. It extends from the sternum to the head of the humerus, enabling us to flex the arm across the chest. The intercostal muscles lie beneath the pectoralis major, between the ribs. These serve as accessory muscles to the diaphragm by enlarging the thoracic cavity during inspiration.

The abdomen is covered by three main muscle layers that run in different directions to make a strong wall to protect the abdominal organs. The external oblique is first, with the internal oblique beneath, and the transversus abdominis the innermost layer. A long, narrow muscle, the rectus abdominis, extends from the pubis to the bottom of the rib cage in the center of the abdomen. It overlies and is surrounded by connective tissue layers from the other three muscles.

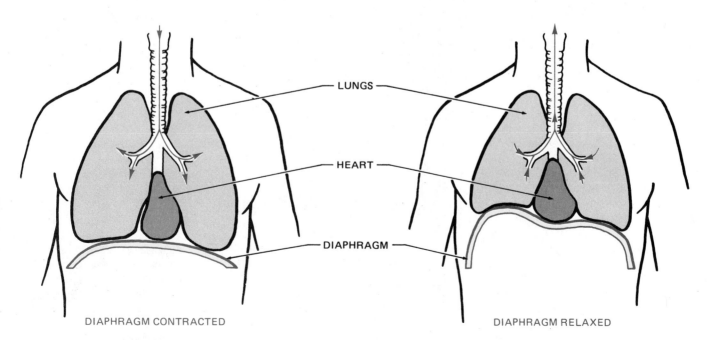

LUNGS

HEART

DIAPHRAGM

DIAPHRAGM CONTRACTED

DIAPHRAGM RELAXED

FIGURE 13–64   The action of the diaphragm muscle

The back is covered by a large muscle called the **latissimus dorsi.** Its main function is to extend and adduct the arm, as when swimming. Thick vertical groups of four different muscles overlap and extend from the sacrum and loser vertebrae to the occipital bone and upper cervical vertebrae to support and move the spinal column.

The shoulders are protected by a triangle of muscle called the **deltoid,** which abducts the arm. The deltoid, if of adequate size, may be used for small injections of medication that must be given intramuscularly.

Lower Extremity Muscles

The muscles of the lower extremities involve about one-half of the body's total muscle mass. The buttocks are formed by the large **gluteus maximus** muscles, which support much of the body's weight and enable us to stand erect. The upper outer quadrant of the buttocks is the site of choice for intramuscular injections, especially for large amounts of a slowly absorbing material.

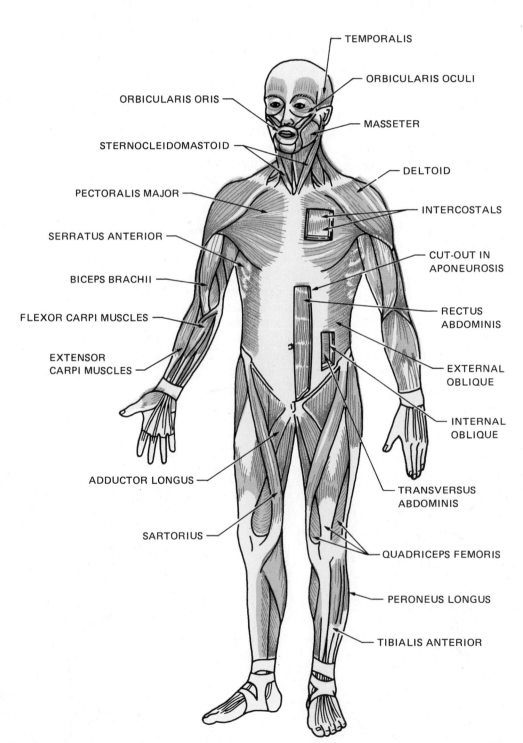

TEMPORALIS
ORBICULARIS OCULI
ORBICULARIS ORIS
MASSETER
STERNOCLEIDOMASTOID
DELTOID
PECTORALIS MAJOR
INTERCOSTALS
SERRATUS ANTERIOR
CUT-OUT IN APONEUROSIS
BICEPS BRACHII
RECTUS ABDOMINIS
FLEXOR CARPI MUSCLES
EXTENSOR CARPI MUSCLES
EXTERNAL OBLIQUE
INTERNAL OBLIQUE
ADDUCTOR LONGUS
TRANSVERSUS ABDOMINIS
SARTORIUS
QUADRICEPS FEMORIS
PERONEUS LONGUS
TIBIALIS ANTERIOR

FIGURE 13–65 Principal muscles (anterior view) (Copyright by Johnson. From Fong, Ferris, & Skelley, *Body Structures and Functions,* 7th ed. Copyright 1989, Delmar Publishers Inc.)

The front of the thigh has the longest muscle of the body, the **sartorius.** It anchors on the iliac spine and crosses diagonally down the front of the thigh to insert on the medial surface of the tibia. The sartorius flexes the hip and knee joints to turn the thigh outward, making it possible to sit cross-legged on the floor. The **quadriceps femoris,** with four separate parts (rectus femoris, vastus lateralis, vastus medialis, and vastus intermedius) makes up the bulk of the anterior thigh musculature. It is a powerful extensor of the knee and is used when we rise from a sitting position, kick a ball, or swim.

The **tibialis anterior** is in the front of the leg. When it is flexed, it is possible to walk on your heels with the rest of the foot off the ground. It also serves to invert the foot, turning it toward the other foot.

The posterior thigh is the site of the **hamstring** group, which includes the biceps femoris, semitendinosus, semimembranosus, and a portion of the adductor

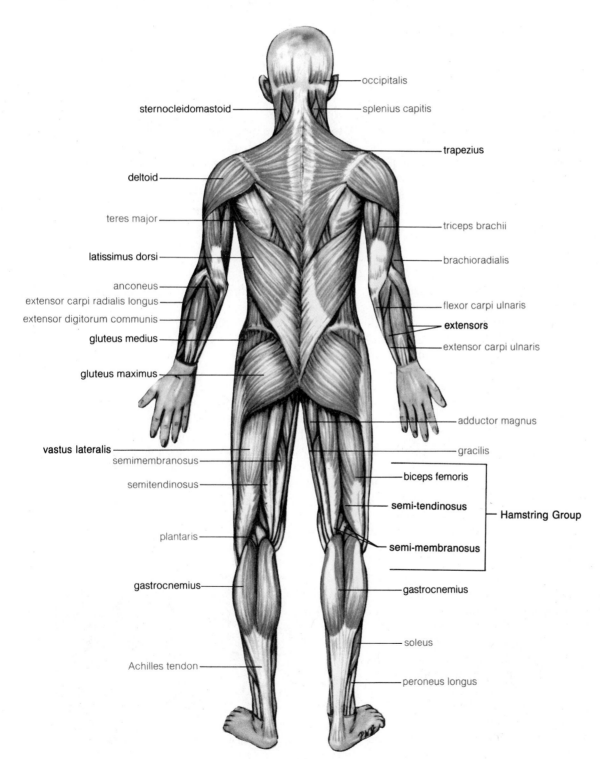

FIGURE 13–66
Principal muscles (posterior view) (Copyright by Johnson. From Fong, Ferris, & Skelley, *Body Structures and Functions,* 7th ed. Copyright 1989, Delmar Publishers Inc.)

magnus. Their primary function is to flex the knee by pulling on the insertion at the fibula and tibia. The tendons are easily identified by palpation behind the knee. The gastrocnemius is the main muscle in the calf of the leg. Its tendon, the Achilles, has been mentioned. Contraction of the gastrocnemius permits you to stand to tiptoe since it acts as the flexor of the plantar surface (sole) of the foot.

Muscles of Expression

A number of muscles in the face enable us to show our feelings. The frontalis (forehead) can be raised to express surprise or lowered to show a stern glance. Raising one side of the obicularis oris about the upper lip will result in a sneer. The obicularis oris also allows us to whistle, kiss, smile, grin, grimace with pain, or pout.

The obicularis oculi around the eyes help complete the frown as well as enabling us to squint or wink. The large muscle of the lower jaw, the masseter, in cooperation with other smaller muscles, opens and closes the mouth to express emotions of surprise and disbelief but also is powerful and is responsible for our ability to chew and grind the food we eat.

Muscle Strain and Cramps ....

Occasionally, too much stress is applied to skeletal muscles while exercising or participating in athletic activities. This may result in a strain, but the muscles will recover with a period of rest. Athletes frequently "pull" their hamstring group during strenuous competition. Another frequent occurrence is a muscle cramp or spasm, caused by a muscle that has contracted but cannot relax. It can usually be treated by working the extremity or rubbing the muscle.

Muscle Fatigue

Prolonged strenuous exercise can result in muscle fatigue. Muscles require large amounts of oxygen to sustain the conversion of glycogen stored in the muscle into energy (adenosine triphosphate or ATP), a function of the many mitochondria within muscle cells. Vigorous exercise is believed to cause an oxygen deficit within the muscle because the body cannot take in and circulate oxygen fast enough to keep up with the demand. When this occurs, lactic acid begins to accumulate, the glycogen is depleted, and the muscle's supply of ATP runs low. The muscle loses its ability to contract effectively and finally becomes incapable of reacting at all to the stimulus to contract. This occurs primarily in marathon runners who sometimes even collapse from muscle fatigue. Most of us simply stop our activities long before this happens.

Oxygen debt is "paid back" by the rapid and deep breathing that follows exercise. When the accumulated lactic acid is removed and the amount of oxygen restored

to once again produce ATP, the muscle can again respond to a stimulus and contract.

Smooth Muscle Action ....

Smooth, involuntary muscles can be found throughout the internal organs and structures of the body. They are controlled automatically by signals from the autonomic nervous system.

In the esophagus (the structure that connects the mouth with the stomach), the muscle tissue changes from voluntary muscles at the top that assist in swallowing, to smooth, involuntary muscles that move the food to the stomach. A two-layer muscle structure in the lower esophagus continues into the stomach and intestines. One layer of smooth muscle is circular and contracts to narrow the tube. Another layer is longitudinal and contracts to shorten the tube. The alternating action of both layers, contracting and relaxing, works the food through the body in a wave like action called peristalsis, Figure 13–67. The stomach has a third layer in the muscle wall because of its need to break up and churn the food that is swallowed, which must be in a near-liquid state before it can be passed on to the small intestine.

Sphincters

Throughout the digestive system and inside the blood vessels of the body are smooth, donut-shaped muscle structures called sphincters. These pinch shut intermittently to control the flow of food, liquid or blood. Sphincters in the digestive system are capable of remaining contracted for hours if necessary. Both ends of the stomach have sphincter muscles to hold the contents securely inside while muscular action and chemical processes digest food. When the food is in the proper state, the lower sphincter opens slightly to allow small amounts of the liquid to escape into the small intestine.

An example of smooth muscle sphincter action that can be easily observed is the pupil of the eye. When

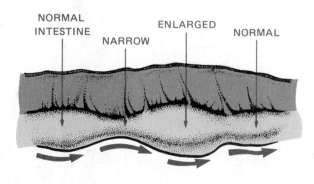

NORMAL INTESTINE   NARROW   ENLARGED   NORMAL

PERISTALTIC WAVE

FIGURE 13–67   Peristaltic action (From *The Wonderful Human Machine*, copyright 1979, American Medical Association)

available light is decreased, the radial muscles of the iris contract to enlarge the pupil, permitting more light to enter, thereby increasing the ability to see. When light is focused on the eye, the circular sphincter muscles of the iris that surround the pupil contract, making the pupil smaller, thereby limiting the amount of light striking the retina. The physician will usually check light reflex action of the eyes in assessing the condition of the brain and autonomic nervous system.

Disorders and Diseases ....

Bursitis/Tendonitis. (See Unit 5.). Tendonitis is a painful inflammation of the tendon and tendon–muscle attachments to bone, usually at the shoulder, hip, heel, or hamstrings. Bursitis is an inflammation of the bursa that covers and lubricates the muscles and tendons, and occurs most often at the shoulder, elbow, or knee. Both conditions are painful and result in limited movement of the extremities.

Tendonitis normally follows a sports-related activity that damages the muscle–tendon structure. It can also result from misaligned posture and other musculoskeletal disorders. With injury, apply ice initially for the first 12 to 24 hours. Later, applications of heat will usually aid in relief of the joint pain. If calcium deposits have formed within the tendon it becomes weak, and the condition will be aggravated by heat. The calcium deposits are visible on X ray to confirm the diagnosis. Application of ice packs will help relieve discomfort from calcified tendonitis.

Both conditions may be treated by resting the joint, oral does of pain medication, and intraarticular injections of a mixture of corticosteroid and a local anesthetic. If fluid has accumulated within the area, it may require aspiration prior to the injection treatment. When pain has subsided, a physical therapy regime may be indicated to maintain joint function and prevent muscular atrophy.

Epicondylitis (Tennis Elbow) (See Unit 5). This is inflammation of a forearm tendon at the attachment on the humerus at the elbow. The initial elbow pain gradually worsens and often involves the forearm and the back of the hand when an object is grasped or the elbow is twisted. There is tenderness over the head of the radius and the projection of the humerus at the elbow joint. Epicondylitis probably begins as a partial tear of the tendon from its attachment.

Injection of the area, as with tendonitis, is effective. Immobilization, heat therapy, and manipulation of the tendon attachment are used before resorting to surgical excision of the tendon for recurring and continual inflammation.

Fibromyositis. This is inflammation of the soft tissue, which results in painful muscles. Often the cause is unknown. It is believed to be stress and tension related. Headaches usually occur as well. The main diagnostic finding is the presence of a "trigger point" which causes pain when pressed. Treatment consists of nonsteroid drugs, muscle relaxants, exercise, and physical therapy.

Muscular Dystrophy. This group of congenital disorders results in progressive wasting away of skeletal muscles. There are several types of muscular dystrophy. Duchenne's, which represents 50% of the cases, is an X-linked chromosome disorder affecting only males. The onset is usually in early childhood, ages 3 to 5, with death occurring after 10 to 15 years. Initially the leg and pelvic muscles are affected, making all activities involving the lower extremities difficult. Children are usually confined to a wheelchair by ages 9 to 12. The disease progresses from skeletal to smooth muscles, affecting the heart and diaphragm and eventually resulting in cardiac or respiratory failure.

Erb's or juvenile muscular dystrophy and a similar type do not reduce life expectancy. These forms progress much more slowly and occur later in childhood or adolescence. Weakness of the facial muscles and inability to raise the arms are among the main symptoms.

The fourth is a mixed type of dystrophy occurring generally between ages 30 and 50, affecting all voluntary muscles and resulting in rapid, progressive deterioration. Death usually results in about 5 years from onset.

A positive diagnosis of dystrophy can be made from a typical medical history and evaluation of voluntary muscle movements. Confirmation is possible by a biopsy of the muscle tissue, which shows characteristic deposits of fat and connective tissue. There is no treatment to stop the progression of the disease.

Torticollis (Wryneck). This neck deformity is caused by shortening or spasm of the sternocleidomastoid neck muscle, which bends the head to the affected side and rotates the chin toward the opposite side. It can be congenital or acquired. The congenital form usually follows a difficult (breech) birth and occurs mostly in firstborn females. It is thought to develop from malposition before birth, prenatal injury, or the rupture of muscle fibers with resulting scar tissue development. Acquired torticollis results from muscle damage by disease, a cervical spine injury, or muscle spasms due to a CNS disorder. It can also result from hysteria.

Treatment of the congenital type consists of stretching the shortened muscle through passive exercises and positional arrangement of the head during sleeping. Surgical correction of the muscle can be accomplished if conservative methods are not effective. Acquired torticollis is treated by correcting the underlying cause whenever possible. Application of heat, cervical traction, a neck brace, exercise, psychotherapy (if hysteria-related), and massage are indicated.

Complete Chapter 13, Unit 6 in the workbook to help you meet the objectives at the beginning of this unit and therefore achieve competency of this subject matter.

U N I T 7

The Respiratory System

OBJECTIVES ....

Upon completion of this unit, the student will meet the following terminal performance objectives by verifying knowledge of the facts and principles presented through oral and written communication at a level deemed competent.

1. Describe the source and importance of oxygen.
2. Trace the path of oxygen to the internal cell.
3. Describe the structure and function of the nose, pharynx, epiglottis, larynx, trachea, bronchus, bronchiole, and alveolus.
4. Explain how voice sounds are produced.
5. Differentiate between external and internal respiration.
6. Describe the structure and function of the pleural coverings of the lungs and chest cavity.
7. Describe the relationship of the diaphragm and brain to breathing.
8. Discuss five normal occurrences that alter breathing patterns and explain why they occur.
9. Identify ten diagnostic examinations for respiratory assessment.
10. Explain the role of surfactant in the lungs.
11. Differentiate between perfusion and ventilation scans.
12. Describe 26 diseases or disorders of the respiratory tract.
13. Spell and define, using the glossary at the back of the text, all the words to know in this unit.

WORDS TO KNOW ....

allergic rhinitis
alveoli
angiography
apnea
arteriography
asthma
atelectasis
bronchi
bronchiole
bronchitis
carbon dioxide
chronic obstructive
 pulmonary disease
cilia
cyanosis
dyspnea
emphysema
empyema
epiglottis
epistaxis
expectoration

expiration
hemothorax
hiccoughs
hiccup
histoplasmosis
hyaline membrane disease
hypoxia
influenza
inspiration
intubation
laryngectomy
larynx
Legionnaires' disease
liter
lung
orthopnea
oxygen
perfusion
pharynx
pleura
pleurisy

pneumoconiosis
pneumonia
pneumothorax
pulmonary
pulmonary edema
pulmonary emboli
respiratory
rhinitis
septum
sinusitis
spirometer

spontaneous
sputum
sudden infant death
 syndrome
surfactant
trachea
tracheotomy
tuberculosis
upper respiratory infection
ventilation
vital capacity

Oxygen (O_2) is provided continuously by plants on land and in the sea. Plants use sun, water, and **carbon dioxide** (CO_2) to make oxygen, which they release into the air. Humans breathe O_2 and exhale CO_2 and water. This cycle provides the means for supporting life.

Oxygen in the air is essential to the survival of living cells. An adult human being carries 2 quarts of O_2 in the blood, lungs, and tissues. This supply is adequate for about 4 minutes. The respiratory system is responsible for taking in air, removing the oxygen content, and sending it in the blood to the cells of the body. The oxygen content of inhaled air is about 24%.

The respiratory system must also take from the blood the waste product CO_2 and exhaust it from the lungs. Exhaled air still contains about 16% oxygen. When the level of CO_2 in the blood rises to a certain point, the respiratory center in the brain is triggered and a breath is taken. This function is so vital to life that its interruption for just a few minutes will result in death.

The Pathway of Oxygen ....

The Nose

Air enters the body through the nose, Figure 13–68. Here the air is filtered, warmed, and moistened by the structures within the nasal cavity. The nose is divided by a wall of cartilage called the **septum.** Near the middle of the nasal cavity, on each side, are a series of three scroll-like bones called conchae or turbinates. The conchae are covered with mucus-producing epithelium, which adds moisture to the air, and are supplied with abundant blood vessels, which warm the air. Just inside the nostrils are hairs called **cilia,** which trap particles in the air so they do not enter the lungs.

The mucus from the lining also helps trap dust and bacteria. When irritating substances come in contact with the lining, extra mucus is produced to dilute the irritant. This is why sneezing occurs and the nose "runs." Both actions are methods of removing irritants.

Ciliated mucosa in the posterior portion of the nose and in the pharynx (throat) help propel inhaled particles into the back of the pharynx to be swallowed. Particles in the trachea and bronchi must first be propelled upward past the epiglottis, in an action called *mucus streaming.* The particles can then be directed toward the esophagus and

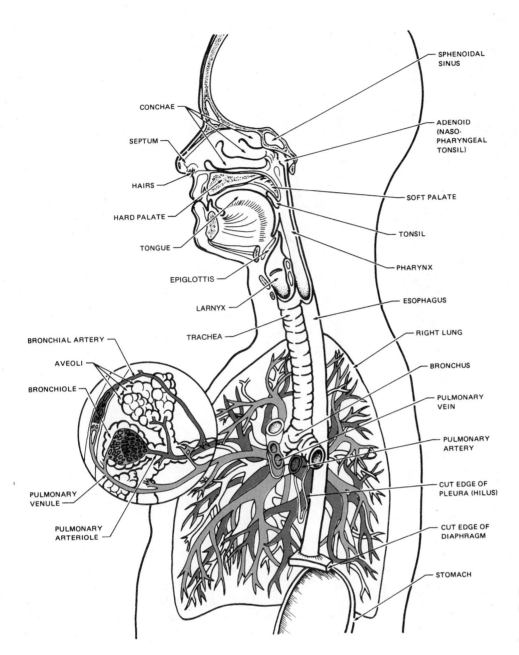

Labels on figure:

SPHENOIDAL SINUS

CONCHAE

SEPTUM

HAIRS

HARD PALATE

TONGUE

EPIGLOTTIS

LARNYX

TRACHEA

BRONCHIAL ARTERY

AVEOLI

BRONCHIOLE

PULMONARY VENULE

PULMONARY ARTERIOLE

ADENOID (NASO-PHARYNGEAL TONSIL)

SOFT PALATE

TONSIL

PHARYNX

ESOPHAGUS

RIGHT LUNG

BRONCHUS

PULMONARY VEIN

PULMONARY ARTERY

CUT EDGE OF PLEURA (HILUS)

CUT EDGE OF DIAPHRAGM

STOMACH

FIGURE 13–68 The respiratory system (From *The Wonderful Human Machine*, Copyright 1979, American Medical Association)

swallowed. The constant beating action of the cilia and the flow of the mucus secretions cleanse the air passages. This beneficial function is temporarily halted by the effect of smoking, which paralyzes the cilia and mucus streaming action, thereby allowing foreign particles to enter the lungs. The paralysis lasts for several minutes.

The sinuses of the head are lined with the continuation of the nasal membranes, Figure 13–69, page 278. This explains why sinusitis occurs frequently with nasal infections, usually the result of spreading the organism by blowing the nose too forcefully.

The Pharynx, Larynx, and Epiglottis

After the air is filtered, warmed, and moistened in the nose, it enters the pharynx. The pharynx serves as a pas-

sageway for both air and food. Except for an occasional mistake, it is not possible to swallow food and breathe at the same time. When this does occur, the result is choking, which can be very serious.

Normally, when food is swallowed, a cartilage "lid" called the epiglottis is pushed by the base of the tongue to cover the opening into the larynx. At the same time, the larynx moves up to help close the opening. With the opening to the larynx covered by the epiglottis, food is directed down the esophagus into the stomach.

When air passes under the open epiglottis, it enters the larynx, commonly called the voice box. The larynx is a tube with a series of nine separate cartilages to maintain its opening, Figure 13–70, page 278. The thyroid cartilage is the largest and is located anteriorly. Its prominent projection is known as the Adam's apple, and

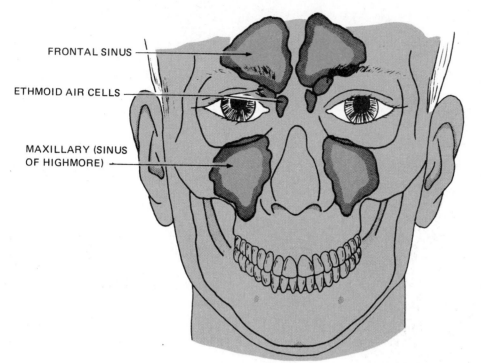

FRONTAL SINUS

ETHMOID AIR CELLS

MAXILLARY (SINUS OF HIGHMORE)

FIGURE 13–69 Paranasal sinuses (frontal view) From Anderson & Burkard, *The Dental Assistant*, copyright 1978, Delmar Publishers, Inc.)

its action can be observed when a person swallows. The larynx is lined with mucous membrane, which also forms two folds called the vocal cords. The cords are attached to the front of the larynx wall by cartilage. Muscles attach to the cartilage, and when they contract or relax the vocal cords move either toward or away from the center of the larynx, Figure 13–71.

During breathing, the vocal cords are near to the wall of the larynx so that air can pass freely in and out. When speaking, the vocal cords move across the larynx and are held tense by the contracting muscles. The degree of tension and the length of the cords determine the pitch of

the voice. The tighter and longer the cords the higher the pitch. The pressure on the air being expelled from the lungs determines the volume or loudness of the voice as it vibrates the vocal cords. Note that speech is most easily accomplished during the exhaling of air. Inhaling does not create sufficient air pressure, nor can it be sustained long enough to produce speech.

Part of the mucous membrane lining of the larynx is loosely attached and of a different type of epithelium. It may become swollen, actually preventing respirations. In this emergency situation, an airway may be achieved by **intubation** (passing a tube through the mouth into the larynx) or by making an external opening into the **trachea,** called a **tracheotomy,** and inserting a tube to permit air to enter.

The Trachea, Bronchi, and Bronchioles

The next passageway for air is the trachea, Figure 13–72. It is commonly called the windpipe and extends from the neck into the chest, directly in front of the esophagus. The trachea is held open by a series of C-shaped cartilage rings. The wall between the rings is elastic, enabling the trachea to adjust to different body positions.

About the middle of the sternum, the trachea divides into two sections called the right and left **bronchi.** The structure of the two main bronchi is similar to that of the trachea, with incomplete cartilage rings to maintain the air passageway. Each bronchus divides and subdivides into many increasingly smaller bronchi, each with the cartilage-ringed structure, until they are barely visible without a microscope. These tiny air passageways have walls of muscle cells and are called **bronchioles.**

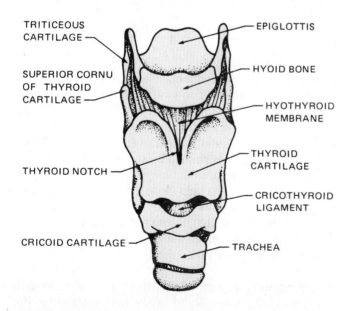

TRITICEOUS CARTILAGE

SUPERIOR CORNU OF THYROID CARTILAGE

THYROID NOTCH

CRICOID CARTILAGE

EPIGLOTTIS

HYOID BONE

HYOTHYROID MEMBRANE

THYROID CARTILAGE

CRICOTHYROID LIGAMENT

TRACHEA

FIGURE 13–70 Larynx (anterior view)

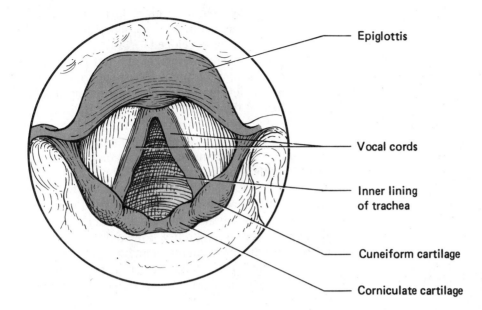

Epiglottis

Vocal cords

Inner lining
of trachea

Cuneiform cartilage

Corniculate cartilage

FIGURE 13–71   The vocal cords in the larynx (From Kinn, *Medical Terminology, Building Blocks for Health Careers*, copyright 1990, Delmar Publishers Inc.)

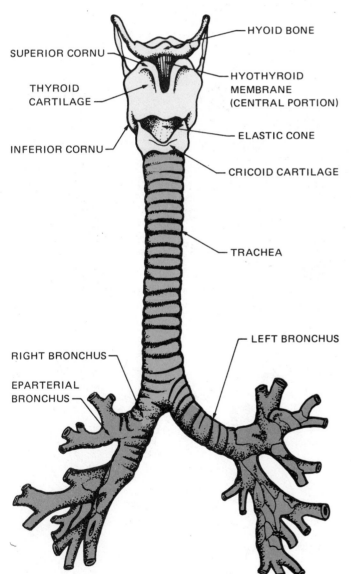

HYOID BONE

SUPERIOR CORNU

THYROID CARTILAGE

HYOTHYROID MEMBRANE (CENTRAL PORTION)

ELASTIC CONE

INFERIOR CORNU

CRICOID CARTILAGE

TRACHEA

LEFT BRONCHUS

RIGHT BRONCHUS

EPARTERIAL BRONCHUS

FIGURE 13–72   The larynx, trachea and bronchi

The Alveoli

Each bronchiole ends in a grapelike cluster of microscopic air sacs called **alveoli.** It is estimated that the body contains about 500 million alveoli, approximately three times the amount necessary to sustain life. The membrane walls of the alveoli are only one cell thick and are surrounded by a network of microscopic blood vessels called capillaries, Figure 13–73, page 280.

Respiration ....

The structure of the **respiratory** apparatus has been compared to an upside down tree, with the trunk, branches, twigs, and leaves corresponding to the trachea, bronchi, bronchioles, and alveoli.

On **inspiration,** air enters the body, eventually arriving in an alveolus. Here O_2 passes through the wall of the alveolus into the surrounding capillary as CO_2 leaves the capillary and enters the alveolus. When **expiration** occurs, CO_2 exits from the bronchial tree and is exhaled from the body. The process of getting O_2 from the nose to the alveolus and into the capillary and the return of CO_2 to the nose is known as *external respiration,* Figure 13–74(a), page 280.

At the same time, oxygen from the alveolus is circulating through the body to every cell. First the oxygen enters the capillary surrounding the alveolus, then it circulates through a venue, a vein, back to the heart, out an artery, to an arteriole, and into a capillary next to a body cell. Here the O_2 in the blood is given to the cell while CO_2 from the cell is picked up by the capillary. The exchange of O_2 and CO_2 at the cell is known as *internal respiration,* Figure 13–74(b), page 280.

Oxygen and carbon dioxide in the alveolus and the cell exchange by the process of *diffusion.* It should be remembered that materials move across a membrane from an area of higher concentration to an area of lower concentration. In the alveoli of the lung, O_2 concentra-

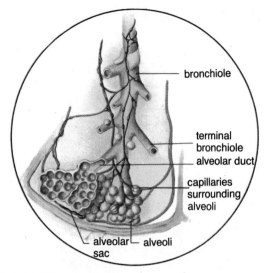

FIGURE 13–73 Alveoli (Adapted from Smith, *Medical Terminology, A Programmed Text*, 6th ed. Copyright 1991, Delmar Publishers Inc.)

tion is greater than in the surrounding capillary, so it diffuses into the blood. At the same time, CO_2 is in higher concentration in the blood than in the alveolus so it leaves the blood and enters the alveolus and is exhaled during the next respiration. At the cell the O_2 content in the capillary is greater than that within the cell, so the O_2 leaves the blood and enters the cell. On the other hand, CO_2 level within the cell is greater than in the capillary, so CO_2 diffuses out of the cell into the blood. This process of external and internal respiration is continuous throughout the life span of a person.

The Lung and the Pleura

The structures of the bronchial tree are contained in an organ known as the lung. The tissue of the lung is so filled with the alveoli that it is spongy and extremely light. It will float if placed in water. Prior to birth and breathing, the lung is solid and will sink in water. At birth, the lungs begin to fill with air, inflating the alveoli. The degree of inflation depends on the presence of surfactant, a fatty molecule on the respiratory membrane. The surfactant maintains the inflated alveolus so it does not collapse between breaths. About 2 weeks are required to completely inflate the lungs. Surfactant is not present in sufficient amounts to cause adequate inflation in premature infants and sometimes also in those born with other conditions. This results in *respiratory distress syndrome* (RDS), which is characterized by labored breathing with resulting exhaustion from the expenditure of energy required to reinflate alveoli after each breath. Many infants die each year even though current technology can supply continuous positive pressure to maintain open alveoli and therefore accomplish O_2 and CO_2 exchange. The lungs continue to mature throughout childhood, with additional alveolar formation until the

young years. It has been determined that smoking at an early age retards the maturing of the lungs and the additional alveoli are never developed.

The lung is divided into a right and left lung, Figure 13–75. The right lung has three lobes: superior, middle, and inferior. The left lung has two: superior and inferior. The heart lies on the medial surface of the left lung in a space called the *cardiac notch*. Each lung with its blood vessels and nerves is enclosed in a membrane called the visceral pleura. A membrane also lines the thoracic cavity, and is called the parietal pleura. The airtight space between the pleural membranes is known as the pleural space or cavity. It contains a lubricating fluid to prevent friction as the membranes rub together during respiration. The "space" is virtually nonexistent in healthy lungs because the lungs fill the thoracic cavity within the rib cage, pressing the visceral against the parietal pleura. However, as will be discussed later, certain conditions and diseases cause an abnormal presence or fluid or air within the pleural space.

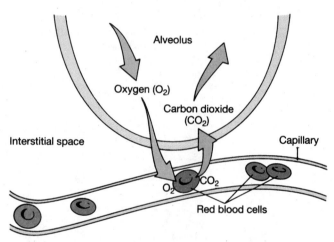

a. External respiration in the lungs

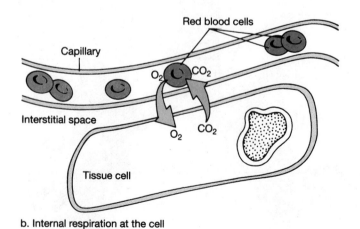

b. Internal respiration at the cell

FIGURE 13–74 Simplified external and internal respiration

The Muscles of Breathing ....

The action of the diaphragm and the muscles of the rib cage were discussed in Unit 6. It is important to remember that the lung itself is not capable of any breathing action. It is acted on primarily by the contraction of the diaphragm producing a vacuum within the thoracic cavity to draw in air. At this time there is a negative pressure within the lungs; the pressure inside is less than the atmospheric pressure outside. When the inside pressure exceeds outside atmospheric pressure, it becomes positive and causes expiration to again equalize inside/outside pressure. When the diaphragm returns to its relaxed state, air is forced out of the lungs, Figure 13–76.

Breathing action is controlled by the respiratory center in the brain. An increase of CO_2 or a lack of O_2 in the blood will trigger the center. Since we can somewhat voluntarily control breathing, it is possible to force rapid respirations and deplete the CO_2 in the blood, temporarily interrupting breathing and possibly losing consciousness. Children will occasionally hold their breath to frighten their parents and receive concessions. Usually, there is no need to be overly concerned because sooner or later a breath has to be taken. If consciousness is lost, the automatic system resumes control and breathing returns to normal.

Other situations can alter a breathing pattern for perfectly normal reasons, such as:

- Coughing—When a deep breath is taken followed by a forceful exhalation from the mouth to clear something from the lower respiratory structures.
- Hiccoughs (also spelled hiccups)—Caused by a spasm of the diaphragm and a spasmodic closure of the glottis (space between the vocal cords). It is believed to be the result of an irritation to the diaphragm or the phrenic nerve, which innervates its muscle.

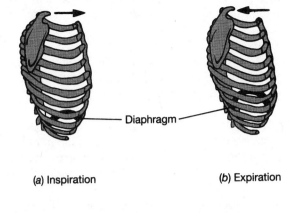

(a) Inspiration   **(b) Expiration**

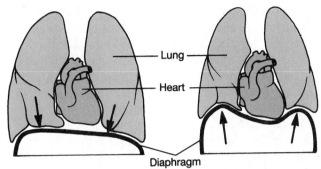

FIGURE 13–76   Position of diaphragm and ribs during inspiration (a) and expiration (b)

- Sneezing—Occurs like a cough except air is forced through the nose to clear the upper respiratory structures. Usually results from mucous membrane contact with an irritant.
- Yawning—A deep prolonged breath that fills the lungs, believe to be caused by the need to increase oxygen within the blood.
- Crying (or laughing)—Alters the breathing pattern in response to emotions.

Diagnostic Examinations ....

- Arterial blood gases—Blood taken directly from an artery to evaluate the exchange of O_2 and CO_2 in the lungs. The test measures the partial pressures of both gases and determines the pH of the blood. The PaO_2 (partial pressure of oxygen) indicates how much oxygen the lungs are delivering to the blood. The $PaCO_2$ (partial pressure of carbon dioxide) indicates how efficiently the lungs eliminate carbon dioxide. The pH determines the acid-base level, which indicates the hydrogen (H_+) ion content. If acid, there is excess hydrogen ion; alkalinity indicates a deficit. Results aid in the diagnosis and treatment of many disorders and conditions such as CNS depression from drugs or injury, hypoventilation, hyperventilation, anxiety, certain kidney diseases, and many others.

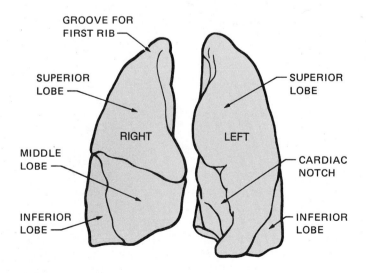

FIGURE 13–75   Anterior lung surface

- Bronchoscopy—The insertion of an instrument, the bronchoscope, into the trachea and bronchial tree to view the tissues, obtain a secretion or tissue sample, or remove a foreign body.
- Chest X ray—A radiological examination to determine the general health of lung and surrounding tissues or to identify a disease process.
- Lung perfusion scan—An examination of the lung following intravenous (IV) injection of a radioactive contrast medium to provide a visual image of pulmonary blood flow. It is useful in diagnosing blood vessel obstruction such as pulmonary emboli (foreign substance in an artery).
- Lung ventilation scan—An examination following the inhalation of a mixture of air and radioactive gas from a mask and bag. The test indicates the areas of the lung that are ventilated during respiration. It determines the distribution pattern of the gas and illustrates obstructed airways or areas of consolidation such as with pneumonia.
- Pulmonary angiography/arteriography—A radiological examination of the pulmonary circulation following the injection of a radiopaque iodine material through a catheter that is placed in the pulmonary artery or one of its branches. The catheter is inserted into a vein at the inner surface of the elbow or in the groin, and passed through the veins and through the first half of the heart into the pulmonary artery. The test aids in diagnosing pulmonary emboli, especially when the lung scan was not conclusive. It is also used to evaluate pulmonary circulation in certain heart conditions before surgery.
- Pulmonary function tests—To measure lung volume in a normal breath, lung capacity when forcing air into and out of the lungs, and other variables during a specified period of time. Many tests can be performed in a specialized hospital pulmonary laboratory; however, the most common test and one that is appropriate to the physician's office, is the spirometer to measure ventilation function. The spirograph reveals the patient's normal breathing capacity volume, the extra forced expiration volume possible, the extra forced inspiration volume possible, and the total extra forced inspiration and expiration volume possible. The total volume exchange achieved is called the vital capacity of the lung. (See Chapter 18 for additional information.)
- Pulse oximeter—The pulse oximeter is a small electronic device that fits over the end of the index finger and is connected by a wire to a machine. The device determines the amount of oxygen in the blood and displays it digitally in the window of the machine. Frequently, postoperative patients are monitored for oxygen content as are patients with cardiac and respiratory conditions. If the pulse oximeter indicates the oxygen level is too low, oxygen will be administered

at a proper amount to supplement that being circulated by the body.
- Sputum analysis—A laboratory examination of material coughed up from the bronchial tree and/or trachea. If properly prepared it can aid in the diagnosis of infectious organisms or cancer cells.
- Thoracentesis—Withdrawing of fluid from the pleural space by needle aspiration following local anesthetic, Figure 13–77. Fluid may be present as a result of excessive production or inadequate reabsorption of the pleural fluid that may be associated with cancer, tuberculosis, or a blood or lymphatic disorder. A specimen is often withdrawn for analysis to determine the presence of organisms, malignant cells, blood, or lymph fluid properties.

Disorders and Diseases

Allergic Rhinitis. A reaction to airborne allergens, causes sneezing, profuse watery nasal discharge, itching of the eyes and nose, red and swollen eyelids, and nasal congestion. Allergic rhinitis may be seasonal, as with hay fever, or perennial, caused by house dust, mold, cigarette smoke, and the like.

Treatment consists primarily of administering antihistamines and avoiding the allergens. The use of air conditioning filters allergens, keeps down dust, and removes excess moisture from the air. The use of steroid nasal sprays may also be helpful. Desensitizing injections of the allergens before or during the season is indicated for long-term management. In severe or persistent cases, it may be necessary to relocate to a relatively pollen-free environment.

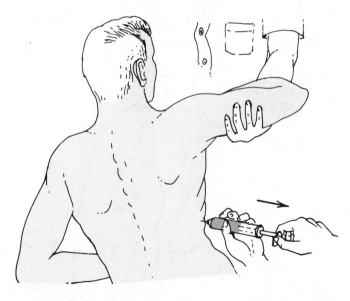

FIGURE 13–77 Thoracentesis. Fluid is being removed from the pleural cavity (From Burke, *Human Anatomy and Physiology for the Health Sciences*, 3d ed. Copyright 1992, Delmar Publishers Inc.)

Asthma. This chronic allergic disorder results from sensitivity to allergens such as pollen, dust, animal dander, certain foods, and a number of other substances. It can also develop from an infectious process or from unknown causes. Asthma is characterized by bronchospasms, which narrow the bronchioles, increased mucus secretions that block passageways of air, and edema of the mucosal lining. These reactions decrease the lung's capacity to exchange air. Symptoms usually occur as a sudden onset of wheezing, dyspnea, and tightness of the chest. They are often accompanied by coughing and expectoration of thick sputum. The patient may become frightened and experience feelings of suffocation to the point that speech is nearly impossible. The symptoms of airway obstruction may be present to some extent between acute attacks.

Determination of the offending allergens is usually accomplished with a series of skin tests. Minute amounts of the most common causative agents are introduced just below the skin by a needle prick or applied as patches to the skin surface. The presence of a reddened area about a site after a specified amount of time is evidence of sensitivity.

The treatment of choice for asthma is prevention by eliminating allergens. However, this is not always possible. Desensitization to specific allergens through injections may be helpful. During attacks, limited inhalation of specific bronchodilating drugs and administration of epinephrine, followed by corticosteroids, should alleviate symptoms. With severe attacks, O_2 administered at approximately 2 liters per minute helps to ease breathing and increase O_2 within the arteries.

Atelectasis. The lack of air in the lungs due to the collapse of the microscopic structures of the lung; atelectasis may occur following abdominal or thoracic surgery or with pressure from pleural effusion (fluid, air, pus, blood, or lymph) in the pleural cavity. It can be chronic, caused by mucous plugs in the bronchial tree in patients with cystic fibrosis and obstructive pulmonary disease and in heavy smokers. Bronchial occlusion can also result from cancer or inflamed tissues. Acute (sudden) atelectasis may occur with any condition that causes pain on deep breathing such as rib fractures, traumatic injury, surgical procedures, or pleurisy.

Chronic Obstructive Pulmonary Disease (COPD). A condition characterized by chronic obstruction of the airways resulting from emphysema, chronic bronchitis, asthma, or any combination of these disorders. Usually, there is more than one condition, most often a combination of bronchitis and emphysema.

Bronchitis is an inflammation of the bronchial walls with distortion and narrowing of the airways. The presence of mucus results in a productive cough and dyspnea on exertion. Bronchitis can be an acute disease, caused by an infection, or a chronic disease, caused by damaged cilia, enlarged mucous glands, and chronic inflammation. The severity of chronic bronchitis is related to the amount and duration of smoking. Wheezing and prolonged expiration time may be observed.

Acute bronchitis is managed with antibiotics to treat the infection, expectorants to help remove excessive mucus, and avoiding smoking. Chronic bronchitis also requires bronchodilators, respiratory therapy to loosen mucous secretions, and corticosteroids in some cases. Adequate fluid intake is important.

Emphysema is an irreversible enlargement of the air spaces in the lungs due to destruction of the alveoli wall. Emphysema results in the inability to exchange O_2 and CO_2 in the affected areas and to exhale stale air from the lungs. Symptoms include a chronic cough, weight loss, barrel chest, the use of accessory muscles to breathe, prolonged expiration, rapid pursed-lip breathing, cyanosis, and, eventually, respiratory failure and death. Treatment and control are the same as those for COPD.

The incidence of COPD is increasing. Until recently, it occurred most often in men, primarily due to their heavier smoking habits. With increased use of tobacco by women, the difference is decreasing. Other causes of chronic obstructive pulmonary disease are chronic respiratory infections and allergies. However, smoking is the most important factor because it impairs ciliary action, causes inflammation in airways, destroys alveolar walls, and results in peribronchiolar fibrosis (formation of scar tissue around the bronchioles).

COPD is a progressive disease; symptoms occur gradually and become worse with age. Initially there is a productive cough and a decline in the ability to exercise. As the disease progresses, the individual becomes dyspnic with minimal exertion, has frequent respiratory infections, develops thoracic deformities (usually barrel chest from muscular changes caused by attempting to breathe), suffers severe respiratory failure and hypoxemia (insufficient O_2 in the blood), and eventually dies.

Treatment consists of methods to halt the progression of the disease and control its present state. Damaged structures cannot be restored. Prime emphasis is placed on avoiding smoking and other respiratory irritants. In addition, the use of bronchodilators, prompt treatment of respiratory infections, effective breathing and coughing instructions, proper diet, and the use of O_2 are indicated. The most important factor in prevention is *not* smoking.

Epistaxis (Nosebleed). (See Unit 3.) Nosebleeds usually follow injury, either external or internal, such as a blow to the nose, nosepicking, or foreign body insertion. Less frequent causes of epistaxis are chronic conditions such as nasal or sinus infection that results in capillary congestion and bleeding, or the inhalation of irritating substances. Predisposing systemic factors include high blood pressure, anticoagulation drugs, chronic aspirin use, and blood diseases such as anemia, hemophilia, and leukemia.

Treatment varies depending on the cause, location, and severity. Even moderate bleeding is considered severe if it persists longer than 10 minutes after pressure is applied. Symptoms may include lightheadedness, a drop in blood pressure, rapid pulse, dyspnea, pallor, and other indications of shock. Initial first aid treatment may consist of: elevating the head; compressing nostrils against the septum continuously for 5 to 10 minutes; applying ice or cold compresses to nose and back of neck; preventing the swallowing of blood (to determine the amount lost); avoiding talking or blowing the nose; and observing for amount of blood loss and signs of shock.

Advanced treatment includes: for anterior bleeding, applying epinephrine-saturated cotton ball or gauze to the bleeding site and the use of external pressure, followed by cauterization by electric cautery or silver nitrate; for posterior bleeding, the insertion of a nasal pack for 48 to 72 hours may be required. If necessary, anterior bleeding can be treated by packing for 24 to 48 hours. Other treatment may include supplemental vitamin K, blood transfusions, and surgical ligation (tying) of the bleeding artery.

Histoplasmosis. A fungal infection, occurring worldwide, histoplasmosis is caused by an organism found in droppings from birds or bats, or in soil near their roosts, as in barns, caves, chicken coops, around buildings, and under bridges. It has also been determined to come from cat feces due to ingested birds.

In the United States, histoplasmosis occurs in three forms: primary acute, progressive disseminated, and chronic pulmonary. Symptoms vary with the form contracted. The primary acute resembles a severe cold. The progressive involves the liver, spleen, and lymph glands, and may cause inflammation of the heart muscle and the pericardium (covering membrane), as well as the meninges of the brain and spinal cord. The chronic form resembles tuberculosis, causing a productive cough, dyspnea, weakness, and cyanosis.

Hyaline Membrane Disease (HMD). This condition results from immature alveolar and bronchiolar development and a weak intercostal musculature in premature infants (before week 37 of gestation). If untreated, 14% of infants weighing less than 5.5 pounds will die within 72 hours. Incidence in the United States alone is 40,000 newborn deaths per year. Hyaline membrane disease occurs more frequently in infants born to diabetic or smoking mothers and those delivered by cesarean section or whose birth is precipitated by hemorrhage.

HMD causes respiratory distress due to the collapse of the alveoli and the immature capillary system resulting in an inadequate oxygen supply. Frequently the infant breathes normally at first, but as the collapse progresses, respirations become rapid and shallow. The intercostal muscles and the sternum retract, and the nostrils flare, providing evidence of increased breathing difficulty. A characteristic "grunting" on expiration can be heard. With progression the heart rate decreases and respirations stop. Low body temperature, due to inadequate body fat, and an immature nervous system add to the difficulties.

Aggressive treatment is required, preferably in a neonatal intensive care unit. Heat is supplemented by an isolette and O_2 is supplied as needed. Fluids are given intravenously or directly by catheter into the stomach, when the infant is too weak to eat. A few of the infants who survive will still have abnormally developed bronchopulmonary tissue.

Influenza (flu). This acute, highly contagious respiratory infection usually occurs in colder months and in infrequent epidemics (widespread incidence, not of local origin). It is more prevalent in school children aged 6 to 14 and adults over age 40. Influenza can be fatal to the elderly or people with chronic heart, lung, or kidney disease. The disease is directly transmitted by droplets inhaled from an infected person's sneezing or coughing, or by indirect contact with contaminated objects such as a drinking glass. Influenza viruses have the ability to alter their influence on the population. As people develop immunity to a virus after having contact with it, the virus alters its composition and a new strain results to which people have little or no resistance. Hence an epidemic or pandemic (present in many areas of the world at the same time) develops.

Influenza viruses are classified into three types:

■ Type A—the most lethal, occurring every 2 to 3 years with a major new strain developing every 10 to 15 years
■ Type B—occurring every 4 to 6 years resulting in epidemics
■ Type C—endemic (of local origin) and causing infrequent cases.

Symptoms of flu are the sudden onset of chills and a fever of 101° to 104°F (38° to 40°C), headaches, muscle aches, a nonproductive cough, and rhinitis. Pneumonia is the most common complication, developing 3 to 5 days after infection begins.

Treatment consists of bed rest, adequate fluid intake, and aspirin or similar medication to relieve the pain and fever. Antibiotics have no effect on the virus and should not be used except for secondary bacterial infection. Flu immunizations, which provide protection for 3 to 6 months, are recommended for the high-risk population. However, the vaccine is only 75% effective because the serum is determined by the previous year's strain.

Laryngectomy. This is surgical removal of the larynx, usually the result of cancer caused by smoking. The earliest symptom of internal disease of the larynx is persistent hoarseness. With involvement externally, it is a lump in the throat or pain, or burning when drinking hot liquids or citrus juices.

Diagnosis can often be made by viewing with a laryngoscope. This examination is often followed with radio-

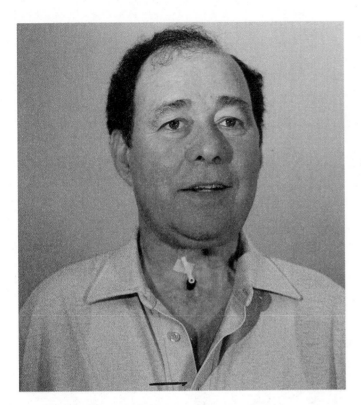

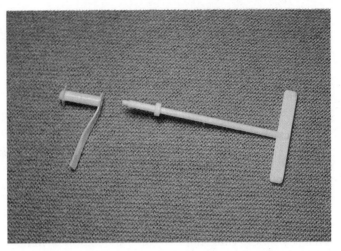

FIGURE 13–78 Laryngeal stoma (a) with voice prosthesis and (b) inserter, following laryngectomy

logical studies to confirm. With positive diagnosis, the larynx may be partially or totally removed. With total removal, a permanent opening called a stoma is made in the neck through which air can be taken in and exhaled, Figure 13–78. Coughing results in material being expelled through the stoma.

A great deal of patient support is necessary to assist in developing alternative methods of communication prior to surgery. The patient may need psychiatric assistance to cope with the loss of speech, sense of smell, ability to blow the nose, and related problems. Much support can be obtained from organizations established to aid in rehabilitation of laryngectomy patients. Local chapters of the "Lost Chord Club," made up of persons who have lost their larynx, volunteer their services to speak with new patients and help them learn techniques of producing speech. The American Cancer Society and the International Association of Laryngectomies also provide assistance with speech methods which use esophageal air that is swallowed and released slowly, the artificial larynx, and other mechanical devices.

The individual in Figure 13–78 has a voice prosthesis inserted into the stoma. By placing his finger over the opening in the prosthesis, he is able to produce a good quality of speech. A "patch" of thin foam is placed over the opening to prevent inhaling foreign materials. The foam is porous and permits easy exchange of air.

Laryngitis. This inflammation of the vocal cords occurs in both acute and chronic forms. Acute laryngitis usually results from an infectious process, excessive use of the voice, inhalation of smoke or fumes, or accidental aspiration of chemicals. Chronic laryngitis develops from other preexistent chronic conditions such as sinusitis, bronchitis, and allergies or from smoking, abuse of alcohol, and continual exposure to irritants.

Laryngitis is treated by resting the voice, using medication for underlying infection, if present, and eliminating coexistent causes (in the case of chronic laryngitis).

Legionnaires' Disease. This acute bronchopneumonia derived its name from a highly publicized incident in which 182 people developed the disease at an American Legion Convention in Philadelphia in 1976. Legionnaires' disease usually occurs in late summer or early fall.

The bacillus is probably transmitted through the air. In past epidemics, it was spread through air conditioning systems and cooling towers. It does not spread person to person. Symptoms include nonspecific signs such as diarrhea, lack of appetite, headache, chills, weakness, and an unremitting fever that develops within 12 to 48 hours. Temperature may reach 105° F (40.5° C). A cough then develops, which becomes productive, with grayish sputum. Other symptoms are nausea, vomiting, confusion, dyspnea, chest pain, and, in 50% of the patients, a slow pulse rate. Severe symptoms are evidence of complications and include low blood pressure, irregular heart beat, respiratory failure, kidney failure, and shock (which is usually fatal). Smokers are three to four times more likely to develop Legionnaires' disease than nonsmokers.

Treatment consists of antibiotics, medication to reduce the fever, maintaining fluid balance, and measures to support adequate respiration, such as oxygen and mechanical ventilation by inhalation therapy.

Lung Cancer. This is the leading cause of cancer deaths among men and increasingly prevalent in women, despite the fact that it is largely preventable. It is attributed to inhalation of carcinogens in tobacco and the environment. The inhalation of carcinogens causes a progressive destruction of the cells in the lungs. There is a correlation between the risk of cancer and the number of cigarettes smoked daily, the depth of inhalation, the age at which smoking began, and the nicotine content of the tobacco. An individual over 40 who began smoking as a teenager and has averaged a pack a day for at least 20 years is most susceptible. Lung cancer can take 20 to 30 years to develop. An estimated 85% of lung cancer in men and 75% in women is caused by cigarette smoking. Less than 10% of lung cancers occur among nonsmokers.

Other inhalants that increase *susceptibility* are industrial air pollutants such as asbestos, arsenic, iron oxides, chromium, radioactive dust, vinyl chloride, and coal dust. There also is an indication that there is a familial tendency link to lung cancer. The combination of industrial pollutants and cigarettes is very risky. For example, asbestos workers who also smoke increase their risk of developing lung cancer by 60 times.

Involuntary smoking, that which the nonsmoker gets "second hand" from a spouse or others, though less concentrated, still contains the same harmful substances. For example, wives exposed to husbands who smoke 20 or more cigarettes a day at home, have double the risk of lung cancer when compared to wives of nonsmokers. Children of smoking parents are also affected. They are more prone to respiratory infections and more likely to develop lung diseases later in life.

The prognosis for lung cancer patients is very poor, because by the time a diagnosis is made, two-thirds of the patients have passed the stage where it might be curable. Only 13% of all lung cancer patients (all races and all stages) live 5 or more years after diagnosis. This is primarily due to delayed diagnosis because of lack of symptoms. The first indication of squamous or oat cell carcinoma is a smoker's cough, wheezing, dyspnea, and hemoptysis (spitting of blood). If the carcinoma is anaplastic or adenocarcinoma, the symptoms are fever, weakness, weight loss, and anorexia. The disease metastasizes to many other sites within the thoracic cavity and throughout the entire body.

Treatment consists primarily of surgical excision when appropriate, radiation, and chemotherapy. Usually since the disease is advanced before treatment begins, little more than temporary reduction in symptoms and discomfort is expected. The best treatment is obviously prevention. Quitting smoking or never starting is the best defense against lung cancer.

Figure 13–79 is a reprint of a brochure distributed by the American Cancer Society that illustrates the effects of emphysema and cancer on the tissues of the lung.

Pleurisy. An inflammation of the visceral and parietal pleura in the thoracic cavity, **pleurisy** develops as a complication of pneumonia, tuberculosis, chest injury, and other factors. Sharp, stabbing pain is experienced on respiration due to irritation of the pleural nerve endings as the lungs move, rubbing against the inner chest wall.

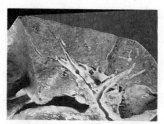
NORMAL LUNG

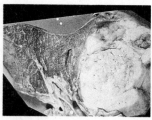
CANCER

The lung is our breathing machine. It draws in air, filters it, separates out life-giving oxygen for the body's use and expels what is left over—mostly carbon dioxide. The normal adult lung is about the size of a football.

When we inhale, air enters the lung through tubes, or passageways, called bronchi. These bronchi are lined with vibrating hairlike structures called cilia, which whip back and forth some 900 times a miunute, to help keep solid pollutants in the air from entering the lung. The air is carried down through smaller and smal-ler bronchi until it reaches tiny air sacs which are uniform in size. This is where the oxygen/carbon dioxide exchange takes place.

Unfortunately, damage to the lung often takes place before there are any symptoms.

Cancer ravages the lungs with an army of wildly multiplying cells. It begins most often with the constant irritation of the lining of the bronchi by cigarette smoke.

Under the onslaught of this irritation, the hairlike cilia which filter the air we breathe disappear from the lining of the bronchi. Although extra mucus is secreted to substitute for the cilia and trap pollutants, this mucus itself becomes a problem. It remains trapped until finally forced out of the lung by a "smoker's cough."

If a smoker quits before cancerous lesions are present, the bronchial lining will return to normal. If not, the abnormal cell growth spreads, blocking the bronchi and then invading the lung tissue itself.

In the latter stages of lung cancer, abnormal cells break away from the lung and are carried by the lymphatic system to other vital organs, where new cancers begin.

Because lung cancer is difficult to detect early, it is very difficult to treat successfully. It is often fatal. Yet if no one smoked cigarettes, 83% of lung cancers would eventually disappear.

Research now shows that even involuntary smoking exposures result in enough inhaling of smoke to increase the risk of developing lung cancer as well as other respiratory illnesses and risk to the fetus during pregnancy. A new study found that women exposed to husbands who smoked 20 or more cigarettes a day at home had double the risk of lung cancer compared to women married to nonsmokers.

It has been said that if the effects of cigarette smoking appeared on our skin instead of in our lungs—where it can't be seen—no one would smoke. Now you have seen the ugly inside story.

Call your local Unit of the American Cancer Society for information on how to quit smoking.

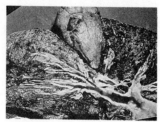
EMPHYSEMA

Emphysema is a disease which destroys the lung's elasticity, and therefore its ability to inhale and exhale properly.

Tissue affected by emphysema can never be repaired or replaced and the disease, progressing slowly but steadily, turns its victims into respiratory cripples. Patients spend years gasping for breath, and when death comes, it frequently is due to an overworked heart.

Emphysema changes the lung's normal appearance. Some of the air sacs burst and collapse, creating tiny craters in the lung, while others balloon in the body's desperate struggle to obtain oxygen and expel carbon dioxide.

Emphysema used to be a relatively rare disease, but today it is becoming increasingly common. It has been stongly associated with the cigarette habit because of the intense air pollution caused by cigarette smoke in the lungs.

AMERICAN CANCER SOCIETY®

FIGURE 13–79 Normal and diseased lung tissue (Courtesy of American Cancer Society)

As a result, lung movement on the affected side may be limited and dyspnea occurs.

Treatment is generally symptomatic, with bed rest and medications to reduce the inflammation and relieve the pain. Some physicians may partially immobilize the chest with a restrictive support to lessen movement of the chest wall and reduce friction. If fluid collects within the pleural space, a thoracentesis is indicated to prohibit lung compression by the fluid or to determine, by laboratory examination, a causative agent (see Figure 13–77).

Paroxysmal Nocturnal Dyspnea (PND). This symptom, associated with chronic lung disease or left ventricular failure (heart disease), occurs at night. Individuals awaken from sleep with a feeling of suffocation. They often run to open a window and gasp for air. Just sitting upright will help some people due to the effect of gravity on fluid in the lungs. The episode will resolve itself usually within a few minutes.

Pleural Effusion. This presence of excess fluid in the pleural space can result from overproduction or inadequate reabsorption of the pleural fluid. Some effusions result from chronic diseases such as congestive heart failure, liver disease, tuberculosis, malignancy, lupus erythematosus, and rheumatoid arthritis. When the effusion becomes symptomatic, depressing lung tissue and reducing the lungs' ability to exchange O_2 for CO_2, resulting in hypoxia (lack of O_2), oxygen will be administered to increase concentration to the remainder of the lung. If the fluid is a result of an infectious process, exudate (pus) and dead tissue will be present and the effusion is known as empyema. Drainage of the material by thoracentesis and insertion of chest tubes may be necessary. Antibiotics are required to destroy the causative organism. Effusion that contains blood is called a hemothorax and will require drainage to prevent fibrothorax (scar tissue) formation.

Pneumoconiosis. These are lung diseases developed after years of contact with environmental or occupational causative agents. Basically, there are three types of pneumoconiosis. One form, *silicosis,* occurs from exposure to silica sand dust in occupations such as sand blaster and foundry worker, in manufacturing of ceramic and sandstone products and construction materials, and in mining of gold, lead, zinc, and iron. Nodules develop where specific disease-fighting cells have ingested the silica particles but then been unable to dispose of the ingested material. The cells die, causing the release of an enzyme that attracts more cells to assist in destroying the invading material. A fibrous (scar) tissue results and the process continues until large areas of the lung tissue are destroyed.

Another form, *asbestosis,* can develop 15 to 20 years after regular exposure to asbestos has ended. Asbestosis is most prevalent in the construction, fireproofing, and textile industries, and in brake and automotive occupations dealing with clutch linings. The general public may also develop the condition from exposure to fibrous dust or the waste piles of asbestos factories. Asbestosis is the result of inhaling minute asbestos fibers, which enter the bronchioles and penetrate the alveolar walls. The fibers become encased and fibrosis of the lung tissue develops, obliterating the air passages. Fibers also cause fibrotic changes in the parietal pleura.

A third type, coal worker's or *black lung disease,* is a progressive nodular form resulting from exposure to coal dust. It is found in two forms: simple, which produces small lung lesions, or complicated, which produces masses of fibrous tissue. The development usually occurs after 15 years or more of exposure and depends to some extent on the amount of dust, the type of coal mined, the silica content, and the location of the mine.

Initially, the body's fighting cells ingest the dust and become filled, forming macules in the terminal bronchioles, which are surrounded by dilated alveoli. The supporting tissue atrophies (wastes away), resulting in permanent dilation of the small airways. When the disease changes from a simple to a complicated form, one or both lungs can become involved. The fibrous tissue masses enlarge, causing destruction of the alveoli and airways.

Treatment of all types is essentially the same: avoiding respiratory infections, use of bronchodilators to aid in respiration, chest vibration, oxygen supplement, and other respiratory therapy to improve removal of bronchial secretions.

Pneumonia. This is an acute infection of the principal tissues of the lungs, which may impair the exchange of O_2 and CO_2. Chances for recovery from pneumonia are good for persons with normal lungs, but pneumonia is the fifth leading cause of death in debilitated (weakened) patients.

Pneumonia is classified in several ways: by microbiological origin (bacterium, virus, fungus, protozoan, etc.); by location (bronchus, lobar, or lobular); or by type (primary, caused by inhaled pathogens, or secondary, following lung damage by an inhaled chemical or by an infection spread from another area of the body).

Pneumonia often occurs with chronic weakening illnesses, such as cancer, or after surgery. It is also associated with malnutrition, smoking, COPD, age, and with a decreased level of consciousness. Symptoms range from coughing, sputum production, and pleural chest pain to chills and fever. Treatment consists of bed rest, an appropriate antibiotic, adequate fluid intake, respiratory support measures such as oxygen or mechanical breathing therapy and medication for pain.

Pneumothorax. In this condition air or gas has accumulated between the parietal and visceral pleurae, causing some degree of collapse of the lung tissue. If it is spontaneous, air has leaked from the lung tissue as the result of a disease process or a ruptured blisterlike lesion. A traumatic pneumothorax results from a penetrating chest wound, as by a knife or gunshot, from thoracic surgery, or from the insertion of tubing into the blood vessels of the chest. Fractured ribs can penetrate the thorax causing collapse of the lung. Since the atmospheric pressure outside is greater than that within the pleural cavity, it compresses the lung tissue as it enters. Frequently blood is also present with an injury and, if located between the pleura, it is referred to as a hemothorax.

In tension pneumothorax, air enters the pleural space as the result of trauma but is unable to leave by the same route. Each inspiration results in additional trapped air being sucked in. Eventually, pressure is exerted against the large chest veins, interfering with blood flow returning to the heart. If severe, the great vessels of the chest and the heart may be pushed toward the uninjured side of the chest.

The primary symptoms of pneumothorax are sudden, sharp pain made worse by breathing or coughing, unequal chest wall movement, shortness of breath, and cyanosis. As the degree of collapse increases, respirations become more stressful, the pulse becomes rapid and weak, and the patient becomes pale. Death may result without prompt treatment.

Treatment varies with the degree of collapse. If it is spontaneous, with 30% or less involvement and no dyspnea or apparent sign of increasing difficulty, it may be treated with bed rest, careful monitoring of vital signs, and perhaps needle aspiration of the air mass. With greater than 30% collapse, the lung is slowly reexpanded by low suction through a tube inserted into the chest. If there is evidence of trauma, the tissue must be repaired, the chest closed, and the wound drained by means of chest tubes.

Pulmonary Edema.

Accumulation within the tissues of the lungs of fluid that has escaped from the blood vessels due to increased pressure, pulmonary edema is common with heart disorders causing left ventricular failure. Symptoms include dyspnea on exertion, coughing, orthopnea (ability to breathe only in an upright position), and rapid pulse and respiration. With progression, respirations become more labored, noisy, and rapid. A cough that produces frothy, bloody sputum may develop. As the condition worsens, the patient becomes cold, clammy, and cyanotic. Confusion and a depressed level of consciousness occur in cases of severe heart failure.

Treatment consists of procedures to decrease the accumulated fluids and improve the exchange of O_2 and CO_2. Diuretics (water pills) bronchodilators, and high concentrations of oxygen may be indicated.

Pulmonary Embolism.

Obstruction of a pulmonary artery or arteriole by a circulating thrombus (blood clot) or another substance such as air, purulent matter, or fatty material is called a pulmonary embolism. The obstruction causes dyspnea, chest pain, rapid heart rate, a productive cough, and a low-grade fever. The symptoms vary with the extent of obstruction. In massive embolism, with over 50% obstruction of arterial circulation, death occurs rapidly.

Predisposing factors include long-term immobility, which permits slow-moving blood to clot within the vessels, varicose veins, surgery, pregnancy, vascular injury, obesity, fractures, and many chronic pulmonary and circulatory diseases.

Treatment consists of measures to maintain adequate heart and lung function while the obstruction is being resolved, usually within 10 to 14 days. Medication is given to inhibit the blood from forming additional clots, as well as break up the present occlusion. Supportive oxygen therapy is used as needed. If the embolus is caused by purulent material from an infectious process, then aggressive antibiotic therapy is indicated.

Sinusitis.

Inflammation of the paranasal sinus cavities, sinusitis, usually results from the common cold organism or chronically from persistent bacterial infection. Symptoms include nasal congestion, low-grade fever, headache pain over cheeks and upper teeth, pain over eyes or eyebrows, and a nonproductive cough. Treatment consists of analgesics for pain, medication to decrease secretions, steam inhalations to encourage drainage, and application of heat to relieve pain and congestion. Surgical drainage of the affected sinus cavity may be necessary in persistent, severe conditions.

Sudden Infant Death Syndrome (SIDS).

This is a mysterious condition that kills apparently healthy infants between the ages of 4 weeks and 7 months. It is unexplainable even after autopsy. Sudden infant death syndrome kills 6000 to 7000 infants annually in the United States. It occurs more frequently in winter, in poorer families, to mothers under 20, and among underweight babies. Study of the syndrome suggests that the infant may have had undetected respiratory dysfunctions which caused prolonged periods of apnea (absence of breathing), resulting in extreme hypoxemia (lack of oxygen in the blood), and serious irregular heartbeat.

Diagnosis of SIDS requires an autopsy to rule out other causes of death. Several characteristics of the syndrome confirm the diagnosis. Parents need a great deal of support to deal with the death, as they often feel they were somehow to blame. There is a National Sudden Infant Death Foundation with local chapters of parents whose babies have died of the syndrome. Many local health organizations provide counseling and information services. These resources can be of great assistance.

Tuberculosis (TB).

An acute or chronic infection causing nodular lesions and patchy infiltration of the lung tissue is known as tuberculosis. The body reacts to the invading causative organism by converting the destroyed tissue into a cheeselike material. This material may localize and become fibrotic or it may develop into cavities within the lung tissue. The cavities are filled with the multiplying bacilli and the infected debris spreads throughout the tracheobronchial tree.

On initial contact with the tubercular bacillus, most people's immune defense system kills the organism or walls it off in a nodule. These dormant organisms may become active later causing an acute phase.

Symptoms of primary infection include fatigue, weakness, lack of appetite, weight loss, night sweats, and low-grade fever. On reactivation, symptoms may include a productive cough characterized by purulent mucus, occasionally mixed with blood, and chest pains.

Treatment consists of isolation until the contagious phase has passed. Care must be taken in handling the nasal and expectorated discharges. Bed rest and an adequate diet are very important. Medication specifically for TB must be continued for a year or more to effect a cure. After 2 to 4 weeks, the disease is no longer infectious and the person can resume a normal life-style.

Upper Respiratory Infection (URI). This term is used to refer to symptoms associated with the common cold. An **upper respiratory infection** may be caused by several different viruses and be transmitted by respiratory droplets, contaminated objects, or hands. Children are the main transmitters of the organism. The disease is usually self-limiting after a 1- to 4-day incubation period. It is characterized by sore throat, nasal congestion, headache, burning and watery eyes, fever, and general lethargy. A cough may be present, which is nonproductive and hacking, often at night. Symptoms usually persist for a week before subsiding. Secondary bacterial infections affecting the lower respiratory tract are uncommon.

Complete Chapter 13, Unit 7 in the workbook to help you meet the objectives at the beginning of this unit and therefore achieve competency of this subject matter.

U N I T 8

The Circulatory System

OBJECTIVES

Upon completion of this unit, the student will meet the following terminal performance objectives by verifying knowledge of the facts and principles presented through oral and written communication at a level deemed competent.

1. Name the four main parts of the circulatory system.
2. Describe the anatomy of the heart, identifying the internal and external structures.
3. Differentiate between pulmonary, systemic, and portal circulation.
4. Describe the heart sounds, including the actions producing the sounds and where they can be ausculated.
5. Locate the pacemaker, explain its action, and tell how the heart rate is influenced by the body.
6. Explain how the cardiac conditions of heart block and fibrillation relate to the pacemaker.
7. Explain the purpose of an artificial pacemaker and how it functions.
8. Name the five types of blood vessels and their purpose and structure.
9. Describe the function of a capillary bed.
10. Trace the pathway of blood through the pulmonary and systemic circulation.
11. Explain the function and structure of the lymphatic system.
12. Name the components of whole blood and the role of each.
13. Describe the clotting process.
14. Name the blood types and explain their importance to recipients of transfusions.
15. Explain the importance of the Rh factor in pregnancy and transfusions.
16. Identify eight cardiovascular tests and the reasons for giving them.
17. Describe 25 diseases or disorders of the circulatory system.
18. Spell and define, using the glossary at the back of the text, all the words to know in this unit.

WORDS TO KNOW

accelerator	leukemia
adenitis	leukocyte
ambulate	lubb dupp
anemia	lymph
aneurysm	lymphatic system
angina	lymphocyte
angioplasty	metastasize
anticoagulant	mitral
aorta	MUGA scan
arrhythmias	murmur
arterioles	myocardial infarction (MI)
arteriosclerosis	myocardium
artery	nodes
atherosclerosis	pacemaker
atrium	papillary muscles
AV node	pericardium
bicuspid	phlebitis
bradycardia	plasma
capillary	platelet
cardiac	portal
cardiovascular	Rh factor
cerebrovascular accident	SA node
compatible	semilunar
congestive heart failure	septum
coronary	sickle cell
cross-match	spleen
diastole	stasis ulcer
electrocardiograph (ECG)	systole
embolism	tachycardia
endocardium	thrombophlebitis
erythrocyte	thrombosis
exudate	transfusion
fibrillation	transient ischemic attack
heart block	tricuspid
hemoglobin	vagus
hemorrhage	valve
Holter monitor	varicose
hypertension	vein
hypotension	vena cava
infarction	ventricle
ischemia	venule

The circulatory system transports oxygen and nutrients to the body's cells and carbon dioxide and other waste products from the cells, to be eliminated from the body. The blood, which flows through a closed circuit of vessels, is the transportation vehicle. A very efficient muscle, the heart, is the force behind the system. A few minutes' interruption of the circulatory system can result in death.

The circulatory system is composed of four main parts: (1) a pump, the heart; (2) the plumbing, the blood vessels; (3) the circulating fluid, the blood; and (4) an auxiliary fluid system, the lymphatic system. Each day the heart pumps the equivalent of 4000 gallons of blood, at 40 miles per hour, through an estimated 70,000 miles of blood vessels. To achieve this, the heart must forcefully contract, squeezing out blood, at an average rate of 72 times per minute, or about 100,000 times each day. In a year's time, the heart will contract 40 million times, resting only a fraction of a second between beats. To appreciate this phenomenal organ, alternately open and close your fist a little more often than once a second for just one minute by the clock. You will notice that not only your hand but also your forearm muscles begin to tire. Scientists have estimated that the work of the heart is about equal to the energy needed to lift a 10-pound weight 3 feet off the floor twice a minute for a lifetime. The condition of the blood vessels and the composition of the blood are major factors in the amount of force the heart must exert to circulate the blood.

The Heart ....

The heart is about the size of a clenched fist and is located behind the sternum, between the lungs, with two-thirds of it on the left side of the chest. It is constructed of several layers of muscles arranged in both circular and spiral fashion. When the muscles contract, blood is squeezed out of the heart chambers. During the relaxation phase, the heart fills with blood entering from the great veins. There is a considerable difference in the size of the heart during the phases, as shown in Figure 13–80.

The contraction phase is known as systole and the relaxation phase is called diastole. Systole is the period when the heart exerts the greatest pressure on the blood. This corresponds to the beat phase of the heart and can be heard over the heart with a stethoscope or felt as the pulse in an artery. The systolic pressure can be determined by measurement with blood pressure equipment and is represented by the larger or top number of the blood pressure reading. Diastole is the period of least pressure and is the time when the heart rests. This phase cannot be felt as a beat, but the diastolic pressure can be heard and determined by measurement. It is represented by the smaller or bottom number of the blood pressure reading.

External Heart Structures

The outer wall of the heart is surrounded by a sac called the pericardium. Like the pleura of the lungs, the pericardium has one layer called the parietal, which lines the sac, and another layer, the visceral, which covers the

heart itself. The pericardial fluid between the layers prevents friction when the heart beats. The heart structure does not receive its blood supply from the blood pumped through its interior, but from a number of small blood vessels which cover the surface of the heart, Figure 13–81. These blood vessels, called the coronary arteries and veins, carry oxygen, nutrients, and waste products to and from the heart muscle. The right and left coronary arteries enter the top of the heart from the aorta. Blood from the coronary veins returns to the right atrium by a small opening called the coronary sinus.

The muscle wall of the heart is called the myocardium. The wall of the left lower chamber is thicker because it must pump blood through the entire general or systemic circulation, as discussed later.

Internal Heart Structures

A tissue known as endocardium lines the interior surface of the heart, Figure 13–82, page 292. The lining also covers the heart valves and the interior surface of the blood vessels to allow for the smooth flow of blood. Internally, the heart is a double pump, divided into a right and left side by a muscular wall called a septum. The septum prevents the blood on the right side from mixing with that on the left. The sides are further divided into upper and lower chambers. The right upper chamber is called the right atrium, the lower, the right ventricle. The left side is similarly divided into a left atrium and left ventricle.

The chambers are separated by one-way valves which keep the blood flowing in the right direction. The tricus-

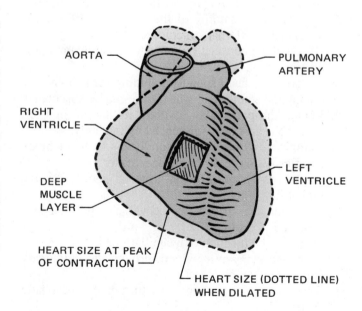

FIGURE 13–80 Heart size during contraction and filling actions (From *The Wonderful Human Machine*, copyright 1979, American Medical Association)

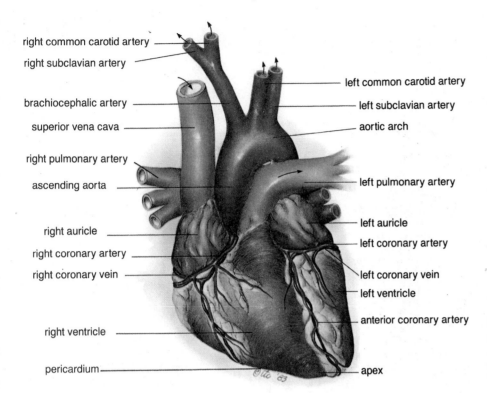

right common carotid artery

right subclavian artery

brachiocephalic artery

superior vena cava

right pulmonary artery

ascending aorta

right auricle

right coronary artery

right coronary vein

right ventricle

pericardium

left common carotid artery

left subclavian artery

aortic arch

left pulmonary artery

left auricle

left coronary artery

left coronary vein

left ventricle

anterior coronary artery

apex

FIGURE 13–81 External heart structures (From Smith, *Medical Terminology, A Programmed Text*, 6th ed. Copyright 1991, Delmar Publishers Inc.)

pid valve is between the right atrium and ventricle, and the **bicuspid** or **mitral** valve is between the left atrium and ventricle. **Papillary muscles** are attached by cords to the undersurfaces of the valve cusps or leaflets. When the atria contract, the papillary muscles also contract to pull open the valves, allowing the blood from the atria to enter the empty ventricles. Then the muscles relax, which allows the valves to close as the atria refill. The closed valves prevent the blood from reentering the atria when the ventricles contract.

At the contraction of the ventricles, blood is forced out to the great arteries of the body. The right ventricle sends the blood through a **semilunar** valve into the pulmonary artery on its way through the pulmonary circulation in the lungs for a supply of oxygen. The left ventricle forces the blood past a semilunar valve into the aorta to be distributed throughout the general or systemic circulation of the body.

A specific sequence of events occurs within the body as the blood is circulated. Blood flow occurs in two distinct patterns, *pulmonary circulation* between the heart and the lungs and *systemic circulation,* between the heart and the rest of the body. Figure 13–83, page 292, and the following material describe the flow of blood through the pulmonary system.

Pulmonary Circulation

1. Deoxygenated (without O_2) blood carried in the superior vena cava from the arms, neck, and head and carried in the inferior vena cava from the lower extremities and internal organs (except the heart itself) enters the right atrium. Circulation from the heart also empties into the atrium by way of the coronary sinus.

2. The right atrium contracts, squeezing blood through the tricuspid valve, which is opened by the papillary muscles, into the right ventricle. Then the valve closes.

3. The right ventricle contracts, sending blood out through the semilunar valve into the pulmonary artery. (Remember, this artery carries deoxygenated blood but is still an artery because it is leaving the heart.)

4. The pulmonary artery divides into a right and left branch, one going to each lung. The division continues into smaller arteries, arterioles, and then to the capillaries in the alveolar sacs. Here the deoxygenated blood gives up its CO_2 and picks up O_2.

5. With a fresh supply of O_2, the capillaries join the venules, then become veins and reenter the heart as four pulmonary veins, two from each lung, emptying into the left atrium. (This is the only time veins carry oxygenated blood, but they are still veins because they are returning to the heart.)

6. The left atrium contracts, forcing blood through the mitral or bicuspid valve into the left ventricle, and the valve immediately closes.

7. The left ventricle contracts forcefully, sending blood racing out of the heart past the semilunar valve into the aorta.

The action of the chambers of the heart just described occurs simultaneously in both sides of the heart. In other words, both atria contract at the same time, as do the ventricles. The chambers must work in unison or blood being pushed forward would have no place to go (this situation does occur in certain cardiovascular disorders and will be discussed later). The total action just described occurs each time the heart beats.

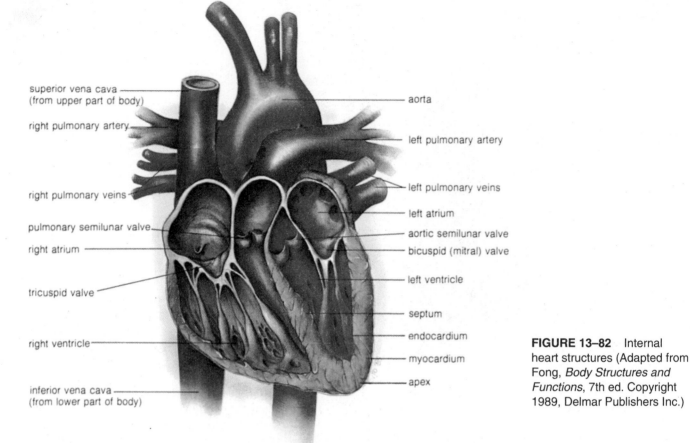

superior vena cava
(from upper part of body)

right pulmonary artery

right pulmonary veins

pulmonary semilunar valve

right atrium

tricuspid valve

right ventricle

inferior vena cava
(from lower part of body)

aorta

left pulmonary artery

left pulmonary veins

left atrium

aortic semilunar valve

bicuspid (mitral) valve

left ventricle

septum

endocardium

myocardium

apex

FIGURE 13–82 Internal heart structures (Adapted from Fong, *Body Structures and Functions*, 7th ed. Copyright 1989, Delmar Publishers Inc.)

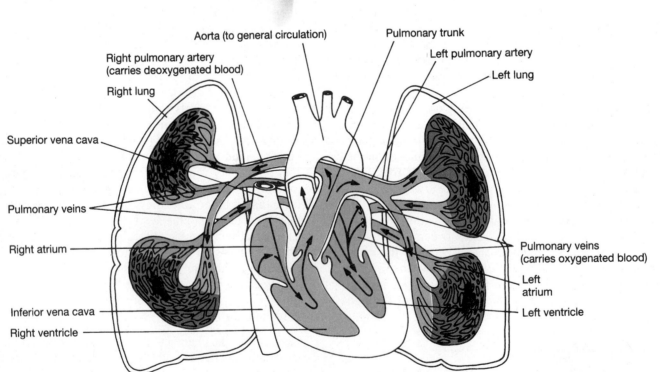

Aorta (to general circulation)

Pulmonary trunk

Right pulmonary artery (carries deoxygenated blood)

Left pulmonary artery

Right lung

Left lung

Superior vena cava

Pulmonary veins

Right atrium

Pulmonary veins (carries oxygenated blood)

Left atrium

Inferior vena cava

Left ventricle

Right ventricle

FIGURE 13–83 Pulmonary circulation. (Copyright by Johnson. From Fong, Ferris, & Skelley, *Body Structures and Functions*, 7th ed. Copyright 1989, Delmar Publishers Inc.)

Heart Sounds

The physician listens at specific locations on the chest wall to hear specific functions of the heart. Figure 13–84 illustrates the anatomical location of the valves and the corresponding auscultatory areas. When a stethoscope is used to listen to the heartbeat, two distinct sounds can be heard. They are referred to as the **lubb dupp** sounds. The lubb sound which is heard first, is caused by the valves slamming shut between the atria and the ventricles. The physician refers to this sound as the S_1. It is heard loudest at the apex of the heart.

The dupp, heard second, is shorter and higher pitched. It is caused by the semilunar valves closing in the aorta and the pulmonary arteries. This sound is known as the S_2. It is loudest at the second intercostal space on each side of the sternum. With a little practice, the valves' condition and level of function can be evaluated from their sounds.

Certain conditions cause changes in the action of the heart valves. Normally the right heart valves close a fraction of a second before the left, due to the lower pressure in the right side of the heart. When the ventricles are distended, an audible vibration may occur, which is referred to as an S_3 or a ventricular gallop. Occasionally, just before S_1, at the end of diastole, the atria may contract, forcing blood into an already filled ventricle. This causes a rise in the ventricular pressure and vibrations known as atrial gallop or S_4.

The Pacemaker

The normal heart beats rhythmically as long as the cells receive the correct balance of sodium, calcium, and potassium and an adequate supply of oxygen and nutrients. Another essential element is the "spark" from the group of nerve cells in the right atrium called the sinoatrial or **SA node,** also called the **pacemaker,** Figure 13–85, page 294. The node generates the electrical impulse that starts each wave of muscle contraction in the heart. The impulse in the right atrium spreads over the muscles of both atria, causing them to contract simultaneously, sending blood into the ventricles. The impulse apparently triggers the atrioventricular or **AV node,** located between the atria and the ventricles, even though there is no direct connection between the nodes. The AV node has nerve fibers which extend through the septum and are called the *bundle of His.* The bundle divides into a right and left branch, infiltrating the muscles of each ventricle with a system of Purkinje fibers. The AV node causes the contraction of the ventricles.

Rhythm Disorders

The self-generating impulse of the heart is one of the body's miracles. Even if the heart were removed from the body it would continue to beat as long as it was supplied with the necessary nutrients. In a **cardiac** condition known as **heart block,** there is an interruption in the

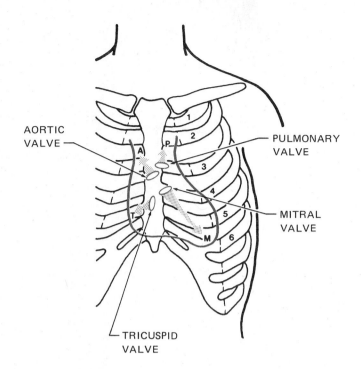

FIGURE 13–84 Anatomical location of the heart valves and the accompanying auscultatory location. Valves are shown as oval structures and the auscultatory location by the letters A, T, M, and P. The rib levels are numbered.

message from the SA node to the AV node. The interruption can occur in varying degrees. The abnormal rhythm patterns can be viewed on an **electrocardiograph** (heart action recording or **ECG**). *First degree block* is characterized by a momentary delay at the AV node before the impulse is transmitted to the ventricles. *Second degree block* can be of two forms. One occurs in cycles of delayed impulses until the SA node fails to conduct to the AV node, then returns to near normal. A second form is characterized by a pattern of only every second, third, or fourth impulse being conducted to the ventricles. This causes a marked decrease in heart output and is usually progressive to the third degree. *Third degree heart block* is known as "complete heart block." There is no impulse carried over from the pacemaker. Because the heart is essential to life, there is a built-in safety factor. The atria continue to beat at 72 times per minute, while the ventricles contract independently at about half the atrial rate, adequate to sustain life but resulting in a severe decrease in cardiac output.

Other rhythm disorders are known as **arrhythmias** (absence of rhythm). Premature contractions cause arrhythmia and occur when an area of the heart, not the SA node, "sparks" and stimulates a contraction of the rest of the myocardium. This area is known as an ectopic (abnormal place) pacemaker. There are three types of premature contractions, each identified by the area of its location; atrial, ventricular, or AV junctional.

Atrial are known as PACs, *premature atrial contractions,* and cause the atria to contract ahead of the antici-

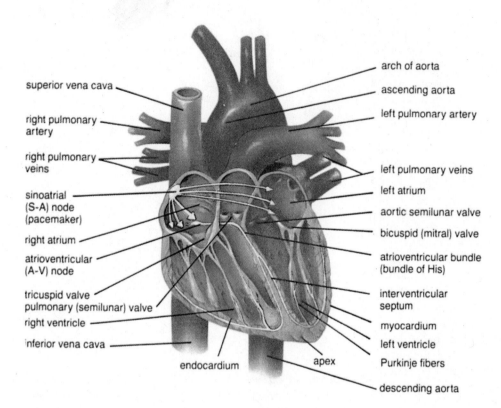

superior vena cava

right pulmonary artery

right pulmonary veins

sinoatrial (S-A) node (pacemaker)

right atrium

atrioventricular (A-V) node

tricuspid valve

pulmonary (semilunar) valve

right ventricle

inferior vena cava

endocardium

apex

arch of aorta

ascending aorta

left pulmonary artery

left pulmonary veins

left atrium

aortic semilunar valve

bicuspid (mitral) valve

atrioventricular bundle (bundle of His)

interventricular septum

myocardium

left ventricle

Purkinje fibers

descending aorta

FIGURE 13–85 SA and AV nodes and the conduction pathway of the heart's electrical impulse (Adapted from Smith, *Medical Terminology, A Programmed Text*, 6th ed. Copyright 1991, Delmar Publishers Inc.)

pated time. *Premature junctional contractions* (PJCs) have the ectopic pacemaker focused at the junction of the AV node and the bundle of His. Usually PACs and PJCs are of no clinical significance and are usually caused by nicotine, caffeine, fatigue, or tension.

Premature ventricular contractions (PVCs) are a different matter. They originate in the ventricle and cause contraction ahead of the next anticipated beat. They can be benign or deadly. If frequent, 5 to 6 per minute or in pairs, they may require immediate intervention to decrease the irritability of the cardiac muscle to maintain cardiac output. If the PVCs occur every other beat, it is a *bigeminal rhythm;* if they occur every third beat, it is a *trigeminal rhythm.* PVCs can be caused by electrolyte and acid-base imbalance, drug therapy, myocardial infarction (see diseases), or oxygen deficit.

In another malfunction of the impulse mechanism known as fibrillation, the rhythm breaks down and the muscle fibers contract at random without coordination. This results in very ineffective heart action and is a life-threatening condition. An electrical device called a *defibrillator* is used to discharge a strong electrical current into the patient's heart through electrode paddles held against the bare chest wall. The shock should interfere with the uncoordinated action and allow the SA node to resume its control.

Artificial Pacemaker

When the natural pacemaker of the heart fails to maintain a normal heart rate and cardiac drug therapy designed to cause effective, regular beats fails to correct the situation, an artificial pacemaker may be indicated.

The device consists of a small battery-powered pulse generator with an electrode catheter, Figure 13–86. The electrode is inserted into a vein and threaded through the vena cava, the right atrium, and into the right ventricle at the apex. The procedure is accomplished while observing the path of the electrode by fluoroscopy. The action of the heart throughout the procedure, and for at least the first 24 hours following, is monitored carefully by frequent electrocardiograph (ECG) tracings. The stimulation threshold of the pacemaker to maintain myocardial contractions is determined by noting the number of milliamperes (MA) which produce the desired QRS complex (ECG tracing of contraction). This MA and the desired rate can be set in the pacemaker.

It should be noted that when the heart is totally dependent on artificial pacing, the heart rate will always be that which is artificially set, regardless of the level of activity. The artificial pacemaker will not increase the rate to meet the needs of increased activity.

A pacemaker can be attached temporarily to the chest wall, upper arm, or waist. It can also be "permanently" inserted surgically into a muscular pocket on the chest wall. Permanent units are self-contained and will operate for about 3 to as many as 20 years. Pacemakers can also be of either the fixed or the demand type. Fixed units fire continuously at a predetermined rate. Demand types sense the person's own rate and fire only when required. An external unit can be programmed to change the mode of firing of some implanted types.

Pacemakers are of benefit to patients with a slow, irregular heart rhythm, complete heart block, or a slow ventricular rate due to congenital or disease conditions.

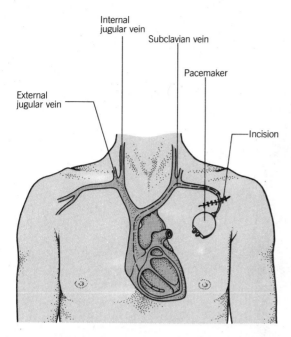

Internal jugular vein

Subclavian vein

Pacemaker

External jugular vein

Incision

FIGURE 13–86 Artificial pacemaker (From Burke, *Human Anatomy and Physiology in Health and Disease*, 3d ed. Copyright 1992, Delmar Publishers Inc.)

Controlling the Rate

Two nerves, the **vagus** and the **accelerator,** have fibers in the muscle of the heart and have some control over the natural rate of the heartbeat, Figure 13–87. The vagus nerve, also called the decelerator, slows down the heart rate while the accelerator nerve increases the rate. The nerves, however, are stimulated by many things. Heart rate can increase as the result of fear, anger, or excitement and can decrease with severe depression. The amount of oxygen, carbon dioxide, and electrolytes (sodium, potassium, magnesium, phosphates, and chlorides) present in the blood affect the rate of the heart. A heart rate which is consistently rapid (over 100 beats per minute) is known as **tachycardia.** When the rate is consistently slow, less than 60 beats per minute, it is referred to as **bradycardia.**

The Blood Vessels ....

Blood vessels are divided into three main types: arteries, veins, and **capillaries,** Figure 13–88, page 296.

Arteries

An artery always carries blood *away* from the heart and usually carries fresh, oxygenated blood. The one exception is the pulmonary artery, which leaves the right ventricle of the heart on its way *to* the lungs to pick up oxygen. Arteries are constructed with layers of elastic fibers that allow the walls to expand and recoil in

response to the injection of blood when the ventricles contract. In the systemic circulation, this action causes a wavelike effect within the arteries, which can be felt as the pulse at the pulse points of the body. Figure 13–89, page 297, shows the main arteries of the human body. In areas where arteries lie over firm or bony structure, such as at the wrist, the side of the neck or inner elbow surface, the pulse can be felt if the artery is pressed against the underlying structure.

As the arteries divide and branch off into smaller and smaller vessels, they become known as **arterioles.** Eventually, the arterioles join the microscopic blood vessels known as capillaries. When the blood enters the vast network of capillaries, called a capillary bed, it is so dispersed that the rate of flow is reduced to a slow trickle, permitting time for O_2 and nutrients to enter the cells in exchange for CO_2 and waste products, Figure 13–90, page 298.

Capillary walls are thin, one-cell structures that allow the passage of molecules into the fluid-filled tissue spaces surrounding the cells. The molecules pass through the fluid to enter either the cell or the capillary. Tiny openings in the capillary walls permit white blood cells to leave the blood and enter the fluid of the tissue spaces to destroy bacteria. **Plasma** also seeps through the capillary walls, adding to the amount of tissue fluid. Excess fluid, certain waste products, and other substances are removed by an adjoining capillary of the lymphatic system, an action that will be discussed later in this unit.

The vast number of capillaries within the body would be more than capable of holding all the body's supply of blood. Therefore, an automatic system is in effect that permits a group of cells being served by one section of a capillary bed to receive blood for only a short period of time. Then another section is served and the first section must wait for another turn. This control is maintained by a series of capillary sphincters, which open and close the entrances to the capillary beds.

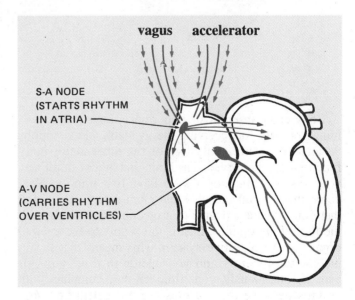

vagus   accelerator

S-A NODE (STARTS RHYTHM IN ATRIA)

A-V NODE (CARRIES RHYTHM OVER VENTRICLES)

FIGURE 13–87 Nerves influencing the heart rate

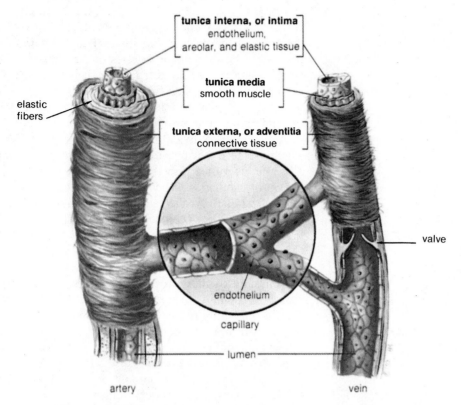

tunica interna, or intima
endothelium,
areolar, and elastic tissue

tunica media
smooth muscle

tunica externa, or adventitia
connective tissue

elastic
fibers

valve

endothelium

capillary

lumen

artery

vein

a. Types of blood vessels and their general structure

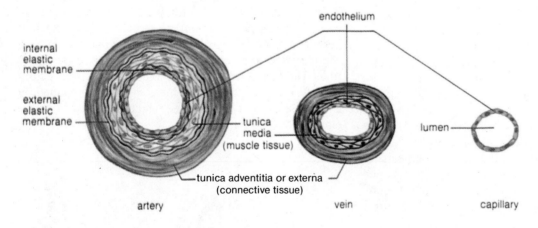

endothelium

internal
elastic
membrane

external
elastic
membrane

tunica
media
(muscle tissue)

tunica adventitia or externa
(connective tissue)

artery

lumen

vein

capillary

FIGURE 13–88
Comparative structure of
blood vessels (From Fong,
*Body Structures and
Functions*, 7th ed. Copyright
1989, Delmar Publishers
Inc.)

Body cells, in order of importance, have a predetermined priority for receiving the available blood supply. At any given time, only two of the three major body functions can be served. The brain and other central nervous system structures always have first priority. Next come the skeletal muscles that enable us to move and therefore provide a degree of protection to the body with the flight/fight options. Last is the supply to the internal organs of the digestive system. This means that if you have eaten recently and you decide to run, swim, or exercise strenuously, your stomach may complain with cramps because the muscles are not getting enough blood supply to digest its contents.

When the blood leaves the capillary bed, it is carrying CO_2 and waste products from the cells to be circulated to the proper organ for disposal. Capillaries join with **venules,** which are tiny branches of the veins. As they return blood toward the heart, venules join together forming veins, which eventually enter the heart, from the lower body by the inferior **vena cava** and from the upper body by the superior vena cava.

Veins

Veins are similar to arteries in construction except that the walls are thinner and they lack the elastic fiber lining that

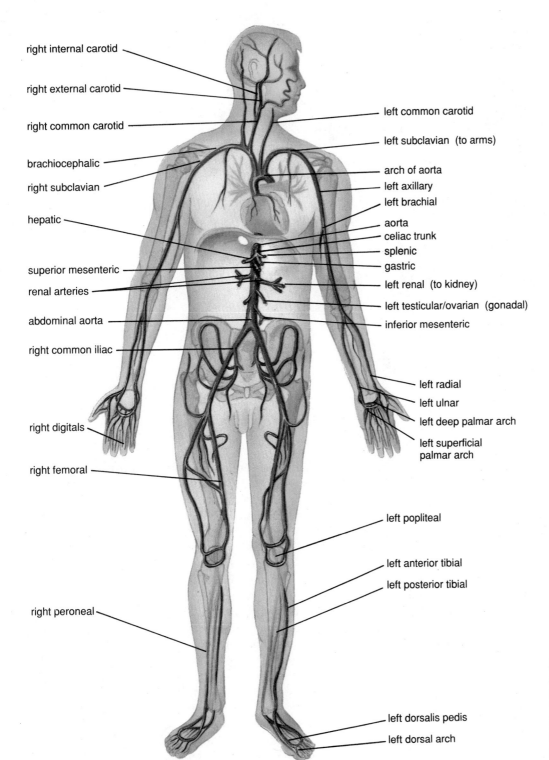

right internal carotid

right external carotid

right common carotid

brachiocephalic

right subclavian

hepatic

superior mesenteric

renal arteries

abdominal aorta

right common iliac

right digitals

right femoral

right peroneal

left common carotid

left subclavian (to arms)

arch of aorta

left axillary

left brachial

aorta

celiac trunk

splenic

gastric

left renal (to kidney)

left testicular/ovarian (gonadal)

inferior mesenteric

left radial

left ulnar

left deep palmar arch

left superficial palmar arch

left popliteal

left anterior tibial

left posterior tibial

left dorsalis pedis

left dorsal arch

FIGURE 13–89 Major arteries of the body (From Smith, *Medical Terminology, A Programmed Text*, 6th ed. Copyright 1991, Delmar Publishers Inc.)

lets arteries alter the size of their openings. The pressure that is present in arteries is absent in veins, and therefore they can collapse when they are not filled. The major veins of the body are shown in Figure 13–91, page 299.

Veins carry deoxygenated blood back to the heart to be sent to the lungs for exhaling of CO_2 and to pick up a new supply of O_2. Every time the heart beats, blood is forced through the arteries and arterioles to the capillaries, where the pressure from the heart is dissipated in the vast capillary network. With each successive beat, additional blood is forced through the capillaries into the venules and veins, which move it back toward the heart. Special valve structures are located throughout the veins to maintain the flow of blood in the proper direction, Figure 13–92, page 300. Veins in the lower extremities especially contain many valves since they are returning blood "uphill" so to speak. During the relaxation phase of the heartbeat, the venous blood could flow back

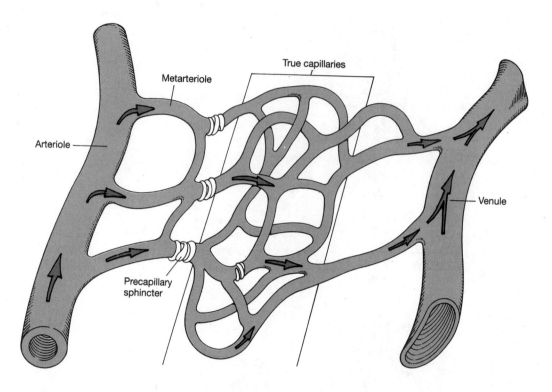

FIGURE 13–90 Capillary bed connecting an arteriole with a venule (Copyright by Richardson. From Fong, *Body Structures and Functions*, 7th ed. Copyright 1989, Delmar Publishers Inc.)

toward the capillaries, but the valves close as relaxation begins, and the blood is trapped in the veins until the following beat forces it to move forward.

Another factor helps move blood in veins back to the heart. The veins of the extremities are located in and around the large skeletal muscles. When the muscles contract, they squeeze the veins, thereby aiding in the movement of the blood, Figure 13–93, page 300.

Blood flows to every cell in the body through the systemic circulation. Refer to Figures 13–89 and 13–91, as you read the following description of the flow through the major arteries and veins.

Systemic Circulation

1. As the blood leaves the left ventricle, it enters the huge aorta. Immediately, the right and left coronary arteries to the heart exit from the aorta at its arch. Other great arteries, the common carotid, the subclavian, and the innominate, which becomes the brachial and radial arteries of the arm, also exit from the arch, divide into right and left branches and supply blood to the head, neck, and upper extremities.
2. As the aorta descends through the body, the thoracic and abdominal portions give origin to the large arteries supplying the organs of the thorax and abdomen.
3. When the aorta reaches the level of the fourth lumbar vertebra, it divides into two large common iliac arteries with the external branch descending down the legs and the internal branch leading to the pelvic organs and genitalia (external sex organs).
4. The external branch of the iliac artery becomes the femoral artery in the thigh and continues down the leg as the tibial branch.
5. Eventually all systemic arteries throughout the body subdivide until they become arterioles and then join the capillaries. In this circuit, the capillaries deliver the O_2, water, and nutrients to the body's cells and pick up the cells' CO_2 and wastes.
6. Upon leaving the capillaries, the blood is considered deoxygenated. The capillaries join venules, which eventually become veins.
7. The major lower extremity veins are the anterior and posterior tibial, the small and great saphenous, the popliteal, and the femoral. These join with pelvic veins and enter the inferior vena cava.
8. The major veins of the upper extremities are the basilic, median, and cephalic. These join with the subclavian, internal and external jugular, the innominate, and the sinuses from the head to enter the superior vena cava.
9. The superior vena cava and inferior vena cava empty into the right atrium of the heart and systemic circulation is completed.

Portal Circulation

The preceding was a simplified description of the body's general circulation. However, there is another "circuit"

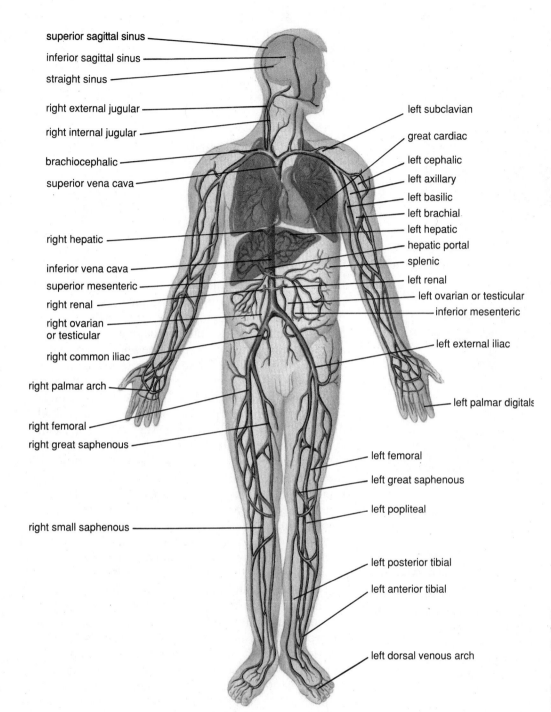

superior sagittal sinus

inferior sagittal sinus

straight sinus

right external jugular

right internal jugular

brachiocephalic

superior vena cava

right hepatic

inferior vena cava

superior mesenteric

right renal

right ovarian or testicular

right common iliac

right palmar arch

right femoral

right great saphenous

right small saphenous

left subclavian

great cardiac

left cephalic

left axillary

left basilic

left brachial

left hepatic

hepatic portal

splenic

left renal

left ovarian or testicular

inferior mesenteric

left external iliac

left palmar digitals

left femoral

left great saphenous

left popliteal

left posterior tibial

left anterior tibial

left dorsal venous arch

FIGURE 13–91 Major veins of the body (From Smith, *Medical Terminology, A Programmed Text*, 6th ed. Copyright 1991, Delmar Publishers Inc.)

that leaves and reenters the system just described. It is called the portal circulation, Figure 13–94, page 301. The details of its function are beyond the scope of this text but it can be described in general terms.

As the aorta descends through the abdomen, arteries branch off to the internal organs: the stomach, liver, spleen, pancreas, kidneys, etc. Each organ receives substances on which it reacts. These substances may be sugar, salt, hormones, a toxic chemical, nutrients, waste products from the cells of other organs—everything you eat, drink, inhale, or inject into your body eventually enters the circulatory system.

The blood leaving certain organs (ones without a pair) empties into the special portal circulation and eventually becomes the portal vein. This vein goes to the liver to permit the blood from the large and small intestines, stomach, pancreas, and spleen to come into contact with the liver's specialized cells. Many life-preserving functions are performed by these liver cells. For example, here nutrients that enter the blood from the digestive system are altered, stored, and/or released into the main circulatory system, as needed. After passing through the liver, the blood is carried by the venous system to the inferior vena cava and is recirculated.

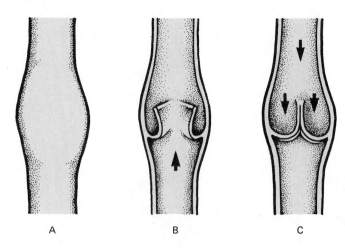

FIGURE 13-92 Vein valves (a). External view shows dilation at site of valve (b). Vein opened and valves opened (c). Valves closed to prevent backflow of blood.

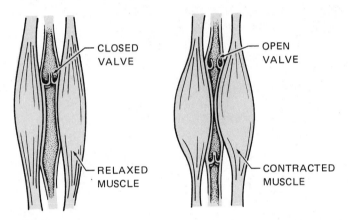

CLOSED VALVE

OPEN VALVE

RELAXED MUSCLE

CONTRACTED MUSCLE

FIGURE 13-93 How muscles help move blood through internal veins

The Lymphatic System ....

The lymphatic system consists of lymph, a straw-colored fluid similar to blood plasma; lymph nodes; lymph vessels; and the spleen. In addition, the lymphatic tissue, which produces lymphocytes (a type of blood cell), is often considered to be part of the system. This includes the tonsils, the thymus gland, and the intestinal lymphoid tissue.

Lymph

Lymph is composed of blood plasma that filters out of the capillaries, lymphocytes, hormones, and many other substances, which are the products of cellular activity, such as water, digested nutrients, salts, oxygen, carbon dioxide, and urea. It is a continuous-forming process. Lymph fills the spaces between the cells and is also referred to as intercellular or *interstitial fluid*. Lymph acts as the "bridge" between cells and capillaries. Lymph is moved through the body primarily by contraction of the skeletal muscles. There is no pump like the heart to move lymph. Lymph vessels are constructed like veins, however, with valves to prevent the backflow of fluid.

Lymph Vessels

Vessels carrying lymph are located throughout the body, somewhat like veins. Lymphatic capillaries absorb fluid and other substances from the tissues and return it to the circulatory system, Figure 13-95. However, it is a one-way system only, from the cells toward the heart. There are no separate vessels bringing lymph to the cells.

The vast network of lymph capillaries joins to form small lymph vessels that in turn form larger vessels called *lymphatics*. Lymphatics eventually form two main ducts. The right lymphatic duct receives lymph from the right side of the head, the right arm, and the upper right trunk. The thoracic duct receives lymph from the rest of the body, Figure 13-96, page 302.

Lymph Nodes

Lymph nodes are small round or oval structures located usually in clusters along the lymph vessels at various places in the body. Lymph enters the nodes from four afferent lymph vessels, filters through a mesh of sinuses, and leaves by way of a single efferent vessel. Lymphocytes, a type of white blood cell, are derived from stem cells in the bone marrow. They enter the blood stream and go to the lymph tissue to "live." Their action is essential to the immune system of the body. When needed, they divide by mitosis, greatly increasing in number. Phagocytes, another type of white blood cell, can also be found in lymph nodes. The structure of the nodes and the cell's function purify the lymph by removing harmful substances such as bacteria or malignant cells. The nodes increase and decrease in size in relation to the amount of material being filtered. In acute infections, they become swollen and tender due to the collection of cells gathered to destroy the invading substances. This condition is known as adenitis. With extensive involvement, the node may break down and an abscess will form.

Physicians palpate for nodes when patients have infectious conditions or when a malignancy is known or suspected. With malignancy, the cancer cells are abnormal and so are identified by the cells in the lymph node to be removed from the circulating fluid. As more cells accumulate, the node becomes enlarged and is therefore palpable. Early detection of lymph node involvement is critical to the prognosis of patients with cancer, for it is through the lymphatic system that a malignancy often metastasizes (spreads) to other sites. The extent of lymph node involvement is an important indicator of the ultimate prognosis of the patient.

The Spleen

The spleen is an organ composed of lymphatic tissue, lying just beneath the left side of the diaphragm, in back of the upper portion of the stomach. The spleen produces lymphocytes, stores red blood cells, keeps the appropriate balance between cells and plasma in the

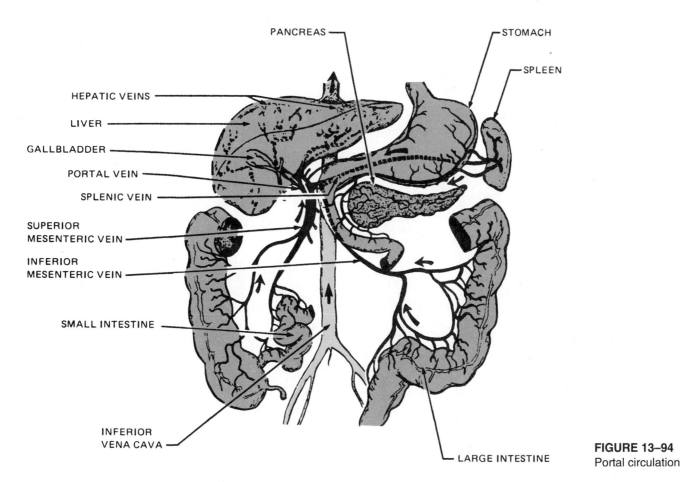

PANCREAS — STOMACH

SPLEEN

HEPATIC VEINS —

LIVER —

GALLBLADDER —

PORTAL VEIN —

SPLENIC VEIN —

SUPERIOR MESENTERIC VEIN —

INFERIOR MESENTERIC VEIN —

SMALL INTESTINE —

INFERIOR VENA CAVA —

LARGE INTESTINE

FIGURE 13–94
Portal circulation

blood capillary

red blood cells

white blood cell

lymph

cells

© *N. B. Richardson*, *1983*

lymph capillary

FIGURE 13–95 Lymph capillary (From Ehrlich, *Medical Terminology for Health Professions*, copyright 1988, Delmar Publishers Inc.)

blood, and removes and destroys worn-out red cells. The organ functions like a large lymph node. It is soft and elastic and varies in size according to the flow of blood through the organ. During an acute infection, it will become enlarged and tender. Patients with leukemia may have an enlarged, firm spleen that is palpable on examination. The spleen is filled with excess immature cells to be destroyed.

The Blood

Blood is the life-giving fluid of the body. It flows through the blood vessels transporting substances essential to the maintenance of life. The average adult has 8 to 10 pints of blood. A loss of 2 pints, or about 20%, is cause for concern. The blood carries oxygen from the lungs to the cells, nutrients from the digestive system to the cells, and cellular wastes from the cells to the appropriate organ for excretion. It picks up hormones excreted from endocrine glands and distributes them throughout the body to the appropriate receiving organ. Blood also delivers the minerals necessary for muscular contraction, heartbeat, stimulation of the respiratory system, and the homeostasis of cells. This vital substance is composed of only two main parts—the plasma and the cells—but each part has many essential components.

Plasma

Plasma is a straw-colored liquid that makes up a little over half the volume of blood. It is about 90% water, the remainder consisting of minerals such as calcium, sodium, potassium, phosphorus, and bicarbonates. The minerals are commonly referred to as *electrolytes*. These

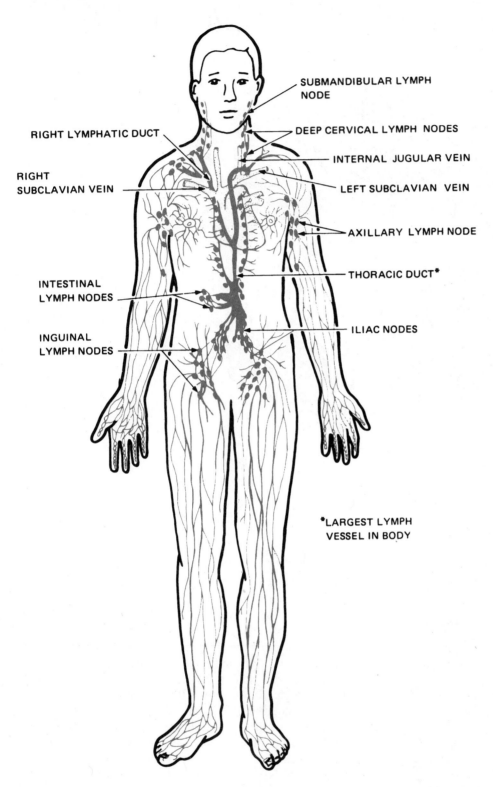

SUBMANDIBULAR LYMPH NODE

DEEP CERVICAL LYMPH NODES

INTERNAL JUGULAR VEIN

RIGHT LYMPHATIC DUCT

LEFT SUBCLAVIAN VEIN

RIGHT SUBCLAVIAN VEIN

AXILLARY LYMPH NODE

THORACIC DUCT*

INTESTINAL LYMPH NODES

ILIAC NODES

INGUINAL LYMPH NODES

*LARGEST LYMPH VESSEL IN BODY

FIGURE 13–96   The lymphatic system

elements are processed by the body from the foods that are eaten and play a major role in maintaining the acid–base balance of the blood.

Plasma contains other vital substances such as vitamins; hormones; enzymes; nutrients absorbed from the digestive system, such as glucose, fatty acids, and amino acids. Oxygen, carbon dioxide, and other waste products from the cells are also carried in the plasma.

In addition, three important proteins are found in plasma: fibrinogen, which is necessary to clot blood; serum albumin, which aids in maintaining blood pressure by regulating the exchange of water between the cells and the blood; and serum globulin, which assists in the formation of antibodies. A substance called pro-thrombin is a type of globulin formed by the liver, with the aid of vitamin K. It plays an important role in the clotting of the blood.

Cells

The cellular portion of the blood can be divided into three types of cells: red, white, and platelets, Figure 13–97.

Red Blood Cells. **Erythrocytes** (red blood cells) are biconcave disks with very thin centers to enable them to fold over if necessary to pass through a narrow opening. Red cells number about 25 trillion in the body or about 5 million to a cubic millimeter of blood. It is the red cells which give blood its color. A red blood cell lasts about 4 months. They are produced in the bone marrow at a rate of about a million a second, the same rate at which they wear out.

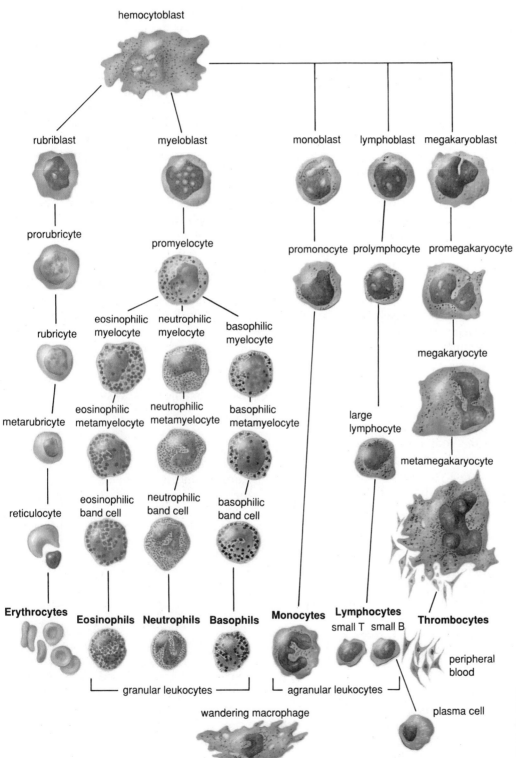

FIGURE 13–97 Types of blood cells (Adapted from Smith, *Medical Terminology, A Programmed Text*, 6th ed. Copyright 1991, Delmar Publishers Inc.)

Erythrocytes obtain their color from hemoglobin, which is a combination of a protein and an iron pigment. It is hemoglobin that attracts and carries the oxygen and carbon dioxide in the blood. When hemoglobin is carrying a lot of oxygen it is bright red in color. As the oxygen is given up to the cells and exchanged for carbon dioxide, the color changes to the dark reddish blue that is visible in surface veins.

White Blood Cells. White blood cells are called leukocytes. Leukocytes are present in the blood at approximately 5000 to 9000 per cubic millimeter, or about one white cell for every 600 to 700 red blood cells. White cells are about twice the size of red blood cells. Leukocytes play a vital role in defending the body against invasion, moving through capillary walls into the tissue fluid to chase down bacteria.

Leukocytes are divided into two major groups, granuocytes and agranulocytes, depending upon the presence of granules and certain staining characteristics.

Granulocytes are produced in red bone marrow and last for only a few days. There are three types. *Neutrophils* phagocytize (destroy) bacteria by surrounding, swallowing, and digesting them. *Eosinophils* are thought to consume the toxic substances in tissues since they are found in increasing numbers when the body has had a foreign protein injected or an allergic reaction or has been infected by a parasite. The third type, the *basophils,* are also thought to participate in phagocytosis since their numbers increase with chronic inflammation or during healing from an infection.

Agranulocytes are of two types: *lymphocytes,* which are produced by bone marrow and lymphoid tissues such as the nodes and spleen; and *monocytes,* which are formed in the bone marrow. Lymphocytes primarily specialize in providing immunity for the body by attaching themselves to foreign bodies and destroying them, and by developing antibodies. The monocyte assists with phagocytosis. Some enlarge greatly when they enter tissue and become fixed.

When an inflammation occurs, white cells can divide and proliferate into capsulelike structures around foreign objects that cannot be digested, such as silica dust and carbon particles, or causative organisms of infections such as tuberculosis. This action effectively walls off involved tissue in an attempt to contain the foreign material or prevent the spread of disease. The evidence of a phagocytic reaction to invading bacteria or a foreign object is the presence of exudate (pus). Exudate is composed of lymph, bacteria, and dead white cells.

Platelets. The third kind of cell is the platelet. These cells are the smallest of the three and are present in the blood at a rate of 200,000 to 400,000 per cubic millimeter. They are also formed in the bone marrow from cell fragments.

Platelets function in the life-saving process of clotting blood. When a blood vessel is cut or damaged it is believed that the rough surface may catch and/or attract platelets to the area. This reaction occurs only when there is an incidence of bleeding; otherwise the clotting process would stop circulation within the blood vessels. When there is a cut, platelets pile up at the site to form a small mass. Once attached firmly to the damaged area, they release the chemical, serotonin, which causes the blood vessel to spasm, resulting in a narrowing of the vessel and a decrease in blood loss until the clot can be formed, Figure 13–98. At the same time, platelets and injured tissues release thromboplastin, which triggers the clotting process to begin. The thromboplastin cooperates with calcium ions and other blood clotting factors in the blood, to convert prothrombin (present in plasma) into thrombin. The thrombin acts on another protein in the plasma called fibrinogen. This reaction results in the formation of fibrin, tiny threads which form a network of fine mesh fibers over the cut. This net begins to catch the red blood cells, other platelets, and plasma, forming the clot. It should be remembered that unless the cut blood vessel is small, a clot may not be able to form. The force of the flow of blood will wash away the body's efforts to form fibrin nets, and therefore will be unable to collect the ingredients of the clot. Clotting can be assisted by applying pressure over the area to stop the blood flow until a clot can form. When major vessels are cut, it may be necessary to surgically close the opening with sutures to control the bleeding. Fortunately, internal bleeding vessels can also undergo the clotting process. Complications can occur from the clotted mass, especially if the clot or its fragments break loose and enter the circulation before the body's natural "housekeeping" function can gradually remove it from the blood vessel.

Bleeding Time

The length of time required for blood to clot from an induced puncture wound is useful information when preparing a patient for a surgical procedure or evaluating the effects of certain disorders or medications. The normal range of bleeding time for the template puncture method is from 2 to 8 minutes. The length of time varies with the method used.

Blood Types

There are four types of blood: A, B, AB, and O. The type of blood a person has depends on the presence of a protein factor called agglutinogen or antigen on the surface of the red blood cell. Type A blood has an A agglutinogen, type B has a B agglutinogen, type AB has both agglutinogens, and Type O has neither, Figure 13–99.

Similarly, a protein is present in blood plasma known as agglutinin or antibody. Type A blood has a b agglutinin, type B blood has an a agglutinin, type AB has no agglutinins, and type O has both a and b.

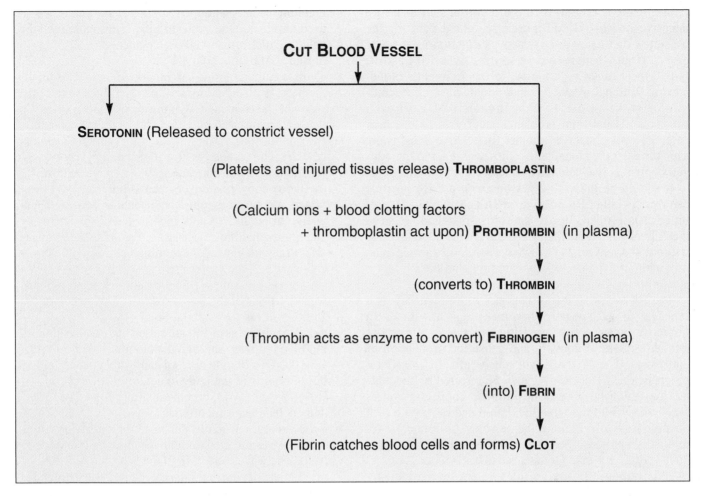

FIGURE 13–98   Process of blood clot formation

The term *agglutinate* refers to the process of clumping or sticking together. Blood clumps and forms clots in the blood vessels if agglutinins and agglutinogens of the same type are mixed together. This reaction can be fatal. Therefore, it is extremely important to determine the blood types of both the recipient and the donor when blood transfusions are required. A laboratory test known as type and cross-match is necessary to make this determination prior to the administration of either whole blood or packed cell transfusions. Not only is the blood typed,

but it is also mixed and observed to assure that agglutination does not occur. Cross-matching will also detect the presence of subtypes and an agglutinogen known as H.

Rh Factor

Red blood cells may have another factor known as the Rh factor. It is an antigen that was first detected in the blood of a Rhesus monkey, therefore the name Rh. If the red cell has the factor it is said to be Rh positive or Rh+.

FIGURE 13–99
Blood types

Blood Type	Percent of Population	Antigen/Agglutinogen on Red Blood Cells	Antibody/Agglutinin in Plasma	Can Receive	Can Donate To
A	41%	A	Anti-b	A or O only	A or AB only
B	12%	B	Anti-a	B or O only	B or AB only
AB	3%	A and B	none	A, B, AB, O Universal recipient	AB only
O	44%	None	Anti-a and b	O only	A, B, AB, O Universal donor

If the factor is absent, then the blood is said to be Rh negative or Rh–. Blood must also be checked for the presence of this antigen when a transfusion is to be given. If an Rh negative person receives Rh positive blood, the antigen is "foreign" to the recipient's bloodstream. Within 2 weeks, the individual will produce antibodies in response to this invasion of a foreign substance. Usually no problems occur unless, at a later date, the person receives another Rh positive transfusion. This time the developed antibodies will react to the antigen being received and may cause serious complications.

It should be noted that persons who are Rh positive can receive either Rh positive or Rh negative blood, provided it is properly typed and cross-matched, because they already have the factor and the Rh negative blood is without the antigen. When the two blood samples can mix without evidence of any clumping and the Rh factor is appropriate, the blood is said to be compatible.

The Rh factor is also of concern with pregnancy. If a female who is Rh negative becomes pregnant with an Rh positive baby, a few positive cells may enter the mother's blood at delivery and cause the production of antibodies. The firstborn will not be affected, but later pregnancies, if Rh positive, may be affected by the antibodies which have been developed. These antibodies slowly filter into the fetal circulation and destroy the Rh positive red cells, making the newborn profoundly anemic and jaundiced. The situation must be treated vigorously, with steps taken to alter the infant's blood.

This potentially fatal situation can be avoided by determining the Rh factor of the mother. If she is negative, then the father's factor must be determined before the first child is born. At the time of delivery, if the baby is positive, the Rh negative mother is given an injection of an Rh(D) immune human globulin, which prohibits the production of antibodies against the baby's Rh positive blood. Only when the mother is negative and the fetus positive is there cause for concern. If the father also happens to be negative, there is no need to treat for the antibodies unless the mother could have, at some previous time, received an Rh positive blood transfusion.

In the next unit on the immune system, we will take a deeper look into the function of leukocytes and how they maintain our immunity. We will also learn more about the antigen/antibody process.

Cardiovascular Tests

Many sophisticated tests can be performed on the circulatory system, but most of them are best studied at a more advanced level. A few of the more frequently encountered cardiovascular diagnostic procedures will be discussed briefly here. Common studies done on blood are discussed in Chapter 17.

- Arteriograph (angiograph)—a radiological examination of an artery or arteries after injecting a contrast medium, usually into the femoral artery. The test is used to indicate the status of blood flow, collateral circulation, malformed vessels, an aneurysm, or the presence of hemorrhage.

- Cardiac catherization—A catheter to the right side of the heart is inserted into a vein at the antecubital space of the right arm. A catheter to the left side of the heart is inserted into the brachial artery at the left antecubital space. The femoral artery or vein may also be used. The catheter is passed through the blood vessels until it reaches the heart. When it is determined, by fluoroscopy, that the catheter is properly positioned, a contrast medium is injected to permit visualization of the heart's activity. The heart's chambers and valves and the coronary arteries or the pulmonary artery may be viewed, depending on the side being catheterized. The procedure can also be used to measure blood pressure within the pulmonary artery and some portions of the heart.

- Doppler ultrasonography—Sound waves are transmitted through the skin and are reflected by the cells in the blood moving through the blood vessels, Figure 13–100. This diagnostic tool can evaluate the major blood vessels of the body to determine deep vein thrombosis (DVT), peripheral arterial aneurysms, and occluded carotid arteries.

- Echocardiograph—A test using ultrahigh-frequency sound waves directed through the chest wall into the heart. The waves reflect from the heart through a mechanical device to produce a record of the structures of the heart and its chambers. The test evaluates cardiac

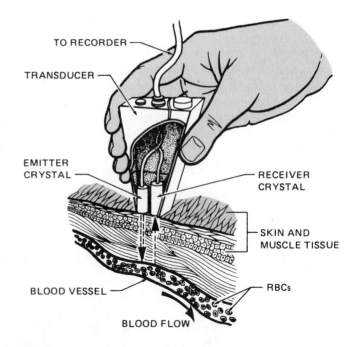

HOW THE DOPPLER PROBE WORKS

TO RECORDER

TRANSDUCER

EMITTER CRYSTAL

RECEIVER CRYSTAL

SKIN AND MUSCLE TISSUE

BLOOD VESSEL

RBCs

BLOOD FLOW

FIGURE 13–100 Doppler ultrasound

function and structure and can reveal valve irregularities, defects in the interior walls, and the presence of fluid between the layers of the pericardium.

- Electrocardiograph (ECG)—This test is also called EKG, usually when referred to verbally; it can be written in either form. It is perhaps the most common tool used to evaluate heart performance. The ECG is a graphic recording of the electrical activity of the heart. It identifies rhythm, abnormalities in conduction, and electrolyte imbalance. The graph is useful in documenting diagnosis and provides a method of measuring progression of cardiac disease conditions. The ECG also helps evaluate the effectiveness of an artificial pacemaker and cardiac medications.

  The test may be taken while the patient is lying in a comfortable position, or in an exercise mode such as bicycling or walking a treadmill. The exercise mode measures the effects of controlled physical stress and is referred to as a *stress ECG*. Frequently, abnormalities of cardiac action are more evident upon exertion.

  Another type of ECG is called the Holter Monitor or ambulatory (walking) ECG. The ECG electrodes are attached to the patient's chest wall and a portable cassette recorder (monitor) is placed in a belt about the waist. For a 24-hour period the patient's heart action is recorded and a diary is kept of daily activities and any associated symptoms. At the end of the test, the recording is analyzed by computer and a report is printed. This type of test is most beneficial for symptoms which occur irregularly or to evaluate the status of recovering cardiac patients. Another version permits the patient to activate the recording device only when experiencing symptoms. This patient-activated monitor can be worn for several days. (See Chapter 18.)

- MUGA scan—MUGA is an acronym for MUltiple Gated Acquisition; it is a test to evaluate the condition of the myocardium of the heart. The test can be done in a resting or exercise mode. Isotopes are injected intravenously and are taken up by the myocardium. The scintillation camera records the motion of the heart. The test permits measurement of ventricular contractions to evaluate the strength of the heart wall. Patients who receive a chemotherapeutic drug that has cardiac toxicity side effects are monitored periodically by MUGA scans due to the drug's tendency to damage the myocardium.

- Stress thallium ECG—A test to evaluate myocardial blood flow and the condition of the cells. The ECG electrodes are attached to the patient before performing the stress test on either a treadmill or a bicycle. The blood pressure and pulse rate are carefully monitored. When the patient reaches peak stress, the thallium is injected intravenously into the anticubital vein and the exercise continued for an additional minute to ensure circulation of the isotope to the heart. The ECG electrodes are removed, and within 3 to 5 minutes the patient is positioned under the scintillation camera. The scanner records the amount of thallium uptake by the heart over the next several minutes. Areas of the heart with normal blood supply and healthy cells rapidly take up the isotope. Areas of poor blood flow or damaged cells do not take up the material and appear as dark spots on the scan; these are known as cold spots.

  The test is indicated for assessing myocardial condition, demonstrating the location and extent of a myocardial infarction (MI), diagnosing coronary artery disease, and determining the effectiveness of artery grafts and angioplasty procedures.

- Venogram—A radiographic examination using a contrast medium to determine the condition of the deep veins of the legs. It is especially useful in determining the presence of deep vein thrombosis (DVT), which may occlude the vein systems and lead to pulmonary embolism, a potentially lethal situation. DVT may result from vein injury, prolonged bed rest, surgery, childbirth, irregularity in the coagulation process, and the use of oral contraceptives.

Diseases and Disorders ....

Anemia. This term indicates that certain elements are lacking in the blood. There are various types of anemias. The most common form of anemia is iron deficiency anemia, or the presence of an inadequate supply of iron to form normal red blood cells. When the body's supply of iron decreases, so does the number of red blood cells and as a result, the hemoglobin. This reduces the body's ability to carry oxygen to the cells and causes symptoms of fatigue, listlessness, pallor, inability to concentrate, and difficulty in breathing on exertion. Iron deficiency anemia develops from an inadequate dietary intake of iron or inability of the body to absorb iron, as the result of diarrhea, partial or total removal of the stomach, or certain diseases. It can also be caused by intestinal bleeding, heavy menstruation, colon cancer, or bleeding ulcers. It is most common among premature infants, children, adolescents (especially girls), and women before menopause. Iron deficiency anemia can be treated, once the cause is determined, by oral iron preparations.

Another form of anemia is known as aplastic. It is a disease resulting from injury or destruction of the blood cell formation function of the bone marrow. This disease generally produces a fatal bleeding episode or a systemic infection, often as a result of infectious hepatitis.

Anemia is a term that is used to describe conditions of low red blood cell count occurring over extended periods of time. However, low red blood cell count can also occur following an acute blood loss and is referred to by some as acute blood loss anemia. In this instance, there is a sudden loss of red blood cells and therefore hemoglobin and iron. The rapid loss of blood volume can be fatal.

Acute blood loss can result from severe trauma, the inability to coagulate the blood, ruptured gastric or intestinal ulcers, postoperative bleeding, postpartum (after birth) hemorrhage, or a ruptured aneurysm. A loss of 20% to 30% of blood volume causes circulatory insufficiency with symptoms of shock; restlessness; low blood pressure; rapid pulse; perspiration; and cool, clammy skin. With a loss greater than 30%, the circulatory system may fail and be followed by shock and then coma. Blood loss beyond 40% is life-threatening, and the patient will die unless blood volume is immediately replaced.

Aneurysm. The ballooning out of the wall of an artery is due to a weakening of the wall structure. Often an aneurysm is associated with atherosclerosis or arteriosclerosis and the resulting hypertension. A slight break or weakness in the muscular layer of an artery allows the pressure of the blood to push the walls of the blood vessel out, Figure 13–101. The larger the bulge, the thinner the arterial wall becomes. Eventually, the wall gives way and a hemorrhage occurs. The extent of the bleeding and its effects on the body depend to a great extent on the location of the aneurysm and the size of the involved blood vessel.

Aneurysms are found primarily in cerebral arteries, the thoracic or abdominal section of the aorta, and the femoral and popliteal arteries of the leg. Some aneurysms are without symptoms and are discovered by accident or an X ray.

A cerebral aneurysm, depending on its location, may rupture and cause bleeding within the subarachnoid space, or an artery within the brain tissue itself may rupture. If the hemorrhage is not too massive the blood clots. Later the body will slowly reabsorb the blood clots and function will return. Hemorrhage may be fatal, however, due to increased intracranial pressure from the blood, which compresses and damages brain tissue. Remember, the skull is a solid structure that does not stretch; therefore when bleeding occurs the delicate tissues of the brain are displaced and damaged. Cerebral aneurysms are graded from I to V depending on the amount of bleeding. Rebleeding after 7 to 10 days is not uncommon. When the initial blood has clotted, the body resumes its normal function of removing clotted material, which may lead to a renewed and often fatal recurrence.

Aneurysms of the aorta occur due to the great pressure in the artery. Rupture of the aorta is usually fatal. If the thoracic aneurysm begins by "splitting" of the wall, the person may experience a tearing or ripping sensation accompanied by chest pain, pallor, rapid pulse, shortness of breath, loss of pulses below the neck, and other symptoms. Surgery can be accomplished to remove the damaged segment of the aorta and replace it with a Dacron or Teflon blood vessel graft.

An abdominal aneurysm is usually without symptoms but is detectable on palpation as a pulsating mass in an area around the umbilicus (navel). If it ruptures, the patient may experience pain similar to that of kidney spasms. About 20% of such patients die immediately; however, if the bleeding is in the retroperitoneal space (behind the peritoneal lining of the abdomen) the limited space puts pressure on the tear as it fills with blood, closing off the opening. An abdominal aneurysm is repaired like an aneurysm of the thoracic aorta. In addition, an external Dacron prosthesis (artificial part) may be applied around the aneurysm and sutured into place to support the weakened wall.

Aneurysms in the lower extremities may interfere with circulation and result in severe ischemia (lack of blood) and gangrene (tissue death), which may require amputation.

Angina. This heart condition causes severe chest pain that radiates down the inner surface of the left arm, usually associated with emotional stress and/or physical exertion. The pain is believed to be caused by a spasm of one or more coronary arteries, which results in ischemia to a portion of the heart muscle. The episode may last from a few seconds to several minutes. Symptoms, in addition to the pain, include irregular heart rate, lowered blood pressure, anxiety, and perspiration. The treatment consists of nitroglycerin, in a tablet form, placed under the tongue or applied to the body in a paste form. The nitroglycerin dilates the constricted artery or arteries to permit the flow of blood to the heart tissue. When angina pain persists after 10 minutes and the use of three sublingual tablets, the patient should go directly to the nearest hospital emergency room.

The patient must be instructed to have nitroglycerin available at all times. Tablets must be kept in a dark, tightly closed bottle, without cotton, and be protected from heat and sunlight. Tablets over 3 months old should be discarded. Nitroglycerin has recently been produced in a Band-aid form to permit prolonged release of the drug in measurable doses. It is also available as an oral spray.

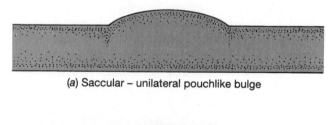

(a) Saccular – unilateral pouchlike bulge

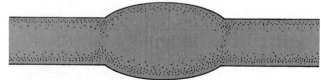

(b) Fusiform – a spindle-shaped bulge of the entire artery wall

FIGURE 13–101 Types of aneurysms

Arrest (Cardiac). This is complete, sudden cessation of heart action. The condition is rapidly fatal, producing irreversible brain damage after 5 minutes. It is believed to result from a failure in the body's ability to transport calcium, which interferes with its electrical and mechanical functions. It is associated with severe lack of blood to the myocardium. Cardiac arrest can also be caused by heart failure, electrical shock, fibrillation, drowning, anesthetics, respiratory failure, and severe electrolyte imbalances.

Arrest is treated initially by external cardiac massage (CPR or cardiopulmonary resuscitation technique), then supplemented by defibrillation, IV drug therapy, and ventilation procedures. Death is certain if function cannot be restored quickly.

Arrhythmia. This term is used to identify any abnormal changes in the heart rhythm. Arrhythmias vary in severity from mild to life-threatening, as with fibrillation. They are classified according to the origin of the irregularity; for example, PVC or atrial flutter. The more the heart action is affected, the greater the consequences on the cardiac output and the blood pressure, which in turn determines the clinical significance.

Arteriosclerosis. A "hardening" of the arteries and arterioles is caused by changes in their structural walls. The muscular and elastic tissue is gradually replaced by fibrous tissue and calcification. Since the vessels are no longer capable of expanding and recoiling with each heartbeat, the heart must exert more pressure on the blood to pump it through the more rigid vessels. Arteriosclerosis results in high blood pressure and may lead to an aneurysm and cerebral hemorrhage.

Atherosclerosis. This condition is characterized by the deposit of fatty material along the linings of the arteries, Figure 13–102. As the material builds up, the opening of the artery may become partially or totally closed, thereby reducing or eliminating the flow of blood to the area. Atherosclerosis can also result in elevated blood pressure, but the greatest danger results from the atherosclerotic plaque deposits breaking loose and circulating through the blood stream as emboli.

Athletic Heart Syndrome. This is a series of cardiac changes resulting from strenuous exercise. Primarily the heart enlarges (cardiomegaly), particularly the ventricles, because of its adaptive ability to meet the body's need for increased output. Since the heart is a muscle, it reacts just as the biceps do to physical endurance training. This syndrome is increasing due to the emphasis on physical fitness.

The athletic heart usually produces no symptoms except perhaps pounding or irregularity after strenuous activity. Bradycardia of 40 beats per minute is common and may be considered "normal" due to the heart's increased efficiency upon contraction.

Carditis. Literally, inflammation of the heart, the term is usually used with one of three prefixes that define the portion of the heart that is involved. The inflammation results from an infectious process caused by a viral, fungal, or bacterial invasion. Other causes vary with the form of inflammation, as follows.

■ *Pericarditis*—An inflammation of the pericardium, the fibroserous tissue sac which covers the heart. It may result in a purulent or bloody exudate forming within the sac, or the tissue may become thickened and fibrous, constricting the filling action of the heart. Pericarditis can follow injury to the heart, an infarction, or cardiac surgery.

Acute pericarditis typically causes sharp, sudden pain that begins at the sternum and radiates across the back to the shoulders and arms. It is similar to pleurisy, becoming more intense on inspiration but decreasing when sitting upright and leaning forward. A very serious condition will occur if the collection of fluid within the pericardium is rapid. Pressure within the sac prevents ventricular filling during diastole, thereby severely decreasing cardiac output and resulting in pallor, hypotension, and eventually cardiovascular collapse and death. Emergency treatment to remove the fluid by needle aspiration or surgical incision will result in a dramatic improvement.

Pericarditis that causes a gradual fluid accumulation allows time for the pericardium to stretch, often to hold 1 to 2 liters of fluid. Chronic pericarditis that results in constriction or recurrent collection of fluid may necessitate partial removal of the pericardium to allow escape of the fluid or, if constriction, a total pericardectomy (removal of the pericardium).

■ *Myocarditis*—An inflammation of the myocardium (heart muscle). It can occur in both acute and chronic forms. Symptoms produced are generally nonspecific, such as fatigue, palpitations, fever, and dyspnea. It is usually an uncomplicated disease and is self-limiting in nature. Normally, it is associated with a recent upper respiratory infection (URI) and fever.

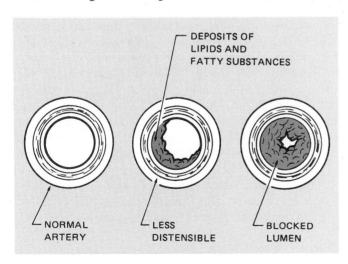

DEPOSITS OF LIPIDS AND FATTY SUBSTANCES

NORMAL ARTERY

LESS DISTENSIBLE

BLOCKED LUMEN

FIGURE 13–102 Atherosclerosis of an artery

Myocarditis may produce mild chest soreness and a feeling of pressure but not the anginal type of pain. Occasionally, myocarditis may initiate a degenerative process of the tiny fibrils (small fibers) in the muscular tissue. This may result in heart failure, enlargement, and arrhythmia. Myocarditis is treated with antibiotics, bed rest, and appropriate measures for complications that may develop.

- *Endocarditis*—Infection of the endocardial lining, heart valves, tissue adjoining artificial valves, or the blood vessel linings. The infecting organism in acute endocarditis is usually a streptococcus, staphylococcus, or pneumococcus. The gonococcus is also capable of causing endocarditis. Intravenous drug abuse may lead to infections from staph or fungi normally present on the skin surface. A subacute form may affect persons with valve or other cardiac lesions that may be acquired or congenital. In the infectious process, fibrin and platelets collect where the invading circulating organisms have produced wartlike vegetations on the valves and often the surrounding structures. The vegetative growths may cause serious complications if they embolize to the spleen, kidneys, or lungs.

If endocarditis is left untreated it usually results in death. Recovery is improved to 70% with proper treatment. When severe valve damage occurs, resulting complications may include insufficient cardiac action and congestive failure due to improper valve function. Damaged valves can be surgically removed with open heart surgery and replaced with artificial valves. If the infection involves an artificial valve, surgery to replace the prosthesis will be required.

Cerebrovascular Accident (CVA). A condition commonly known as a stroke, CVA is the sudden impairment of the flow of blood to the brain, thereby diminishing or interrupting the supply of oxygen and causing serious damage or destruction of brain tissue. A **cerebrovascular accident** is the result of high blood pressure, which ruptures an artery; artherosclerosis, which occludes an artery; or thrombosis (a blood clot), which interrupts the flow of blood. When a large enough area is involved, death will result.

CVAs are classified according to their course of progression. *Transient ischemic attacks* (TIAs) are small, temporary interruptions of blood flow. A progressive stroke is one which is in progress, such as with a thrombosis. It begins with some neurological symptoms and worsens within a day or two. A complete stroke is at its maximum when it occurs. Approximately one-half of CVA patients die as a result of the condition.

Symptoms vary with the area of the brain that is involved. CVAs involving posterior cerebral arteries affect the vision and often result in coma. Anterior artery involvement results in confusion, weakness, loss of coordination, personality changes, and numbness, especially in the legs. If the CVA occurs in the right hemisphere of the brain, symptoms are produced on the left side of the body, and if in the left hemisphere, on the right side. A CVA may leave the patient with many varied symptoms, which may include: slurred speech, amnesia, dizziness, paralysis (one extremity, one side, or total), inability to speak, coma, double vision, incontinence (inability to control bladder and bowels), and rigidity.

Congestive Heart Failure (CHF). This group of cardiac dysfunctions results in poor performance of the heart with related congestion of the circulatory system. Usually the myocardium of the left ventricle is affected, often as a result of prolonged high blood pressure. **Congestive heart failure** can also be a complication of coronary artery disease or a result of a mechanical disorder involving the heart's valvular functions.

With left-sided heart failure, cardiac output is decreased due to poor emptying of the ventricle. However, the left atrium continues to force blood into the ventricle resulting in increased pressure and volume within the ventricle. As this backup continues, the left atrium becomes congested, backing up blood into the pulmonary veins and then the pulmonary capillary beds. The fluid in the capillaries fills the alveolar spaces, resulting in pulmonary edema. There is a lack of oxygen exchange, and a decrease in the emptying capability of the right ventricle. Symptoms of left-sided failure are shortness of breath, inability to breathe while lying down, periods of gasping for air, weak and rapid pulse, cool and clammy skin, and an ashen gray or cyanotic skin coloring. Often a cough produces pink, frothy sputum.

Right-sided heart failure is usually a result of failure on the left side. However, it can occur in isolation as a result of pulmonary disease, a malfunctioning tricuspid valve, or a congenital defect. With right-sided failure, returning blood flow becomes congested in the systemic circulation, eventually causing fluid to enter the interstitial spaces. Initially, the fluid can be viewed as edema in the lower extremities, but as the failure continues edema is present in the upper extremities and in various organs throughout the system. Right-sided failure symptoms include swelling of the extremities, enlarged liver and spleen, and ascites (fluid in the abdominal cavity) due to filtration from portal circulation venous pressure.

Heart failure is extremely serious. Treatment involves the use of drugs to quickly increase cardiac output and remove congested fluids. Arterial vasodilators increase the efficiency of heart action. Bed rest is enforced and antiembolism stockings are used to prevent thromboembolism due to venous stasis. Continued treatment involves the use of cardiac drugs, frequent periods of rest, the use of elastic support stockings, skin care of the lower extremities, and dietary adjustments to reduce sodium intake and ensure proper nutrition.

Coronary Artery Disease. This disease of the arteries that surround the heart, carrying oxygen and nutrients to the myocardium, characteristically results from atherosclerosis, which narrows the vessel openings, thereby reducing the volume of blood flow to that portion of the heart muscle served by the arterial branch. Consequent lack of oxygen causes the typical symptoms of angina: tightness of the chest and crushing substernal chest pains radiating to the left arm, neck, and shoulder blades. Other symptoms may be nausea, vomiting, fainting, and perspiring. When angina pain persists, it suggests an infarction.

Coronary artery disease may be diagnosed by the ECG during an attack or during a treadmill or exercise bicycle test. An angiograph, also called an arteriograph, allows visualization by X-ray examination of the arteries following injection of a contrast medium into an artery.

Narrowed, clogged arteries can be treated by three methods. First is the use of nitrates to dilate the vessel. Nitroglycerin in tablet form is placed under the tongue or can be applied in an ointment form to the skin surface. Second, an angioplasty can be performed during catheterization of the heart. A balloonlike device is inflated to compress the fatty deposits against the arterial walls thereby opening the constricted vessel, Figure 13–103. A third method is coronary bypass surgery. This entails bypassing clogged arteries by redirecting blood through vein grafts surgically transplanted from the legs to the heart's surface.

Coronary artery disease is best treated by prevention, which includes weight control; a diet low in salt, fats, and cholesterol; regular active exercise; reduction of stress; and refraining from smoking.

Embolism. An embolus is defined as foreign matter that enters and circulates in the blood stream. Emboli (more than one) can result from various situations. A thrombus that forms within a blood vessel becomes an embolus when it breaks loose and begins to circulate. When the embolus obstructs a blood vessel it is called an embolism. An embolus can also result from air introduced into a blood vessel. An infection may produce a circulating clump of exudate, as discussed under endocarditis. Skeletal fractures are known to cause the formation of fat emboli. One theory holds that minute fat globules from the bone marrow enter the damaged blood vessels at the fracture site. The greatest danger of fat emboli is that they may circulate to the capillary beds in the lungs and block the alveolar exchange, resulting in an insufficient supply of oxygen.

An embolus of any type is potentially lethal if the circulating mass is of adequate size to obstruct the blood supply to a significant portion of an organ. The resulting infarction (interference with circulation) is especially rapid when it occurs within a major pulmonary artery or in one of the coronary arteries, and it can prove fatal. Infarction of a kidney, the spleen, or the brain will produce symptoms related to the degree of tissue damage. If a nonvital organ is extensively destroyed, surgical removal may be indicated.

Hypertension. In this condition, blood pressure is consistently elevated above 140/90 for persons under age 50 and 150/90 for those over 50. The severity can be gauged by the diastolic pressure, or the least amount of pressure present during the resting phase of the heartbeat. Mild hypertension diastole is about 100 mm Hg, moderate is 110, and severe is over 120 mm Hg.

Hypertension may be classified as *essential* (unknown cause) or *secondary* (resulting from another disease or disorder). Essential hypertension is correlated with family history, race (higher among blacks), obesity, stress, a diet high in saturated fats and salt, oral contraceptives, and aging.

Secondary hypertension may be the result of kidney disease; thyroid, pituitary or parathyroid dysfunction; or neurological disorders that interfere with blood pressure

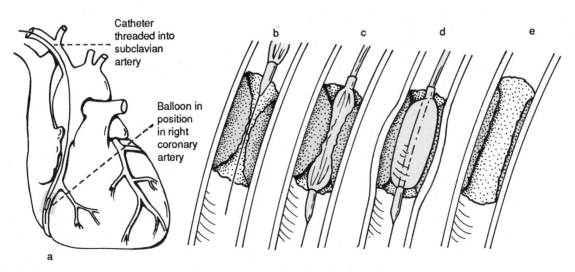

FIGURE 13–103 Balloon angioplasty (From Burke, *Human Anatomy & Physiology in Health and Disease*, 3d ed. Copyright 1992, Delmar Publishers Inc.)

regulation. Treatment of the primary cause will reduce the blood pressure.

Hypertension may also be classified as *benign* or *malignant.* In the benign form, the pressure rises moderately over a fairly long period of time. Malignant hypertension is characterized by an accelerated, rapid, and severe increase, which may not respond to treatment.

Hypertension is the foremost contributing factor to CVAs, kidney damage, and various cardiac conditions. It is predictably more severe among individuals who smoke, because the nicotine in tobacco causes constriction of the blood vessels.

Treatment of hypertension is directed at reducing the elevated pressure and maintaining an acceptable level. It is of great importance to prevent complications of the disease. Treatment focuses around diet, the control of sodium (currently being questioned), the use of diuretics to encourage elimination of retained body fluids, and antihypertensive drugs to reduce vasoconstriction and/or increase kidney filtration. It is of the utmost importance that the patient maintain the treatment regimen, since hypertension is not curable, only treatable. Patients must be encouraged to continue with their medication even though they have no symptoms of hypertension. Compliance with dietary and drug therapy is the only means of preventing life-threatening complications.

Hypotension. Defined as blood pressure below the normal range, hypotension can result from an acute blood loss, heart failure, shock, kidney failure, thyroid disease, and certain other infectious conditions. Hypotension may become life-threatening when the circulation of blood becomes impaired and the exchange of gases is inadequate. The treatment of hypotension is determined by the underlying cause. Options include transfusion and intravenous fluid replacement, cardiac stimulants, thyroid medication, and other appropriate drugs.

Leukemia. This is a malignant disease of the bone marrow (myelogenous) or lymphatic tissue (lymphocytic). Leukemia can be present in either an acute or chronic form. In the acute phase, a great number of immature white blood cells are produced in the bone marrow or lymph tissue. The excessive amount of white cells cause pressure and discomfort within the bones, swelling and pain in the lymph nodes, and greatly elevated white cell count in the blood. The earliest symptoms of the disease are fever, pallor, fatigue, swelling of lymphoid tissue (spleen, liver), and a tendency toward large bruises.

Even in the presence of great numbers of leukocytes and lymphocytes, the body has little defense against infection due to the immaturity of the cells. The major complication of leukemia is infection. The disease process may progress to produce bleeding within the brain and other vital organs. In acute leukemia, the onset is rapid and death occurs within a few months unless treated aggressively with chemotherapy. Acute lympho-cytic leukemia is the form common in children. Typically it is approximately 30% into its course before it is diagnosed. Acute myelogenous leukemia is more common in adults. Both acute forms are ultimately fatal, but long-term remissions in the childhood form and approximately 50% cures are now being reported.

Chronic leukemia differs from acute only in that its onset is more insidious (slow), and its course is more prolonged. The median survival rate is 3 to 4 years. Often the first symptoms are a general malaise (vague discomfort, feeling "bad") and weight loss. Anemia, fatigue, and greatly enlarged spleen and lymph nodes are typical symptoms. Chronic myelogenous leukemia is almost always associated with a chromosome irregularity known as the Philadelphia chromosome. Chronic myelogenous leukemia is characterized by two distinct phases: the chronic phase, which is insidious, lasting an average of 3 to 4 years; and the eventual acute phase, an immature cell crisis, lasting only a few weeks or months before death occurs.

Diagnosis can be confirmed initially by blood studies in addition to typical clinical findings. Differentiation of type and positive identification of acute or chronic forms is possible through cellular and chromosomal analysis of bone marrow aspirates. The bone marrow sample can be withdrawn through a large-gauge needle introduced into the sternum or preferably the posterior superior iliac spine.

Treatment varies with the type and form of leukemia. Systemic chemotherapy is used to destroy abnormal white cells and induce a remission so that more normal function of the bone marrow will occur. The side effects of the drugs are loss of hair, nausea, vomiting, gouty arthritis, and a number of other complications. Some success has been achieved with bone marrow transplants among siblings, particularly twins. This procedure is especially indicated in treatment of children and younger adults. Before the marrow is given, the patient is medicated with large doses of drugs to completely suppress the body's ability to react to foreign material. Total bone radiation treatments are used to induce marrow aplasia (lack of function) and aid in lowering the body's resistance to the transplant. Approximately 500 to 750 ml of bone marrow is removed from the pelvic bones of the donor. The marrow is processed and then given to the recipient intravenously. To prevent contact with any microorganisms, the patient is placed in a reverse isolation unit. The patient is in an extremely vulnerable state and a prolonged hospital stay is inevitable. Barring complications, which are numerous, chances for recovery are good.

Murmur. The abnormal sound of blood flowing through a heart valve can be heard with a stethoscope and is known as a murmur. The murmur is named for the valve which is "leaking." The mitral valve is the one most frequently affected and the gurgling or swishing sound is called a mitral murmur. Murmurs are further identified as systolic or diastolic. This classification specifies whether the sound is heard during the contraction or relaxation phase of the heartbeat.

Valve damage that results in murmurs can be caused by rheumatic fever, an inflammatory disease which follows a streptococcal infection. The valves may become inflamed and in time thicken and develop scar tissue. Hence the valves lose their flexibility and no longer close completely.

Endocarditis is another condition that may lead to valve damage. As previously discussed, bacteria circulating through the heart collect on the valvular surfaces causing the growth of vegetation and resulting in ulceration and death of some tissue. In its damaged state, the valve is no longer capable of normal function. Preexisting valve damage from rheumatic fever, especially of the mitral valve, is quite common in endocarditis. Artificial valve replacement may be indicated to alleviate the problem.

Myocardial Infarction (MI). A complication of coronary artery disease that results from occlusion (partial or complete) of the artery causing myocardial tissue destruction. It is characterized by severe, crushing pain, which radiates through the chest to the neck and jaw and down the left arm. It is not relieved by rest, as with angina, and is accompanied by nausea, perspiration, a change in blood pressure, hypo- or hypertension, and dyspnea. MIs are one of the leading causes of death in the United States. Mortality is high when treatment is delayed; approximately 50% of patients die within an hour after symptoms develop.

Predisposing factors include sedentary life-style, stressful occupation, obesity, cigarette smoking, hypertension, aging, positive family history, and elevated levels of cholesterol and triglycerides in the blood. An attack can often be precipitated by a heavy meal, physical exertion, or exposure to cold weather.

Treatment of MI is directed at relieving the pain with strong analgesic drugs such as demerol or morphine and administering extra oxygen to maintain an adequate supply to the tissues. It is important to prevent complications. Heart rhythm must be stabilized to prevent arrhythmia, which can lead to congestive heart failure. Complete bed rest must be enforced to decrease cardiac workload and a possible additional infarction. Anticoagulant drugs are given to reduce the tendency to develop thromboembolism.

Severe complications may occur in the damaged ventricular area in addition to the systemic threat of embolism and heart failure. Unusual and potentially lethal conditions may develop. The ventricular septum may rupture, causing a circulatory defect in which blood flows between the ventricles. The ventricular wall may weaken due to necrosis following infarction. The wall may develop an aneurysm, leading to a ventricular rupture.

The patient who survives an MI will be faced with a lengthy recovery period. Life-styles may need to be altered and dietary and smoking habits changed. An exercise rehabilitation program must be initiated and adhered to, to promote optimum recovery and maintenance of a healthy state.

Phlebitis. This localized inflammation of a vein causes an alteration in the epithelial lining, which is predisposing to the formation of a thrombus. Phlebitis can occur in deep or superficial veins (see thrombophlebitis).

Sickle Cell Anemia. This is a congenital anemia occurring primarily among blacks, about 1 in 10 of whom carry the abnormal gene. When two carriers have children, there is a 25% chance that each child will have the disease. When two persons with the disease sickle cell anemia have children, all children will have the disease. If only one has the disease and the other is normal, all children will be carriers of the trait.

Sickle cell anemia is characterized by red blood cells with a hemoglobin defect in their molecular structure that causes the cells to become sickle shaped. Cells of this shape cannot pass easily through blood vessels and they tend to interfere with circulation.

Symptoms are tachycardia, cardiomegaly, cardiac murmurs, chronic fatigue, unexplained dyspnea, chest pain, enlarged liver, jaundice, pallor, swollen joints, aching bones, and leg ulcers. These symptoms begin after about 6 months of age, when the protective excess amounts of hemoglobin present at birth are exhausted.

The most common feature of the disease is a painful crisis, which usually appears first at about age 5. Sickled red blood cells become tangled, causing blood vessel obstruction and a lack of oxygen to the tissues, with possible destruction of the involved area. This tissue infarction causes severe pain to the affected area. Usual sites are the lungs, liver, bones, and spleen. The spleen, particularly, is affected so frequently that the resulting damage and scarring cause it to shrink and become useless. A crisis usually lasts from 4 days to several weeks and recurs cyclically.

Diagnosis can be made from a positive family history and the typical clinical features. It is confirmed by a blood smear that shows the sickled cell structure. At present, research has failed to discover a means to prevent the sickling alteration. Treatment focuses on alleviating the symptoms of the disease and on transfusions with packed red cells when an aplastic crisis occurs (depression of bone marrow activity and destruction of RBCs).

The disease produces long-term complications such as delayed puberty and a tendency toward delayed growth. If the patient survives to adulthood, the body is described as spiderlike, with a narrow trunk and long extremities, curved spine, elongated skull, and barrel-shaped chest. Premature death may result from repeated infarctions within vital organs or from an infectious process. The most successful treatment may be prevention through genetic counseling of persons known to be carriers. Information is provided to allow individuals to arrive at informed decisions regarding the conception and birth of children.

Stasis Ulcer.   This is a secondary condition resulting from chronic venous insufficiency, a lower extremity trauma, or a skin irritation. The most common site of stasis ulcers is the ankle at the internal malleous area. Stasis ulcers develop following deep vein thrombophlebitis which destroys the valve structures. Communicating veins in the affected area fail to compensate for the damaged vein. The venous pressure increases, causing fluid to enter the interstitial tissues and produce edema. The tissue swelling leads to fibrosis and skin discoloration from blood entering the subcutaneous tissues. The poor condition of the skin and the inadequate circulation from the area lead to a breakdown of the surrounding tissues, Figure 13–104.

Treatment of small ulcers involves elevation of the affected extremity, warm soaks, bed rest, and the use of drugs to counteract infection. When the swelling subsides, pressure is applied by a sponge rubber dressing or an Unna's boot (zinc gelatin boot). Large stasis ulcers not responding to treatment may require removal of the ulcer site followed by a skin graft.

Thrombophlebitis.   This is an acute condition in which the lining of the vein wall becomes inflamed and a thrombus forms. Thrombophlebitis can develop within small superficial veins and is usually self-limiting. DVT can affect small or large veins. When there is an alteration of the vein lining, platelets begin to collect at the area. The platelet fibrin catches red blood cells, white blood cells, and additional platelets, forming a blood clot. The thrombus enlarges rapidly, particularly if the blood flow is slow, causing an inflammation which becomes fibrotic. The enlarging clot may completely fill the vein opening, occluding the vessel, or it may break loose becoming an embolus.

DVT usually results from lining damage, but it can also follow accelerated blood clotting and a slow, reduced flow of blood. Conditions that precipitate thrombophlebitis are prolonged bed rest, trauma, childbirth, surgery, and the use of oral contraceptives.

Symptoms of deep thrombophlebitis include severe pain, fever, chills, and possibly edema, with discoloration of the affected extremity. When superficial veins are involved, visible and palpable signs may include heat, swelling, tenderness, redness and discoloration, and induration (hardening) along the affected portion of the vein.

Treatment is directed toward preventing complications, controlling the development of thrombi, and relieving the discomfort. The patient is maintained on bed rest, with the affected extremity elevated to aid circulation. Warm, moist soaks are applied to the affected area. Medication is given to relieve pain, and frequently anticoagulants are used to reduce the blood's clotting ability. Antiembolism stockings (tight-fitting, elastic, knee- or thigh-length hose) are indicated to assist the return of blood from the legs to the heart. Individuals who are prone to develop thrombophlebitis should avoid prolonged periods of sitting or standing, especially with little movement, to help eliminate pooling of blood in the lower extremities. When sitting, the legs should be resting on a support that does not cause pressure to interfere with return circulation.

Varicosities.   Veins which become dilated, twisted, and inefficient are known as varicose veins. The condition usually results from weakness of the valves in the saphenous vein and its branches, which permits blood to leak backward due to incomplete closure. As the blood accumulates, the veins become dilated, the valve is no longer capable of reaching across the opening of the vein, and the situation becomes worse. This stasis (stagnation) of blood is often the result of occupations requiring long periods of standing or of other factors interfering with circulation, such as pressure against the veins during pregnancy.

Symptoms include a feeling of heaviness, night leg cramps, aching, and a feeling of fatigue. With deep vein involvement, edema may accumulate in the feet and ankles, often associated with the discoloration that precedes stasis ulcers. Superficial varicosed veins can often be seen or palpated behind the knees or on the medial surface of the calf. Varicosed veins are not to be confused with the tiny purplish red surface veins seen on the skin of most adults. These are commonly referred to as spider veins and are evidence of increased venous pressure. They are often associated with varicosities.

Treatment for mild to moderate varicosities includes an exercise program to improve circulation; use of antiembolism stockings; attention to sitting position; and the elimination of tight-fitting or constricting clothing such as girdles, garters, elastic bands of clothing, and knee-high or thigh-high hose. More severe varicosities may require injection of a sclerosing agent into small venous areas to scar and harden the vein. Larger involvement will necessitate surgical ligation (tying off) of the involved vein from its branches and stripping the vein from the leg.

Complete Chapter 13, Unit 8 in the workbook to help you meet the objectives at the beginning of this unit and therefore achieve competency of this subject matter.

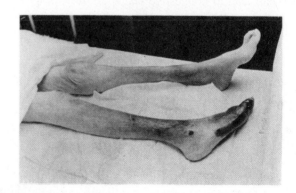

FIGURE 13–104   Stasis ulcer and gangrene (From Burke, *Human Anatomy & Physiology in Health and Disease*, 3d ed. Copyright 1992, Delmar Publishers Inc.)

U N I T   9

The Immune System

Upon completion of this unit, the student will meet the following terminal performance objectives by verifying knowledge of the facts and principles presented through oral and written communication at a level deemed competent.

1. Relate the origin and maturation of blood cells.
2. List the organs of the immune system and identify their locations.
3. Explain how the immune system differentiates between "self" and "non-self."
4. Differentiate between the roles of B cells and T cells.
5. Discuss the three types of T cells describing their roles.
6. Tell how NK cell action differs from phagocytic action.
7. Discuss complement and what it does.
8. Explain what causes an inflammatory response.
9. Differentiate between antibody-mediated and cell-mediated immune response.
10. Tell how immunizations and vaccines work.
11. Explain how the AIDS virus destroys the immune system.
12. Identify ways to acquire the AIDS virus.
13. List four high-risk behaviors to avoid.
14. Discuss how an allergen causes an immune response.
15. Explain how cancer develops and what might be some causative factors.
16. Identify the characteristics of a cancerous cell.
17. List the six factors that interfere with or prohibit immune response.
18. Discuss eight diagnostic procedures used to determine the presence of cancer.
19. Discuss the three major methods of treating cancer.
20. Discuss 10 new investigative treatments for cancer.
21. Discuss chronic fatigue syndrome, its symptoms and treatment.
22. Discuss how lupus affects the immune system and the major body organs it may effect.
23. Differentiate between discoid, systemic, and drug-induced lupus.
24. Identify the general and suggestive symptoms of lupus.
25. Discuss how lupus is treated.
26. Discuss how rheumatoid arthritis may be connected to the immune system.
27. Describe the beginning and eventual symptoms of rheumatoid arthritis.
28. Spell and define, using the glossary at the back of the text, all the words to know in this unit.

abstinence	immunosuppressed
acquired	interferon
allergens	interleukin
allergies	intracellular
anaphylaxsis	lupus erythematosus
antibody	lymphocyte
antibody-mediated	lymphokine
antigen	macrophage
autoimmune	malignant
autologous	metastasis
basophil	monoclonal
benign	monokine
biopsy	monocyte
cancerous	monogamous
carcinoembryonic antigen	mutation
carcinogensis	neoadjuvant
carcinoma	neoplastic
cell-mediated	neutrophils
chemotherapy	oncogenes
clone	opportunistic
complement	permeable
corticosteroids	phagocyte
cytotoxic	prostaglandin
debilitating	psychoneuroimmunology
desensitization	radiation
discoid	Raynaud's phenomenon
eosinophils	remission
extracellular	retrovirus
heterosexual	sarcoma
histamine	suppressor
homosexual	syndrome
humoral	thymus
hyperthermia	transmission
immune	vaccine
immunodeficiency	virus
immunoglobulin	

The **immune** system is not a true body system, but rather a function of the white blood cells of the circulatory system. However, because of its essential role in the health and well-being of humans and the severity of the consequences when it fails, it is considered to be of sufficient significance to warrant individual emphasis.

The immune system is the body's way of defending itself against the environment of microbes in which we live. There are several **antigens** (foreign materials) in the environment that are capable of causing an immune response, such as a virus, a bacterium, a fungus, a parasite, or even only a portion or product of these organisms. Tissues or cells from another individual in transfusions or organ transplants are also "foreign" as are the proteins we eat until they are properly processed by the body. Particles in the air or foods we eat, which cause reactions, are also antigens but are called **allergens.** One's own cells, which become malignant, are likewise targeted as "different."

The body's first line of defense against disease is the protective barrier of the skin and the mucus secreted by the mucous membranes. While they are intact, antigens on their surfaces cannot enter. Various body secretions provide bactericidal components such as acid in the gastric juice, lysozme in tears and saliva, and certain "normal" bacteria that control potential pathogenic bacteria and fungi in the vagina and intestines. The immune system is composed of billions of cells and an even a greater number of protein molecules known as antibodies and complement, which can be directed toward foreign invaders.

Scientists have made great progress in understanding the function of the many components of the immune system, but a great deal still remains a mystery. The immune response is an unbelievably complicated interaction between cells, antibodies, and proteins against antigens and allergens. Recently, it has been recognized that the brain and nervous system also have an effect on the immune system. A new science, psychoneuroimmunology, is researching the connection between the brain, behavior, and immunity.

This unit introduces the basics of immunity—the cells, their function, the process of developing immunity, and the destruction of antigens. There are great numbers of immune cells. Some are for general defense, others are highly specific, but to be most effective they must work together. They can communicate through direct contact or chemical messengers. When an antigen appears, the specifically matched cells are stimulated to undergo mitosis and multiply rapidly to destroy the invader. When the attack has succeeded, another message stops the activity. A look at some of the diseases resulting from ineffective or inappropriate immune response and how science is using its knowledge of the immune system to try to control their outcome will prove most interesting.

Origin of Cells

To understand immunity, it is necessary to learn about the structure and function of its component parts. In the last unit, it was stated that cells within the blood are of three types—red, white and platelets. The leukocytes (white cells) were identified as playing a vital role in defending the body. It is these cells in cooperation with protein molecules that are responsible for immunity.

All blood cells originate in the bone marrow and initially develop from stem cells, Figure 13–105. They progress through stages on their way to maturity. Erythrocytes (RBCs) develop from erythroid stem cells and mature in the bone marrow. White blood cells (WBCs) which become the granulated eosinophils, neutrophils and basophils, develop from myeloid stem cells. One type of agranulocyte, the lymphocyte, develops from a lymphocyte stem cell into two major classes, B cells that mature in the bone marrow and T cells that mature in the thymus. Mononuclear phagocyte stem cells become the

monocytes, which circulate in the blood then enter into the tissue to become macrophages. Phagocytes are cells that engulf and destroy antigens. Several cells have this capability, mainly the monocytes and macrophages. Neutrophils are also phagocytic but in addition carry granules with potent chemicals to destroy microorganisms. They are key players in acute inflammatory reactions. Eosinophils and basophils, also granulated cells, release their chemicals to effect cells or microbes in their environment.

Organs of the Immune System

The organs of the immune system are located throughout the body and are generally known as lymphoidal organs because they are where lymphocytes develop, grow, or perform their functions. These organs include the bone marrow, the thymus, lymph nodes, spleen, tonsils, adenoids, appendix, and clumps of lymphoid tissue in the small intestine called Peyer's patches, Figure 13–106, page 318. The blood and lymphatic vessels are also considered to be lymphoid organs. When the B and T lymphocytes leave the bone marrow and thymus they travel throughout the body in the blood and lymphatic vessels. All along the lymphatic vessels are clusters of lymph nodes. Each node contains specialized compartments that store large numbers of B and T cells as well as others that are capable of trapping antigens to present to the T cells for destruction, Figure 13–107, page 318.

The spleen likewise provides a place for antigen destruction to occur. It also has compartments for different types of cells. As the lymph flows around the cells and through the body, it carries the lymphocytes, macrophages, and antigens to the lymph nodes where the antigens are filtered out and shown by the macrophages to the immune cells to be destroyed. Then the lymphocytes and other immune cells go back into circulation to search for more foreign materials, gradually working their way back to the lymphatic vessels and nodes and another cycle is completed.

Cell Markers

Basic to the immune system is the ability of cells to distinguish between self and non-self. Immune cells are also able to remember previous encounters and react accordingly. All body cells carry molecules that are encoded by a group of genes contained in a specific chromosome known as the *major histocompatibility complex* (MHC). This allows immune cells to recognize and communicate with each other. The body's immune defenses do not normally attack cells carrying this "self" marker. But when they meet molecules carrying foreign markers, they move quickly to destroy them. Any substance capable of triggering an immune response is considered to be an antigen. An antigen announces its foreignness by carrying perhaps several hundred different kinds of characteristic shapes called *epitopes,* which

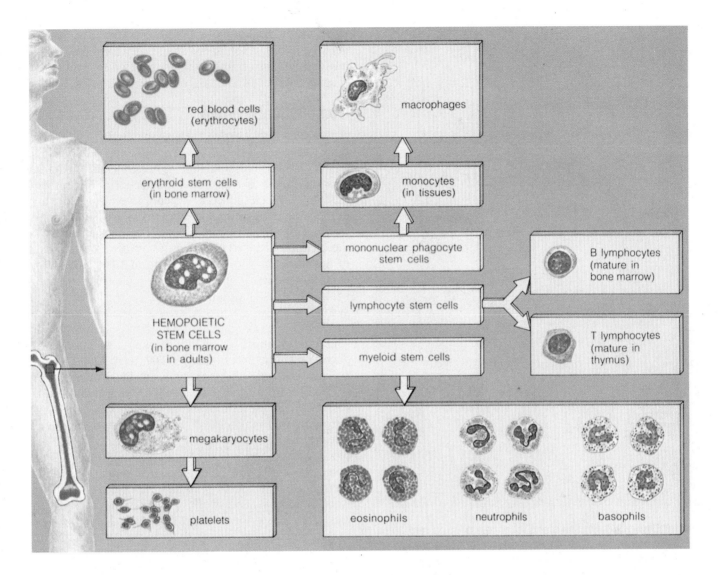

FIGURE 13–105 Origin of cells (From Starr & Taggart, *Biology, The Unity and Diversity of Life*, 5th ed. 1989, Wadsworth Publishing Co.)

stick out from its surface. The immune system is capable of recognizing millions of non-self molecules or it can produce molecules and cells that can match to and counteract against each one.

Lymphocytes

Lymphocytes are the small white cells charged with immunity functions. Both B cells and T cells are able to recognize specific antigen targets. When B cells are maturing, they go through two stages of development beginning before birth and lasting for the first few months of an infant's life. Each immature cell inserts numerous molecules of one specific kind of antibody into its cytoplasmic membrane. Antibodies belong to a family of large molecules known as immunoglobulins, which are protein substances that have two areas on their surface to uniquely match the surface of an antigen molecule. Scientists have identified nine distinct

classes of human immunoglobulins (Ig). IgG coats microorganisms to speed up the uptake by other immune system cells. IgM is very effective in killing bacteria. IgA is concentrated in body fluids to guard the entrances of the body. IgE is effective against parasites but also is the "problem" in allergies. IgD is found in the membranes of B cells and is thought to regulate the cell's activities.

When B cells come into contact with antigens, they undergo a second change. When the combining site of a B cell's surface "fits" one of the variety of antigen's shapes, they join and are changed into an antigen-antibody complex. The antibody can then perform its duty or cause the antigen to stick to other antigens forming clumps so the large macrophages can destroy large numbers of them at one time.

After B cells have undergone antigen-antibody complex, they begin to divide, rapidly producing many clone cells with the same antibody. Later the cells divide into

Organs of the Immune System

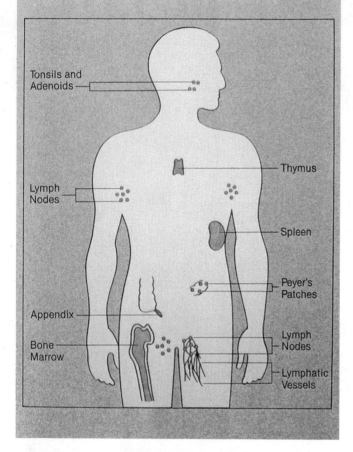

FIGURE 13–106 Organs of the immune system, (From Schindler, *Understanding the Immune System*, 1990, U.S. Department of Health and Human Services)

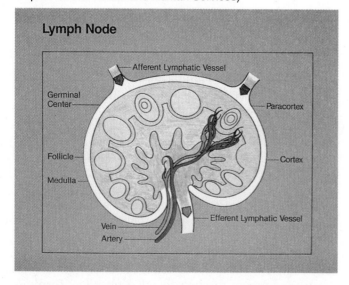

FIGURE 13–107 Lymph node. T cells concentrate in the paracortex, B cells in and around the germinal centers, and plasma cells in the medulla. (From Starr & Taggart, *Biology, The Unity and Diversity of Life*, 5th ed. 1989, Wadsworth Publishing Co.)

memory or plasma cells, Figure 13–108. The memory cells go to the lymph nodes to stand by for the next same antigen invasion while the plasma cells continue to secrete millions of identical antibody molecules.

Complement System

Antibodies may change their shape slightly when they bind with antigens. This change will expose two regions called complement-binding sites. Complement is a group of about 20 *inactive* enzyme proteins normally present in the blood. When one complement protein meets an antibody–antigen complex, it will *activate* and begin a chain reaction of attracting the others. The consequences are the creation of lethal chemicals to attract the phagocytes to the scene, coat the target cell to make it more recognizable, or destroy the antigen by puncturing its membrane. In this way, antibodies and the complement system work together to destroy antigens by **antibody-mediated** response also known as **humoral** immunity. This type of immunity is the resistance to disease produced by antibodies, Figure 13–109, page 320.

The events set off by antibody-mediated response and other chemicals help to develop an inflammatory response. When complement proteins begin to act, basophils and mast cells are also activated. Both cells release the substance called **histamine,** which dilates blood vessels and makes the vessel walls more **permeable.** This slows down the rate of flow and allows fluid to seep into the surrounding tissues. The result is localized warmth, redness, and swelling. The complement proteins and other factors in the fluid can easily leave the blood vessels and attract the phagocytes to fight the intruders.

T cells, in contrast to B cells, interact directly with their targets in what is called cellular immunity or **cell-mediated** response. T cells function in two major ways. Some are vital to the operation of other cells. B cells cannot make antibodies against most substances without a regulatory T cell assistance. One type of cell is known as the helper T and is identifiable by the T4 cell marker. Helper T cells are essential for activating B cells and other T cells as well as the natural killer (NK) cells and macrophages. A subset of T cells acts to turn off or "suppress" these cells. **Cytotoxic** (killer) T cells act directly on infected or malignant cells, as well as any other body cell that has a target antigen and an MHC marker. These cells usually carry the T8 marker and are called killer T cells (refer to Figure 13–108). One type can attach tightly to its target, secrete perforin and other chemicals, which make holes in the cell membrane, destroying it before it can reproduce. Unfortunately, killer cells can also cause rejection of tissue and organ transplants because of non-self markers.

Cytokines

Cytokines are non-antibody proteins that regulate the immune response. One type are **lymphokines,** which are

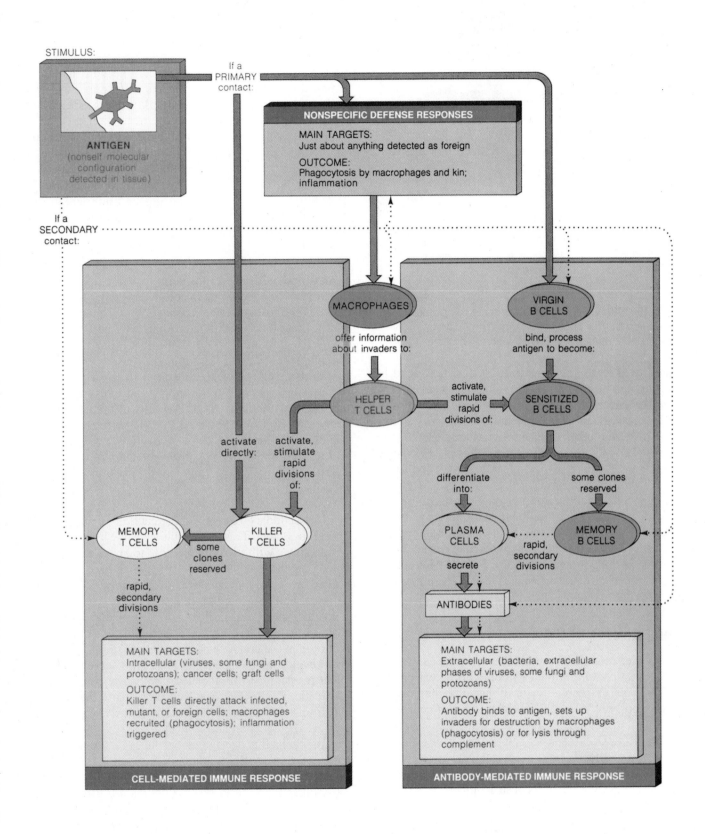

FIGURE 13–108 The development of B cells in antibody-mediated immune response and T cells in cell-mediated immune response (From Starr & Taggart, *Biology, The Unity and Diversity of Life*, 5th ed. 1989, Wadsworth Publishing Co.)

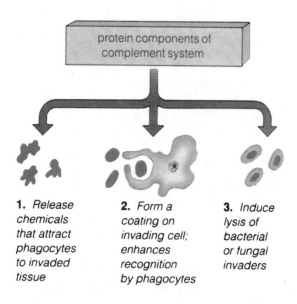

protein components of
complement system

1. *Release chemicals that attract phagocytes to invaded tissue*

2. *Form a coating on invading cell; enhances recognition by phagocytes*

3. *Induce lysis of bacterial or fungal invaders*

FIGURE 13–109 Function of proteins in the complement system (From Starr & Taggart, *Biology, The Unity and Diversity of Life*, 5th ed. 1989, Wadsworth Publishing Co.)

secreted by T cells, and the monokines, produced by monocytes and macrophages. These substances are diverse and potent chemical messengers. Lymphokines bind to specific receptors on target cells and set off other actions such as involving other cells and substances, encouraging cell growth, and stimulating macrophages. Two other cytokines are lymphotoxin from lymphocytes and tumor necrosis factor from macrophages. Both of these cytokines kill tumor cells. Many cytokines have been renamed as interleukins (IL), which means "messengers between leukocytes." IL-1 from macrophages helps to activate B and T cells. IL-2 is produced by antigen-activated T cells and promotes rapid growth of mature B and T cells and the development of different types of T cells. There are three other types of interleukins.

Natural Killer (NK) Cells

Natural killer cells (NK) are another type of deadly lymphocytes that contain granules filled with potent chemicals. They get the name "natural" because they do not need to recognize a specific antigen to kill a cell. They target tumor cells and protect against a wide variety of microbes. In AIDS, this killer cell activity is deactivated. NK cells, like killer Ts bind to their targets and deliver a lethal burst of chemicals to produce holes in the target cell's membrane leading to its destruction.

Immune Responses

The immune response system has two branches, one resulting from B cell activity, antibody-mediated immune response and one resulting from T cell activity, cell-mediated immune response (review Figure 13–108).

The response can also be primary, the first encounter with the antigen, or a secondary response with subsequent encounters. In primary antibody-mediated response, an antigen enters the body and goes undetected past "virgin" B cells until it meets one with matching antibody sites. The B cell connects (becomes sensitized) and processes the antigen, displaying its fragments bound to its MHC molecule to attract helper T cells. When the sensitized B cell and the helper T combine, interleukins are released, which cause the cell to begin mitosis. At the same time, other similar antigens have been engulfed and displayed by the macrophages. Helper T cells bind with the macrophages and interleukins are secreted. The secretion of interleukin stimulates the helper T cells to mature and secrete lymphokines to cause a rapid growth and division of the B cells. This produces a group of clones that release identical antibodies to bind with more antigens to be recognized and destroyed. Some of the B cells convert to memory B cells and go to lymphoidal tissues.

The immunoglobulins get other cells and substances involved. IgM and IgG activate macrophages and the complement system. IgE stimulates mast cells to release histamine. IgA causes secretions in the first line of defense in the saliva, tears, lungs, and intestines to protect the body's entrances. IgD works in the cell's membranes to regulate activity. A full primary immune response requires 5 to 6 days to develop.

Antibody-mediated responses act against bacteria and extracellular viruses, fungi, and parasites. It *cannot* react to an invader already within a cell's cytoplasm, only those in circulation or attached to a cell's surface.

In a secondary response, the reaction is much faster, only 2 to 3 days. This is possible because leftover clonal lymphocytes with memory are able to attack the antigen. Once one of the cells meets the same antigen, mitosis is immediate and large numbers of appropriately matched cells and antibodies are produced.

Primary response of T cells in cell-mediated response has already been described. The action is direct and quick. After the initial contact with an antigen, some T cells will also develop memory and are held in reserve for subsequent invasions. Cell-mediated immune responses attack intracellular viruses, fungi and protozoans, cancer cells, and transplant tissue cells. T cells will destroy any cell with an MHC marker and a target antigen.

Killer cells that cause rejection of organ transplants do so because the MHC markers of the donor cells are not identical self-markers unless from an identical twin. Individuals who are to receive organs are usually given drugs to destroy the killer Ts to prevent rejection but that leaves the recipient without the ability to have a full immune response to other invaders and can lead to death from infections such as pneumonia.

Both antibody-mediated and cell-mediated immune responses are controlled reactions. When the "battle" is won, binding sites are saturated with antibodies and the

suppressor T cells stop the attack. Without this feedback, immune reactions would go out of control.

There is a recognition of a connection between nutrition, mental and emotional health, and physical activity to the status of the immune system. There also seems to be a significance in the appropriate amounts of zinc, iodine, fats, sugars, and fiber. Some vitamins appear to reduce chronic stress, which is an immune depressor. The personality, coping style, quality of life, exercise, support of loved ones, and optimism, to name a few, all appear to greatly influence the effectiveness of the components of the immune system.

The following material is taken from a presentation by Elaine Glass, RN, MS, OCN; Clinical Nurse Specialist in Medical Oncology and Hematology at The Arthur G. James Cancer Hospital and Research Institute. She explains the functions of the components of the immune system and relates them to the familiar roles of a police and military force. She also interjects emotions and activities that affect the action of the components. This provides a good summary of the immune system.

COMPONENTS OF THE IMMUNE SYSTEM
AGRANULOCYTES
A. Macrophages/Monocytes
The cop on the beat
Monocytes circulate in the blood; macrophages infiltrate the tissues. They engulf antigens and summon other cells to analyze them.
(Stress causes release of cortisol that renders the macrophage unresponsive.
Exercise increases endorphins [natural brain analgesic] which may increase macrophage activity.)
B. Lymphocytes
A collective label for T and B immune cells
1. T CELLS
Involved in the cellular immune system response. Mature in the thymus gland.
   a. Helper T cell
   The detective
   Identifies the antigens trapped by macrophages or monocytes and stimulates other cells to destroy them. Does not attack or destroy by itself.
   b. Activated helper T cell
   Helps destroy identified antigens by producing interleukin-2, which stimulates other helper and killer T cells to multiply.
   c. Killer T cell
   SWAT team member
   Destroys cells that have been invaded by antigens. They can trigger a process that punctures a cell membrane and destroys it before the invading virus inside has a chance to grow.
   d. Natural killer T cell
   Rambo or a vigilante
   Attacks cancerous or virus-infected cells without previous exposure to the antigen. NKs are stimulated by interferon. They can recognize artificial antigens created in a lab to which humans have never come into contact.

(In one study, patients with a lot of support from their "significant others" and doctors, had higher levels of NK cells.)
   e. Suppressor T cell
   The police chief
   Slows down or stops other immune cell activity after antigens are destroyed.
2. B CELLS
Produces antibodies against antigens; involved in the humoral immune response.
   a. Plasma cell
   The army sergeant
   Descends from B cells to produce antibodies. They make thousands of antibodies per second.
   b. Antibodies
   The foot soldiers
   Proteins that neutralize antigens and destroy other cells where the antigen has invaded.
      1) IgG
      The most common protein antibody in the blood and tissue spaces where it coats antigens speeding their uptake by other immune cells.
      2) IgM
      A protein antibody that circulates in the bloodstream in star-shaped clusters, very effective in killing bacteria.
      3) IgA
      A protein antibody in body fluids (tears, saliva, respiratory and digestive tracts) to guard body entrances.
      (College students who watched a video of Mother Theresa had higher levels of IgG and A than students who watched a video that did not stimulate positive emotions.)
      4) IgE
      A protein antibody that attaches itself to mast cells and basophils. When it encounters its matching antigen, it stimulates the cell to pour out its contents. It provides protection by coating bacteria and viruses.
      5) IgD
      A protein antibody that inserts itself into the membrane of the B cell to regulate the activation of the cell.
   c. Complement
   Flying Aces
   A series of 20 proteins that circulate in the blood in an inactive state until they are triggered by contact with antigen-antibody complexes or by contact with the cell membrane of an invading organism.
3. MEMORY CELLS
   T cells = Police chief with a history on the force
   B cells = Army sergeant with a history in the service
   T and B cells that have been activated by an antigen and continue to circulate within the body, ready to attack an antigen if it reinvades. (These cells are the basis of how vaccines work.)
GRANULOCYTES
A group of immune cells filled with granules of toxic chemicals that enable them to digest microorganisms.
A. Neutrophil

Like cop on beat but more heavily armed.

A circulating WBC that destroys foreign matter and cell debris by phagocytosis, by digesting cellular membranes, and by releasing chemotactants and pyrogenic substances that cause fever.

B. Basophil

A firefighter

A circulating WBC that is responsible for allergy symptoms by releasing heparin, histamine, bradykinin, and serotonin from its granules, to cause vasodilation and permeability.

C. Eosinophil

A circulating WBC that can digest microorganisms, especially parasites, and assists in allergic reactions by detoxifying some of the inflammation-inducing substances to prevent the spread of the local inflammatory process.

D. Mast cells

Special member of police force that is armed with chemicals

Special cells found in tissues that contain granules of chemicals that produce redness, warmth, and swelling (allergy symptoms).

CYTOKINES

All non-antibody proteins that regulate the immune response. Cytokines produced by T cells are called *lymphokines*. Cytokines produced by macrophages/monocytes are called *monokines*.

A. Lymphokines

A number of proteins produced by T cells

1. GM-CSF

Granulocyte-macrophage colony-stimulating factor stimulates the growth of neutrophils, eosinophils, and macrophages. It increases the ingestion of bacteria and the killing of tumors coated with antibody. It activates mature granulocytes and macrophages.

2. Interferons

A class of lymphokines with important immunoregulatory functions, especially improving the activities of macrophages and NK cells. Exercise may increase the production of interferon.

a. Alpha (IFN-α)

Is produced by leukocytes in response to viral infections. It also increases NK activity and the numbers of cytotoxic T cells, and starts the tumoricidal activity of macrophages.

b. Beta (IFN-β)

Its activity is similar to IFN-α

c. Gamma (IFN-γ)

Is produced by T and NK cells. It (1) activates killer T cells; (2) increases the ability of B cells to produce antibodies; (3) keeps macrophages at the site; (4) assists them in digesting bacteria and cancerous cells they engulf. IFN-γ also regulates other lymphokines, increases NK activity, and starts the production of T cell suppressor factor.

(Interferon is now produced synthetically and is being used as an anticancer drug. It has shown promise in the treatment of some types of malignancies.)

3. IL-2 (Interleukin-2)

Is produced by helper T cells and NK cells, which stimulates other helper, killer, and suppressor T cells to multiply. It starts cytokine production by T cells and monocytes. It improves NK cell activity.

4. IL-3

Is produced by activated T cells. It is a growth factor for mast cells and most bone marrow progenitor (after stem) cells.

5. IL-4

Is called B cell growth factor, causes B cells, mast cells and resting T cells to multiply. It increases toxicity of killer T cells and macrophages. It is produced by helper T cells.

6. IL-5

Is produced by activated T cells. It is an important factor in the final differentiation of eosinophils and activated B cells. It increases IgA, IgM, and IgE development and secretion. It begins the appearance of IL-2 receptors on B cells.

7. SIRS

Soluble immune response suppressor is released by suppressor T cells and may slow down immune cell activity.

B. Monokines

Proteins produced primarily by monocytes

1. G-CSF

Granulocyte colony-stimulating factor stimulates the growth and activity of neutrophils. It is produced by monocytes and some other nonblood cells.

2. M-CSF

Macrophage colony-stimulating factor stimulates the growth and activity of macrophages. It is also produced by monocytes and other nonblood cells.

C. Other Cytokines

(Produced by both lymphocytes and macrophages/monocytes)

1. IL-1

Is produced by macrophages, T cells, granulocytes, and NK cells. It activates helper T cells and raises the body's temperature. (Fever increases immune cell activity). It stimulates the production of lymphokines and activates macrophages to immobilize cancer cells. It starts the differentiation of stem cells and activated B cells and increases the number of activated B cells. Exercise may increase IL-1 production.

2. IL-6 (BCDF)

Is called B cell differentiation factor, which causes some B cells to stop dividing and to start making immunoglobin and antibodies. Improves the differentiation of killer T cells. Is produced by helper T cells, monocytes, and fibroblasts. It also stimulates the production of platelets.

3. TGF-β

Tumor growth factor-beta is produced by T cells, macrophages, and tumor cells. It suppresses T and B cell growth and differentiation and antibody secretion.

4. TNF-B

Tumor necrosis factor-B, also known as lymphotoxin, is produced by B cells, T cells, mast cells, and macrophages. It makes some cells more vulnerable to lysis by NK cells.

5. TNF

Tumor necrosis factor is produced by monocytes, activated macrophages, NK cells, and mast cells. It can kill tumors or retard their growth. It causes some tumors to bleed and die. It stimulates the production of lymphokines and activates macrophages.

I'm certain by now you are amazed at the complexity and function of the immune system. The previous outline of the duties of its components causes one to wonder how all that coordinated effort ever gets accomplished. And yet, so much more is not understood.

To give an overall picture of what happens during an immune process, Elaine outlines the following, which is demonstrated with a series of cartoon slides:

Immune System Surveillance Process

1. A macrophage (or complement protein, NK cell, or memory cell) recognizes an antigen.
   (*A cop begins to struggle with an alien.*)
2. Helper T cells bind to the macrophage and become activated by the cytokine, IL-1, which also causes fever.
   (*The detective sees the cop and alien struggling and calls for help.*)
3. Activated helper T cells produce a lymphokine, IL-2, which stimulates other helper and killer T cells to multiply.
   (*Help arrives, detectives, SWAT team, and a few army sergeants.*)
4. Helper T cells also secrete a lymphokine, IL-4, which causes B cells to multiply.
   (*The detective decides more army personnel are needed and calls in the troops. The army comes marching in.*)
5. Helper T cells also secrete a lymphokine, IL-6, which causes some B cells to stop dividing and start making antibodies.
   (*The sergeant calls the foot soldiers into duty.*)
6. Helper T cells also produce the lymphokine interferon, which activates killer T cells, increases the ability of B cells to produce antibodies, and keeps macrophages at the site and assists them in digesting the cells they engulf.
   (*The detective calls out words of encouragement to the SWAT team, the sergeants and the street cops.*)
7. Killer T cells destroy the cells where antigens have invaded.
   (*The SWAT team member nails an alien inside a phone booth.*)
8. Antibodies neutralize the antigen and destroy other cells that have also been infected.
   (*A foot soldier punches out an alien.*)
9. Complement proteins, triggered by antigen-antibody complexes, or the cell membranes of some invading microorganisms:
   (*The flying aces come into the action.*)

   - Cause chemotaxis of macrophages and neutrophils to the area. (*An ace calls in the street cop.*)
   - Increase phagocytosis of macrophages and neutrophils. (*The street cops look mean and ugly.*)
   - Activate basophils and mast cells to release immobilizing chemicals and other products that increase inflammation. (*The firefighters and cops with chemicals soak the aliens.*)
   - Change the invader's cell surface, causing them to stick together. (*The aliens get stuck.*)
   - Attack the invader's structure and make it inactive. (*The aces crop-dust the aliens.*)

   - Rupture the invader's cell membrane. (*The ace's gunner blows a hole through the alien.*)
10. Suppressor T cells halt the immune response after the antigen is destroyed.
    (*The police chief enters the scene and halts the action once the aliens are destroyed.*)
11. Memory T and B cells are left in the blood and lymph system to defend against another attack.
    (*The detectives and the army sergeants have the alien's ID in case future attacks occur.*)

Figure 13–110 (a) and (b), page 324, illustrates a portion of the B and T cell activities.

Elaine points out that study is just beginning on the connection between the brain and immunity. Scientists have discovered the brain produces over 50 neuropeptides that have receptors on WBCs which can affect the cell's activity. For example, people who feel hopeless have sluggish macrophages. Laughter increases NK activity, lymphocyte proliferation, migration of monocytes, and the production of IL-2 and IgA. It would seem we have the power to improve our own immune system if we can learn how.

Immunization

With the knowledge of immune reactions, it is easy to understand how immunizations (shots) and vaccinations provide protection against antigens. The smallpox **vaccine,** for instance, is deliberately introduced into the body in a state that causes only minor reaction but is sufficient for the body to produce an antigen-antibody complex and eventually memory cells against the disease. Other examples of purposeful antigen introduction are measles, mumps, diphtheria, and pertussis given routinely to infants and children and tetanus toxoid given to selected individuals.

Vaccines are often given in initial and "booster" doses to provide additional memory cells and antibodies for a longer period of time. These methods provide *active immunity* because the recipients make their own immunity. Another form is known as *passive immunity* and is given to people already exposed to a disease such as tetanus. Antibodies from another source are injected into the person to provide a temporary immunity to counter the immediate attack of pathogens. This immunity is short lived.

Diseases and Disorders

The following diseases are illustrative of what happens when the immune function for some reason fails to operate properly.

Acquired Immunodeficiency Syndrome (AIDS). The beginning of **acquired immunodeficiency syndrome** (AIDS) in the United States is well documented. Between October 1980 and May 1981, five young, previously healthy

homosexual men were treated for a pneumonia caused by a parasite, *Pneumocystis carinii.* They were treated at three different hospitals in Los Angeles. Doctors and health care professionals were curious because usually *P. carinii* pneumonia occurred only in **immunosuppressed** patients, especially those receiving cancer therapy. At the same time, a rare and unusual blood vessel malignancy called Kaposi's sarcoma was being diagnosed with increasing frequency in young homosexuals in California and New York. By July 1981, 26 cases of Kaposi's sarcoma had been diagnosed. Seven of these men also had serious infections; four had *P. carinii* pneumonia. These cases were an early indication of an epidemic of a previously unknown disease. Later it was called the acquired immunodeficiency syndrome.

AIDS is an infectious disease caused by the human immunodeficiency **virus** (HIV), which renders the body's immune system ineffective. The virus has been found in many body fluids but survives well only in those with numerous WBCs such as blood, semen, and vaginal secretions. The virus invades the helper T cells and macrophages, hiding within their membranes. Since both stimulate one another at different times in the immune response, when the helper Ts are "disabled" they do not cause the macrophages to act, which results in the diversion of B cell antibody production and the absence of NK cell formation. HIV is a **retrovirus;** therefore, its genetic material is RNA instead of DNA. Its core is wrapped in a lipid envelope from the host helper T cell membrane. Once inside the host, an enzyme uses the viral RNA as a "pattern" for making DNA and inserts it into the host's chromosome.

From 2 weeks to 3 months following infection and thereafter, antibodies to several HIV proteins can be detected in the body, BUT, they do not eliminate the infected cells. Several variations of the disease are possible. Some individuals remain well but are still carriers and capable of infecting others. Some people will develop a less serious disease than AIDS called *AIDS-related complex* (ARC). Persons with ARC will present

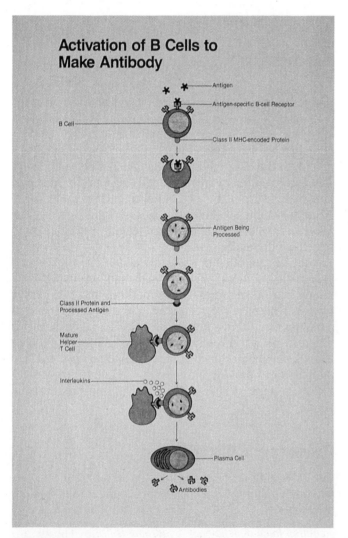

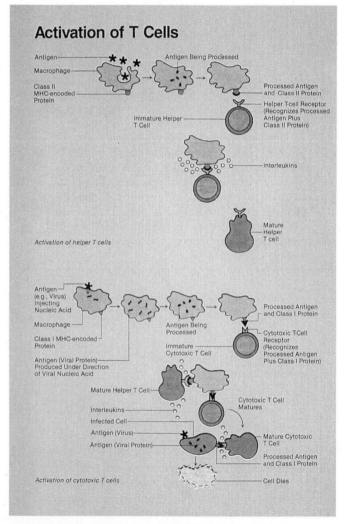

FIGURE 13–110 (a) and (b) B cell and T cell function (From Schindler, *Understanding the Immune System*, 1990, U.S. Department of Health and Human Services)

a set of less severe clinical symptoms than those with AIDS. The symptoms include loss of appetite, weight loss, fever, night sweats, skin rashes, diarrhea, fatigue, lack of resistance to infection, and swollen lymph nodes. Unfortunately, these are also signs of many diseases.

The virus stays in the cells for months to years. At some time, the body makes a secondary response and the infected cells are activated. They copy their new DNA with the viral RNA and new virus particles are assembled. They form "buds" on the helper T cell membrane and separate, and the cell is destroyed. This process continues until the helper T cells are depleted and the body cannot mount an immune response. Even though its effects are devastating, the virus is fragile outside the body and cannot survive. It is easily destroyed by alcohol, hydrogen peroxide, lysol, heat of 132°F (56°C) for 10 minutes, or a solution of 1:10 household bleach.

Symptoms of AIDS include:

- Unexplained fatigue
- Unexplained weight loss of 10 to 15 pounds in less than 2 months
- Unexplained fever, chills, and night sweats for more than 2 weeks
- Unexplained swollen lymph glands or nodes
- Unexplained diarrhea or bloody stools for more than 2 weeks
- Unexplained persistent dry cough (not from smoking), shortness of breath, or difficult breathing
- Creamy white patches on the tongue or mouth that cannot be scraped off

Without an intact immune system, **opportunistic** infections, those not likely to cause disease normally, are contracted. The most common are *P. carinii* and Kaposi's sarcoma. AIDS patients also develop other forms of pneumonia, meningitis, encephalitis, esophagitis, persistent diarrhea, and skin inflammation. These are often resistant to treatment. About 60% of AIDS patients have neurological symptoms including motor problems, inability to concentrate, memory loss, and progressive mental deterioration. It is believed to be caused by brain infection or cancer.

AIDS is diagnosed from careful assessment of the symptoms and the presence of opportunistic diseases. No blood test verifies the disease. However, two types of AIDS tests can be helpful. The ELISA (enzyme-linked immunosorbent assay) test is an AIDS antibody indicator. It can detect antibodies the body has developed to fight the AIDS virus but NOT the virus itself. A positive test may not mean you are infected because some false results do occur. A follow-up test called the Western blot and another called IFA (immunofluorescent antibody) are used to confirm a positive ELISA. A negative test, on the other hand, is also not conclusive. There may not have been enough time to develop antibodies since becoming infected. Once infected, a person remains so

throughout life, capable of transmitting the virus to others even though it may take years to begin to show the classical symptoms of AIDS.

The incidence of AIDS among the population increases daily. In 1991 it was estimated over 1 million people in the United States were infected with the AIDS virus and assumed capable of spreading it to others. Of this number, an estimated 200,000 will develop ARC. (Estimation is difficult because it may take as long as 10 years to develop symptoms). Scientists predict 20% to 30% of the infected will develop an illness meeting the description of AIDS within a period of 5 years. The number of known persons with AIDS in the United States up until February 1992 was over 206,678 with 136,473 (about 66%) having died of the disease. With no cure, the others are also expected to eventually die. The Centers for Disease Control in Atlanta (CDC) estimates by the end of 1993 between 390,000 and 480,000 Americans will be diagnosed with AIDS and between 285,000 to 400,000 deaths will occur. **Heterosexual transmission** is on the rise, though still relatively a small percentage. AIDS is rising sharply among American women, especially poor blacks and Hispanics. Death rate among women aged 15 to 44 quadrupled between 1985 and 1988. By the year 2000, there will be 25 to 30 million people worldwide infected with HIV, 10 million of whom will be infants.

AIDS is not transmitted by casual, nonsexual contact. Even family members have not developed the disease from sharing food, dishes, towels, toothbrushes, or kissing each other. Health care workers, however, must take precautions in caring for AIDS patients. The virus has been found in tears, saliva, urine, and other body secretions, but there is no evidence that the virus is transmitted by fluids other than blood, semen, vaginal secretions, and breast milk. It may be that concentrations of the virus are not sufficient in other body fluids. But because of the severity of the consequences, activities known as *Universal Precautions* must be taken to protect oneself (see Chapter 14). Through the use of aseptic procedures, gloves, and care with syringes and needles to avoid accidental puncture, contracting the virus can be prevented.

A lot of controversy has surfaced recently regarding mandatory testing of health care providers for the AIDS virus. People are afraid they may contract the disease from their physician or dentist. Two cases in particular have caused this concern: One was a hospital OB/GYN resident who later developed and died from AIDS. Of the 1,100 patients he had treated, nearly half have been tested and none have contracted the disease. The other was a dentist. He had infected five of his patients, presumably from suffering injury to his hands while providing dental care, which caused his blood to come into contact with open areas in the patients' mouths. Health care professionals have argued that the risks of them acquiring the virus from caring for patients far exceeds the danger of patients acquiring the disease from them. Prior to 1990, about twelve cases had developed among health care workers; 7 from needle sticks, 1 from contaminated blood coming into contact with an open wound, 2 from providing prolonged unprotected personal care, 1 from accidentally splattering blood into the mouth, and 1 from blood contact with severely chafed hands. As of October 1991, that number has increased to 28 known infected on the job. This is extremely low incidence among nearly 7 million health care and related (eg: housekeeping) workers. The use of universal precautions is essential to controlling the spread of the disease.

According to data from the Center for Disease Control, there are about 7,000 health care workers who have AIDS. Of that number, 761 are physicians and 1,539 are nurses. All persons, health care providers and patients who know they have the virus should reveal their condition to others who might be at risk from contact. Because of the implications upon the practice of physicians and dentists, it presents a very real dilemma which has ethical and legal implications.

AIDS is primarily acquired from two main ways:

- Having sexual intercourse (oral, vaginal, or anal) with an infected person, male or female
- Sharing drug needles and syringes with an infected person. (A drop of blood from an infected person left in the needle will infect the next user.) One research team tested known IV drug users in a northeastern city and discovered all were HIV positive.

The virus can also be transmitted in other ways. Another group of infected individuals are the newborns who acquired the virus from their mothers during pregnancy or at the time of birth and through breast milk afterward. About one third of the babies born to HIV-positive mothers will become infected. Most babies with AIDS have been born to women who are IV drug users, prostitutes or are a sexual partner of an IV drug user. Women who have had sex with someone in the high-risk group should consult a physician before beginning a pregnancy.

A small number of infected people are hemophiliac men, their sexual partners, and other transfused patients who have acquired the virus in donated blood, especially prior to 1985 when blood banks began testing for the virus.

It is also possible to acquire AIDS from previously used needles with ear piercing or tattooing. The use of a new needle for each person would eliminate this concern. Another area requiring surveillance and screening for antibodies are sperm obtained from sperm banks and organs used in transplant operations.

AIDS can be prevented by practicing personal measures to protect oneself. The disease is contracted primarily through contact with an infected person's blood, semen, or vaginal secretions. The virus enters through the vagina, penis, rectum, or mouth (in oral sex). The safest life-style is sexual **abstinence** or a faithful **monogamous** relationship. If absolute certainty is not known, then precautions must be taken.

1. Avoid high-risk sexual activities. Behaviors that may cause you to acquire the virus are clear:
   - Having unprotected sex, homosexual or heterosexual, with an HIV-infected person; oral, vaginal, or anal
   - Using IV drugs and sharing needles
   - Having many sexual partners; risk increases with number of partners
   - Having other sexually transmitted diseases, such as gonorrhea, syphilis, or genital herpes
2. Use a latex condom *properly* to maintain a barrier to the transmission of the virus. It must stay intact and be in place from the beginning to the end of vaginal, anal, or oral sex. The use of a spermicide provides additional protection. The condom must be carefully removed and disposed of properly. Condoms must never be reused.

Unfortunately, no vaccine, antitoxin, or drug "cures" AIDS. The current best line of treatment is a drug called Zidovudine (formerly AZT). It boosts the immune system to stay stronger. Many patients cannot tolerate the side effects and bone marrow toxicity. Another drug, dd I, has been released by the government and is being used to treat patients with advanced AIDS who are rapidly deteriorating or with those patients who cannot tolerate Zidovudine. Experimental agents include another drug dd C, interferon, IL-2, and vaccines. Often, supportive measures to help control the symptoms of AIDS are all that can be offered the patient.

AIDS must be of concern to everyone. The full impact of the virus is yet to come. It is anticipated that mental disturbances due to the virus's effect on the brain will develop even in the carriers over time. Economically, the cost of care to AIDS patients will strain the health care delivery system. Currently the cost per patient can range from $50,000 to $150,000 or more. In 1991, 145,000 patients were estimated to need health care and supportive services at a cost of $8 to $16 *billion* dollars. AIDS is preventable. The best line of defense is education for prevention. Everyone must become personally responsible for eliminating the transmission of AIDS.

Information presented in the following tables was obtained from a publication titled *HIV/AIDS Surveillance* issued in March 1992 by the U.S. Department of Health and Human Services, Public Health Service Centers for Disease Control, Center for Infectious Diseases, Division of HIV/AIDS.

Incidence is usually reflected by population and the presence of large cities within a state, but from reviewing the figures, it is apparent this is not always true. Table 13–5 shows the number of cases and the rate in incidence per 100,000 population during one of the same

TABLE 13–4

Number of new adult and adolescent AIDS Cases in the 10 States with the Highest Incidence from March 1991 to February 1992 and the Comparative Incidence from March 1990 to February 1991

State	Number of Cases Mar. 1991– Feb. 1992	Mar. 1990– Feb. 1991
1. New York	7910	7841
2. California	8317	7212
3. Florida	5585	4625
4. Texas	3061	3239
5. New Jersey	2212	2397
6. Puerto Rico	1554	1724
7. Illinois	1641	1293
8. Georgia	1392	1208
9. Pennsylvania	1256	1092
10. Maryland	988	976

time periods. It is clear, that the rate is more of an indication of the extent of the disease among a given population. The higher the percentage, the greater the chance of acquiring the AIDS virus.

Another interesting look at AIDS incidence is shown in Table 13–6. The metropolitan areas in the US with the highest rate per 100,000 population have been listed. Table 13–6 also shows the total number of cases for a time period plus the total cumulative cases to date. Again, the higher the percentage within a population, the greater the chance of acquiring AIDS or knowing someone who is infected.

Other data giving information about the increased incidence and the ultimate outcome of the disease shows:

TABLE 13–5

The 10 States with the Highest Rate in Incidence per 100,000 Population

State	Mar 1991–Feb 1992 Number	Rate
1. Dist of Columbia	707	177.1
2. New York	7910	43.9
3. Puerto Rico	1554	43.7
4. Florida	5585	42.1
5. New Jersey	2212	28.8
6. California	8317	27.4
7. Georgia	1392	21.2
8. Nevada	257	20.7
9. Maryland	988	20.4
10. Texas	3061	17.7

- Overall fatality rates for adolescents and adults since records have been kept is 65% of the 210,043 AIDS cases reported.
- Rates for children under 13 show 53.4% of the 3598 cases have died.
- The incidence of infection in 1981 was only 299 people; however, 272 (91%) of those have died during the past 10 years. Children under age 13 diagnosed during the same year numbered 15 with 13 (90%) having died as of February 1992.
- In 1991, 33,242 adult and adolescent cases were reported with 23,999 having died during the year. There were 428 children under age 13 diagnosed with 249 having died during the year.
- Seventy-four percent of all diagnosed males and females are between the ages of 25 and 44.

TABLE 13–6

The Top 12 Cities in the US with the Highest Rate of AIDS, the Incidence for March 1991 to February 1992, and the Cumulative Totals to Date

Metropolitan Area	Mar 1991– Feb 1992 No.	Rate	Cumulative Totals
1. San Francisco, CA	1970	122.0	11,648
2. Miami, FL	2001	101.7	6303
3. New York, NY	6807	79.4	37,952
4. Fort Lauderdale, FL	953	74.5	3606
5. Jersey City, NJ	408	73.8	2162
6. San Juan, PR	901	52.8	4233
7. Newark, NJ	915	50.3	5412
8. W. Palm Beach. FL	393	44.0	1883
9. New Orleans, LA	488	39.4	1993
10. Atlanta, GA	1054	36.3	4481
11. Houston, TX	1139	33.9	6118
12. Washington, DC	1332	33.4	6091

A March 26, 1992 news release from Louis W. Sullivan, M.D., secretary of US Department of Health and Human Services, was alarming. It included the following statements:

- Over a million Americans are currently infected with HIV; this represents about 1 in every 100 adult males and about 1 in every 800 adult females.
- Another person is infected about every 13 minutes
- During 1992 alone, 40,000 Americans will be infected and as many as 40,000 will die as a result of AIDS
- The number of *reported* AIDS cases just surpassed 200,000; the epidemic is increasing. It took 8 years to reach the first 100,000, only two years to reach the second.
- AIDS is now the third leading cause of death among adults 25–44.

AIDS must be prevented. To obtain a free brochure, materials and confidential AIDS counseling, call the toll-free National AIDS Hotline (1–800–342–AIDS).

Allergies. Sometimes the immune system can damage instead of protect the body. A secondary response to a normally harmless substance is seen in allergies and may actually damage tissues. About 15% of human beings are predisposed to become sensitive to dust, animal dander, certain food, pollen, insect stings, drugs, and other substances.

When exposed to the sensitive allergens, the antibody IgE is produced, resulting in allergic symptoms. Other factors such as emotional state, air pressure or temperature change, and infections can either trigger or complicate allergic reactions. With each additional exposure to the allergen, IgE antibody is produced and becomes attached to the mast cells or basophils, which in turn release histamine and prostaglandins, Figure 13–111. The histamine causes the mucous membranes to secrete and capillaries to become more permeable. Prostaglandins constrict smooth muscle in some organs such as the bronchioles of the lungs. The two initiate a local inflammatory response. With hay fever or asthma, for example, there is sneezing, runny nose, congestion and difficult breathing.

Exaggerated reactions to allergens can be life-threatening. For instance, some people are very sensitive to bee stings and certain drugs. The histamine and prostaglandins cause extensive bronchial constriction, mucous production, and excessive capillary permeability. Breathing is difficult and extensive loss of blood plasma drastically lowers the blood pressure leading to circulatory collapse and death. This reaction is known as anaphylaxis and the situation is called *anaphylactic shock.*

Diagnostic tests to confirm allergies consist of blood counts to determine eosinophil numbers (increase denotes allergy); chest X ray to determine congestion and perhaps focal atelectasis (mucous plugs with asthma); and pulmonary function test to evaluate lung condition. Often there is a family history of sensitivity. A series of skin tests can identify allergic substances (see Chapter 18).

Treatment consists of eliminating contact with allergens and other causative factors as much as possible. Desensitization to specific allergens may be helpful. By injecting minute amounts of the allergen intradermally and gradually increasing the amount, the body can be caused to produce IgG antibodies, which circulate and bind with the allergen prohibiting its interaction with IgE. In addition, antihistamines, bronchial dilators, antibiotics for secondary infection and sometimes corticosteroids, are helpful.

Cancer. Cancer is a large group of diseases characterized by uncontrolled growth and spread of abnormal cells. Cancer cells might arise at any time as a result of mutations induced by an event such as viral infection (especially the Epstein–Barr virus that causes infectious mononucleosis), irradiation, chemicals, genetic predisposition, diet, and immunological factors. The malignant transformation of cells is known as carcinogenesis. A *carcinogen* is anything that is capable of causing cancer. Radiation is the most dangerous because it damages the DNA, which could lead to abnormal cells. Other known substances are asbestos, vinyl chloride, chemicals in polluted air, and cigarettes. Cancers of the colon seem related to dietary causes such as a high protein and fat intake; liver tumors may arise from nitrate additives.

A cancer cell is one that has begun reproducing irradically at a rapid rate and continues to grow until it interferes with surrounding cells and the function of tissues. Normal cells have a built-in mechanism that permits controlled division. Tumor cells do not, and continue to divide as long as growth conditions are favorable. Some of the tumors are "clonal," meaning all their cells are genetically identical to the parent cell. Tumor cells that divide but stay in one place forming a mass are known as benign. Tumor cells that spread into surrounding tissue and migrate to other organs are said to be malignant. To be considered a malignant cell, it must have certain characteristics:

- Profound abnormalities in the plasma membrane (absence or change in surface proteins)
- Extreme changes in the cytoplasm
- Abnormal growth and division; proteins formed that cause extensive growth of capillaries to service the mass
- Loss of capacity to hold cells in the parent tissue

With the change in membrane proteins, cells do not "know" each other and fail to bind together as tissues. This allows cells to travel from the primary site through the blood and lymph to start new secondary growths in other tissues. This process is known as metastasis.

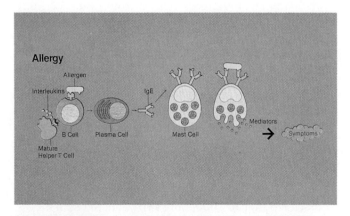

FIGURE 13–111 Response to allergens (From Schindler, *Understanding the Immune System*, 1990, U.S. Department of Health and Human Services)

Cancers can be classified according to their cellular origin. Malignant tumors from epithelial tissues are known as carcinomas, those from connective, muscle, or bone tissue are called sarcomas. Cancer cells are also called neoplastic: they are larger than normal, divide quickly, and serve no useful purpose.

Theoretically, the body develops cancer cells continuously, but the immune system recognizes them as foreign and destroys them. The cellular response causes T cells to become sensitized to the antigen (cancer cell). The sensitized T cells release lymphokines to destroy the antigen and transform some Ts into killer T cells. At the same time, the plasma cells release antibodies and the complement system activates to destroy the cell. The difficulty arises from opposing immune factors, the "blocking antibody," which actually enhances tumor growth by protecting cells from immune destruction. Factors that prohibit immunity are:

- Aging cells that begin to err in copying their genetic material causing mutants the aging immune system fails to recognize
- A decrease in antibodies and lymphocytes due to cytotoxic drugs or steroids
- Stress, which stimulates production of *cortisol,* a lymphocyte destroyer
- Severe systemic infection, which depresses the immune system
- Cancer itself causes suppression of the immune system and eventual exhaustion of a response
- Increased infection due to radiation, toxic drug therapy, and bone marrow depression, which interferes with leukocyte production

Some scientists believe that the mutated cell's surface markers either did not change (still say self), are disguised, or even are released and cause immune fighters to follow them instead of destroying the cell.

Diagnostic Procedures. Currently diagnostic procedures from simple to complex include thorough medical history, physical examination, X rays, computerized axial tomography (CAT) scans, magnetic resonance imaging (MRI), and biopsy of the suspected tissue. A more recent blood test carcinoembryonic antigen (CEA), a tumor marker, can detect malignancies involving the large intestine, stomach, pancreas, lungs, breast, and sometimes sarcomas, leukemias, and lymphomas. CEA presence above a certain level indicates suspicion or confirmation if higher. The test is also used to determine tumor extent, degree of treatment response, and tumor recurrence, but it is not organ specific. A similar new test is specific. Prostate-specific antigen is capable of measuring the presence and extent of disease in the prostate gland. This is possible because the specific antigen markers have been identified. Ultrasound, a probe used to produce images on a screen, is being used rectally to view the prostate gland to increase early detection of occult (before suspected, hidden) cancer.

Genetic researchers have identified genes in tumor cells call oncogenes. Their activity is associated with the transformation of normal to cancer cells. This is beneficial in predicting which family members are likely to be at risk, due to similar genes.

Treatment. Treatment consists primarily of three major therapies: surgery, radiation, and chemotherapy (potent drugs), either individually or in combination. The choices depend upon the type of cancer. If the tumor is contained within an organ such as the uterus or prostate, surgical removal is indicated, usually followed by chemotherapy. However, when cancer affects bone marrow or the lymphatic system, which is spread throughout the body, chemotherapy becomes the principal method. Unfortunately, chemotherapy and radiation cannot distinguish between regular and cancerous cells so both are destroyed. In some instances with leukemia, surgery in the form of a bone marrow transplant, as described in the last unit, may be an option. Then the bone marrow is purposely destroyed before new is transplanted. Several new techniques and treatments are being investigated and tried:

- Taxol, a new drug which is extracted from the bark of yew trees. In clinical trials it has been effective in the treatment of ovarian cancer.
- Neoadjuvant chemotherapy, given to shrink the cancer before surgery has been successful in certain types of cancers.
- IL-2 stimulates cells to fight cancer directly. It is being researched for use in kidney cancer and melanoma.
- The use of a patient's own bone marrow, autologous bone marrow transplant, removes a portion of the marrow before treatment, saves it, and later gives it back to the patient. This eliminates the need for donor matching and makes it possible to give the patient larger doses of chemotherapy and radiation. Obviously, this will not work if the bone marrow is the source of the cancer.
- The use of heat, hyperthermia, to increase body temperature. It is known heat of 45°C (113°F) kills cancer cells and temperature of 42° to 43°C (107.6° to 109.4°F) makes the cell more susceptible to the effects of radiation. Studies are being conducted to see if hyperthemia can increase the effect of radiation and chemotherapy.
- Immunotoxins are antibodies that are targeted against cancer cells and can be coupled with toxins, drugs, or radioactive substances and delivered directly to the cancer cell.
- New immune therapy is being researched and is in the experimental state. This form of treatment uses the body's immune system to direct its effects to the cancerous cells. Some therapy stimulates the immune mechanisms to produce additional antibodies and lymphocytes. It can be directed specifically to a par-

ticular tumor antigen or nonspecifically to multiple antigens. Stimulation also helps combat the immuno-suppressive effects of cancer and its treatments.

- Interferons are lymphokines produced by leukocytes following viral infections. They improve the activity of macrophages and NK cells. Interferon can be administered to patients and has been shown to be effective with certain cancers but not universally beneficial as hoped.

- Perhaps the most exciting immune therapy is **monoclonal** antibodies. Scientists implanted specific cancer cells (antigens) into a mouse, Figure 13–112. The mouse made antibody-producing plasma cells specific to the antigens, which were then extracted from its spleen and fused with a malignant plasma cell. These new "hybrid" cells multiplied rapidly in a culture producing the same antibodies as the mouse cells. These clone cells will continue indefinitely making the same identical antibody, therefore the name "monoclonal" antibody.

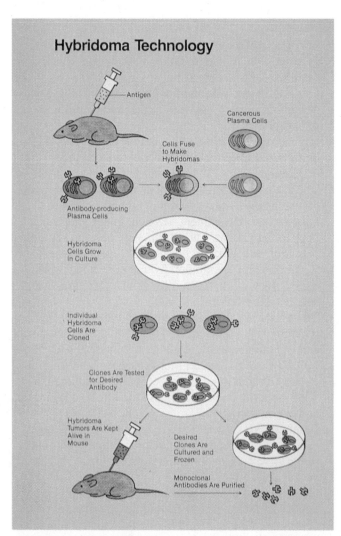

FIGURE 13–112 Producing monoclonal antibodies (From Schindler, *Understanding the Immune System*, 1990, U.S. Department of Health and Human Services)

Monoclonal antibodies may be effective for use as passive immunization for flu and hepatitis B. Theoretically, they can be cloned for various diseases. With cancer, the hope is to attach highly toxic drug molecules to the antibodies so they can be specifically targeted to the cancerous cell and avoid damage to healthy cells. Scientists have since devised human monoclonal antibodies that eliminate the recipient's reaction to mouse proteins. Uses for these engineered antibodies are just beginning to be tested but the future looks promising.

Monoclonal antibodies are also being used in radioimmunology. The antibodies are "labeled" (treated) with a radioactive substance specific for certain tissues. The cells "take up" the substance and can be detected by scanning equipment. This makes it possible to determine the location and size of a tumor.

Surgeons at The Ohio State University Medical Center are using a small hand-held scanner called a Neoprobe during surgery. The scanner connects to a monitor that produces audible beeps and digital readouts of radiation levels. Patients, primarily with colon cancers, are given radioactive-labeled antibodies over a specified period just before surgery. On the day of surgery, external probe counts are taken and recorded over the heart, liver, and perineal areas. When the abdomen is opened, probe counts are taken and recorded at the tumor site(s), lymphatic drainage areas, and any identifiable metastatic sites. Then appropriate resection (removal) of all identifiable disease is completed. The abdomen is again scanned with the probe to locate any other areas of radioactive concentration that may have been missed. If found, they are first biopsied and the specimen sent immediately for frozen section evaluation. If tumor is verified, further resection is carried out.

The use of the Neoprobe has helped surgeons locate disease that was neither visible nor palpable. It is capable of finding minute segments of the tumor as well as ruling out suspicious areas, which prove to be nonmalignant, that could have been unnecessarily removed. This process, known as "second look surgery," is also being used in rectal, primary breast, and pancreatic cancer surgery.

Another researcher funded by the American Cancer Society is studying the chemicals in the cells that are required to begin the mitosis process. If these can be isolated, blocked, labeled with chemotherapy and targeted toward cancer cells, they can be prevented from completing division to multiply. The researcher is studying drugs that will block the chemical changes.

Hopefully more effective means of treatment and even cures will soon be discovered to control this devastating disease. Currently the outlook for some patients is guarded at best. The following data were obtained from *Cancer Facts and Figures—1992,* a publication of the American Cancer Society. Note the estimates for incidence and deaths by cancer site, Figure 13–113, and the increase in 5-year survival by site and race, Figure 13–114, page 332. It is plain to see the odds are still poor

CANCER INCIDENCE AND DEATHS BY SITE AND SEX—1992 ESTIMATES

CANCER INCIDENCE BY SITE AND SEX*

PROSTATE 132,000	BREAST 180,000
LUNG 102,000	COLON & RECTUM 77,000
COLON & RECTUM 79,000	LUNG 66,000
BLADDER 38,500	UTERUS 45,500
LYMPHOMA 27,200	LYMPHOMA 21,200
ORAL 20,600	OVARY 21,000
MELANOMA OF THE SKIN 17,000	MELANOMA OF THE SKIN 15,000
KIDNEY 16,200	PANCREAS 14,400
LEUKEMIA 16,000	BLADDER 13,100
STOMACH 15,000	LEUKEMIA 12,200
PANCREAS 13,900	KIDNEY 10,300
LARYNX 10,000	ORAL 9,700
ALL SITES 565,000	ALL SITES 565,000

*Excluding nonmelanoma skin cancer and carcinoma in situ.

CANCER DEATHS BY SITE AND SEX

LUNG 93,000	LUNG 53,000
PROSTATE 34,000	BREAST 46,000
COLON & RECTUM 28,900	COLON & RECTUM 29,400
PANCREAS 12,000	PANCREAS 13,000
LYMPHOMA 10,900	OVARY 13,000
LEUKEMIA 9,900	UTERUS 10,000
STOMACH 8,000	LYMPHOMA 10,000
ESOPHAGUS 7,500	LEUKEMIA 8,300
LIVER 6,600	LIVER 5,700
BRAIN 6,500	BRAIN 5,300
KIDNEY 6,400	STOMACH 5,300
BLADDER 6,300	MULTIPLE MYELOMA 4,500
ALL SITES 275,000	ALL SITES 245,000

FIGURE 13–113 Estimates of cancer incidence and deaths by site and sex (From American Cancer Society, Cancer Facts & Figures—1991. Reproduced with permission.)

in cancers of the esophagus, stomach, liver, pancreas, and lungs.

In 1992, it was estimated that about 1,130,000 people were diagnosed as having cancer. In addition, over 600,000 people developed cancer in situ, basal, or squamous cell skin cancer. About 520,000 died, or about 1400 per day. One of every 5 deaths from all causes is cancer. The rate per 100,000 people has been increasing. In 1930 it was 143 people; in 1940 it was 152; by 1950 the rate had risen to 158 and has remained at 171 since 1984. The major cause of this increase is cancer of the lung, ironically, the major one that could be drastically reduced by doing just one thing—stop smoking. Cigarette smoking is responsible for 83% of lung cancer cases and 30% of all cancer deaths. About 76 million Americans now living will eventually have cancer, about one in three, at the present rate. Cancer will strike in three of every four families. A study from the National Cancer Institute put overall costs for cancer at $104 billion in 1990: $35 billion for direct medical costs, $12 billion for lost productivity, and $57 billion for mortality costs. The cost for detection activities, mammograms, Pap smears, and colorectal screening adds another $3 to $4 billion to the overall costs.

KNOW THE SEVEN WARNING SIGNALS OF CANCER
1. Change in bowel or bladder habits
2. A sore that does not heal
3. Unusual bleeding or discharge
4. Thickening or lump in breast or elsewhere
5. Indigestion or difficulty in swallowing
6. Obvious change in wart or mole
7. Nagging cough or hoarseness

IF YOU OR SOMEONE YOU KNOW HAS A WARNING SIGNAL, SEEK MEDICAL ADVICE

The most effective means of dealing with cancer is prevention first and early detection second. The following information from the American Cancer Society identifies factors to avoid and actions to follow to increase the odds against its development.

PREVENTION
AVOID THOSE FACTORS THAT MIGHT LEAD TO THE DEVELOPMENT OF CANCER (PRIMARY PREVENTION)

SMOKING   Cigarette smoking is responsible for 90% of lung cancer cases among men and 79% among women—about 87% overall. Smoking accounts for about 30% of all cancer deaths. Those who smoke two or more packs of cigarettes a day have lung cancer mortality rates 15 to 25 times greater than nonsmokers.

SUNLIGHT   Almost all of the more than 600,000 cases of basal and squamous cell skin cancer diagnosed each year in the US are considered

TRENDS IN SURVIVAL BY SITE OF CANCER, BY RACE
Cases Diagnosed in 1960-63, 1970-73, 1974-76, 1977-80, 1981-87

SITE	WHITE RELATIVE 5-YEAR SURVIVAL					BLACK RELATIVE 5-YEAR SURVIVAL				
	1960-63[1]	1970-73[1]	1974-76[2]	1977-80[2]	1981-87[2]	1960-63[1]	1970-73[1]	1974-76[2]	1977-80[2]	1981-87[2]
All sites	39	43	50	51	53*	27	31	39	39	38
Oral cavity & pharynx	45	43	55	54	54	–	–	35	34	31
Esophagus	4	4	5	6	9*	1	4	4	4	6*
Stomach	11	13	14	16	16*	8	13	16	16	17
Colon	43	49	50	53	58*	34	37	46	48	47
Rectum	38	45	49	51	55*	27	30	41	37	44
Liver	2	3	4	3	5	–	–	1	3	5
Pancreas	1	2	3	2	3*	1	2	2	5	4
Larynx	53	62	66	67	68	–	–	59	58	54
Lung & bronchus	8	10	12	13	13*	5	7	11	12	11
Melanoma of skin	60	68	80	82	82*	–	–	69†	51‡	70
Breast (female)	63	68	75	75	78*	46	51	63	63	63
Cervix uteri	58	64	69	68	68	47	61	63	62	57
Corpus uteri	73	81	89	86	84*	31	44	62	56	56
Ovary	32	36	36	38	39*	32	32	41	40	36
Prostate gland	50	63	67	72	76*	35	55	58	62	63*
Testis	63	72	79	88	93*	–	–	77†	73†	94
Urinary bladder	53	61	74	76	79*	24	36	48	55	59*
Kidney & renal pelvis	37	46	52	51	53	38	44	49	57	52
Brain & nervous system	18	20	22	24	24*	19	19	27	28	33
Thyroid gland	83	86	92	92	94	–	–	87	92	94
Hodgkin's disease	40	67	71	73	77*	–	–	68	73	74
Non-Hodgkin's lymphoma	31	41	47	49	51*	–	–	48	49	45
Multiple myeloma	12	19	24	25	26*	–	–	27	32	28
Leukemia	14	22	34	36	36*	–	–	31	30	29

Source: Cancer Statistics Branch, National Cancer Institute.

[1] Rates are based on End Results Group data from a series of hospital registries and one population-based registry.

[2] Rates are from the SEER Program. They are based on data from population-based registries in Connecticut, New Mexico, Utah, Iowa, Hawaii, Atlanta, Detroit, Seattle-Puget Sound and San Francisco-Oakland. Rates are based on follow-up of patients through 1988.

* The difference in rates between 1974-76 and 1981-87 is statistically significant (p < 0.05).

† The standard error of the survival rate is between 5 and 10 percentage points.

‡ The standard error of the survival rate is greater than 10 percentage points.

– Valid survival rate could not be calculated.

FIGURE 13–114 Cancer five-year survival rates by site and race (From American Cancer Society, Cancer Facts & Figures—1991. Reproduced with permission.)

to be sun-related. Epidemiologic evidence shows that sun exposure is a major factor in the development of melanoma and that the incidence increases for those living near the equator.

IONIZING RADIATION Excessive exposure to ionizing radiation can increase cancer risk. Most medical and dental x-rays are adjusted to deliver the lowest dose possible without sacrificing image quality. Excessive radon exposure in homes may increase risk of lung cancer, especially in cigarette smokers. If levels are found to be too high, remedial actions should be taken.

NUTRITION AND DIET Risk for colon, breast, and uterine cancers increases in obese people. High-fat diets may contribute to the development of cancers of the breast, colon, and prostate. High-fiber foods might help reduce risk of colon cancer. A varied diet containing plenty of vegetables and fruits rich in vitamins A and C may reduce risk for a wide range of cancers. Salt-cured, smoked, and nitrite-cured foods have been linked to esophagus and stomach cancer.

ALCOHOL Oral cancer and cancers of the larynx, throat, esophagus, and liver occur more frequently among heavy drinkers of alcohol especially when accompanied by cigarette smoking or chewing tobacco.

SMOKELESS TOBACCO Use of chewing tobacco or snuff increases risk of cancer of the mouth, larynx, throat, and esophagus and is a highly addictive habit.

ESTROGEN Estrogen treatment to control menopausal symptoms increases risk of endometrial cancer. However, including progesterone in estrogen replacement therapy helps to minimize this risk. Consultation with a physician will help each woman to assess personal risks and benefits.

OCCUPATIONAL HAZARDS Exposure to several different industrial agents (nickel, chromate, asbestos, vinyl chloride, etc.) increases risk of various cancers. Risk from asbestos is greatly increased when combined with cigarette smoking.

ACTIONS TO DIAGNOSE A CANCER OR PRECURSOR AS EARLY AS POSSIBLE (SECONDARY PREVENTION/EARLY DETECTION).

BREAST CANCER DETECTION The American Cancer Society recommends that screening mammography begin by age 40. Women age 40–49 should have mammography every 1–2 years, depending on physical and mammographic findings. Women age 50 and older should have mammograms yearly. The ACS recommends the monthly practice of breast self-exam (BSE) by women 20 years and older as a routine good health habit. Clinical examination of the breast should be done every three years from ages 20–40 and then every year.

COLORECTAL The American Cancer Society recommends three tests for the early detection of colon and rectum cancer in people without symptoms. A digital rectal examination by a physician during an office visit, should be performed every year after the age of 40; the stool blood test is recommended every year after 50; and the proctosigmoidoscopy examination should be carried out every 3 to 5 years, based on the advice of a physician.

PAP TEST For cervical cancer, women who are or have been sexually active, or have reached age 18, should have an annual Pap test and pelvic examination. After a woman has had three or more consecutive satisfactory normal annual examinations, the Pap test may be performed less frequently at the discretion of her physician.

Chronic Fatigue Syndrome (CFS). This **debilitating** disorder was officially recognized and reported in 1984 by two doctors near Lake Tahoe, Nevada. It was officially declared a disease in 1988. The CDC started a surveillance program costing $1.5 million to track the frequency and impact of the disorder. They also established the following guidelines to help physicians diagnose the condition.

- Persistent overwhelming fatigue for at least 6 months, that does not go away with rest
- Low grade fever
- Sore throat and/or swollen lymph nodes
- Headaches
- Lingering fatigue after levels of exercise that would normally be easily tolerated
- Unexplainable muscle weakness or pain
- Pain in joints without swelling
- Forgetfulness, irritability, confusion, inability to concentrate, depression, sensitivity to light, and impaired vision
- Sleep disturbances

Patients experience varying levels of ability to perform activity from profound fatigue to being completely bedridden. CFS affects twice as many women as men, particularly between 25 and 45 years old. However, children and senior citizens have also been diagnosed.

The disorder begins suddenly like the common flu, but the CFS symptoms last for 3 to 4 years. Only about 15% to 20% seem to recover fully; 5% are homebound or bedridden.

The cause of the disorder appears to be genetically predisposed. About 79% to 80% of CFS patients have allergies. Current theories suggest that a virus, bacteria, allergen, or environment chemical enters the body but does not set off the normal immune response to fight the invasion. Instead, the system continues to make symptom-producing chemicals. A second theory suggests that some unidentified organism weakens the immune system, allowing normally dormant viruses to become activated. This theory is supported by the presence of high levels of antibodies to Epstein–Barr virus and others.

Physicians still do not know much about the disorder; some deny its existence because it cannot be detected by a blood test. Diagnosis requires a thorough physical examination and laboratory tests to rule out other conditions with similar symptoms.

Treatment consists of analgesics for pain, antihistamines for allergic symptoms, antidepressants to improve sleep and fatigue. Patients should avoid emotional and physical stress and have good nutrition. Exercise must be appropriate. Psychological counseling may be required to help a patient deal with the changes caused by CFS.

Lupus Erythematosus. **Lupus erythematosus** is a chronic disease of unknown cause in which striking changes occur in the immune system. It causes inflammation of various parts of the body. It can involve only a few body organs or cause serious life-threatening problems. Lupus can affect the skin, joints, kidneys, lungs, heart, nervous system, and other body organs and systems.

In lupus, the usually protective antibodies are produced in large quantities but react against the person's own normal tissue; therefore, it is called an **autoimmune** disease. There are three main types of lupus:

- Cutaneous or **discoid** lupus which is confined to the skin and causes a persistent flush of the cheeks or disclike lesions on the face, neck, scalp and other areas exposed to ultraviolet light. The rash is usually scaly and red but not itchy. If not treated, scarring may result and if on the scalp, bald spots.
- Systemic lupus erythematosus (SLE) inflames the organs of the body. Some persons also have skin and joint involvement, others, skin and lungs or kidneys and blood. The disease is characterized by periods of **remission** when few if any symptoms are evident and other periods of active disease and symptoms.
- Drug-induced lupus can be caused by certain medications and is similar to SLE. The most common offenders are hydralazine for hypertension and procainamide for cardiac arrhythmia. The symptoms fade when the drugs are stopped.

The incidence of SLE in the US is approximately 500,000 people. SLE effects women nine times more often than men, most frequently during the childbearing years. Lupus is more common in blacks, Asians and certain Indian tribes. About 16,000 new cases are diagnosed each year.

General symptoms of beginning lupus are:

fever	loss of appetite
weight loss	nausea and vomiting
headache	easy bruising
fatigue	hair loss
swollen glands	edema
depression	

Suggestive symptoms of lupus include:

A rash over cheeks and bridge of nose	Discoid lupus lesions
	Ulcers inside mouth
Rashes developing after being in the sun	Pleurisy
	Anemia
Arthritis in two or more joints	**Raynaud's phenomenon** (fingers turn white or
Seizures	blue in the cold)
Bald spots	

Diagnosis is made on the strength of symptoms and blood tests showing low cell counts. Urine is checked for protein, RBCs and WBCs. A specific antibody test ANA (antinuclear antibody) looks for antibodies to the nuclei of cells. Over 99% of people with lupus will have a positive test; however, only 33% of people with a positive ANA have SLE.

Treatment of SLE consists of assuring patients they can live near-normal lives. Limits on activities are dictated by the disease. Rest when needed but otherwise engage in normal employment and exercise. Sun exposure should be avoided at peak hours (10:00 A.M. to

2:00 P.M.), otherwise as tolerated. Sunscreens of at least SPF 15 are advisable. No medication has been developed to cure lupus. Joint and muscle pain is controlled with anti-inflammatory and analgesic drugs such as aspirin, ibuprofen, Naprosyn, and Tylenol. During flare-ups or if major organs are involved, steroids such as prednisone are often used to suppress inflammation. The steroid also interferes with the proliferation and interaction of the cells in the immune system and causes T cells to gather in the lymph nodes, which removes them from concentrating at the inflammation sites. The drugs chloroquine and Plaquenil (antimalarials) are valuable in managing the skin lesions and also help control arthritis symptoms.

Many new treatments are being tested, several dealing with self-antigens, immunoreplacement therapy, and even plasmapheresis (the removal of blood plasma, and hence antibodies). It is believed with further understanding of the immune system, an effective treatment of lupus will be discovered.

Rheumatoid Arthritis. This chronic systemic inflammatory autoimmune disease affects the joints and surrounding muscles, tendons, ligaments, and blood vessels. It affects women three times more often than men. It occurs primarily between the ages of 20 and 60 with a peak onset period between 35 to 45. This disease was discussed in the skeletal system; however, it is believed there is a connection to the immune system. Recent findings suggest a link to genetic defects, which cause the cells to display a specific cell marker. Patients may also have an autoantibody known as *rheumatoid factor,* which locks onto the body's own IgG molecule as if it were an antigen. These antigen–antibody complexes seem to be deposited on the synovial membranes of the joints and are the targets of the inflammatory response.

When the complement system is activated, the macrophages gather at the joint. The inflammatory response dilates the blood vessels and fluid accumulates in the joint cavity. The cells of the membrane proliferate in response, thickening the joint membrane causing more swelling. These events continue in cycles and result in the destruction of the joint.

The symptoms develop insidiously, then become localized in joints, usually bilaterally. The affected joints stiffen following inactivity, swell, and may show beginning signs of deformity. They eventually become tender, painful, hot and enlarged, have marked deformities, and decreased function.

Treatment consists primarily of salicylates to reduce inflammation. Corticosteroids (prednisone), anti-inflammatory agents such as ibuprofen, gold salts, and antimalarial drugs may prove helpful. Patients need periods of rest during the day and 8 to 10 hours of sleep every night. Activities such as range of motion exercises, application of heat during chronic episodes and ice packs with acute

phases may be helpful. Advanced disease may necessitate total joint replacement or joint fusion to relieve pain.

Complete Chapter 13, Unit 9 in the workbook to help you meet the objectives at the beginning of this unit and therefore achieve competency of this subject matter.

U N I T 1 0

The Digestive System

OBJECTIVES ....

Upon completion of this unit, the student will meet the following terminal performance objectives by verifying knowledge of the facts and principles presented through oral and written communication at a level deemed competent.

1. Define digestion.
2. Name the raw materials required for a healthy body.
3. Trace the pathway of food through the alimentary tract.
4. Describe the structures of the mouth and the digestive processes that occur there.
5. Explain the process of swallowing.
6. Describe how the esophagus propels food toward the stomach.
7. Describe the structure and function of the stomach.
8. Describe the structure and function of the small intestine.
9. Tell why the duodenum is such a vital link in the digestive system.
10. List the functions of the liver, including the portal circulation connection.
11. Describe the role of the gallbladder and its association with the liver.
12. Describe the location and function of the pancreas.
13. Explain how and where nutrients are absorbed.
14. Name the sections of the colon and describe its function.
15. Describe the function of the rectum.
16. Describe the structure and function of the anal canal.
17. Describe 11 diagnostic examinations of the digestive tract.
18. Discuss 26 disorders of diseases of the digestive system.
19. Spell and define, using the glossary at the back of the text, all the words to know in this unit.

WORDS TO KNOW ....

alimentary canal	bile
anal	bolus
anus	cardiac sphincter
appendectomy	cecum
appendicitis	cholecystectomy
ascending	cholelithiasis

chyme
cirrhosis
colitis
colon
colostomy
common bile duct
constipation
Crohn's disease
cystic
defecate
descending
diarrhea
digestion
digestive
diverticulitis
duodenum
emesis
enzyme
esophagus
fecal
fissure
fistula
flatus
gallbladder
gastric
gastrointestinal (GI)
gastroscopy
hemorrhoidectomy
hemorrhoids
hepatic
hepatitis
hernia
herniorrhaphy
hiatus
hydrochloric acid
ileocecal
ileostomy

ileum
impaction
incontinent
insulin
intestine
jaundice
jejunum
liver
mesentery
mouth
nausea
pancreas
pancreatitis
paralytic ileus
peptic
peristalsis
polyp
proctoscope
pruritus ani
pyloric
rectum
saliva
salivary glands
sigmoid
sigmoidoscopy
spastic colon
stenosis
stomach
stool
tongue
transverse
ulcer
varices
vermiform appendix
villi
villous adenoma
vomit

The **digestive** system is the group of organs that changes food eaten into a form that can be used by the body's cells. The system is also known as the **gastrointestinal (GI)** tract or system, and the connecting chain of organs is sometimes referred to as the **alimentary canal.** The digestive process can be divided into four phases: *ingestion, digestion, absorption,* and *elimination.* Food which is consumed is acted on by various mechanical and chemical means as it progresses through the body. Each organ, whether main or accessory, plays an important role in physically or chemically altering the composition of the food, selectively absorbing the elements, or eliminating the remains.

The main organs of the system are those through which the food passes. These organs form a continuous tube from the entrance to the exit of the body. They are the mouth, pharynx, esophagus, stomach, small intestine, and large intestine. As important as these organs are, it is the accessory organs which play a major role in the digestive process. In the mouth there are the teeth, sali-

vary glands, and tongue. The liver, gallbladder, and pancreas have access to the small intestine, Figure 13–115, page 336.

Digestion is the activity performed by the organs of the digestive system, and is defined as the process by which food is broken down, mechanically and chemically, in the gastrointestinal tract and converted into an absorbable form that can be used by the cells of the body. This process cannot occur within the digestive system alone. As with all body functions, an interrelationship of systems is required to achieve the desired results. Digestion requires cooperation from the nervous system, the muscular system, the circulatory system, and the endocrine system.

The human body can be compared to an engine that needs appropriate fuel to operate. The energy we need to function must come from the foods we eat. The right fuel will not only supply the body with energy, but also provide the materials necessary to build and repair the body so that it can operate efficiently. If the wrong fuel is used too often, the machine will eventually break down.

The human body can manufacture the appropriate fuel if it receives an adequate supply of the right raw materials, mainly carbohydrates, proteins, fats, minerals, vitamins, water, and roughage. All these raw materials are available from the basic food groups and should be eaten daily.

Carbohydrates supply about two-thirds of the energy calories needed each day. Fats are also an excellent source of energy; in fact, an ounce of fat yields about three times the calories of an ounce of carbohydrate. Unfortunately, the body does not waste excess energy-producing calories but stores them instead. Therefore, when all the calories eaten are not used for energy they are stored as excess body tissue we may not desire.

Proteins are obtained primarily from plant and animal sources but are not stored by the body. It is especially important that they be eaten daily because they are the main ingredients needed to build and repair cells and tissue.

Other raw materials required for a healthy body are vitamins and minerals. Vitamins are regulating chemicals needed for growth and control of body activities. For instance, the chemical that becomes vitamin D must be absorbed by the body and then become activated in the skin by contact with the sun. The body needs vitamin D to absorb and use calcium. Calcium and another mineral, phosphorus, are needed by the body for the muscles, nerves, and blood as well as the teeth and bones. The formation of red blood cells requires iron and copper. We have already learned that the combination of an iron pigment and a protein forms the hemoglobin of the red blood cells, which enables them to attract O_2 and CO_2 as they move through the body.

All the raw materials the body needs are altered by the digestive system to provide the essential elements necessary for good health. The various stages in this process will become clearer by tracing the pathway of food through the alimentary canal.

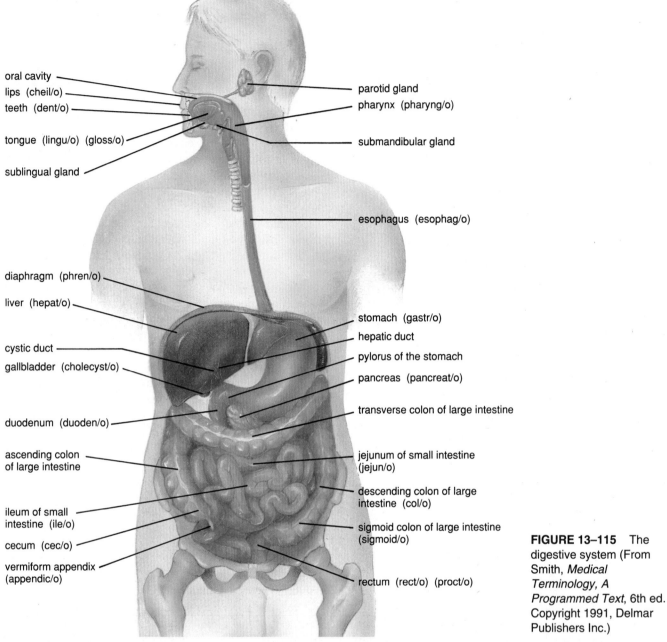

oral cavity
lips (cheil/o)
teeth (dent/o)
tongue (lingu/o) (gloss/o)
sublingual gland

parotid gland
pharynx (pharyng/o)
submandibular gland

esophagus (esophag/o)

diaphragm (phren/o)
liver (hepat/o)
cystic duct
gallbladder (cholecyst/o)
duodenum (duoden/o)
ascending colon of large intestine
ileum of small intestine (ile/o)
cecum (cec/o)
vermiform appendix (appendic/o)

stomach (gastr/o)
hepatic duct
pylorus of the stomach
pancreas (pancreat/o)
transverse colon of large intestine
jejunum of small intestine (jejun/o)
descending colon of large intestine (col/o)
sigmoid colon of large intestine (sigmoid/o)
rectum (rect/o) (proct/o)

FIGURE 13–115 The digestive system (From Smith, *Medical Terminology, A Programmed Text*, 6th ed. Copyright 1991, Delmar Publishers Inc.)

The Mouth ....

Food enters the body through the mouth. It is held in the oral cavity while the initial digestive process is begun. Teeth break up food into small pieces to make it easier to swallow and also to prepare it for more effective action by digestive enzymes. "Baby" teeth are called *deciduous* and begin to appear at about 6 months of age. They are gradually exchanged for permanent teeth beginning at about age 6 years. Different teeth have specific duties to perform. The incisors bite food with their sharp edges. The canines or cuspids are pointed to puncture and tear. The premolars or bicuspids and the molars are for grinding and crushing, Figure 13–116. The tongue aids in the process by moving the food around within the mouth, bringing it into contact with the teeth. The tongue is a

muscle and can alter its shape to reach all areas of the mouth. The surface of the tongue contains the taste buds, located within the papillae projections.

The salivary glands excrete the fluid known as saliva. It is released from three pairs of glands: the parotid, the submandibular, and the sublingual, Figure 13–117, page 338. Certain foods cause the glands to excrete profusely, often producing some discomfort, as when eating something sour. The disease called mumps is the inflammation of the parotid glands. A virus causes the glands to enlarge and become painful. With mumps, mastication (chewing) causes great discomfort, because the muscle action squeezes the swollen glands.

Saliva contains an enzyme called ptyalin. This chemical begins the breakdown of carbohydrates into sugar. Saliva also provides moisture that enables the taste buds to perceive the sensations of sweet, sour, bitter, and salty. In addition, saliva aids in cleansing the teeth by washing away food particles that might allow bacteria to grow. The presence of saliva in the oral cavity keeps the surfaces moist and flexible, which aids in the production of speech.

The combination of mashed food substances and saliva is called a bolus. When it has been mixed well and contains sufficient moisture, it can be easily swallowed. For this to occur several muscles must work together. The tongue presses upward and backward against the palate (roof of the mouth) while the muscles in the cheeks help in the formation of a chute to direct the bolus toward the back of the mouth and into the pharynx, Figure 13–118, page 338. At this point, the bolus could go in three different directions: into the nasal cavity, down and forward into the trachea, or down into the esophagus.

The directing of the bolus is accomplished by a complex combination of "lids" and muscles, which operate automatically. As the bolus is swallowed, it raises the

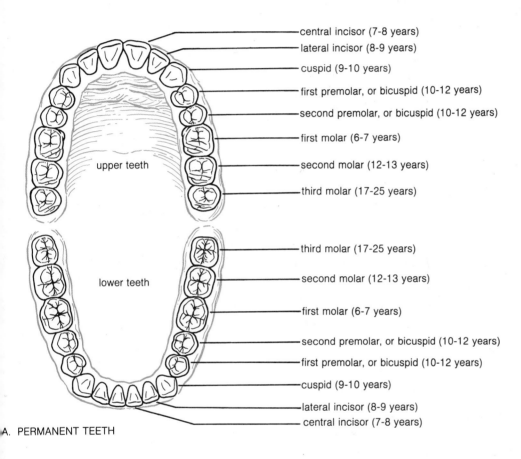

- central incisor (7-8 years)
- lateral incisor (8-9 years)
- cuspid (9-10 years)
- first premolar, or bicuspid (10-12 years)
- second premolar, or bicuspid (10-12 years)
- first molar (6-7 years)
- second molar (12-13 years)
- third molar (17-25 years)

upper teeth

lower teeth

- third molar (17-25 years)
- second molar (12-13 years)
- first molar (6-7 years)
- second premolar, or bicuspid (10-12 years)
- first premolar, or bicuspid (10-12 years)
- cuspid (9-10 years)
- lateral incisor (8-9 years)
- central incisor (7-8 years)

A. PERMANENT TEETH

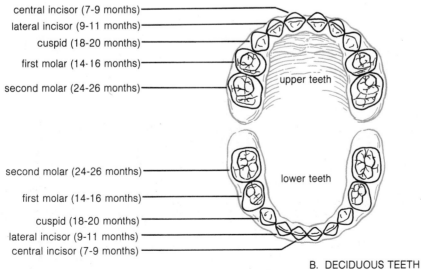

central incisor (7-9 months)
lateral incisor (9-11 months)
cuspid (18-20 months)
first molar (14-16 months)
second molar (24-26 months)

upper teeth

second molar (24-26 months)
first molar (14-16 months)
cuspid (18-20 months)
lateral incisor (9-11 months)
central incisor (7-9 months)

lower teeth

B. DECIDUOUS TEETH

FIGURE 13–116 Deciduous and permanent teeth (From Fong, *Body Structures and Functions*, 7th ed. Copyright 1989, Delmar Publishers Inc.)

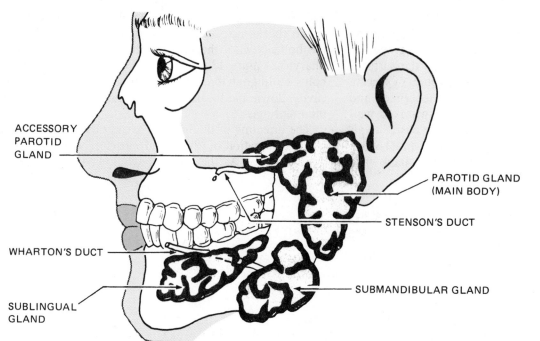

FIGURE 13–117
Salivary glands (From Anderson & Burkard, *The Dental Assistant*, copyright 1987, Delmar Publishers Inc.)

soft palate, closing off the nasal cavity. At the same time, the epiglottis, a cartilage lid attached at the top of the larynx, moves across the opening into the larynx when the tongue pushes the bolus against the palate. At the moment of swallowing, the larynx moves upward against the epiglottis to close the opening. Usually, this reflex action works perfectly, but when the timing is slightly off, food may enter the larynx, triggering the cough reflex (to remove the material). We say, "It went down the wrong pipe."

The Esophagus

Once food is swallowed, its movement through the body is maintained by the smooth, involuntary muscle action called **peristalsis.** The esophagus has two layers of involuntary muscles. The inner layer forms circles around the esophagus, while the outer layer runs longitudinally along its approximately 10-inch length. When food enters the esophagus, the muscles alternately contract and relax, squeezing the bolus. Together they create the peristaltic "milking action," which moves the bolus to the **stomach.** The whole process only requires about 5 seconds. Because peristaltic action moves material in one direction only, and this process does not depend on gravity, it is possible to drink a glass of water while standing on your head.

The Stomach

The upper opening to the stomach is controlled by a circular muscle called the **cardiac sphincter.** As the peri-

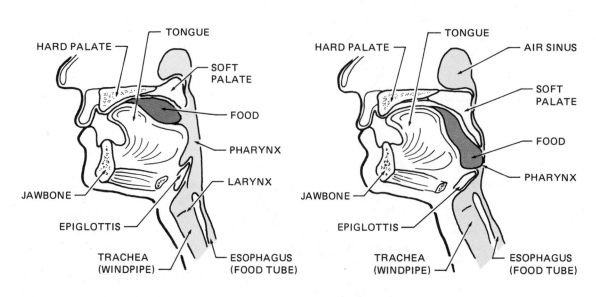

FIGURE 13–118 The process of swallowing

staltic wave approaches, the sphincter dilates, allowing the food to enter. Once the food is inside, this one-way "gate" closes to prevent its escape.

The stomach is a 10-inch-long, J-shaped organ constructed of three layers of strong muscle tissue, Figure 13–119. It lies just beneath the diaphragm. The inner lining of the stomach is thick and full of folds called *rugae*. Because muscle tissue is elastic and the folds in the lining can straighten out, the stomach is capable of expanding. It can hold about half a gallon of food and liquid.

Once the material has entered the stomach, the muscular layers begin to contract. A circular layer, a longitudinal layer, and an oblique layer work together in a strong rhythmic motion to break up the food into tiny particles. The stomach continues the digestive process that began in the mouth. The churning action is prolonged and made more difficult by poorly chewed food.

The mechanical digestive process is assisted by a chemical process. The stomach lining is formed of mucous membrane, whose glands secrete mucus. The stomach lining also has about 35 million gastric glands, which secrete hydrochloric acid and several enzymes. As the stomach contents are being kneaded, acid and enzymes are excreted by the gastric glands and thoroughly mixed into the bolus. One enzyme, rennin, curdles milk. Another enzyme, lipase, splits certain fats, while pepsin

digests the milk curds from the rennin. The hydrochloric acid unites with protein to form another chemical, which in turn is split by the pepsin.

Since hydrochloric acid burns holes in most things it touches, you may wonder why it doesn't destroy the stomach. This is because the lining also secretes small amounts of ammonia, which is capable of counteracting normal amounts of the acid. However, when a sufficient amount of excess acid is present for a sufficient length of time, an ulcer (open sore) will develop, usually along the posterior wall near the pylorus. An ulcer in the stomach is known as a gastric (stomach) or peptic ulcer.

The partially digested food in the stomach is changed into a semiliquid state called chyme in 3 to 5 hours. Liquids, on the other hand, pass through the stomach in a matter of minutes. Of the solid foods, carbohydrates are digested first, proteins second, and fats last. When the consistency of the chyme is right, the pyloric sphincter, at the end of the stomach, allows the chyme to spurt through the sphincter into the small intestine.

Because of the two sphincters, food is held in the stomach until it is properly prepared to leave. But occasionally when you suffer from nausea and vomit, it is obvious the material did not go in the right direction. This action is accomplished by the contraction of the abdominal muscles, forcefully squeezing the stomach as it is pushed downward by the diaphragm. With this pressure and

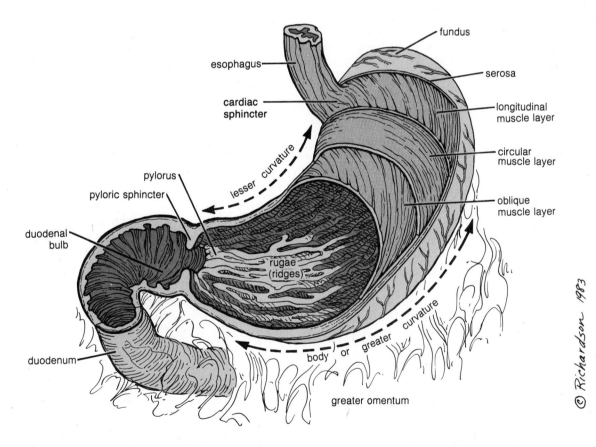

FIGURE 13–119   The stomach (From Fong, *Body Structures and Functions*, 7th ed. Copyright 1989, Delmar Publishers Inc.)

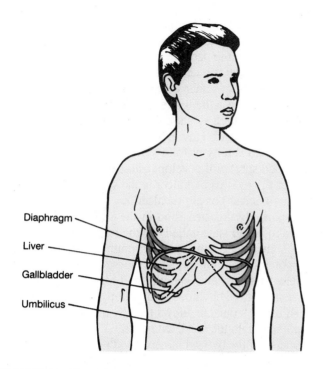

Diaphragm

Liver

Gallbladder

Umbilicus

FIGURE 13–120 The liver and gallbladder

reverse peristaltic waves, the contents of the stomach are forced out and emesis (vomiting) occurs.

The Small Intestine ....

The small intestine is a tube about 1 inch in diameter and about 20 feet in length. It completes the digestive process and absorbs the nutrients from the chyme.

The small intestine is divided into three sections. The first is a C-shaped segment, about 9 inches long, called the duodenum (see Figure 13–119). Since this area receives the highest concentration of acid from the stomach, it is especially prone to the development of ulcers. An ulcer in this area is called a duodenal ulcer.

The next segment, the jejunum, is about 8 feet in length. The last segment, about 12 feet long, is called the ileum. The jejunum and ileum are suspended in the abdominal cavity by the mesentery, a fan-shaped fold of tissue which is attached to the posterior abdominal wall.

The ileum is reduced to about half an inch in diameter by the time it joins the large intestine in the right lower quadrant of the abdomen. The junction is marked by a sphincter called the ileocecal valve, which allows the chyme to enter the cecum (first segment of the large intestine) but prohibits anything from returning to the ileum.

The small intestine completes the digestive process with the aid of accessory organs and intestinal juice secreted by the glands of the small intestine.

The Liver and Gallbladder

The liver is the largest gland in the body. It lies below the diaphragm in the upper right quadrant of the

abdomen, extending into the upper left quadrant, Figure 13–120. The liver is a vital organ performing several functions for the body. It secretes bile at a rate of over a pint a day, and the bile is continuously excreted through bile passages to the bile duct. Unconcentrated liver bile is a bitter, yellow-orange liquid that is required to digest fats. Bile is composed primarily of water and contains pigment from red blood cells that have been destroyed (carried to the liver from the spleen in the portal vein). The pigment is changed in the intestines and excreted in fecal material, giving it its yellow-brown color. The iron from the destroyed cells is reabsorbed into the body.

The liver also stores glycogen, a form of glucose (carbohydrate). When the body needs additional blood sugar, it changes the glycogen back to glucose and releases it. In addition, the liver processes proteins from amino acids and either burns fats as fuel or stores them. The liver performs the life-essential service of manufacturing fibrinogen, prothrombin, and other substances required for the process of clotting blood. Antibodies to counteract certain disease organisms are produced in the liver. Also, toxins (poisons) that have been absorbed from the intestine, inhaled, injected, or otherwise taken into the body are circulated in the blood to the liver, where for the most part they are rendered harmless. The liver is also an important storage area for blood and body fluid, because of its large size.

The liver receives blood from two separate systems. It receives arterial blood for its own support and preservation from the hepatic artery. It also receives blood from the portal vein that conveys absorbed nutrients and other substances from all the abdominal organs for processing.

The gallbladder is a small sac attached to the underside of the liver, Figure 13–121. Its sole purpose is the concentration and storage of bile. When the body needs bile to digest food, the gallbladder releases the concentrated bile to supplement that being currently produced by the liver. Concentrated bile is very bitter and is green-yellow in color. The gallbladder empties its contents via the cystic duct. The cystic duct from the gallbladder and the hepatic duct from the liver combine to form the common bile duct. This combined duct empties the bile directly into the duodenum to be added to the chyme during the digestive process. The duodenum is a very vital segment of the digestive system. Not only does it receive chyme from the stomach and bile from the liver and gallbladder, but as we will soon see, it also receives pancreatic juices from the pancreas.

Obstruction of the bile ducts by cholelithiasis (gallstones) is not uncommon. Bile contains certain mineral salts that can become crystallized into "stones" in the gallbladder, perhaps from poor drainage or extended storage. Frequently the stones will be expelled into the cystic duct where they become lodged, causing pain, an inadequate supply of bile, and frequently requiring surgical removal. If the stone reaches the common bile duct before becoming lodged, a much more serious situation results. Now

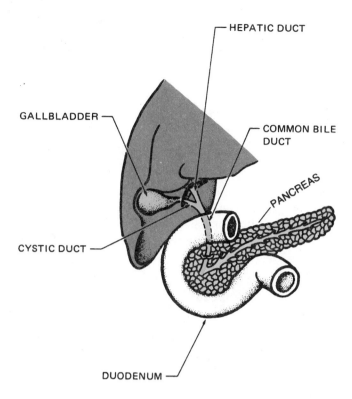

HEPATIC DUCT

GALLBLADDER

COMMON BILE DUCT

PANCREAS

CYSTIC DUCT

DUODENUM

FIGURE 13–121 The gallbladder and cystic, hepatic, and common bile ducts on the undersurface of the liver

neither the gallbladder nor the liver can empty its bile. The liver maintains its production, but now the bile is absorbed into the bloodstream, producing the yellow discoloration of the sclera, mucosa, and skin known as **jaundice.** The gallbladder itself may become infected or filled with stones and nonfunctional. Periodic "gallbladder attacks" will usually prompt a **cholecystectomy** (surgical removal). The hepatic duct and the common bile duct must remain for the liver to function, however.

A new surgical procedure to remove cholelithiasis has revolutionized the way cholecystectomies are performed. The procedure is accomplished with the use of three laparoscopes inserted into the abdomen. One is placed in the RUQ, one at the umbilicus, and one mid-upper abdomen. One scope serves as the light source, another to supply air to manipulate tissues, and one through which the operation is performed. The gallbladder and its contents, if any, are excised and removed through the operative scope. Following surgery, only a few sutures are required to close the small abdominal openings. Previous surgery resulted in a long incision extending down the right side of the abdomen and a considerably uncomfortable postoperative period. The new laparoscopic surgery has shortened recovery to 2 weeks or less from about 6 weeks.

The Pancreas

The **pancreas** lies behind the stomach, with its head in the curve of the duodenum, Figure 13–122. The pancreas, like the liver, is a gland but it secretes substances in two different ways. Functioning as an *exocrine gland* (secreting through ducts), the pancreas secretes pancreatic juice via the pancreatic duct directly into the duodenum. The three powerful enzymes in pancreatic juice react chemically on all three types of nutrients to break them down for absorption into the bloodstream. Most of the chemical changes that occur in the intestinal tract are due to pancreatic juices, which are probably sufficient to digest all foods by themselves. If pancreatic juice is absent, serious digestive problems occur.

Functioning as an *endocrine* (ductless) *gland,* the pancreas also secretes directly into the bloodstream a substance called **insulin.** This function will be covered in Unit 12, The Endocrine System.

It should be clear now why the duodenum is such a critical segment of the digestive tract. Since it receives

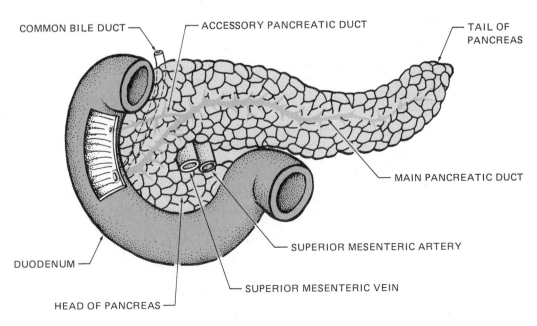

COMMON BILE DUCT

ACCESSORY PANCREATIC DUCT

TAIL OF PANCREAS

MAIN PANCREATIC DUCT

DUODENUM

HEAD OF PANCREAS

SUPERIOR MESENTERIC VEIN

SUPERIOR MESENTERIC ARTERY

FIGURE 13–122 The duodenum and pancreas. A window has been cut in the anterior wall of the duodenum to show the openings of the common bile duct and the pancreatic ducts into the lumen of the duodenum.

products from four organs—stomach, liver, gallbladder, and pancreas—it is a vital connective link. When ulceration occurs or a tumor develops in this area, it may interfere drastically with the digestive process. Involvement of the duodenum is a cause for concern.

The Absorption Function

When all the digestive juices and enzymes have been added and the chyme passes into the jejunum, digestion has progressed to the point where absorption of some nutrients and other substances can begin. Absorption is a vital function of the small intestine, occurring primarily in the jejunum and gradually decreasing toward the end of the ileum.

Absorption is accomplished through millions of microscopic structures known as villi, Figure 13–123. The villi project from the lining of the major part of the small intestine. These fingerlike structures serve a dual purpose. First, they move continuously swinging back and forth keeping the chyme thoroughly mixed with the digestive juices. Second, each projection is equipped with blood capillaries and a lacteal (intestinal lymphatic capillary) from the lymphatic system. The external cells of the villi absorb the nutrients, minerals, and water from the chyme. Some fats and all carbohydrates and proteins, in the form of sugar and amino acids, are absorbed into the capillaries of the villi, to be sent by way of the portal vein to the liver. Here, the products are processed and released into the body or stored in reserve. Many fats are absorbed into the lacteals of the lymphatic system, to be processed through the lymph nodes and eventually returned to the circulatory system for distribution.

The Large Intestine

With digestion completed and the useful nutrients and other substances absorbed from the chyme, the waste products, any undigestible material, and the excess water are sent on to the large intestine through the ileocecal valve. The large intestine is only about 5 feet long but it is approximately 2 inches in diameter. The colon, as it is also called, frames the abdomen, Figure 13–124.

The large intestine absorbs the excess liquid from the chyme through capillaries in the lining. There are no villi in the large intestine. The absorbed water, plus some salts and proteins, are later filtered out of the blood by the kidneys to be eliminated in the urine. The remaining fibrous waste materials are formed into semisolid feces to be eliminated through the rectum.

The Cecum and Appendix

When material leaves the ileum it enters a small, pouch-like segment of the colon called the cecum. A small projection, the vermiform appendix, extends from the cecum. The appendix is a blind worm-shaped structure about the size of the little finger. It tends to become filled easily but drain rather slowly. Occasionally, a substance causes irritation to the lining, resulting in a painful, inflammatory process known as appendicitis. If it persists or progresses, a surgical procedure called an appendectomy is indicated.

The Ascending, Transverse, and Descending Colon

The large intestine is divided into ascending, transverse, and descending sections as a means of identifica-

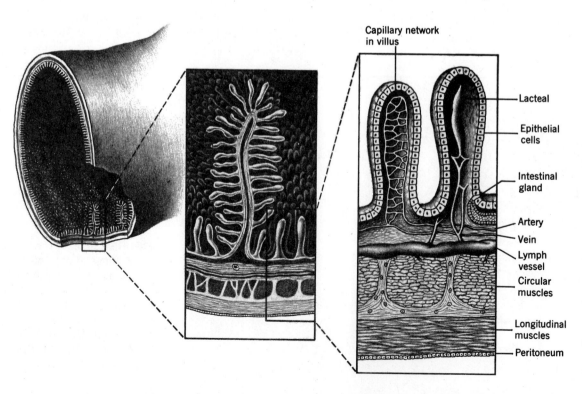

Capillary network in villus

Lacteal

Epithelial cells

Intestinal gland

Artery

Vein

Lymph vessel

Circular muscles

Longitudinal muscles

Peritoneum

FIGURE 13–123 A magnified view of the inner lining of the small intestine, showing the villi with blood and lymphatic capillaries for the absorption of the products of digestion (From Burke, *Human Anatomy and Physiology for the Health Sciences,* 3d ed. Copyright 1992, Delmar Publishers Inc.)

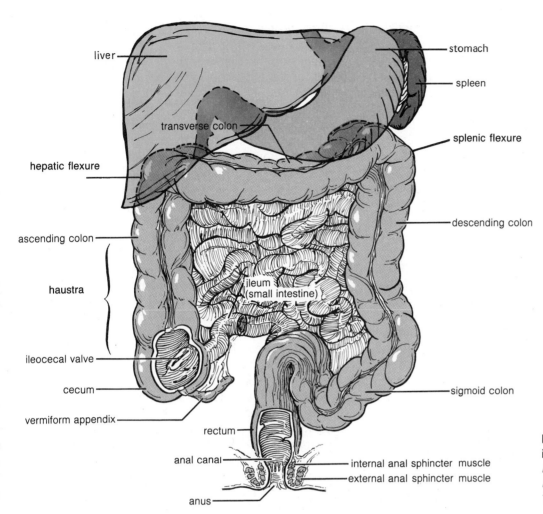

liver
stomach
spleen
transverse colon
splenic flexure
hepatic flexure
descending colon
ascending colon
haustra
ileum
(small intestine)
ileocecal valve
cecum
sigmoid colon
vermiform appendix
rectum
anal canal
internal anal sphincter muscle
external anal sphincter muscle
anus

FIGURE 13–124 The large intestine (Adapted from Fong, *Body Structures and Functions*, 7th ed. Copyright 1989, Delmar Publishers Inc.)

tion. The ascending section joins the cecum at the level of the ileocecal valve and continues upward along the right side of the abdomen to the hepatic flexure (bend at the liver). It is generally a little larger in diameter than the descending section. The upper right corner, the hepatic flexure, lies in front of the right kidney and behind the right lobe of the liver. The transverse section begins at the hepatic flexure and extends in a loop across the abdominal cavity to a point below the spleen, the splenic flexure (bend at the spleen). The center section is attached to the mesentery but can move freely. Both the hepatic and splenic flexures are firmly attached to the rear of the abdominal wall with the splenic attachment being slightly higher.

The descending section begins at the splenic flexure and extends downward along the left side of the abdomen until it reaches the edge of the pelvic cavity. This section is somewhat smaller in diameter. It is firmly anchored to the abdominal posterior wall to maintain its position.

The Sigmoid, Rectum, and Anal Canal

After the large intestine enters the pelvic cavity, it makes two bends suggestive of an *S* and is therefore labeled the **sigmoid** section of the colon. The sigmoid section

extends from the left iliac crest over and back to join the rectum. The rectum is 6 to 8 inches long. It serves as a collecting area for the remains of digestion. When enough material is accumulated, sensors are activated and the urge to **defecate** is felt.

The **anal** canal is a narrow passageway about an inch long, extending from the rectum to the **anus** (opening from the body). Both ends of the anal canal are controlled by sphincter muscles. The internal anal sphincter is an involuntary muscle. When defecation occurs, the nerve endings in the rectum are stimulated to contract and the internal sphincter is relaxed, allowing the fecal material to enter the anal canal. The external anal sphincter is a voluntary muscle and can be consciously controlled to prevent the rectum from emptying when it is inappropriate. It is unwise to make a habit of delaying defecation unnecessarily, however, as this tends to a lessening of the urge, which can result in **constipation.**

When a patient's condition interferes with the ability to control the anus, as in a stroke with paralysis, and the rectum empties whenever the nerve impulse is triggered, the patient is said to be **incontinent** of feces. This situation can be extremely embarrassing to a patient who is still capable of being aware of this occurrence. The opposite problem is often the result of prolonged or serious illness causing a loss of muscle tone so that the patient is too weak to expel the contents of the rectum. This results in material becoming more and more solid as fluid content is lost and the mass becoming of such size that it cannot be expelled. This condition in known as a fecal impaction. The best solution is manual breakup of the mass followed by an enema to irrigate the rectum and remove the material. A patient may attempt to remove the impaction by taking a laxative. Laxatives work either by increasing the rate of passage through the tract, therefore reducing the water absorption time, or by stimulating the secretion of fluid into the tract. Regardless, the results will not help an impaction but only cause an uncontrollable flow of liquid stool around the mass.

The proper function of the digestive system is essential to health. If raw materials cannot be digested and absorbed, the patient will starve. If waste products are not adequately removed, toxins may accumulate and cause illness and even death. This vital function requires a total of about 36 hours from the mouth to the anus. Of course, this time period is influenced by the type of foods eaten and the rate of the peristaltic action.

Diagnostic Examinations ....

A great many studies can be done on blood to determine the function of the digestive organs. Also chemical analysis can be performed on secretions withdrawn by catheter from the stomach or small intestine. However, six other types of examinations will be discussed here because they are so frequently used in diagnosis.

■ Cholecystography—An X-ray examination of the gallbladder following oral administration of a contrast medium. The patient is instructed to take the tablets, one at a time, 5 minutes apart, about 2 hours after dinner the evening before the examination is scheduled. After the tablets are taken, the patient must refrain from any food or drink. The medium is digested and absorbed by the small intestine and sent to the liver by the portal vein. The liver processes the blood, excreting the medium in the bile. The gallbladder concentrates the bile. X rays taken 12 to 14 hours after ingestion of the pills will show the gallbladder filled with the medium. If a fatty substance is then given to the patient to eat or drink, the gallbladder should contract and empty bile into the duodenum. This study allows the physician to determine if the gallbladder is functioning properly. A nonfunctioning gallbladder will neither absorb nor empty the dye properly. The presence of cholelithiasis and/or obstruction of the bile ducts can be determined.

■ Colonoscopy—An examination to view the entire large intestine using a flexible fiberoptic scope. It is indicated in patients with complaints of diarrhea, constipation, bleeding, or lower abdominal pain. It is usu-

ally indicated following negative or inconclusive results from barium enema studies or sigmoidoscopy examination. Preparation for the examination is like that for sigmoidoscopy. The patient is positioned on the left side and the scope is guided and advanced through the large intestine. The physician may insert air to distend the walls of the intestine to facilitate passage. Manipulation of the abdomen also assists with insertion as well as the repositioning of the patient to facilitate passage through the splenic and hepatic flexures. It is possible to obtain tissue samples and secretions through the scope to provide cytology studies. Polyps can also be snared and electrocautery can be performed through the instrument.

■ Gastrointestinal series (X rays)—Radiological studies of the GI tract are indicated for a wide variety of reasons and concentrated on various portions of the system.

Barium swallow—If the condition or function of the esophagus is in question, the patient may be asked to drink a radiopaque liquid called barium while the action of the esophagus is observed by fluoroscope. This test is known as a barium swallow. It aids in diagnosing conditions such as hiatus hernia, diverticulosis, and varices. It also detects strictures, tumors, ulcers, and functional disorders. The barium swallow is usually included as part of the more complete GI series.

Upper GI series—A barium swallow is performed initially to evaluate the esophagus. Then 16 to 20 ounces of additional barium are drunk as the progress of the medium is observed by fluoroscope. X-ray films are taken at specific time periods to permit further evaluation. The stomach is compressed to ensure that the barium coats the entire lining. As the barium enters the small intestine, the radiologist manipulates the abdomen to obtain distribution of the barium throughout the bowel loops. The patient is rotated to several positions to record pertinent areas. Spot films may be taken at 30- to 60-minute intervals until peristalsis carries the barium to the ileocecal valve.

An upper GI series is not painful, but the chalky taste and consistency of barium are unpleasant. Preparation for the test may require a 2- to 3-day diet of low-residue foods before the examination. All oral intake must stop at least 8 hours before it is scheduled. The patient must also refrain from smoking. Both a laxative and a cleansing enema may be ordered the evening before the procedure to be certain the tract is empty.

An upper GI series aids in the diagnosis of gastric ulcers, tumors, strictures of the sphincters, inflammation of the lining, motility irregularities, duodenal ulcers, tumors, filling defects, and the like. Following the exam, another laxative may be ordered to aid in removal of the barium from the intestines. Retained barium may cause constipation, obstruction, or fecal impaction.

Lower GI series—To permit viewing of the entire large intestine, the barium mixture is administered as an enema. The medium outlines the interior wall of the colon for detection of mucosal changes, tumors, polyps, ulcerated sites, diverticulitis, and structural irregularities. The patient must be carefully prepared with a restrictive, low-residue diet for about 2 days, followed by liquids only the day before examination. A cathartic (strong laxative) is ordered the afternoon preceding the test and the colon is thoroughly emptied with tap water enemas until no more fecal material is expelled.

A barium enema of 1000 to 1500 cc is administered through a tube inserted into the rectum. This tube is often capable of being inflated with a balloonlike section to aid in retention of the medium until the examination is completed. As the medium is instilled, the filling is observed by fluoroscope. The patient is rotated on the X-ray table to assist the flow of the barium. The patient is placed on the left side to fill the descending, on the back to fill the transverse, and on the right side to fill the ascending colon. Periodic X-ray films are taken.

When the procedure is completed, the balloon is deflated and the tube is removed. The patient is instructed to expel as much barium as possible. An additional X ray may be taken to record the ability of the colon to empty.

■ **Gastroscopy**/Esophagogastroduodenoscopy—Viewing of the esophagus, stomach, and upper duodenum through a flexible scope which is lighted by fiberoptics. This permits observation of the inside of the organs without an exploratory operation. If an unusual area or growth is seen, a biopsy (small piece) can be removed through the scope. The procedure is also used to remove small foreign objects, obtain cells from the lining, and, with the attachment of a camera, to photograph suspicious areas for later study.

The patient is prepared by spraying the back of the throat with local anesthetic to block the gag reflex and given a sedative to produce drowsiness. The patient must be awake to swallow the scope. As it is passed into the patient, air is instilled to expand the pathway or flatten out folds. Water may also be instilled to wash off the lens and is removed, along with the air and any other secretions, by suction.

The examination is especially helpful in diagnosing tumors, ulcers, structural abnormalities, damage from ingested chemicals, and esophogeal varices.

■ Nuclear medicine study—Scanning of structures such as the liver or spleen is made visible by radioactive materials. A special camera or scanning device may be used to screen the liver for disease processes, infarcts, cysts, tumors, and organ size. The patient is given an intravenous injection of a radioactive material which the body will absorb in the cells of the liver. The scanner is positioned above the patient and passes slowly back and forth in a descending pattern over the area being examined. The resulting pictures outline the organ and indicate irregularities in its composition. A gamma camera is capable of producing images instantly without the scanning procedure.

Similar studies are accomplished with different types of equipment. Computerized axial tomography studies (CAT scans) are multiple X-ray beams passed into tissue to be interpreted and reconstructed by a computer into a three-dimensional picture on a screen. This type of study can be done on the liver, the ducts, and the pancreas.

■ Occult blood test—When bleeding from the intestinal tract is not visible because of the small quantity, it can be detected through analysis of the feces. Visible blood in the stool has a characteristic coloration that suggests the approximate location of the bleeding. Basically, the nearer the rectum, the brighter red the blood. Dark maroon stool is an indication of bleeding in the ileum or jejunum. Bleeding from the stomach or esophagus will be acted on by gastric juices, which cause it to turn black, resulting in a tarry looking stool. Occult blood studies are frequently used to identify bleeding associated with colorectal malignancy.

■ Proctoscopy—An examination of the lower rectum and anal canal through a 3-inch-long proctoscope. It is preceded by a digital examination to determine anal sphincter condition. The proctoscope permits detection of hemorrhoids, polyps, fissures, fistulas, and abscesses. The patient may need an enema if fecal material is obstructing the view.

■ **Sigmoidoscopy**—An examination to view the lower portion of the sigmoid and rectum through a 10- to 12-inch sigmoidoscope. A longer flexible fiberoptic scope is capable of manipulation into the descending colon. A digital examination to determine anal sphincter condition precedes insertion of the scope. The patient is examined, preferably on a special jackknife table, otherwise in the less comfortable knee–chest position. Sigmoidoscopy aids in the diagnosis of inflammation, infection, or ulcerative conditions. It also permits viewing of tumors, polyps, and other disease processes. Biopsy through the scope permits confirmation of a diagnosis without surgery. The patient must be prepared for the examination with an enema administered a short time before. Soap or other irritants must not be added to the water because they may affect the appearance of the lining.

■ Ultrasound—Ultrasonography uses high-frequency sound waves directed toward the liver, gallbladder, or pancreas. The waves create echos of varying degrees, which are changed into patterns of dots on a screen. The patterns reveal the size, shape, and position of the organ being studied. Ultrasonography is especially useful when liver and gallbladder functions are impaired and the use of contrast media is ineffective.

Disorders and Diseases ....

Anorectal Abscess and Fistula. This localized infection is due to a collection of exudate in the soft tissue adjacent to the anus or rectum. It is characterized by a throbbing, painful lump, which makes sitting, coughing, etc., very uncomfortable. The abscess may be initiated from within the rectum due to a sharp object in the feces, such as a piece of seashell or bone, penetrating the surrounding tissue. Because the feces contain bacteria, an infection develops and an abscess results. The exudate may develop an escape route into the rectum, anal canal, or skin surface, which will periodically relieve the pain and excess pressure. Such a tract is known as a fistula. Surgical intervention is indicated to correct the condition by incision and drainage of both the abscess and the tract.

Occasionally, an abscess occurs without a fistula. It may appear on the surface of the perineum as a large, firm, red mass, with or without a yellow center. This abscess requires incision to promote drainage and eventual expression of the solid core of material. The application of heat by sitting in a tub of warm water aids in the drainage process and relieves discomfort.

Appendicitis. An acute inflammation of the appendix probably is due to an obstruction of the intestinal lumen. When obstruction occurs, an inflammatory process begins and leads to infection, thrombosis, destruction of tissue, and eventually perforation of the appendix. On rupture, the infectious material spills into the abdominal cavity and initiates peritonitis, a serious complication. If left untreated, it is fatal.

Symptoms of appendicitis begin with generalized abdominal pain that later localizes in the lower right abdomen at a site known as McBurney's point. Increased tenderness, anorexia, nausea, vomiting, and rebound tenderness (produced by slowly compressing abdomen over site then suddenly releasing the pressure) occur.. A slight fever may be present. A moderately elevated white blood cell count (12,000 to 15,000) in addition to the physical findings supports the diagnosis. The sudden cessation of symptoms is an indication of infarction or rupture.

The only effective treatment for appendicitis is surgical removal, an appendectomy. When appendicitis is suspected, abdominal heat, enemas, or laxatives must never by administered because of the risk of causing perforation. Usually pain medication is avoided to prevent masking of the symptoms. Positioning patients on their right side with the knees flexed will usually help to reduce the discomfort.

Cirrhosis. This chronic disease of the liver causes destruction of the liver cells. The destruction leads to impaired blood and lymph circulation and interferes with the life-preserving functions of the liver. The most frequent cause of cirrhosis is malnutrition associated with alcoholism. Other causative factors are hepatitis or the suppression of bile flow due to a disease of the ducts.

Early symptoms include a variety of GI tract signs such as lack of appetite, indigestion, nausea, vomiting, constipation, and diarrhea. Later, nosebleeds, bleeding gums, and anemia may develop. The liver becomes enlarged, jaundice is present, and ascites (collection of fluid) occurs within the abdomen. Because the disease interferes with portal circulation, hypertension occurs in the portal system causing esophageal varices that eventually rupture and bleed.

Various blood tests support the diagnosis of cirrhosis, but positive confirmation can be obtained through a liver biopsy. A liver scan will detect abnormal thickening and a mass. Treatment consists of measures to prevent further damage or complications, and dealing with the underlying cause. Dietary changes, supplemental vitamins, rest, and appropriate exercise are indicated. Extra care is required when prescribing drugs because the damaged liver may not be able to process them. Alcohol must be prohibited. It is also important to avoid contact with infections. Mortality is high, with many patients dying within 5 years of diagnosis.

Colitis. This inflammation of the colon causes tenderness and discomfort. It may be acute, occurring as the result of a bacterial invasion, or chronic, associated with allergy, emotional stress, or other diseases. (See ulcerative colitis.)

Colostomy. This is an artificial opening of the colon, allowing fecal material to be excreted from the body through the abdominal wall. Colostomies are classified according to the portion of the colon involved; for example, transverse colostomy. The terms *single* and *double barrel* tell whether only the proximal loop is involved or both the proximal and distal loop. A colostomy can also be temporary or permanent. If a disease process could improve if the colon were not constantly irritated by passing feces, then a temporary colostomy is indicated. By surgically providing for the fecal material to empty through an opening in the colon before reaching the affected area, the area is allowed to rest and heal. After an adequate period, surgery is performed to reattach the ends of the colon.

A colostomy is also indicated when an obstructive growth process, such as a tumor, prohibits the passage of feces. When the growth is close to the end of the rectum, there may not be enough healthy tissue remaining to which a segment of the colon can be attached. There may also be evidence that removal of the affected area, even if possible, would be to no advantage. In these cases a colostomy will be performed, in order for elimination to occur until the disease process results in death.

The colostomy patient has a major emotional as well as physical adjustment to make. The alteration in body image may be difficult to accept. The thought of fecal material being expelled into a pouch attached to the abdomen may be very unappealing. Consider also that there is no control over the expulsion of flatus (gas) or stool and it is easy to understand the new patient's rejection. However, with time, diet control, and the use of irrigation, a colostomy can be regulated so that its emptying is at the patient's convenience. Support groups of colostomy patients provide emotional and physical assistance to help new ostomy patients adjust to their changed life-style.

Constipation. This condition is characterized by dry, hard, infrequent bowel movements. To have normal elimination of body wastes, three things are necessary: a proper diet including bulk, adequate fluid intake, and exercise. When one or more of these elements is missing, constipation is likely to occur. Other contributing factors are habitual disregard of the impulse to defecate and the chronic use of laxatives or enemas, which dulls the impulse stimulation. Constipation is common among the elderly, persons with paralysis, and the chronically ill or bedridden, due to lack of activity.

Treatment varies with the cause and condition of the patient. If possible, increasing the dietary bulk, fluid intake, and amount of exercise will usually solve the problem. Prompt response to the urge to defecate is necessary. Normally, a person's body will establish a routine schedule given the opportunity. The habitual use of laxatives and enemas must be stopped. The use of bulk-forming products and glycerin suppositories can be substituted until new bowel habits are learned.

Crohn's Disease. This is an inflammation of any portion of the GI tract, most common in the terminal ileum. The inflammation involves all layers of the intestinal wall leading to edema, ulceration, narrowing, and the formation of abscesses and fistulas. Symptoms vary according to the location of the disease. An acute episode often causes appendicitis-type complaints of pain, cramping, and tenderness in the right lower quadrant with flatulence, nausea, fever, and diarrhea. Bloody stools are also possible. Chronic disease is characterized by diarrhea of four to six stools daily, marked weight loss, weakness, and difficulty in coping with everyday stress. The exact cause of Crohn's disease is unknown. Some feel it is caused by allergies or immune disorders, obstruction of the lymphatics, or infection.

Diagnosis is made after positive blood tests showing increased white blood cells, decreased hemoglobin, and other specific abnormalities. Barium enema studies showing segments of stricture separated by normal bowel known as *string signs* supports the diagnosis. Sigmoidoscopy, which reveals patchy areas of inflammation, helps to differentiate Crohn's disease from ulcerative colitis.

Treatment is mainly symptomatic and may include dietary supplements, steroids to reduce the inflamma-

tion, and the use of antibacterial agents. Most important are changes in life-style to obtain more rest and dietary adjustments to eliminate contributing agents. The ingestion of fruits and vegetables must be restricted with intestinal stenosis (narrowing). Surgery may be necessary if certain conditions develop such as a fistula, bowel perforation, hemorrhage, or obstruction. With extensive disease of the colon, a colectomy with ileostomy may be required (see Ileostomy).

Diarrhea. This condition is characterized by frequent, liquid stools. It can be very serious in infants and small children due to the excessive loss of body fluid. Diarrhea can be caused by a bacterial, viral, or amebic organism. It can also result from a poor diet, toxic substances, foods such as prunes that stimulate peristalsis, or an irritated colon. Basically, diarrhea occurs because the chyme is moved too rapidly through the colon without sufficient time for the water to be absorbed. When the lining is inflamed, as with colitis, rapid peristalsis occurs as soon as material reaches the affected area. In addition, the lining secretes excess mucus to counteract the irritating material. This response results in a liquid stool with shreds of mucus. Diarrhea can also result from nervousness or anxiety. Again, the peristaltic action is stimulated and the waves move rapidly. Diarrhea is best treated by providing an adequate intake of liquids and taking care of the underlying cause. Medication to slow down peristalsis is helpful but it will not treat the underlying cause.

Diverticulosis. This is the presence of bulging pouches in the wall of the GI tract where the lining has pushed into the surrounding muscle. The sigmoid colon is the most common site but diverticuli can occur anywhere from the esophagus to the anus. They are believed to be caused by a high degree of internal pressure and an area of weakness in the intestinal wall. There is a theory that lack of roughage in the diet permits the bowel lumen (opening) to narrow, resulting in higher pressure developing during defecation. The disease is much less common in nations where more natural food and fiber are eaten.

Diverticulitis develops when undigested food mixes with the bacteria normal to the tract and collects in a diverticular sac, forming a hard mass. The mass shuts off the blood supply to the thin-walled sac, followed by inflammation, possibly perforation (a hole), abscess, or hemorrhage.

Symptoms of diverticulitis include irregular bowel movements, lower left abdominal pain, nausea, flatus, low-grade fever, and an increase in WBCs. Chronic diverticulitis may result in fibrosis and adhesions (tissues growing together) that severely limit or obstruct the lumen. Symptoms progress from constipation to ribbon-like stools, diarrhea, distention (swelling up) of the abdomen, nausea, vomiting, pain, and abdominal rigidity.

Treatment initially consists of preventing constipation and combating infection. A liquid diet, antibiotics, and one medication to soften the stool and another to relieve pain and relax muscle spasms are called for. When conservative measures fail, the affected colon section may need to be removed.

Esophageal Varices. Dilated, tortuous veins in the lower section of the esophagus are called esophageal **varices** and are the result of hypertension within the portal vein. The blood flowing through the portal system in the liver meets with resistance due to cirrhosis, a tumor, thrombosis, or occlusion of the veins. As a result, blood backs up to the spleen causing it to enlarge, and the blood flows through other veins. The number of platelets decreases, and the other veins dilate. This results in fluid entering the abdominal cavity causing ascites. With the veins dilated and therefore thinner, and the number of platelets reduced, hemorrhage occurs readily and is often the first sign of the condition. Often massive hemorrhage occurs, producing bloody emesis and stools.

Treatment is limited. To control bleeding, a tube may be inserted into the esophagus to put pressure against the bleeding site. In addition, iced salt water may be instilled into the tube. A drug may be given to control bleeding temporarily. Surgical bypass procedures to correct venous flow may cause from 25% to 50% mortality, and the patient may still die eventually from liver complications instead of hemorrhage. Blood transfusions are also temporary measures. At best, the patient can be kept comfortable until the inevitable massive hemorrhage or coma from liver damage occurs.

Fissure of the Anus. An anal **fissure** is a crack or tear in the lining of the anus, usually the result of passing large, hard stools that stretch the lining beyond its capacity. Symptoms of acute fissure are a burning pain and a few drops of blood on the toilet tissue or underwear. The fissure may develop a swelling at the lower end known as a *sentinel pile.* This protrusion may ulcerate, resulting in painful anal sphincter spasms.

A fissure may heal completely or become chronic due to partial healing and retearing. Later, scar tissue develops in the area, narrowing the passageway. Since the anus must stretch each time stool is passed, healing is difficult.

Treatment consists of digital dilation to prevent stricture, a low-residue diet, stool softeners, adequate liquid intake, hot sitz baths, and a local medication for pain. A chronic condition will require surgical excision of the scar tissue, providing two fresh surfaces that can heal by a gradual regrowth of tissue. Fissures can be prevented by drinking plenty of fluids (eight glasses of water a day), eating a proper diet, and passing stool promptly when indicated.

Gastroenteritis. An inflammation of the stomach and intestines, this term may be applied to such conditions as intestinal flu, traveler's diarrhea, and food poisoning. The inflammation usually subsides within a couple of days and poses no threat to persons in good general health. However, the very young, the elderly, and the generally debilitated are at risk due to the loss of intracellular fluid.

Gastroenteritis is characterized by fever, nausea, abdominal cramping, diarrhea, and vomiting. It is treated with bed rest, increased fluid intake, and diet. Antibiotics may be indicated for the person at risk, as well as intravenous fluids to combat dehydration. Medication may be needed to control vomiting and diarrhea.

Hemorrhoids. The anal canal and the lower portion of the rectum contain vertical folds of mucous membrane called anal and rectal columns. The veins in the mucosa of the folds frequently become dilated, resulting in internal or external **hemorrhoids.** Hemorrhoids can result from long periods of sitting or standing, diarrhea, constipation, vomiting, coughing, hepatitis, alcoholism, loss of muscle tone, pregnancy, or anorectal infections. Any condition that increases portal pressure, such as pregnancy or hepatitis, or that leads to a trapping of blood in the veins, as when stool is being expelled, interferes with the return flow of blood. As more blood enters the veins, it causes dilation and the veins bulge into the anal canal or protrude to the outside, resulting in hemorrhoids. With protrusion comes the possibility of developing a thrombosis. The blood may become trapped externally, forming a painful, hard lump. Once this occurs, it will probably need to be incised to remove the clotted blood.

Treatment of mild to moderate hemorrhoids involves regulating bowel habits; limiting sitting time on the toilet; increasing intake of water, raw vegetables, fruits, and fiber; and applying local heat. When swelling and discomfort persist, with pain and bleeding on defecation, additional treatment is indicated. A sclerosis agent can be injected into internal hemorrhoids, which causes scar tissue to develop, thus reducing the dilation. More severe involvement requires surgical removal of the dilated vein and the surrounding stretched mucosa in a procedure called a **hemorrhoidectomy.**

Hepatitis. This three-stage viral infection of the liver results in cell destruction, which causes jaundice, hepatomegaly (enlarged liver), and loss of appetite. **Hepatitis** occurs in three forms called type A, infectious, type B, serum, and a type non-A, non-B hepatitis that is being called type C. All three types are found throughout the world. Type A tends to be self-limiting and rather benign. Type B is extremely contagious and has a higher mortality rate. Type C is the mildest of the three. Type A is also highly contagious and is usually transmitted by the fecal-oral route, meaning organisms from sewage, human, or animal wastes get into the food chain. It is usually transmitted through ingestion of food, water, or milk that has been contaminated, and from seafood taken from contaminated water. Type B is usually transmitted parenterally (other than by mouth). Health care workers are especially prone to it, due to contact with human secretions and feces. Universal precautions are indicated when caring for all patients to prevent acquiring or spreading the disease. Like AIDS, hepatitis B can be acquired through sexual intercourse and contaminated needles, including ear piercing and tattooing. It can also be passed from mother to newborn during delivery. But it can be spread by more casual contact through cuts in the skin and in saliva.

In most patients, involved cells will repair themselves leaving little damage, and in the case of type A hepatitis only, confers a lifelong immunity. When other disorders are present, such as congestive heart failure, diabetes, severe anemia, cancer, and advanced age, complications are more likely and the prognosis is poor.

Hepatitis produces a variety of additional symptoms, which appear suddenly with type A; type B & C symptoms are insidious. Clinical features of stage one include: fatigue, malaise, headache, anorexia (lack of appetite), sensitivity to light, sore throat, cough, nausea, vomiting, frequently a fever of 100° to 101°F (37° to 38°C), and possibly liver and lymph node enlargement. These symptoms occur during the preicteric (before jaundice) stage and disappear when jaundice begins. About 6% to 10% of adults and 25% to 50% of children become chronic carriers. These individuals are infectious and can develop potentially fatal complications due to liver degeneration and cancer.

The second, icteric, stage has begun once the urine becomes dark, the stool is clay-colored, the sclera and skin yellow, and a mild weight loss has occurred. The liver remains enlarged and tender, and the spleen and cervical nodes swell. The jaundice may continue for 1 to 2 weeks. Then liver enlargement subsides, but the fatigue, flatulence (intestinal gas), abdominal tenderness, and indigestion continue. The third stage, posticteric, usually lasts for 2 to 6 weeks. Full recovery requires 6 months.

Complications may develop leading to a chronic hepatitis, which occurs in benign or active forms. The active, known as chronic aggressive hepatitis, has about a 25% fatality rate due to liver failure from cell destruction.

Diagnosis is made based on history that reveals recent exposure to drugs, chemicals, a jaundiced person, or a recent blood transfusion and the presence of typical symptoms. Blood tests revealing hepatitis B antigens and the presence of B antibodies confirm type B hepatitis. Antigens are present only in the early phase of the disease, so a false negative result may occur if the blood is drawn too late.

Presence of the antibody (anti-HAV) indicates type A hepatitis. If these antigens and antibodies are absent, but the patient still exhibits appropriate symptoms, then type C hepatitis is confirmed.

A vaccine has been developed to prevent hepatitis B and is recommended for the following groups of people:

- IV drug users
- Health workers
- Individuals living with an infected person
- Sexually active homosexuals
- Heterosexuals with multiple partners
- Recipients of certain blood products
- Children born to immigrants from regions where hepatitis B is common, such as Southeast Asia
- Infants born to infected women. (Up to 90% of children born to infected mothers become infected and suffer a high death rate.)
- Travelers spending more than 6 months in an area with high incidence

The main problem with the vaccine is it requires three shots over an 8-month period and costs approximately $120 in the US. Many of the targeted groups of people, except for health care workers and infected mothers, are difficult to reach. It is interesting to note several developing countries are immunizing newborns and others at a cost of about $1.

There is no specific treatment nor cure for hepatitis B. Patients are expected to rest and eat small meals with high calorie and protein content. Medication to help relieve nausea and vomiting may be necessary. An effort is made to determine the source of infection or contagion. Hepatitis is one of several contagious diseases that are to be reported to the local public health department.

Health care workers should protect themselves from suspected or confirmed disease by wearing gloves to handle body secretions or draw blood. Hospitalized patients are isolated, with strict techniques utilized to prevent the spread of the disease.

Hernia (Hiatus). The protrusion of an internal organ through a natural opening in the body wall is known as a hernia or rupture. One form of hernia involves a defect in the diaphragm that allows a portion of the stomach to move up into the chest cavity through the opening for the esophagus. It is called a **hiatus** or **hiatal hernia.** There are three types of hiatal hernias: sliding, which is most common; rolling or paraesophageal (alongside the esophagus); and mixed, which is a combination of both. This condition is found in up to 50% of the population over 50 years old. If no symptoms occur, no treatment is required.

In all forms of hiatal hernia, some portion of the stomach, the end of the esophagus, or both slips through the diaphragmatic opening, Figure 13–125, page 350. In paraesophageal, a portion of the stomach "rolls" through the opening into the chest but causes few symptoms except a feeling of fullness in the chest and anginalike pain. This type of hernia needs surgical repair. A sliding hernia may cause symptoms such as heartburn from 1 to 4 hours after eating, which is often aggravated by reclining and occasionally results in regurgitation or vomiting; chest pain, caused by the reflux (return) of gastric juices; distention and spasms of the stomach; difficulty swallowing, due to inflammation of the esophagus, or an ulcer. The most serious symptom is severe pain and shock, which result from incarceration when a large portion of the stomach is trapped above the diaphragm cutting off circulation to that part of the organ. Since strangulation leads to tissue death, immediate surgery is indicated.

Conservative treatment for uncomplicated hiatal hernia involves medication to strengthen the esophageal sphincter muscle, using gravity to decrease the reflux of gastric juices, and a diet of small, frequent, bland meals. Other helpful measures include waiting at least 2 hours after eating to lie down, eating slowly, and avoiding spicy foods, fruit juices, alcohol, and coffee. Smoking is discouraged because it stimulates the production of gastric acid.

Hernia (Inguinal). The wall of the abdominal cavity has normal openings through which blood vessels or other body structures pass. For example, the male's spermatic cords pass through the inguinal rings of the lower abdominal wall to reach the testes, which are external to the body. When the surrounding structure of fibrous tissue, the fascia, becomes weak, it allows a loop of small intestine to protrude through the ring, following the path of the spermatic cord. This type of hernia is called an inguinal hernia, and it often extends into the scrotum when the patient stands. Diagnosis of a smaller hernia can be made on manual examination of the inguinal ring while the patient

is asked to cough. If the examiner feels something touch the examining finger, the patient has a hernia.

A protruding hernia can usually be reduced, or pushed back into place. Some patients may wear a device called a truss, which exerts pressure directly over the herniated opening, to hold the protruding mass inside the cavity. Occasionally, the mass cannot be reduced and will remain in the hernial sac. It is then possible for additional intestine to enter the sac and/or the contents to become twisted or trapped, interfering with the circulation of blood to the intestine. This condition is referred to as a *strangulated hernia* and requires a surgical procedure known as herniorrhaphy as quickly as possible. The procedure replaces the contents of the sac within the abdominal cavity and closes the opening.

Hernias can be the result of weak abdominal muscles due to a congenital condition or the natural process of aging. Hernias can also develop from increased abdominal pressure due to heavy lifting, pregnancy, obesity, or straining.

Other types of hernias are: femoral, which occurs where the femoral artery exits the abdomen to the legs; umbilical, involving the structure around the umbilicus; and incisional, in an area of previous surgery.

Ileostomy. This surgical opening of the ileum allows the chyme of the small intestine to empty through the abdominal wall. An ileostomy is similar to a colostomy except that the chyme is liquid and highly caustic to the skin due to the digestive juices. The patient with an ileostomy has no control over its function and must wear an ostomy appliance (collection bag) attached to a donutlike disk that perfectly surrounds the stoma (mouth or opening). A protective adhesive creates a watertight seal. A belt attached to the disk supports the device. A permanent type of bag may be attached, which must be emptied and cleaned periodically. Disposable plastic bags can also be used. Some disposable types incorporate a deodorizing material; the permanent type requires instillation of a deodorizer.

The patient with an ileostomy must accept a great alteration in body image and function. The passing of flatus and the gurgling of liquid stool being expelled occurs without warning and cannot be controlled. Most patients who have had ileostomy surgery feel better off than before surgery. Many had extensive ulcerative colitis with much pain, bleeding, and excessive, sudden, and frequent diarrhea, and were in poor physical condition from the debilitating effects of the disease. The removal of the diseased colon necessitates the ileostomy. Other patients may have been affected by Crohn's disease, which causes inflammation, scarring, and near or complete obstruction of the bowel. These patients experienced pain, nausea, fever, cramping, bleeding, and diarrhea, occurring four to six times a day. The freedom from pain and relative increase in control over excretion are often considered to make an ileostomy worthwhile. Many times, these patients have been nearly confined to

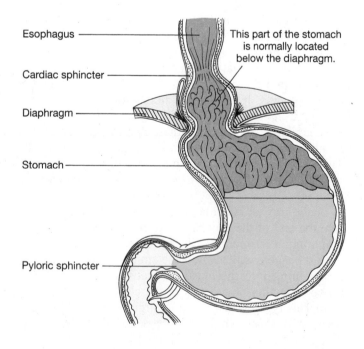

Esophagus

Cardiac sphincter

Diaphragm

Stomach

Pyloric sphincter

This part of the stomach is normally located below the diaphragm.

FIGURE 13–125 Hiatal hernia

their homes because of their weakness and the characteristics of the disease. With an ileostomy they can regain fairly good health and live a nearly normal life.

Oral Cancer. The mouth should be examined for oral cancer every time a visit is made to a dentist for routine cleaning and examination. It should also be inspected by the physician as part of a physical examination. People who do not visit a dentist or physician frequently should observe their own mouths for oral cancer warning signals:

- Swelling, lump, or growth anywhere in or about the mouth
- White scaly patches inside the mouth
- Any size sore that does not heal
- Numbness or pain anywhere in the mouth area
- Repeated bleeding in the mouth without cause

Any of these signals should be examined by a physician or dentist. Oral cancer can result in a disabling and disfiguring condition when areas are excised. If the tongue is involved, speech and the process of eating become difficult.

Pancreatitis. This is inflammation of the pancreas, which occurs in both acute and chronic forms. The most frequent predisposing factors are alcoholism, trauma to the pancreas, reaction to certain medications, and pancreatic carcinoma. It may also develop as the result of a duodenal ulcer. **Pancreatitis** progresses in an unusual manner. The enzymes normally produced and excreted into the pancreatic duct remain and digest the pancreatic tissue. If the cells that produce insulin are destroyed, the condition will be complicated by diabetes.

Mild pancreatitis is characterized by epigastric pain not relieved by vomiting. A severe attack causes extreme pain, persistent vomiting, a rigid abdomen, and rales (noisy, ausculated breath sounds) at the lung bases with pleural fluid on the left side. Tachycardia may occur, and a fever of from 100° to 102°F (38° to 39°C) with cold, perspiring extremities. Rapidly progressing pancreatitis can cause massive hemorrhage, which results in shock and coma. Mortality is as high as 60% when there is tissue destruction and hemorrhage.

The complicated treatment consists of methods to decrease pancreatic secretions and relieve pain while maintaining adequate fluids. Shock is treated vigorously by replacing electrolytes and proteins IV to prevent death. After the emergency passes, IVs containing electrolytes and proteins that do not stimulate the pancreas are continued for 5 to 7 days. This may be followed by tubal feeding if the patient is unable to take enough nutrients by mouth. In extreme cases, a pancreatectomy, the removal of the pancreas, may be indicated.

Paralytic Ileus. A physiological intestinal obstruction, a **paralytic ileus** usually occurs in the small intestine. Peristalsis is either drastically reduced or totally absent. This results in severe abdominal distention and distress, frequently accompanied by vomiting. The condition is often precipitated by manipulation of the bowel during abdominal surgery or the paralyzing effects of the anesthesia. The ileus usually disappears after 2 to 3 days. If it continues for more than 48 hours, it may be necessary to insert a weighted tube into the small intestine to remove the accumulated fluids and gas. Medication to stimulate colon action may be given.

Peptic Ulcer. This encircled lesion in the mucous membrane lining of the stomach, lower esophagus, duodenum, or jejunum is caused by contact with gastric juices, especially hydrochloric acid. Predisposing factors include long-term overproduction of secretions due to emotional stimulation; damage from chemical irritants (alcohol and aspirin); stimulation of secretions by tobacco; reflux (backflow) of bile into the stomach through a relaxed pylorus; and an overactive vagus nerve, increasing secretions that damage the duodenum.

Gastric (stomach) peptic ulcers are often associated with older men who are undernourished and chronic users of aspirin and alcohol. Duodenal peptic ulcers account for approximately 80% of peptic ulcers. They often become chronic, recurring after a time of remission. About 10% of these patients will require surgical treatment.

Duodenal peptic ulcers cause heartburn, epigastric pain that is relieved by food, a weight gain (due to extra eating), and a strange feeling of bubbling hot water in the back of the pharynx. Attacks occur whenever the stomach is empty or after drinking alcohol, juice, or coffee. Complications that may develop with either type of ulcer are perforation, hemorrhage, and pyloric obstruction.

Treatment consists of diet, drugs, rest, and informed patient cooperation. Medications are used to reduce gastric secretions, with antacids to help neutralize the acidity. Sedatives and tranquilizers are given for gastric ulcers. Drugs that inhibit the vagus nerve are used for duodenal ulcers. Surgical cutting of the branches of the vagus nerve may be indicated to correct excess secretion. Partial removal of the diseased portion of the stomach may be required as a final measure.

Polyp. This is a mass of tissue that results from an overgrowth of upper epithelial cells of the mucosal membrane of the GI tract. There are five varieties, some hereditary, others of common adenoma structure. Most are benign, but **villous adenoma** and hereditary polyps show a tendency to become malignant. Most types develop in adults over 45 years old. Predisposing factors are age, heredity, diet, and infection.

Polyps are difficult to diagnose because they are almost always asymptomatic. They are usually discovered accidentally during a rectosigmoidoscopy or lower GI series X ray. The most common symptom is rectal bleeding. The structure of the polyps varies from small lesions covering the surface of the rectum or sigmoid to large lesions attached by long, thin stalks. The type of polyp determines its physical characteristics.

Treatment consists of surgical removal often by electrocautery, especially if benign and pedunculated (on a stalk). If they are villous adenomas, which are invasive and therefore malignant, treatment usually involves abdominoperineal resection (removal of the colon and rectum, including the area around the anus), with a resulting permanent ileostomy. Each type of polyp is dealt with in relation to its current state or its tendency to become malignant.

Pruritus Ani.

This is itching of the area surrounding the anus, often associated with irritation and burning. The main contributing factors for pruritus ani are harsh, vigorous rubbing with soap and a washcloth; poor hygiene; spicy foods; anal skin tags (small pieces of suspended extra skin); excessive perspiration; a systemic disease such as diabetes; the use of perfumed or colored toilet paper; coffee, alcohol, or food preservatives; a fungus or parasitic infection; an anorectal disease such as fissure, fistula, or hemorrhoids; and certain skin cancers.

Classical symptoms are itching after a bowel movement or at night. Scratching can cause reddened, weeping skin or thickened, leathery, darker tissue.

Treatment consists of removing the underlying cause, such as a rectal tag, and eliminating irritants to the skin such as soaps, powders, and colored tissue. The area should be kept clean and dry. Witch hazel applied on wiping pads or cotton balls is soothing. Steroid creams aid in reducing inflammation and controlling itching.

Pyloric Stenosis.

This narrowing of the pyloric sphincter interferes with the emptying of the stomach. Stenosis can be caused by scar tissue developed during healing of a gastric ulcer. It can also be a congenital condition in infants. The sphincter is enlarged and often cartilagenous, causing a narrowing of the opening, which results in the dilation of the stomach. Forceful vomiting will develop by the third week after birth and lead to a serious dehydration problem.

Congenital stenosis often corrects itself in time if the vomiting is not so intense as to require surgical correction. In adult stenosis, the patient may be able to alter the diet and use medication for some time; however, surgical correction will probably be required eventually.

Spastic Colon.

This common condition is characterized by alternating periods of constipation and diarrhea. A spastic colon is a functional disorder, often associated with stress. However, it can also be caused by physical conditions such as diverticulitis, food poisoning, cancer of the colon, and eating certain irritants such as raw fruits or vegetables.

The condition is characterized by lower abdominal pain, which is relieved by expelling flatus or stool, and the occurrence of diarrhea during the daytime. This pattern alternates with constipation or normal function. Sometimes the stool contains mucus.

Treatment consists of therapy to relieve symptoms such as counseling for stress, dietary restriction of known irritant foods, rest, heat to the abdomen, and the use of sedatives for a short period of time.

Ulcerative Colitis.

An inflammatory disease, often chronic, that affects the mucosa of the colon. It usually begins in the sigmoid and rectum, extending upward to involve the whole colon. The small intestine is seldom involved. The disease produces congestion followed by edema, which makes the mucosa fragile. As the lining breaks down, ulcers are formed, which eventually develop into abscesses. The disease can be confined to one area and be known as segmented colitis or it can spread throughout the colon. Severe colitis may cause a perforation of the colon, which can result in a life-threatening infection called peritonitis, as well as toxemia (blood poisoning).

Ulcerative colitis primarily affects young adults, mostly female. Predisposing factors are a family history of colitis, a bacterial infection, overproduction of enzymes that damage the mucous membrane, emotional stress, an autoimmune reaction, and allergic reactions to some foods.

The prime symptom of ulcerative colitis is recurrent bloody diarrhea, often containing exudate and mucus. The frequency and intensity will vary with the extent of the disease. Other symptoms include weight loss, weakness, anorexia, nausea, vomiting, irritability, and abdominal pain. The disease leads to other complicating conditions such as anemia, coagulation defects, liver damage, arthritis, loss of muscle mass, hemorrhoids from frequent stools, and stricture due to no solid stool, perforated colon, and toxemia.

Treatment consists of controlling inflammation, maintaining nutrition and blood volume, and preventing complications. Patients are usually placed on bed rest, IV fluid replacement, and a clear liquid diet. Drug therapy is used to control the inflammatory process and combat infection. Severe involvement may necessitate antispasmotics and pain medication to relieve the cramping and discomfort. If the patient fails to respond to medical treatment and the symptoms become intolerable, surgical resection (removal) of the colon is indicated, with an ileostomy as previously described. Patients who develop colitis before age 15, which persists for at least 10 years, are especially prone to colorectal cancer. Figure 13–126 illustrates some of the disease conditions of the colon and may help in the visualization of their characteristics.

Complete Chapter 13, Unit 10 in the workbook to help you meet the objectives at the beginning of this unit and therefore achieve competency of this subject matter.

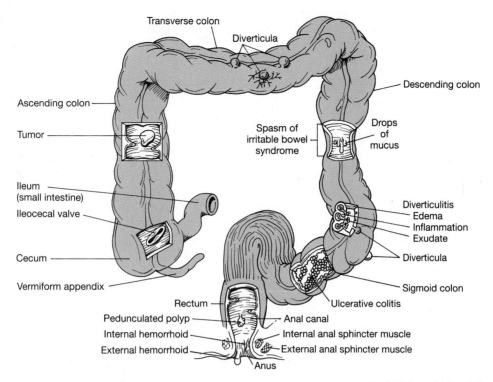

FIGURE 13–126 Common conditions of the colon (Courtesy of Lakeside Pharmaceuticals Division of Murell Dow Pharmaceuticals, Inc.)

UNIT 11

The Urinary System

OBJECTIVES

Upon completion of the unit the student will meet the following terminal performance objectives by verifying knowledge of the facts and principles presented through oral and written communication at a level deemed competent.

1. Explain the three main functions of the urinary system.
2. Identify the organs of the urinary system and describe their physical characteristics.
3. Explain how the urinary system functions with other systems.
4. Describe the interior structure of the kidney.
5. Name the parts of a nephron and explain how each part functions.
6. Describe the process of dialysis and name two types.
7. Discuss the likelihood of success with a kidney transplant.
8. List the two main categories of diagnostic examination and give examples, explaining briefly how each test is performed and for what purpose.
9. Describe 10 diseases or disorders of the urinary system.
10. Spell and define, using the glossary at the back of the text, all the words to know in this unit.

WORDS TO KNOW

anuria
bladder
Bowman's capsule
calculi
calyces
calyx
catheterization
cortex
cystitis
dialysis
dribbling
dysuria
elimination
excretion
fistula
frequency
glomerulonephritis
glomerulus
graft
hematuria
hemodialysis
hesitancy
hilum
intravenous pyelography
kidney
lithotripsy

medulla
nephron
nephrotic syndrome
nocturia
oliguria
peritoneal
polycystic kidney disease
polyuria
ptosis
pyelonephritis
renal
renal failure
residual
retention
secretion
stricture
suppression
uremia
ureter
urethra
urgency
urinary
urinary meatus
urine
void

The urinary system removes nitrogenous waste products, certain salts, and excess water from the blood and eliminates them from the body. At the same time, it evaluates the body's acid–base balance and selectively reabsorbs the elements needed to maintain the proper ratio.

The urinary system performs three main functions. The first is excretion, the process of removing waste products and other elements from the blood. The second is secretion, by which it produces urine. The third is elimination, or emptying of the urine from its bladder storage.

The major work of the system is performed by two organs called the kidneys, Figure 13–127. The well-being of the human body depends heavily on the function of the kidneys. When waste products are not removed from the blood, they build up, producing potentially fatal toxicity. After the kidneys have performed their functions, the waste material, urine, is carried through the ureters, one for each kidney, to temporary storage in the bladder. When an adequate amount has been accumulated, the bladder expels the urine through the urethra, eliminating it from the body.

As we have said before, no system can function by itself. The urinary system is no exception. Waste products and other substances that are filtered out of the blood must first have been ingested, digested, and absorbed by the digestive system into the circulatory system, to be delivered in the blood to the kidneys. The peristalsis of the muscular system moves the urine through the ureters. The nervous system, in cooperation with a muscular sphincter, controls elimination. The respiratory system and the urinary system cooperate to control the body's acid–base balance and the amount of fluid retained. Pulmonary action influences the amount of O_2–CO_2 exchange as well as the amount of fluid loss through respiration. Hormones from the endocrine system also influence the amount of urine excreted. And the integumentary system works in close relationship to the urinary system to remove or retain body fluid as required. Once again it is apparent that the body is a complex, interdependent organism.

The Kidneys

The kidneys are shaped like a lima or kidney bean. Each kidney is about $4\frac{1}{2}$ inches long, from 2 to 3 inches wide, and about an inch thick, and weighs about $\frac{1}{4}$ pound. The kidneys are located on each side of the vertebral column, high up on the posterior wall of the abdominal cavity, between the muscles of the back and the parietal peritoneum that covers the abdominal organs. Because they are not within the area occupied by the organs, the kidneys are said to be retroperitoneal (behind the peritoneum). The left kidney is slightly higher than the right, which is displaced by the liver. Normally, a heavy cushion of fat helps keep the kidneys in their proper position.

A condition known as ptosis (dropping) occurs in very thin persons due to an inadequate fatty cushion.

Externally the kidney is covered with a tough, fibrous capsule. The concave border has a notch called the hilum through which the renal (kidney) artery enters and the renal vein and renal pelvis of the ureter exits. Internally the kidney is divided into two sections, an outer layer, the cortex, and an inner, the medulla, Figure 13–128. The medulla is divided into triangular-shaped wedges called renal pyramids with bases toward the cortex and "tops," or renal papillae, emptying into cavities called calyces (singular, calyx). The pyramids have a striated (striped) appearance; the cortex appears smooth. The cortex extends inward between the pyramids in sections called renal columns.

The Nephrons

The life-preserving service of the kidney is performed by microscopic units called nephrons. Each kidney has over 1 million of these units, which altogether contain roughly 140 miles of filters and tubes. Each minute, the kidneys filter over 1000 cc's of blood, producing about 60 cc's of urine per hour. In an average day, a person takes in 2500 cc of fluid ($2\frac{1}{2}$ quarts) and generates another 300 cc (10 ounces) of water, which is formed by the cells in the process of combining oxygen and other materials. About 1500 cc ($1\frac{1}{2}$ quarts) is eliminated as urine each day. Additional fluid is lost through feces and respiration. Some moisture is also lost through the skin, especially when perspiring. Despite the amount of liquid consumed, the kidneys maintain a constant amount of fluid in the body's tissues, excreting the excess as urine. The concentration of the urine is in direct relationship to the amount of liquid consumed.

The process by which the nephrons produce urine is complex. The nephron is a peculiarly shaped structure resembling a funnel with a long, twisted tail, Figure 13–129, page 356. The top of the funnel is a double-walled hollow capsule called the Bowman's capsule. Each capsule contains a cluster of about 50 capillaries called the glomerulus. The Bowman's capsule and the glomerulus together are known as the renal corpuscle.

Blood enters the glomerulus by way of an afferent arteriole, flows through the glomerular capillaries, and leaves through the efferent arteriole. The efferent arteriole branches into capillaries that surround the renal tubule. The capillaries come back together in tiny veins, which join a branch of the renal vein.

Beyond the Bowman's capsule is a twisted section of tubule called the *proximal convoluted tubule*. The capsule and this section of tubule descend into the medulla and are called the *loop of Henle*. This loop has a straight descending and ascending limb, but when it returns to the cortex it changes into another twisted section called the *distal convoluted tubule*. Several distal tubules join into a straight collecting tubule, which empties into the calyx.

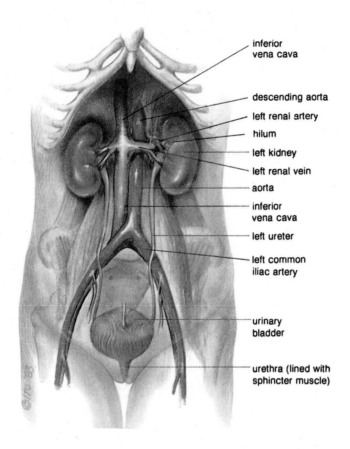

FIGURE 13–127 The urinary system (From Fong, *Body Structures and Functions*, 7th ed. Copyright 1989, Delmar Publishers Inc.)

Filtration and Reabsorption. Filtration is the first process in the formation of urine. Blood enters the capsule by way of the afferent arteriole, carrying waste products, water, salt, urea, and glucose. The arteriole divides, forming approximately 50 glomerular capillaries. Because so many capillaries are emptied by a single efferent arteriole, blood pressure increases significantly. This higher pressure forces the fluid to leave the blood by filtration and enter the Bowman's capsule at the rate of about 125 mL a minute. This equals a rate of 60,000 mL (60 liters, or 56.8 quarts) in an 8-hour period.

By a reabsorption process, 99% of the filtrate is returned to the bloodstream. Not only fluid but also useful substances such as glucose, vitamins, amino acids, electrolyte salts, and bicarbonate ions (base) are reabsorbed. As the filtrate enters the proximal tubule, about 80% of the water is reabsorbed into the surrounding peritubular capillaries along with other substances the body needs to maintain a proper balance. For example, the filtrate contains glucose, which is normally completely reabsorbed. However, when levels exceed normal limits, the selective cells lining the tubules no longer reabsorb glucose but allow it to remain in the tubule to be eliminated in the urine. The term used to describe the limit of sugar reabsorption is the *threshold*. Passing this level is referred to

as *spilling over the threshold*. Patients who have diabetes spill sugar frequently and therefore test its presence in their urine to determine the need for additional insulin.

A final reabsorption takes place in the distal tubule. The remaining 10% to 15% of water may be reabsorbed depending on the body's need. The process is controlled by a hormone that acts upon the nephron.

Secretion. The secretion function of the nephron moves substances directly from the blood in the peritubular capillaries into the urine in the distal and collecting tubules. The substances secreted directly are ammonia, hydrogen ions, potassium ions, and drugs. The elements are selectively secreted to maintain the body's acid–base balance.

Urinary Output. Anything that increases the volume of blood in the capillaries increases the output of urine; conversely, the urine output decreases with a lessening of blood volume. For example, a large fluid intake increases the volume of blood and the output of urine. Hemorrhage or dehydration decreases blood volume and urine output.

Another factor regulating secretion is the amount of solutes in the filtrate. Again considering the diabetic, when there is an increase in the amount of glucose, it spills over into the urine, increasing the urine volume eliminated that day because more liquid is allowed to pass through to dilute the glucose content.

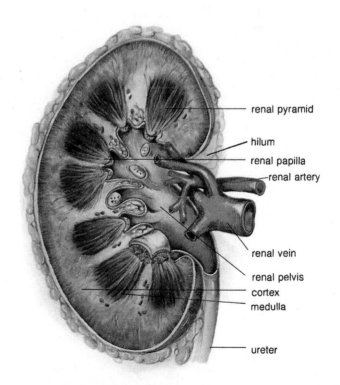

FIGURE 13–128 Internal structure of the kidney (From Fong, *Body Structures and Functions*, 7th ed. Copyright 1989, Delmar Publishers Inc.)

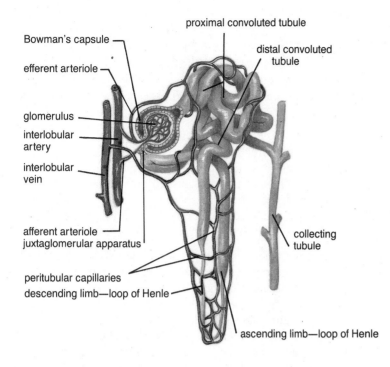

Bowman's capsule

efferent arteriole

glomerulus

interlobular artery

interlobular vein

afferent arteriole
juxtaglomerular apparatus

peritubular capillaries
descending limb—loop of Henle

proximal convoluted tubule

distal convoluted tubule

collecting tubule

ascending limb—loop of Henle

FIGURE 13–129 A nephron unit and related structures. (The collecting tubules, which are not microscopic, give the pyramids of the medullary portion of the kidney a striated appearance. As shown, there are some collecting tubules in the cortical portion of the kidney) (From Burke, *Human Anatomy and Physiology for the Health Sciences*, 3d ed. Copyright 1992, Delmar Publishers Inc.)

The functional capacity of the healthy kidney is so great that removal of one kidney poses no problem to the body in removing liquid wastes.

The Ureters

The urine secreted by the nephrons drops out of the collecting tubules into the calyces, then enters the renal pelvis and continues down the ureters into the urinary bladder, Figure 13–130. The ureters begin with a widened upper portion, continuing as a long, slender, muscular tube approximately 10 to 12 inches in length. Peristaltic waves, at a rate of one to five a minute, move the urine down the ureter to enter the lower posterior wall of the bladder. Because of the solutes in urine, some persons tend to form renal calculi (stones). As the calculi form in the renal pelvis, they are washed into the ureter by the urine. When a stone is large enough to become lodged in the ureter, severe pain results. Frequently, removal of the stone may be required if it cannot be passed into the bladder. (See Renal Calculi in Diseases and Disorders.)

The Urinary Bladder

The bladder is a collapsible bag of muscular tissue lying behind the symphysis pubis. The lining has many folds, giving it the ability to expand. The bladder serves as a reservoir for urine, collecting approximately 250 cc before the urge to void (urinate) is felt. The capacity of the bladder is two to three times this amount, and in instances of retention (inability to empty bladder), may

be in excess of 1000 cc. In such instances, urine must be removed by inserting a catheter through the urethra into the bladder to relieve the distention and discomfort. This procedure is known as catheterization.

The Urethra

The urethra is a tube leading from the bladder to an exit from the body. In the female, it is a straight tube about $1\frac{1}{2}$ inches in length. It opens externally between the clitoris and the vagina within the folds of the labia minora. The opening is called the urinary meatus. Only urine passes through the female urethra. In the male, the urethra is about 8 inches long, extending internally from the bladder down through the prostate gland and out through the penis to the meatus. The male urethra also serves as a passageway for semen.

A circular muscle sphincter within the urethra permits voluntary control of bladder function. This control, however, requires an intact nerve supply and motor area of the brain. Involuntary emptying of the bladder is known as *incontinence*.

Other medical terminology commonly used to describe urinary output includes: anuria, an absence of urine; dysuria, pain or discomfort associated with voiding; hematuria, blood in the urine; nocturia, having to urinate at night; oliguria, a scanty urinary output; and polyuria, excessive urination. Descriptive words used to clarify symptoms are: dribbling, the involuntary loss of drops of urine; frequency, the necessity to void often; hesitancy, difficulty in initiating urination; and urgency, the sudden need to void.

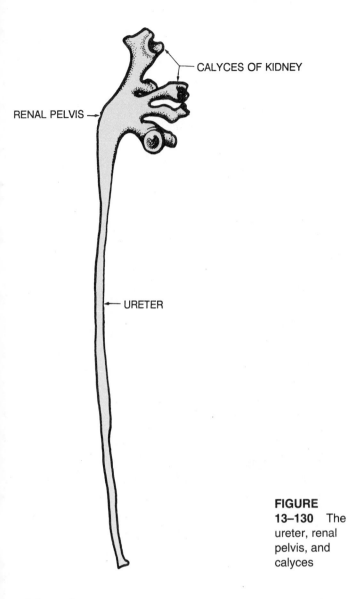

RENAL PELVIS →

CALYCES OF KIDNEY

← URETER

FIGURE 13–130 The ureter, renal pelvis, and calyces

Dialysis

Dialysis is the mechanical process of removing waste products from the blood normally removed by the kidneys. Basically it is a process for purifying blood by passing it through thin membranes and exposing it to a solution which continually circulates around the membranes. The solution is called *dialysate*. Substances in the blood pass through the membrane into the lesser concentrated dialysate in response to the laws of diffusion. This is called hemodialysis.

The term artificial kidney is often used to refer to the kidney dialysis unit. However, the part of the unit that actually substitutes for the kidney is a glass tube approximately 8 inches long and about $1\frac{1}{2}$ inches in diameter. The tube, called the dialyzer, is filled with thousands of minute hollow fibers attached firmly at both ends, Figure 13–131. Blood from the patient flows through the fibers, which are surrounded by circulating dialysate. The dialysate can be individualized for each patient to provide the appropriate levels of sodium, bicarbonate, and

other substances. These cross the membrane and enter the blood. At the same time, extra water and waste products leave the blood to enter the dialysate.

The patient is connected to the dialysis unit by means of needles and tubing that take blood from the patient, circulate it through the machine and return it to the patient. New programmable dialysis management systems, as seen in Figure 13–132, page 358, can monitor blood pressure; allow variable control of solution substances; adjust temperature, flow, and filtration rate of the blood; and preset the length of treatment time, plus other functions, all automatically. (On the system pictured, the dialyzer is located just left of center; it has black ends with tubing attached to both ends.)

A fistula (opening between an artery and vein), or a graft (vein inserted between an artery and a vein) is surgically constructed in the patient to provide a site for inserting the large needles required in dialysis, Figure 13–133, page 358. The fistulas and grafts are artificial veins that can withstand repeated needle insertions. They lie just under the skin surface and require 2 to 4 weeks for a graft and 8 to 12 weeks for a fistula to completely heal before they can be used. There is considerable amount of pressure within the blood vessels, which could rupture new sites.

The initial site is the nondominant forearm, usually at the radial artery. When this begins to fail, sites are constructed at the brachial artery, then in the dominant arm, and finally grafts at the femoral artery in the groin area.

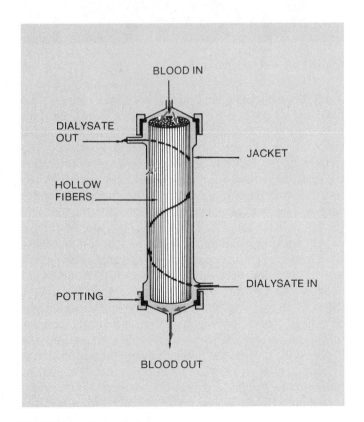

BLOOD IN

DIALYSATE OUT

JACKET

HOLLOW FIBERS

DIALYSATE IN

POTTING

BLOOD OUT

FIGURE 13–131 Dialyzer

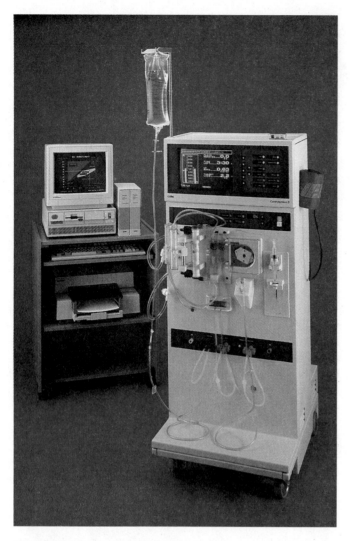

FIGURE 13–132 Hemodialysis unit

require dialysis two to three times per week, for 3 to 5 hours each time.

An alternative to hemodialysis is continuous ambulatory peritoneal dialysis, Figure 13–134. Instead of an artificial dialyzer to cleanse the blood, the patient's own peritoneal membrane is used (the peritoneum covers the abdominal organs and lines the abdominal cavity). The dialyzing solution is introduced into the peritoneal cavity where it comes into contact with blood vessels. The solution enters through a catheter permanently implanted into the abdomen. The solution tubing is aseptically attached and approximately 2 liters of dialyzing solution are infused by the process of gravity by suspending the bag at shoulder level. Then the empty bag is rolled up and placed around the waist under the clothing. The solution attracts the waste products and water from the blood and they are suspended in the solution. After approximately 4 to 6 hours, the bag is unrolled, placed lower than the abdomen, and the waste-bearing dialyzing solution is drained out. Another fresh bag is infused and the dialysis continues. The exchange process of draining the solution and infusing fresh solution requires from 30 to 45 minutes. This is repeated about every 4 to 6 hours during the day and for an 8 hour period at night.

Another form of peritoneal dialysis is called *automated peritoneal dialysis*. This is more acceptable to some individuals because the dialysis is accomplished during 6 to 8 hours every night while they sleep. This is especially well-suited for children. The patient can completely control peritoneal dialysis, permitting greater freedom of activity; however, solution exchanges approximately 4 times daily do create some inconvenience.

Artificial veins last from 3 to 5 years. Some patients who have had a graft constructed from one of their own veins have had unusually successful sites for as long as 10 years, but this is not the norm. Since dialysis occurs so frequently, the multiple needle insertions not only affect the grafts or fistulas but the overlying skin as well. When too much damage has occurred, the site is no longer usable. The patient must learn to care for the site and protect it from damage. This is truly the lifeline for the patient with renal failure. Nothing, such as tight clothing or elastic cuffs, must constrict the site area. The patient is not allowed to sleep on the involved arm. Women cannot have purse straps across the forearm. Care must be taken when carrying any objects in the arms such as grocery bags, boxes, firewood, books, and similar articles that could damage the site.

Since the rest of the patient's life depends on dialysis, access to a machine becomes critical. Most patients are assigned to dialysis centers for periodic treatment. However, equipment can be obtained for home dialysis when the patient and the family are willing to assume the responsibility. Patients usually

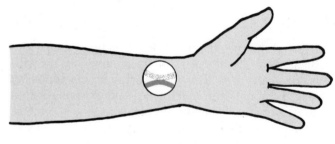

ARTERIOVENOUS FISTULA

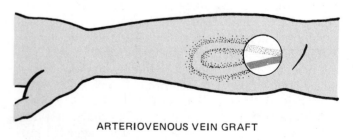

ARTERIOVENOUS VEIN GRAFT

FIGURE 13–133 Hemodialysis sites

The main complication of peritoneal dialysis is peritonitis, an inflammation of the peritoneum from accidental contamination of the tubing when connecting and disconnecting solutions. Users of the method must be meticulous in performing the procedure. Peritonitis is painful and can cause scarring of the peritoneum, making it no longer useful for dialysis. Peritonitis can be fatal.

Many considerations must be weighed when dialysis becomes necessary. Routine procedures such as taking medications, for example, must be timed after dialysis to prevent removing them from the bloodstream. For additional information about this life-prolonging procedure, contact your local branch of the National Kidney Foundation; inquire at a dialysis center, or consult your physician.

Kidney Transplant

The transplantation of body organs is always at risk of recipient rejection; however the kidney appears to be fairly successfully transplanted. Transplantation is indicated in cases of prolonged chronic debilitating disease and renal failure involving both kidneys. It is usually done following an extended period of time on dialysis waiting for a compatible organ.

The demand exceeds the supply for healthy organs. In addition, blood and other cellular structure must "match" to ensure the greatest probability for a functioning transplanted organ. There is an anticipated percentage of success within immediate family members. A twin provides the greatest likelihood, with a brother or sister, parent, or child providing decreasing percentages of success in that order. The surgical procedure itself is well established and presents virtually no concern as far as the success of the transplanted kidney. The patient, however, is almost always in a state of relatively poor physical condition due to the effects of the extended illness. This status plus the tendency of the body to reject a "substance" that is foreign and not of the same cellular structure sometimes results in the organ not surviving in its new host. The use of drugs to control the body's natural defensive mechanism of rejection increases the rate of success. Research into new and more effective drugs is a continuing process.

Diagnostic Examinations

Several procedures and tests are used to determine the physical characteristics of the urinary system and assess its function. Analysis of the blood can determine levels or uric acid and the amount of urea nitrogen present. Urinalysis (analysis of the urine) can determine presence of blood cells, bacteria, acidity level, specific gravity (weight), and physical characteristics such as color, clarity, and odor.

- Noninvasive procedures—Procedures that attempt to evaluate function deal with urinary output. An intake–output measurement involves keeping a record of all fluid, or food that melts to liquid, that is consumed, along with all urine or other fluid loss, be measured or estimated. For example, emesis would be measured; perspiration estimated as slight, moderate, or profuse; diarrhea indicated as to frequency; and any other loss such as bleeding; drainage through a stoma, or excessive respiratory activity, evaluated. Hence, intake is compared to output to evaluate fluid balance within the body.

A 24-hour urine test collects all urinary output, from a specified hour one day until the same time the next day, in a special container under specific conditions (see Chapter 17). Urine can be collected by various methods, depending to some degree on the purpose for collection. A routine specimen, preferably the first of the morning, is simply voided into a clean container. A clean catch specimen, usually for culture

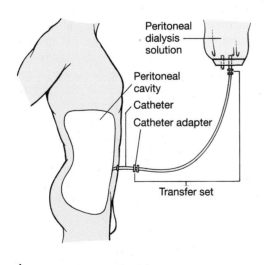

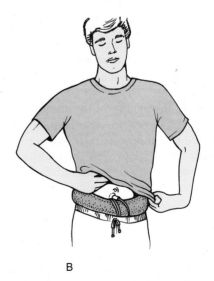

A

B

FIGURE 13–134   Peritoneal dialysis. (a). Infusion of the solution. (b). Rolled empty solution container is hidden under clothing.

purpose, pregnancy determination, or microscopic examination, involves specific cleaning of the meatal area and catching the specimen midstream in a sterile container.

An X ray or plain film of the abdomen may be taken to determine size, shape, and position of the urinary organs. It may also indicate the presence of calculi. This is usually referred to as a KUB (kidney, ureters, and bladder) series.

The kidney is also frequently examined by ultrasound to detect abnormalities or to clarify findings from other tests. It is a safe, painless procedure that can be used especially in cases where sensitivity to the radiological opaque materials prohibits other tests. Examinations for kidney function that use a contrast medium are of little value when there is renal failure. Ultrasound, however, can be used to at least view the structure of the kidney in these instances.

■ Invasive procedures—Another means of collecting a urine specimen is to withdraw it directly from the bladder through a catheter into a sterile container by strict aseptic (sterile) technique.

One of the most common diagnostic procedures is an X-ray series called IVP (intravenous pyelography). The patient is required to fast (no food or water) for approximately 10 hours beforehand. A laxative and/or cleansing enema removes from the colon any fecal material that might obscure the urinary organs. A contrast medium is injected into a vein, usually at the antecubital space of the arm. After a period of time, a film is taken to demonstrate the function, location, and position of the kidneys, as determined by the presence of the dye. Subsequent films outline the ureters and bladder as the dye is processed by the system. The film is taken at specific intervals to assess the efficiency of the kidney function. Because the contrast medium is iodine based, it is extremely important to determine if the patient has an allergic response to iodine or seafood before the injection.

Cystourethroscopy is an examination using lighted instruments inserted into the urethra and bladder to view the interior surfaces. A local anesthetic (sometimes a general) is given. Then the urethroscope is inserted into a lubricated sheath. As the scope and sheath are inserted, the interior of the urethra is observed. The scope is then advanced into the bladder. The urethroscope is withdrawn and the cystoscope inserted through the sheath to view the interior of the bladder. A solution is instilled to distend the bladder lining for observation and to make the ureteral openings visible. At this point, based on findings, other procedures can be performed such as: catheterization of the kidney(s) by inserting a catheter up through the ureter(s); biopsy of a tumor; or removal of calculi in the bladder. It may be possible to crush larger calculi with an instrument and irrigate the pieces out through the scope. When examination of the bladder is com-

pleted, the cystoscope is withdrawn and the urethroscope reinserted. Both the scope and the sheath are slowly withdrawn while the neck of the bladder and the interior of the urethra are examined.

Other standard procedures performed initially during cystourethroscopy are obtaining a sterile specimen for culture and sensitivity testing and measuring the amount of residual urine left in the bladder after the patient has voided, just prior to the examination.

Other X-ray examinations can be performed in connection with endoscopic examinations. When a catheter is inserted into the ureters and passed into the pelvis of the kidney, any urine present can be removed and a radiopaque medium instilled. This procedure, known as *retrograde ureteropyelography,* is especially useful for viewing the renal structure when poor kidney function prohibits an IVP procedure. The structure of the ureters can be seen by an additional dye injection as the catheter is withdrawn.

Fluoroscopy as well as X-ray films aid in determining abnormalities. A delayed film, 15 to 20 minutes following instillation of the dye, can be taken to check for retention indicative of urinary stasis (stagnation). If an obstruction of the kidney is observed, it can be located by the film to be corrected. When an obstruction prohibits urinary function, the catheter may be left in position temporarily to ensure adequate drainage. A kidney can be severely, if not permanently, damaged in a relatively short period of time if pressure from urine builds up due to the inability to drain.

Diseases and Disorders ....

Cystitis. This inflammation of the bladder usually results from an ascending organism introduced through the meatus. The most common cause in women is *E. coli* from the rectum, which is carried to the meatus by improper cleansing following defecation. Women should be instructed to always cleanse from front to back when washing, wiping, or drying the perineal area. Cystitis can also be caused by organisms from the vagina or a sexual partner. Women are far more prone to infection than men, presumably because the urethra is so short. Also the prostatic fluid in the male acts as an antibacterial shield.

Symptoms of cystitis are frequency, dysuria, spasms of the bladder, nocturia, and often fever and hematuria. Nausea, vomiting, chills, tenderness over the bladder area, and lower-back pain may occur. A frequent complaint is sharp, stabbing pain when voiding, especially at the end of the stream. This discomfort, together with the urge to void small amounts frequently, prompts the patient to seek medical help.

Diagnosis is confirmed by clinical characteristics and the presence of organisms in the urine in excess of normal amounts. Cystitis is treated with antibiotics sufficient to sterilize the urine. Usually, medication is given for approximately 5 days. A culture of the urine after 3 days should show no organisms. If bacterial resistance to a certain medication has developed, the drug of choice will need to be changed. The sensitivity studies performed on the urine culture will identify appropriate alterations.

Urinary tract infections (UTI) are particularly common in patients with neurogenic bladders. The problem stems from the loss of innervation to the bladder, which can cause incontinence, residual retention, spasticity, or flaccidness. Bedfast patients or those confined to wheelchairs are especially susceptible. The use of indwelling catheters to deal with incontinence or the inability to void frequently results in UTI due to the direct entrance route for bacteria into the bladder.

Glomerulonephritis. This inflammation of the glomerulus of the nephron occurs in both acute and chronic forms. Acute glomerulonephritis (AGN) always follows a streptococcal infection, usually of the respiratory system. It affects boys ages 3 to 7 most frequently, but can strike either sex at any age. Up to 95% of children and 70% of adults recover fully, with the remainder developing chronic renal failure. AGN results from a collection of antigen–antibodies from the streptococcal infections, which become entrapped in the glomeruli membranes. The entrapment causes interference in the glomerular function, damaging the membrane and resulting in the loss of its ability to selectively filter solutes. Red blood cells and protein molecules are allowed to filter out and the filtration rate drops. Uremic poisoning may result. (See Uremia.)

AGN usually begins from 1 to 3 weeks after an untreated throat infection. Symptoms include moderate edema, protein in the urine, hematuria, oliguria, and fatigue. Hypertension may develop due to retention of sodium or water from the decreased glomerular filtration rate. Diagnosis is made following a detailed history and clinical assessment. Laboratory findings confirm elevated electrolytes, BUN (blood urea nitrogen), and creatinine in the blood as well as red and white blood cells, and protein in the urine. A throat culture may show a streptococcal organism.

Treatment consists of bed rest, fluid and salt restriction, and correction of the electrolyte imbalance. Diuretics (water pills) may be used to reduce the accumulation of cellular fluid. At this time the use of antibiotics is controversial. The course of AGN usually resolves in about 2 weeks.

Chronic glomerulonephritis is a slow, progressive disease that results in scarring and sclerosing of the inflamed glomeruli, gradually leading to renal failure. Unfortunately, sufficient symptoms are not produced to cause early clinical investigation. The first symptoms are proteinuria (protein in the urine), hematuria, and a specific form of a urine cast. By the time it is diagnosed, chronic glomerulonephritis is usually irreversible. Occasionally, the chronic form follows AGN, but most frequently it is an insidious disease precipitated by other primary renal disorders or systemic syndromes.

The chronic stage can be asymptomatic for many years, suddenly becoming progressive and producing hypertension, proteinuria, and hematuria. In the later stages, uremic symptoms occur, such as nausea, vomiting, pruritus, dyspnea, fatigue, mild to severe edema, and anemia. Severe hypertension may cause enlargement of the heart, congestive heart failure (CHF), and eventually renal failure.

Treatment consists of measures to treat the symptoms only, such as a diet to restrict sodium, antihypertensive drugs, correction of the electrolyte imbalance, reduction of edema, and prevention of cardiac failure.

Nephrotic Syndrome. (Nephrosis). This noninflammatory disease involving the glomerular membrane allows a large number of protein molecules to leave the blood and enter the urine. As a result, large amounts of water accumulate in the body causing generalized dependent edema. This often leads to pleural effusion, swollen external sex organs, and ascites (fluid within the abdomen). Nephrotic syndrome occurs most often in children, but adults can contract the disease as well.

The underlying cause of the disease is usually glomerulonephritis (75% of the cases). The remaining 25% are associated with diabetes; circulatory diseases such as sickle cell anemia, CHF, and renal vein thrombosis; toxins that affect the nephrons such as mercury, bismuth, or gold; allergic reactions; and systemic infections such as tuberculosis. Symptoms range from the dominant clinical feature of edema to hypotension, especially on standing, lethargy, fatigue, lack of appetite, pallor, and depression.

Diagnosis can be confirmed with consistently elevated proteinuria over a 24-hour period, the presence of characteristic fatty casts and oval fat bodies in the urine, and increased serum cholesterol levels with decreased albumin levels.

Treatment consists of correcting the underlying cause whenever possible. Supportive treatment involves a high-protein diet, restrictive sodium intake, diuretics for edema, and antibiotics to combat infection. Some favorable results have occurred with the use of corticosteroids, but they are limited to specific uses.

Polycystic Kidney Disease. An inherited disorder, polycystic kidney disease is characterized by bilateral, grapelike clusters of fluid-filled cysts. The presence of the cysts greatly enlarges the size of the kidney externally and also compresses the nephrons inside, eventually replacing the functioning renal tissue. The disease appears in an infantile form, which results in stillbirth or early newborn death. Occasionally, an infant will survive for about 2 years before developing renal failure. The adult form has an insidious onset, usually apparent between ages 30 to 50. The deterioration of the kidney is slower but is nevertheless fatal unless treated by dialysis.

Symptoms of the infantile form include a pointed nose, small chin, floppy low-set ears, and folds in the inner eyelids. The kidneys become huge bilateral masses between the bottom of the ribs and the top of the ileum and are symmetric, firm, and dense. Usually there is evidence of CHF and respiratory distress. Adult polycystic disease initially presents nonspecific symptoms such as hypertension, polyuria, and UTI. Eventually additional symptoms appear relating to enlarged kidney masses, such as lumbar pain, widened body, and a swollen, tender abdomen. As the disease advances, the patient develops recurrent hematuria, life-threatening bleeding from cyst rupture, proteinuria, and pain due to ureteral spasm from the passing of clots or calculi. After approximately 10 years, the insufficiency of the kidney results in failure and uremia.

Polycystic disease is not curable but it can be managed, to a certain degree, by controlling hypertension and urinary infections. Treatment is like that for any chronic, destructive kidney disease, and includes dialysis.

Pyelonephritis. One of the most common kidney diseases, acute pyelonephritis is caused by bacteria that normally inhabit the intestines. The bacteria typically spread from the bladder up the ureters and into the pelvis, causing the development of colonies of bacteria within 24 to 48 hours. Pyelonephritis may also result from urinary stasis, the inability to empty the bladder completely, or urinary obstruction due to strictures, tumors, or enlarged prostate in males.

Symptoms associated with pyelonephritis include urgency, dysuria, burning during urination, nocturia, and hematuria. The urine may have an ammoniac or fishy odor and is usually cloudy in appearance. Other common symptoms include fever of 102°F (39°C) or higher, chills, lack of appetite, flank pain, and fatigue. The symptoms generally develop rapidly and may subside within a few days. However, a residual bacterial infection may recur at a later time.

Diagnosis is confirmed by urinalysis, which shows sediment containing leukocytes and possibly a few red blood cells. Culture reveals a significant population of bacteria. Specific gravity is below normal due to the temporary inability to concentrate urine. Treatment consists of antibiotics determined by culture and sensitivity tests. A course of treatment is usually 10 to 14 days even though urine becomes sterile after 2 to 3 days.

Reculturing is done 1 week after treatment and periodically for the next year to observe for residual infection, Mechanical problems causing urinary stasis, such as strictures, "dropped" bladder (positioned so that it cannot totally empty), or tumors should be corrected.

Renal Calculi. Kidney calculi (stones) are formed from chemicals in the urine forming crystals that stick together. They may be as small as a grain of sand or as large as a golf ball. Small stones pass out of the kidney with the urine. Some that are larger become caught in a ureter where they cause severe pain. Still others may pass into the bladder where they continue to enlarge and will again cause pain if they get washed into the urethra and become lodged.

Kidney stones affect primarily young to middle-aged adults, with men being affected four times as often as women. The condition tends to recur. The causes of calculi formation are not always clear; however, certain factors seem to contribute to their development.

- Drinking too little fluid
- Chronic UTIs
- Blockage of the urinary tract
- Prolonged limited activity
- Misuse of certain medications
- Certain genetic and metabolic diseases
- Specific foods in certain susceptible people

Symptoms of renal calculi are:

- Severe pain, starting suddenly in the kidneys or lower abdomen moving to the groin area. It may last for minutes or hours alternating with periods of relief.
- Nausea and vomiting
- Burning and frequent urge to urinate
- Chills, fever, and weakness, probably from infection
- Cloudy or foul-smelling urine
- Blood in the urine
- Blocked urine flow

Diagnosis is made based on symptoms, X rays such as KUB or IVP, and ultrasound. Once size and location are determined then an appropriate course of action can be selected. About 90% can be passed without requiring special treatment or surgery. Often increasing fluids and a specific medication to dissolve the stone is sufficient. However, calcium-containing stones, the most common type, cannot be dissolved.

The simplest treatment is chosen first. Many stones, if in the bladder or ureters, can be removed through the ureterocystoscope either directly or following crushing or breaking up with laser or sound waves. Stones in the kidney may still be removed through a scope inserted through the side into the kidney proper to remove stones whole or break them up by crushing, sound waves, or other methods and allowing them to pass normally in the urine within a few weeks.

A relatively new method of stone removal is called extracorporeal shock-wave lithotripsy (ESWL). Shock waves (high-energy pressure waves) similar to sonic booms generated by aircraft are produced outside the body by an electrical spark. The patient, in a disposable swimsuit, is positioned and strapped into a hydraulic chair. IV sedation is given to make the patient comfortable. The chair is lowered into a tank of warm water and the shock wave-producing device is positioned to focus on the stone. The waves travel through the water and the body without damaging living tissue.

It takes about 2000 shock waves to break up the average stone and requires about 1 hour to complete the treatment. Most describe the shock feeling as a slapping or tapping sensation. Patients are fitted with headphones to listen to music while the procedure is being done. About an hour after the treatment, most patients are allowed to leave. The remaining small fragments of the stone can be easily passed in the urine. It may take several weeks to completely pass all the fragments.

Most patients experience some abdominal discomfort with or without bruising on the abdomen or back. Frequent urination with burning and slight tinge of blood is common. Patients are instructed to collect passed stone fragments for analysis and to see their urologists as a follow-up to be certain there is no kidney blockage from the fragments.

Occasionally people do not qualify for ESWL due to stone location or one of the following:

- Weight in excess of 295 pounds
- Height over 6 foot 6 inches
- Involved kidney has little or no function
- Uncontrolled urinary infection
- Cardiac pacemaker or severely irregular heartbeat
- It is the urologist's opinion that another form of treatment is more appropriate

If no other method can be used, the stone will be removed by surgical incision into the kidney. This is now considered the final choice to solve the problem because of the risks involved with any major surgical procedure and the length of recovery time required.

Renal Failure (Acute and Chronic). A critical illness, acute renal failure results in the sudden cessation of kidney function. Renal failure may be caused by an obstruction, inadequate circulation, or damage to the nephrons. Effective medical treatment usually can overcome the problem. If not, however, it will progress to uremia and death. Failure due to bilateral obstruction is usually associated with calculi, blood clots, tumors, strictures, an enlarged prostate, or urethral edema. Inadequate blood flow results from low blood pressure, as well as volume, in the arteries, which eliminates the force required for the kidney to filter out water and solutes from the blood. This can result from shock, embolism, hemorrhage, loss of fluid due to burns, congestive heart failure, and arrhythmias. Nephron damage, which may cause failure, can result from acute glomerulonephritis, sickle cell anemia, bilateral renal vein thrombosis, acute pyelonephritis, renal myeloma (tumor), or toxic substances.

Symptoms initially apparent are oliguria and azotemia (nitrogenous products of protein metabolism in the blood). Without filtration the waste products and excess solutes quickly collect in the blood, resulting in severe electrolyte imbalance, acidosis, and uremia, which interfere with the function of the other body systems. A vast number of other symptoms develop, listed here by body system and in ascending order within the system: gastrointestinal: anorexia, nausea, vomiting, hematemesis (bloody vomitus); nervous: headache, drowsiness, confusion, convulsion, coma; integumentary: dryness of the skin, pruritis, pallor, uremic frost (powdery white crystals of urea on the skin); circulatory: hypotension initially, then hypertension, cardiac rhythm irregularities, CHF, edema, anemia, pulmonary edema; respiratory: Kussmaul's respirations (fast, deep respirations, over 20 per minute and usually sounding labored, resembling sighs). Fever and chills, indicators of infection, are an expected complication.

Diagnosis of renal failure is confirmed by blood test findings of greatly elevated quantities of urea, nitrogen, and creatinine and urine samples with casts, protein, and altered specific gravity. Additional verification with diagnostic examinations such as KUB, IVP, and retrograde pyelography may be indicated.

Treatment consists of a high-calorie diet that is low in protein, sodium, and potassium. Fluids are controlled. Dialysis may be required.

Chronic renal failure occurs as an end result of the progressive loss of kidney function. Symptoms do not develop significantly enough to warrant investigation until almost 75% of glomerular function is gone. The remaining normal nephrons gradually deteriorate, causing symptoms of renal failure and other system involvement.

Chronic failure can be the result of many preexisting conditions, such as chronic glomerular disease, chronic infections, obstructions, endocrine diseases, vascular diseases, and chronic overdose of toxic agents. Signs and symptoms initially are related to the loss of sodium, which causes hypotension, dry mouth, listlessness, fatigue, and nausea. Later the patient will begin experiencing mental dullness and confusion. Symptoms increase as more nephrons fail. Muscular irritability results from potassium retention and eventually changes to weakness.

Additional systems involvement is similar to that described with acute failure, but a few specific differences do occur with the slower progressive course. Children with chronic failure show stunted growth patterns due to endocrine abnormalities. Infertility and amenorrhea (lack of menses) in women, impotence in men, and impaired carbohydrate metabolism also result from improper endocrine action. The skeletal system develops a mineral imbalance that results in bone pain due to parathyroid hormone imbalance. This in turn allows the minerals to be withdrawn from the bones causing fractures. Calcifications develop in the brain, eyes, joints, myocardium, and blood vessels.

Diagnosis is made in the same manner as for acute renal failure. Treatment is almost exclusively dependent on dialysis to eliminate or decrease the effects of the disease. Other treatment is required for the complications developed in the other body systems. Long-term dialysis also requires specific physical as well as psychological therapy. Patients must be meticulous in their personal care. The skin must be clean and lotions applied to combat dryness and itching. Good oral hygiene is a must to alleviate bad breath and counteract excessive dryness and bad taste. Diet is extremely critical and requires individual adjustments in relation to dialysis. Daily records of intake and output aid in determining fluid status. If urine is not being excreted, fluid builds up within the body's tissues. Dialysis removes this fluid causing the patient to express feelings of being "wrung out."

Stricture. Narrowing of a passageway interferes with the movement of substances through its interior. For example, the **stricture** of a ureter interferes with the flow of urine to the bladder. A more common stricture occurs in the urethra, particularly in male children. It may be a congenital abnormality or, in either sex, the result of scarring following infection. Symptoms of urethral stricture are indicative of a decreased passageway, such as a small urine stream and prolonged urination time. Stricture of a ureter may not be evident until distention occurs due to the buildup of pressure, or until kidney stones develop from urinary stasis. Complete stricture of a ureter will destroy the function of the affected kidney.

Urethral strictures can be readily treated by dilation to open up the narrowed passageway. Increasingly larger dilators are inserted into the urethra to stretch the constricted area. The procedure often needs to be repeated periodically to maintain patency (openness), especially with the growing child.

Suppression. This term is used to describe the complete failure of a natural secretion or excretion. In the context of the urinary system, it refers to the failure of the kidneys to secrete urine. When anuria occurs, catheterization is indicated to determine if urine is present in the bladder but cannot be expelled. The absence of bladder urine indicates no production by the kidneys. Therefore the patient has **suppression.**

Uremia. This term describes the presence in the blood of products normally found in the urine. It is a toxic condition leading to coma and death if not treated. As previously described, it can be the end result of many acute and chronic kidney diseases. Any condition which renders the kidney unable to regulate the chemical composition of the blood by excretion of waste products causes the wastes to accumulate, slowly building to a toxic level. When renal failure exists, **uremia** is inevitable. Dialysis is the only substitute for kidney function, except for surgical transplantation of another kidney.

Complete Chapter 13, Unit 11 in the workbook to help you meet the objectives at the beginning of this unit and therefore achieve competency of this subject matter.

UNIT 12
The Endocrine System

OBJECTIVES
Upon completion of the unit the student will meet the following terminal performance objectives by verifying knowledge of the facts and principles presented through oral and written communication at a level deemed competent.

1. Differentiate between endocrine and exocrine glands and give an example of each.
2. Give examples of body functions affected by hormones.
3. Name and locate the nine glands discussed in the unit.
4. Describe the structure and function of the pituitary, thyroid, parathyroid, adrenal, pancreas, and thymus glands.
5. Describe the hormones and functions of the pineal body and the gonads.
6. Explain the hormone secretion abnormalities that cause: gigantism, dwarfism, acromegaly, goiter, tetany, diabetes, cretinism, Cushing's syndrome, and myxedema.
7. Describe the interrelationship of the hormonal secretions.
8. Identify the diagnostic examinations used to confirm diabetes, thyroid function, pregnancy, and Cushing's syndrome.
9. Describe briefly the symptoms, characteristics, and the usual course of action of five endocrine disorders presented in the unit.
10. Spell and define, using the glossary at the back of the text, all the words to know in this unit.

WORDS TO KNOW

acromegaly	hormone
adrenal	hyperglycemia
adrenaline	hyperthyroidism
adrenocorticotropic hormone (ACTH)	hypoglycemia
	hypothyroidism
aldosterone	islet of Langerhans
cretinism	luteinizing
Cushing's syndrome	myxedema
diabetes mellitus	ovary
dwarfism	parathyroid
endocrine	pineal body
epinephrine	pituitary
estrogen	progesterone
exocrine	puberty
exophthalmia	testes
gigantism	testosterone
glycosuria	tetany
goiter	thymus
gonad	thyroid
gonadotropic	thyroidectomy

The **endocrine** system is a group of glands that secrete substances directly into the bloodstream. Endocrine glands are ductless; in other words, their secretions do not drain into the body by way of a duct but are secreted directly into the capillaries of the circulatory system. Glands secreting substances through ducts are **exocrine** glands. The liver secretes bile through the hepatic duct; therefore it is an exocrine gland. Similarly, the pancreas secretes pancreatic juices by way of a duct into the duodenum, so it is an exocrine gland. However, the pancreas also secretes insulin directly into the blood, which also makes it an endocrine gland.

The secretions from endocrine glands are called **hormones.** A hormone is a complex chemical which influences and controls body functions. Hormones are chemical messengers that cause changes which persist for a considerable length of time, in the activity of other glands or organs. Examples of body functions affected by hormones are growth and development, metabolism, the composition of the blood and bones, sexual maturity, and the function of all endocrine glands.

Nine glands or groups of glands will be discussed: the **pituitary, thyroid, parathyroids,** pancreas (introduced in Unit 10, The Digestive System), **adrenals, ovaries, testes, thymus,** and the **pineal body,** Figure 13–135. Each gland performs a specific function. The hyper- or hypoactivity of the gland causes changes in the body, often altering its appearance, always altering its function,

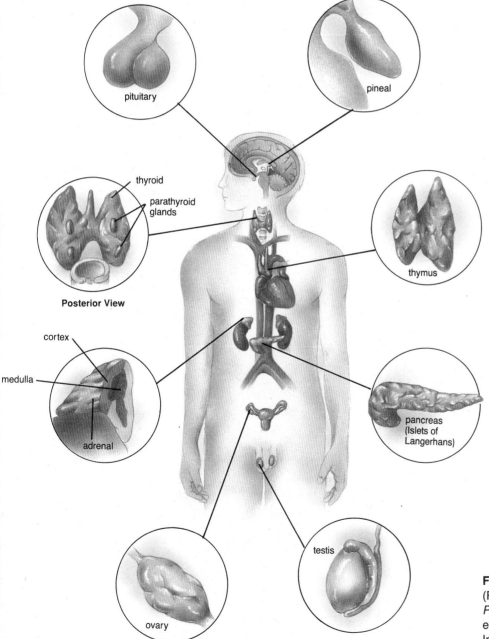

pituitary

pineal

thyroid

parathyroid glands

Posterior View

thymus

cortex

medulla

adrenal

pancreas (Islets of Langerhans)

testis

ovary

FIGURE 13–135 The endocrine system (From Burke, *Human Anatomy and Physiology for the Health Sciences*, 3d ed. Copyright 1992, Delmar Publishers Inc.)

even to the point of death in specific hormonal crises. Hormones either stimulate or inhibit glandular function to maintain homeostasis. See Table 13–7, page 368 for a summary of the glands and their functions.

Pituitary Gland ....

The pituitary gland is considered to be the "master" gland of the body, secreting a large number of hormones that affect other glands, growth, and development.

The gland is attached by a thin stalk to the undersurface of the brain. It is so vital to the body that it is protected within a bony cradle deep within the skull. It sits in a bony depression of the spheroid bone of the skull, called the *sella turcica,* behind the bony orbits of the eyes at about the level of the bridge of the nose. This tiny gland, not much larger than a pea, secretes nine known hormones.

The pituitary is constructed of a large anterior and a small posterior lobe, each producing specific hormones. A thin sheet of tissue lies between the two lobes. The production of pituitary hormones is under the control of the hypothalmus of the brain by way of a feedback mechanism that senses the level of all hormones available to the body and the need for hormones to be released in response to stimuli.

Anterior Lobe

The hormones of the anterior lobe are as follows:

1. Growth hormone (GH)—Essential for normal growth of the body's tissues, affects the length of long bones and therefore height. Insufficient production during childhood results in **dwarfism,** whereas overproduction produces **gigantism,** Figure 13–136. Overproduction in adulthood will produce a condition known as **acromegaly,** which is characterized by overgrowth of cartilagenous and connective tissue resulting in a bulky appearance, protrusion of the eyebrow area, enlargement of the hands and feet, and deformation of the features, Figure 13–137.
2. Thyrotropin, the thyroid-stimulating hormone (TSH)—Increases the growth and activity of thyroid cells to produce thyroid hormone.
3. **Adrenocorticotropic hormone (ACTH)**—Stimulates the cortex of the adrenal gland.
4. Melanocyte-stimulating hormone (MSH)—Increases skin pigmentation.

The following three **gonadotropic** hormones control the development of the reproductive system in both males and females, including the female menstrual cycle. If production fails before **puberty,** sexual maturity will not occur. If it fails after puberty, secondary sexual characteristics regress.

5. Follicle-stimulating hormone (FSH)—Enlarges the graafian follicle of the ovary to the point of rupture and stimulates the follicle to produce estrogen in the

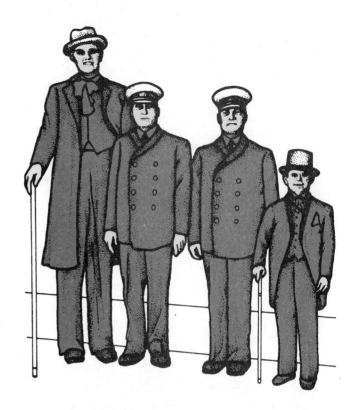

FIGURE 13–136 The effect of growth hormone—a giant, a dwarf and a normal-sized person. (From C.P. Anthony and G. Thibodeau, *Textbook of Anatomy and Physiology.* St. Louis: C.V. Mosby. Reproduced with permission.)

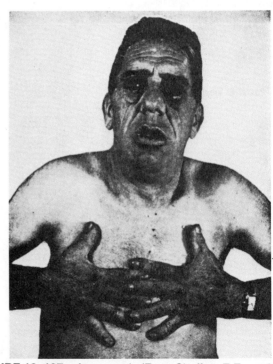

FIGURE 13–137 Acromegaly (From Chaffee, E.E., and Lytle, I.M., *Basic Physiology and Anatomy,* 4th ed. Philadelphia: J.B. Lipincott, Co., 1980.)

female. FSH stimulates the production of the sperm in the male.

6. **Luteinizing** hormone (LH)—In the female causes the ruptured ovarian follicle to become a corpus luteum that in turn secretes the hormone progesterone. Interstitial cell stimulating hormone (ICSH) in the male stimulates the interstitial cells in the testes to produce testosterone.
7. Prolactin (PR)—Responsible for breast development and the production of milk.

Posterior Lobe

The hormones of the posterior lobe are as follows:

1. Oxytocin—Stimulates the contractions of the uterus, especially during childbirth; it also is responsible for the flow of milk from the breast.
2. Vasopressin, or the antidiuretic hormone (ADH)—Acts on the kidney tubule cells to concentrate urine and conserve water within the body. It also stimulates the smooth muscles of blood vessels to constrict.

Thyroid Gland ....

The thyroid gland has two lobes, one on each side of the larynx, with a connecting central section called the isthmus, Figure 13–138. It is located in front of the upper portion of the trachea in the lower part of the neck. The gland is encased in a capsule of connective tissue.

The thyroid gland produces three hormones: thyroxine (T_4), triiodothyronine (T_3), and thyrocalcitonin. Thyrocalcitonin causes calcium to be stored in the bones to reduce the level of calcium in the blood. The other two hormones strongly affect metabolism, which influences both the physical and mental activity necessary for normal growth and development. When thyroid activity is below normal it is called **hypothyroidism,** indicating a decrease in the basal metabolic rate. An overactive thyroid is called **hyperthyroidism** and indicates an increased metabolic rate.

The thyroid gland requires iodine to form the thyroid hormones. Iodine is obtained by eating vegetables grown in soil containing iodine or by eating seafood. Lack of the element causes the thyroid gland to enlarge because of the feedback mechanism. When the pituitary receives information that the level of thyroid hormones is too low it sends out TSH to stimulate the thyroid cells. The cells in turn enlarge, trying to increase output, and eventually enlarge the entire gland. An enlarged thyroid gland is commonly known as a **goiter.**

A person who has hypothyroidism feels fatigued, has low blood pressure and pulse rate, often a subnormal temperature, and may be overweight due to decreased metabolism. The hyperthyroid patient is nervous, restless, and irritable, with heart rate above normal and elevated blood pressure. The patient may lose weight despite a good appetite. Occasionally the eyes protrude dramatically in a condition called **exophthalmia,** Figure 13–139.

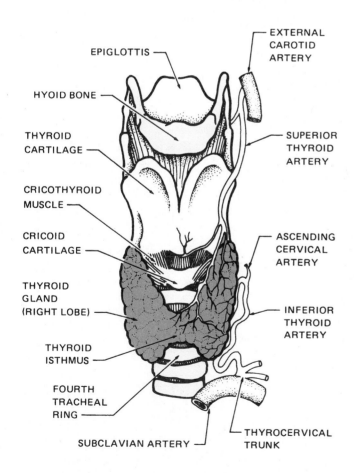

FIGURE 13–138 The thyroid gland

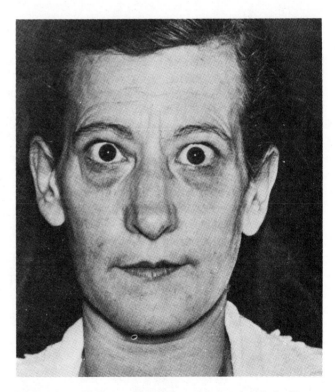

FIGURE 13–139 Hyperthyroidism with exophthalmia (From DeGroot, *The Thyroid and Its Diseases,* 4th ed. New York: John Wiley & Sons, Inc., 1975.)

TABLE 13–7
Endocrine Glands

Gland	Location	Hormone	Principal Effects
PITUITARY Anterior lobe	Undersurface of the brain in the sella turcica of the skull	Growth hormone (GH)	Normal growth of body tissues
		Thyroid stimulating hormone (TSH) (Thyrotropin)	Stimulates growth and activity of thyroid cells to produce thyroid hormone
		Adrenocorticotropic hormone (ACTH)	Stimulates the cortex of the adrenal gland
		Melanocyte-stimulating hormone (MSH)	Increases skin pigmentation
		Follicle-stimulating hormone (FSH)	Stimulates the maturity of the graafian follicle to rupture and to produce estrogen in the female. In the male it stimulates the development of the testes and the production of sperm
		Luteinizing hormone (LH) Interstitial-cell stimulating hormone (ICSH)	Causes the development of the corpus luteum, which then secretes progesterone in the female. ICSH in the male stimulates the interstitial cells of the testes to produce testosterone.
		Prolactin (PR)	Develops breast tissue and stimulates secretion of milk from mammary glands
Posterior lobe		Oxytocin	Stimulates contraction of uterus, especially during childbirth; causes ejection of milk from mammary glands
		Vasopressin or Antidiuretic hormone (ADH)	Acts on cells of kidney tubules to concentrate urine and conserve fluid in the body. Also acts to constrict blood vessels.
THYROID	Lower portion of the anterior neck	Thyroxine (T_4) and Triiodothyronine (T_3)	Increases metabolism; influences both physical and mental activity; promotes normal growth and development
		Thyrocalcitonin	Causes calcium to be stored in bones; reduces blood level of calcium
PARATHYROID	Posterior surface of thyroid gland	Parathormone	Regulates exchange of calcium between the bones and blood
ADRENAL Medulla	Superior surface of each kidney	Adrenaline (Epinephrine)	Increases heart rate, blood pressure, and flow of blood; decreases intestinal activity
		Aldosterone (Mineral corticoid)	Controls electrolyte balances by regulating the reabsorption of sodium and the excretion of potassium
Cortex		Glucocorticoids	Affect the metabolism of protein, fat, and glucose, thereby increasing blood sugar
		Sex hormones (Androgens)	Govern sex characteristics, especially those that are masculine
PANCREAS	Behind the stomach	Insulin	Essential to the metabolism of carbohydrates; reduces the blood sugar level
		Glucagon	Stimulates the liver to release glycogen and convert it to glucose to increase blood sugar levels
THYMUS	Under the sternum	Thymosin	Reacts upon lymphoid tissue to produce T lymphocyte cells to develop immunity to certain diseases
PINEAL BODY	Third ventricle in the brain	Melatonin	Controls onset of puberty
OVARIES	Female pelvis	Estrogen	Promotes growth of primary and secondary sexual characteristics
		Progesterone	Develops excretory portion of mammary glands; aids in maintaining pregnancy
TESTES	Male scrotum	Testosterone	Develops primary and secondary sexual characteristics; stimulates maturation of sperm

Treatment of hypothyroidism is relatively simple: the thyroid hormone is taken orally as a supplement. Hyperthyroidism may initially be treated with supplemental iodine to prohibit or control gland enlargement. With progressive disease, it may be necessary to remove part or all of the gland or limit its function by radiation. The surgical removal of the thyroid is called a thyroidectomy.

A thyrotoxic crisis or thyroid storm is the extreme clinical development of hyperthyroidism. It produces a greatly accelerated metabolism, severe nervous system malfunction, overheating, and heart failure. The situation is precipitated by stress or a severe infection and is usually fatal. The vigorous use of antithyroid drugs can frequently prevent the complication from occurring.

Parathyroid Glands

The parathyroid glands, usually two pairs, are embedded on the posterior surface of the thyroid gland. Their number and size vary greatly, but normally they resemble grains of wheat. The parathyroids are responsible for regulating the calcium content of the blood. The hormone parathormone cooperates with vitamin D to balance the level of calcium in the blood by stimulating the bones to release stored calcium and phosphate into the circulation.

Hyperparathyroidism results in increased levels of calcium in the blood, which causes lethargy and the excretion of large quantities of calcium salts in the urine, leading to the formation of kidney stones. The condition leads progressively to decalcification of the bones and is usually associated with a tumor of one of the glands. Decalcified bones are prone to pathological fracture.

Hypoparathyroidism is dramatically demonstrated by a condition known as tetany, an uncontrollable twitching of the muscles of the body. This results from hyperirritability of the nervous system in response to the lowered concentration of calcium throughout the body. The condition is easily treated by the addition of calcium. Hypoparathyroidism occurs following damage to or accidental removal of the parathyroids during a thyroidectomy.

Adrenal Glands (Suprarenal)

The adrenal glands sit atop each kidney, hence the additional name of *suprarenal.* Each gland is contained in a fibrous capsule and is composed of two parts, each of which acts separately. The outer glandular tissue is called the *cortex,* while the inner tissue is referred to as the *medulla.*

The principal hormone of the medulla is adrenaline, also called epinephrine. Another hormone, norepinephrine, has a similar action on the body. Together they are considered to be the "flight or fight" hormones because of their effects in emergency situations. The hormones cause an increase in the heart rate, blood pressure, and flow of blood, and a decrease in intestinal activity. The adrenal medulla is considered to be nonessential to life.

The cortex of the adrenal gland, however, is essential to life. The cortex produces steroid hormones in three categories: mineral corticoids, glucocorticoids, and sex steroids. The mineral corticoids, of which aldosterone is the principal one, control electrolyte balances through regulating the reabsorption of sodium in the kidney tubules and the excretion of potassium. The glucocorticoids affect the metabolism of protein, fat, and glucose. They stimulate the liver to convert protein into glycogen and then break it down into glucose, thereby increasing blood sugar level. This change is seen when the body is subjected to stressful situations. The hormone level is increased, which in turn accelerates the conversion process to allow the body to cope.

The sex steroids govern certain sexual characteristics, especially those that are male oriented. These steroids are referred to as *androgens.* Excessive secretions cause the virilization and development of masculine secondary sex characteristics in the female and immature male, Figure 13–140. A mature female's voice will deepen, a growth of beard will appear, menstruation will become irregular, and sterility will result.

Pancreas

The pancreas is a dual-function organ. It has an exocrine function, producing pancreatic juices excreted by way of

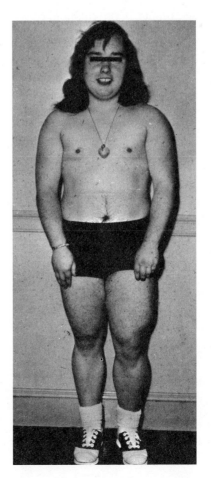

FIGURE 13–140
Effects of excess androgens on young female (Adapted from Anthony & Thibodeau, *Textbook of Anatomy and Physiology,* 11th ed. 1983. St. Louis, C.V. Mosby Co.; courtesy Dr. William McKendree Jefferies, Case Western Reserve University School of Medicine, Cleveland, Ohio)

the pancreatic duct into the duodenum to become part of the digestive juices. It is also an endocrine gland. The hormone *insulin* is secreted by the B cells of the islet of Langerhans, often called beta cells, Figure 13–141. They are one of four cell types, A, B, C, and D, located in the pancreas. It is known that the A cells secrete glucagon, but the exact function of this substance is uncertain. It may stimulate the liver to release glucogen, converting it to glucose to raise the blood sugar level.

Insulin is necessary for the metabolism of carbohydrates. With reduced islet function, the level of blood sugar rises to an abnormal amount and is referred to as hyperglycemia. Conversely, an abnormally low level of blood sugar is known as hypoglycemia. When excess glucose is present in the blood, it is excreted in the urine, a finding known as glycosuria. Hyperglycemia and glycosuria are the two outstanding characteristics of diabetes mellitus.

The exact function of insulin and its relationship to diabetes are not clearly understood. It is believed that insulin makes it possible for the cells to use the glucose present in the body tissues. Without the ability to burn glucose, it cannot be changed into energy and is therefore passed on to the kidneys for excretion. Insulin is also required for the metabolism of fat and protein.

Thymus Gland

The thymus gland is a two-lobed structure, located under the sternum. It is composed primarily of lymphoid tissue and enclosed in a fibrous capsule. The thymus is fairly large during childhood, but begins to disappear with the onset of puberty, becoming a small mass of connective tissue and fat in adulthood. It appears to produce a hormone known as thymosin, which is believed to react on lymphoid tissue to produce T lymphocytes and develop immunity against certain diseases.

Pineal Body

The pineal body is a small mass of tissue attached by a slim stalk to the roof of the third ventricle in the brain. The pineal body is believed to produce a substance called melatonin. This substance combines with a hypothalamic substance to delay puberty until the normal time.

Gonads (Testes and Ovaries)

The ovaries in the female and the testes in the male are called the gonads, or sex glands. The ovaries are located in the pelvic cavity, one on each side of the uterus. The testes are located outside the body of the male, suspended in the scrotum. Both gonads secrete hormones that control the development of secondary sex characteristics.

In the female, the ovaries secrete estrogen, which reacts on the lining of the uterus, promotes growth and development of the primary and secondary sex organs,

and maintains them throughout adult life. Estrogen also affects the release of other hormones from the pituitary. Another hormone, progesterone, is also secreted by the ovaries. It affects the uterine lining as well as the development of the secretory portion of the breasts. It aids in maintaining pregnancy.

In the male, the testes produce a hormone known as testosterone. This hormone develops the primary male sexual characteristics as well as the secondary characteristics of a deep voice, muscular development, and body hair distribution. It stimulates maturation of sperm cells.

The gonads are the organs of fertility and reproduction in both sexes. The maturity of the organs and the proper balance of hormonal secretions creates the desire for and ability to engage in sexual activity.

Interrelationship of the Glands

As stated previously, hormonal secretion is regulated by a feedback mechanism. When the hormone is present or the substance produced by the effect of that hormone on another gland or organ is present, further secretion is affected. For example, the parathyroids increase secretion of parathormone to raise the serum calcium level to be withdrawn from the bones. When the serum level rises, a negative feedback message is signaled and the secretion of parathormone is decreased. A more complicated feedback involves both positive and negative action. For example, the pituitary gland secretes TSH, which causes the thyroid gland to increase the production of hormones. When the appropriate level is reached, TSH secretion is inhibited, a negative feedback. The hypothalamus produces a thyrotropin-releasing hormone (TRH), which is stimulated by low levels of thyroid hormone. Therefore, when the level again drops, the hypo-

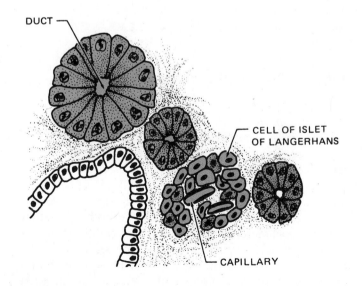

FIGURE 13–141 Pancreatic structure

thalmus secretes TRH, which stimulates the pituitary to release TSH, which in turn stimulates the production of the thyroid hormones, a positive feedback mechanism.

In the next unit, the interrelationship of the pituitary and the ovary will be discussed to explain how this complex balance prepares the female for pregnancy and then either sustains that hormonal state or allows it to alter, all in response to the feedback mechanism.

Diagnostic Examinations ....

A great variety of diagnostic tests can be performed on blood and urine, which either measure the amount of specific hormones present in the body or measure the effectiveness of their function. A few of the more common tests are:

- Blood sugar, frequently measured after fasting (FBS)—To assess the function of the pancreas, including insulin production and utilization.
- T_3 and T_4—To measure the level of the thyroid hormones.
- Urine human chorionic gonadotropin (HCG) (pregnancy test)—To measure the presence of a hormone secreted by the placental cells
- Glucose tolerance—To measure the body's ability to process a large dose of glucose. Multiple blood and urine samples are taken at specific intervals following ingestion.

There are also specific tests measuring hormone levels in the blood to aid in confirming diagnoses, such as:

- ACTH, FSH, LH, and TSH—When acromegaly or dwarfism is suspected.
- FSH, LH, estrogen and testosterone—When sex organs fail to develop properly.
- ACTH, cortisol—When Cushing's syndrome (chronic excessive glucocorticoids) is suspected.
- PTH—When hypo- or hyperparathyroidism is suspected.

Scanning Tests

The thyroid gland is probably the one most frequently scanned.

- Radioactive iodine uptake test—An oral dose of radioactive iodine is given to the patient. After intervals of 2, 6, and 24 hours, an external detector (scintillation counter) measures the amount of the original dose that is present in the gland. Thyroid function can be determined by the gland's ability to absorb and retain iodine.
- Thyroid scan—The thyroid gland is viewed by a scintiscanner camera following either an oral or IV dose of a radioactive iodine. The scan is indicated by discovery of a palpable nodule or mass, enlarged thyroid gland, or asymmetric goiter. The camera is capable of photographing the isotopes, which identify the size of the gland, position, and uniformity of absorption. A nodule with poor or no uptake capability shows as a "cold spot," suggesting a possible malignancy. A "hot spot" indicates a hyperfunctioning nodule, possibly a toxic nodular goiter. A total gland picture that shows little uptake is indicative of hypothyroidism; an enlarged gland showing uniformly increased uptake is indicative of hyperthyroidism.

Diseases and Disorders ....

Cretinism. This condition results from serious lack of the thyroid hormone thyroxine beginning in the early stages of life. Cretinism is characterized by lack of mental and physical growth resulting in mental retardation and a characteristic dwarflike appearance, Figure 13–142, page 372. If thyroid replacement is initiated early enough, a degree of normal development may be achieved, but once cretinism has developed, total normal development is not possible. An infant born without thyroid hormones of its own must be treated within a few weeks to prevent irreversible mental retardation.

Cushing's Syndrome. This disorder is characterized by a group of symptoms that result from the hypersecretion of glucocorticoids from the adrenal cortex due to excess ACTH production. Cushing's syndrome may also be directly related to a tumor of the cortex of the adrenal gland. Symptoms include hypertension, obesity, weakness of the muscles, and a tendency to develop bruises. Typical characteristics result from the rapid deposit of body fat: a deposit of fat between the shoulders, referred to as "buffalo hump," and a rounded face referred to as "moon face," Figure 13–143, page 373. Purple streaks develop in the skin, called striae (stretch marks). The trunk becomes obese, yet the arms and legs are slender.

The excess amount of glucocorticoids, which metabolize protein into glucogen and then into glucose, results in a "steroid diabetes" with hyperglycemia and glucosuria. The urinary system is affected by the hormone imbalance and excretes excessive amounts of potassium, which results in hypokalemia. The lack of potassium results in muscular weakness. Muscle mass slowly wastes away. The decreasing amount of bone minerals results in pathological fractures.

Treatment is related to the underlying cause. If there is an adrenal tumor, then the adrenal gland must be removed. If both adrenals are removed, replacement steroid therapy must be instituted. If the adrenals are being stimulated because of a pituitary tumor, then the pituitary gland must be irradiated or removed. Afterwards rigorous hormone therapy would be required to replace all the pituitary's secretions. Many drugs, some experimental, are used to suppress adrenal function and destroy adenocortical cells.

Diabetes Mellitus. A chronic disease of insulin deficiency or resistance, diabetes mellitus interferes with the metabolism of carbohydrates, proteins, and fats. Insulin in the blood "carries" glucose into the cell to be used for energy or stored as glycogen. It also stimulates the formation of proteins and free fatty acid storage. Without sufficient insulin being secreted by the pancreas, the body's tissues do not have access to essential nutrients for fuel or storage.

The cause of diabetes is unknown but certain factors contribute to its development:

- Heredity—There is a tendency among family members.
- Weight—Weight plays an important role because obesity causes resistance to insulin. Eighty percent of all diabetics are overweight when diagnosed.
- Pregnancy—Pregnancy adds extra demands on the body. Increased levels of estrogen and other hormones antagonize insulin. Women who deliver large babies or have repeated miscarriages may be diabetic.
- Physical trauma or emotional stress—Crisis, emotional tension, a major illness, or physical trauma from surgery or an accident can lead to development of diabetes because of prolonged elevation of stress hormones raising demands on the pancreas.
- Virus—Certain cases of insulin-dependent diabetes are viral in origin.

Diabetes mellitus affects an estimated 5% of the US population or approximately 12 million people. About one-half are unaware they have diabetes.

There are two forms of diabetes: a juvenile or insulin-dependent diabetes mellitus (IDDM), and a mature-onset or noninsulin-dependent form (NIDDM). IDDM usually occurs before age 30. The patient is thin and requires insulin support therapy and diet control. NIDDM occurs most frequently among obese adults and responds to diet with or without oral hypoglycemics and/or insulin.

Signs and symptoms of diabetes include fatigue, due to the lack of energy production, and hyperglycemia, because the glucose cannot be utilized. The elevated glucose level in the blood causes fluid to be withdrawn from the body's tissues. The excess fluid in the blood causes polyuria and dehydration of the cells. The diabetic patient is frequently thirsty and has dry mucous membranes. The lens of the eye becomes affected by deposits of sugar and edema, which results in visual difficulties. Characteristically, glycosuria is present, as the body tries to eliminate excess glucose from the blood. This wasting of sugar causes the weight loss and hunger of the IDDM patient.

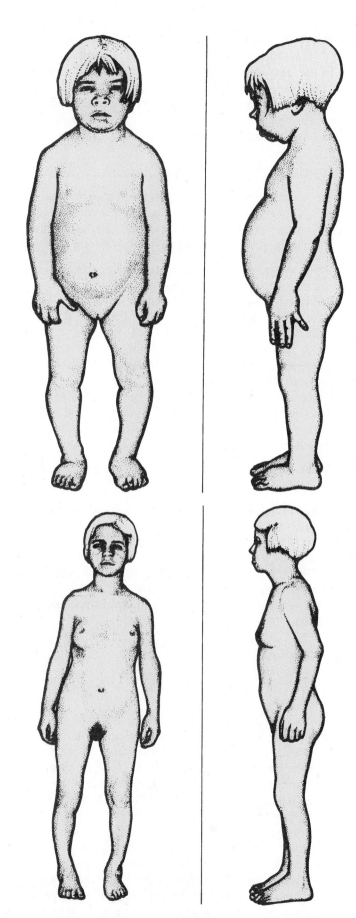

FIGURE 13–142 (Top) Cretinism of a 16-year-old female due to lack of thyroid hormone. (Bottom) Same female after two years of treatment with thyroid extract. (From Anthony, *Textbook of Anatomy and Physiology*, 6th ed. 1963, St. Louis, C.V. Mosby Co; courtesy Dr. Edward E. Beard)

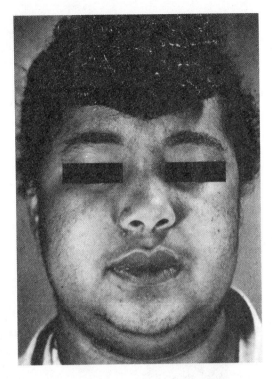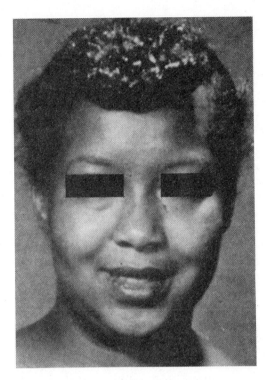

FIGURE 13–143 Cushing's syndrome from excessive glucocorticoids. (a). preoperatively. (b). 6 months postoperatively. (Adapted from Anthony & Thibodeau, *Textbook of Anatomy and Physiology*, 11th ed. 1983. St. Louis, C.V. Mosby Co.; courtesy Dr. William McKendree Jefferies, Case Western Reserve University School of Medicine, Cleveland, Ohio)

There are many long-term effects of diabetes. Patients are prone to myocardial infarction and stroke and deteriorating disease of the retina and nerves. It contributes to renal failure, peripheral vascular disease, and blindness. Approximately 50% of patients who have had myocardial infarctions and 75% who have had cerebrovascular accidents are also diabetic. It also interferes with resistance to organisms, which may result in skin and bladder infections because the glucose content of the epidermis and urine are conducive to bacterial growth. Diabetic retinopathy results from circulatory changes in the retina of the eye in the poorly controlled diabetic. In patients who have had diabetes for 20 or more years, 80% develop retinopathy. It is the leading cause of adult acquired blindness.

Treatment begins with a strict diet, planned to meet the nutritional needs of the individual patient and to control the blood sugar level. When diet alone is inadequate, insulin injections or the use of an oral hypoglycemic drug are indicated. Injections may be necessary only once a day, using a long-acting insulin; when control is more difficult, a regular insulin, injected at specific times, may be used. Diabetic patients are taught to evaluate their glucose level by performing a urine test for sugar or a finger stick for blood analysis. The amount of the insulin injected is based on the findings. Hypoglycemic drugs are taken orally to aid in the metabolism of sugar. Oral therapy is usually adequate only for NIDDM patients.

The glucose level of the blood can be affected by circumstances other than food or insulin. For example, the diabetic will require either less insulin or more food when engaging in a high level of physical activity. Adjustments are also required with illness. A patient who has diarrhea and/or vomiting requires less insulin. Pregnancy, the use of contraceptives, a fever, and periods of stress, all influence the diabetic's need for supplemental insulin or hypoglycemic therapy.

Diabetic patients must be encouraged to maintain their optimal level of health. They must guard against injury, especially to the lower extremities, because of difficulty healing. They must use extreme caution when cutting toenails and must never try to remove corns or calluses themselves. Diabetics frequently suffer amputations as a result of infection from an injury that would not heal or from the loss of peripheral circulation, which causes tissue death.

Patients should be encouraged to visit an ophthalmologist regularly to detect the possibility of retinal changes. Blindness will result from uncontrolled diabetes. The physician must be alert to signs of cardiovascular complications as well as urinary tract involvement. Cerebral vascular disease, coronary artery disease, and renal failure due to vascular deterioration in the kidney are not uncommon.

Graves' Disease. This condition, caused by the overproduction of the thyroid gland, is the most common form of hyperthyroidism. The thyroid gland enlarges, the patient becomes nervous; has an intolerance to heat; loses weight; sweats; and may have diarrhea, tremors, and palpitations. The increased thyroxine may also cause difficulty in concentrating because of the accelerated cerebral functioning. Mood swings and emotional instability may occur. The cardiovascular system is also affected and results in tachycardia, increased cardiac output and blood volume, cardiomegaly, and possibly atrial fibrillation (especially in the elderly). The patient may experience dyspnea and an array of musculoskeletal symptoms ranging from weakness and fatigue to localized or generalized paralysis. The dominant feature of exophthalmus may also be present.

The patient can get into serious difficulty if the hyperthyroidism escalates into a thyroid storm. The symptoms persist and others develop, such as hypertension, extreme irritability, vomiting, high fever, delirium, and eventually coma.

Myxedema. This condition is caused by hyposecretion of the thyroid gland in adulthood. Clinically, myxedema's characteristics are in relation to the degree of hypothyroidism. If it is mild, the patient will probably complain of forgetfulness, dry skin, and an intolerance for cold. With more severe myxedema, the decreased metabolism and vital functions will become more evident. Decrease in heat production (because of decreased metabolism) causes a marked intolerance for cold. There is a noticeable weight gain. The motor function and reflex actions are slowed. The voice becomes low and husky. A characteristic yellowish discoloration of the skin, called *carotenemia,* results from reduction in the conversion of carotene to vitamin A. Levels of cholesterol are increased and may also produce atherosclerosis. Since cardiac function is depressed, the myocardium becomes flabby and weak. Protein and certain electrolytes accumulate in the tissue spaces, causing edema. Myxedema patients have a characteristic drowsy appearance, with puffiness about the eyes, Figure 13–144. There is a marked degree of fatigue and weakness. The temperature, pulse, respiration, and blood pressure are all below normal.

Treatment consists primarily of thyroid hormone replacement to a level necessary to maintain normal balance.

Diagnosing, treating, and maintaining hormonal balance in patients with endocrine gland malfunctions is an involved and challenging endeavor because of the hormone interactions. What may appear to be a simple overproduction by the thyroid may actually be a pituitary malfunction, a failed hypothalamus, or an inhibitor that did not cause the pituitary to stop secreting a thyroid stimulant. Many possibilities must be considered to explain the symptoms presented by a patient with endocrine dysfunction.

Complete Chapter 13, Unit 11 in the workbook to help you meet the objectives at the beginning of this unit and therefore achieve competency of this subject matter.

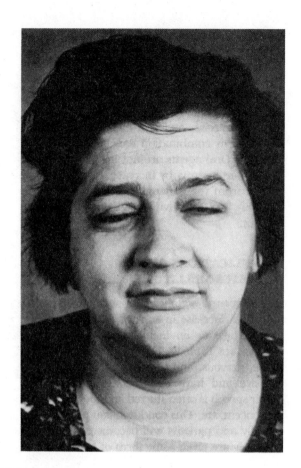

FIGURE 13–144 Myxedema (From Burke, *Human Anatomy and Physiology for the Health Sciences,* 3d ed. Copyright 1992, Delmar Publishers Inc.)

U N I T 1 3

The Reproductive System

OBJECTIVES ....

Upon completion of this unit, the student will meet the following terminal performance objectives by verifying knowledge of the facts and principles presented through oral and written communication at a level deemed competent.

1. Differentiate between sexual and asexual reproduction.
2. Describe the differentiation of reproductive organs.
3. Explain how sperm are able to fertilize an egg.
4. Describe male prenatal development.
5. Name the male sex organs and describe their location and function.
6. Explain how pituitary hormones affect the functions of the testes.
7. Identify the male secondary sex characteristics.

8. Trace the pathway of sperm from production to expulsion.
9. Name the components of semen.
10. Describe four diseases and disorders of the male reproductive system.
11. Name the female sex organs and describe their location and function.
12. Explain the interaction of pituitary hormones with the ovaries and other organs.
13. Identify the female secondary sex characteristics.
14. Describe the maturation and release of an ovum.
15. Compare the internal and external sexual organs of the male and female.
16. Describe the phases of the menstrual cycle and the purpose of menstruation.
17. Explain how fertilization occurs.
18. Discuss the events occurring during each trimester of pregnancy as they relate to the woman and the embryo/fetus.
19. Discuss the events that occur in the three stages of labor.
20. List eight reasons for practicing contraception.
21. Identify 10 contraceptive methods, stating their relative effectiveness.
22. Describe eight diagnostic tests of the female reproductive system.
23. Describe 20 diseases or disorders of the female reproductive system.
24. Identify the characteristics of eight sexually transmitted diseases.
25. Spell and define, using the glossary at the back of the text, all the words to know in this unit.

WORDS TO KNOW ···

ablation	dysmenorrhea
abortion	ectopic
amniotic	effacement
areola	ejaculation
Bartholin's glands	ejaculatory duct
benign hypertrophy	embryo
bulbourethral glands	endometrium
cervix	epididymis
cesarean	episiotomy
chlamydia	erectile
circumcision	fallopian tubes
clitoris	fertilization
coitus	fetus
colposcopy	fibroid
conceive	foreskin
conception	gamete
contraception	genital herpes
contraction	genitalia
corpus luteum	gonorrhea
cryptorchidism	graafian follicle
dilation and curettage	gynecology

hydrocele	placenta
hymen	pregnancy
hysterectomy	prolapse
hysteroscopy	prostate
impotence	prostatectomy
inguinal canal	rectocele
inguinal hernia	reproductive
labia majora	retroflexed
labia minora	retroverted
ligation	salpingo-oophrectomy
mammary glands	scrotum
mammogram	semen
mastectomy	sperm
menarche	spermatazoan
menopause	suprapubic
menorrhagia	syphilis
menstruation	transurethral
mons pubis	trichomoniasis
myometrium	trimester
nonspecific urethritis	uterus
os	vagina
ovulation	vaginitis
ovum	vas deferens
Papanicolaou (Pap) smear	vasectomy
penis	vulva
perineum	womb
phimosis	zygote

The **reproductive** system consists of the organs that are capable of accomplishing reproduction, the creation of a new individual. All living organisms reproduce, some very simply by an asexual method, or without the need of sexual contact. An example of asexual reproduction is one of the simplest forms of life, a single cell. In binary fusion, a cell divides into two cells by simple cleavage. In mitosis, a single cell rearranges its chromatin into chromosomes and then divides into two cells (the method by which human cells reproduce). Both methods require that the "parent" become the "children"; therefore both parent and child cannot exist at the same time.

Sexual methods of reproduction are found in multi-celled forms of life, including humans. The methods may vary but certain characteristics are common to all. In each species, there are sexes, namely a male and a female. Each sex has special sex glands, or gonads, which produce sex cells (**gametes**). In humans, the union of the male gamete (a **spermatozoan**) with the female gamete (an **ovum**) forms a new one-celled structure called a **zygote.** The zygote then undergoes mitosis repeatedly to form a new individual.

In Unit 1, the cell was described as having 46 chromosomes, or 23 pairs. Each chromosome has a partner of the same shape and size. One pair of chromosomes are the sex chromosomes. In the female, both chromosomes in the pair are X chromosomes, but in the male, one is an X and one is a Y. When the gonads produce the ovum and spermatozoan cells, the number of chromosomes is reduced to 23 (one-half). When the two cells unite as fertilization occurs, the new cell, a zygote, will again have 46 chromosomes. If the spermatozoan carries an X chromosome, the embryo will develop female characteristics. If it carries a Y chromosome the embryo will develop as a male.

The reproductive organs are the only organs in the human body which differ between the male and female, and yet there is still a significant similarity. This likeness results from the fact that male and female organs develop from the same group of embryonic cells. For approximately 2 months, the embryo develops without sexual identity. Then the influence of the X or Y chromosome begins to make a differentiation.

Differentiation of Reproductive Organs

The gonads of the embryo begin to evolve into the sexual organs of the female at about the tenth or eleventh week of pregnancy. The ovaries of the embryo develop high in its abdomen from the same type of tissue as the testes. However, the testes evolve from the medulla of the gonad, while the ovaries develop from the cortex. Figure 13–145 illustrates how the undifferentiated external genitalia develop into fully differentiated structures. In the male, the tubercle becomes the glans penis, the folds become the penile shaft, and the swelling develops into the scrotum. In the female, the tubercle becomes the clitoris, the folds the labia minora, and the swelling the labia majora.

Internally, there is also a similarity of structures. The embryonic müllerian ducts degenerate and the wolffian ducts become the epididymis, vas deferens, and ejaculatory duct in the male. In the female, the wolffian ducts degenerate and the müllerian ducts develop into the fallopian tubes, the uterus, and the upper portion of the vagina. It is believed that the presence of the testes in the male is the differentiating factor in the development. Without the androgens (male hormones) from the testes, a female develops. With the androgens, a male develops. Another substance called the müllerian inhibitor works in partnership with the androgens to produce the sex dif-. ferentiation.

Male Reproductive Organs

When the zygote contains a Y chromosome, a male child will develop. About the seventh or eighth week of pregnancy, the testes begin to develop within the abdominal cavity at about the level of the ileum of the pelvis bone. The sex of the fetus is evident by about the fourth month.

During the eighth and ninth months of pregnancy, the testes move from the abdomen through the inguinal canal into the external pouch called the scrotum, Figure 13–146, page 378. After the testes pass, the canal closes to prevent the descent of other structures into the scrotum or the return of the testes into the abdomen. When a loop of small intestine descends through the canal due to improper closure or later in life due to relaxed inguinal structures, it in known as an inguinal hernia, Figure 13–147, page 378.

If the testes fail to descend or if they return to the abdomen, a condition known as undescended testicle (unilateral or bilateral) exists, which must be corrected or sterility will result. An undescended testicle is known medically as cryptorchidism. The testes normally produce sperm, but sperm cannot be produced or survive in the internal heat of the body. It is this characteristic that necessitates their location outside the body.

The scrotum, which contains the testes, has another function as well, which is to regulate the temperature of the testes' environment. Sperm are most effectively produced at temperatures 1.5° to 2°C below body temperature. To maintain this difference, the scrotum contains many sweat glands that perspire profusely to dissipate heat. The scrotum also has cremasteric muscles, which can contract to draw the testes closer to the body and increase the temperature or relax to lower them away from the body and reduce it.

Testes

The testes or testicles are the primary sex organs of the male. They are of equal size, oval in shape, about 2 x 1 x $1\frac{1}{2}$ inches in size, and are suspended in the scrotum, with the left testis usually somewhat lower than the right. A testis has two functions, to produce sperm and to secrete testosterone, the male hormone. These functions begin to occur about age 10 when the hypothalamus releases a hormone that initiates puberty. The hormone stimulates the anterior pituitary gland, which then releases the gonad-stimulating hormones to effect change in the testes.

Male gonadotropic hormones secreted by the pituitary are FSH (follicle-stimulating hormone) and ICSH (interstitial cell-stimulating hormones). FSH causes sperm to develop in the male and ova to mature in the female, a very similar function.

Sperm Production. Sperm develop and mature in microscopic tubes in the testes known as *seminiferous tubules,* Figure 13–148, page 379. FSH stimulates the production of sperm in the cells that line the tubules. There are about 300 sections of coiled tubules which, if uncoiled, it is estimated, would extend over a mile. As the sperm develop, they are released into the tubules to start their journey from the testes. Sperm formation in an adult male requires about 74 days to maturity. The function normally begins to develop at about age 12, and the first mature sperm are ejaculated at about age 14.

Testosterone. As sperm are developing, ICSH is causing the interstitial cells in the network of structures around the tubules to secrete testosterone. Testosterone aids in the maturing of sperm and also causes many changes in

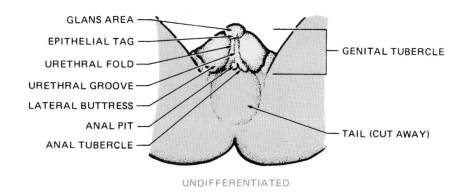

GLANS AREA
EPITHELIAL TAG
URETHRAL FOLD
URETHRAL GROOVE
LATERAL BUTTRESS
ANAL PIT
ANAL TUBERCLE

GENITAL TUBERCLE

TAIL (CUT AWAY)

UNDIFFERENTIATED

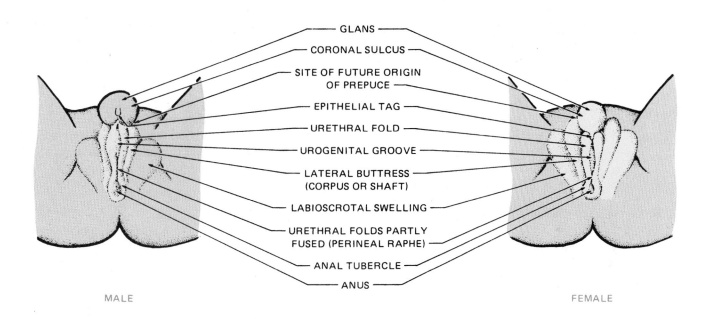

GLANS
CORONAL SULCUS
SITE OF FUTURE ORIGIN OF PREPUCE
EPITHELIAL TAG
URETHRAL FOLD
UROGENITAL GROOVE
LATERAL BUTTRESS (CORPUS OR SHAFT)
LABIOSCROTAL SWELLING
URETHRAL FOLDS PARTLY FUSED (PERINEAL RAPHE)
ANAL TUBERCLE
ANUS

MALE

FEMALE

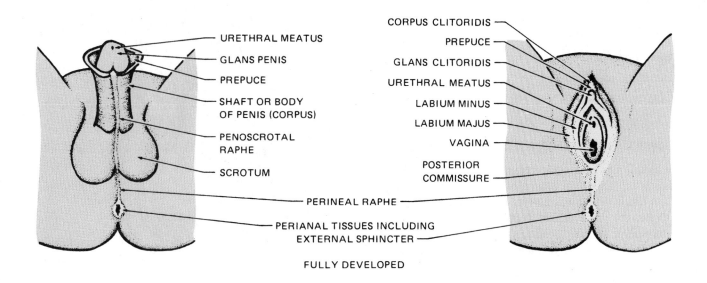

URETHRAL MEATUS
GLANS PENIS
PREPUCE
SHAFT OR BODY OF PENIS (CORPUS)
PENOSCROTAL RAPHE
SCROTUM

CORPUS CLITORIDIS
PREPUCE
GLANS CLITORIDIS
URETHRAL MEATUS
LABIUM MINUS
LABIUM MAJUS
VAGINA
POSTERIOR COMMISSURE

PERINEAL RAPHE

PERIANAL TISSUES INCLUDING EXTERNAL SPHINCTER

FULLY DEVELOPED

FIGURE 13–145 Sexual differentiation before birth

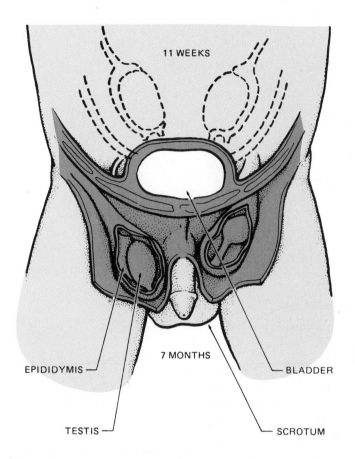

FIGURE 13–146 The descent of the testes

vas deferens joins one epididymis extending upward for about 45 cm through an inguinal canal to the base of the urinary bladder. Each vas joins with a duct from a seminal vesicle to form a common ejaculatory duct, Figure 13–151, page 381.

The seminal vesicles are a pair of convoluted tubes lying posterior to the bladder. They also empty into the ejaculatory duct. The vesicles secrete a fluid that contains fructose, a simple sugar, which provides nutrition for the sperm. The fluid makes up a major portion of the ejaculant. The ejaculatory duct is a short straight tube that passes through the prostate gland to join the urethra.

Prostate Gland, Bulbourethral Glands, and Urethra

The prostate gland is a donut-like-pyramidal structure with the urethra extending through its center, Figure 13–151. The gland is positioned just beneath the bladder. It produces secretions that are drained through tiny tubules into the prostatic section of the urethra. The fluid secreted is alkaline in nature. Its addition to the ejaculant stimulates sperm motility and preserves their life by neutralizing the acidity of the vagina. The prostate is also constructed of muscular tissue that contracts during ejaculation to empty the semen (ejaculant fluids and sperm) into the urethra to be propelled from the body.

the male body as it circulates in the blood stream. These changes are referred to as the development of secondary sex characteristics, Figure 13–149.

In the male, secondary sex characteristics are:

1. Longer and heavier bone structure
2. Larger muscles
3. Deep voice
4. Growth of body hair
5. Development of the genitalia (external sex organs)
6. Increased metabolism
7. Sexual desire

Epididymis, Vas Deferens, and Seminal Vesicles

The epididymis is a coiled structure about 20 feet in length. It is shaped like a half-moon and sits with its head on top of the testes and its tail extending down the side to join the vas deferens, Figure 13–150, page 380.

After sperm are produced in the tubules they pass into the epididymis where a small number are stored. The sperm mature in the epididymis for about 18 hours. The fluid secreted by the epididymis adds to the volume of ejaculant.

The vas deferens serves as the passageway for sperm to exit the body from the epididymis. On each side, one

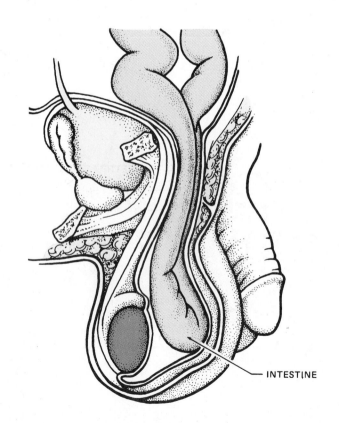

FIGURE 13–147 Inguinal hernia

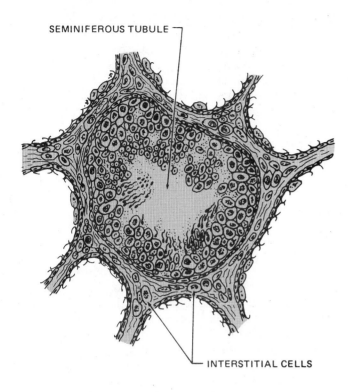

SEMINIFEROUS TUBULE

INTERSTITIAL CELLS

FIGURE 13–148 The production of sperm in the seminiferous tubules and the secretion of testerone by the interstitial cells

The **bulbourethral glands** lie beneath the prostate and empty their contents into the urethra. The fluid the glands secrete aids in the movement of sperm as well as making the normally acid male urethra alkaline just prior to ejaculation. The secretions may also serve as a lubricant for intercourse. Bulbourethral glands are sometimes called Cowper's glands.

Semen

The combined secretions from all the glands and ducts along with the sperm is called the seminal fluid or semen. Approximately 3.5 mL of total fluid is expelled per orgasm (series of rhythmic muscular contractions). Semen is composed of:

- Fluids from the testes and epididymis containing about 350 million sperm (5%)
- Fluid secreted by the seminal vesicles (30%)
- Fluid secreted by the prostate gland (60%)
- Fluid secreted by the bulbourethral glands (5%)

Penis

The penis is constructed of three columns of spongelike **erectile** tissue surrounded by a layer of subcutaneous tissue and covered with skin. The distal end of the penis enlarges to form the glans. A circular fold of skin that extends down over the glans is called the prepuce or **foreskin.** A number of small glands in the foreskin

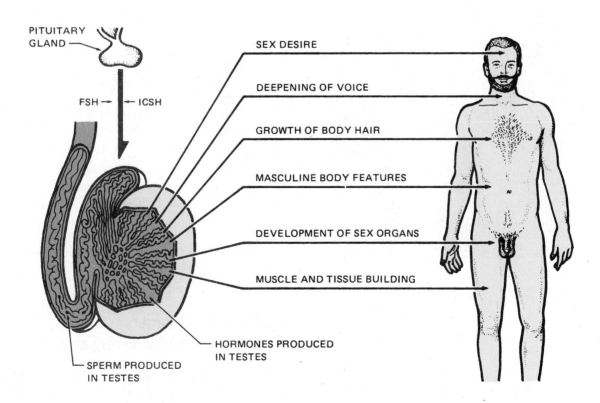

PITUITARY GLAND

FSH → ← ICSH

SEX DESIRE

DEEPENING OF VOICE

GROWTH OF BODY HAIR

MASCULINE BODY FEATURES

DEVELOPMENT OF SEX ORGANS

MUSCLE AND TISSUE BUILDING

HORMONES PRODUCED IN TESTES

SPERM PRODUCED IN TESTES

FIGURE 13–149 Secondary sex characteristics of the male

secrete a waxy, odoriferous substance called smegma onto the glans. A circumcision (surgical removal of the foreskin) is performed on most male infants to prevent accumulation of the smegma. It has also been observed that circumcised men have a lower incidence of cancer of the penis and that women married to circumcised men have a lower incidence of cancer of the cervix. Circumcision is also indicated to correct phimosis, a narrowed opening of the foreskin, which prohibits its retraction over the glans. Phimosis also contributes to the accumulation of smegma. Many men also feel that sexual sensations are heightened when the glans is not covered or restricted by the foreskin.

Erection and Ejaculation

The urethra extends down the length of the penis, opening at the urinary meatus of the glans. The urethra serves two purposes, to empty urine from the urinary bladder and to expel semen. Sexual intercourse becomes possible due to the columns of erectile tissue in the penis. When a male is sexually aroused, nerve impulses cause the erectile tissue to engorge with blood, which makes the erec-

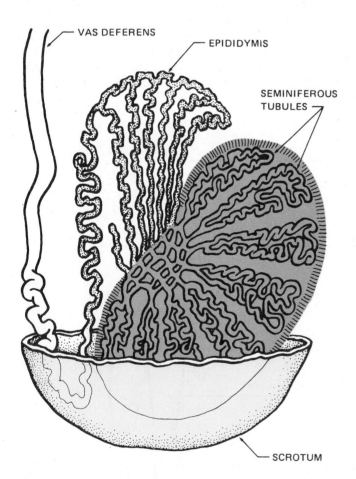

FIGURE 13–150 Seminiferous tubules, epididymis, and vas deferens

Labels: VAS DEFERENS, EPIDIDYMIS, SEMINIFEROUS TUBULES, SCROTUM

tile tissue increase in size and become firm. Blood entering the dilated arteries squeezes the veins against the penile structures prohibiting venous return.

After stimulation of the glans results in maximum stimulation of the seminal vesicles, impulses are sent to the ejaculatory center and orgasm occurs. Orgasm is the result of muscular contractions from the vas deferens, seminal vesicles, ejaculatory ducts, and prostate gland. Secretions produced and stored in these structures, along with the sperm, are forcefully expelled through the urethra after which the engorgement gradually subsides.

Vasectomy

Vasectomy is a simple surgical procedure to prohibit the ejaculation of sperm and effect sterilization of the male. It has become a popular means of birth control. The procedure involves making a small incision in each side of the scrotum near the attachment to the body. The vas deferens on each side is grasped and a loop is withdrawn through the incision. The physician ties off the duct in two places and removes a piece of the duct between the ties. The cut ends may be turned back and sewn. The ends are placed back in the scrotum and the small incision is closed with sutures. The procedure can be performed in the physician's office under local anesthesia or in a hospital outpatient clinic. It is a much simpler means of sterilization than the surgery required to perform a similar procedure on a female.

Vasectomy does not interfere with the ability to have intercourse. The sperm are still produced but there is no place for them to go. The testosterone is an endocrine function so it is not altered. Most men report as much or more sexual activity after as before their surgery. The only negative factor is that the procedure is likely to be permanent. Recently, success at restoring fertility has been achieved by surgical repair in about one out of five attempts. However, the patient may have developed autoantibodies toward his own sperm and may no longer be fertile.

Testicular Self-examination. The American Cancer Society recommends that men perform routine testicular self-examination (TSE) as a means of early identification of testicular cancer. The testicle is the most common site of cancer in men from 29 to 35 years of age. It tends to occur primarily in men from 20 to 40 years of age. The society recommends monthly TSE beginning at 15 years of age (see Chapter 16).

Diseases and Disorders of the Male Reproductive System ....

Epididymitis. This is an infection of the epididymis and is a common infection of the male reproductive tract. It may spread to the testicle, causing *orchitis* (inflamma-

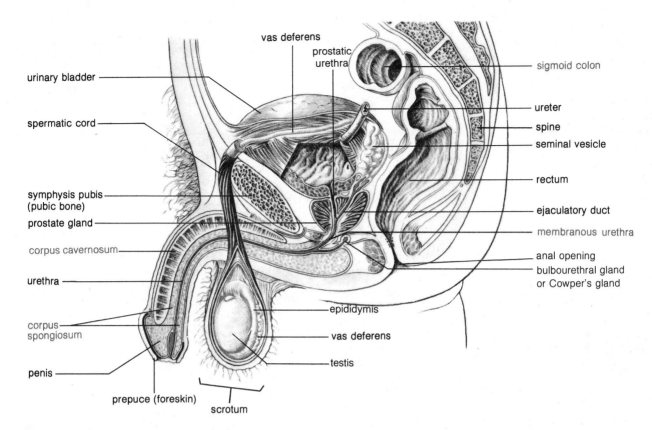

FIGURE 13–151   Longitudinal section of the male reproductive system (From Creager, *Human Anatomy and Physiology*, copyright 1983, Wadsworth Publishing Co. Reprinted with permission.)

tion of the testicle). The causative organism is usually staph or strep and generally follows urinary or prostatic infections. Other causes include trauma, gonorrhea, or syphilis. The primary symptom is intense pain with swelling in the groin and scrotum. Other symptoms include fever, malaise, and a characteristic waddle when walking.

Treatment consists of bed rest, elevation of the scrotum on towel rolls, and ice to relieve pain and swelling. A broad-spectrum (inclusive) antibiotic and pain medication are indicated. Therapy must be initiated immediately, especially if there is bilateral involvement, due to the threat of sterility.

Hydrocele.   The presence of an excessive amount of normal fluid within the structures of the scrotum is called **hydrocele** and may occur following injury or inflammation or may develop as a result of the aging process. It is usually caused by excess production of fluid, lack of reabsorption, or blockage of the circulatory process. If the excess fluid that collects causes discomfort, it may be necessary to aspirate the liquid to temporarily relieve the situation. Surgical correction is indicated with continued involvement.

Impotence.   This is an inability to have or sustain an erection to complete intercourse. Primary **impotence** refers to the patient who has never had an erection. Secondary impotence refers to the patient who is currently

impotent but has had intercourse in the past. Transient periods of impotence are not considered a dysfunction and probably occur in half the adult male population. The incidence of impotence increases with age.

Impotence is approximately 80% psychogenic in origin. The usual causes are anxiety, fear of failure, depression, parental rejection, and previous traumatic sexual experiences. Occasionally, impotence may result from stress. Interpersonal factors such as insufficient knowledge of sexual function or lack of communication with partner may cause impotence. Organic dysfunction may result from a chronic illness such as diabetes, renal failure, or cardiopulmonary disease. Spinal cord trauma, the effects of alcohol, or the results of certain drug therapy may also cause organic dysfunction.

Treatment of impotence consists primarily of sexual therapy to reduce the anxiety and usually involves both partners. The type of therapy chosen depends on the specific cause of the dysfunction. Most often it involves improving communication, reevaluating attitudes toward sex, restricting sexual activity, and encouraging attention to the physical sensations of touching. Patients with organic impotence need to develop alternative means of sexual expression. Some patients may benefit from surgically inserted inflatable penile implants. Such implants can be operated by the patient to effect an erection by releasing fluid from a reservoir to distend the implant. A noninflatable type provides a constant state of firmness.

Because of the negative connotation of the word "impotent," some physicians and sex therapists are now using the term *erectile dysfunction* to identify the occurrence.

Prostatic Hypertrophy. This enlargement of the prostate gland common in men over age 50 may be caused by inflammation, a tumor, nutritional disturbances, or a change in hormonal activity. In **benign** (nonmalignant) **hypertrophy,** the prostate may enlarge sufficiently to constrict the urethra, making it difficult to empty the bladder. Surgery may then be indicated to remove the obstructive gland. A malignant prostate is one of the most common forms of cancer found in men.

Symptoms of hypertrophy vary with the extent of involvement. Usually the initial symptoms are reduced force and size of urinary stream, difficulty in starting a stream, dribbling, a feeling of incomplete voiding, nocturia (having to void at night), and frequent urination. As the hypertrophy increases, symptoms become more pronounced, and eventually hematuria and retention may develop. Diagnosis of hypertrophy can be confirmed by a digital examination to palpate the prostate through the rectal wall, Figure 13–152.

Treatment of benign hypertrophy of the prostate will be conservative until the gland squeezes the urethra and interferes with voiding. Sitz baths, prostatic massage,

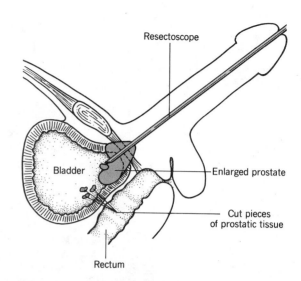

FIGURE 13–153   Transurethral prostatectomy (From Burke, *Human Anatomy and Physiology in Health and Disease*, 3d ed. Copyright 1992, Delmar Publishers Inc.)

and fluid restriction (for a short time) can be used, with the addition of antibiotics if an infection develops due to urine retention. Prostatic congestion may benefit from regular sexual intercourse. Conservative therapy is usually only temporary, with a more permanent surgical solution required to effectively relieve urinary retention and other symptoms.

A **prostatectomy** (removal of the prostate) can be performed by different methods. A **suprapubic** (above the pubis bone) is indicated with a large prostate or advanced malignancy. An incision is made through the pubic area and the total gland is removed. Another common method is the **transurethral** prostatectomy (TUR). In this procedure, a resectoscope is inserted into the urethra and the prostate is approached through an incision in the wall of the urethra, Figure 13–153. A wire loop with electric current removes a segment of the gland, thereby interrupting the integrity of the prostate and prohibiting its constricting action.

When hypertrophy is due to malignancy, symptoms are the same and unfortunately are not apparent before the disease is in the advanced stages. A rectal examination that identifies a small, firm nodule would be the first finding. Physical examinations of men over age 40 should always include a routine prostatic screening examination. There is a 5-year survival rate in 70% of the patients without metastasis and in less than 35% after metastasis. The usual site of a fatal secondary involvement is bone. Typically, primary prostatic cancer spreads along the ejaculatory ducts, in the space between the seminal vesicles.

Treatment is determined by clinical assessment, expected life span, the stage of the disease, and tolerance for the therapy. Usually, patients are older men with complicating conditions of hypertension, diabetes, or heart disease. Normally radiation, a prostatectomy, an orchidec-

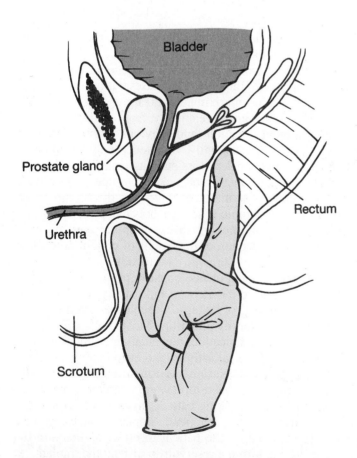

FIGURE 13–152   Digital examination of the prostate gland

tomy (removal of testes to reduce hormone production), and oral doses of female estrogen are used alone or in combinations, according to the stage of the involvement, to arrest and control the malignancy, Favorable results are obtained from high doses of radiation. Not only does the cancer go into remission but the associated metastatic skeletal pain, if present, is also relieved.

Female Reproductive Organs ....

Since the similarity in function of the male and female reproductive organs is another indication of their common origin, a comparison will be made, when appropriate, as each organ or structure is presented. The order of presentation will be, as with the male, from the formation of the sex cell to its exit from the body.

Ovaries

The embryonic gonadal tissue that is to become the ovaries begins to develop about the tenth or eleventh week of pregnancy. The ovaries of the fetus develop high in the abdominal cavity near each kidney, but descend to the pelvis as the time for delivery nears. Ovaries are small, almond-shaped glands measuring about $1\frac{1}{2}$ x 1 x $\frac{1}{4}$ to $\frac{1}{2}$ inch, Figure 13–154. They are supported by the ligaments, which attach to the uterus and tubes to ensure their position near the fimbriated (fringelike projections) ends of the fallopian tubes. These two organs play a significant role in the life of every female. They have two main roles: to produce the sex cell, the ovum, and to secrete hormones. These functions parallel the role of the testes in the male.

It is estimated that at birth the ovary has between 200,000 and 400,000 primary graafian follicles (podlike structures), which contain immature ova. Many follicles never mature and degenerate by puberty. During the reproductive life of a female, about 375 will develop and mature, releasing an ovum. By age 50, most of them have disappeared.

The ovaries are the primary sex organs of the female. When the female is about age 8, the pituitary gland begins to send hormonal messages that puberty is approaching. Within a few years, the messages get stronger, and the pituitary hormone causes the ovaries to begin releasing estrogen into the blood. Estrogen affects the development of the sex organs such as: (the fallopian tubes, the uterus or womb, and the vagina) causing them to increase in size and maturity, Figure 13–155, page 384.

Estrogen also produces secondary sex characteristics, which alter the shape and appearance of the female body, Figure 13–156, page 384. In the female, secondary sex characteristics are:

1. Broadening of the pelvis, making the outlet broad and oval (to permit childbirth). (The male pelvic outlet is oblong and narrow.)
2. The epiphysis (growth plate) becomes bone and growth ceases. In the absence of estrogen, females continue to grow, becoming several inches taller than normal
3. Development of softer and smoother skin
4. Development of pubic hair in a flat upper border pattern
5. Deposits of fat in the breasts and development of the duct system
6. Deposits of fat in the buttocks and thighs
7. Sexual desire

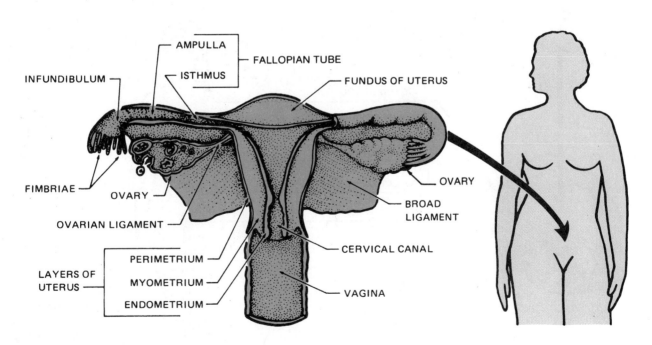

FIGURE 13–154 Female internal reproductive organs

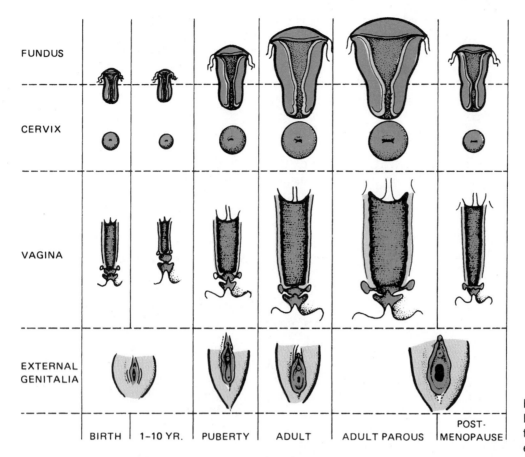

FIGURE 13–155
Development and maturity of the uterus, vagina, and external genitalia

FUNDUS					
CERVIX					
VAGINA					
EXTERNAL GENITALIA					
BIRTH	1–10 YR.	PUBERTY	ADULT	ADULT PAROUS	POST-MENOPAUSE

In addition to physical changes, two physiological functions begin to occur, namely ovulation and menstruation. Ova are produced in the germinal epithelium layer of the ovary, Figure 13–157. There a "nest" of cells undergo change with some cells forming a wall around a liquid-filled cavity. Other cells join to thicken one area of the wall. This structure is known as a primary follicle. One of the inner cells will become the ovum. Under the continued influence of FSH and LH from the pituitary, the follicle and ovum mature. Additional fluid collects

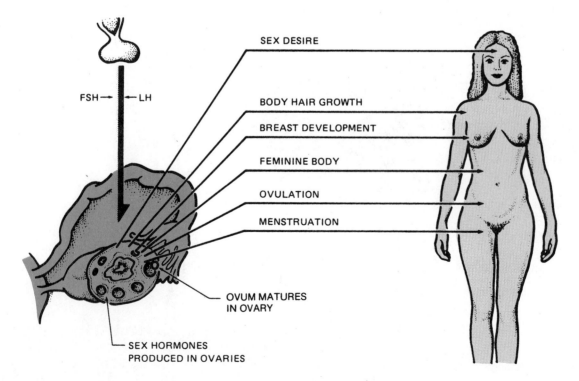

SEX DESIRE

BODY HAIR GROWTH

BREAST DEVELOPMENT

FEMININE BODY

OVULATION

MENSTRUATION

FSH → ← LH

OVUM MATURES IN OVARY

SEX HORMONES PRODUCED IN OVARIES

FIGURE 13–156
Secondary sex characteristics of the female

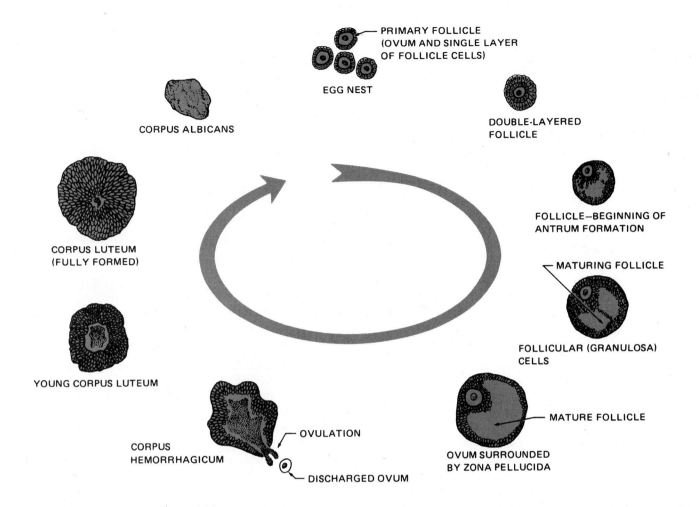

FIGURE 13–157 The life cycle of an ovarian follicle and the ovum

within the follicle and it begins to resemble a blister. The follicle moves toward the surface of the ovary and develops a small protrusion called a stigma.

The maturing follicle, called a graafian follicle, produces estrogen, which in turn stimulates the pituitary to release increasing amounts of FSH and LH. When maturity has been achieved and the amount of LH is high, the stigma disintegrates, allowing the follicle to rupture and release the egg into the surrounding area. This action is known as ovulation. At this point, the follicle undergoes change to provide support to the ovum. Under the influence of LH, the follicle fills with a yellow material and begins to function as a temporary endocrine gland, secreting a hormone called progesterone. The follicle is now called a corpus luteum (yellowish body).

The high levels of FSH and LH act as a feedback mechanism to prevent the pituitary gland from secreting FSH to mature an additional follicle. The corpus luteum continues to secrete estrogen and progesterone, which prepare the uterus for reception of a fertilized ovum. If fertilization does not occur, the ovum will pass from the body through the vagina, and the corpus luteum, after 10 or 12 days, degenerates and becomes inactive, causing a sharp decline in the hormonal level. This decline stimu-

lates the pituitary to again begin releasing FSH and LH and the cycle starts again.

Fallopian Tubes

The fallopian tubes extend about 4 inches from the superior lateral surface of the uterus and are attached to the broad ligament, see Figure 13–154. The vas deferens and ejaculatory ducts of the male can be compared to the fallopian tubes of the female. The ducts provide a passageway for sperm as the fallopian tubes provide a passageway for the ovum to reach the uterus.

The fallopian tubes are constructed of four layers, including a muscle layer and ciliated mucosal layer. The distal ends of the tubes expand into funnel-shaped openings with many fingerlike projections (fimbriae). Upon ovulation it is believed the fimbriae move the ovum toward the opening of the tube. At the same time, the muscular layer of the tube contracts to produce a vacuum within the tube, and the cilia beat to create a current moving towards the uterus.

The ovary and fallopian tubes lie close together but are not connected. An ovum may be lost within the surrounding abdominal space. Occasionally, sperm will locate and fertilize such an ovum, which will then attach itself to a nearby structure and develop into an abdominal pregnancy. At term, surgical removal of the baby is necessary because no outlet for delivery exists.

Normally, conception (fertilization) takes place in the outer third of the fallopian tube. Upon union, the two cells begin to multiply. The corpus luteum causes secretions to be released from glands within the mucosa of the tubes. The secretions provide nutrition for the new zygote, which must now move into the uterus within 3 to 7 days for implantation and development. However, the opening of the tube narrows in the isthmus section, to about 1 mm in diameter near the entrance to the uterus. If the zygote is unusually large or slow, or if there is any constriction of the tube, the zygote may not be able to pass through the opening and an ectopic (abnormal location) tubal pregnancy develops. Since there is no space for growth, pain and discomfort will develop within a few weeks. Surgical removal of the embryo is imperative to prevent rupture of the tube.

Uterus

The uterus is a thick-walled, hollow, muscular organ lying within the pelvis, behind the urinary bladder, and in front of the rectum. It is shaped like an upside-down pear, measuring, before pregnancy, about 3 x 2 x 1 inch, Figure 13–158. The uterus is divided into three parts: the fundus, or rounded upper portion where the fallopian tubes are attached; the body, or middle and main portion; and the cervix, or narrowed section that opens into the vagina. The cervix has an internal and an external os (opening), with the cervical canal between them. The cavity within the uterus is a small triangular opening.

The uterus has three layers within its walls. The innermost is called the endometrium. The structure of the

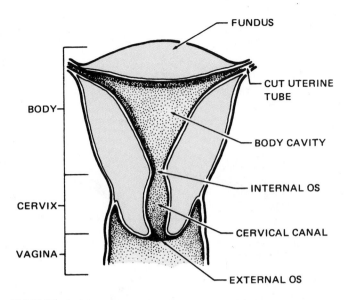

FIGURE 13–158 The uterus

endometrium changes considerably in response to the influence of hormones, as will be discussed under menstruation. The myometrium is made up of three layers of muscle fibers running circularly, longitudinally, and diagonally. The outer layer consists of the serous membrane, which covers most of the body and fundus of the uterus.

The uterus has a great capacity for expansion. During pregnancy, its thick walls stretch and thin out until the fundus touches the diaphragm. Even at this great overextension, the powerful uterine muscles are still able to contract forcefully to produce labor and delivery. In addition, the uterus is flexible in its position, being easily moved in all directions. It is pressed posteriorly when the bladder fills and anteriorly when the rectum is full.

Certain uterine positions are considered to be abnormal, however. When the uterus is horizontal, at right

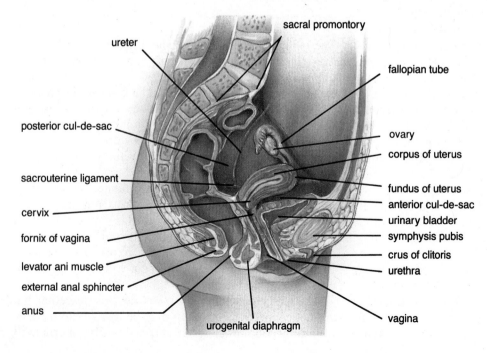

FIGURE 13–159 Female internal reproductive organs with uterus in normal position. (From Burke, *Human Anatomy and Physiology for the Health Sciences*, 3d ed. Copyright 1992, Delmar Publishers Inc.)

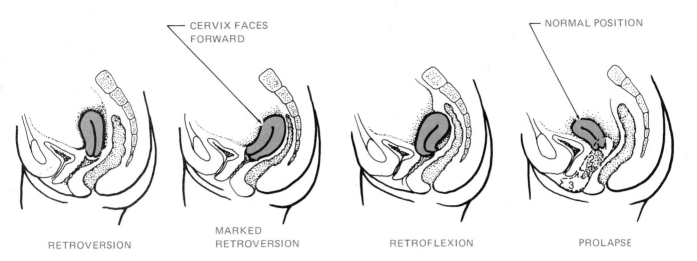

CERVIX FACES FORWARD

NORMAL POSITION

RETROVERSION

MARKED RETROVERSION

RETROFLEXION

PROLAPSE

FIGURE 13–160 Abnormal uterine positions

angles to the vagina, it is in its normal position, Figure 13–159. When only the body is tilted posteriorly and the cervix is still in its normal position, the uterus is said to be **retroflexed,** Figure 13–160. When the entire uterus tilts posteriorly, either moderately or markedly, it is said to be **retroverted.** When the supporting structures become weakened, the uterus may **prolapse** (drop) from its normal position. The extent of prolapse is specified as first, second, or third degree. Once the prolapse passes the introitus (vaginal opening), the uterus and a portion of the vagina are exterior and it is considered to be a third-degree prolapse.

Vagina

The vagina is a collapsible muscular tube lined with mucous membrane, which is arranged in folds. The walls of the vagina lie in contact with each other. The posterior wall is 3 to 4 inches long. The anterior wall extends about $2\frac{1}{2}$ or 3 inches to the cervix. The vagina is capable of great expansion. It serves as the passageway for menstruation, an organ of sexual intercourse, and the birth canal for delivery of an infant.

Behind the vagina and anterior to the rectum is a rectouterine pouch, a space called the cul-de-sac or pouch of Douglas. Infection occasionally develops in this area and necessitates draining. A surgeon can make an incision through the vaginal wall, eliminating the need for abdominal surgery. This is also the area where abdominal ectopic pregnancies usually occur. Though rare, this type of ectopic pregnancy occurs because the fertilized ova goes out the open end of the fallopian tube instead of descending into the uterus. It falls naturally by gravity into the cul-de-sac.

Near the outlet of the vagina is a muscular sphincter that can be detected when inserting tampons or upon examination. The sphincter will maintain a tampon within the vagina and provides a "snugness" for sexual intercourse. The vaginal canal is kept moist by secretions

from the uterus and by droplets of mucoid material from the vaginal walls.

Up to this point, all the structures discussed have been internal. While the external genitalia of the male are quite visible, those of the female are practically hidden from sight. Many authorities recommend that a woman become familiar with her genitalia by making a thorough examination using a mirror and a good light. It is almost inevitable that you will be assisting with the examination of female patients, and it would be to your advantage to be aware of the structures.

The vagina opens onto the surface of the body at the **perineum,** posterior to the urinary meatus and anterior to the anus, Figure 13–161. The external opening is par-

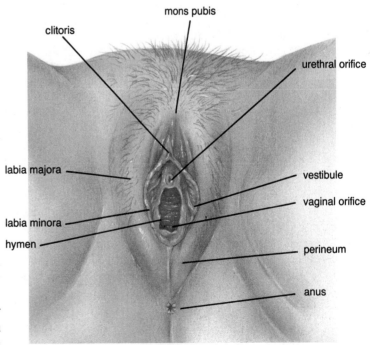

clitoris

mons pubis

urethral orifice

labia majora

vestibule

labia minora

vaginal orifice

hymen

perineum

anus

FIGURE 13–161 Female external genitalia (From Burke, *Human Anatomy and Physiology for the Health Sciences,* 3d ed. Copyright 1992, Delmar Publishers Inc.)

tially covered by folds of mucous membrane called the **hymen,** which border the edges prior to intercourse. Occasionally, the hymen is thicker than normal or covers the entire opening (imperforate hymen). The tissue must be removed prior to menstruation when imperforate. It occasionally requires surgical removal (hymenectomy) to permit intercourse when the narrowing tissue cannot be stretched naturally.

Vulva

The **vulva** is the area of the female external sexual structures. The large pad of fat that is covered with course hair on the mature female and overlies the symphysis pubis is known as the **mons pubis.** The labia majora (large lips) are a pair of rounded folds of skin on each side of the vulva and are continuous with the mons pubis. The labia are covered with hair on the exterior surface but with pigmented smooth skin on the inner surface. The labia are composed mainly of fat and numerous glands. The labia majora develop in the female from the same embryonic tissue that becomes the scrotum in the male.

The labia minora (small lips) lie within the labia majora and come together anteriorly in the midline continuous with the prepuce which covers the glans of the clitoris. The labia minora are covered with mucous membrane that is continuous with the lining of the vagina. The female labia minora develop from the same embryonic tissue as the male penile shaft.

The term vestibule is used to denote that portion of the vulva that lies inside the labia minora and posterior to the clitoris. It contains the opening to the urethra and the vagina. The ducts to the vestibular glands (**Bartholin's glands**) open at the base of the labia minora. They secrete a fluid which serves as a lubricant for **coitus** (intercourse). Posteriorly the labia minora are connected by a thin piece of tissue called the fourchette, which is just posterior to the vaginal opening. The fourchette is destroyed by the birth of the first child.

Clitoris

The clitoris is a rounded mass composed of two small columns of erectile tissue. The clitoris develops in the female similarly to the glans and penis of the male, except that the urethra does not descend through its interior. The clitoris and the glans penis are very sensitive and provide for heightening of sexual excitement. The clitoris becomes enlarged and engorged with blood and is involved in the orgasmic response to sexual arousal.

Perineum

The perineum is identified in two different manners. Some physicians consider the entire pelvic floor as the perineum and apply the term to both male and female.

But in **gynecology** (the study of female diseases), the perineum refers to the area posterior to the vaginal introitus and anterior to the anus. In the male, the perineum in this sense is posterior to the scrotum and anterior to the anus. The perineal area is composed of muscles that form a sphincter for the vestibule. During childbirth, the perineum must stretch adequately to permit the delivery of the infant. If it appears the tissue might be torn, the physician will surgically cut the perineum to avoid a ragged tear. This procedure is known as an **episiotomy.** Following delivery, the straight, clean cut is sutured (sewn closed). When the repair heals, the perineum is much smoother, with less scar tissue, than if torn tissue had healed.

Mammary Glands (Breasts)

The mammary glands are secondary sexual structures that develop and function only in the female. The breast consists of lobes separated into sections by connective tissue, somewhat like the structure of a grapefruit half. Each lobe has several lobules composed of connective tissue with grapelike clusters of secreting cells (alveoli) embedded in the tissue. The glandular clusters are drained by minute ducts that unite into a single duct for each lobe for a total of about 15 to 20 in each breast, Figure 13–162. The ducts are arranged like the spokes of a wheel, meeting at the nipple. Here they enlarge slightly to form small reservoirs. The main ducts exit on the surface of the nipple through tiny openings.

Fatty tissue is deposited around the surface of the gland, between the lobes and beneath the skin. A darkened area called the **areola** surrounds the nipple. The color of the areola varies from pink in light blonds and redheads to brown in brunettes. A pink areola will turn

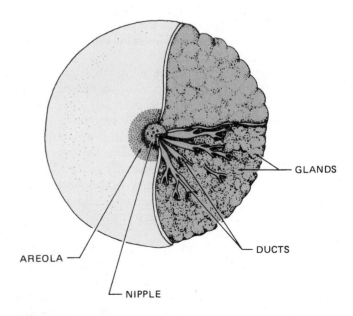

FIGURE 13–162 The structure of the breast

brown early in pregnancy and regress somewhat after delivery, but will not return to pink. About 3 days after delivery, the glands begin to secrete milk due to hormonal stimulation from the pituitary. The hormone prolactin stimulates the production of milk while oxytocin causes it to be ejected in response to the infant's sucking.

Menstruation

When the ovum is not fertilized and therefore the uterine structures prepared for reception of the embryo are not needed, the lining deteriorates and is discharged from the body in the process called menstruation. Menstruation begins at menarche (first cycle) and ends with menopause (last cycle). A complete cycle is approximately 28 days in length. If menarche occurs at age 13, the female will experience approximately 455 cycles over the following 35 years. A 28-day cycle is based on a lunar month, not a calendar month; therefore, there are 13 cycles (lunar months) per year.

The menstrual cycle is a result of the interaction of hormones and the endometrium of the uterus. Normally, menstruation is interrupted only by pregnancy or severe illness. The interrelated effects of the hormones and their effects on the sex organs are illustrated in Figure 13–163, page 390. The menstrual cycle can be divided into four phases, each characterized by hormonal, ovarian, and uterine changes.

Phase I—The Follicular Phase. Beginning about day 5 in the cycle (counting from the first day of menstruation), the pituitary secretes high levels of FSH to stimulate the ovarian follicles. One follicle ripens an egg and brings about ovulation, at the same time secreting estrogen. About day 10, the pituitary begins to secrete LH in large amounts to react on the follicle. As the estrogen increases, the FSH slows down. The follicle continues to move its maturing egg toward the ovarian surface. At the same time, the endometrium of the uterus has been stimulated by the high level of estrogen and grown a thick lining in preparation for receiving a fertilized egg. This change in the lining in known as *proliferation.*

Phase II—Ovulation. The follicle releases the matured ovum. Estrogen is at a high level; FSH is reduced just prior to ovulation. The high level of estrogen stimulates the release of LH by the pituitary, which causes the follicle to rupture about day 14 in the cycle. The endometrium has continued to grow a thick lining.

Phase III—The Luteal Phase. After the egg is released, the empty follicle undergoes a rapid change due to the influence of LH. It becomes a glandular mass of cells called the corpus luteum and begins to release progesterone as well as estrogen. The progesterone reacts on the glands in the endometrium to begin secreting a nourishing substance for the egg. The corpus luteum continues to secrete progesterone for about 12 days, until approximately day 26 of the cycle. As the level of progesterone rises, LH is inhibited and the LH level falls. When LH drops, the corpus luteum degenerates, causing the levels of progesterone and estrogen to decline sharply.

Phase IV—Menstruation. With hormonal support gone, the lining buildup in the uterus begins to slough off (shed), causing menstruation from day 1 to 5. The excess endometrium and a small amount of blood pass out through the cervix. Estrogen and progesterone levels are low, but the FSH level is rising to start the next cycle, preparing the uterine lining and the next ovum for the opportunity of pregnancy.

Fertilization ....

The miracle of reproduction begins with fertilization. In the process of sexual intercourse, sperm at the rate of about 360 million per ejaculation are deposited into the female vagina. From here the microscopic sperm begin an incredible journey toward a single female ovum, which will normally be in the outer one-third of one of the fallopian tubes. The ovum must be fertilized within 24 hours after expulsion from the ovary, or fertilization will have to be postponed until the next ovum is ready in approximately 1 month.

The sperm travel at a rate of about 1 to 5 millimeters per minute; their course seems to be in a straight line but in a random direction. Studies on humans are difficult to do, but some research has been conducted. In one study, it was found that sperm deposited in the vagina of a woman just prior to surgery had migrated through the fallopian tubes by 30 minutes later. This finding could not be explained based on sperm motility alone. It is hypothesized (suggested) that intercourse or artificial insemination causes the release of a hormonal substance that increases uterine contractions, propelling sperm toward their destination.

The ovum is considerably larger than the sperm, yet it is still only about 1/125 of an inch in diameter, Figure 13–164, page 391. When the sperm reach the egg, they surround its outer surface attempting to enter. Only the strongest sperm are able to survive the acidity of the vaginal secretions to attack the protective corona radiata that surrounds the ovum. In repeated attacks, the sperm release an enzyme called hyaluronidase, which gradually breaks down the ovum's protection. Eventually, an exposed area of membrane will allow one spermatozoan to penetrate the ovum. The head and middle of the sperm enter the ovum while the tail drops off outside. Immediately, the membrane becomes sealed against additional sperm. The nucleus of the sperm moves to combine with the ovum nucleus and a zygote is formed. At this time, the traits which are inherited, as well as the sex of the new individual, are determined and cannot be altered. The father has determined the sex, but the other charac-

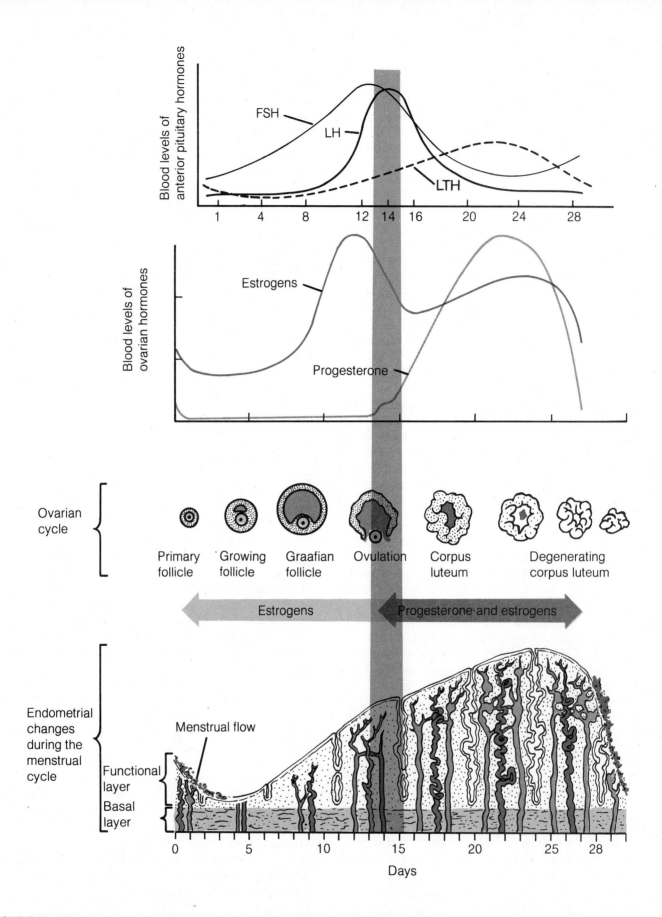

FIGURE 13–163 Menstrual cycle illustrating the levels of pituitary and ovarian hormones, ovarian cycle, and endometrial changes (From Burke, *Human Anatomy and Physiology for the Health Sciences*, 3d ed. Copyright 1992, Delmar Publishers Inc.)

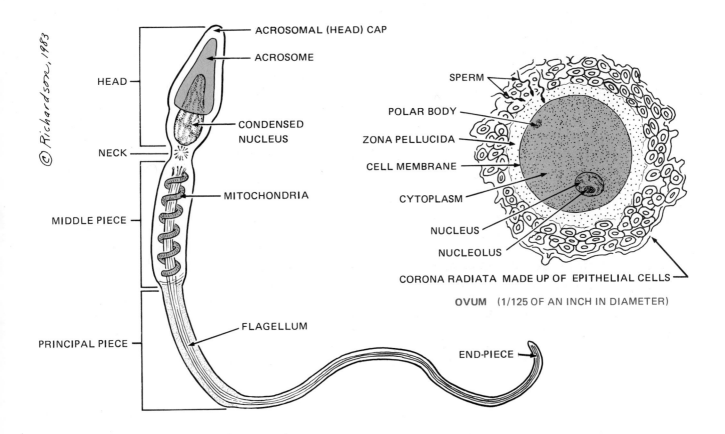

FIGURE 13–164 Sperm and ovum. NOTE: actual size comparison of sperm entering ovum. (Copyright by Richardson, from Fong, Ferris, & Skelley, *Body Structures and Functions*, 7th ed. Copyright 1989, Delmar Publishers Inc. Used with permission.)

teristics are contributed by both parents. At this point, conception has occurred.

Following fertilization, the zygote begins the journey to the well-prepared uterus, arriving about 6 days after ovulation. There it implants itself in the thick wall and a change in the menstrual cycle begins. At this point, phase III is at about day 20. The endometrium is at its peak. The levels of estrogen and progesterone are high. LH and FSH are low due to the feedback of adequate amounts of hormones; this is preventing stimulation of new follicle maturity. The secretions from the fallopian tubes and the uterine glands are providing nutrition for the embryo.

The high level of progesterone inhibits the myometrium from contracting; therefore, the embryo cannot be expelled. Progesterone also stimulates development of the ducts of the mammary glands (breasts). These effects must be continued to maintain the implantation. If the corpus luteum fails, so does the production of progesterone. Therefore, the developing placenta (afterbirth) secretes a hormone, human chorionic gondadotropin (HCG), which maintains the corpus luteum during the early stages of pregnancy. This is the hormone that is detectable on urine pregnancy tests. As the embryo develops, the placenta begins to secrete

progesterone and estrogen, and the corpus luteum degenerates and disappears.

The placenta maintains its high level of hormone output throughout pregnancy. When the time for delivery nears, the placenta decreases production of progesterone, which allows the myometrium to begin contracting, and labor begins. With progesterone diminished, the release of prolactin from the pituitary can occur. Prolactin stimulates the mammary glands to produce, for the first few days, *colostrum,* a thin nutritious liquid, and later, milk. The continued production of milk depends on stimulation from the regular sucking of the infant or the removal of milk by pumping.

Pregnancy

About 36 hours after fertilization occurs, the zygote begins to grow from its one-cell beginning. It is almost beyond comprehension to realize that everything necessary to the formation of a new life, the bones, muscles, blood vessels, the brain, all the organs, and the skin and hair are all contained in one microscopic cell. In addition, the life-support system of the placenta and umbilical cord and the protective membranes and amniotic fluid, also develop from this single cell. By about day 6, the small cluster of cells firmly implant within the uterine wall and it enters the embryonic period (8 weeks) of development when most of the major organ systems are formed at an amazing speed. The group of cells arrange themselves into three layers from which the various organs are formed. One layer, the *ectoderm,* becomes the nervous system, skin, hair, and parts of the eye. The *endoderm* layer becomes the digestive and respiratory systems. The skeletal, muscular, connective tissue, reproductive, and circulatory systems develop from the *mesoderm* layer.

The embryo develops from the head down which explains why in Figure 13–165 the head is so large when compared to the rest of the body. By the end of the tenth week of pregnancy, all systems are completed, even to nails on the fingers. Many of the organs begin limited function by the seventh week. After 8 weeks, the embryo is called a fetus. By week 12 the sex can be determined and the fetus is about 4 inches long and weighs about 2/3 ounce. This marks the end of the first trimester or one-third the total pregnancy period.

It is obvious the fetus has a lot of growing to do and it does so rapidly. By week 14, movement can be felt and by week 18, the heartbeat is detectable with a stethoscope. By now the pregnancy is about half way. A fetus must be carried past the next several weeks to survive. If born in week 23, a little past 5 months, it will weigh less than 2 pounds and has a 1 in 10,000 chance or surviving.

By the twentieth week, the fetus opens its eyes and by week 24, it can hear sounds from inside the uterus. The movements are very vigorous by now and there are periods of sleep and wakefulness as the second trimester ends.

During the last trimester, the fetus adds greatly to its size. By the end of the seventh month, it has assumed a head-down position and if born would have over a 50% chance of survival. The odds increase to about 95% at 8 months when weight reaches 5 pounds to 99% at full-term 9 months with average weight being 7 1/2 pounds and a length of 20 inches.

The pregnant woman also undergoes body changes during pregnancy. Initially the first sign is a missed menstrual period. This is a time of joy for couples who have been trying to conceive but may be less than welcome to others. Another early sign is breast tenderness due to the stimulation of hormones. Some women will experience "morning sickness" especially for the first 6 to 8 weeks.

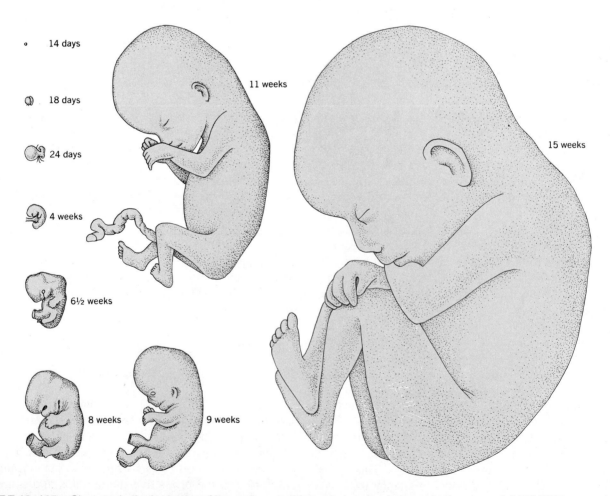

FIGURE 13–165 Changes in the body size of the embryo and fetus during development in the uterus (all **FIGURE**s natural size). (From Burke, *Human Anatomy and Physiology for the Health Sciences*, 3d ed. Copyright 1992, Delmar Publishers Inc.)

Usually there is more frequent urination, fatigue, and the need for additional sleep. By the sixth to eighth week, pregnancy can be detected by manual pelvic examination and the bluish hue of the formerly pale pink cervix. Once pregnancy is confirmed, the woman is usually interested in the expected delivery date. It is calculated using Nagele's rule which states: take the first day of the last menstrual period, subtract 3 months, and add 7 days plus a year. For example, if the first day of the last period was September 1, 1992 the expected day of delivery would be June 7, 1993. Remember, this is only the "expected" date. Babies have a habit of being born when they are "ready." On a percentage basis, 39% are born within 5 days of the projected date and another 55% are within 10 days. The rest obviously are either early or late.

It is important to confirm pregnancy early so that good prenatal care is started. Proper nutrition, vitamin supplements, and exercise are extremely important. It is also critical to the health and welfare of the fetus that the mother refrain from the use of tobacco, alcohol, and drugs, all of which cause problems such as low birth weight, drug addiction, and birth defects. The added insult of AIDS, hepatitis, or the effects of genital herpes from an infected mother is a terrible inheritance. Every pregnant woman should consider it her responsibility to do everything possible to ensure the birth of a healthy baby. A child born with any condition that the mother could have prevented must suffer its lifetime from her negligence and probably succumb to an early death.

Other symptoms experienced with pregnancy develop as the weeks pass. Usually there are psychological changes, such as the stereotypes of "being radiant," happy and having "cravings," such as for dill pickles at unusual times of the day. However, the symptoms of depression and fatigue are also common. In general, the symptoms are influenced by the attitude toward the pregnancy. If there are marriage conflicts or economic problems, or it's an unwanted pregnancy, it can hardly be a time of joy and anticipation.

As the pregnancy continues, the morning sickness disappears and edema of the hands, face, feet, and legs appears. There may also be constipation due to pressure on the rectum. Urinary frequency is universal due to the bladder being limited in its expansion. As the third trimester progresses, the size of the uterus causes shortness of breath and indigestion because of pressure from displaced organs and the uterus against the lungs and stomach. Hemorrhoids are common due to the constipation and pressure on the blood vessels of the rectum.

Weight gain continues throughout pregnancy. Most physicians prefer to establish a set amount of permissible gain. The total weight of the baby (7 1/2 pounds), placenta (1 pound), enlarged uterus (2 pounds), enlarged breasts (1 1/2 pounds), and additional fat and water (about 6 pounds) add up to about 18 pounds, so 20 pounds is sometimes the recommended amount of gain. Excess weight causes complications such as hypertension, increased stress on the heart, and the problem of weight to be lost after delivery.

The Birth Process

The beginning of the birth process is usually signaled by a show of bloody mucus. This is from the mucous plug that was in the cervix to protect the fetus from organisms in the vagina. There may also be a slow leak or a gush of the amniotic fluid. Irregular contractions of the uterus will begin and stimulation from prostaglandin may initiate labor.

Labor is divided into three stages. The first begins when uterine contractions become regular and proceeds through cervical dilation and effacement (thinning out). The cervix must dilate to about 10 centimeters (4 inches) in diameter before the baby can be delivered. Contractions increase in frequency and intensity until they become very strong, uncomfortable, and exhausting. First stage labor varies between as little as 2 to as long as 24 hours; 12 to 15 hours is average for a first pregnancy.

The second stage of labor begins with complete dilation and the entrance of the head (or another part) into the vagina. Continued contractions and bearing down by the woman push the baby through the vagina until it is visible at the entrance; this in known as *crowning* (if it is a head presentation). Strong contractions and pushing force the head through the vaginal opening, then the baby rotates to the side so the shoulders can be delivered. The rest is easily passed and the second stage is completed.

The baby is suctioned to remove mucus from its mouth and nose and crying begins to inflate the lungs. The baby's body function changes dramatically. For the first time it must breathe on its own to take in oxygen and begin to circulate its own blood. It changes from a bluish color to a healthy skin tone within a couple of minutes. As soon as baby's condition is satisfactory, the umbilical cord is clamped, tied, and cut.

To help assess a newborn's condition, a universally accepted evaluation technique called the Apgar scoring system is used. Observation of the newborn is made at one and five minutes following delivery. The ratings are entered on a chart and the scores totaled. A score of 10 is considered the best possible condition. A score of 7 to 9 is considered adequate and no treatment is required. A score of 4 to 6 indicates close observation and some intervention, such as suctioning, is necessary. A score below 4 requires immediate intervention and continued evaluation. Table 13–8, page 394, is an example of the Apgar scoring system.

The third state of labor begins with the detachment of the placenta from the uterine wall and the *afterbirth* (placenta and its membranes) are expelled. Usually a few more contractions are required to accomplish this stage. After it has emptied, the muscles of the uterus maintain a level of contraction to close off open blood vessels and control bleeding.

TABLE 13–8
Apgar Scoring System

Sign	0	1	2	Rating 1 min	5 min
Heart rate	Not detectable	Below 100	Over 100		
Respiratory effort	Absent	Slow, irregular	Good, crying		
Muscle tone	Flaccid	Some flexion	Active motion of extremities		
Reflex irritability (response to flick on sole)	No response	Grimace, slow motion	Cry		
Color	Blue, pale	Body pink, extremities blue	Completely pink		
			TOTAL		

Scoring system developed by Dr. Virginia Apgar

In some cases such as inadequate pelvic outlet, breech presentation (other than head), large baby, ineffective labor or the development of a serious complication, the baby may need to be removed by cesarean section. This involves cutting through the abdomen and into the uterus to remove the baby and the afterbirth. About 10% of all deliveries are cesarean. Repeated pregnancies may be delivered normally; however, if there are structural problems, then as the old saying goes, "once a cesarean, always a cesarean."

Contraception

The authors acknowledge that some religious and ethnic groups oppose birth control and this text does not ignore that issue; however, this subject matter is presented factually, from a clinical viewpoint, as information required for practice as a medical assistant. As the word implies, contraception is literally "against" conception. Several reasons may be given to avoid pregnancy:

- Avoid health risks to the woman. A woman in poor health may not survive a pregnancy.
- Spacing pregnancies. Some women are very fertile and conceive every year or less. The infant death rate is reported to be 50% higher at 1-year intervals than at 2 or more years.
- Avoid having babies with birth defects. Some women have chromosome defects or are genetic disease carriers (or married to carriers) and choose not to risk pregnancy.
- Delay pregnancy early in marriage to allow a time for adjustment to avoid additional stress in the new relationship and establish a strong marriage.
- Limiting family size. It is sometimes a personal decision and other times a reality of limited resources.

- Avoid pregnancy among unmarried couples. Single parenthood is difficult.
- Permit the woman to develop a successful career with planned pregnancies to integrate motherhood. A career can be useful if the woman is left to raise the child alone.
- Curbing population growth. The concern over worldwide food supply and supportive environment prompts some to promote contraception. It is anticipated the population will double between 1960 and the year 2000, only 40 years. Each successive doubling time becomes shorter.

Several methods to prevent conception and their relative percentage of effectiveness are listed in Table 13–9. Selection is usually made by the woman in consultation with her doctor. The cost, ease of use, degree of effectiveness, and likelihood of side effects, must be taken into consideration when selecting a method.

Diagnostic Tests of the Female Reproductive System

- **Colposcopy**—An examination of the cervix using a colposcope. It is used to rule out cancer when there are questionable pap smear results prior to performing a biopsy. Often cell structure may be temporarily altered by antibiotics, yeast infections and other reasons which might give a false positive pap smear. The cervix is cleansed with a solution of acetic acid and the scope introduced. The cervix can then be viewed through the colposcope which magnifies the mucosa making cellular structure visible.
- **Diaphanogram**—A study that uses light and sound waves and the detection of malignancy of the breast. Diagnostic accuracy is similar to mammography and it can be repeated as often as desired without patient risk from radiation. Diaphanography uses infrared light, which is directed through the breast and photographed. Dense tissue shows as darker areas on the film, healthy tissue is translucent, fluid cysts are bright spots, benign tumors are red, and malignant growths are dark brown or black. The test is not always reliable, because certain structures may be falsely interpreted; therefore it is not used very often.
- **Hysteroscopy**—A hysteroscope is inserted vaginally into the uterus. It is connected to a monitor that permits viewing of the endometrium. By using instruments through the scope it is possible to biopsy suspicious areas and remove polyps and fibroid. It is possible to take photographs or make a videotape for documentation of findings.
- **Mammogram**—An X ray of the breast for the detection of malignancy. A mammogram is indicated whenever there are palpable breast masses, breast pain, or nipple discharge. The film can also help differentiate between benign breast disease or breast malignancy. The American College of Radiologists

TABLE 13–9
Different methods of preventing conception

% Effective	Method	Description/Comments
100%	Abstinence	Refraining from sexual intercourse; absolutely most effective
100%	Sterilization	Tubal **ligation** (cutting of the fallopian tubes) in the female. The cut ends can be sewn back in opposite directions or cauterized. The surgical procedure is done through a laparoscope inserted into the abdomen. The procedure is considered permanent. A vasectomy in the male, with the ends being sewn in opposite directions. The surgery is performed through a small incision at the base of the scrotum. Vasectomies are usually not reversible; however, in some instances, reconstructive surgery has been successful, especially in cases of shorter duration; sperm production is usually significantly decreased in time. Usually a second marriage and the desire for another child prompt the attempt. The method is relatively expensive initially.
95%–99%	Birth control pills	Many different kinds are available. They are a combination of hormones that prevent ovulation; no ovum, therefore no pregnancy. Failure occurs when pills are not taken as prescribed. Side effects can be prohibitive for some women. Available only by prescription and requires regular visits to a physician. Cost is a factor to consider.
93%–99%	IUD	The intrauterine device is a small piece of plastic or coiled material inserted into the uterus to prevent implantation of a fertilized egg, presumably by providing irritation to the endometrium. Failure can occur if the device is expelled and during the first few months after being inserted. Initial insertion costs involved, and cost of removal. Side effects bother some women.
90%–99%	Diaphragm	A thin piece of dome-shaped rubber with a firm ring, which is inserted into the vagina to cover the cervix and provide a barrier to sperm. It is most effective when used in combination with a contraceptive cream placed into the dome before inserting. Failure usually results from improper insertion, a defect in the rubber, such as a hole, failure to insert before any penile penetration, or failure to maintain in place at least 6 hours following intercourse, Initial cost to examine and fit and purchase. No side effects. Requires cleaning and inspection after each use.
85%–97%	Condom	A thin sheath of rubber or latex that fits over an erect penis to catch the semen. A properly used condom is very effective. It must be unrolled onto an erect penis *before* any penetration occurs. It is important to leave about 1/2 inch of free air space at the tip (unless the condom is constructed with a tip) to catch the semen; otherwise, the force of the ejaculant may burst the condom. It must also remain in place throughout intercourse. After ejaculation has occurred, care must be taken to withdraw with the condom in place. It may require grasping with the fingers. This is the only contraceptive that also provides a level of protection against sexually transmitted diseases. It is relatively inexpensive, easy to use, and readily available. Remember, only a latex condom is also effective against the AIDS virus.
70%–75%	Spermicides	Contraceptive foams, jellies, and creams with *sperm-killing* ingredients, inserted by applicator, deep into the vagina before intercourse. It must remain for at least 6 to 8 hours afterward. Each application is good for only one act of intercourse. They should not be relied on alone as an effective contraceptive. Combined with a diaphragm or condom, they are effective. Few side effects (some report allergic reactions), easily used, and readily available. Must not be confused with lubricants such as K-Y or Lubafax, which contain *NO* spermicide.
?%	Douching	Absolutely not reliable. It only takes a couple of minutes for sperm to enter the cervix. In all reality, douching cannot be accomplished quickly enough. In fact, it may even assist sperm towards the cervix.
70%–80%	Withdrawal	This method has been practiced since Biblical times. It simply requires that the penis be withdrawn and ejaculation occur outside the vagina. It is not very effective because some sperm are deposited in the vagina before ejaculation occurs. In addition, the man may not be able to withdraw in time. It requires a lot of concentration to control. It is also not advised because it may lead to a sexual dysfunction if practiced for a prolonged period of time.
65%–85%	Rhythm	Is the practice of abstinence during an 8-day period from day 10 to 17 of the menstrual cycle when conception is theoretically possible. The method works fairly well for women who are extremely regular in their cycles and couples who can practice strong self-control. However, it requires a careful assessment of at least 6 months of cycles to establish ovulation days. If cycles vary in length, the period of abstinence must be increased to cover the longest possible period of time.

recommends a single baseline mammogram for all women between ages 35 and 40. All women over age 50 should have an annual mammogram. Women at risk require earlier and more frequent examinations. Risk-related factors are: fibrocystic disease; history of breast, uterine, ovarian, colorectal, or salivary gland cancer; or a family history of breast malignancy.

- Maturation index—A means of determining hormonal level by examining the percentage of certain types of cells in scrapings taken from the lateral vaginal walls.
- Papanicolaou (Pap) smear (test)—A routine examination done on secretions removed from the cervix and upper vagina to determine the presence of cancerous cells.
- Pregnancy test—Conducted on a first voided morning urine specimen to determine presence of the hormone human chorionic gonadotropin (HCG), which is produced by the developing placenta at the onset of pregnancy.
- Ultrasonography—A test for malignancy. A transducer is used to focus a beam of high-frequency sound waves through the skin into the breast. Sound waves bounce back echos, which are displayed on a computer screen for diagnosis. Ultrasound can detect tumors less than 1/4 inch in diameter and can distinguish between cysts and solid tumors. It is anticipated that ultrasonography will eventually replace mammography in breast cancer screening programs.

Diseases and Disorders of the Female Reproductive System ....

Abortion (Miscarriage). This is the spontaneous (unforced) or induced (therapeutic) loss of a pregnancy of less than 20 weeks' gestation. A spontaneous abortion usually results from one of three factors: (1) *fetal:* defective implantation or development of the embryo (most common cause); (2) *placental:* premature separation or abnormal implantation of the placenta; or (3) *maternal:* endometrial rejection, infection, malnutrition, trauma, drug reaction, endocrine difficulties, or blood group incompatibility. Spontaneous abortions occur in about 30% of all first pregnancies and up to 15% of all pregnancies.

Symptoms of spontaneous abortion are a pink or brownish discharge for several days followed by uterine cramping and increasing vaginal bleeding. When contractions are sufficient, the cervix dilates and the fetus is expelled. A complete abortion includes expulsion of the fetus, placenta, and membranes, resulting in the end of cramping and minimal bleeding because the uterus contracts to close off the blood vessels. An incomplete abortion results from the retention of some or all of the placenta. If the placenta (or a portion) adheres to the uterine wall, bleeding will persist, necessitating a D & C (dilation and curettage) to scrape out the retained placenta and permit the uterus to close off the blood vessels.

A therapeutic abortion is one performed to preserve the mother's mental or physical health in such instances as rape, unplanned pregnancy, or an existing medical condition such as cardiac or kidney disease.

Cervical Erosion. Ulceration of the epithelium on a portion of the cervix usually results from chronic cervicitis. The area bleeds easily when touched during examination, and may cause intermenstrual bleeding. Erosion is treated locally by cauterization (burning) to destroy the abnormal tissue growth. Cauterizing agents used can be chemical, such as silver nitrate sticks, or electrical, such as the electrocautery. The treatment is administered through a vaginal speculum and produces immediate cramping, which subsides quickly. Vaginal discharge will increase for a few days as the tissue sloughs off.

Cervicitis. This inflammation of the cervix is caused by an invading organism. Often the only symptoms are a purulent discharge and a tenderness of the cervix. Treatment consists primarily of antibiotics to destroy the organisms.

Cystitic Breast Disease (Fibrocystic). This is the presence of multiple lumps within the breast tissue. The lumps may be fibrous tumors that have degenerated or cysts (sacs) containing fluid. They may occur singularly or in multiple clusters. Fibrous tumors are either round or lobular. They are usually firm, well-defined (with definite borders), freely moveable, and painless. Cysts are also round, soft to firm, elastic, well-defined, moveable, and often tender. Neither type is attached to underlying tissues or to the skin to cause signs of retraction. Treatment may include needle aspiration of cystic fluid followed by instillation of a steroid. Often the cyst will not refill. Women with fibrocystic disease are believed to be at greater risk of developing a malignancy in one of the masses.

Many women naturally have "lumpy" breasts and should not be classified as having a "disease." Young women often have dense breast tissue that feels lumpy all over. This is just a condition of being fibrocystic. Often breasts become fibrocystic as a woman ages. Only professional examination and mammography can accurately diagnose a fibrocystic condition.

Cystocele. This bulging of the anterior wall of the vagina and the bladder into the vaginal canal, sometimes into the introitus, can be demonstrated by asking the patient to bear down or strain as the vaginal opening is observed. Cystocele appears in older women due to poor musculature from aging and the effects of childbearing. Other predisposing factors are obesity, lifting of heavy objects, instrument deliveries, and chronic coughing. The displacement of the bladder contributes to improper emptying, which results in cystitis, frequency (because some urine is always in the bladder), urgency, and incontinence, particularly stress incontinence as a result of coughing, sneezing, or laughing.

Dysmenorrhea. This lower abdominal and pelvic pain associated with menstruation is common among young females and tends to decrease with maturity, particularly after pregnancy. Dysmenorrhea in women in their late 20s or early 30s may be a symptom of an organic disease such as cervical stenosis, pelvic congestion, or endometriosis. Dysmenorrhea typically begins 12 to 14 hours before the onset of the menses and lasts between 24 to 48 hours. It may be associated with headache, nausea, vomiting, fatigue, and diarrhea. Occasionally, pain may be felt in the back and upper legs.

Treatment consists of analgesics, heat, drugs to decrease uterine contractions, and the use of hormonal therapy to suppress ovulation. When discomfort has an organic cause, the underlying condition must be corrected.

Endometriosis. The presence of endometrial tissue outside the uterus is most commonly found in the pelvic area, affecting the ovaries, ligaments, and peritoneal tissues. The cause of endometriosis is unknown, but, it is believed to be the result of the following:

- Recent surgery that opened the uterus
- Endometrial fragments expelled through the fallopian tubes at menstruation
- Alteration in the epithelium by inflammation or hormones that changes it to endometrium

The condition is characterized by dysmenorrhea, with constant pain in the lower abdomen, pelvis, vagina, and back beginning about a week before menses and lasting 2 to 3 days after onset. The degree of pain depends on the location of the endometrial tissue. Other symptoms include excessive, profuse menses when ovarian; hematuria when located in the bladder; rectal bleeding when located in the colon; and nausea, vomiting, and abdominal cramps when located in the small intestine.

Treatment consists of conservative methods in younger women, using androgens or progesterone to produce temporary remission by false pregnancy. When ovarian masses exist, they may be surgically removed. In women who no longer desire children, the treatment of choice is hysterectomy (removal of the uterus) and bilateral salpingo-oophorectomy (removal of both fallopian tubes and ovaries). The condition is not life-threatening, but pain and anemia must be controlled. Since the disease may cause sterility, childbearing should be accomplished as soon as convenient. Endometriosis generally subsides with menopause if surgery is ruled out.

Fibroids. Known technically as uterine leiomyomas or myomas, they are a common benign, smooth tumor formed of muscle cells, not fibrous tissue as suggested by the name. Usually fibroids do not occur singly and are located most often in the body of the uterus.

The cause of leiomyomas is unknown but it is believed they are cells that have grown into a tumor, probably stimulated by estrogen and the growth hormone, because following menopause they usually shrink in size and disappear. The primary symptom associated with leiomyomas is menorrhagia (excessive menstruation). Other characteristics are pain, a feeling of heaviness in the abdomen if the mass is large, discomfort from pressure against other organs, possible urinary frequency or constipation, and an irregular enlargement of the uterus. When a leiomyoma is attached to the lining by a stalk and is suspended within the uterine cavity, pain will occur due to the uterus contracting in an attempt to expel the mass. The patient is frequently anemic due to excessive bleeding. The diagnosis is usually confirmed by a D & C showing cells from leiomyoma in the scrapings from the endometrium.

Treatment depends on several factors, such as the patient's age, general health, and desire for children; the size of the tumors; and the severity of the symptoms. Small masses can be surgically removed, but a complete hysterectomy is indicated with greater involvement. The ovaries are left intact if possible to maintain hormone levels naturally. Uterine leiomyomas occur in about 20% of all women over age 35, with leiomyosarcoma (malignancy) developing in only about 0.1% of the patients.

Hysterectomy. This is surgical removal of the uterus, and is one of the most common procedures performed on female patients. It is not done on an elective or request basis but as a solution to a problem such as endometriosis, leiomyomas, uterine rupture, or malignancy. A hysterectomy can be performed in different ways, depending on the situation. Figure 13–166 illustrates the extent of surgery. Removing the uterus through an abdominal incision is termed an abdominal hysterectomy. When the uterus is positioned appropriately, it can be removed through the vagina, termed a vaginal hysterectomy.

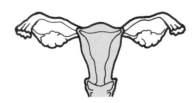

TOTAL HYSTERECTOMY

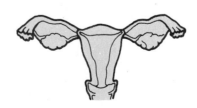

TOTAL HYSTERECTOMY WITH A SALPINGO-OOPHORECTOMY

FIGURE 13–166 Types of hysterectomies

A recent controversial alternative procedure has been developed. It is called endometrial ablation. It is used in cases of excessive bleeding from the buildup of endometrium or benign fibroid. A pen-sized instrument called a resectoscope is inserted into the uterus through the cervix. The procedure removes the lining by electrical cautery using a loop or rollerball attached to the end of the scope. It requires about 20 minutes to perform, is relatively painless, avoids surgery, takes only a few days' recovery time, and is a fraction of the cost of a hysterectomy. In contrast, a hysterectomy is major surgery, requiring well over an hour to perform, approximately 6 weeks to recover, and costing between $4000 and $7000. The ablation is probably an alternative for 20% to 50% of the annual 600,000 hysterectomies done mainly to stop uncontrollable bleeding. The procedure almost always results in sterilization, which of course would also happen with a hysterectomy. There is a slight chance of perforating the uterine wall, which may then lead to a hysterectomy.

Malignancy of the Breast. This is the most common malignancy among females and the number two cause of death. It is most common in women over age 35. The cause is not known, but estrogen is believed to be in some way responsible. Other predisposing factors include: a family history of breast cancer; long menstrual cycles; early menarche or late menopause; first pregnancy after age 35; race (white); socioeconomic status (middle to upper); stress; and previous cancer of the other breast, endometrium, or ovary.

Breast cancer is more common in the upper outer quadrant and in the left breast. It spreads through the lymphatic and circulatory system by way of the right side of the heart to the lungs, liver, bone, adrenal glands, kidneys, and brain. Cancer may be classified according to its location and cellular type as adenocarcinoma (from the epithelium) or Padget's disease (cancer of the nipple). In addition, most cancers are classified according to stages, to identify the amount of tumor, node, and extent of metastasis.

Specific warning signals which may indicate breast cancer are:

- A lump or mass in the breast tissue
- Change in breast size or shape
- Change in appearance of the skin
- Change in skin temperature (a warm, hot, or pink area)
- Drainage or discharge from a nonnursing woman or discharge produced by manipulation
- Change in the nipple, such as itching, burning, erosion, or retraction

Pain should be investigated but is not usually an early symptom.

Diagnosis is most often made by mammography, ultrasonography, and surgical biopsy. The best and most reliable means of detecting breast cancer is through routine monthly breast self-examination (see Chapter 16). Almost all initial findings of breast cancer (over 90%) are made by the patient. Statistics indicate that 67,000 American women develop breast cancer each year and about one-half die within 5 years. If the malignancy is discovered very early, surgery can save 70% to 80% of the patients. Though uncommon, breast cancer can also occur among males. The technique for self-examination is the same but is much easier to complete.

The type of surgical treatment selected for breast cancer takes into consideration, first of all, the stage, the woman's age, and her menstrual status. These factual items alone, however, do not totally influence the medical team. They have become aware, during the course of their investigation, of the woman's fears, attitudes, and feelings about the disfigurement of her body, and will, if possible, choose the least radical method of surgery.

A lumpectomy (removal of the tumor only) can be done on a small mass when there is no evidence of lymph node involvement. The next step would be a lumpectomy and removal of axillary lymph nodes but not the breast itself. With additional breast involvement, but no node enlargement, a simple mastectomy would remove just the breast and no underlying muscles. A modified radical mastectomy removes the breast and axillary nodes. A radical mastectomy removes the breast, axillary lymph node, and muscles from the chest wall. Radical mastectomies are seldom performed, because of the lack of statistical data to verify their additional survival benefit.

Recent advances have been achieved in mastectomy surgery. Reconstruction of a breast mound can be provided for most patients. A prosthesis may be implanted after underlying tissues are excised with the skin and breast surface structures being maintained. The approach is determined by the extent of involvement. A mastectomy is disfiguring surgery that may alter the patient's body image drastically. Because it can affect a woman's opinion of her sexuality and her relationship with her sexual partner, numerous volunteer support groups and other services are available to assist with the problems of adjustment.

Surgical treatment is usually combined with chemotherapy and/or radiation in an attempt to destroy cells within other structures of the body. Hormone therapy involves the use of androgens, estrogen, progesterone, or an antiestrogen, depending on the hormone-receptive nature of the tumor.

Malignancy of the Reproductive Organs ....

Cancer of the other reproductive organs is all too common. *Cervical* malignancy is a common cancer of the female reproductive system. It produces no symptoms until the cancer cells penetrate through the membranes and begin to travel through the lymphatic vessels or spread directly to nearby structures. The earliest symptoms are abnormal vaginal bleeding, persistent discharge, and pain and bleeding after intercourse. Cervical cancer can be detected very early by a Pap smear before any clinical evidence is observable. For this reason, the American Cancer Society recommends that all adult women under 40 [and sexually active teens] have smears done at least every 3 years and women over 40 be checked annually. The Pap test is not a reliable diagnostic tool for uterine cancer, only cervical. Women at risk require more frequent evaluation.

Uterine cancer is the most common gynecologic malignancy, affecting, usually, the postmenopausal woman between ages 50 and 60. The first signs of uterine cancer are uterine enlargement and unusual premenopausal or any postmenopausal bleeding. It may begin as blood-streaked watery discharge but changes gradually to more bloody drainage. The only reliable diagnostic test is biopsy, with a follow-up D & C if the biopsy is negative. Surgery is the treatment of choice, removing all reproductive organs. Radiation, either by an implanted internal device or externally administered, is indicated before surgery if the tumor is poorly defined. Chemotherapy may be used as well as hormonal therapy with progesterone. Both cervical and uterine cancers are rated by stages from 0 to IV with 0 being suspicious and IV-b indicating metastasis to distant organs.

Vaginal cancer is far less common, occurring primarily in women in their early to mid-50s. It occurs most often in the upper third of the vagina and, like cervical cancer, begins in the epithelial layer, then deepens. It spreads very slowly. Symptoms include vaginal discharge and bleeding, with an ulcerated, usually firm, lesion of the vagina. Diagnosis is made by the presence of abnormal vaginal cells on a Pap smear. Any visible lesion is biopsied. Involvement of the cervix must be ruled out. Lesions of the vagina are often difficult to visualize because of its physical structure and the presence of the vaginal speculum blades, which obstruct the view. Treatment of early stages may be confined to the area alone. Surgery or radiation varies according to the involvement. With extensive disease, surgical exenteration (removal of all pelvic organs) may be required, with construction of a colostomy and an ileal conduit (ureter emptying into the ileum). Radiation is the preferred treatment for vaginal cancer.

Ovarian cancer is one of the most common causes of cancer deaths among American women. Prognosis varies with the stage and type of tumor, but only about 25% of patients survive for 5 years. One type, primary epithelial, accounts for about 90% of the cases. Another form strikes children. It is more prevalent in higher socioeconomic women between 40 and 65 and in single women. Ovarian cancer spreads rapidly by local extension and occasionally through the blood or lymphatics. The most common metastasis is through the diaphragm into the chest cavity. Because of its location, early diagnosis is difficult. Symptoms are confined to vague abdominal discomfort and mild gastrointestinal disturbances. With progression, urinary frequency, constipation, pelvic discomfort, and distention develop. Symptoms may be confused with appendicitis. Diagnosis requires careful evaluation, complete history, surgical exploration, and lab studies on tissue samples. Treatment generally involves aggressive surgery to remove all reproductive organs, affected lymph nodes, the omentum (the apron of tissue covering the organs), and the appendix. Chemotherapy may be beneficial in early stages, to extend the survival time. Recent therapy is resulting in prolonged remissions in some patients.

Cancer of the *vulva* accounts for 5% of gynecologic malignancies. It occurs usually among older women, most often in their mid-60s, but can occur at any age, even in infancy. Early diagnosis and treatment greatly enhance survival. A 5-year survival rate is possible in 85% of patients without lymph node involvement, 75% when removed nodes are positive. Symptoms often begin with pruritis, bleeding, and a small surface ulcer that becomes infected and painful. Diagnosis is tentatively made from abnormal cells on a Pap smear and the typical clinical findings. Firm diagnosis requires biopsy of the suspected lesion.

Treatment consists of surgery, which varies with the extent of involvement. Small, confined lesions without lymph node involvement are treated by simple vulvectomy, perhaps on only one side. With node involvement in advanced stages a radical vulvectomy is required. This involves the vulva, as well as superficial and deep inguinal lymph nodes. With adjoining tissue metastasis, it may be necessary to excise the urethra, vagina, and rectum, leaving an open perineal wound requiring 2 to 3 months to fill in and heal. If surgery is prohibited, radiation may be used to make the patient more comfortable.

Ovarian Cyst. A sac of fluid or semisolid material on an ovary, it is usually nonmalignant, small, and produces no symptoms. Common cysts include follicular and lutein types that occur in the follicle or the corpus luteum. They can occur any time between puberty and menopause, including during pregnancy.

Follicular cysts develop as a result of an overdistended follicle that fails to close off properly. They secrete excessive amounts of estrogen in response to the FSH hormone. Granular lutein cysts are enlargements of the ovaries caused by excessive accumulation of blood during the bleeding phase of the menstrual cycle. Another form of lutein cyst is usually found bilaterally and contains clear, straw-colored liquid.

An ovarian cyst may cause an acute abdomen (a sudden condition, probably requiring surgical treatment) if the ovary is twisted by the cystic mass or the cyst ruptures. Large or multiple cysts may cause pelvic discomfort, lower-back pain, and abnormal uterine bleeding.

PMS (Premenstrual Syndrome). This combination of characteristics appears from 7 to 14 days before menstruation and usually subside with the onset. It is estimated that the syndrome occurs in 30% to 50% of women, particularly between the ages of 25 and 40. The cause of premenstrual tension is unknown. For whatever reason, intravascular fluid enters the body tissues and results in secretion of an antidiuretic hormone. This causes fluid retention with characteristic bloating. The tissue edema results in headaches and alterations in mood due to central nervous system changes.

Symptoms include any or a combination of the following:

- Behavioral changes such as nervousness, irritability, fatigue, and depression
- Neurological changes including headache, dizziness, numbness of extremities, and fainting
- Respiratory changes including increase in colds, exacerbation (aggravation or increase) of allergic rhinitis, and asthma
- Gastrointestinal changes such as constipation, diarrhea, abdominal bloating, and change in appetite
- General symptoms of backache, palpitations, temporary weight gain, increase in acne, or breast tenderness and enlargement

Treatment basically is symptomatic. Medication can be used to help relieve emotional symptoms as well as the physical manifestations. Many physicians prefer not to use drug therapy because the underlying cause for PMS is unknown.

Polyp. This is a growth with a slender stem attachment usually arising from the mucous membranes. Polyps of the cervix can often be visualized protruding from the external cervical os. They are red, soft, and rather fragile. If only the tip can be seen, it cannot be differentiated from a polyp of the endometrium. Depending on the location, size, and attachment, removal may be a simple office procedure or an outpatient surgical procedure.

Rectocele. This is bulging of the posterior vaginal wall, by the rectum, into the vagina. Inspection of the introitus may disclose a posterior mass, or it may be demonstrable on requesting the patient to bear down. It is most common in postmenopausal women. Contributing factors are believed to be pregnancies, prolonged labor, instrument deliveries, obesity, chronic coughing, and lifting of heavy objects. A rectocele of advanced degree may cause difficulty in emptying the rectum.

Sexually Transmitted Diseases ....

AIDS—Acquired Immune Deficiency Syndrome. Refer to Unit 9, The Immune System, for an in-depth look at this disease.

Chlamydia. This disease is caused by a specialized bacterium that lives as an intracellular parasite. There are two types of bacteria, both of which are pathogenic to humans. One strain causes a type of pneumonia. The other, chlamydia trachomatis, lives in the conjunctiva of the eye and the epithelium of the urethra and cervix. It is one of the most frequent sexually transmitted diseases in North America and affects between 3 and 10 million people each year. Approximately 10% of all college students are infected. It is probably present in half the patients with pelvic inflammatory disease (PID).

Symptoms do not easily lead to diagnosis. Men experience burning on urination and a mucoid discharge from the penis and are often misdiagnosed as having gonorrhea. Women experience a vaginal discharge mimicking gonorrhea and have frequent painful urination associated with urinary tract infections. When misdiagnosed, penicillin is given (for gonorrhea) or a medication for urinary infection and the chlamydia remains unaffected. Proper treatment requires repeated doses of tetracycline or erythromycin for at least a week to destroy the organism. If left untreated, or mistreated, men usually have no lasting effect but carry the organism and infect their sexual partners. In women, the bacteria will travel up the reproductive tract, causing inflammation of the fallopian tubes and eventual scarring. Some develop severe pain; others are barely aware of the infection. The scarring can interfere with pregnancy by causing tubal implantation of the fertilized ova due to the narrowed opening. Complete blockage may also occur, which prevents conception.

The disease, if contracted during pregnancy, will be transmitted to the baby during birth. The infant may develop conjunctivitis or pneumonia. Some evidence suggests that the infection may cause an increase in premature and still births. Two recently developed tests, which are inexpensive and quick to perform, accurately diagnose the disease. Because of its widespread incidence, many physicians routinely treat patients with symptoms and evidence of PID or gonorrhea even without positive chlamydia test results, due to the risk of sterility.

Gonorrhea. An infection caused by the gonococcus bacteria is known as gonorrhea. The organism is fragile and can survive only in a moist, dark, and warm area within the body. The most common sites are the vagina, penis, rectum, mouth, and throat. Since the organism dies almost immediately on exposure to air, it can be spread only by direct sexual contact.

Symptoms vary between the male and female. Men notice burning, itching, or pain on urination; a sore throat with gland involvement; discharge from the anus; or penile drainage that begins as a clear, watery fluid but changes to a thick, milky consistency. Women are usually asymptomatic, but they often develop an inflammation with a greenish yellow discharge from the cervix. Other common symptoms are similar to those experienced by men, including sore throat, anal discharge, and swollen glands. Women may also develop lower abdominal pain, especially if fallopian tubes and other structures become involved (see PID). Diagnosis can usually be made on visual inspection but confirmation depends on a positive culture of the gonococcus organism from the discharge. Treatment is necessary; gonorrhea will not go away by itself.

Large doses of penicillin or tetracycline are required to destroy the organism. A follow-up examination after treatment is important because strains of the gonococcus organism have become so resistant to the drugs that one course may not be sufficient. Untreated or undertreated gonorrhea can continue to spread, causing much damage. Men may develop chronic urethritis, long-term urinary tract inflammation, and sterility. Women may develop PID, which damages the reproductive organs and results in sterility.

Women who are infected with gonorrhea when giving birth pose a grave danger to the newborn. The gonococcus organism can infect the delicate tissues of the newborn's eyes and cause permanent blindness. Because of this needless happening, all newborns routinely receive silver nitrate solution in their eyes as part of immediate after-birth care.

Although gonorrhea can be controlled and prevented with proper education and treatment, using common sense—such as a knowledge of his or her sexual frequency with others—before engaging in sexual activity can prevent a person from becoming infected in the first place. Since the advent of the contraceptive pill and the IUD, the use of condoms, diaphragms, and foams has diminished. These chemical and mechanical barriers, especially the condom, somewhat deterred the spread of the disease.

Herpes. The virus causing herpes has two strains, type I and type II. Type I is the typical cold sore on the lip or at the edge of the nose. Type II is the form that appears on the external genitalia, mouth, or anus. Herpes is passed by direct skin-to-skin contact with your own or someone else's lesions, even 24 hours before they erupt. It is possible to spread your own herpes without being aware of its presence.

Herpes takes from 3 to 7 days to erupt. With **genital herpes,** fluid-filled vesicles appear on the cervix (primary site), labia, vulva, vagina, or perianal skin of the female. The male lesions appear on the glans, foreskin, or penile shaft. Nongenital lesions may cause complications such as herpetic keratitis of the eye, which may lead to blindness. Vesicles are usually painless at first, but may rupture and develop into shallow, painful ulcers with edema, redness, and tender inguinal lymph nodes.

Diagnosis is made by observation and from patient history. Confirmation of type II herpes is possible from a culture of the vesicle fluid. Treatment with the usual antiviral medications is ineffective. Sulfa-based creams help reduce edema and ease discomfort. Antibacterial agents help combat secondary infections.

After lesions heal, the virus becomes dormant. It may never recur, but about two-thirds of herpes sufferers have additional attacks, some within a few months. Future recurrences decrease in frequency and severity. The best defense is a healthy, well-rested body that can fight the disease organism with its natural defense mechanisms.

Other complications demand attention. Newborns can be infected with herpes during vaginal delivery. Some infants survive, but others develop a brain infection that rapidly leads to death. If a woman has active herpes II lesions at the time of birth, a cesarean section delivery is indicated. Women with herpes genitalis also have a higher-than-usual rate of spontaneous abortion. One major long-term risk associated with the disease is cervical cancer; therefore, women infected with or exposed to herpes II should have a Pap smear every 6 months.

Nongonococcal Urethritis (NGU). Sometimes also called NSU, or **nonspecific urethritis,** this is usually the result of a bacterial infection. In men it causes urethral inflammation; in women, vaginitis. NGU is transmitted by sexual intercourse. Men can also develop inflammation or allergic reactions from vaginal creams, contraceptive foams, soaps, douching solutions, and deodorants used by their sexual partners.

Symptoms are similar to cystitis: burning on urination, frequency, itching (penile or vaginal), and possibly a thin discharge (penile or vaginal). Treatment is normally with tetracycline or a similar antibiotic because NGU does not respond to penicillin therapy. If untreated it may lead to complications like those associated with gonorrhea. The most serious complication is a scarred urethra, which results in problems with urination. In addition, some strains can cause birth defects in newborns whose mothers have the disease.

Differential diagnosis between NGU and gonorrhea must be made because the symptoms are similar, but the treatment is different. Confirmation is made by absence of the gonococcus from the culture of the discharge.

Pelvic Inflammatory Disease (PID). This is any acute or chronic infection of the reproductive tract, including the cervix (cervicitis), uterus (endometritis), fallopian tubes (salpingitis), and ovaries (oophoritis). It can also involve the surrounding tissues. Early treatment is important to prevent reproductive damage, infertility, pulmonary emboli, septicemia (blood poisoning), and death.

PID is caused by an infection from aerobic or anaerobic organisms. The gonorrhea coccus is the most common aerobic organism. It can rapidly destroy the bacterial barrier of the cervical mucus. With the barrier gone, the bacteria present in the vagina can ascend into the uterus and cause infection. Uterine infection can also develop following insertion of an IUD (intrauterine device), which accidentally introduces contaminated cervical mucus into the uterus. Other factors causing PID are abortion, tubal examinations that test patency by inserting air, pelvic surgery, and infection associated with pregnancy. Organisms can enter from the blood stream, an abscess, an infected tube, or a ruptured appendix.

Symptoms include purulent vaginal discharge, fever, and malaise (especially if gonorrhea-related). There is lower abdominal pain, with severe pain on manipulation of the cervix and adjoining structures. PID can be treated with antibiotics to prevent progressive involvement. Culture of the drainage to identify the organism is important to be certain the appropriate drug is being used. Improper treatment will result in a chronic disease state. If the causative organism is gonorrhea, syphilis may also be present and require treatment. Bed rest, analgesics, and IV therapy may be indicated. Pelvic abscesses may develop, which require drainage. If permitted to rupture, they may cause a life-threatening situation.

Pediculosis Pubis (Pubic Lice). Little yellowish-gray insects, about the size of a pinhead, can attach themselves to the moist hair roots in the pubic area of humans. They feed on the blood of their host and hop from person to person during sexual contact. It is possible, however, to get lice from contaminated towels, upholstery, clothing, or bedding, because they can survive for about a day without a supporting host. The prime symptom is an intense itching which can't be ignored. They are visible on close inspection.

Treatment is quite simple with a product called Kwell, which is applied to the infected area. All clothing, bedding, and linens must be washed in very hot water and detergent to destroy the nits (eggs) and lice. Nonwashable items can be drycleaned or ironed with a hot iron. Lice eggs can survive for a week, so uncleaned items must be avoided.

Syphilis. The disease is caused by a delicate bacteria called a spirochete that inhabits the warm, moist areas of the genitals and rectum. The organism can be viewed by dark-field microscope examination. Syphilis is spread by direct sexual contact during either the primary, secondary, or early latent stages of infection. Prenatal transmission to the fetus across the placental barrier is possible, resulting in an infant with congenital syphilis. If the mother is in the primary or secondary stage, the infant will probably die before or shortly after birth. If syphilis is diagnosed and treated before the fourth month of pregnancy, the fetus will not develop the disease. Therefore, a blood analysis for syphilis is routinely performed as part of early prenatal care.

Symptoms vary according to the stage of involvement. Primary stage syphilis begins with entrance of the organism through the mucous membrane of the genitals as the result of contact with an infected person. After 3 to 4 weeks, a lesion called a *chancre* appears at the point of entrance. It is an ulcerlike area with a raised, hard edge, which looks painful but is not. In the female it often appears on the cervix and is therefore hidden from sight and unknown. It may also develop on the vulva and be visible on examination. In the male, the usual site is the glans or corona (ridge) of the penis. It may also develop on the penile shaft or scrotum. The bacteria can also enter the mucous membranes of the mouth or rectum during nongenital intercourse, causing chancres to develop on the lip, tongue, tonsils, or around the anus.

The disease progresses through four stages. The primary stage chancre, even if untreated, disappears within 1 to 5 weeks, giving the infected person a false sense of having healed. Actually, the disease enters an asymptomatic period during which the bacteria circulate through the body in the blood. About 1 to 6 months later a secondary stage begins. This stage is characterized by a generalized painless, nonitching rash. It is particularly distinctive because of its appearance on the soles of the feet and palms of the hands. Hair loss may occur during this stage as well as a sore throat, headache, loss of appetite, nausea, constipation, persistent fever, and pain in the bones, muscles, or joints. These symptoms could be indicative of any number of illnesses. If the disease is diagnosed accurately and treated, it can be cured without permanent effects. Without treatment, the disease again "goes away" in 2 to 6 weeks, leading to the belief that nothing is wrong, while, on the contrary, a dangerous stage is approaching.

The third stage is the latent stage, which may last for years. There are no symptoms during this stage, but the organism is at work, burrowing into blood vessels, the spinal cord, the brain, and the bones. After the first year, the disease is no longer infectious except to a fetus. About 50% of those who contract syphilis move into the dangerous late or tertiary stage. This stage is further categorized according to the type of involvement: benign late (affecting internal organs); cardiovascular late (affecting the heart and major blood vessels); or neurosyphilis (affecting the brain and spinal cord). Cardiovascular forms can lead to death; neurosyphilis is almost always fatal.

Diagnosis is difficult by history alone, and physical examination at certain periods would be negative. However, a definitive blood test has been developed and is used routinely for suspected infection and as a mass screening test by some states for persons seeking a marriage license. The test is known as a VDRL, named for the Venereal Disease Research Laboratory of the US Public Health Service. The blood test is fairly accurate, cheap, and easy to perform; however, it does not give accurate results until 4 to 6 weeks after initial infection. About 25% of the tests will be false negatives during the primary stage, but they are completely accurate in the secondary phase.

Penicillin is the treatment of choice for syphilis, which is relatively easily destroyed. Since some of the bacteria may survive, a large initial dose of long-acting penicillin (1.2 million units) is divided into two injections, one in each buttock. Much greater doses are required for latent, late, or congenital syphilis. A follow-up exam should be done to confirm freedom from organisms.

Trichomoniasis. This is an inflammation caused by the single-celled parasitic organism called *Trichomonas vaginalis.* It is oval in shape, with four hairlike strands protruding from it which whip back and forth to propel the organism. **Trichomoniasis** can be passed back and forth between sexual partners; therefore, treatment must involve both persons. The organism can also be transmitted by toilet seats and washcloths.

The prime and discriminating symptom is abundant, frothy, white or yellow vaginal discharge, which irritates the vulva and has a characteristic foul odor. There are usually no symptoms in the male. Diagnosis is made by placing a drop of the secretion on a slide and identifying the organism by microscope. This confirmation rules out ordinary vaginitis from female hygiene products or the presence of rectal *Escherichia coli* in the vagina. Treatment of choice is a product called Flagyl, which is taken orally. However, there is some controversy regarding its safety. If left untreated, the female may develop an inflamed cervix and urethra and exhibit abnormal Pap smears. Damaged cells of the cervix may make it more susceptible to cancer. Men develop an infected prostate, testicles, or bladder.

Vaginitis. This is an inflammation of the vaginal mucosa. There are several causes of vaginitis.

1. Allergic reaction—this usually happens as a result of douche solutions, (especially those that are scented), spermicidal materials, deodorant treated tampons, or other materials inserted into the vagina. This can be treated easily by discontinuing the causative agent.
2. Non-specific—this can be the result of a pH imbalance, bacteria, and any number of other causes not meeting other categories. Treatment is determined by the etiology of the infection.
3. Yeast—specifically, a type known as Monilia, which is a fungus that requires glucose for growth. It is the most common form, often caused by birth control pills and may be secondary to antibiotic therapy. It also affects pregnant women twice as often as non-pregnant women, and commonly affects diabetics. Many women have yeast infections frequently and the cause is not readily known. This form of vaginitis causes intense itching and can be treated successfully with over-the-counter vaginal preparations.
4. Vaginal mucosa atrophy—this occurs in menopausal women due to decreased levels of estrogen, which predisposes to bacterial infection.

REFERENCES

American Cancer Society. Atlanta, GA: *What You Should Know About Melanoma.* 1985;
The Decision is Yours. 1986;
Cancer Facts & Figures. 1992;
Open Wide.
Facts on Testicular Cancer.
For Men Only. 1989.

American Medical Association. *The Wonderful Human Machine.* Chicago: American Medical Association, 1977.

Anderson, Pauline C., and Burkard, Martha R., *The Dental Assistant.* Albany: Delmar, 1987.

Anthony, Catherine Parker, and Thibodeau, Gary A. *Structure and Function of the Body,* 7th ed. St. Louis: C.V. Mosby, 1984.

Anthony, Catherine Parker, and Thibodeau, Gary A. *Textbook of Anatomy and Physiology,* 11th ed. St. Louis: C.V. Mosby, 1983.

Bates, Barbara. *A Guide to Physical Examination.* Philadelphia: J.B. Lippincott, 1974.

Burke, Shirley R. *Human Anatomy and Physiology for the Health Sciences,* 3rd ed. Albany: Delmar, 1992.

Burt, John J., and Meeks, Linda Brower. *Education for Sexuality,* 2nd ed. Philadelphia: W.B. Saunders, 1975.

Caldwell, Esther, and Hegner, Barbara. *Nursing Assistant,* 6th ed. Albany: Delmar, 1992.

Chlamydia: The silent epidemic. *Time* Magazine, February 4, 1985.

Ehrlich, Ann. *Medical Terminology for Health Professions.* Albany: Delmar, 1988.

Fong, Elizabeth, Ferris, Elvira B., and Skelley, Esther G. *Body Structures and Functions,* 7th ed. Albany: Delmar, 1989.

Francis, Carl C., and Martin, Alexander. *Introduction to Human Anatomy,* 7th ed. St. Louis: C.V. Mosby, 1975.

Groer, Maureen E., and Skekleton, Maureen E. *Basic Pathophysiology,* 2nd ed. St. Louis: C.V. Mosby, 1983.

Guyton, Arthur C. *Basic Human Physiology,* 2nd ed. Philadelphia: W.B. Saunders, 1977.

Haslam, Robert H.A., and Valletutti, Peter J. *Medical Problems in the Classroom.* Baltimore: University Park Press, 1978.

Hohwald, Diane RN, CNN. Educational Coordinator, Riverside Outpatient Dialysis Center. Interview. Columbus, 1991.

Human Sexuality Supplement of *Current Health* 10 (1): (September 1983).

Hyde, Janet Shibley. *Understanding Human Sexuality.* New York: McGraw-Hill, 1979.

Kinn, Mary E. *Medical Terminology: Building Block for Health Careers.* Albany: Delmar, 1990.

Krames Communications. *Laser Eye Surgery* (pamphlet). Columbus: Grant Laser Center, 1991.

Krupp, Marcus A., et al. *Physician's Handbook,* 18th ed. Los Altos, CA: Lange, 1976.

Lithotripsy. Columbus: Ohio Kidney Stone Center, 1991.

Lyme disease opens new opportunities and new risks for pest control industry. *The Bell Report,* 8 (3). Madison, WI: Bell Laboratories, Inc., June/July 1989.

Majzesik, Cathy, RN, MS. et. al. Radioimmunoguided surgery in primary colon cancer. *Cancer Detection and Prevention,* 14 (6). CRC Press, Inc.

Marieb, Elaine N. *Essentials of Human Anatomy and Physiology.* Menlo Park: Benjamin/Cummings, 1984.

Memmler, Ruth L., and Wood, Dena L. *Structure and Function of the Human Body,* 4th ed. Philadelphia: J.B. Lippincott, 1987.

Morris, Getta. Lyme disease: Summer's scourge. *New Choices,* 31 (6). New York: Retirement Living Publishing Co., June 1991.

Nurses Reference Library. *Assessment.* Springhouse, PA: Springhouse, 1983.

Nurses Reference Library. *Diagnostics.* Springhouse, PA: Springhouse, 1983.

Nurses Reference Library. *Diseases.* Springhouse, PA: Springhouse, 1983.

Nurses Reference Library. *Procedures.* Springhouse, PA: Springhouse, 1983.

91 Questions and Answers About AIDS. Columbus: The Columbus Health Department Medical Services/AIDS Program, 1991.

Roitt, Ivan. *Essential Immunology,* 7th ed., Oxford: Blackwell, 1991.

Schindler, Lydia Woods. *Understanding the Human Immune System.* US Department of Health and Human Services, NIH Publication No 90–529. Washington: National Cancer Institute, 1990.

Smith, Genevieve L., Davis, Phyllis E., and Dennerll, Jean Tannis. *Medical Terminology,* 6th ed., Albany: Delmar, 1991.

Starr, Cecie. and Taggart, Ralph. *Biology, The Unity and Diversity of Life,* 5th ed. Belmont: Wadsworth, 1989.

Taber, Clarence. W. *Taber's Cyclopedic Medical Dictionary,* 14th ed. Philadelphia: F.A. Davis, 1981.

The National Kidney Foundation. New York:
CAPD, a New Alternative to Dialysis. 1990.
About Kidney Stones. 1990.

U.S. Public Health Service. *Surgeon general's report on Acquired Immune Deficiency Syndrome.*
Understanding AIDS. HHS–88–8404.
HIV/AIDS Surveillance Report. March 1992.

University of California at Berkeley, School of Public Health. *Wellness Letter:*
Hepatitis B: Despite an effective vaccine, the spread of the disease isn't slowing. Vol. 7, No. 8, April 1991.
Lyme disease. Vol. 7, No. 10, July 1991.
Preventing carpal tunnel syndrome. Vol. 7, No. 7, April 1991.
Progress on the mystery disease (CFS). Vol. 7, No. 9, June 1991.
Skin cancer: As the ozone layer thins, the risk of cancer goes up. Vol. 7, No. 10, July 1991.
Why call it a disease when it's not? Vol. 7 Issue 8, May 1991.

Yoffe, Emily. An alternative to hysterectomy. *Newsweek,* October 1990.

The Clinical Medical Assistant

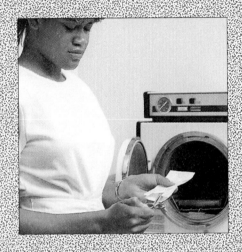

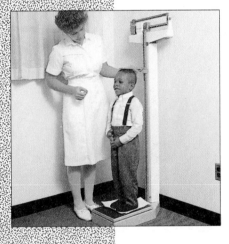

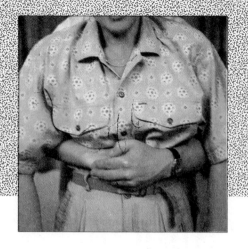

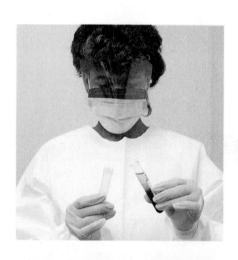

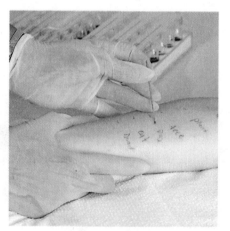

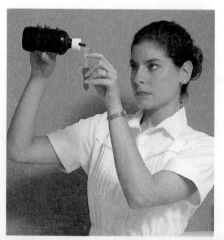

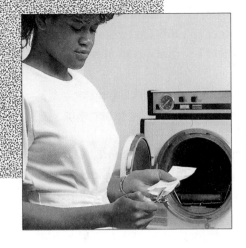

C H A P T E R 1 4

The Medical Assistant as Clinical Assistant

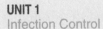

UNIT 1
Infection Control

To be a valuable employee, the clinical assistant must be proficient in many skills. Patients will ask many questions regarding their illnesses and treatments. You should be able to reply with correct and understandable information. You are also expected to be knowledgeable about office policies. And because health care costs are so high, you must perform tasks in a minimal amount of time while also conserving supplies. It is up to each medical assistant to practice the necessary skills. Patience and perseverance are necessary to reach the goal of proficiency.

You will be assisting in many procedures that are extremely personal in nature. Considering the patient's feelings and emotions will help in dealing with these delicate matters. The procedures patients must experience are sometimes painful, often discomforting, and may be embarrassing for them. You must always try to ease the patient's fears and anxieties. Always ask patients if they have any questions concerning the examination or procedure for which they are scheduled. Procedures that have become routine to you and other medical personnel may be new or at least unfamiliar to patients. Patients may be apprehensive not only about the procedure itself, but about what the physician may find. Finally, patients usually do not feel well and are not themselves. Empathy and understanding in handling patients will make tasks much more pleasant.

Patients who are intellectually impaired or developmentally disabled, hearing impaired or deaf, sight impaired or blind, elderly, senile, or non-English speaking may need the undivided attention of the medical assistant during their visit and may take considerably more time than the average patient. Make appropriate adjustments in scheduling whenever necessary. Any significant information should be noted on the schedule and in the patient's chart to avoid awkward situations. Kindness and patience are important qualities to use especially with these patients. Assistance should be offered, but not imposed.

You should make an effort to speak directly to the patient, but you may also communicate necessary instructions to the person who accompanies the patient. Writing instructions down for these patients is one way to eliminate uncertainties concerning the patient's care. If the patient seems to be in need of a service that you know is available, your suggestion may be well received. Some people are unaware of community services and are grateful for advice.

Being friendly is a sure way to gain rapport with patients. Even the blind will hear a smile in your voice. All people smile in the same language.

For vision-impaired or blind patients, it is appropriate to offer to take their arm to guide them. You must also explain what is going on and describe floor plans and furniture arrangements to help the patient feel more comfortable especially during times when you are not present.

In communicating with the deaf or hearing-impaired patient, you should speak clearly in a normal tone of voice while facing the patient so that your lips can be read. If the patient does not read lips, you can write notes to explain procedures and other important information.

Patients who have physical disabilities are usually self-sufficient and will need little if any assistance in getting around. Try to make them feel comfortable and do not dwell on their disabilities.

All of us can learn a great deal from patients who have a disability, no matter what it may be, for they have learned to accept life and make the best of it.

In addition to giving special regard to patients, health care workers have the responsibility of self-protection. It is recommended that universal blood and body fluid precautions be used for all patients, especially when the infection status of the patient is unknown. Appropriate protection against exposure to blood and body fluids should be routine practice for all health care workers. Gloves should be worn when in contact (direct or indirect) with blood or any body fluids, mucous membranes, or nonintact skin; in handling items or surfaces soiled with blood or body fluid; and when performing venipuncture or any other surgical procedure. After each patient contact, gloves should be changed. If procedures could possibly generate droplets of blood or other body

fluids, the health care worker should wear shields to protect the eyes or face in addition to gloves and gown. This will protect the mucous membranes of the eyes, mouth, and nose.

After gloves are removed, hands should be thoroughly washed. If hands and/or other skin surfaces have been in contact with blood or other body fluids, they should be washed immediately.

At all times, extreme caution must be used by health care workers in handling needles, scalpels, and other sharp instruments to avoid self-injury. To prevent possible self-injury, it is recommended that needles should never be recapped, broken off, or removed from disposable syringes by hand after use. They should be carefully placed in puncture-proof containers near the area for practical purposes. Reusable needles should be placed in a receptacle (puncture-proof) for sanitization and sterilization.

All infectious waste must be disposed of by placing each contaminated item in its appropriate hazardous waste container provided by the agency specified by your employer. Any disposable material that has even a trace of human tissue, blood, or other body fluid on it must be considered as infectious and must be treated with extreme caution. Latex gloves must be worn when handling any contaminated item to reduce the possibility of disease transmission, especially acquired immunodeficiency syndrome (AIDS) and hepatitis B virus. The precautions are recommended for all health care professionals by the Centers for Disease Control (CDC) and the United States Public Health Service.

U N I T   1
Infection Control

OBJECTIVES ....

Upon completion of this unit, the student will meet the following terminal performance objectives by verifying knowledge of the facts and principles presented through oral and written communication at a level deemed competent, and will demonstrate the specific behaviors as identified in the terminal performance objectives of the

procedures, observing all aseptic and safety precautions in accordance with health care standards.

1. Describe methods of control of growth of microorganisms.
2. List the growth requirements of microorganisms.
3. Describe the infection cycle of disease transmission.
4. Describe the body's defenses against infection.
5. Demonstrate the proper procedure for handwashing.
6. Identify disinfectants and antiseptics commonly used in the medical office.
7. Explain the difference between sanitization, disinfection, and sterilization.
8. State the purpose of autoclaving.
9. Demonstrate the procedure for wrapping items to be autoclaved. (Note: Many different types of autoclaves or sterilizers are on the market; all have cleaning and operating instructions prominently displayed.)
10. Locate and interpret from the communicable disease chart the means of transmission, incubation time, symptoms, and treatment for a given disease.
11. Explain the reasons for sterilizing all used items, even disposables, before discarding.
12. Discuss the recommended universal precautions in regard to human tissue, blood, and body fluids.
13. Spell and define, using the glossary at the back of the text, all the words to know in this unit.

WORDS TO KNOW ....

aerobe	fungi	petechial
anaerobes	heterotrophs	*p*H
asepsis	hygiene	protozoa
autotrophs	incinerate	pruritic
bacteria	inorganic	pustular
biohazardous	malaise	resistance
coma	microorganism	seizures
confinement	morphology	spores
contaminate	nits	sterile
debilitated	obligate	susceptible
droplet	organic	vulnerable
facultative	parasite	virulence
fecal	pathogen	virus

One potential problem in any medical practice is disease transmission, and precautions must be taken to reduce this possibility. Microorganisms have certain requirements for growth. Making sure those requirements are not met will maintain asepsis, so that disease transmission need not be a concern.

Handwashing ....

The first responsibility of the medical assistant is to perform the handwashing procedure before beginning the

The medical assistant has a perfect opportunity to instruct patients in the area of basic aseptic technique. During the patients' scheduled appointments it is appropriate to inform patients about proper handwashing and other methods to use at home, especially when one is sick, in preventing the transfer of disease to others. Good personal hygiene practice should be stressed to patients. The following general guidelines are suggested to help decrease the possibility of disease transmission among family members and others who share living/work/social facilities:

1. Frequent handwashing before and after: especially when taking care of one who is ill, eating, using the toilet, touching soiled objects, or being in direct contact with any body fluids.
2. Encourage daily personal hygiene: shower/bath, dental care, clean clothes/bedding.
3. Always properly wash glasses, dishes, and utensils before reuse (when one is ill with a highly contagious disease, it is best to use disposable items to decrease the possibility of spreading the disease). Remind patients *not* to share their germs by eating, drinking, or smoking after one another.
4. Instruct patients to cough/sneeze into a disposable tissue, use once, and discard in a paper or plastic bag and dispose of properly.
5. Advise patients about the importance of proper ventilation and light (microorganisms do not prosper in a lighted and well-ventilated area).
6. Remind patients to wash hands after touching door knobs, railings, handles, and so on, to avoid the possibility of getting or giving invisible microorganisms.
7. Advise patients to use a commercial disinfectant routinely to clean bathrooms and kitchens (as well as other rooms in the house as necessary) to eliminate germs and discourage insects and rodents that carry disease.
8. Urge sexually active patients of adolescent age and older to use condoms properly to prevent spread of sexually transmitted diseases, AIDS and hepatitis B (discretion must be used).
9. Remind patients about immunization schedules and urge them to follow them carefully.

As item number 6 advises, all microorganisms are invisible to the naked eye. Therefore, it is easy to forget that they are everywhere. The medical assistant can be most influential in educating others in ways to reduce the threat of disease by following these basic guidelines.

HANDWASHING

TERMINAL PERFORMANCE OBJECTIVE: Provided with liquid hand soap in a dispenser, cuticle stick, nail brush, paper towels, and waste receptacle, the student will stand at a sink with hot and cold faucets and demonstrate each step in the handwashing procedure as specified in the procedure sheet.

EQUIPMENT: A liquid soap dispenser is desirable. It eliminates the possibility of dropping a bar of soap in the sink or on the floor during the procedure. It is also more economical and more attractive. Bar soap is often wasted as it becomes soft and starts to separate. The water that collects in the soap dish is also a good environment for microorganisms and therefore cancels the effort made in removing them from the hands.

1. Remove all jewelry: rings, bracelets, watches (wedding rings may be left on but must be scrubbed). **Key Point: If next procedure to be performed requires sterile technique, jewelry may not be replaced until after sterile procedures are completed.**

2. Stand at sink and turn faucets on using paper towel to avoid direct contact with faucets, Figure 14–1. Adjust water temperature to moderately warm and discard paper towel. Leave water running at desired temperature. **Key Point: Be careful not to touch sink with any part of the body.**

3. Wet hands and press soap dispenser to obtain approximately 1 teaspoon of soap in palm of one hand. Work soap into lather and distribute soap over both palms and backs of hands in circular motions constantly and vigorously for 2 minutes.
   Key Points:
   a. **Use nail brush on nails and all areas of hands and fingers, rubbing with approximately a dozen motions.**
   b. **Use a cuticle stick to remove material brush may not reach under nails.**

4. Rinse well being careful not to touch inside of sink or faucets during procedure. **Key Point: Lab area will have a "clean" sink for washing hands, but it is not sterile and therefore will contaminate hands. "Dirty" sink is used for contaminated items.**

5. Reapply 1 teaspoon of soap from dispenser into palm of one had and begin lathering up to elbows of both arms. Key Point: Use nail brush in circular motion to scrub forearms, approximately a dozen motions, and rinse well.

6. Rinse hands thoroughly. Leave water running and reach for sufficient paper towels to dry hands and arms completely. Turn off water, touching faucets with paper towels.

Refer to the patient education section for guidelines that all health care professionals should also follow.

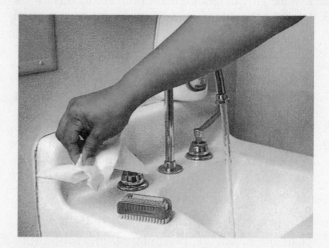

FIGURE 14–1a A dry paper towel should be used to turn the faucet on.

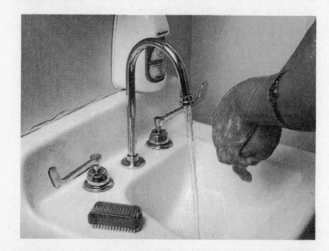

FIGURE 14–1b Fingertips should be pointed down while washing hands. Use the palm of one hand to clean the back of the other hand.

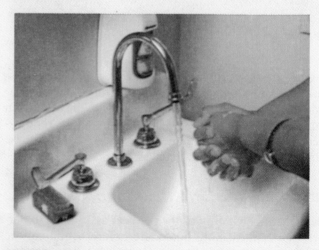

FIGURE 14–1c Interlace the fingers to clean between them.

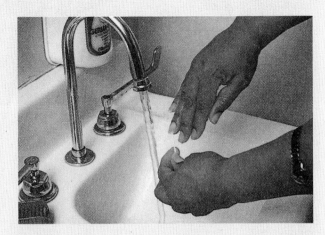

FIGURE 14–1d Use the blunt edge of an orange cuticle stick to clean the nails.

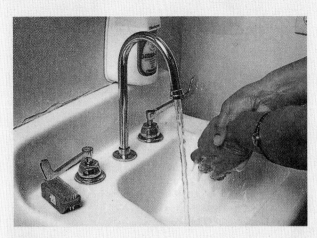

FIGURE 14–1f Rinse the hands thoroughly with the fingertips down.

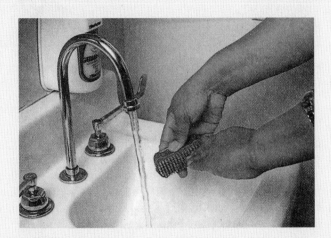

FIGURE 14–1e Another way to clean under the fingernails is to use a hand brush.

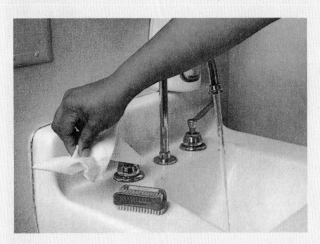

FIGURE 14–1g Use paper towels to dry hands and to turn off water faucets.

(Photos from Henger and Caldwell, *Nursing Assistant: A Nursing Process Approach,* 6th ed. Copyright 1992, Delmar Publishers Inc.)

daily routine. It is also important to repeat this procedure after breaks, lunch, and after any other procedure that may contaminate the hands and therefore allow disease to be transmitted.

Disease Transmission ....

Microorganisms cannot be seen with the naked eye. Commonly known microorganisms are viruses, bacteria, protozoa, fungi, and parasites. Disease-producing microorganisms are called pathogens.

Bacteria are unicellular microorganisms that vary in their morphology. Figure 14–2, page 412, shows the various forms of bacteria. Many different species of bacteria are pathogenic to humans and animals. Some examples: *Escherichia coli* causes urinary tract infections (among other illnesses) in humans; *Bordetella pertussis* causes whooping cough, which is transmitted by droplet

infection; and *Vibrio cholerae* causes cholera in humans who ingest contaminated food and water.

Viruses, which are the smallest of the microorganisms, may be viewed only by an electron microscope. Figure 14–3, page 413, shows a magnified view of a virus. Viruses can only reproduce themselves within a host. Commonly known viruses are: herpes virus, most childhood diseases, the common cold, and influenza virus.

Protozoa are complex single-celled microorganisms that attach themselves to other organisms, Figure 14–4, page 413. Amebic dysentery, malaria, and trichomonas vaginalis are diseases caused by protozoa.

Fungi are simple parasitic plants (molds) that depend on other life forms for a nutritional source. They reproduce by budding. Multicellular fungi reproduce by spore formation. Approximately 100 fungi are common in humans; however, only 10 of these are pathogenic. Some

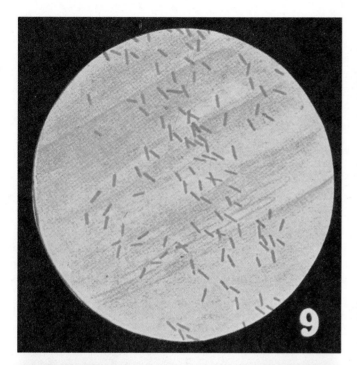

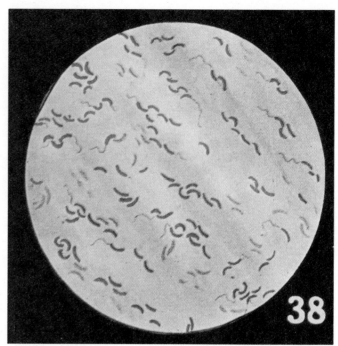

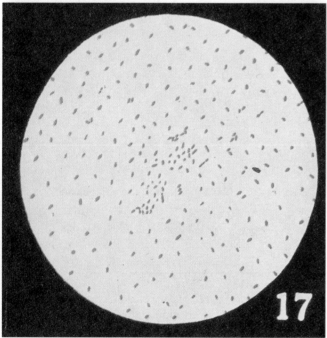

FIGURE 14–2a–c Bacterial forms: (a). *Escherichia coli.* (b). *Hemophilus pertussis.* (c). *Vibrio cholerae.* (Courtesy of the Centers for Disease Control, Atlanta, GA)

examples of pathogenic fungus conditions are histoplasmosis caused by *Histoplasma capsulatum,* and tinea pedis (athlete's foot), Figure 14–5.

Parasites are organisms that depend on another living organism for nourishment. An obligate parasite is one that depends completely on its host for survival. Facultative parasites are able to live independently from their hosts at times. Protozoa mentioned earlier are internal parasites for they live within the body of a human or an animal. *External parasites* are those that attach themselves on the outside of the body, such as fleas and ticks

on animals. Humans are sometimes troubled with the itch mite (scabies), pinworms (*Enterobius vermicularis*) and hookworms (*ancylostomiasis*), Figure 14–6. Other microorganisms are helpful and necessary to normal flora in humans and animals for they provide a balance in the body and destroy pathogens.

Microorganisms that feed on organic matter are called heterotrophs; those that feed on inorganic matter are called autotrophs. Those that need oxygen to grow are called aerobes and those that grow best in the absence of oxygen are called anaerobes. Microorganisms grow best at the average body temperature (98.6°F or 37°C). The human body has not only a desirable temperature for microbial growth, but also furnishes darkness and moisture, other growth requirements. In addition, the body has a neutral pH, making it a prime target for infection. An environment that is too acid or too alkaline will not support microbial growth.

Disease begins when a pathogen finds a body (a host) that offers it the conditions necessary for growth, Figure 14–7, page 415. Microorganisms, in the proper growth environment, can be extremely virulent, particularly for debilitated, aged, or young vulnerable patients. When the microorganism has reached the stage of causing an infection, the host should take precautions against transmitting it to another. Confinement is the best way, but many patients insist on taking their colds and flu to work or play. The next step in the cycle, then, is transmission to another by way of body openings. The microorganisms leave the host through the discharge of body secretions and make either direct or indirect contact with another host. When a patient with a cold coughs or sneezes, for example, the vapor contains the microorgan-

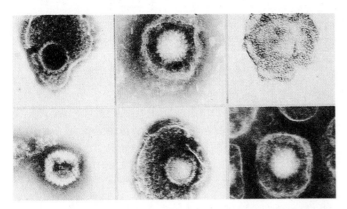

FIGURE 14–3 Electron micrographs of the various types of herpes simplex virus. (Courtesy of the Centers for Disease Control, Atlanta, GA)

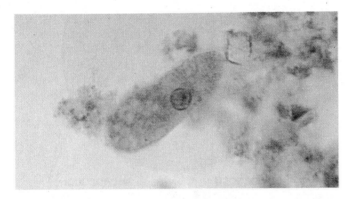

FIGURE 14–4 Intestinal protozoa *Entamoeba coli* (Courtesy of the Centers for Disease Control, Atlanta, GA)

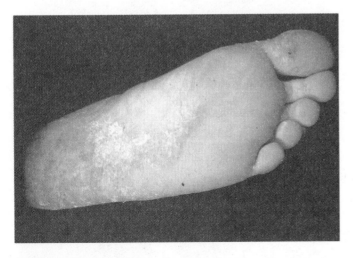

FIGURE 14–5 Ringworm of foot (tinea pedis) (Courtesy of the Centers for Disease Control, Atlanta, GA)

ism that is causing the infection, Figure 14–8, page 416. Someone else may then breathe in that microorganism. This is called *droplet infection* and is a form of indirect contact. Direct contact is through touch. The growth requirement is then a susceptible host, or one whose body resistance is low because of poor nutritional habits, or poor hygiene.

Disease Prevention

To prevent the spread of diseases caused by microorganisms it is necessary to provide a defense against them. Becoming aware that the threat of disease is always present will assist you in taking the necessary precautions. Routine cleaning procedures, such as disinfecting room equipment and surfaces, are one means of disease control. Patients should be educated in this area, and it is the responsibility of the medical assistant and the other members of the health care team to see that it is practiced. Refer to Table 14–1, pages 415-16, to learn the common communicable diseases, means of transmission, incubation time, symptoms, and treatment.

Another defense against disease is maintenance of good health through good health habits of proper rest, nutrition, and hygiene. Exercise is most helpful in resisting disease because it promotes circulation, encourages nutrition, and reduces stress.

The body also has defense mechanisms. In the respiratory tract are hairlike cilia that filter out invading pathogens. Coughing and sneezing are reflexes to rid the body of invaders. Body secretions such as tears, sweat, urine, and mucus also wash pathogens from the body.

The body secretions have a low *p*H, which discourages bacterial growth. In the digestive tract, hydrochloric acid discourages the growth of pathogens with its low *p*H.

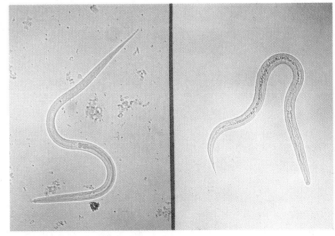

FIGURE 14–6 Strongyloides—filariform larvae of hookworm and strongyloides. (Courtesy of the Centers for Disease Control, Atlanta, GA)

TABLE 14–1
COMMUNICABLE DISEASES

Disease	Means of Transmission	Incubation	Symptoms	Treatment
AIDS (Acquired immunodeficiency syndrome)*	Direct contact: sexual, anal, or vaginal intercourse, sharing IV drug needles, infected mother to child (childbirth), blood to blood (from cuts, scrapes, punctures of skin) Indirect contact: blood transfusions	Onset of AIDS following infection with human immunodeficiency virus (HIV) from 6 months to 10 years +	Early—loss of appetite, weight loss, fever, night sweats, skin rashes, diarrhea, fatigue, poor resistance to infections, swollen lymph notes Later—cough, fever, shortness of breath, dyspnea, purple blotches on the skin	Research and new developments continue in the search for a cure and/or a vaccine. Current treatment most commonly used is zidovudine (AZT)
Chickenpox* (Varicellazoster virus)	Direct or indirect contact, droplet, or airborne secretion of infected person	2—3 weeks, usually 13—17 days	Crops of pruritic vesicular eruptions on the skin, slight fever and headache, malaise	Bed rest, topical antipruritics
Common Colds (Upper respiratory infection—URI)	Direct or indirect contact with infected person	12—72 hours (some viruses 2—7 days), usually 24 hours	Slight sore throat, watery eyes, runny nose, sneezing, chills, malaise, low–grade fever	Rest, decongestant mild analgesics, increased fluid intake
Conjunctivitis* (Pink eye)	Direct or indirect contact with discharge from eyes or upper respiratory tract of infected person	Viral: 24 hours to days Bacterial: 24—72 hours	Redness of eyes, itching, burning of eyes, matted eyelashes	Antibacterial agents, antibiotics, corticosteroids depending on causative agent
Head Lice* (Pediculosis)	Direct contact with infected person; indirect contact, rare	1 week (nits, or eggs, hatch in 1 week, mature in 2 weeks)	Itching of scalp, presence of small light gray lice and nits (eggs) at the base of hairs	Topical use of 1% lindane: shampoo, lotion, or cream (7—10 days); comb nits from hair; launder washable items in hot water with hottest drying cycle, dry–clean or seal in plastic bags nonwashable items (2 weeks); Thoroughly vacuum the environment
Haemophilus influenzae Type b Hib (H-flu)*	Direct and indirect contact and droplet infection from respiratory tract	3 days+	URI symptoms, fever, aches, sleepiness, no appetite; as disease progresses, child is irritable and fussy	Antibiotics, increased fluid intake, antipyretics, rest, analgesics
Hepatitis A* (Acute infective hepatitis)	Direct contact or by fecal–contaminated food or water	14—50 days, avg. 25—30 days	Slow onset, fever, malaise, loss of appetite, nausea, vomiting, jaundice, weakness, dark urine, whitish stool	Bed rest, increased fluid intake, proper nourishment (no fats or alcohol)
Hepatitis B* (Serum hepatitis)	Contaminated serum in blood transfusion or by use of contaminated needles or instruments	14—50 days	Same as above, of rapid onset, of acute symptoms	Same as above
Herpes Simplex Virus (HSV) (Cold sores, fever blisters)	Direct contact with infected person	2—14 days, usually 4—6 days	Painful blisters on lips, which turn pustular and then form crusted scabs; oral lesions are small ulcerated areas	Topical applications of drying medications. Antibiotics for secondary infections
Impetigo	Direct contact with draining sores	2—10 days	Blisterlike lesions (later become crusted), itching	Cleansing of areas with antibacterial soap and water, topical and/or oral antibiotics
Influenza*	Direct and indirect contact and by airborne secretions.	1—3 days	Sudden onset of fever, chills, headache, sore muscles, malaise, (commonly runny nose, sore throat, and cough)	Bed rest, increased fluid intake, antipyretics
Meningitis* (Aseptic)	Direct contact, fecal–oral route, and respiratory secretions	2—21 days	Sudden or gradual fever, intense headache, nausea, vomiting, stiff neck, irritability, sluggishness	Hospitalization, bed rest, increased fluid intake, antipyretics, analgesics

Meningitis* (Bacterial) Haemophilus and Meningococcal	Direct contact and droplet infection from respiratory tract	1—10 days, usually 3—4 days	Sudden onset, fever, intense headache, nausea, vomiting; sometimes petechial rash, irritability, sluggishness (possible seizures and/or coma)	Same as above plus antibiotics, by intravenous and/or oral administration
Pinworms (Enterobius vermicularis)	Direct transfer of eggs from anus to mouth; indirect contact with eggs in clothing, bedding	3 weeks—3 months	Anal itching, insomnia, irritability	Anthelmintics, initiate scrupulous personal hygiene, shorten fingernails. Launder washable items in hottest or boiled water
Scabies*	Direct contact or indirect contact with infected clothing/bedding	2—6 weeks	Intense itching of small raised areas of skin that contain fluid or tiny burrows under the skin, resembling a line—may be anywhere on the body	Topical scabicide, oral antihistamines, and sabicylates to reduce itching
Strep Throat	Direct contact	1—3 days	Fever, red and sore throat, pus spots on back of throat, tender and swollen glands of neck	Antibiotics, analgesics, antipyretics, increase fluid intake
Scarlet Fever* (Scarlatina) (Streptococcal)	Direct or indirect contact	1—7 days	Same as above, plus strawberry tongue, rash of skin and inside mouth, high fever, nausea, and vomiting	Same as above, plus bed rest

*Report these diseases to local health department. Refer also to sexually transmitted diseases in Chapter 13, Unit 13.

Source: *Medical Assisting*, Delmar Publishers Inc.

The methods of preventing disease transmission in the medical practice are many. Sanitization is one that has already been described. *Sanitization* is washing and scrubbing to remove such material as body tissue, blood, or other body fluids. You should wear gloves during this process to protect your hands from dryness, which may result in chafing and cracking of the skin and possibly lead to infection. Items should be rinsed in cool water, soaked in a detergent solution, usually for 20 minutes, washed thoroughly with a brush, rinsed in warm to hot water to remove the detergent, and dried.

Disinfection is a process by which disease-producing microorganisms are killed. There are many disinfectant solutions in use. The most common are zephirin chloride and chlorophenyl. Disinfectants are used on objects, not patients. They are chemical solutions that must be changed often to ensure their effect. Antiseptics are used in preparing the patient's skin for injection or surgical procedures. The most commonly used are alcohol and betadine.

Disinfectants and antiseptics do not always kill spores, however. Spores are thick-walled hard capsules formed

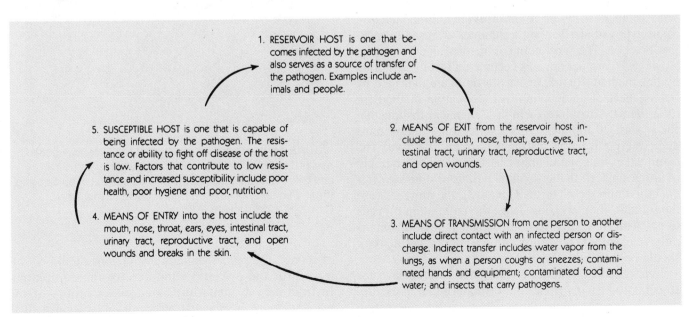

FIGURE 14–7 The infection cycle

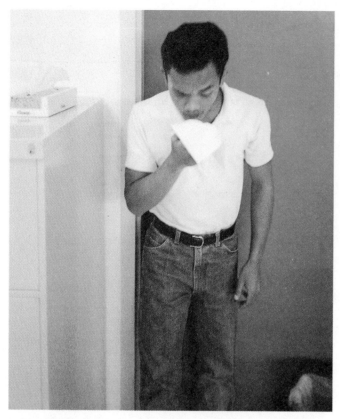

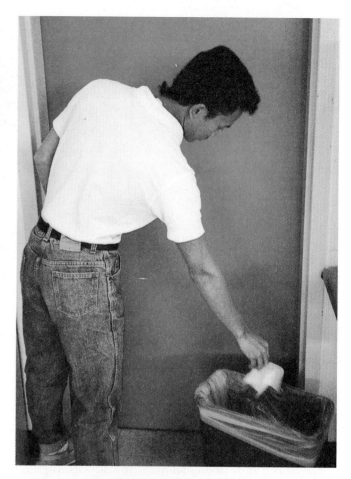

FIGURE 14–8 (a) Patient coughing/sneezing into a tissue to prevent the spread of microorganisms to others. (b). Patient properly discarding used tissue into waste receptacle.

by some bacteria when conditions for growth are poor. When the proper growth requirements are present the bacteria break out of the capsule, grow, and multiply to start infection. An example of bacteria that produce spores is *Clostridum tetani,* the cause of tetanus, or lock jaw.

Something that is free of all living microorganisms and spores is considered sterile. *Sterilization* is the process that destroys all forms of living microorganisms. Many types of sterilization techniques are used in medical practice. The most common method is autoclaving. However, sharp instruments become dull from sterilizing by this method. Rubber or vinyl articles are damaged by intense heat of autoclaving. An alternative method for these items is to place them in a chemical disinfectant for at least 20 minutes. This disinfectant solution must completely cover the instruments to be effective. The disinfectant must be changed periodically. The number of articles placed in this solution will determine how frequently it must be changed. Obviously, the more you use the solution for sterilizing items, the more often it needs to be changed. If this means of sterilizing instruments is only occasional, changing the solution once a week should be sufficient, Figure 14–9.

Every medical practice should have an autoclave for sterilization of instruments by steam under pressure, which is the only method that guarantees the destruction

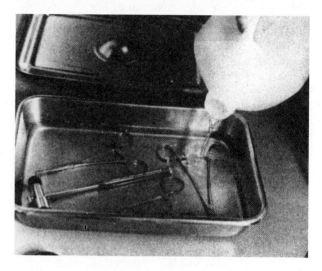

FIGURE 14–9 Chemical disinfectant solutions are used for aseptic control of sharp instruments (dulled by autoclaving) and other articles damaged by the intense heat of autoclaving. (From Simmers, *Diversified Health Occupations,* 2d ed. Copyright 1988, Delmar Publishers Inc.)

of spores. The manufacturer's instructions should be followed for the operation and care of the equipment. Instructions are usually printed either on top of the machine or on a tray that pulls out underneath it. It is

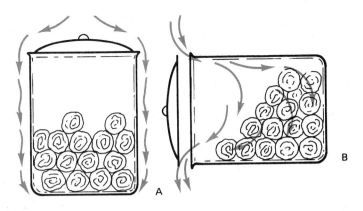

FIGURE 14–10 The (a) incorrect and (b) correct way to place jars of dressing in the sterilizer

TABLE 14–2
STERILIZATION TIMES AND TEMPERATURES

Articles	Time 250° to 254° (121° to 123°C)
Glassware. empty. inverted	
Instruments. metal in covered or open tray. padded or unpadded	15 minutes
Needles. unwrapped	
Syringes. unassembled. unwrapped	
Flasked solutions. 75–250 ml	
Instruments. metal combined with other materials in covered and/or padded tray	
Instruments wrapped in double-thickness muslin	20 minutes
Rubber gloves. catheters. drains. tubing, etc. unwrapped or wrapped in muslin or paper	
Dressings. wrapped in paper or muslin—small packs only	
Flasked solutions, 500–1000ml	
Needles. individually packaged in glass tubes or paper	
Syringes. unassembled. individually packed in muslin or paper	30 minutes
Sutures. silk. cotton, or nylon. wrapped in paper or muslin	
Treatment trays. wrapped in muslin or paper	

Source: *Medical Assisting*, Delmar Publishers Inc.

STERILIZATION OF SYRINGES, ETC.
CAT. NO.1866-0103   10 & 20cc

"ANOTHER □ A.P.S □ PRODUCT"
FOR -

THE PINK
ARROWS
TURNS
BROWN ▶
WITH PROPER
AUTOCLAVING

THE PINK
"BULLS-EYE"
TURNS
BROWN ▶
WITH PROPER
AUTOCLAVING

DATE_____

NEEDLE_____

SYRINGE   (Circle One)
2cc
5cc
10cc
20cc

_____APPLICATORS_____
_____CLAMPS_____
_____FORCEPS_____
_____INSTRUMENT_____
_____
_____
_____
_____PADS_____
_____SCISSORS_____
_____SPONGES_____
_____TONGUE BLADES_____

FIGURE 14–11 Envelope-type packaging for autoclaving

important that the desired temperature of the sterilizer be maintained for the proper amount of time. Table 14–2 lists the most commonly used articles and the desired times and temperatures for sterilization.

In the process of sterilization the autoclave exerts approximately 15 pounds of steam pressure per square inch at a temperature between 250° and 254°F. The steam flows through the items and destroys all microorganisms and spores, Figure 14–10.

Articles to be autoclaved must be sanitized and then wrapped in a double thickness of paper or muslin. Envelope packaging is manufactured for some instruments such as scissors, Figure 14–11. Figure 14–12, page 418, shows a medical assistant inserting an instrument into an envelope type of packaging in preparation for autoclaving. A section on the paper envelope permits recording the instrument name, the date, and the initials of the person who sterilized it. Sterilization indicators register proper and complete sterilization, Figure 14–13, page 418. Autoclave tape has an indicator stripe that changes

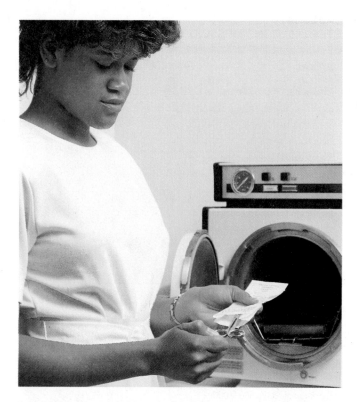

FIGURE 14–12 Placing an instrument into an envelope package for autoclaving

color when the proper temperature has been maintained for a long enough time for sterilization to have taken place. The same principle applies to indicators placed inside the wrapped package.

Some offices or medical centers use the autoclaving service of a hospital. In this case, minimum cleaning is all that is necessary, for all items are properly sanitized before autoclaving.

With the identification of the disease AIDS, precautions must be taken to eliminate the transmission of this virus. Extreme caution must be practiced whenever the medical assistant, or any member of the health care team, comes into contact with any body fluid. Appropriate barriers, such as latex gloves, goggles, masks, or other protective coverings must be worn when procedures performed on patients could cause possible contamination.

All items, whether disposable or reusable, must be properly autoclaved. The sterilized disposables may then be discarded in proper receptacles without fear of transmitting the AIDS virus. Blood and other body fluid specimens must also be sterilized before discarding.

Many companies provide this service for medical facilities with large volumes. They supply containers in various sizes for disposables and schedule periodic pickup of these biohazardous items to take back to the company for sterilization before discarding in general city trash dumps.

Any disposable items, such as needles (never recap), scalpels, suture removal forceps and scissors, and the like, must be placed in the container, Figure 14–14, for

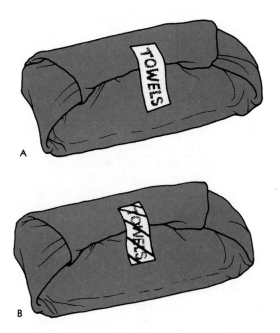

FIGURE 14–13 Package of towels (a) before and (b) after autoclaving. Note that the sterilized package has diagonal lines on the tape, a positive sign that autoclaving has been done correctly.

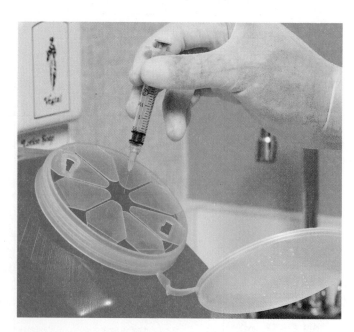

FIGURE 14–14 Discard the entire disposable syringe with used needle intact in the biohazardous sharps container.

WRAP ITEMS FOR AUTOCLAVE

PURPOSE: To wrap items to be autoclaved so that they will be protected from contamination after the sterilization process is completed for storage and handling.

EQUIPMENT: muslin/autoclave paper/disposable paper bags/envelopes, autoclave tape, items to be sterilized/autoclaved, sterilization indicator, pen.

TERMINAL PERFORMANCE OBJECTIVE: Provided with several items, to be autoclaved/sterilized, the student will wrap each in autoclave paper/muslin, in preparation for the sterilization process. Each item must be wrapped neatly and snugly but not too tightly; the instructor and student will jointly determine if each wrapped item is suitable for autoclaving.

After the paper wrapping procedure is demonstrated and checked, the paper should be removed from each item and discarded. The above-stated procedure will be repeated using muslin cloth (Note: when the muslin cloth wrapping procedure is completed, the muslin cloth is retained).

1. Wash hands and assemble all necessary items. **Key Point: Work in a clean area where there is sufficient work space.**

2. Check items for flaws and to make sure that they function properly. **Key Point: Items must be sanitized before wrapping for autoclave process.**

3. Wrap item(s) in desired wrap so that there is a double thickness of protection. Make sure that there is no opening and seal with autoclave tape. Wrap item(s) snugly but not too tightly, Figure 14–15.

Key Points:

a. **Double thickness and complete covering protect item from pathogenic entry.**

b. **Wrapping items too tightly will prevent steam from freely penetrating during sterilization process.**

c. **For envelope wrap, place item into envelope, seal, and label.**

d. **Place spinal needles (small items) in glass test tube with cotton or gauze padding at bottom. Wrap autoclave tape around top to seal, with a pull tab for ease in opening. Label contents on a piece of tape secured to glass. (Note: including, but not limited to, forceps, hemostats, needle holders, and towel clamps.) (This performance may also be extended to include autoclave envelopes/bags; office policy differs with preference.)**

e. **All hinged instruments must be autoclaved open.**

4. Make a tab for ease in opening wrapped packages after autoclaving by taping 1 to 2 inches of tape to itself at edge of package.

5. Label contents, write date and your initials on tape. **Key Point: Refer to Table 14–2 for proper time and temperature for items to be autoclaved.**

6. Return all items to proper storage area when finished.

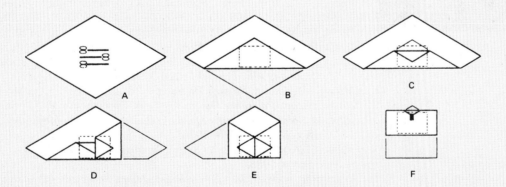

FIGURE 14–15 To wrap instruments for autoclaving: (a) place items in center of wrap, (b) fold the material up from the bottom, (c) double back a small corner, (d) fold the right and then (e) left edges in, again leaving corners doubled back, (f) fold the pack up from the bottom and secure with pressure-sensitive tape.

company sterilization or wrapped and sterilized before discarding in a general trash receptacle.

Another type of sterilization is by flame. This is a method for completely destroying disposable items by **incineration.** Items that will be treated in this way must be properly bagged for the procedure so that anyone handling the contaminated articles will not be affected.

Still another method of sterilization is the *dry heat oven.* Instruments with sharp blades, such as scissors or scalpels, are sometimes sterilized in this way. It is not the most desirable sterilization method, because it is time-consuming. The process takes 1 to 2 hours at a temperature of 350°F, depending on the article. It is *not* a way to sterilize items made of rubber. For rubber articles, thorough washing and rinsing is the first step in preparing them for reuse. They must be completely dry before being placed in a disinfectant for chemical sterilization. Spores may still be a threat with this method. Finally, in every medical practice the policy of the establishment must be followed.

Complete Chapter 14 in the workbook to help you meet the objectives at the beginning of this unit and therefore achieve competency of this subject matter.

MEDICAL-LEGAL ETHICAL HIGHLIGHTS

Mr. Right...

is always careful when handling specimens and follows all universal precautions when assisting with invasive procedures. He remembers to wash his hands and glove properly before and after each patient with which he comes in contact. He places all waste in the appropriate receptacles.

Promotion outlook: Excellent

Ms. Wrong...

is careless about following universal precautions and frequently forgets to wear gloves or other protective coverings when assisting with invasive procedures. Other health care team members are tiring of reminding her about disposing of waste appropriately.

Promotion outlook: Poor

REFERENCES

Fong, Elizabeth, and Ferris, Elvira. *Microbiology for Health Careers*, 4th ed. Albany: Delmar, 1987.

Garza, Diana, and Becan-McBride. *Phlebotomy Handbook.* 2d ed. East Norwalk, CT: Appleton and Lange, 1989.

Miller, Benjamin F., and Keane, Claire Brackman. *Encyclopedia and Dictionary of Medicine and Allied Health*, 3d ed. Philadelphia: W.B. Saunders, 1983.

Mosby's Medical & Nursing Dictionary, 3d ed. St. Louis: C.V. Mosby, 1990.

Nurse's Ready Reference Diagnostic Tests. Springhouse, PA: Springhouse, 1991.

Raphael, Stanley S. Lynch's Medical Laboratory Technology, 3d ed. Windsor, Ontario: W.B. Saunders, 1976.

Taber, Clarence W. *Taber's Cyclopedic Medical Dictionary*, 14th ed. Philadelphia: F.A. Davis, 1983.

Ware, Barbara E. *CLIA '88 Physician's Office Laboratory, Are You Ready?* June 1991.

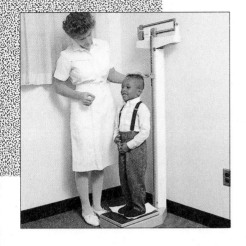

C H A P T E R 1 5

Beginning the Database

Establishing an accurate data base is a most important duty. When you assist the physician in collection of vital information about patients, you must keep in mind that patients have feelings and empathy is essential in your communication with them. You must realize that patients may be seeing a physician for the first time, or may have fear and anxiety about what the outcome of their visit might be. Even though you must be efficient and use your time well to help patient flow run smoothly, you should not rush patient care. You should treat each patient as an individual. Gaining the patient's trust will yield better compliance in treatment.

Accuracy is extremely important in recording information. As you learn to assist with beginning the database in the following text, you will gain a better understanding of how valuable you can be to both physician and patient as a medical assistant, a most versatile health care team member.

U N I T 1

Medical History

OBJECTIVES ....

Upon completion of this unit, student will meet the following terminal performance objectives by verifying knowledge of the facts and principles presented through oral and written communication at a level deemed competent, and will demonstrate the specific behaviors as identified in the terminal performance objectives of the procedures, observing all aseptic and safety precautions in accordance with health care standards.

1. Complete a medical history form.
2. Discuss the parts of a medical history form.
3. List the guidelines in regard to patient education.
4. Measure height of patients accurately.
5. Weigh patients accurately.
6. Record pediatric measurements on growth charts.
7. Spell and define, using the glossary at the back of the text, all the words to know in this unit.

WORDS TO KNOW ....

abnormalities	remedy
dispatch	stature
elicit	symptom
over the counter (OTC)	triage
recumbent	vertex

Patient's Medical History ....

Information needed for administrative purposes is obtained from the patient by the medical assistant in the receptionist's role. The clinical medical assistant then escorts the

Patient education is a primary function of the medical assistant. Most patients are not trained health professionals and are somewhat confused by medical terminology, tests, procedures, and medications they encounter. Therefore, patient education becomes an important part of their medical care.

Whenever possible, the patient should be involved in making decisions about treatment or care. This will encourage the patient to participate more fully in the procedure. Patients will be more willing to cooperate if they understand the necessity for a particular procedure or treatment. Your careful and clear explanations of these procedures will encourage the patient to be more cooperative. If patients sense that you are truly concerned about their well-being, this will stimulate more cooperation. Always offer encouragement and praise where appropriate, even for the smallest accomplishment.

To properly instruct a patient, the medical assistant must know the material. Be prepared to answer any questions from the patient. If you cannot answer one of the patient's questions, tell the patient that you do not know the answer but will ask the physician. Never try to answer a question that you are not prepared to discuss. You could give incorrect information that could harm the patient's well-being. Never give information that is beyond your scope of practice.

In teaching a patient about health care and all that is involved in medical well-being, the primary goal of the medical assistant should be good communication. This means that each patient must be treated as an individual with particular needs. As the patient educator, you will have to meet these needs. You must communicate in the most efficient and effective manner for each individual. Listening is vital to this education. Patients may be shy or embarrassed by their problems or questions and may not ask direct questions. Therefore, you must listen carefully to the patient's comments and questions. Be familiar with information about the patient before proceeding with an explanation. This will help determine how to communicate best with each individual.

Never assume that a patient already knows the information you are conveying. Sometimes a patient will state that he understands something to keep from being embarrassed. If you sense that this is the situation you should briefly repeat the information and provide printed material for the patient to take home to read. Printed materials, such as one-page handouts, brochures, pamphlets, and booklets on various procedures and examinations, as well as diseases, conditions, and treatment plans, should be clear and concise in content. These informative materials should be appropriately distributed routinely to patients.

One very important aspect of patient teaching is your attitude toward the patient. The medical assistant must be open when approaching patients. This means that you must accept each patient as an individual who needs your help. There is no room in the medical office for prejudice. All patients should be treated with respect regardless of their financial status, race, religion, age, or station in life. Remember, your job is to provide assistance. If the patients sense any negative feelings on your part, then they will be less likely to pay attention to your instructions and suggestions.

Most patients are interested in getting better and staying healthy. Patient education involves not only instructing those who are sick, but helping healthy patients say well. By following current trends in wellness and prevention of medical problems, you can help patients help themselves to a healthier life.

The following are some general guidelines for patient education:

1. Become familiar with your office's or clinic's policy concerning patient care.
2. Thoroughly read all handout information given to patients to explain procedures, examinations, or treatment plans so that you can intelligently answer patients' questions.
3. Make yourself available to patients for answering questions. Always remember to ask patients if they have any questions about their treatment or diagnosis.
4. Always take the opportunity to explain procedures to patients and offer additional information, when appropriate, at the time of their visits. For example, be sure to explain warmup and stretching exercises to the weekend athlete with a sprained ankle.
5. Attend continuing education programs to keep abreast of the latest medical information to pass on to patients.
6. Post charts, posters, and other information that will benefit the patient. Be sure that this information is kept current and is posted in areas where patients may spend time waiting.
7. Have current health-conscious magazines available in the reception area.
8. Post meeting times and information for patient support groups (weight control groups, stop smoking groups, tough love meetings) and encourage their participation. Keep this information current.

patient to a private area away from distractions to assist the patient in completing the medical history form. Keeping the patient out of earshot of others will allow the patient to answer personal questions without stress. It is up to you to reassure and put the patient at ease.

It is a common practice to ask the patient to fill out this form, but most patients will appreciate help because of terminology they may not understand or the manner in which questions are asked. In some cases the patient may be too ill or lacking in basic reading skills and will obviously need assistance. Assistance should always be offered but not insisted on. In some practices the medical history and patient information forms are mailed to a new patient before the initial visit. This is a most convenient practice because it not only gives patients adequate time to gather all the necessary information about their health history, but it helps with keeping the medical office on schedule by eliminating unnecessary time in completing the sometimes lengthy form during the appointment.

This completed medical history provides the physician with vital information to assist in making decisions about the diagnosis and course of treatment for the patient. Thereafter, when the patient comes in for an appointment, this data may be used time and time again as an essential reference in that patient's health care plan.

When the patient arrives for the next appointment, the assessment of the complaint is taken by the medical assistant. This should be done away from others in a private area so that the patient's disclosure to you is given in confidence. Screening the symptoms of patients and assessing their needs is called triage. It is a term that originated during wartime when injured soldiers were assessed as to how serious their wounds were and where to dispatch them for treatment. Today it is a term used in nursing and in medical facilities to determine what patients are being seen for and the procedures they will most likely need to have performed. This practice helps expedite patient flow in and through the medical facility much more efficiently.

The following terms are found on most medical history forms.

P R O C E D U R E

Interview Patient to Complete Medical History Form

PURPOSE: To obtain important information about the patient in assessment and plan of the treatment and total care of the patient.
EQUIPMENT: Medical history form, clipboard, pen (blue, black, and red ink).
TERMINAL PERFORMANCE OBJECTIVE: Using copies of the medical history forms included in this text and a pen (blue/black ink), the student will obtain and record a medical history from another student within a set time as specified by the instructor. *All* items should be appropriately marked. (Note: the only exception to this is in items the instructor has specified that only the physician should complete.)

1. Assemble clipboard, medical history form, and pen.
2. Escort patient to private area where you can both sit comfortably.
3. Sit opposite patient. **Key Point: Gain eye contact.**
4. Ask necessary questions of patient and record answers neatly and accurately.
   Key Points:
   a. **Speak in a clear and distinct voice so that patient can easily understand you.**
   b. **Give patient time to answer before going on to next question.**
   c. **Explain any terms that patient may not understand.**
   d. **Avoid getting off subject.**
   e. **Since the AIDS and hepatitis B viruses, as well as other dangerous diseases, have been made apparent as a serious threat to health, additional questions must be asked concerning the**

history of IV drug use and of sexual activity of the patient to determine if further investigation should be made as to the health status of that patient. This is a delicate subject and must be handled with the greatest degree of tact and diplomacy.

5. Forms have spaces to make check marks or write in answers. If further explanation is needed, use section for comments. If there is not an appropriate space to enter information, write a note on a separate sheet of paper to alert physician. For example, a recent death in the family or loss of a job are stress-inducing situations that could influence care and treatment of patient. Patients do not always mention these types of problems to physician.
6. You may be instructed to make certain notations about a patient's medical history in red ink to alert physician. **Key Point: Patient's chief complaint should be obvious to physician before entering examination room to see patient.**
7. When finished with form, thank patient and explain next step in examination. Ask if the patient needs to empty the bladder and if a urinalysis is to be performed as a part of the physical examination, obtain a urine specimen at this time. Having the patient empty the bladder helps to make the examination more successful and more comfortable for the patient. Make patient comfortable by offering reading material if there will be a wait.
8. Gather all necessary forms into patient's permanent chart and give it to physician to use during examination.

NAME		AGE	SEX	S M D W

ADDRESS	PHONE	DATE

SPONSOR	ADDRESS

OCCUPATION	REF BY	ACKN

COMPLAINTS

HISTORY

PRESENT CONDITION	PULSE	TEMP	RESP	B P	HEIGHT	WEIGHT

PHYSICAL FINDINGS

LAB TESTS

DIAGNOSIS

TREATMENT

REMARKS

FIGURE 15–1 General medical history form

Patient's Name _____ Date _____

Address: _____ Ins. _____

Home Phone: _____ Business Phone: _____

Occupation: _____

Referred By _____ Age_____ B.D._____ Sex_____ S M W D

Family History: Father_____ Mother_____
Brothers _____ Sisters _____ Cancer_____
Tuberculosis_____ Insanity _____ Diabetes_____
Heart Disease _____
Rheumatism_____ Gout _____ Goiter_____
Obesity_____ Nephritis _____ Epilepsy_____
Other_____

Past History: Diphtheria _____ Measles _____ Mumps_____
Chicken -Pox _____ Scarlet Fever_____ Smallpox _____ Thyroid_____
Infantile Paralysis_____ Malaria _____ Pneumonia _____
Dysentery_____ Jaundice _____ Boils_____ Rheumatic Fever_____
Tuberculosis_____ Asthma_____ Heart Disease _____
Hypertension_____ Diabetes _____ Infections _____
Gonorrhea _____ Syphillis_____ Tonsillitis_____
Nephritis_____ Operations _____

Menstrual: Onset _____ Frequency_____ Type_____
             Duration_____ Pain_____ L.M.P._____
Marital: Miscarriages_____ Abortions_____ Sterility_____
           Children_____
Habits: Alcohol_____ Tobacco _____ Drugs_____ Coffee_____
          Tea_____ Meals_____ Water_____ Sleep_____
          Bowel Movements_____ Exercise_____
          Amusements or Hobbies_____

Injuries:_____

Allergies:_____

Present Illness:_____

PHYSICAL EXAMINATION: Ht._____ Wt._____ Temp._____ B.P._____
Pulse_____ Respirations_____ General Appearance_____
Skin_____ Mucous Membranes_____
Eyes: Vision: O.D._____ O.S._____ O.U._____
Ishihara_____ Near Vision_____

FIGURE 15–2   In-depth medical history form

Pupil_____ Fundus_____

Ears_____ Nose_____

Chest_____ Breasts_____

Heart_____

Lungs_____

Abdomen_____

Genitalia_____

Rectum_____

Vagina_____

Extremities_____

Lymph Nodes: Neck_____ Axilla_____ Inguinal_____

Abdominal_____ Reflexes_____

REMARKS:_____
_____
_____
_____

DIAGNOSIS:_____
_____
_____

TREATMENT:_____
_____
_____

FIGURE 15–2   (Continued)

- Chief Complaint (CC)—Gives a description of why the patient has come to seek medical attention. Asking an open-ended question such as "What brings you here to see the doctor today?" will **elicit** an answer that will furnish you with the main reason for the office/clinic visit. The response to your question from the patient should be in quotation marks. The following are examples: (you should ask the length of time that the patient has had the complaint and it should then be added if the patient does not include it in responding to your question).

CC—"I think I have the flu," past 3 days

CC—"I have pain when I urinate," 2 days' duration

CC—"I fell and twisted my left ankle this morning."

If the patient has no complaints or symptoms to list and has an appointment to see the physician for a checkup or a report of a physical examination or consultation, that should be noted on the chart as well. Examples of charting other reasons for appointments are as follows:

Patient states that he is here for a physical examination and has no complaints.

Patient says that she is here for annual Pap test; reports that she has no physical complaints.

Patient said that this visit is for a routine checkup and that he feels fine.

It is recommended that you write exactly what the patient complains of in the patient's own words. If there are several chief complaints, you should make a list of the **symptoms.**

- Present Illness (PI)—A detailed description of the patient's chief complaint, including what the patient has done for the symptoms, if it has helped or not, how long it has been since the symptoms first occurred, and if the patient has ever experienced the symptoms before. Any medications the patient is taking to relieve the symptoms should be listed, whether prescription, **over the counter (OTC),** or home **remedy.**

MEDICAL HISTORY FORM

Date _____

Patient's name _____

Age	Date of birth	Sex	

Address _____ City _____ State _____ Zip code _____

Phone ( ) _____

Insurance company _____ Policy number _____

Place of employment _____ Address _____

Phone ( ) _____ Job responsibilities _____

Parent/Guardian if minor _____

Address _____ City _____ State _____ Zip code _____

Phone ( ) _____

Family History:

List family members: (mother, father, brothers, sisters, grandparents, etc.)—ages and health status (if deceased write their age at the time of their death and the cause). List allergies and/or any conditions or diseases they may have or have had, such as asthma, arthritis, tuberculosis, diabetes, cancer, heart disease, hypertension, kidney disease, mental illness, depression, or any other health problems that you know of in your family.

_____

_____

Patient's Past History: Mark the boxes to the right either "yes" or "no" for the following questions:*

Do you ever have or have you ever had any of the following: **(yes) (no)**

SKIN

Rashes, hives, itching or other skin irritations ( ) ( )

EYES, EARS, NOSE, THROAT

Headaches, dizziness, fainting ( ) ( )

Blurred or impaired vision ( ) ( )

Hearing loss or ringing in the ears ( ) ( )

Discharge from eyes or ears ( ) ( )

Sinus trouble/colds/allergies ( ) ( )

Asthma or hay fever ( ) ( )

Sore throats/hoarseness ( ) ( )

CARDIOPULMONARY

Shortness of breath ( ) ( )

Persistent cough or coughing up blood or other secretions ( ) ( )

Chills and/or fever ( ) ( )

Night sweats ( ) ( )

Tuberculosis or exposed to TB ( ) ( )

Scarlet fever or rheumatic fever ( ) ( )

Chest pain ( ) ( )

Heart palpitations or rapid heartbeat or pulse ( ) ( )

High blood pressure ( ) ( )

Swelling of hands and/or feet ( ) ( )

GASTROINTESTINAL

Heartburn or indigestion ( ) ( )

Nausea and/or vomiting ( ) ( )

Loss of appetite ( ) ( )

Belching or gas ( ) ( )

Peptic ulcer, gallbladder or liver disease ( ) ( )

Yellow jaundice or hepatitis ( ) ( )

Diarrhea or constipation ( ) ( )

Dysentery ( ) ( )

Rectal bleeding, hemorrhoids (piles) ( ) ( )

Tarry or clay-colored stools ( ) ( )

GLANDS

Weight gain or loss ( ) ( )

Diabetes ( ) ( )

Thyroid or goiter ( ) ( )

Swollen glands ( ) ( )

GENITOURINARY

Kidney disease or stones, or Bright's disease ( ) ( )

Painful, frequent or urgent urination ( ) ( )

Blood or pus in urine ( ) ( )

Sexually transmitted disease (venereal disease) ( ) ( )

Been sexually active with anyone who has AIDS or HIV or hepatitis ( ) ( )

NEUROMUSCULAR

Problems with becoming tired and/or upset easily ( ) ( )

Nervous breakdown/depression ( ) ( )

Poliomyelitis (infantile paralysis) ( ) ( )

Convulsions ( ) ( )

Joint and/or muscular pain ( ) ( )

Back pain or injury/osteomyelitis/rheumatism ( ) ( )

Are you currently taking any medications? Yes ( ) No ( )

If yes, please list them _____

Have you ever had or been treated for cancer or any tumors? ( ) ( )

Are you anemic or have you ever had to take iron medication? ( ) ( )

Do you use tobacco? ( ) ( )

What type? _____

Do you use IV drugs or alcohol? ( ) ( )

WOMEN ONLY

Painful menstrual periods ( ) ( )

Pregnancy/abortion/miscarriage ( ) ( )

Vaginal infection or discharge/abnormal bleeding ( ) ( )

Last menstrual period _____

Birth control _____

List dates of all operations/surgeries, injuries, and illnesses that required hospitalization:

_____

Did you ever receive benefits from a medical insurance claim due to illness or injury? Yes ( ) No ( )

Were you ever rejected from the military or for employment? ( ) ( )

Were you absent from school/work in the past 10 years because of illness or injury? ( ) ( )

Did you ever file a Workers' Compensation claim? ( ) ( )

Did you ever seek psychological or psychiatric treatment? ( ) ( )

*Please use the back of this form to explain any "yes" answers. Thank you.

FIGURE 15–3 Medical history form

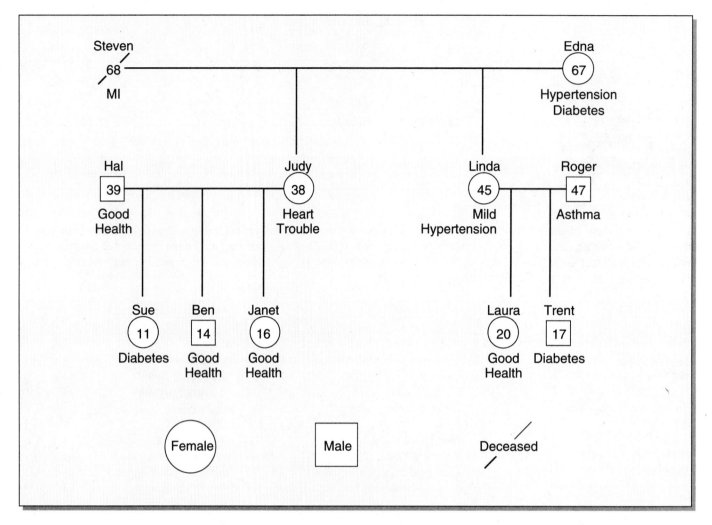

FIGURE 15–4 Example of a genogram

- Review of Systems (ROS)—A systematic review of all body systems to detect any problems the patient may not yet be aware of.
- Past History (PH) or Past Medical History (PMH)—Includes Usual Childhood Diseases (UCHD), major illnesses, surgeries, allergies, injuries, immunizations, and medications that the patient has taken, past and present.
- Family History (FH)—Past and present health of the patient's biological mother, father, and siblings; if they are deceased, the cause and their age at the time.
- Personal/Sociocultural History (PSH)—Refers to a profile of the patient's personal life history. It includes the patient's self-concept, role relationships, coping patterns, and life-style. Risk factors are also identified. This is most helpful to the physician in planning treatment programs for patients. (Confidentiality must be practiced in regard to the information disclosed by patients to all health care professionals.)

Medical history forms vary with the type of practice. Some forms are short; others are quite extensive and time-consuming, Figures 15–1 to 15–3, pages 424–427.

A relatively new concept of recording a family health history is by using the genogram, Figure 15–4. This method shows a diagram of the family's medical history over several generations. Most genograms include at least three generations. This is most helpful to the physician in reviewing the patient's chances of developing particular hereditary diseases. The diagram makes it easy to check the family history at a glance to detect genetic tendencies. Specialized printing companies can assist in designing a form for a particular practice. Forms may be color coded for easy identification.

Height and Weight

The patient's height and weight must be recorded at the initial visit to serve as a reference point. Accuracy is important both in measuring and in recording this information. Infants and small children should have height and weight measured and recorded routinely for growth and development patterns to be established.

Using Figure 15–5, page 429, as an example, you will see that the age of infant males ranges from birth (B) to

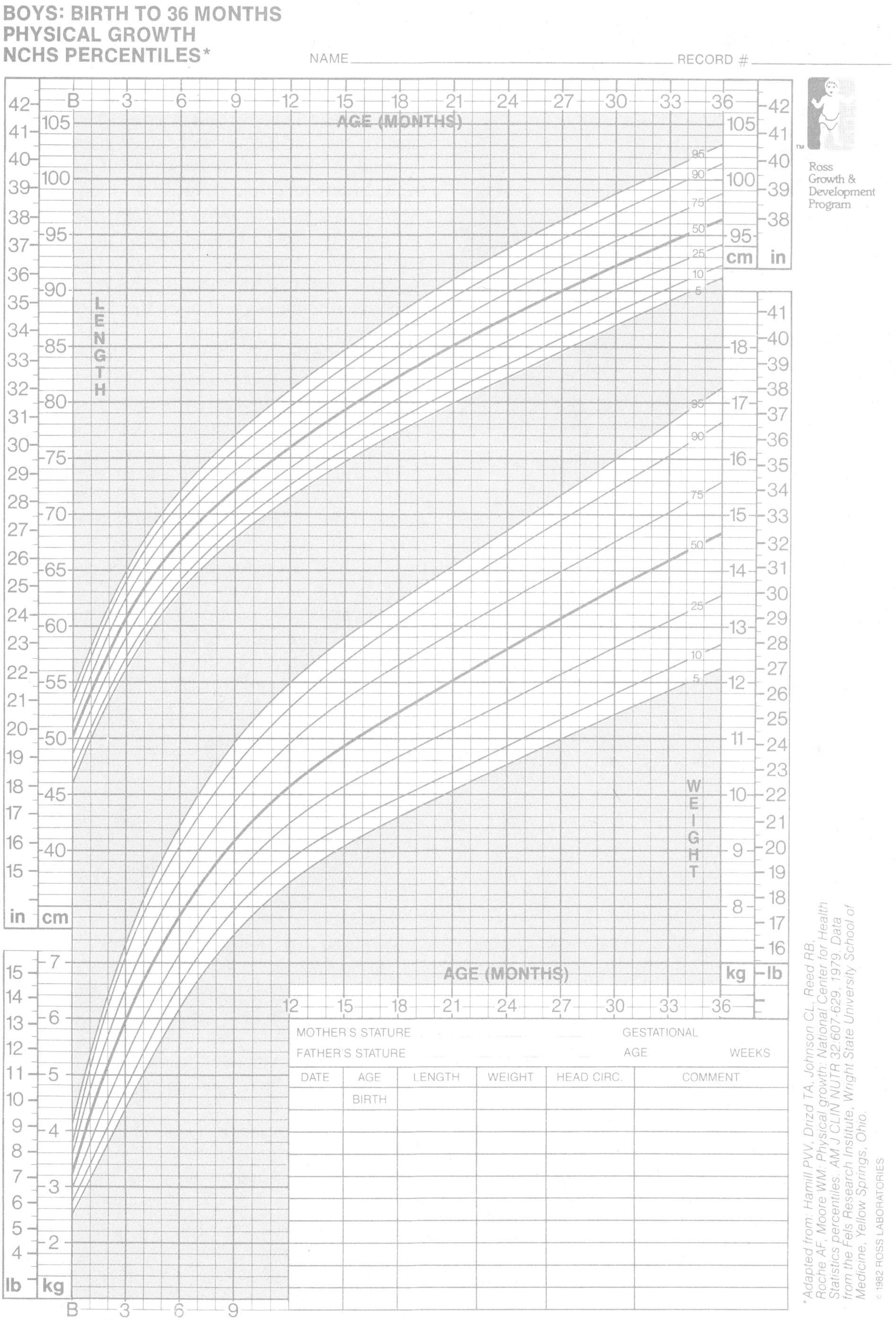

NAME_____ RECORD #_____

FIGURE 15–5 Growth chart for boys height and weight, age birth to thirty-six months

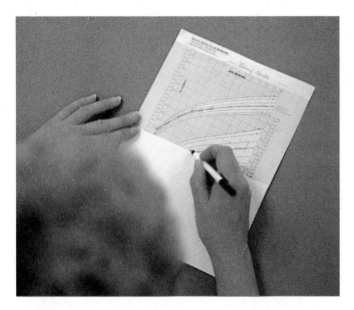

FIGURE 15–5A Medical assistant plotting measurement on growth graph

36 months across the top of the chart (it is also printed across the bottom). Each of the squares across the graph represents one month. After the measurements of the infant have been obtained at each checkup, they are plotted on this graph. The recumbent length of the child is recorded in either inches or centimeters, and the weight in pounds or kilograms. One must be consistent in measuring the child in the same manner to avoid discrepancies. To record these measurements, follow the age line (vertically) down to the child's length measurement on the left and follow the horizontal line to the point at where the two intersect and place a dot with your pen (or pencil); stay on the vertical (age) line and look to the right side of the chart for the weight of the child. Following the horizontal line from right to left, place a dot at the intersection of the weight and age line.

Record the head circumference in the same fashion by following the vertical age line down to the corresponding horizontal measurement (to the left of the chart) in inches or centimeters and place the dot with pen or pencil where the two lines intersect. It is helpful to place a plain sheet of paper over the graph while finding the intersecting lines to avoid errors, Figure 15–5 (a).

The dots are connected by drawing a straight line with a ruler from one point to another providing a neat and concise appearance.

The curved lines printed across the growth charts show the normal range of growth of infants and children in the United States. The numbers to the right of the chart in the boxes vertically between age 34 and 35 months show the percentiles of other children the same age. The National Center for Health Statistics (NCHS) growth charts become a permanent record of the child's development, Figures 15–5 to 15–8, pages 429–434. These give the physician a quick way to check the child's growth in relation to that of other children the

---

P R O C E D U R E

Measure Height

PURPOSE: To obtain an accurate measurement of a patient's height.

EQUIPMENT: Upright scale with extension measuring bar, patient's chart, pen (a measuring scale may be fixed to the wall)

TERMINAL PERFORMANCE OBJECTIVE: After the instructor has measured and recorded the height of all students, each student will, in turn, select five other students. The student will demonstrate on five other students each step in the height measurement procedure to determine the precise height of each of the other five students. The height measurements obtained should agree with the heights for those five students as measured and recorded by the instructor ± 1/8".

1. Raise measuring bar higher than apparent height of patient. **Key Point: Raising measuring bar before patient steps on to scale will prevent possible injury.**

2. Ask patient to remove shoes. (Patients ready for physical exams will not have shoes on.) Place a paper towel on platform of scale. **Key Point: Shoes must be removed to get a true measurement.**

3. Help patient onto scale facing you with his or her back to measuring device. Advise patient to stand erect.

4. Slide measuring bar down slowly and carefully to rest on top of patient's head, gently compressing hair. **Key Point: Measurement of height is from the top of the head not the hair. This can cause a discrepancy in the reading.**

5. Read measurement in inches or centimeters and tell patient what it is.

6. Help patient down from scale. Tell patient to put shoes back on unless ready for physical exam.

7. Place measuring extension bar back in place and discard paper towel.

8. Record height measurement on patient's chart.

P R O C E D U R E

Measure Recumbent Length of Infant

PURPOSE: To obtain an accurate measurement of recumbent length of an infant up to 36 months of age.

EQUIPMENT: Ruled measuring tape/yard/meter stick, patient's chart, parent's record booklet, growth graph, pen

TERMINAL PERFORMANCE OBJECTIVE: Provided with at least three lifelike clinical or toy dolls (or an infant or small child under the close supervision of the parent/guardian and/or the instructor) and a pediatric table or examining table along with a ruled measuring device, the student will demonstrate each step required in measuring recumbent length of infants/small children and obtain a length measurement for each doll; each length measurement must be within ± 1/8" of each doll's actual length as determined by the instructor beforehand.

1. Wash hands and ask parent to remove infant's shoes and socks or booties.
2. Ask parent to place infant on examination table with its head against (end) headboard of table at zero mark of ruler. Gently straighten infant's back and legs to line up along ruler. Ask parent to hold infant's head against (end) headboard of table while you place infant's heels against footboard. If there is no footboard (to place the infant's feet against) use your right hand as one, Figure 15–11, page 437. Place your left hand over the child's legs at the knees to secure the child in place and straighten the legs so you can read the recumbent length from the head (vertex) to the heel.
3. Read length in inches or centimeters from ruler. **Key Point: There may be discrepancies with measurement at birth or from another facility because of difficulty in getting an accurate reading. Infants are so used to fetal position that it is difficult to straighten the legs. Placing your fingers behind knees with your thumb over the kneecap applying gentle pressure will help to keep the legs straightened out for the procedure. The former reading may have been from measuring the infant's length from head to toe making the measurement of the recumbent length up to a few centimeters longer or more.**
4. Return infant to parent.
5. Record measurement on growth chart, patient's chart, and parent's booklet of child's growth and development.

same age. Growth charts aid in the diagnosis of growth abnormalities and nutritional disorders and diseases. Of course, hereditary factors also influence growth patterns, hence the importance of having the family history in the medical record.

In measuring stature (standing height), all patients over 3 years of age should be asked to stand tall and hold still until the measurement has been obtained. Children under 3 can be measured in either a standing or recumbent position. A child's length in the recumbent position will be nearly an inch greater than when standing, so it is necessary to be consistent in the method of measurement. Make a notation of which method is used when recording the measurement. It is recommended that a right-angle headboard be used to ensure accuracy in measuring children, Figure 15–9, page 436.

Since either the gaining or the losing of weight can change the course of a patient's diagnosis and treatment, proper balancing of the scales should be a routine practice.

Most physicians require that patients are weighed routinely at each visit. Measuring the height of patients should be done periodically after age 18 years of age because of certain degenerative conditions and anatomical changes of the body from aging. Patients are weight conscious, so the remarks of the medical assistant should be positive ones, if any. A chart of desirable weight of men and women may be posted above the scale for patient education, Figure 15–10, page 437.

If there is no measuring device for use in obtaining the recumbent length of a baby, you may measure the length of the child by using a flexible measuring tape. Place the child on her back on the examination table and mark on the table paper with a pen the top (vertex) of the head and the bottom of the feet (the heel). Then measure the distance between the two marks with the tape measure to obtain the length of the child. Be sure that the baby was straight and still while marking the positions of head and heel for the measurement.

Head Circumference ....

Head circumference is a measurement that is routinely recorded on an infant's chart to alert the physician to any abnormal development. This procedure should be performed during routine visits until the child is 36 months old. Head circumference procedure requires a flexible measuring tape, Figure 15–16, page 439. Plotting the measurement on a growth chart is the most efficient way to keep records, Figures 15–17 and 15–18, pages 440–441.

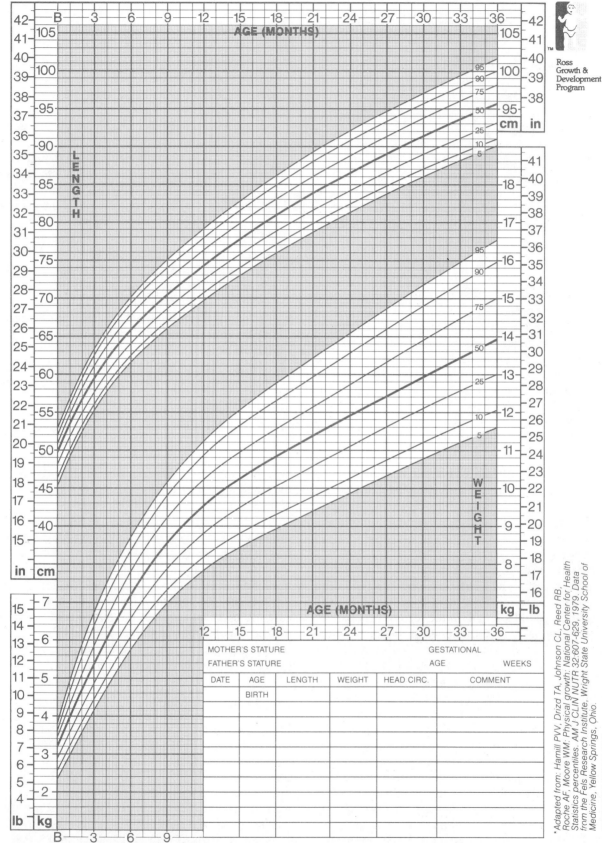

FIGURE 15–6   Growth chart for girls height and weight, age birth to thirty-six months

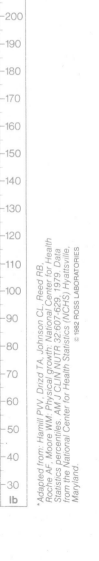

BOYS: 2 TO 18 YEARS
PHYSICAL GROWTH
NCHS PERCENTILES*

NAME_____

RECORD #_____

*Adapted from: Hamill PVV, Drizd TA, Johnson CL, Reed RB, Roche AF, Moore WM: Physical growth: National Center for Health Statistics percentiles. AM J CLIN NUTR 32:607-629, 1979. Data from the National Center for Health Statistics (NCHS) Hyattsville, Maryland.

© 1982 ROSS LABORATORIES

Ross
Growth &
Development
Program

FIGURE 15–7 Growth chart for boys height and weight, age 2 to 18 years

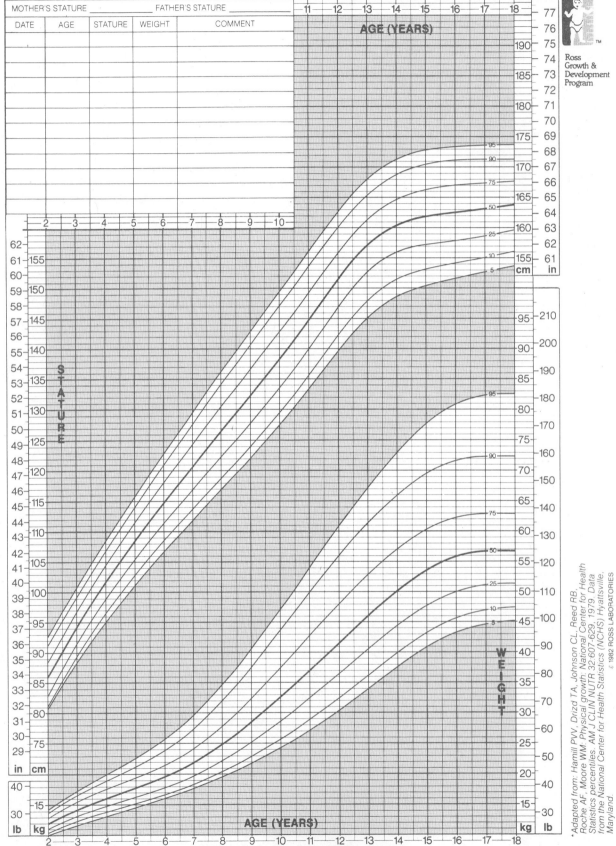

FIGURE 15–8 Growth chart for girls height and weight, age 2 to 18 years

P R O C E D U R E

Weigh Patient on Upright Scale

PURPOSE: To obtain an accurate measure of the patient's weight.

EQUIPMENT: Upright balance scales, Figure 15–12, page 438, patient's chart, pen

TERMINAL PERFORMANCE OBJECTIVE: After the instructor has measured and recorded the weight of all students, each student will, in turn select five other students. The student will demonstrate on five other students each step in the weight measurement procedure to determine the accurate weight of each of the five students. The weight measurements obtained should agree with the weights for those five students as measured and recorded by the instructor ± 1/4 lb.

1. Wash hands and balance scales.
2. Ask patient to remove shoes. *Some patients prefer to be weighed in a paper gown to give lowest weight.*
3. Place a paper towel on base of scale.
4. Help patient onto scale.

5. Make sure patient is in center of platform. Ask patient to stand still while you adjust balance and read weight, Figure 15–3, page 427. **Key Point: If patients are weighed with their clothes on, it is common to allow at least 3 pounds for women's clothing and 5 pounds for men's.** If you are to obtain both the height and weight of a patient, it is best to have the patient remain on the scales. Raise the bar by pushing it up with one hand and holding the extension of the bar with the other hand protecting the patient from possible injury (the patient is still facing the measuring device). Refer to Step 4 of the procedure for measuring height to complete.
6. Help patient from scale and discard paper towel.
7. Record weight on patient's chart. Be sure to record whether patient was wearing street clothing or gown.
8. Return scale to balance at zero.

P R O C E D U R E

Weigh Infant

PURPOSE: To obtain an accurate weight measurement of an infant.

EQUIPMENT: Infant balance scales, towel, patient's chart, growth graph, parent's record booklet, pen

TERMINAL PERFORMANCE OBJECTIVE: Provided with at least three lifelike clinical or toy dolls (or an infant or very small child under the close supervision of the parent/guardian or the instructor) and an infant scales, the student will demonstrate each step required in weighing infants and very small children by weighing each of the dolls; each weight must be within ± 1/8 lb. of each weight as determined by the instructor beforehand.

1. Wash hands.
2. Ask parent to remove infant's clothing.
3. Place a clean towel on scale cradle to avoid disease transmission and to decrease shock of cold metal for infant. This will lessen chance that infant will move because of being uncomfortable or afraid. Keep diaper or towel over infant's genital area in case of an elimination.
4. Balance scale at zero with towel in place.
5. Place infant on scale holding one hand over infant

(almost touching) to give a sense of security. Talking in a quiet tone will also help keep infant still until reading has been taken. The age of the baby may determine how the child is placed on the scales. Small infants will be easier to weigh lying down; those who can sit up on their own will most likely be more cooperative sitting on the scales, Figures 15–14 and 15–15, page 438. In either case the safety of the baby is primary.

6. Slide weight easily until scale balances, which determines weight of infant. Read scale in pounds and ounces or kilograms.
7. Return infant to parent.
8. Remove towel from scale, place it in proper receptacle, and balance scale at zero mark.
9. Record weight on growth chart, patient's chart, and parent's booklet. Note: If infant is unruly when weight is attempted, a notation should be made on chart that weight is approximate. Other attempts can be made at same visit. If weight is needed to determine nutritional needs or medication dosage you may have to weigh parent holding infant, then weigh parent, and subtract to get approximate weight of child.

PROCEDURE

Measure Head Circumference

PURPOSE: To obtain an accurate measurement of infants' and small children's head circumference in screening for head growth abnormalities.

EQUIPMENT: Flexible tape measure without elasticity, growth graph, patients's chart, pen

TERMINAL PERFORMANCE OBJECTIVE: Provided with at lease three lifelike clinical or toy dolls and a flexible tape measure, the student will demonstrate each step required in measuring the circumference of heads of infants/small children on each of the three dolls; each circumference measurement must be within ± 1/8" (0.2 cm) of each doll's actual head circumference as determined by the instructor beforehand.

1. Wash hands.
2. Talk to infant to gain cooperation. Infant may be held by parent or lie on examination table for procedure. Older children of 2 or 3 years may stand or sit if they will remain still.
3. Use one thumb or finger to hold tape measure with zero mark against infant's forehead (above eyebrows). With other hand, bring tape around infant's head just above ears to meet in front. **Key Point: Pull tape snugly to compress hair.**
4. Read to nearest 0.1 cm or 1/2 inch.
5. Record on growth chart, parent's record booklet, and patient record.

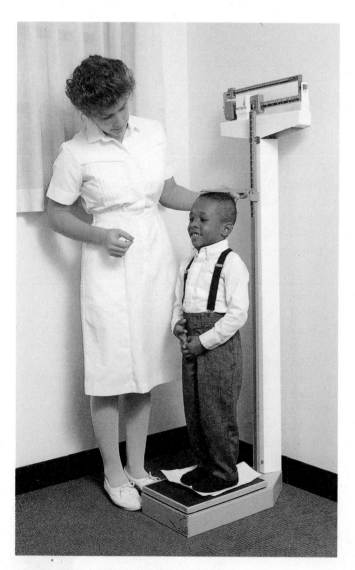

FIGURE 15–9   Measure height of a child

Chest Measurement ....

Many physicians request the chest measurement of infants along with the height, weight, and head circumference at the regularly scheduled visits up to 12 months of age. This is performed to monitor growth abnormalities. Patients of any age may require that this measurement be taken for a particular health history. Because of the extremely strenuous physical demands of some programs, additional body measurements are sometimes necessary to assess the condition of the person before they are accepted. Accuracy is vital in recording these and all measurements. Follow the procedure for obtaining chest measurement for infants and children and adapt for measuring adults. There is usually a request for measuring the chest while the patient inhales deeply, expanding the chest to full capacity.

Complete Chapter 15, Unit 1 in the workbook to help you meet the objectives at the beginning of this unit and therefore achieve competency of this subject matter.

U N I T 2

Vital Signs

OBJECTIVES ....

Upon completion of this unit, the student will meet the following terminal performance objectives by verifying knowledge of the facts and principles presented through oral and written communication at a level deemed competent, and will demonstrate the specific behaviors as identified in the terminal performance objectives of the

MEN			
Height	Small	Medium	Large
5' 2"	128–134	131–141	138–150
5' 3"	130–136	133–143	140–153
5' 4"	132–138	135–145	142–156
5' 5"	134–140	137–148	144–160
5' 6"	136–142	139–151	146–164
5' 7"	138–146	142–154	149–168
5' 8"	140–148	145–157	152–172
5' 9"	142–151	148–160	155–176
5'10"	144–154	151–163	158–180
5'11"	146–157	154–166	161–184
6' 0"	149–160	157–170	164–188
6' 1"	152–164	160–174	188–192
6' 2"	155–168	164–178	172–197
6' 3"	158–172	167–182	176–202
6' 4"	162–176	171–187	181–207

WOMEN			
Height	Small	Medium	Large
4'10"	102–111	109–121	118–131
4'11"	103–113	111–123	120–134
5' 0"	104–115	113–126	122–137
5' 1"	106–118	115–129	125–140
5' 2"	108–121	118–132	128–143
5' 3"	111–124	121–135	131–147
5' 4"	114–127	124–138	134–151
5' 5"	117–130	127–141	137–155
5' 6"	120–133	130–144	140–159
5' 7"	123–136	133–147	143–163
5' 8"	126–139	138–150	146–167
5' 9"	129–142	139–153	149–170
5'10"	132–146	142–156	152–173
5'11"	135–148	145–159	155–176
6' 0"	138–151	148–162	158–179

FIGURE 15–10 Chart of desirable weights for men and women

procedures, observing all aseptic and safety precautions in accordance with health care standards.

1. Identify the four vital signs and the body functions they measure.
2. Explain how the body controls temperature.
3. Describe the different designs of glass clinical thermometers and their appropriate uses.
4. Demonstrate the cleaning and storing of mercury thermometers.
5. Accurately measure oral, rectal, and axillary temperature, identifying the normal temperature value and relative accuracy of each.
6. Explain situations when oral measurement is contraindicated.

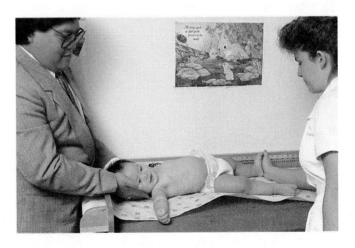

FIGURE 15–11 Measuring recumbent length of infant

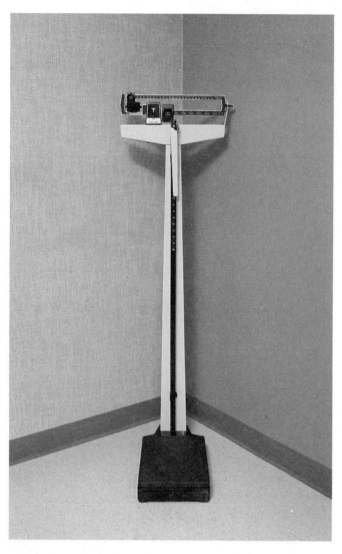

FIGURE 15–12   The traditional beam balance scale with measuring bar

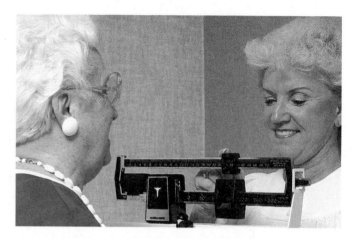

FIGURE 15–13   The weight of the patient may be read on either side of the scales.

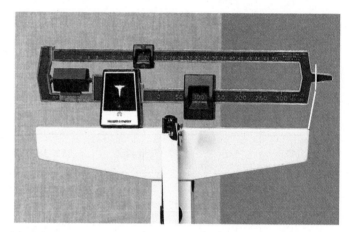

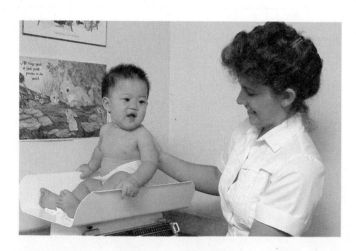

FIGURE 15–14   Weighing an infant sitting on scale

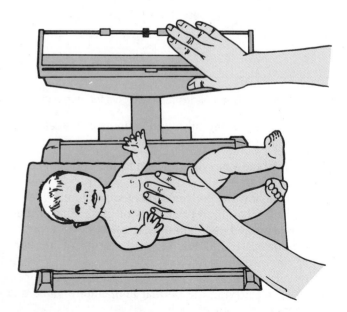

FIGURE 15–15   Weighing an infant lying on scale

PROCEDURE

Measure Chest of Infant

PURPOSE: To obtain an accurate measurement of infants' and small children's chests in screening for growth abnormalities.

EQUIPMENT: Flexible tape measure without elasticity, patient's chart, pen

TERMINAL PERFORMANCE OBJECTIVE: Provided with at least three lifelike clinical or toy dolls and a flexible tape measure, the student will demonstrate each step required in obtaining the chest measurement of infants and small children on each of the three dolls; each chest measurement must be within ± 1/8" (0.3 cm) of each doll's actual chest measurement as determined by the instructor beforehand.

1. Wash hands.
2. Talk to infant/child to gain cooperation. Infant/child may lie down on examination table or be held by parent/guardian for the procedure. Children of 2 or 3 years and older may sit or stand on their own if they will cooperate and remain still for the procedure.
3. Use one thumb to hold tape measure with zero mark against the infant's chest at the midsternal area. With the other hand, bring the tape around/under the back to meet the zero mark of the tape in front. Take the measurement of the chest just above the nipples with the tape fitting around the child's chest under the axillary region. If you need assistance in holding the child still, ask the parent or another assistant. The measurement should be taken when the child is breathing normally, not with forced inspiration or expiration, Figure 15–19, page 442.
4. Read measurement to the nearest 0.1 cm or 1/2 inch.
5. Record on patient's chart and in parent's record booklet.

Note: This procedure can be used for obtaining the chest measurement of patients of all ages.

---

7. Describe what causes pulse, why it can be felt, and name and locate five pulse points.
8. Identify normal pulse rates and describe five factors that affect the rate.
9. Measure radial and apical pulse and describe the quality characteristics to be observed.
10. Define pulse deficit, explaining its significance and how it is measured.
11. Measure respiration, identifying the normal rate and describing the quality characteristics to be observed.
12. Describe normal respiration and explain four abnormal breathing patterns.
13. List the five circulatory factors reflected by the measurement of blood pressure.
14. Explain how the body maintains blood pressure.
15. Identify the phases of blood pressure, comparing them to the action of the heart.
16. Measure blood pressure by palpation and auscultation, explaining pulse pressure and normal findings.
17. Explain an auscultatory gap.
18. Spell and define, using the glossary at the back of the text, all the words to know in this unit.

WORDS TO KNOW ....

afebrile
aneroid
antecubital
apex

apical
apnea
arrhythmia
auscultate

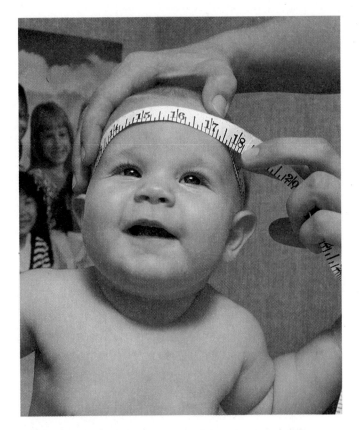

FIGURE 15–16 Measuring head circumference of infant

NAME_____   RECORD #_____

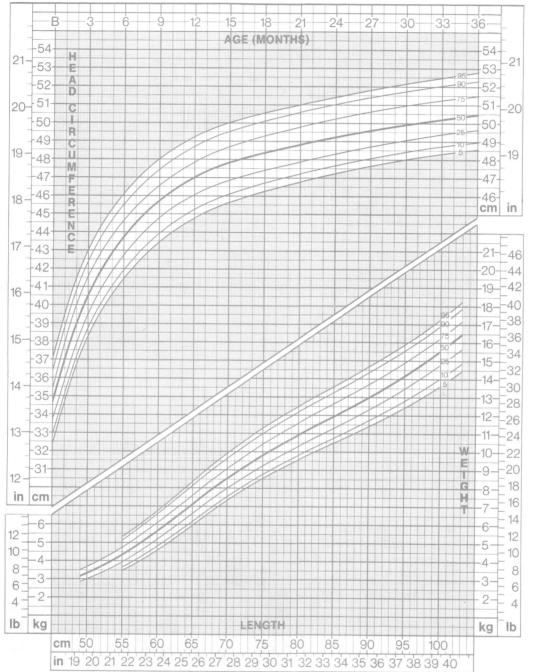

AGE (MONTHS)

HEAD CIRCUMFERENCE

WEIGHT

LENGTH

*Adapted from: Hamill PVV, Drizd TA, Johnson CL, Reed RB, Roche AF, Moore WM. Physical growth: National Center for Health Statistics percentiles. AM J CLIN NUTR 32:607-629, 1979. Data from the Fels Research Institute, Wright State University School of Medicine, Yellow Springs, Ohio.

© 1982 ROSS LABORATORIES

DATE	AGE	LENGTH	WEIGHT	HEAD CIRC.	COMMENT

Recommend the formulation you prefer
with the name you trust

SIMILAC®
SIMILAC® WITH IRON
SIMILAC® WITH WHEY
Infant Formulas

The ISOMIL® System of
Soy Protein Formulas

ADVANCE®
Nutritional Beverage

ROSS LABORATORIES
COLUMBUS, OHIO 43216
Division of Abbott Laboratories, USA

G105/JUNE 1983   LITHO IN USA

FIGURE 15–17 Growth chart for boys head circumference, birth to 36 months

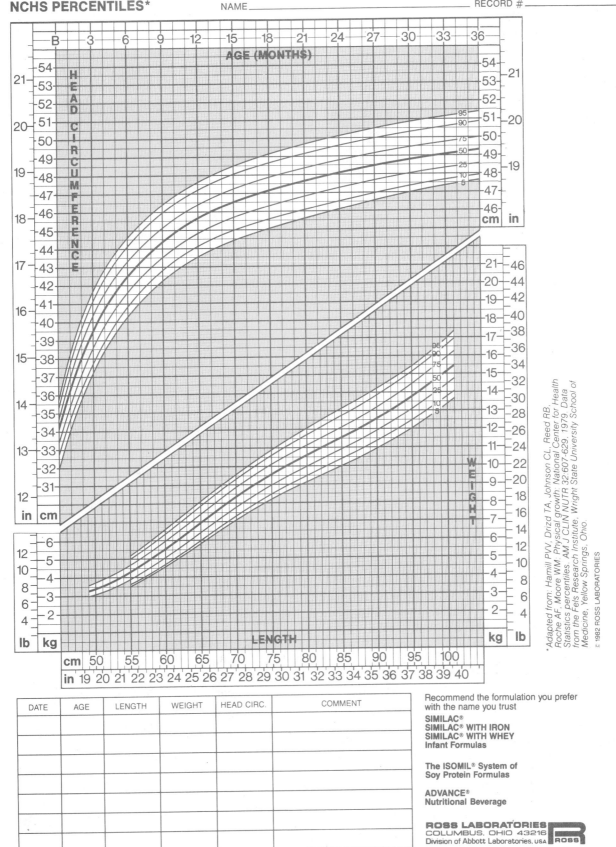

GIRLS: BIRTH TO 36 MONTHS
PHYSICAL GROWTH
NCHS PERCENTILES*

NAME _____ RECORD # _____

*Adapted from: Hamill PVV, Drizd TA, Johnson CL, Reed RB, Roche AF, Moore WM. Physical growth: National Center for Health Statistics percentiles. AM J CLIN NUTR 32:607-629, 1979. Data from the Fels Research Institute, Wright State University School of Medicine, Yellow Springs, Ohio.

© 1982 ROSS LABORATORIES

DATE	AGE	LENGTH	WEIGHT	HEAD CIRC.	COMMENT

Recommend the formulation you prefer with the name you trust

SIMILAC®
SIMILAC® WITH IRON
SIMILAC® WITH WHEY
Infant Formulas

The **ISOMIL®** System of
Soy Protein Formulas

ADVANCE®
Nutritional Beverage

ROSS LABORATORIES
COLUMBUS, OHIO 43216
Division of Abbott Laboratories, USA

FIGURE 15–18 Growth chart for girls head circumference, birth to 36 months

G106/JUNE 1983   LITHO IN USA

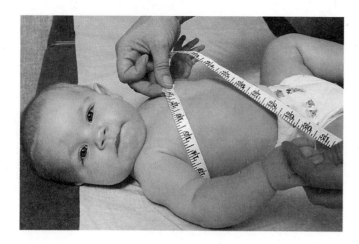

FIGURE 15–19 Measuring chest of infant

axillary
blood pressure
brachial
cardinal signs
carotid
Cheyne–Stokes
dorsalis pedis
dyspnea
essential
exhale
fatal
febrile
femoral
groin
hyperventilation
idiopathic
infrared
inhale
mercury

oral
palpate
pulse
pulse deficit
pulse pressure
pyrogen
radial
râles
rectal
rhythm
sphygmomanometer
stethoscope
sublingual
temperature
thermometer
thready
vital
volume

The term **cardinal signs** or **vital** signs is used by health care personnel to identify the measurement of body functions that are essential to life. The four vital indicators are **temperature, pulse,** respiration, and **blood pressure,** commonly referred to as TPR, and B/P. They indicate the body's ability to control heat; the rate, volume, and rhythm of the heart; the rate and quality of breathing; and the force of the heart and condition of the blood vessels. The vital signs give the physician an assessment of the status of the brain, the autonomic nervous system, the heart, and the lungs.

The correct measurement of vital signs is extremely important. Proper technique and attention to details are essential. Findings should be recorded immediately following measurement to avoid a memory error. Always repeat the procedure if you think you may have made a mistake in measuring or recording. Occasionally, you may have a problem measuring a vital sign because of a patient's unusual physical condition that makes measurement difficult. Inform the physician of your problem and follow the course of action advised. Avoid alarming the patient. *Never* estimate the measurement. The physician's choice of treatment and medication is often based on the findings; therefore, they must be accurate.

Temperature

The temperature of the body indicates the amount of heat produced by the activity of changing food into energy. The body loses heat through perspiration, breathing, and the elimination of body wastes. The balance between heat production and heat loss determines the body's temperature.

Conditions affecting body heat include metabolic rate, time of day, and amount of activity. Body temperature is usually lower in the morning following a period of rest. In the afternoon and evening, body temperature rises due to the heat produced by activity and the metabolism of food. These activities warm the blood that circulates though the body. "Normal" body temperature for an individual is that temperature at which his or her body systems function most effectively. Not all people have the same normal oral temperature. An *average* normal temperature is 98.6°F (Fahrenheit) or 37°C (centigrade), Figure 15–20. Normal oral temperature of patients may vary from 97.6° to 99.6°F. A person with a temperature above normal is said to be **febrile** or to have a temperature elevation. A person with a temperature which is normal or subnormal is said to be **afebrile.**

TABLE 15–1
Temperature Variations Considered "Normal"

	Oral	Axillary	Rectal
Average Temperature	98.6°F (37°C)	97.6°F (36.5°C)	99.6°F (37.5°C)
Range	97.6–99.6°F (36.5–37.5°C)	96.6–98.6°F (36–37°C)	98.6–100.6°F (37–38.1°C)

Controlling Body Temperature

The temperature regulating center in the body is located in the hypothalamus of the brain. The action of the hypothalamus can be compared to a thermostat that turns the furnace in your home off and on to keep the room temperature at the set number of degrees. As discussed previously, the brain, autonomic nervous system, blood vessels, and skin cooperate to regulate temperature. This is achieved through a feedback mechanism from temperature receptors. In the body, the hot and cold peripheral receptors in the skin send messages to the hypothalamus about the environment surrounding the body. Temperature receptors in the spinal cord, abdomen, and other internal structures send messages about the internal body temperature. One section of the hypothalamus also has many heat-sensitive neurons, which increase their output

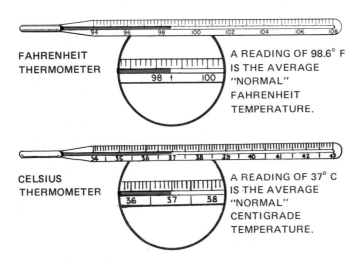

FAHRENHEIT THERMOMETER

A READING OF 98.6° F IS THE AVERAGE "NORMAL" FAHRENHEIT TEMPERATURE.

CELSIUS THERMOMETER

A READING OF 37° C IS THE AVERAGE "NORMAL" CENTIGRADE TEMPERATURE.

FIGURE 15–20 Normal body temperature on Fahrenheit and Celsius thermometers

of impulses when temperature rises and decease their output when it drops. The signals from this section of the hypothalamus merge with those received in another section, along with the internal and skin receptors, to evaluate the situation and send signals to control heat loss or production. Therefore, this central center is referred to as the *hypothalamic thermostat.*

The hypothalamic thermostat is very effective. When receptors sense the body is too warm, they send a message to the brain, which in turn acts on the sweat glands of the skin to produce moisture. The moisture evaporates from the skin's surface and cools the body. At the same time, nerve impulses are sent to the surface blood vessels to dilate, which brings more blood in contact with the surface of the skin. The blood gives up heat, which cools the blood within the vessels and therefore cools the body.

When the body senses coolness, the opposite activities occur. Surface blood vessels constrict to keep the blood away from the surface of the skin and prevent the loss of heat. Impulses to the sweat glands are stopped when temperature falls below normal. The small papillary muscles around the hair follicles contract causing gooseflesh. Heat is produced by the activity of the papillary muscles, thereby helping to warm the body. In addition, a portion of the hypothalamus becomes active when cold signals are received. Now hypothalamic messages are sent to skeletal muscles throughout the body, causing increased muscle tone that produces heat. When the muscle tone rises above a certain level, shivering results and heat production is raised dramatically. The results are evident with an infectious process such as influenza. Microorganisms cause the patient to experience chills and shivering until the temperature rises to warm the body and a fever develops.

During an infectious process, the presence of microorganisms cause **pyrogens** to be secreted, which raise the

"set point" of the hypothalamic thermostat. Pyrogens are toxins from bacteria or a by-product of degenerating tissues. When the set point is higher than normal, the body's heat production and conservation processes are activated. Surface blood vessels constrict, causing the person to feel cold even though the temperature is above normal. No sweat is secreted. Increased white blood cell activity from fighting bacterial invasion also produces heat. Chills and shivering begin and continue until the temperature reaches the higher set point where the hypothalamus will continue to operate until the infectious process is reversed. Once this occurs, the hypothalamic thermostat is reset to a lower or normal value and the body's temperature reduction process results in profuse sweating and a hot, red skin from general vasodilation. After this onset reaction, the temperature will begin to fall.

The extent of the infection determines the amount of heat (fever) generated. A mild infection may cause the temperature to rise to 100°F. A moderate infection may elevate the temperature to 102°F. Fevers are categorized by the degree of body heat present as slight, moderate, severe, dangerous, or **fatal,** Table 15–2. Temperatures below normal are called subnormal. Collapse will occur at about 96.0°F, and death follows if temperature goes below 93.0°F except briefly. Fatality-associated elevated temperature also depends on the extent of time the fever is present. Fevers of short duration well above 106.0°F have not proved fatal, but immediate measures to reduce body temperature must be administered.

TABLE 15–2
Classification of Fevers

	Fahrenheit	Celsius
Slight	99.6°–101.0°	37.5°–38.3°
Moderate	101.0°–102.0°	38.3°–38.8°
Severe	102.0°–104.0°	38.8°–40.0°
Dangerous	104.0°–105.0°	40.0°–40.5
Fatal	over 106.0°	41.1°

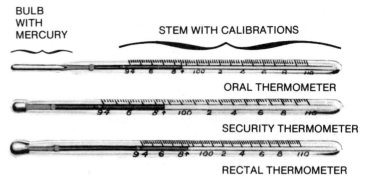

FIGURE 15–21   Types of mercury thermometers

Thermometer Types and Designs

Body temperature is measured by means of a thermometer in scales of Fahrenheit or the metric system equivalent, Celsius. Thermometers are of the following main types: glass mercury, also called clinical; disposable, in the form of plastic strips; a self-contained digital, battery-operated electronic; and the most recent, a tympanic infrared thermometer. The mouth (oral), underarm (axillary), rectum (rectal), and ear (aural) may be used to measure body temperature. The large variety of thermometers, each with its own advantages and disadvantages, allow for personal preference in equipment selection for the physician's office. Table 15–3 briefly outlines the main features for each type.

Glass mercury thermometers are of three designs to measure the temperature by oral, rectal, and axillary method, Figure 15–21. An oral thermometer has a long slender bulb to fit under the tongue. A rectal thermometer has a fat rounded bulb that is stronger and safer to insert into the anus. An oral thermometer that is constructed with a rounded bulb is known as a stubby or security thermometer, and is suitable for oral or axillary measurement. Many thermometers are further identifiable by a color-coded dot at the stem end. Blue indicates

oral; red indicates rectal. Usually the word *oral* or *rectal* is inscribed on the stem.

It is extremely important that thermometers be used for their intended purpose. It is not safe to insert an oral thermometer into the rectum. The slender bulb may perforate (puncture) the tissues, and it is more easily broken. Be equally careful that a rectal thermometer is *never* used to measure an oral temperature.

Reading a Mercury Thermometer and Recording Measurements

Clinical thermometers are slender glass rods with a hollow central cavity extending from a bulb reservoir of mercury. The stem of the Fahrenheit thermometer is calibrated in even tenths, [.2,.4,.6,.8] (Figure 15–22). The whole degrees are marked with long lines, but only the even-numbered degrees are printed on the thermometer. There is also a long line at 98.6° with an arrow, because

TABLE 15–3
Comparison of Thermometer Types

Type	Advantage	Disadvantage
Glass mercury	Accurate, inexpensive, familiar	Slow, somewhat difficult to read, easily broken, requires cleaning and plastic cover
Plastic disposable	Single use avoids cross-contamination, no cleaning, relatively fast	Must protect from heat, somewhat unpleasant for patient; storage and inventory costs
Digital	Quick, signals when registered, easily read, self-contained	Moderate initial cost, plastic cover and battery expenses
Electronic probe	Quick, signals when registered, easily read, self-contained	Fairly expensive, cumbersome cord, requires recharging, probe cover costs; may cause inaccurate readings if patient bites too hard on probe
Tympanic infrared	Instant results, easily read, core temperature, individualized probe cover, eliminates mucous membrane concerns	Expensive, probe cover costs, replacement battery costs

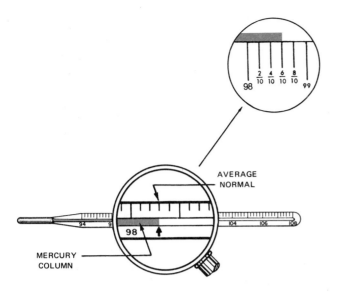

FIGURE 15–22 Reading a thermometer. This thermometer reads 98.6F.

this is the average normal body temperature when it is measured orally.

To view the numbers, lines, and column of mercury, hold the thermometer at eye level, between the thumb and index finger of the right hand, by the stem end only. Look directly at the edge of the glass triangle with the lines at the top and the numbers at the bottom. Rotate the stem slightly back and forth until you see the silver mercury column in the middle, Figure 15–23. The point where the mercury stops is read and recorded as the body temperature. When the mercury is between tenth markings, it is read to the next highest two-tenths of a degree, Figure 15–24. Many thermometers have markings printed in blue below the normal arrow and in red above to make temperature identification easier.

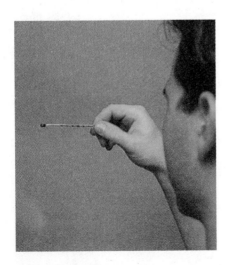

FIGURE 15–23 Hold the thermometer at eye level to read. (From Caldwell & Hegner, *Nursing Assistant*, 6th ed. Copyright 1992, Delmar Publishers Inc.)

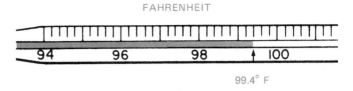

99.4° F

FIGURE 15–24 A temperature reading of 99.4 F. When the mercury is between the tenth markings it is read to the next higher tenth. (From Caldwell & Hegner, *Health Care Assistant*, 5th ed. Copyright 1989, Delmar Publishers Inc.)

It is extremely important that you not only read the thermometer accurately but that you also record the findings accurately. Remember that every line on a Fahrenheit thermometer represents two-tenths of a degree. Note the difference between 100.2°F and 102.0°F. For example, Figure 15–25. When reporting verbally, 100.2° is referred to as "one hundred and two-tenths" or "one hundred point two." A temperature of 102.0° is reported as "one hundred two" or "one hundred two point zero." It is good practice to read the thermometer and record the temperature as soon as possible after measuring. After you have written it down, read the thermometer again and check what you wrote to be certain you are accurate. The implications of an error in reporting should be obvious.

PRECAUTION: Taking temperatures requires contact with mucous membranes in the mouth or rectum. Discussion and procedure descriptions will reflect universal precautions. In any clinical setting, it is advisable to eliminate cross-contamination to prevent the spread of disease-producing organisms that cause hepatitis, AIDS, and many other transmittable diseases. Until a method of prevention or effective treatment is discovered, <u>EVERYONE</u> should be considered to be infected.

Care of Thermometers

Each time a temperature is taken, the thermometer must be cleaned and soaked in disinfectant. Even when cov-

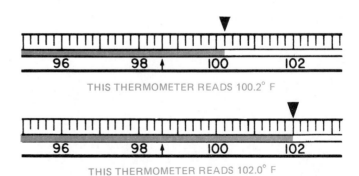

THIS THERMOMETER READS 100.2° F

THIS THERMOMETER READS 102.0° F

FIGURE 15–25 It is important to read and record temperature accurately.

ered with a plastic sheath, it is possible to accidentally contaminate the thermometer, depositing organisms on the bulb or stem. Glass mercury thermometers are extremely fragile, and care must be taken to prevent breakage.

When many thermometers are used daily, they will be processed in quantity. Each thermometer is cleaned and rinsed after use, then placed in a gauze-lined basin filled with disinfectant. Timing must begin after the last thermometer is added. All thermometers must be completely covered by the disinfectant. The thermometers are then removed from the solution, rinsed, and inspected. They may be stored in individual dry containers or placed in individual clean envelopes and stored in a drawer. Solution used in quantity disinfection is discarded after soaking time has elapsed.

An individual container filled with disinfectant solution is not recommended. It is no longer considered safe to use an unsheathed thermometer even when it is cleaned after each use and returned to a solution-filled container. If such an individual storage method is used, wipe the solution from the thermometer with a cotton ball, from the bulb to the stem, and discard cotton in a biohazardous container. Slip a sheath over the thermometer and continue as indicated in the procedure which follows. Stop and think, would **you** like to be your next patient? Remember your responsibility to others in stopping the threat of disease transmission. AIDS and hepatitis are very dangerous communicable diseases. Follow correct procedure each time you measure the temperature of any patient.

Slip-on Thermometer Sheaths

Clear plastic slip-on sheaths must be used when taking oral or rectal temperature with a glass thermometer. This narrow plastic cover slides over the thermometer like a loose skin. The covers come packaged in individualized narrow paper envelopes, Figure 15–26. The clean thermometer is inserted into the open end marked "insert." The opposite end is separated and peeled back revealing the plastic cover. Peel back the envelope to the stem end and snap off the tear tab. Check the cover to be certain it has remained intact before using. The thermometer is

---

PROCEDURE

Clean and Store Mercury Thermometers

TERMINAL PERFORMANCE OBJECTIVE: Given soiled mercury thermometers, cotton balls, soap, water, gloves, and a prepared container, the student will clean, inspect, disinfect, and store the thermometers aseptically, in accordance with procedure technique and observing aseptic and safety precautions. **Key Point: Oral and rectal thermometers are cleaned and disinfected separately.**

1. Wash hands and put on gloves.
2. Take soiled thermometers to sink.
3. Apply soap to cotton ball and add water to make solution.
4. While holding thermometer by stem, rotate and wipe it from stem to bulb with soapy solution.
   Key Point: Apply pressure to force solution into calibration engravings.
5. Discard cotton ball in biohazardous waste container.
6. While holding by stem with bulb pointed downward, rinse in cool running water. **Key Point: Hot water will overexpand mercury and either damage or break thermometer.**
7. Inspect for cleanliness and condition. If still soiled, repeat steps 3 to 6. Discard a chipped or cracked thermometer.
8. Grasp stem firmly between thumb and index finger.

9. Shake mercury down to 95.0° or below. **Key Point: Use a wrist-snapping action. Avoid striking faucet, sink, or counter. Shake to 95.0° or below to prepare for next use to help avoid an error with the next reading should it be below the current level. Remember, the mercury will not go down unless forced.**
10. Place thermometers in gauze-lined container filled with disinfectant. **Key Point: Thermometers must be completely covered and allowed to remain in solution for at least 20 minutes. If additional thermometers are added, timing must begin after last one is placed in the container.**
11. Using correct procedure, remove and discard gloves.
12. Wash hands.
13. Set timer or note time.
14. Following adequate time for disinfection, wash hands. Rinse, inspect, and place clean thermometers in individual envelopes, individual dry holders, or storage container. Remember if stored in individual holders to place a cotton ball in the bottom to prevent breakage of the bulb.
15. Clean area and equipment. Return thermometers to appropriate locations.

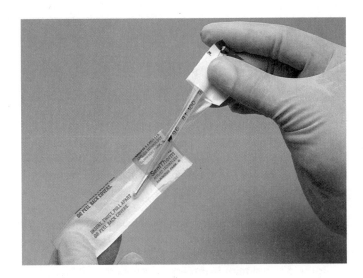

FIGURE 15–26 Slip-on thermometer sheaths

used exactly as if it were not covered. The covering is somewhat undesirable from the patient's viewpoint as it is a rather strange feeling to have a "minibaggie" under one's tongue.

When the temperature has been measured, the cover is simply held by the tear tab, pulled off, and discarded in the biohazardous waste container. The design is such that the sheath inverts itself, thereby reducing the chance of contamination of the thermometer. The temperature is then read and recorded and the thermometer cleaned, ready for use with the application of another sheath. A rectal thermometer *must* always be covered with a sheath and used only for rectal temperatures. It will require lubrication for ease of insertion.

Measuring Oral Temperature

Measuring temperature orally is the method of choice because it is relatively convenient, quick, and accurate. The oral clinical thermometer is placed in sublingually (under the tongue) and for a *minimum* of 3 minutes, Figure 15–27. (A study recently conducted indicated that 8 minutes was necessary to obtain the most accurate oral measurement.) Remember that a reading of 98.6°F or 37°C is considered normal.

Temperature readings will be inaccurate if the patient has smoked or had either a hot or cold drink within the previous 10 minutes. Always ask patients about this before placing the thermometer in their mouth. Tell them to keep the thermometer under their tongue with their lips closed around the stem. Readings will also be inaccurate if the patient breathes through the mouth. Caution the patient against biting down on the glass stem. It is possible to break the thermometer with the force of the teeth, cutting the tongue, gums, or inside of the mouth. The possible ingestion of glass fragments and poisonous mercury presents a real hazard.

Note: In temperature procedures, recording of findings is being delayed until after gloves have been removed and hands washed. This seems to be necessary to avoid contamination of pens/pencils, charts, and in turn yourself.

Contraindications to Oral Measurement

Oral temperature measurement is not the method of choice in certain situations, such as with infants and children under 6; patients with respiratory complications that require mouth breathing or the use of oxygen; confused, disoriented, or emotionally unstable patients; patients with oral injuries, recent oral surgery, facial paralysis, nasal obstruction, etc. In such situations, temperature must be measured by either the rectal, axillary or aural (auditory canal) method.

Measuring Rectal Temperature

Rectal temperature is a very accurate measurement, simply because it is taken internally. Rectal measurement is always indicated with babies and with young children who have not yet learned how to keep an oral thermometer in place or who might break it by biting down. Often children complain bitterly about having a rectal tempera-

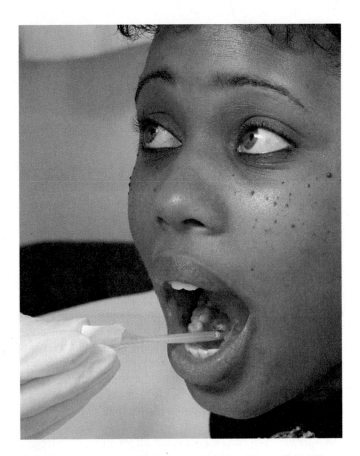

FIGURE 15–27 Place oral thermometer sublingually in a heat pocket.

P R O C E D U R E

Measure Oral Temperature with Mercury Thermometer

TERMINAL PERFORMANCE OBJECTIVE: In a simulated or actual situation, given a patient, an oral mercury thermometer, latex gloves, thermometer sheath, watch, or timer, paper and pen/pencil, the student will measure and record a patient's oral temperature. The procedure will be done with 100% accuracy, within a 6-minute period of time, following correct procedural technique, and observing aseptic and safety precautions.

1. Wash hands, put on gloves.
2. Identify patient. **Key Point: Call patient by name and check chart to avoid error.**
3. Explain procedure.
4. Determine if patient has recently had a hot or cold drink or smoked. **Key Point: If so, allow 10 minutes before measuring.**
5. Remove thermometer from holder or envelope. Avoid touching bulb end with fingers.
6. Inspect thermometer. Discard a chipped or cracked thermometer.
7. Read thermometer and shake down to 95° or below if necessary.

8. Put plastic sheath on thermometer. **Key Point: Check that sheath is intact.**
9. Place bulb sublingually in patient's mouth. **Key Point: Take care not to probe sensitive sublingual tissues.**
10. Tell patient how to maintain proper position of thermometer: to keep lips closed, breathe through nose, and avoid biting.
11. Leave thermometer in position a minimum of 3 minutes. **Key Point.: Time by watch or timer.**
12. Remove and read thermometer. **Key Point: Reinsert for additional minute if reading is less than 97.0°.**
13. Reread thermometer.
14. Holding by stem end, pull off plastic sheath and discard in biohazardous waste container.
15. Follow procedure for soiled thermometers.
16. Remove gloves and discard in biohazardous waste container.
17. Wash hands.
18. Record temperature.
19. Follow procedure to clean thermometer, returning to storage when completed. (Note: If greater accuracy is desired, adjust time and performance objective.)

---

ture taken when they think they are "too big." The physician usually has a policy concerning the age limit for rectal temperatures, which you will follow.

When measuring the temperature of infants, they may be positioned as in Figure 15–28, page 450. If positioning on back, unfasten the diaper to expose the anus. Grasp the ankles securely with one hand, flexing the knees to the abdomen. With the other hand insert the lubricated sheathed thermometer about 1 inch through the anal canal into the rectum. Hold the thermometer securely in place. Maintain your grasp on the ankles so the infant cannot turn over. Be prepared for the procedure to initiate urination or expelling of stool. It would wise to cover the male infant's penis with a diaper to absorb the urine stream. When positioning prone across a person's lap or on a table, be certain to maintain control of the infant or child's position to prevent turning over and causing injury to the rectum from the inserted thermometer. In either position, the thermometer position can be maintained by holding it securely between the index and middle finger with the palm of the hand against the buttocks.

Older children can be positioned either on their abdomen or side, whichever is preferred. Adults would be positioned on their side and draped with a sheet for privacy.

Temperatures measured rectally require a minimum of 3 minutes insertion time (5 minutes for greater accuracy). When recording a rectal measurement, place the letter R in parentheses following the reading, for example, 99.6°(R). Normal rectal temperature is 99.6°F or 37.5°C, one full degree above normal oral temperature. Temperature must never be measured rectally if the patient has had recent rectal surgery. It is possible to damage the operative site or perforate newly sutured lines.

Measuring Axillary Temperature

Temperature can also be measured by placing the thermometer in the axilla (armpit), Figure 15–29, page 450. This method is the least accurate and requires a full 10 minutes. Axillary measurement is appropriate only when oral is contraindicated and rectal is inconvenient, undesirable, or contraindicated. An oral stubby or security design thermometer is best suited for axillary measurement. Normal axillary temperature is 97.6°F or 36.4°C, one full degree *below* normal oral temperature. When recording axillary findings, place the letters *Ax* in parentheses following the reading; for example, 97.6°(Ax).

Measure Rectal Temperature with Mercury Thermometer

TERMINAL PERFORMANCE OBJECTIVE: In a simulated or actual situation, given a patient or manikin, a rectal mercury thermometer, tissue, lubricant, watch or timer, paper and pen/pencil, thermometer sheath and latex gloves, the student will measure and record a patient's rectal temperature. The procedure will be done with 100% accuracy, within an 8-minute period of time, following correct procedural technique, and observing aseptic and safety precautions.

1. Wash hands and put on gloves.
2. Identify patient. **Key Point: Call patient by name and check chart to avoid error.**
3. Explain procedure and what you are going to do, to child, parent, or adult patient.
4. Place a small amount of lubricant on a tissue. **Key Point: Lubricant should be water soluble.**
5. Remove thermometer from holder or envelope. **Key Point: Hold by stem end only.**
6. Inspect thermometer. Discard a chipped or cracked thermometer.
7. Read thermometer and shake down to 95° or below if necessary.
8. Place thermometer in plastic sheath. Check that sheath is intact.
9. Rotate thermometer bulb in lubricant on tissue and place in convenient location. **Key Point: A lubricated thermometer inserts with less discomfort and reduces chance of injury. Note: When performing procedure on an adult patient, proceed with the following steps:**
10. Instruct patient to remove appropriate clothing, assisting as needed. **Key Point: Provide privacy.**
11. Assist adult patient onto examining table and cover with drape. Avoid overexposure.
12. Position on side. Ensure patient's comfort and safety.
13. Arrange drape to expose buttocks.
14. With one hand raise upper buttock to expose anus.
15. With other hand, carefully insert lubricated thermometer into anal canal approximately 1 1/2 inches.
    Key Points:
    a. **Do not force thermometer. Rotating will often facilitate insertion.**
    b. **If opening is not apparent, request patient to bear down slightly; this will usually expose opening. Note: When performing the procedure on infants or small children, ask the parent or accompanying adult to prepare the child while you prepare the thermometer.**
16. Position as to parent's or physician's preference.
17. Ensure safety during procedure by maintaining control of the infant's or child's position. (A parent can be instructed to assist you, as in Figure 15–28(b), especially if it comforts the child.)
18. Expose anus.
19. Carefully insert well-lubricated thermometer one inch into anal canal. (See Key Point in Step 15 a.)
20. Hold thermometer in place for a minimum of 3 minutes (5 minutes for greater accuracy). **Key Point: Time by watch.**
21. Withdraw thermometer. Carefully remove plastic sheath and discard in biohazardous waste container.
22. Read thermometer.
23. Reread to check temperature.
24. Place thermometer on tissue. **Key Point: Never place soiled thermometer directly on unprotected surface.**
25. Remove any excess lubricant from anal area with tissue. Wipe from front to back.
26. Ask parent or accompanying adult to dress infant or child.
27. Assist adult patient from examining table and instruct to redress. **Key Point: Provide privacy as appropriate.**
28. Follow procedure for soiled thermometer.
29. Remove and discard gloves in biohazardous container.
30. Record temperature, placing (R) after the finding.
31. Return thermometer to storage after cleaning.

Disposable Thermometers

Disposable plastic oral thermometers may be used in some offices, urgent care centers, and hospital emergency rooms. Since they are used only once and discarded, they are free from contamination, and no time or equipment is required for cleaning. One disadvantage is the cost factor. The patient's reaction may also be less than enthusiastic. The plastic is thin and almost sharp.

Care must be taken to avoid touching the dot matrix portion, which is placed in the patient's mouth. The dots can be placed up or down. The thermometer must be held under the tongue, as far back as possible in the heat pocket with the tongue pressed against the end and the mouth closed on the stem, Figure 15–30, page 450. Wait 60 seconds, then remove the thermometer. Allow 10 seconds for the dots to stabilize, then read and record the temperature. The heat in the mouth causes a reaction on

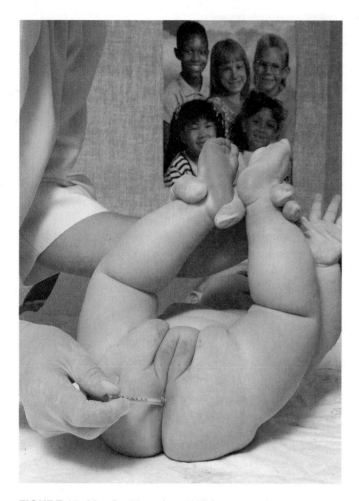

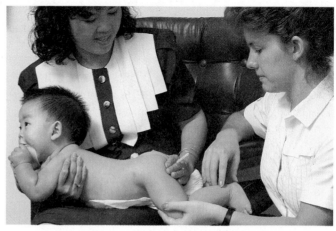

indicates the correct temperature. Then discard the thermometer in a biohazardous waste container. Plastic thermometers are not considered to be precisely accurate; however, for usual temperature determination, their single use and freedom from contamination concerns may outweigh any minor disadvantages.

The disposable plastic thermometer can also be used to measure axillary temperature. The dot matrix portion is placed next to the body, deep in the axillary space, with the handle extending straight down the patient's side. The arm must be held tightly at the side. After 3 minutes, remove the thermometer, wait 10 seconds, then read and record the temperature.

FIGURE 15–28 Positions (a and b) for measuring rectal temperature of infants

the heat-sensitive dots printed on the surface of the plastic strip. Readings are calculated by counting the number of dots that change color within a degree grouping, Figure 15–31, page 452. The last changed dot on the matrix

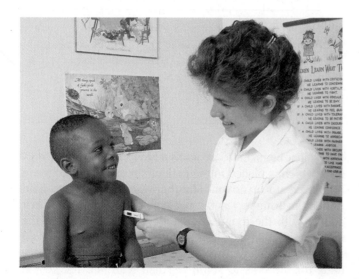

FIGURE 15–29 Measuring axillary temperature

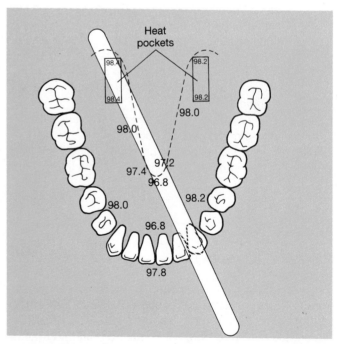

FIGURE 15–30 Dot matrix portion of disposable thermometer must be placed sublingually into a heat pocket. (Illustration courtesy of PhMaH Corporation, Sommerville, NJ)

P R O C E D U R E

Measure Axillary Temperature with Mercury Thermometer

TERMINAL PERFORMANCE OBJECTIVE: In a simulated or actual situation, given a patient, a mercury oral security thermometer, tissues, watch or timer, paper and pen/pencil, the student will measure and record axillary temperature with 100% accuracy, within a 14-minute period of time, following correct procedural technique, and observing aseptic and safety precautions.

1. Wash hands.
2. Identify patient. **Key Point: Call patient by name and check chart to avoid error.**
3. Explain procedure and what you are going to do.
4. Remove thermometer from holder or envelope.
5. Inspect thermometer. Discard a chipped or cracked thermometer.
6. Read thermometer and shake down to 95° or below if necessary.
7 Place thermometer on tissue or in envelope in convenient location.
8. Assist patient, as necessary, to expose axilla. **Key Point: Provide privacy.**
9. Pat axillary space with tissue to remove perspiration. Perspiration prevents thermometer from coming into direct contact with skin. It also makes it more difficult to keep thermometer in place.

10. Place thermometer deep in the axillary space. Position so that the bulb is in direct contact with the top of the axillary space with the stem projecting anteriorly. Note: The thermometer may be placed with the stem extending posteriorly if desired.
11. Hold arm tightly against body. Have patient maintain position for a minimum of 10 minutes.
    Key Points:
    a. **Time by watch or timer.**
    b. **Help weak or confused patient maintain position.**
    c. **Be certain thermometer remains deep in axillary space. Children will require close attention and assistance.**
12. Remove thermometer and wipe with tissue from stem to bulb. **Key Point: Action is from clean to soiled area.**
13. Read and record findings. **Key Point: Place (Ax) after reading.**
14. Reread and check recording.
15. Help patient replace clothing.
16. Follow procedure for soiled thermometer.
17. Wash hands.
18. Return thermometer to storage after cleaning.

P R O C E D U R E

Measure Oral Temperature with Disposable Plastic Thermometer

TERMINAL PERFORMANCE OBJECTIVE: In a simulated or actual situation, given a patient, a disposable plastic thermometer, watch or timer, paper and pen/pencil, the student will measure and record oral temperature with 100% accuracy, within a 4-minute period of time, following correct procedural technique and observing aseptic and safety precautions.

1. Wash hands.
2. Identify patient. **Key Point: Call patient by name and check chart to avoid error.**
3. Explain procedure and what you are going to do. **Key Point: Ensure patient has not smoked or drunk any hot or cold liquids in the past 15 minutes.**
4. Open package by peeling back top of wrapper to expose handle end of thermometer.
5. Grasp handle and remove from wrapper. **Key Point: Do NOT touch dot matrix portion, which will be**

placed in the patient's mouth.
6. Insert thermometer into patient's mouth as far back as possible into one of the heat pockets (see Figure 15–30).
7. Instruct patient to press tongue down on thermometer and keep mouth closed.
8. Maintain position for 60 seconds. **Key Point: Time by watch or timer.**
9. Remove thermometer and wait 10 seconds for dots to stabilize. **Key Point: Take special care to avoid touching the portion that has been in the patient's mouth.**
10. Read thermometer and discard in biohazardous waste container.
11. Wash hands.
12. Record temperature.

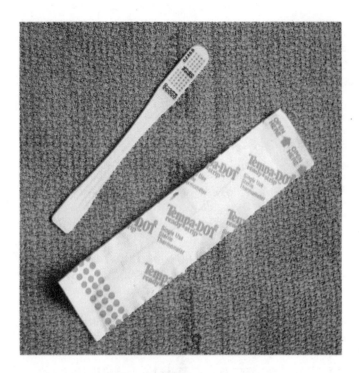

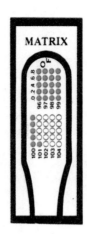

FIGURE 15–31 Disposable plastic thermometer. The matrix in (b) reads 101 F. (Adapted from Caldwell & Hegner, *Health Care Assistant*, 5th ed. Copyright 1989, Delmar Publishers Inc.)

A variation of the disposable thermometer is available for rectal use. It is packaged with a plastic sheath and is not recommended for infants or toddlers. The thermometer must be well lubricated and inserted until the dot matrix is completely covered. After 3 minutes, it is withdrawn and the sheath discarded. After 10 seconds, the temperature may be read and recorded. It would be necessary to wear gloves because the chances are great that you may contact secretions from rectal mucosa.

When exposed to high temperatures the matrix dots will turn blue. If this should occur, place them in a freezer for 1 hour for each box of 100 thermometers. Rectal thermometers will require 2 hours per 100 thermometers. Then let them stand at room temperature for a day. The thermometers will then be ready for use and their accuracy should not be affected.

Electronic Thermometers

The use of electronic thermometers is becoming more common. They are quick, sanitary, easily read, and do not require cleaning. A small, battery-operated unit with a digital read-out window is very accurate and capable of measuring a temperature within a few seconds, Figure 15–32. A metal probe, blue for oral, red for rectal, is used like a mercury thermometer. It is attached by a cord to the battery unit. A disposable cover slips over the probe to provide each patient with an individual thermometer. The covered probe is inserted in the patient's mouth like a mercury thermometer. It is usually held in place by the medical assistant since the time involved is short, and the probe, with its cord, is heavy and somewhat cumbersome. As soon as the temperature level has

been reached, the unit will sound a signal and the final reading will appear in the window of the unit.

Electronic thermometers are time-saving and convenient, but they are somewhat expensive. Care must also be taken to adjust the unit frequently and correctly. It is critical that the dial be observed from a direct view at eye level while making adjustments. The unit must be returned to its charging stand after use to maintain the battery.

Electronic thermometers may also be used to measure axillary and rectal temperature. Use the rectal (red) probe to take a rectal temperature. Remove the rectal probe

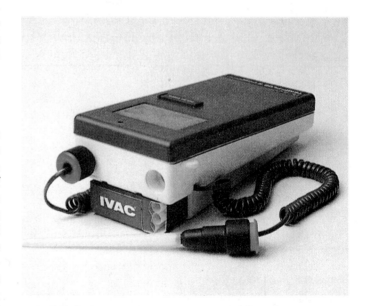

FIGURE 15–32 Electronic thermometer (From Caldwell & Hegner, *Health Care Assistant*, 5th ed. Copyright 1989, Delmar Publishers Inc.)

P R O C E D U R E

Measure Oral Temperature Electronically

TERMINAL PERFORMANCE OBJECTIVE: In a simulated or actual situation, given a patient, an electronic thermometer unit, probe, sheath/cover, paper and pen/pencil, the student will measure the patient's temperature electronically. The temperature will be read and recorded at 100% accuracy, within a 2-minute period of time, following correct procedural technique, and observing aseptic and safety precautions.

1. Wash hands, assemble equipment.
2. Identify patient. **Key Point: Call patient by name and check chart to avoid error.**
3. Explain procedure and what you are going to do.
4. Place probe connector in receptacle of unity base and check to make sure it is properly seated.
5. Holding it by the collar, remove appropriate probe from stored position.
6. Insert probe firmly into probe cover to ensure that it is properly seated.
7. Insert covered probe into mouth. **Key Point: The** probe and connecting cord is rather heavy and cumbersome. It will be necessary to hold the thermometer steady in place.
8. Maintain covered probe in position until unit signals, approximately 10–15 seconds.
9. Remove probe from patient. Do not touch probe cover.
10. Read and record temperature measurement. **Key Point: Temperature is displayed digitally in window of unit.**
11. Recheck your reading and recording.
12. Press the eject button to discard used probe cover into biohazardous waste container. **Key Point: Avoid touching.**
13. Return probe to stored position in unit. Thermometer display will read zero and shut off.
14. Store unit in charging stand. **Key Point: Unit should remain in stand when not in use. A red light in the upper left hand area of the display indicates that the thermometer is charging.**

---

from its holder and attach a probe cover. The probe is inserted into the rectum 1/2" for adults and 1/4" for children. The use of lubricant is optional. The probe should be angled slightly to ensure contact with the rectal mucosa. After the reading is registered, remove the probe and discard the cover in a biohazardous waste container.

When taking axillary temperature, some manufacturers recommend using the rectal probe; others recommend the oral probe. Consult the instructional booklet with your equipment to determine which to use. Apply a probe cover and insert the tip well into the axillary space with the probe extending down and slightly forward along the patient's side. Press gently into the space to establish good tissue contact. Have patient lower arm over probe. Hold probe in position to maintain good contact. Remove and read after unit signals completion. It should be noted that a "normal" axillary temperature is 0.5°F (0.3°C) lower than an oral temperature.

Some units have built-in operator prompts to signal when technique or problems exist. If the phrase OPER ERR 9 (or something similar) shows on the readout window, it means the probe is not in contact with tissue. A readjustment of the thermometer will erase the message and allow the continued measurement of the temperature. A BAT LO (or similar) message indicates the unit's batteries do not have enough charge to take a temperature. The unit must be returned to the charger base for 6 to 8 hours to be fully charged or 45 minutes to permit a limited number of measurements. A PROB BAD (or similar) message indicates the probe is damaged and will not sense temperature properly. This can be corrected only by installing a new probe.

Another electronic thermometer is simple and self-contained. It is also a digital thermometer and is excellent for home use, Figure 15–33. The thermometer will register the temperature in about 60 seconds on an easy-to-read LCD panel that shows the temperature in tenths of degrees. The thermometer can be cleaned with soap and water and sanitized with a disinfectant. Probe covers

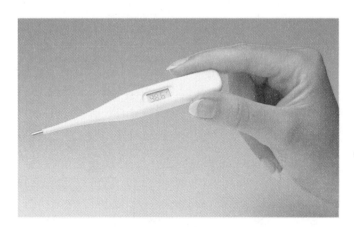

FIGURE 15–33 Electronic digital thermometer (Courtesy, Omron Marshall Products, Inc., Vernon Hills, IL)

are available for clinic or office use. It may be used for oral, axillary, or rectal measurement. Some models have a beeper that sounds when the maximum temperature is reached. This feature is especially appealing to children.

Tympanic Membrane Thermometers

A totally new concept in temperature measurement is the instantaneous tympanic membrane (aural) thermometer. At the present time two manufacturers have models available. The Thermoscan Pro-1 is shown in Figure 15–34. The other, First Temp Genius operates by the same principle. Both instruments measure the strength of the infrared heat waves generated by the tympanic membrane and will digitally display that temperature in less than 2 seconds. Because the tympanic membrane shares the same blood supply as the hypothalamus, it is believed the auditory canal is an ideal site for obtaining an accurate assessment of the body's core temperature. Studies conducted with temperature-sensing devices placed internally in a large blood vessel have shown strong correlation in results.

Although its greatest asset is the instant result, it has become a real benefit to health care professionals in hospital emergency rooms, labor and delivery rooms, and pediatric units because it does not involve contact with mucous membranes and the site is so easily accessible. Another advantage is the readings are not affected by hot or cold liquids or smoking as are oral methods. In addition, the patient does not even need to be conscious.

The thermometer is extremely easy to use. You simply position the covered plastic tip inside the auditory canal, press the scan button, and an infrared beam measures the

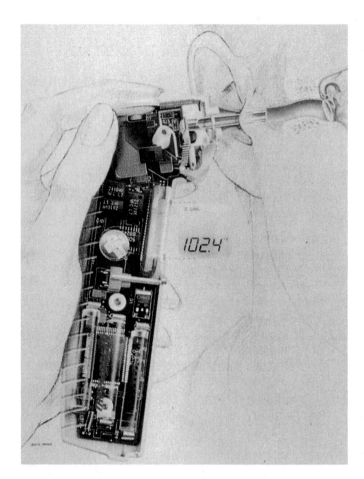

FIGURE 15–34 Tympanic thermometer (Courtesy of Thermoscan Inc., San Diego, CA)

heat waves. The results are displayed digitally on the screen. A release button ejects the probe cover and in 10

  P R O C E D U R E

Measure Core Body Temperature with an Aural Thermometer

TERMINAL PERFORMANCE OBJECTIVE: In a simulated or actual situation, given a patient, an aural thermometer, a probe cover, paper and pen/pencil, the student will measure and record tympanic temperature with 100% accuracy within a 3-minute period of time, following correct procedural technique and observing aseptic and safety precautions.

1. Wash hands.
2. Identify Patient: **Key Point: Call patient by name and check chart to avoid error.**
3. Explain procedure and what you are going to do.
4. Remove aural thermometer from base. The display should read "ready."
5. Attach a disposable probe cover to the ear piece.
6. Insert covered probe into ear canal, sealing opening.
7. Press the scan button to activate the thermometer.
8. Observe the display window, noting the temperature.
9. Withdraw the thermometer.
10. Press the release button on the thermometer to eject the probe cover into a waste basket.
11. Record the temperature using (T) or (Tc) to indicate tympanic or tympanic core temperature.
12. Return thermometer to base.

   Note: Thermometers can be set to correlate with an oral or rectal reading. Usually, the oral mode is used and a reading of 98.6°F is considered "normal."

seconds another temperature can be taken. The method is acceptable to patients and a real time saver to the health care worker. The units operate on three AAA alkaline batteries and will measure at least 10,000 temperatures before needing to be replaced. As the aural thermometer becomes more acceptable and less expensive, many clinics, urgent care centers, and group practices may use the new technology.

Celsius Thermometers

The only difference between Celsius and Fahrenheit thermometers is the calibration. On a Celsius thermometer, each long line represents a degree. They are numbered consecutively, with the nine lines that are between each number representing one-tenth of a degree, Figure 15–35.

Temperature can be converted from one scale to another by a mathematical calculation. To convert Celsius to Fahrenheit, multiply the degrees by 9/5 and add 32. To change Fahrenheit to Celsius, subtract 32 and multiply by 5/9. Table 15–4 shows examples of temperature conversions and compares some common temperatures.

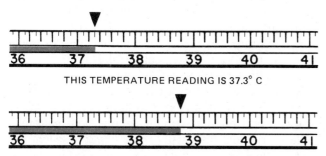

THIS TEMPERATURE READING IS 37.3° C

THIS TEMPERATURE READING IS 38.8° C

FIGURE 15–35   Reading a Celsius thermometer

Pulse ....

Each time the heart beats, blood is forced into the aorta, temporarily expanding its walls and initiating a wavelike effect. This wave continues through all the body's arteries, causing the alternating expansion and recoil of the arterial walls, Figure 15–36. This effect can be palpated (felt) in the arteries that are close to the body surface and that lie over bone or firm structures. When the artery is pressed against the underlying structure, it is possible to feel the rhythmic pulsation, known as the pulse.

Pulse Points

The pulse can be felt in several locations on the body, Figure 15–37, page 456. The radial pulse point is on the thumb side of the inner surface of the wrist, lying over the radius bone. The radial pulse point is used most frequently when measuring pulse rate.

The brachial artery pulse point is on the inner medial surface of the elbow, at the antecubital space (crease of

TABLE 15–4
Temperature Conversion and Comparison
To convert Celsius to Fahrenheit:
$$37°C \times \frac{9}{5} \left(\frac{333}{5}\right) = 66.6 + 32 = 98.6°F$$
To convert Fahrenheit to Celsius:
$$98.6°F - 32 = 66.6 \times \frac{5}{9} \left(\frac{333}{9}\right) = 37°C$$

	Celsius (C)	Fahrenheit (F)
Freezing	0°	32°
Body Temperature	37°	96.6°
Pasteurization	63°	145°
Boiling	100°	212°
Sterilizing (Autoclave)	121°	250°

elbow). This point is used to palpate and auscultate (listen to) blood pressure.

The carotid pulse can be felt in the carotid artery of the neck when pressure is applied to the area at either side of the trachea. It is the carotid pulse that is palpated during the cardiopulmonary resuscitation (CPR) life-saving maneuver.

Two other points often palpated to evaluate circulation in the lower extremities are the femoral, located midway in the groin where the artery begins its descent down the femur, and the dorsalis pedis, on the instep of the foot.

Pulse Rate

The number of times the heart beats per minute is measured by counting the pulse in the radial artery. The average adult pulse rate is 72 beats per minute. The pulse rate is recorded as beats per minute preceded by a capital *P*; for example, P. 72.

The rate of the pulse is influenced by several factors. The most obvious is exercise or activity. With increased activity, the heartbeat increases 20 to 30 beats per minute to meet the body's needs. It should return to normal

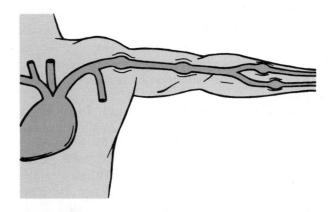

FIGURE 15–36   Blood pumped from the heart causes a wavelike effect in the arteries.

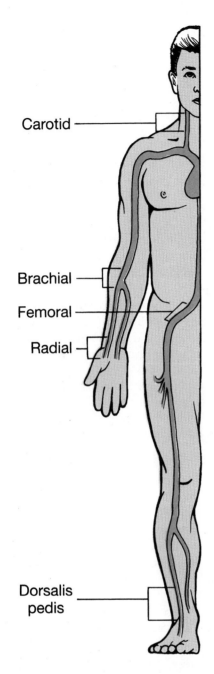

Carotid

Brachial

Femoral

Radial

Dorsalis
pedis

FIGURE 15–37 Pulse points of the upper and lower extremities and the neck.

within 3 minutes after activity has stopped. Of course, the rate of increase will be in proportion to the level of activity.

Age is directly related to pulse rate. The younger the person, the faster the heartbeat. A sample of age-related average pulse rates is shown in Table 15–5.

Pulse rate is also related to the sex of the patient. A female's pulse is approximately 10 beats per minute more rapid than a male's of the same age. Pulse rate is also related to size; therefore the larger male will have a slower rate than a smaller male. The relationship of size is particularly evident in animals. The heart rate of a bird

may be well over 200 beats per minute while an elephant has a rate of about 30.

The physical condition of the body is another factor. Athletes, especially those who run or engage in strenuous sports, have a considerably slower pulse rate due to a more efficient circulatory system.

In general, the heart rate increases when the sympathetic nervous system is stimulated by such feelings as fear, anxiety, pain, or anger. The rate also increases with certain other conditions, such as thyroid disease, anemia, shock, or fever. A rate of over 100 beats per minute is known as *tachycardia.*

When the parasympathetic nervous system affects the heart, it causes the rate to be much slower. A rate below 60 beats per minute is known as *bradycardia.* This may also occur with the use of certain medications, heart disease, emotional depression, and drugs. A rate below 60 beats per minute is also normal for many athletes.

Pulse Characteristics

When measuring pulse rate, two other characteristics must also be observed and recorded. The force or strength of the pulse is referred to as its volume. Words used to describe this quality are: normal, full or bounding, weak, and thready (scarcely perceptible).

The quality of rhythm of the pulse refers to its regularity, the equal spacing of the beats. A pulse which lacks a regular rhythm is said to have arrhythmia. The pulse can be irregular (without a consistent pattern) or regularly irregular (unequally spaced but consistently the same beating pattern). A pulse can also be intermittent and occasionally skip or insert beats. Often caffeine or nicotine react on the heart to cause irregularity and increased rate.

Measuring Radial Pulse

The patient should be completely relaxed and sitting comfortably or lying down when the pulse is measured and evaluated. Ideally the arm should be well supported, with the wrist near the level of the heart. Place the tips of your first three fingers at the wrist area, about an inch above the

TABLE 15–5
Pulse–Age Relationship

Age	Pulse Rate
Less than 1 year	100–170
2–6 years	90–115
6–10 years	80–110
11–16 years	70–95
Midlife adult	65–80
Aged adult	50–65

base of the thumb, Figure 15–38. Never use your thumb to measure pulse rate; there is a chance you may feel and record your own heart rate in your thumb's artery.

An appropriate amount of pressure applied to the artery will permit the pulsations to be felt. Too much pressure will shut off the circulation and therefore eliminate the pulse beat. Too little pressure will not compress the artery sufficiently against the radius. With practice, applying the correct amount of pressure will become routine.

Measuring Apical Pulse

In instances when measuring heart rate by the radial pulse is not appropriate, it is necessary to listen to the heart at its **apex** with a **stethoscope.** This is a very accurate method of measuring heartbeat. The contraction of the atria and the ventricles will be heard as two closely occurring sounds, known as the lubb dupp; however, both contraction phases are counted as only one beat. Whenever a pulse rate is measured at a point other than radial, that fact should be noted when recording the rate; for example, P. 97 (Ap). Note that an **apical** pulse is counted for a full minute, so it is possible to record an uneven number.

Locating the Apex.   The bottom or lower edge of the heart is known as the apex. This is the point of maximum

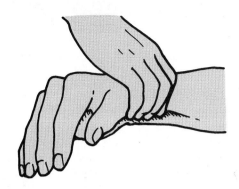

FIGURE 15–38   Measuring radial pulse

impulse of the heart against the chest wall. It can be palpated at the left fifth intercostal space in line with the middle of the left clavicle. This spot may be located by pressing the fingertips between the ribs and counting down five spaces on the left chest wall, Figure 15–39(a), page 459. Often the beat at the apex can be felt with the fingertips.

Another, quicker method for estimating the location of the apex is to place the outstretched left hand on the chest wall with the tip of the middle finger in the suprasternal notch and the thumb at a 45-degree angle, Figure 15–39(b), page 459. The end of the thumb will be approximately over the apex. This is only an approximate

---

P R O C E D U R E

Measure Radial Pulse

TERMINAL PERFORMANCE OBJECTIVE: In a simulated or actual situation, given a patient, a watch with a sweep-second hand, paper and pen/pencil, the student will within a 3-minute period of time, assess and record the quality and measure and record the rate of a patient's radial pulse, within 2 beats per minute accuracy, following correct procedural technique.

1. Wash hands, assemble equipment.
2. Identify patient. **Key Point: Call patient by name and check chart to avoid error.**
3. Explain procedure. Identify what you are going to do.
4. Determine patient's recent activity. Exertion within past 3-5 minutes will cause temporary increase in pulse rate.
5. Have patient assume a comfortable position with arm supported, palm of hand down, wrist near level of heart or placed across upper abdomen if lying down.
6. Locate radial artery on thumb side of wrist. **Key Point:**

Do not use your thumb. Place tips of fingers over artery; exert light pressure.
7. Observe quality of pulse before beginning to count. Determine if regular, strong, weak, thready, etc.
8. Check watch. Begin counting beats when second hand is at 3, 6, 9, or 12 (Note: Makes 30 seconds easier to observe.)
9. Count a *regular* pulse for 30 seconds and multiply results by 2. Note that this will always be an even number. If *irregular,* count for full minute, but do not multiply by 2.
10. Record pulse in beats per minute. **Key Point: Immediate recording helps eliminate errors.**
11. Describe quality characteristics. **Key Point: Usually only abnormal characteristics are noted. In certain situations, noting a normal quality may be important.**
12. Wash hands.

PROCEDURE

Measure Apical Pulse

TERMINAL PERFORMANCE OBJECTIVE: In a simulated or actual situation, given a patient, a watch with a sweep-second hand, stethoscope, alcohol wipe, paper, and pen/pencil, the student will, within a 5-minute period of time, locate the apex of the heart, assess and record the quality and measure and record the rate of a patient's apical pulse. This procedure will be done with 100% accuracy, following correct technique, and observing aseptic precautions.

1. Wash hands.
2. Prepare stethoscope by wiping earpieces and chestpiece with germicidal solution to prevent transfer of organisms.
3. Identify patient. **Key Point: Call patient by name and check chart to avoid error.**
4. Tell patient what you are going to do. If an infant or small child, explain to parent.
5. Provide privacy and a gown or drape if indicated.
6. Uncover left side of chest. Auscultation must be done directly against the skin surface.
7. Place earpieces in ears. Openings in tips should be forward, entering auditory canal.
8. Locate apex by palpating to left fifth intercostal space at midclavicular line. **Key Point: If chestpiece does not have a chill ring, warm in palm of one hand while** locating apex. This also prevents accidental striking against hard surface and resulting noise in ears.
9. Place chestpiece of stethoscope at apex.
10. Determine quality of heart sounds. **Key Point: Concentrate on rhythm and volume.**
11. Concentrate on rate of beats. **Key Point: Be certain of sounds and pattern.**
12. Observe watch and begin counting rate when second hand is at 3, 6, 9, or 12.
13. Count beats for a full minute. **Key Point: Both pulse phases count as one beat.**
14. Remove earpieces from ears.
15. Record rate and quality of heart sounds.
    Key Points:
    a. Immediate recording aids in eliminating errors.
    b. Indicate apical measurement.
16. Assist or instruct patient to dress unless physician also wishes to assess heart action. Determine this by asking physician prior to measurement of if your findings indicate the need.
17. Wipe earpieces and chestpiece of stethoscope with disinfectant. Return to storage.
18. Wash hands.

measurement since the size of the chest and the hand will vary. For a ready reference point, the apex should be just below the left breast. Again, this is a variable, particularly in the female, due to the size and placement of the breast.

Apical Indications. Apical pulse measurement is indicated for infants and small children due to their normally rapid rate, which is easier to hear and count than to palpate. Patients with heart conditions, especially if being medicated with cardiac drugs, will require apical measurement for greater accuracy. Apical measurement is always indicated if you have difficulty feeling a radial pulse and believe you may be missing beats. Other indications are an excessively rapid or slow rate, a thready or irregular quality, or with an existing or suspected pulse deficit.

Measuring Apical-Radial Pulse

Certain heart conditions cause a symptom known as pulse deficit. A patient with a pulse deficit will have a higher apical than radial pulse rate. This difference indicates that some heart contractions are not strong enough to produce a palpable radial pulse. It is important to determine the extent of the deficit by measuring the apical and radial rate at the same time.

A procedure call *apical-radial pulse* requires one person to measure the pulse rate radially while another auscultates the apical rate with a stethoscope, Figure 15–40. The radial rate is then subtracted from the apical, the difference being the pulse deficit. Ideally, two people measure the rate at the same time. If this is not possible, then the apical rate is measured and recorded, followed immediately by the radial. Apical-radial rates are always measured for a full minute.

Respiration

The third vital sign to be measured is respiration. One respiration is the combination of total inspiration (breathing in) and total expiration (breathing out). Other frequently used terms are inhale and exhale.

Respirations are usually measured as one part of total vital signs assessment. Since patients can voluntarily control the depth, rate, and regularity of their breathing to some extent, it is important that they not be aware the procedure is being done. To accomplish this, it is com-

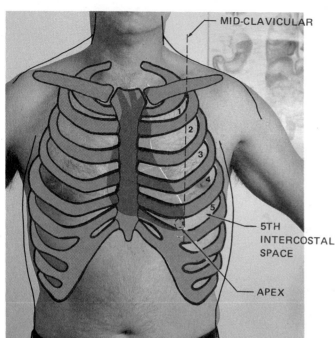
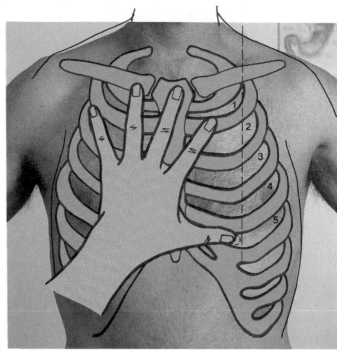

FIGURE 15–39 (a) Locating the apical pulse by counting intercostal spaces. (b). Alternative method for locating the apex of the heart.

mon practice to observe and measure respiration immediately after assessing the pulse, while maintaining your fingers at the radial pulse or auscultating the apex. Using this method, the patient assumes you are still measuring pulse rate.

Quality of Respiration

Respirations should be quiet, effortless, and regularly spaced. Breathing should be through the nose with the mouth closed. Excessively fast and deep breathing, commonly associated with hysteria, is called **hyperventilation.** Difficult or labored breathing is called **dyspnea.** Frequently dyspnea is accompanied by discomfort and an anxious expression, due to fear of being unable to breathe. This patient will use the accessory respiratory muscles of the rib cage, neck, shoulders, and back to assist the breathing process.

The presence of **râles** (noisy breathing) usually indicates constricted bronchial passageways or the collection of fluid or exudate. Râles may be present with pneumonia, bronchitis, asthma, and other pulmonary diseases.

Respirations should be observed for the depth of inhalation. Three words are used to describe this quality: normal, shallow, or deep. Depth of inhalation can be determined by watching the rise and fall of the chest. The rhythm of the respirations must also be assessed. This quality can be described as regular or irregular. Absence of breathing is known as **apnea.** A breathing pattern called **Cheyne–Stokes** occurs with acute brain, heart, or lung damage or disease, and with intoxicants. It is characterized by slow, shallow breaths that increase in depth and frequency to be followed by a few shallow

breaths, and then a period of apnea for 10 to 20 seconds, often more, Figure 15–41, page 460. This type of breathing pattern frequently precedes death.

Respiration Rate

Normal respiration rate for adults is from 16 to 20 times per minute. The respiration rate in infants and children has a greater range and fluctuates more during illness, exercise, and emotion than adult rates do. In the new-

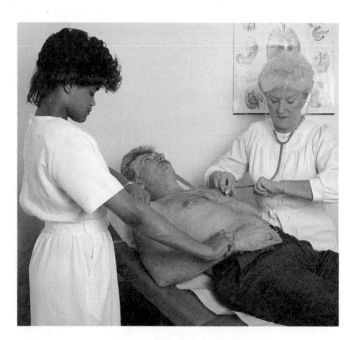

FIGURE 15–40 Measuring apical-radial pulse

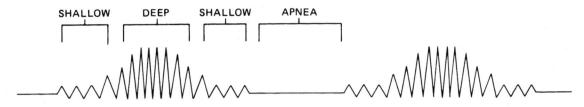

FIGURE 15–41 Cheyne–Stokes breathing pattern

born, the rate per minute may range from 30 to 80; in early childhood, from 20 to 40; and during late childhood from 15 to 25. The rate will reach an adult normal range of 16 to 20 by age 15. An abnormally slow rate of respiration is known as *bradypnea*. A faster than normal rate of respiration is known as *tachypnea*.

Counting Respirations

It is necessary to observe the patient carefully while measuring respiration rate. If the patient is lying on the examination table, position the patient's arm across the upper abdominal area, placing your fingers over the radial pulse point. In this position you cannot only visualize respiration but feel it as well, Figure 15–42. With the patient in a sitting position, you will need to observe more carefully as you count the respirations. Remember, it is also necessary to keep your watch in view as you

observe. With a little practice, you will be able to manage both at the same time.

When counting respirations as part of the TPR assessment, it is very important that you remember the number of heartbeats you have just counted. It may help you to use the following method:

1. Assume the pulse measuring position.
2. Observe, determine the characteristics, and describe to yourself the qualities of both the pulse and the respirations.
3. Count the number of heartbeats during the first 30 seconds.
4. Then repeat the pulse rate to yourself as you count the number of respirations during the second 30 seconds. (Note: You MUST use the word "and" between each respiration so you do not accidentally add counts to the pulse rate.)

 P R O C E D U R E

Measure Respirations

TERMINAL PERFORMANCE OBJECTIVE: In a simulated or actual situation, given a patient, a watch with a sweep-second hand, paper, and pen/pencil, the student will assess and record the quality and rate of a patient's respirations with 100% accuracy, within a 3-minute period of time, following the correct procedural technique.

1. Wash hands.
2. Identify patient. **Key Point: Call patient by name and check chart to avoid error.**
3. In this procedure, it is preferable *not* to explain to the patient what you are about to do. If the patient knows that you will be counting respirations, control of breathing is possible, resulting in an inaccurate measurement.
4. Ask about recent activity level. **Key Point: Patient should have been relatively quiet for past 2-5 minutes.**
5. Place patient in comfortable position, either sitting or lying down.

6. Assume pulse measurement position. **Key Point: Respirations are more easily counted if patient's arm is across upper abdomen.**
7. Assess quality. **Key Point: Determine regularity, depth, quietness.**
8. Count respirations for 30 seconds.
   Key Points:
   a. **One rise and fall of the chest equals one respiration.**
   b. **Maintain radial pulse position.**
   c. **If respirations irregular, count for a full minute; do not multiply results by two.**
9. Multiply results by two and record.
10. Record quality characteristics. **Key Point: Usually only abnormal characteristics are noted. In certain situations, noting a normal characteristic may be important.**
11. Wash hands.

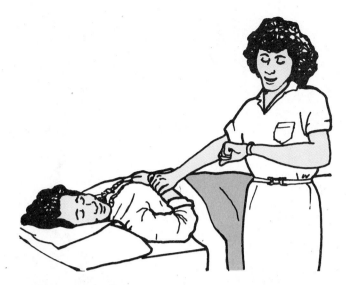

FIGURE 15–42 Measuring respirations

For example, if your patient's pulse rate at 30 seconds is 40, repeat the rate as you count the respirations "40 and 1, 40 and 2, 40 and 3," etc., until the second 30-second period is past. At the end of a minute, you will have both counts, which you will need to multiply by two and record.

Temperature–Pulse–Respiration Ratio

Respiration rate, like pulse, will increase with activity, excitement, fear, and other strong emotions, and certain disease conditions. Respirations are, as is the pulse, in proportion to the degree of fever present. Table 15–6 demonstrates the relationship of the three vital signs.

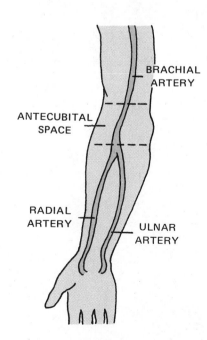

FIGURE 15–43 Blood pressure is measured in the brachial artery at the antecubital space.

Whenever a patient, either child or adult, has been upset and crying, a period of time must pass before an accurate measurement of either pulse or respirations can be made. Strong emotions elevate the vital signs and may make a true measurement impossible.

Blood Pressure

The fourth vital sign is blood pressure. Learning to assess blood pressure accurately requires attention to details, careful listening, and correct technique. The term *blood pressure* means the fluctuating pressure that the blood exerts against the arterial walls as the heart alternately contracts and relaxes. The blood pressure reflects the condition of the heart, the amount of blood forced from the heart at contraction, the condition of the arteries, and to some extent the volume and viscosity (stickiness) of the blood.

Blood pressure is measured in the brachial artery of the arm at the antecubital space, Figure 15–43. It should be measured in both arms, at least initially. There is normally a 5- to 10-mm difference. Subsequent readings should be made on the arm with the higher pressure.

Maintaining Blood Pressure

Two main factors cooperate to maintain a fairly constant blood pressure. The first is the heart or pump, which exerts pressure on the blood. About 100,000 times a day the heart contracts, forcing blood into the aorta and throughout the blood vessels of the body. Without a strong, effective pump, the blood will not flow and the pressure will drop.

The second factor is the brain, which controls, through the autonomic nervous system, the rate of the heart and the size of the opening or caliber of the arteries. When sensors in the arteries detect an increase in arterial pressure, a message is sent to the brain, which in turn directs the arteries to dilate slightly (reducing resistance to the flow of blood) and directs the heart to slow

TABLE 15–6
Temperature–Pulse–Respiration Ratio

Respiration	Pulse	Temperature (F°)
18	80	99
19 (plus)	88	100
21	96	101
23	104	102
25 (minus)	112	103
27	120	104
28 (minus)	128	105
30	136	106

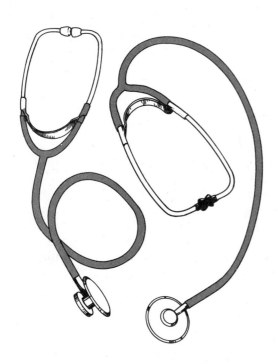

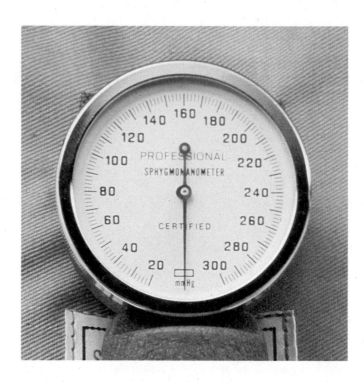

FIGURE 15–44 Blood pressure measuring equipment. (a). Single and dual-head stethoscopes. (b). Mercury sphygmomanometer scale. (c). Aneroid sphygmomanometer dial.

down (reducing the amount of blood being forced out). When the pressure drops too far, the message to the brain results in slightly increased heart action and constriction of the arteries, which cause the pressure to rise. Both actions are needed to maintain homeostasis.

Blood Pressure Phases

The phases of blood pressure are identical to those of the pulse. A contraction phase, known as *systole,* corresponds to the beat phase of the heart, and is the period of greatest pressure. The relaxation phase, known as *diastole,* corresponds to the resting or filling action of the heart, and is the period of least pressure.

Normal Blood Pressure

Blood pressure is measured in millimeters of mercury (mm Hg) using a stethoscope and a sphygmomanometer, which may have either a calibrated column of mercury or an aneroid dial, Figure 15–44. Blood pressure readings are measurements of systolic and diastolic pressure written as a fraction; for example, B/P 120/80, where 120 is systolic and 80 is diastolic pressure.

A normal adult will have a systolic pressure between 100 and 140 mm Hg, and a diastolic pressure between 60 and 90. Blood pressure readings persistently above 140/90 indicate *hypertension* (high blood pressure). Hypertension can result from things such as stress, obesity, high salt intake, sedentary life-style, and aging. Physical conditions that cause hypertension are kidney

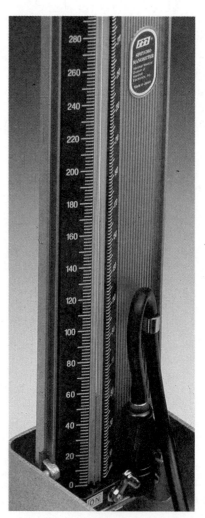

disease, thyroid dysfunction, neurological disorders, and vascular conditions, such as atherosclerosis and arteriosclerosis, which make circulation more difficult, therefore requiring a greater pressure to circulate the blood. An elevated pressure without apparent cause is said to be idiopathic or essential hypertension. A blood pressure consistently below 90/60 indicates *hypotension* (low blood pressure), which may be normal for some persons. Hypotension will be present with heart failure, severe burns, dehydration, deep depression, hemorrhage, and shock.

Pulse Pressure

Pulse pressure refers to the difference between the systolic and diastolic reading and is an indicator of the tone of the arterial walls. For example, when the pressure is 120/80, the pulse pressure is 40, which is a normal finding. A pulse pressure over 50 or less than 30 mm Hg may be considered abnormal. A general rule of thumb is that the pulse pressure should be approximately a third of the systolic measurement. If less, the patient may have an auscultatory gap (absence of sound) and the pressure may have been incorrectly measured. This disorder will be described later.

Equipment Factors

It is important that sphygmomanometers be in proper working order and correctly calibrated. A mercury manometer that leaks mercury or has bubbles rising in the mercury column when used may not measure accurately. If correctly calibrated, the meniscus of the mercury is at 0 when viewed at eye level. The desktop manometer must always be placed on a flat, level sur-

face. Wall mounted units should be at a height permitting eye-level viewing. The medical assistant must either sit down or stoop to view a floor model manometer at eye level. Figure 15–45 shows various types of sphygmomanometers.

The aneroid dial should be calibrated occasionally by attaching it to a calibrated mercury manometer with a Y connector, Figure 15–46, page 465. Elevate the manometers to 250 mm Hg together, then let the pressure fall, noting the reading at four different points. There should be no more than a 3-mm Hg difference according to the National Bureau of Standards. Mercury sphygmomanometers are much more accurate than aneroid models; however, they still need to be checked for faults every 6 to 12 months, depending on use. They should be serviced and calibrated to ensure accuracy in measurement. Aneroid models must

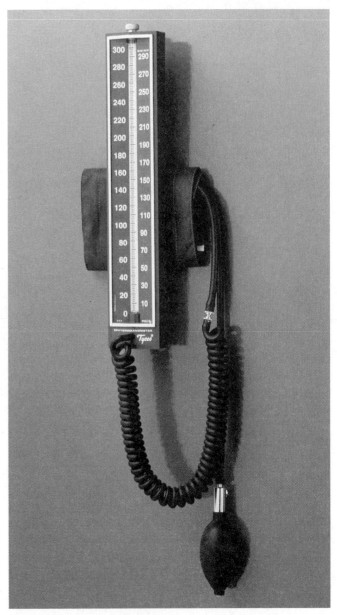

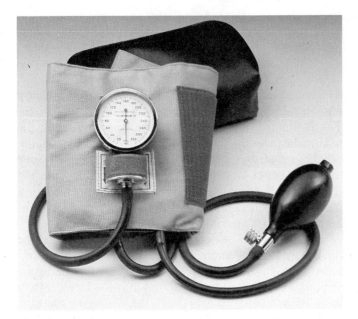

FIGURE 15–45 Types of sphygmomanometers (a). Aneroid. (Courtesy Omron Marshall Products, Inc.) (b). Wall mounted mercury. (Courtesy Tycos.)

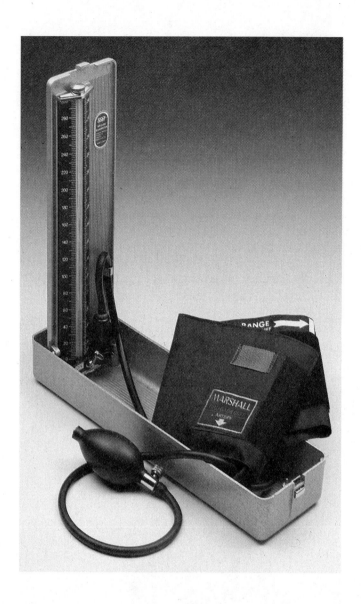

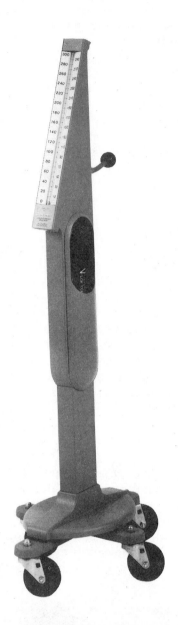

FIGURE 15–45 (continued) Types of sphygmomanometers (c). Desk-type mercury. (Courtesy Omron Marshall Products, Inc.) (d). Standby mercury. (Courtesy WA Baum Co., Inc.)

be checked every 3 to 6 months over the entire pressure range against an accurate mercury manometer. Figure 15–46 illustrates how the manometers are connected together by a "Y" tube and measured simultaneously.

Studies have shown many sphygmomanometers used in family practice to be faulty. The primary areas of failure in both models are in the control valves of the cuffs, which result in leakage and in unsatisfactory condition of the mercury columns either due to inadequate mercury in the reservoir or dirt from oxidation in the glass calibrated tube, which makes reading more difficult. The aneroid models showed a greater problem with accuracy due to dial errors because they are rarely calibrated.

It is important that sphygmomanometers be serviced regularly. Faults in aneroid models have to be corrected by service technicians or the manufacturer. A mercury manometer can be maintained by the owner if desired. The common sources of error—the mercury level, the glass tube, and the air vent—can be solved by topping off the mercury in the reservoir, cleaning the glass tube to permit better viewing and mercury flow, or replacing the chamois leather in the air vent. Because mercury is a harmful substance, it is probably best to use trained technicians to service the equipment.

The cuff is also critical to correct measurement. If the reading is to be accurate, the cuff must be the appropriate size, Figure 15–47. If it is too small for the upper arm, the reading will be falsely high; if too large, falsely low. To determine the proper size, compare the cuff width to the width of the upper arm. The cuff should be

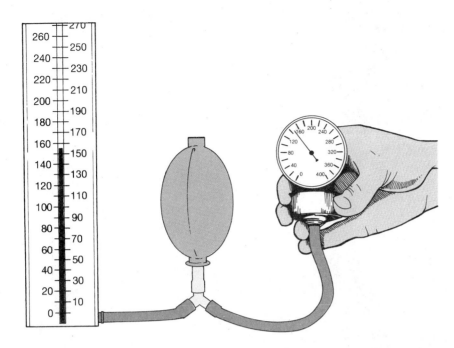

FIGURE 15–46 Testing an aneroid sphygmomanometer

about 20% wider than the arm. When a cuff is too small and you do not have access to a wide adult cuff, measure to the width of the forearm. If the cuff is of adequate size, take the blood pressure reading in the forearm by placing the stethoscope over the radial artery.

Measuring Techniques

Because blood pressure readings are so critical to the determination of hypertension and consequently to the medication given for managing it, strict procedure techniques must be followed. Several factors affect the accuracy of results.

1. The cuff must be completely deflated when applied.
2. The patient must be comfortable, with the arm slightly flexed at the elbow and the brachial artery on a level with the heart. The arm must be bare and free of a constricting sleeve, Figure 15–48, page 466.
3. The center of the bladder in the cuff must be placed over the brachial artery. Fold the bladder area of the cuff in half to locate the center. Many cuffs have improper artery markings.
4. The manometer must be viewed directly from a distance of not more than 3 feet.
5. A palpatory reading should be taken first to determine proper inflation. Afterwards, deflate cuff completely by compressing with hands before reinflation.
6. A minimum of 15 seconds should elapse between inflations (30 is better) to allow blood pressure to normalize.
7. The cuff should be inflated rapidly to 30 mm Hg above the palpatory reading.

To obtain a baseline reading for new patients it may be desirable to measure the pressure twice in each arm, once while the patient is sitting and once while lying down.

Blood pressure has two phases, both of which must be determined. When the cuff is properly inflated, the valve must be opened carefully to allow deflation at a rate of 2-3 mm per beat. Listen for the first sounds of heartbeat and note the reading as the systolic pressure once you have heard at least two consecutive beats. Continue to listen and observe as the cuff is deflated until you hear a sudden change in sound to a softer, muffled tone. Note

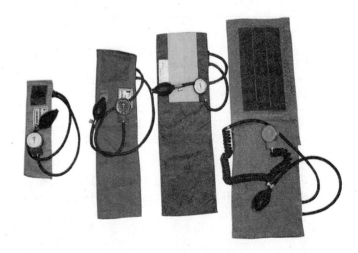

FIGURE 15–47 Blood pressure cuffs in sizes to fit the arm of a small child to an adult thigh (From Caldwell & Hegner, *Nursing Assistant*, 6th ed. Copyright 1992, Delmar Publishers Inc.)

through the cuff tourniquet is striking against the walls of a near empty artery.

Auscultatory Gap. In some patients, usually those who are hypertensive, there is a silent interval between systolic and diastolic pressure, called an *auscultatory gap,* Figure 15–50, page 468. If this is not detected, it may lead to serious undermeasurement of the systolic pressure. For example, the patient's actual systolic pressure is 200, with a gap from 170 to 140, and a diastolic of 120/110. You inflate the cuff to 170 and hear nothing until the manometer reaches 140, which you presume is the systolic pressure. You would continue deflation and record 120/110 as the diastolic; therefore, you would have a pulse pressure of only 20 or 30 mm Hg. Keeping in mind the normal range for pulse pressure, however, you would view 20/30 as suspicious. Taking one-third of 140 would give you about 47. To be certain you had not missed a portion of the pressure, you would remeasure, palpating the systolic and then inflating the cuff

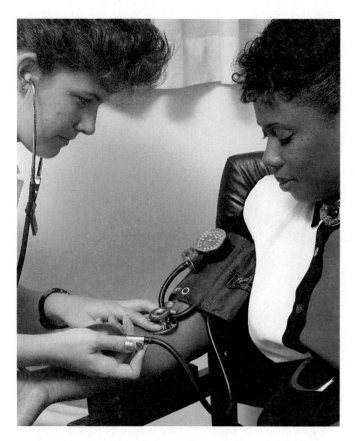

FIGURE 15–48   Measuring blood pressure

this reading as the diastolic pressure. Continue to observe the manometer until the sound disappears. Note this reading also, even if 0. To record, you would write, for example, B/P 140/90/70. You should ask the physician which sound, the change or the absence, you are to record as the diastolic measurement. There are reasons to support either method.

Probably the mistake made most often in measuring blood pressure is reinflating the cuff after only partial deflation or too soon after complete deflation. Either error may cause a false reading and will also cause difficulty in hearing the sound changes because of venous congestion in the forearm.

Augmenting Sound.   To augment heartbeat sounds when they are difficult to hear, use the following technique:

1. With the cuff properly applied and deflated have the patient elevate the arm above the shoulder and make and release a fist a few times to aid in emptying forearm veins, Figure 15–49.
2. With the patient's arm still raised, rapidly inflate the cuff to 30 mm Hg above palpated pulse.
3. Have patient lower arm.
4. Begin deflation, listening for initial beats. The sounds will be intensified because the blood spurting

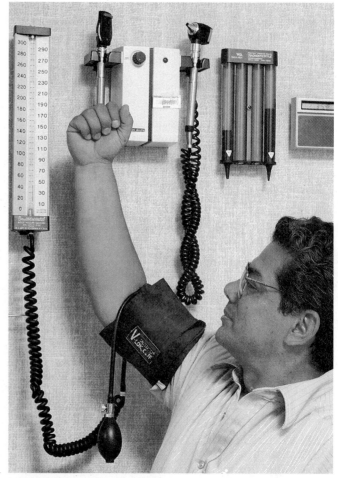

FIGURE 15–49   A technique to augment heart sounds in blood pressure measurement

Measure Blood Pressure

TERMINAL PERFORMANCE OBJECTIVE: In a simulated or actual situation, given a patient, stethoscope, mercury or aneroid sphygmomanometer, alcohol wipe, paper and pen/pencil, the student will measure palpatory and auscultatory blood pressure, recording findings, within a 5-minute period of time, at 4 mm Hg accuracy, following correct procedural technique and observing safety and aseptic precautions.

1. Wash hands.
2. Assemble equipment
3. Clean earpieces and head of stethoscope with antiseptic. **Key Point: This prevents the transference of microorganisms.**
4. Identify patient. **Key Point: Call by name and check chart to avoid error.**
5. Explain procedure. If it is new to a patient, especially if a child, explain that the cuff will squeeze but that they must not move.
6. Place a mercury manometer on a flat, level surface near patient. Put aneroid type within easy reach.
7. Place patient in a relaxed and comfortable sitting or lying position.
8. Expose patient's upper arm well above elbow, extending arm with palm up. If sleeve is tight, remove garment. Arm must be bare for accuracy. **Key Point: Arm must be relaxed, on a supporting surface, slightly flexed at elbow, with brachial artery approximately at level of heart.**
9. With valve of inflation bulb open, squeeze all air from bladder, fold to identify center, placing bottom edge of cuff 1 to 2 inches above elbow. Wrap cuff smoothly and snugly around arm, with deflated bladder centered over brachial artery. If using mercury manometer, cuff and tubing may be disconnected for easier application. If using aneroid, be certain dial can be easily viewed and end of cuff does not interfere. (**Caution:** Be alert to patient's movements. Could pull attached desk-type mercury manometer off table.)
10. Take position with mercury manometer or aneroid dial in a direct line at eye level.
11. With *one hand,* close valve on bulb, clockwise. **Key Point: Do not overtighten or it will be hard to open.**
12. Position other hand to palpate radial pulse.
13. Observing manometer, rapidly inflate cuff to 30 mm above level where radial pulse disappears.

14. Open valve, slowly releasing air until radial pulse is detected. (Note: Provides information for auscultatory measurement.)
15. Observe mercury or dial reading. **Key Point: This is estimated for palpatory systolic pressure, which is recorded, for example, as B/P 120 (P).**
16. Deflate cuff rapidly and completely. Squeeze cuff with hands to empty. Adjust position if necessary.
17. Position earpieces of stethoscope in ears with openings entering ear canal.
18. Palpate brachial artery at medial antecubital space with fingertips.
19. Place head of stethoscope directly over palpated pulse. **Key Point: Stethoscope head must not touch either cuff or clothing (creates static).**
20. Close valve on bulb and rapidly inflate cuff to 30 mm above palpated systolic pressure. **Key Point: A minimum of 15 seconds must have elapsed since previous inflation.**
21. Open valve, slowly deflating cuff. **Key Point: Pressure should drop 2–3 mm Hg per second.**
22. With eyes at level of descending meniscus or directly in line or over dial, note reading at which you hear systolic pressure.
    Key Points:
    a. **Must be at least two consecutive beats.**
    b. **Remember systolic measurement.**
23. Allow pressure to lower steadily until you note a change in sound to a softer, more muffled sound. Note this as diastolic pressure (if so instructed).
24. Continue to release pressure until all sound disappears. Note point as diastolic pressure (if so instructed).
25. Release remaining air. Squeeze cuff between hands.
26. Record systolic and whichever diastolic the physician prefers.
27. Reevaluate if indicated after a minimum of 15 seconds.
28. Remove stethoscope from ears.
29. Remove cuff from patient's arm.
30. Assist patient with clothing, if necessary.
31. Clean tips and head of stethoscope with alcohol to disinfect. Fold cuff properly and place with sphygmomanometer and stethoscope in storage.
32. Wash hands.

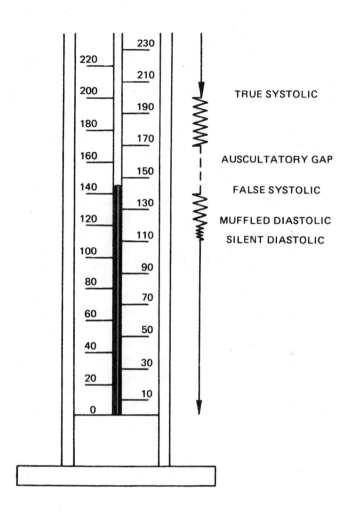

FIGURE 15–50 Auscultatory gap

30 mm above. If sounds were still audible at that point you would reinflate it higher *after complete deflation* until you hear the first sounds of systolic pressure.

When recording a blood pressure with an auscultatory gap, list your complete findings; for example, B/P 200/120/110 with the auscultatory gap from 170 to 140.

Blood Pressure in Children

The blood pressure of infants and children is often omitted from the physical examination because it is so difficult to obtain. Variation in blood pressure due to anxiety and emotional upset make accurate readings very challenging. Basically, the procedure is the same as with adults. Often physicians prefer to do the measurement last after having established some rapport with the child.

The cuff size is important in measuring a child's pressure. It should be appropriate to the size of the arm. The inflatable bag must entirely encircle the extremity.

The level of systolic pressure gradually rises throughout childhood. Normal pressure for a 6-month-old is 70; at 1 year it is 95; and it rises to 100 at 6 years. By age 16, the systolic pressure will be 120, the adult average. The diastolic pressure reaches 65 by age 1 and does not change appreciably during childhood.

Complete Chapter 15, Unit 2 in the workbook to help you meet the objectives at the beginning of this unit and therefore achieve competency of this subject matter.

REFERENCES

Bates, Barbara A. *A Guide to Physical Examination.* Philadelphia: Lippincott, 1974.

Burch, George E., M.D., and Shewey, Lana, M.D. *Sphygmomanometer Cuff Size and Blood Pressure Recordings. JAMA* 225: 1215-1218, 1973.

Caldwell, Esther, and Hegner, Barbara. *Nursing Assistant: A Nursing Process Approach,* 6th ed. Albany: Delmar, 1992.

Diagnostic Tests, Nurse's Ready Reference. Springhouse, PA: Springhouse, 1991.

Fong, Elizabeth, Ferris, Elvira, and Skelley, Esther G. *Body Structures and Functions,* 7th ed. Albany: Delmar, 1989.

Mosby's Medical, Nursing, and Allied Health Dictionary, 3rd ed. St. Louis: C. V. Mosby, 1990.

Nurse's Reference Library, Assessment. Springhouse, PA: Springhouse, 1983.

Ohio's Health. Blood Pressure: Are You Reading it Right? Ohio Department of Health, Division of Chronic Disease, May 1984.

Perlman, Lawrence V., M.D., Chang, Benjamin N., M.D., and Keller, Jacob, MPH. *Accuracy of Sphygmomanometers in Hospital Practice. Arch Intern Med,* 125: 1000-1003, 1970.

Reader's Digest Illustrated Encyclopedic Dictionary. Boston: Houghton Mifflin Lexical Databases, 1987.

Sarason, , and Sarason, . *Abnormal Psychology: The Problem of Maladaptive Behavior,* 5th ed. Englewood Cliffs, NJ: Prentice-Hall, 1987.

Starr, Cecie, and Taggert, Ralph. *Biology: The Unity and Diversity of Life,* 5th ed. Belmont: Wadsworth, 1989.

Taber, Clarence W. *Taber's Cyclopedic Medical Dictionary,* 14th ed. Philadelphia: F.A. Davis, 1983.

Ms. Right... respects the privacy of each patient when obtaining information for medical records. She makes every effort to establish a good rapport with all patients by accepting each individual. She is ever mindful of the importance of confidentiality and obtains the proper authorization before release of information concerning patients. Ms. Right performs procedures and records results carefully and efficiently. She never guesses what a pulse or blood pressure reading is. If she is not sure of a result, she asks a supervisor or physician to check it. She also follows the statutes regarding the rights of minors in their medical treatment, reminding patients under age 18 that a parent or guardian must accompany them for their appointments.

Advancement potential: Excellent

Mr. Wrong... disregards confidentiality, privacy, and respect regarding patients. He has a good rapport only with those patients he likes. He frequently forgets to obtain proper authorization to release information about a patient and often gives it over the telephone. He has told coworkers that sometimes if he cannot hear a blood pressure, he just records the reading from the patient's last visit. He pays little attention to the statutes concerning the rights of minors regarding medical treatment. He frequently has to be reminded by others to follow office policy.

Advancement potential: Poor (employment will most likely be terminated)

The American Medical Association Family Medical Guide. New York: Random House, 1987.

United States Department of Health and Human Services, Public Health Service Centers for Disease Control. *Recommendations for Prevention of HIV Transmission in Health Care Settings.* Atlanta, 1987.

Zakus, Sharron. *Mosby's Fundamentals of Medical Assisting: Administrative and Clinical Theory and Technique,* 2nd ed. St. Louis: C. V. Mosby, 1990.

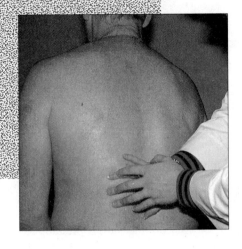

CHAPTER 16

Preparing Patients for Examinations

The Medical Assistant is a significant *liaison* between the patient and the physician. You should be *discreet* and courteous at all times with all patients. You must listen carefully and observe them closely as they disclose their complaints and symptoms to you and while you are performing the many procedures dealing with their care. Some patients (themselves) may not even be aware of a condition or symptom that you could bring to their attention. Often a patient becomes so used to a problem that it may be overlooked, such as clearing the throat, a change in weight, or a skin discoloration. When changes like these happen gradually, sometimes the patient is really not aware of them. You can then alert the physician to initiate treatment for a problem that may have otherwise gone undetected.

In the pages that follow you will learn of many ways to be of assistance to both patient and physician. Pay special attention to the patient education sections for application while performing the many procedures and examination preparations for patients.

The overall preparation of patients for examinations performed by the physician is the responsibility of the medical assistant. To gain full cooperation of the patient for a particular examination the patient must understand completely what is expected. The medical assistant must keep in mind that these procedures and examinations, although routine to the medical staff, are not usually routine to patients.

In this chapter you will learn valuable skills to help you in getting patients ready for the doctor to see them. Patients will have appointments for a variety of reasons. The medical assistant's duty is to ascertain the reason the patient is visiting the physician (triage) and prepare the patient for the appropriate examination.

The patient will want to know: what the particular examination is (a brief definition); why it has to be done; how long it takes; if it hurts; when it must be done; and, of course, preliminary preparation if necessary. Even though the doctor tells the patient about all of these points concerning orders during the

1. While performing procedures involving the eye, the medical assistant may want to remind patients to use eye protection when indicated. You might suggest the use of safety glasses/goggles when working with tools that often make particles of material fly into the air, a potential cause of injury. These safety measures are required at the workplace. Your reinforcement may possibly save someone's sight.

2. Remind patients to wear protective sunglasses when they are out in direct sun for extended periods of time because the eyes can become sunburned as well as the skin.

3. Patients need to be reminded to have routine eye examinations, especially when the family medical history includes glaucoma, cataracts, or diabetes. Tonometry and funduscopy are recommended examinations of the eye that should be performed every 4 years after patients are age 40 and over.

4. Explain to patients that over-the-counter eyedrops should be used carefully and only as directed. The extended use of such preparations could cause tissue damage. They should be used only when necessary and with the advice of the physician.

5. Advise patients not to rub their eyes because further irritation and possibly tissue damage could result. Instruct them to use a cold compress for these minor problems. Itching, burning, or watering eyes can be signs of infection. Rubbing the eyes transmits germs of others, thereby spreading disease.

6. Tell patients that in the event of a chemical splash in the eye, to flush the eye with clear (room temperature) water for 20 minutes (nonstop) and seek medical attention immediately.

UNIT 1
Procedures of the Eye and Ear

OBJECTIVES

Upon completion of this unit, the student will meet the following terminal performance objectives by verifying knowledge of the facts and principles presented through oral and written communication at a level deemed competent, and will demonstrate the specific behaviors as identified in the terminal performance objectives of the procedures, observing all aseptic and safety precautions in accordance with health care standards.

1. Discuss patient education concerning the eye and the ear.
2. Assist with examinations of the eye and the ear.
3. Administer screening tests of visual acuity.
4. List and describe screening tests of auditory acuity.
5. Demonstrate the procedure for eye irrigation.
6. Demonstrate the procedure for eyedrop instillation.
7. Demonstrate the procedure for eardrop instillation.
8. Demonstrate the procedure for ear irrigation.
9. Discuss the purpose of the Pelli–Robson and the Vectorvision visual screening chart.
10. Spell and define, using the glossary at the back of the text, all the words to know in this unit.

WORDS TO KNOW

achromatic	lavage
acuity	liaison
anesthetize	occluder
audiometer	OD
auditory	ophthalmic
cerumen	OS
daltonism	otic
decibel	OU
discreet	pertinent
deuteranopia	protanopia
funduscopy	Snellen chart
instill	tonometry
irrigate	tritanopia
Ishihara	vertex
Jaeger	wick

Eye and Ear Examination

In assisting with eye and ear examinations, you will be expected to hand instruments to the physician as needed. Assembling the instruments in the order of their use will be most helpful. You will be responsible for making sure that the instruments are clean and in working order. Otoscopes and ophthalmoscopes should be checked to be sure that the light bulbs are providing a strong enough light.

course of the visit, the patient may not ask questions (or even know what to ask). Often physicians leave these explanations up to the medical assistant who can review the information with the patient in a more relaxed setting. Usually this allows a few minutes for the patient to think about questions to ask before they leave the office.

As you are getting patients ready for the physician's examination, it is an ideal time to provide them with pertinent information regarding the maintenance of their health.

The units that follow provide valuable information in preparing for and assisting with simple to complex preparations and examinations.

These tiny light bulbs must be changed from time to time because they eventually burn out, as do any other kind of bulbs. If these instruments are the hand-held portable type, the batteries must also be changed periodically. The medical assistant is usually responsible for these minor but important tasks. More popularly used in most medical offices are the wall-mounted units with both otoscope and ophthalmoscope instruments, which have an electrically powered light source.

The ear speculum should be sterilized. Most physicians use the disposable plastic ear speculum, which eliminates the worry of disease transmission. The reusable ones must be washed after every use with a mild detergent and placed in a disinfectant solution for at least 20 minutes before they can safely be reused to examine another patient.

Proper lighting of the examination room is most important, because inspection is a large part of the examination of these sensory systems.

Some patients will need reassurance during the examination because of apprehension caused by an earlier experience or for other reasons. Usually a kind word and a reassuring smile will help them feel at ease, and their cooperation will follow. Remembering their comfort is vital.

Patients with discharge of the ear or the eye will require irrigation (also known as lavage) to remove the matter. The physician will then examine the ear or eye to ensure no damage was done by the discharge. A procedure for this will be given. You may also have the responsibility of instilling drops into a patient's eye or ear. This simply means dropping a solution into the patient's eye or ear to medicate the tissue or to soothe an irritation. Sterile technique should be used. Recording the amount of medication and the organ to which it is administered is a must.

Instillation of the ear is also performed to soften cerumen (ear wax). *Cerumen* is a protective secretion of the ear, produced to ward off invading microorganisms. Patients sometimes try to remove it by using a cotton-tipped swab, but often push it farther into the ear canal, where it becomes lodged and hardens. This buildup can be very uncomfortable and eventually impair hearing.

Procedures for eye and ear instillation follow. Sometimes it is necessary to instill medication into the ear to soften ear wax before an irrigation procedure can be performed. Irrigation of

P R O C E D U R E

Irrigate the Eye

PURPOSE: To irrigate the patient's eye(s) to soothe tissues, relieve inflammation, remove foreign objects, and aid the eye in draining.
EQUIPMENT: Latex gloves, small basin for irrigation solution, towel, emesis basin to catch the solution, bulb syringe or bottle of solution, patient's chart, pen
TERMINAL PERFORMANCE OBJECTIVE: Provided with a mannequin and all equipment required for the eye irrigation procedure, the student will irrigate the eyes of the mannequin; each step of the procedure must be accurately demonstrated in proper order.

1. Wash hands and put on gloves.
2. Assemble items needed for procedure; prepare solution.
3. Identify patient. **Key Point: Call patient by name and check chart to avoid error.**
4. Explain to patient reason for procedure and how it will be done.
5. Ask patient which position would be more comfortable, sitting or lying down, and assist in draping with towel to protect clothing.
6. Ask patient to turn head back and to side. Place emesis basin against head for patient to hold to catch solution during irrigation. Placing a couple of tissues, gauze squares, or a towel between the face and the basin will help prevent the patient from getting wet during the procedure. You may have to hold the basin yourself, Figure 16–1, page 474.
7. Wipe eye with gauze square from bridge of nose out to remove any particles before proceeding with irrigation.
8. Fill bulb syringe with ordered solution.
9. Hold affected eye open with thumb and index finger of one hand or with your little finger of the hand you hold the bottle of solution in and slowly release the solution over the eye gently and steadily. **Key Point: This must be done from inner canthus to outer canthus to prevent any solution from entering other eye, which may not be affected, and for comfort of patient in catching solution at side instead of near nose.**
10. When irrigation is completed, use sterile gauze squares or tissues to blot area dry and make patient comfortable.
11. Record procedure in patient's chart and initial. **Key Point: Be sure to record type of solution that was used, which eye was irrigated, results, and any other important information you may have observed while performing procedure.**
12. Wash items and return them to proper storage area.
13. Remove gloves and wash hands.

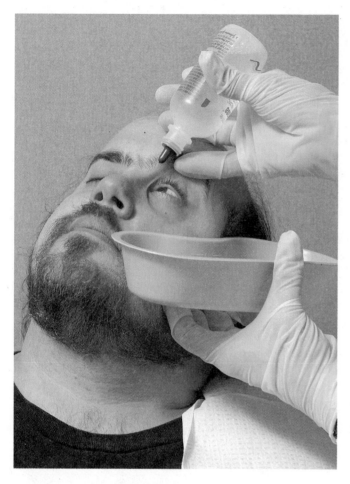

FIGURE 16–1   Irrigation of the eye is also referred to as lavage, which means to wash out.

the eye and the ear may be ordered before a successful examination can be conducted by the physician.

Patients should have impacted cerumen removed by a member of the health care team to avoid further discomfort or possible injury to the ear. Many offices and clinics have adopted the water pic for this purpose because of the gentle flow it produces and its convenience for irrigation procedures. Some patients will need both irrigation and instillation procedures. A softening solution may be instilled into a severely impacted ear, followed by irrigation to remove the excess ear wax.

After having irrigation procedures performed, even with gentle care, many patients feel a little dizziness. You must be sure that patients are completely stable before permitting them to leave.

A simple method of medicating the eye is by placing a small amount of ointment just inside the lower eyelid. The tip of the ointment tube must not touch the eyelid, where its contents would become contaminated by the secretions of the eye. Care must also be taken when instilling eyedrops so that the tip of the dropper does not come in contact with the eye.

Visual Acuity

Measuring visual **acuity** is a diagnostic screening procedure most often done by the medical assistant on the patient's initial visit prior to the physical examination. It should be done in a well-lighted room with no interruptions. Observation of the patient for any conditions or

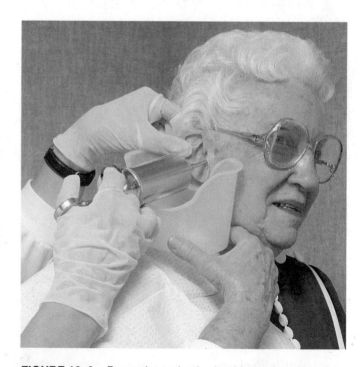

FIGURE 16–2   The examiner is using the otoscope to view the ear canal. This instrument has a light source and a magnifying lens that assists with inspection.

FIGURE 16–3   Drape the patient's shoulder and position the basin under the ear. Ask the patient to hold the basin as you position the syringe and straighten the ear canal.

PROCEDURE

Irrigate the Ear

PURPOSE: To irrigate the ear canal to remove foreign objects, impacted cerumen, or to relieve inflammation and swelling.

EQUIPMENT: Latex gloves, small basin for ordered irrigation solution, towel, ear basin to catch solution, Pomeroy or bulb syringe, gauze squares, otoscope, ear speculum, and tissues.

TERMINAL PERFORMANCE OBJECTIVE: Provided with an anatomical model of the ear or a mannequin, and all equipment required for the ear irrigation procedure, the student will first irrigate the anatomical ear, then the ears of the mannequin; in each process the steps of the procedure must be demonstrated in proper order.

1. Wash hands and put on gloves.
2. Prepare solution as ordered and assemble necessary items for procedure. **Key Point: Solution is usually between 100°F and 105°F for patient comfort.**
3. Identify patient. **Key Point: Call patient by name and check chart to avoid error.**
4. Explain procedure.
5. View affected ear with otoscope to see where cerumen or foreign object is located so flow of solution can be directed properly. The flow should be directed upward and to one side (as you would rinse out a bucket with a hose). To use the otoscope for viewing the ear canal, place one hand gently against the patient's head and grasp the auricle with your thumb and index finger pulling up and back for adults and down and back for babies up to 36 months. Hold the otoscope with the thumb, index, and great finger of your other hand to avoid using too much pressure as you insert the speculum into the ear canal, Figure 16–2.
6. Ask patient to turn head to side and back. Position ear

basin under ear for patient to hold to catch solution as it returns during procedure. Place a towel over patient's shoulder to protect clothing, Figure 16–3. For pediatric patients, ask parent to hold the child on lap and assist you during procedure.

7. Use gauze square to wipe away any particles from outer ear before proceeding.
8. Fill syringe with ordered solution.
9. With one hand, gently pull auricle up and back for an adult (down and back for an infant or small child) to straighten ear canal. With other hand place tip of syringe into canal and aim flow of solution upward so entire ear canal will be irrigated. DO NOT direct the flow of the solution straight into the ear or use force or the result will be quite painful for the patient and will damage the tympanic membrane.
10. Use gauze square to wipe excess solution from outside of patient's ear.
11. Give patient several gauze squares or tissues and have patient hold head tilted to side to allow drainage of excess solution from canal.
12. Inspect ear canal with otoscope to determine if desired results have been obtained. **Key Point: Proceed until desired results are obtained. Patients sometimes feel a little dizzy following this procedure. Allow the patient time to gain balance; assist patient from the examination table.**
13. Record procedure on patient's chart and initial. **Key Point: Note which ear was irrigated, solution that was used, the results of the procedure, and any other important observations.**
14. Wash equipment and return to proper storage area.
15. Remove gloves and wash hands.

behaviors that may indicate visual disturbances is an essential part of the overall examination.

The most common screening device for distance vision is a Snellen chart, which shows at what distance a patient can read. The regular chart has letters arranged in rows from largest to smallest.

Those who may have difficulty with reading, such as preschool children or non-English speakers, should be tested with the chart or cards of the letter *E* arranged in different directions. Figures 16–6, page 477 and 16–7, page 478, show the various Snellen vision screening charts, which are made to standard specifications. These charts are hung on the wall with a mark 20 feet away to show where the patient should stand or sit to read the

chart. The chart should be at the patient's eye level. Charts are available on a lighted view box to increase the visibility of the letters.

Most preschoolers have a short attention span. You may need some assistance in screening them for visual acuity, either by having a parent or guardian help to interpret your instructions to them, or in the positioning and covering of their eyes during the screening process. It is best to familiarize the child with either chart (Big E or Kindergarten) at a short distance before you begin to screen them for visual acuity. This will help you determine whether or not the child is actually having trouble seeing, or if the child simply does not know what to call the letter or symbol you are pointing to on the chart. You can make it fun for the child by taking your turn first to read the chart and then letting the child have a turn to read it to you. Remembering to praise the child will encourage good behavior. Usually it is not recommended to screen 3-year-olds below the 30-foot line. Make sure that you pay close attention to the patient (child or adult) during the procedure. The following are suggestions of what observations you should make while performing the test: tilting the head to the side or forward; blinking or watering of eyes; frowning or puckering of the face; closing of one eye when testing both eyes; or any other signs of straining to see.

Often while you are preparing the child for this procedure, the parent may offer one or more reasons why the child was brought in for the examination. For instance, the child may hold story books too close to the face or rub the eyes frequently. You should record the symptoms on the patient's chart as well as the results of the visual screening. A list of common complaints that may indicate vision problems are in Table 16–1. These complaints pertain to both children and adults.

Patients should be screened with and without their corrective lenses and the results recorded as such on their charts. Note that if visual acuity does not exceed

---

P R O C E D U R E

Instill Eyedrops

PURPOSE: To instill medication (in the form of drops or ointment) into the eye(s) to relieve irritation; treat infection; dilate the pupil; or **anesthetize** the eye in preparation for an examination or for a surgical procedure.

EQUIPMENT: Latex gloves, ordered medication, sterile eyedropper, sterile gauze squares, tissues

TERMINAL PERFORMANCE OBJECTIVES: Provided with an anatomical model of the eye or a mannequin, and all equipment necessary to perform instillation of the eye, the student will instill drops into the eyes of the anatomical model or of the mannequin; in each process the steps of the procedure must be demonstrated in proper order.

1. Verify medication ordered by physician in the patient's chart (check the expiration date) and assemble necessary items for procedure. **Ophthalmic** medications are often kept in the refrigerator after they have been opened, so it is necessary to bring them to room temperature by allowing the drops to set out for a while or running warm water over the bottle before using. This is for the comfort of the patient.

2. Wash hands and put on gloves.

3. Identify patient. **Key Point: Call patient by name and check chart to avoid error.**

4. Explain procedure to patient.

5. **a.** Open the bottle of ophthalmic medication and draw into the dropper the ordered amount of drops for instillation. (Many prepared eye medications have their own dropper. It is vital that this dropper be used very carefully so as to keep it sterile. DO NOT touch the tip of the dropper in the eye!)

   b. If the medication ordered is an ointment, you should open the tube by removing the cap, being very careful not to touch the tip or it will become contaminated. Medication should be placed carefully and sparingly just inside the lower eye lid without touch-

ing the eye tissue.

6. Ask the patient to sit up straight and tilt the head back slightly (some patients may prefer to lie down). If the patient is very young or uncooperative, you may need to have another's help with holding the child during the procedure.

7. With one hand, use a sterile gauze square to touch the patient's skin just under the eye and gently pull down. This will expose a small pocket (a recessed area between the eye just inside the lower lid), Figure 16–4. Hand a couple of tissues to the patient before you begin.

8. Hold the dropper steadily approximately 1/4 inch from the area being careful NOT to touch the tissue. Tell the patient to look up while you gently drop the prescribed amount of drops into the pocket of the patient's eye. Ask the patient to blink to further distribute the medication. Advise the patient NOT to rub the eye and not to squeeze out the medications from the eyes. Remind the patient to use the tissues to gently blot excess medication from eyes and not to touch the eyes with bare hands. (This is an ideal time to go over patient education material concerning the eyes.) Repeat for the other eye if ordered.

9. Close the bottle or tube of medication. Avoid touching the dropper to the outside of the bottle or it will contaminate the contents. If you have touched the patient's eye or anything else with the dropper, it must either be sterilized or replaced before any other doses of medication can be taken from the bottle, otherwise the contents will become contaminated.

10. Remove gloves and wash hands.

11. Record procedure on patient's chart and initial. Be sure to note any complaints of the patient while performing the procedure, i.e., burning or other eye discomfort.

12. Return items to proper storage area.

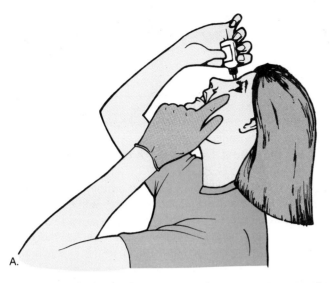
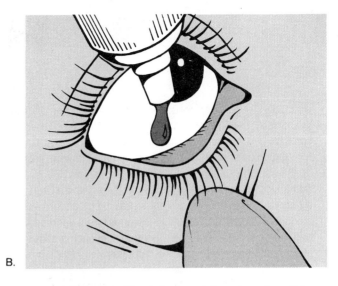

FIGURE 16–4 When instructing patients to use eyedrops at home, tell them to tilt the head back, look up (a), and gently pull the skin down just under the eye (b) to form a small pocket where the drops should be instilled.

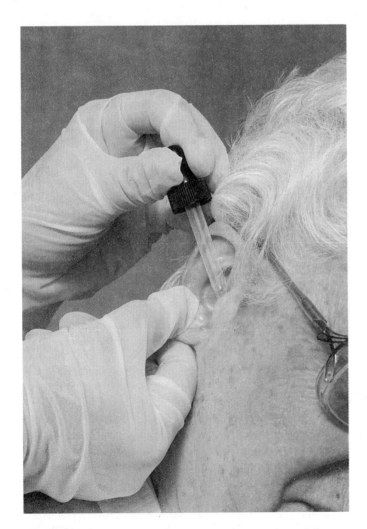

FIGURE 16–5 Instill eardrops into the ear canal carefully.

20/200 in the better eye with corrective lenses, the patient is considered legally blind.

The Jaeger system is a most common method of screening for near vision acuity. The chart used for this procedure is very small compared to the wall mounted charts for distance visual acuity. The card is held by the patient between 14 and 16 inches from the eye. You should measure with a yardstick, meterstick, or a tape measure for accuracy. This is the distance at which one

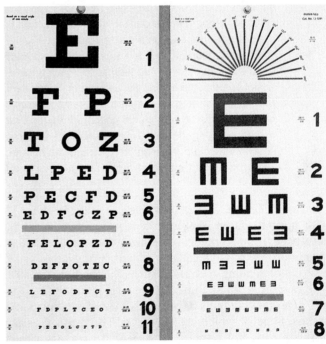

FIGURE 16–6 Snellen visual acuity screening charts. On the left, letters appear in descending sizes; on the right, the letter E appears in various directions and in descending sizes.

Instill Eardrops

PURPOSE: To treat infections, relieve pain, and soften ear wax.

EQUIPMENT: Latex gloves, gauze squares, sterile cotton-tipped applicators and cotton balls, sterile dropper, ordered medication (may be in the form of drops or ointment), tissues.

TERMINAL PERFORMANCE OBJECTIVE: Provided with an anatomical model of the ear or a mannequin, and all equipment required to perform the ear instillation procedure, the student will first instill drops into the anatomical ear model, and then into the ears of the mannequin; in each process the steps of the procedure must be demonstrated in proper order.

1. Verify medication ordered by physician (and check expiration date) in the patient's chart and assemble necessary items for procedure. Otic medications are often kept in the refrigerator after they have been opened, so it is necessary to bring them to room temperature by running warm water over the bottle before using. This is for the comfort of the patient.

2. Wash hands and put on gloves.

3. Identify patient. **Key Point: Call patient by name and check chart to avoid error.**

4. Explain procedure to patient.

5. a. Open the bottle of otic medication and draw into the dropper the ordered amount of drops for instillation. (Many prepared ear medications have their own dropper. It is vital that this dropper be used very carefully so as to keep it sterile. DO NOT touch the tip of the dropper in the ear!) It is a good practice to place the lid *inside* up on a gauze square.

   b. If the medication ordered is an ointment, you should open the tube by removing the cap, being very careful not to touch the tip or it will become contaminated. Medication should be instilled by placing a small amount on the tip of a sterile cotton applicator stick and applying it gently into the ear canal. Use extreme caution to avoid puncturing the tympanic membrane.

6. Ask the patient to sit up straight and tilt the head slightly to the left for instilling the right ear; and to the right for the left ear (some patients may prefer to lie down). If the patient is very young or uncooperative, you may need to have another's help with holding the child during the procedure.

7. Hand a couple of tissues to the patient before you begin. Hold the auricle of the ear *gently* with one hand, while you hold the dropper in the other. To straighten the ear canal to allow the medication to enter, pull up and back for adults, and down and back for infants and children up to 36 months.

8. Position the dropper with the medication into (but not touching) the ear canal, Figure 16–5. Depress the bulb to release the prescribed amount of drops into the ear. Advise the patient to remain in this position for a minute or so to allow the medication to settle. Any excess may be wiped away with the tissues or gauze squares. (This is an ideal time to go over patient education material concerning the ears.) Repeat for the other ear if ordered. Sometimes physicians will request that sterile cotton be inserted into the ear canal to hold the medication in. Simply place a small portion of the sterile cotton ball gently into the canal after instilling the medication; this is sometimes referred to as a wick. It is often saturated with the medication before being placed in the ear canal.

9. Close the bottle or tube of medication. Avoid touching the dropper to the outside of the bottle or it will contaminate the contents. If you have touched the patient's ear or anything else, the dropper must be either sterilized or replaced before any other doses of medication can be taken from the bottle.

10. Remove gloves and wash hands.

11. Record procedure on patient's chart and initial. Be sure to note any complaints of the patient while performing the procedure, i.e., stinging or other discomfort.

12. Return items to proper storage area.

---

with normal vision is able to read printed material (a newspaper), or work on something that requires close attention (sewing). The Jaeger screening test consists of a series of reading material that has ascending sizes of type ranging from .37 mm to 2.5 mm, Figure 16–8, page 481. The test contains excerpts from a variety of paragraphs, none of which are the same. The medical assistant should pay careful attention to observe any difficulty the person exhibits (i.e., holding the chart right in front of the face, squinting, blinking, etc.) while the patient reads this card. The medical assistant records the results on the chart. Record the line number that the patient can read easily. The screening procedure should be conducted in a well-lighted room without interruptions. The patient ought to be tested with and without wearing corrective lenses and each eye separately for a complete assessment to be made by the physician.

Many devices for screening for visual acuity are available besides the methods already discussed in this unit. One compact instrument is the Titmus Vision Tester, Figure 16–10, page 483. In this system of screening, the patient looks into the instrument to view 8 different specialized fields designed to detect all common vision problems. While administering this test, the medical assistant sits or

TABLE 16–1
Possible Indications of Visual Disturbance

During Activities That Require Reading Shows	Illness	Condition	Behaviors	Complaints
1. Difficulty with near or distant vision 2. Avoids reading, writing, and other related activities.	1. Childhood 2. Current infection/condition	1. Redness of the eye(s) or eyelid(s) 2. Crusting/swelling of eyelid(s) or styes 3. Poor eye coordination 4. Watering and/or discharge 5. Accident/injury to the eye	1. Looks cross-eyed 2. Rubbing eyes frequently 3. Confuses letters, i.e., *a* and *c, f* and *t, m* and *n* 4. Turns head or leans forward to see better 5. Blinks continually 6. Irritable at attempting close work	1. Blurriness of vision 2. Nausea 3. Headaches often 4. Dizziness 5. Eyes sensitive to light 6. Feels like something in the eye(s)

If a patient has a past history or a current complaint of any of the areas listed above, a visual disturbance is suggested.

stands next to the patient to operate the selection of visual fields. A vision occluder is within the device for testing each eye individually as the patient reads the various lines. Again, the medical assistant must be alert in observing and listening while the patient completes this test. All complaints or observations should be recorded on the patient's chart along with the results of the test. The instrument comes with forms for recording the results of the test.

Color vision acuity means that one can accurately recognize colors. Deficiency in this ability to perceive colors of the spectrum distinctly is commonly termed *color blindness.* This is due to changes that happen in the pigments of

P R O C E D U R E

Screen Visual Acuity With Snellen Chart

PURPOSE: To measure the visual acuity of a patient.
EQUIPMENT: Patient's chart, pen, Snellen chart, pointer, occular eye occluder, card or paper cup.
TERMINAL PERFORMANCE OBJECTIVE: Provided with the necessary vision screening equipment, the student will measure the visual acuity of at least two other students or visitors by demonstrating each step of the vision screening procedure; the results of each test will be accurately recorded on the individual patient's chart.

1. Explain procedure to patient—that patient is to read each line from the chart as you point to it with pointer.
2. Ask the patient to read the chart with both eyes (OU) first, standing 20 feet from the chart.
3. Have patient cover left eye (OS) with a card or paper cup. If patient wears corrective lenses, procedure should be performed first wearing lenses and then without and recorded as such.
   Key Points:
   a. Chart should be at patient's eye level.
   b. Tell patient to keep both eyes open but to cover one eye. This prevents squinting and blurring.
   c. Record any observations of individual accom-

modations made to read chart, such as squinting, turning head, etc.
   d. Follow office policy in giving test. Asking patients to read only certain lines of chart is sometimes less time-consuming and less tiring for patient. Covering part of chart that is not being read keeps patients from "studying" for their eye test.
4. Record smallest line that patient can read without making a mistake.
5. Have patient cover right eye (OD), and test acuity of left, following same procedure.
6. Record the number of the lowest line that the patient can see. Distant visual acuity is written as a fraction, 20/20, which is average. The numerator is the number of feet, or the distance from the chart; the denominator is the numbered line the patient read. If one's distant visual acuity results are 20/100, it means that the person stood 20 feet from the chart and read the line that should be read at 100 feet. One who has 20/10 acuity can see at 20 feet what should be seen at a distance of 10 feet, or excellent vision.

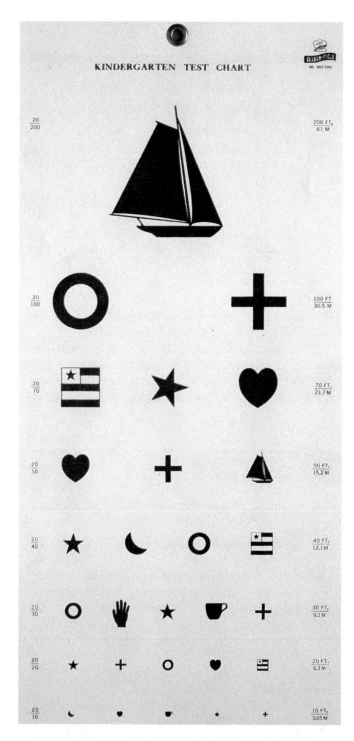

FIGURE 16–7 Kindergarten vision screening chart in descending sizes. Pictures must be reviewed with the child at a short distance before testing to be sure the child know what you are pointing to during the test for accurate results.

the cones in the retina of the eyes as they react to colored lights of red, green, and blue.

There are two primary types of color blindness: (1) daltonism, which is the most common, is a visual disorder in which the person cannot tell the difference between red and green. It is an hereditary disorder; and, (2) achromatic vision, which is total color blindness, and very rare, where the person cannot recognize any color at all. These people see everything in white, gray, and black. The probable cause for this condition is that the cones in the retina are defective or there may be none at all.

Several other conditions involve one's inability or weakness in distinguishing certain colors. In deuteranopia, the person has trouble in telling any difference between varying shades of green and also of bluish reds and neutral shades. Protanopia is partial color blindness. These people have trouble with the perception of reds, and sometimes yellows and greens are confused. This condition is often referred to as red blindness. Tritanopia, which is the rarest, means that the person cannot distinguish blue color.

A method for screening patients for defects in distinguishing color vision acuity is with the Ishihara color plates book. A sample of the series of multicolored charts in the test book is shown in Figure 16–11, page 483. Patients are asked to trace the patterns of color with their finger as you observe them. There are letters and numbers (and curved lines and shapes for nonreaders) that are one color within another. When administering this procedure, make sure that the room is well-lighted, preferably with natural daylight (not direct sunlight), so that the patient is able to follow your instructions without straining to see. Whatever method of color vision assessment is used where you are employed, it is vital that you are accurate in reporting the results. Medical assistants should first be tested to determine if they have normal color vision to administer the test to patients.

All patients with thyroid conditions should routinely be screened for color vision acuity during their scheduled visits. The procedure should include testing with both eyes first, and then each eye separately to see if there is any difference in the perception of color in either eye. The eye not used should be covered and not held shut. Grave's disease patients especially need frequent assessment of their color vision acuity changes to detect possible damage to the optic nerve. In conditions such as this where swelling occurs behind the eye, pressure builds up and hypertrophy of the tissues results. This interferes with the patient's ability to distinguish colors because the optic nerve is being compressed. The color vision test results may lead to earlier diagnosis and treatment of Grave's ophthalmopathy.

Pelli–Robson Contrast Sensitivity Chart

A recent advance in the measurement of visual acuity is the development of the Pelli–Robson contrast sensitivity chart, Figure 16–12, page 483. This chart measures contrast sensitivity by determining the faintest contrast that an observer can see. Recent clinical evidence shows that contrast sensitivity is affected by all of the major eye diseases—diabetic retinopathy, macular degeneration,

No. 1.
.37M

In the second century of the Christian era, the empire of Rome comprehended the fairest part of the earth, and the most civilized portion of mankind. The frontiers of that extensive monarchy were guarded by ancient renown and disciplined valor. The gentle but powerful influence of laws and manners had gradually cemented the union of the provinces. Their peaceful inhabitants enjoyed and abused the advantages of wealth.

No. 2.
.50M

fourscore years, the public administration was conducted by the virtue and abilities of Nerva, Trajan, Hadrian, and the two Antonines. It is the design of this, and of the two succeeding chapters, to describe the prosperous condition of their empire; and afterwards, from the death of Marcus Antoninus, to deduce the most important circumstances of its decline and fall: a revolution which will ever be remembered, and is still felt by

No. 3.
.62M

the nations of the earth. The principal conquests of the Romans were achieved under the republic; and the emperors, for the most part, were satisfied with preserving those dominions which had been acquired by the policy of the senate, the active emulations of the consuls, and the martial enthusiasm of the people. The seven first centuries were filled with a rapid succession of triumphs; but it was

No. 4.
.75M

reserved for Augustus to relinquish the ambitious design of subduing the whole earth, and to introduce a spirit of moderation into the public councils. Inclined to peace by his temper and situation, it was very easy for him to discover that Rome, in her present exalted situation, had much less to hope than to fear from the chance of arms; and that, in the prosecution of

No. 5.
1.00M

the undertaking became every day more difficult, the event more doubtful, and the possession more precarious, and less beneficial. The experience of Augustus added weight to these salutary reflections, and effectually convinced him that, by the prudent vigor of

No. 6.
1.25M

his counsels, it would be easy to secure every concession which the safety or the dignity of Rome might require from the most formidable barbarians. Instead of exposing his person or his legions to the arrows of the Parthians, he obtained, by an honor-

No. 7.
1.50M

able treaty, the restitution of the standards and prisoners which had been taken in the defeat of Crassus. His generals, in the early part of his reign, attempted the reduction of Ethiopia and Arabia Felix. They marched near a thou-

No. 8.
1.75M

sand miles to the south of the tropic; but the heat of the climate soon repelled the invaders, and protected the unwarlike natives of those sequestered regions

No. 9.
2.00M

The northern countries of Europe scarcely deserved the expense and labor of conquest. The forests and morasses of Germany were

No. 10.
2.25M

filled with a hardy race of barbarians who despised life when it was separated from freedom; and though, on the first

No. 11.
2.50M

attack, they seemed to yield to the weight of the Roman power, they soon, by a signal

FIGURE 16–8 The near distance visual acuity screening chart

glaucoma, and cataract. Therefore, measuring contrast sensitivity provides a sensitive screening test for eye disease to provide earlier diagnosis and treatment.

Another contrast sensitivity screening method has been developed by Vectorvision. Even though all patients can be tested in this way, it is especially useful in screening small children, foreigners, and illiterates. This test has a series of four groups of circles. In these rows of circles, some are solid gray colored and some have vertical lines within them. The patient is instructed to look at the first group and tell you which circles have lines within them. The last correctly identified circle in each group is charted on a graph. The results of this test are interpreted by the physician.

Auditory Acuity

The function of the ear is to enable sound to be perceived. If this process is impaired, hearing loss results. Diseases or conditions of the ear, if not treated, can cause damage to nerves and tissues, which may result in

mild to complete deafness. Often patients try to hide a problem such as hearing loss because it is an embarrass-

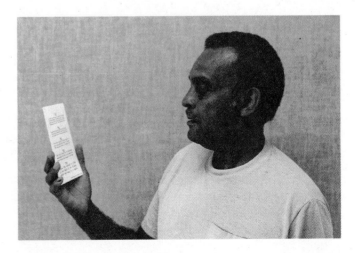

FIGURE 16–9 Patient holds near vision acuity screening card 14 to 16 inches from eyes to read.

PROCEDURE

Screen Visual Acuity With Jaeger System

PURPOSE: To determine near distance visual acuity of a patient using the Jaeger system.

EQUIPMENT: Jaeger near vision acuity chart, pen, patient's chart

TERMINAL PERFORMANCE OBJECTIVES: Using the Jaeger near vision acuity chart, in a well-lighted area, the student will determine the near distance visual acuity of at least two other students or visitors by demonstrating each step of the visual acuity procedure; the results of each test will be accurately recorded on the individual patient's chart.

1. After identifying the patient, explain the procedure. **Key Point: Call patient by name and check chart to avoid error.**
2. Have the patient sit up straight but comfortably in a well-lighted area.
3. Hand the Jaeger chart to the patient to hold, between 14 and 16 inches from the eyes. Figure 16–9 shows proper positioning of the card.
4. Instruct the patient to read (out loud to you) the various paragraphs of the card with both eyes open, first without wearing corrective lenses and then with them on. Each eye should be tested individually having the person cover the left eye first while reading the card and then the other eye. Observe carefully for any difficulty the patient has in reading any of the lines on the card. Listen also to any remarks made by the patient and make a note of it on the chart.
5. Record the results and problems, if any, on the patient's chart to assist the physician in determining the visual acuity of the patient and initial. The smallest line of print that the patient can read should be recorded.
6. Thank the patient for cooperation and answer any questions.
7. Return Jaeger chart to proper storage.

ment to them. They are sometimes afraid they may have to wear a hearing aid or worry that they may need to have an operation. So that they can avoid making a decision, often the patient will try to compensate for the hearing loss by learning to read lips, always turning the best ear toward the sound source (or pretending that they heard), increasingly turning up the volume on audio equipment, standing very close during conversation, and sometimes by withdrawing from others. The family members of the patient may relate this information to

PROCEDURE

Determine Color Vision Acuity by Ishihara Method

PURPOSE: To determine color vision acuity of a patient using the Ishihara method.

EQUIPMENT: Ishihara book, pen, patient's chart

TERMINAL PERFORMANCE OBJECTIVE: Using the Ishihara book, in a well-lighted area, the student will determine the color vision acuity of at least two other students or visitors by demonstrating each step of the color vision screening procedure; the results of each test will be accurately recorded on the individual patient's chart.

1. Obtain chart from back of book. **Key Point: Before administering this screening test, you should first be tested with it.**
2. Explain procedure to patient.
3. Conduct the test by first asking the patient to read the plates with both eyes (if the patient wears corrective lenses, with them on). A common practice is to ask the patient to trace the letters, numbers, or patterns of color printed in the various plates with the index finger. Continue testing by having the patient cover the left eye and test the right one, and then cover the right and test the left. Make sure to note any difficulty or complaint of the patient during the screening process.
4. Compare answers with those given on chart. Record frames patient misses and write down what patient sees so that degree of color impairment may be determined by physician.

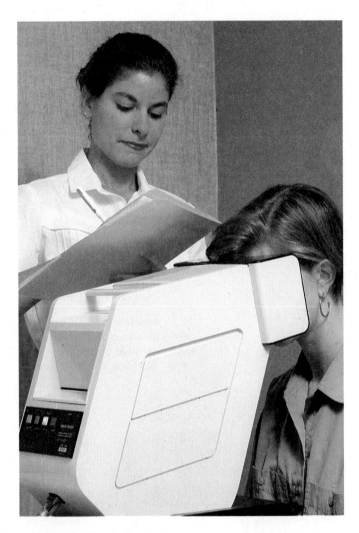

FIGURE 16–10 The medical assistant records the visual acuity as the patient looks into the Titmus Vision Tester.

you. You should advise the person to have the patient schedule a time to have the doctor examine the ears and have a hearing test. You should carefully note the information on the patient's chart and bring it to the physician's attention. The physician will discuss the problem with the patient during the scheduled appointment.

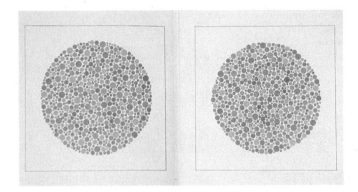

FIGURE 16–11 Sample color plate from Ishihara color acuity test

V R S K D R
N H C S O K
S C N O Z V
C N H Z O K
N O D V H R
C D N Z S V
K C H O
R

FIGURE 16–12 The Pelli–Robson contrast sensitivity chart. The faintest letters that can be read on this chart determine an individual's contrast sensitivity. The use of such a chart is an aid to earlier diagnosis of certain eye diseases.

Sometimes the problem may be as simple as the patient having impacted cerumen, and after an irrigation, the person's hearing usually returns to normal. Sometimes it is not that simple and further measures are necessary. The medical assistant is in contact with the patient usually more than the physician. It is the assistant's responsibility to act in the best interest of the patient in conveying important information observed. You can watch for many behaviors as you are getting patients ready for their scheduled appointments or when you talk to them over the phone. One of your most important duties is relaying information to the physician about patients.

Common behaviors of patients that indicate they may have lost some hearing ability are: (1) you are asked to repeat what you've said frequently during conversation; (2) inappropriately loud voice when speaking to you; (3) does not respond at all when spoken to; (4) does not pronounce words well; and (5) responds only when you speak very loudly. Certain complaints may suggest hearing loss or **auditory** nerve damage. When patients disclose any of the following symptoms you should bring it to the attention of the physician for further assessment:

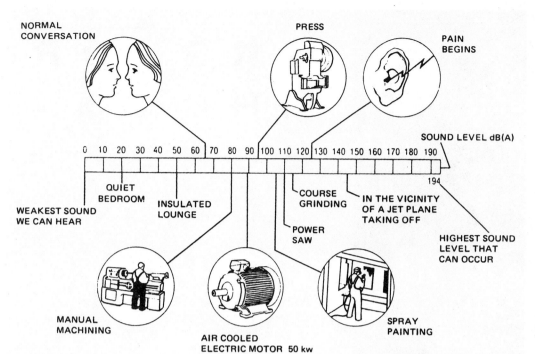

NORMAL CONVERSATION

PRESS

PAIN BEGINS

SOUND LEVEL dB(A)

0 10 20 30 40 50 60 70 80 90 100 110 120 130 140 150 160 170 180 190

194

QUIET BEDROOM

INSULATED LOUNGE

WEAKEST SOUND WE CAN HEAR

COURSE GRINDING

IN THE VICINITY OF A JET PLANE TAKING OFF

POWER SAW

HIGHEST SOUND LEVEL THAT CAN OCCUR

MANUAL MACHINING

AIR COOLED ELECTRIC MOTOR 50 kw

SPRAY PAINTING

FIGURE 16–13 Noise levels associated with selected conditions, locations, and operations

(1) ringing in the ears; (2) decreased hearing in either ear (sometimes caused by impacted cerumen); (3) infection or injury to the ear(s); (4) bleeding or discharge from the ear(s); and (5) any unusual noise or feeling inside the ear(s). These signs, or any others, which patients tell you should be written on the chart during triage. Further examination by the physician is necessary to determine the extent of the problem and its treatment.

An audiometer is an instrument used to measure one's hearing. The audiometer determines the hearing thresholds of pure tones of frequencies that are normally audible by an individual. Some also measure bone and air conduction. The threshold of hearing is the point where a sound can barely be heard. A person with normal hearing should hear all frequencies up to 15 decibels, depending on the surrounding noise levels, Figure 16–13.

Audiometric devices are powered either by batteries or electricity. Whatever type is used in the facility where you are employed should be checked periodically for proper performance and accuracy. If the batteries need to be changed or if a wire is frayed, it should be taken care of before being used with patients, not only for their safety, but to make sure that it works efficiently. Several types of audiometers are available for use in determining hearing acuity. Many are still used requiring that the operator manually turn a dial to emit the various frequencies for the patient to hear during the test. Companies that manufacture audiometers offer in-service demonstrations to make sure their equipment is used properly. Operations manuals should be kept with the instrument for handy reference.

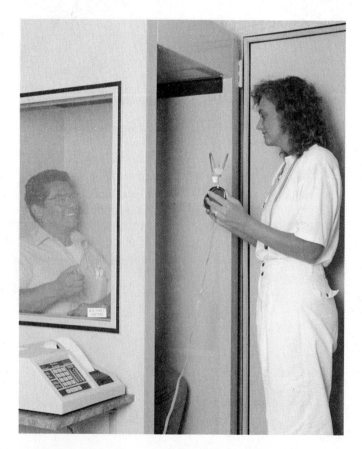

FIGURE 16–14 The patient presses the hand-held control button each time he hears a sound while in the soundproof booth. The signals are transmitted to the computer outside and printed as an audiogram.

1. Advise patients not to put anything into their ears to avoid damaging the tympanic membrane. The ear wax produced by the body has a purpose. It is to protect and moisten the membrane of the ear canal. Many people feel that they must completely remove this daily with a swab, which often results in being packed down into the ear canal where it hardens. This impacted ear wax (cerumen) must be removed by a qualified medical team member.

2. Instruct patients that eardrops and other ear medications should be used only with the advice of their physician. Earache, pain, or discharge should be reported to and examined by the physician as soon as possible.

3. Discuss the possibility of permanent hearing loss with patients who work around extremely loud noise or who have gotten into a habit of turning the volume way up when listening to audio systems/radios/TVs, etc. Explain to these patients that protective ear coverings should be worn while on the job (it is a safety requirement) and advise those who listen to loud music to turn down the volume before their hearing is lost from damage to nerves.

4. Urge patients to have regular hearing tests to detect loss of hearing or other related problems. It is recommended that this be done annually unless otherwise instructed by the physician, or if there is a noticeable difference or problem with hearing. Patients who have a history of ear infections should have periodic hearing tests.

The procedure for every audiometer is basically the same. The patient is instructed to place the earphones (marked red for the right ear and blue for the left ear) over the ears. The medical assistant tells the patient in the soundproof booth how the earphones are to be placed and how to work the control signal, Figure 16–14. The printer on the table next to the booth records the results of the hearing test. The printout is called an audiogram, which is filed in the patient's chart after the physician reads the results of the test and makes an evaluation.

During the procedure in whichever ear that is not being tested, the sound is automatically blocked by the machine. In the ear which is being tested, the machine provides a series of tones. The patient listens and signals (either by raising a finger or by using a hand-held control) to the medical assistant as the various sounds are heard. The tones range in frequencies from very low to very high with a varied level of decibel intensity. After the right ear has been tested, the machine switches automatically to test the left ear. The medical assistant should report any com-

plaints that the patient may have had before or during the hearing test and any unusual behavior to the physician. You should make a note of this information on the patient's chart along with the results of the test and place your initials indicating that you have completed the test.

Physicians use several audiometric assessment procedures to determine the cause of a patient's hearing loss, some of which are a part of the complete or routine physical examination.

During the physical examination the physician will use a tuning fork to test the patient's hearing. A two-pronged metal tuning fork is used, its frequency varying with the size of the instrument. The common tests done are the Rinne and the Weber.

In the Rinne test, the examiner strikes the fork and then holds the shank (stem) against the patient's mastoid bone until the patient no longer hears the sound. The prongs of the tuning fork are then placed about 1 inch from the auditory meatus (opening to the ear) and then next to it. In a

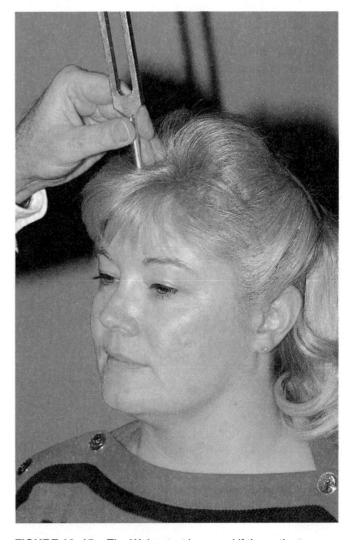

FIGURE 16–15 The Weber test is normal if the patient can hear the sound in both ears equally well as the end of the tuning fork is placed against the skull.

normal ear the sound is heard about twice as long by air conduction as by bone conduction. If hearing by bone conduction is greater, the result is spoken of as a negative Rinne.

In the Weber test the vibrating tuning fork is held against the vertex (crown of the head) or against the skull or forehead in the midline, Figure 16–15, page 484. The sound is heard best by the unaffected ear if deafness is due to disease of the auditory apparatus, by the affected ear if deafness is due to obstruction of the air passages.

A simple means of screening the hearing of infants and small children is to place a ticking watch behind their shoulder, without their seeing it, of course, and see how quickly they become aware of the noise.

A small amount of hearing loss may be temporary due to a patient's physical condition and a recheck in 1 or 2 weeks may be advisable.

Complete Chapter 16, Unit 1 in the workbook to help you meet the objectives at the beginning of this unit and therefore achieve competency of this subject matter.

U N I T   2

Positioning and Draping for Examinations

OBJECTIVES ....

Upon completion of this unit, the student will meet the following terminal performance objectives by verifying knowledge of the facts and principles presented through oral and written communication at a level deemed competent, and will demonstrate the specific behaviors as identified in the terminal performance objectives of the procedures, observing all aseptic and safety precautions in accordance with health care standards.

1. Explain the purpose of each of the examination positions.
2. Demonstrate the proper method of positioning and draping patients for the various examinations.
3. Discuss safety precautions regarding both the medical assistant and patient in positioning for examinations.
4. Spell and define, using the glossary at the back of the text, all the words to know in this unit.

WORDS TO KNOW ....

anterior	dowel
body mechanics	dyspneic
dorsal	fenestrated
flexed	postpartum
genucubital	prone
genupectoral	recumbent
horizontal	shock
incompetent	supine
lithotomy	Trendelenburg
prolapsed	

Positioning and Draping Patient ....

Positioning the patient for examination is an important function of the medical assistant. There are a number of standard positions for specific examinations and treatments, which you should know. If a power table is used, you must learn how to operate it. The power table illustrated in Figure 16–16 is considered to be the most advanced power examination table in America. It is possible to program this table to the best height for the physicians who will use it and to the positions desired. The desired position is then achieved by the press of a button. This table has an optional plug-in foot control that could be used in the event of a failure in the computer circuit. This table also has two rolls of paper under the frame at the head of the table so you should never run out of paper.

Most examination tables are vinyl covered and easily cleaned with antiseptic soap and a sponge or cloth if any body fluids are noted after a patient has been examined. The table needs to be cleaned regularly. The table is covered with a roll of paper, which needs to be the proper width to cover the table. The paper roll is usually inserted on a dowel under the head of the table and is secured at the bottom of the table with a strap. The strap is useful in your practice of tearing off the paper when you pull down a clean paper for the next patient.

A female medical assistant should remain in the room when a female patient is being examined by a male physician. The patient should feel more relaxed and the physician is protected from lawsuits that could result from patients claiming the physician acted improperly during the examination. Patient gowns and drapes are made of cloth or disposable paper. The patient is instructed on the use of the gown to avoid unnecessary exposure. If the examination table is too high for the patient to sit on it comfortably, a foot stool should be provided. A very ill patient or a small child should never be left alone on a table; a member of the family may be asked to sit with them if you must leave the room.

Body mechanics are important. Never try to lift a patient who is obviously more than you can safely handle, but have someone help you. If a patient needs help in moving on the table, reach under the arm at the shoulder and help the person move up. If it is necessary to help a patient out of a wheelchair, position the chair and lock the wheels before trying to help the patient move from the chair to the table. A procedure for this will be given later. The standing erect or anatomical position may be used

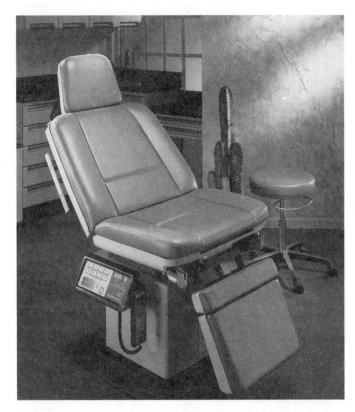

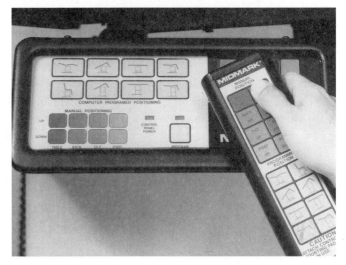

FIGURE 16–16 (a). Midmark power table (b). Control panel (Courtesy Midmark Corporation)

especially for neurological examination, range of motion, and flexibility while the patient is being instructed by the physician in bending and walking. This position begins with the patient standing upright with arms at sides and palms facing forward (see Chapter 13, Unit 1). If the patient is well enough to sit on the edge or end of the table with feet hanging down and no back support this position may be used to begin the examination.

The **horizontal recumbent** or **supine** position is used for examination and treatment of the **anterior** surface of the body and for X rays, Figure 16–17. The term *dorsal* recumbent is used to indicate that the legs are **flexed**. This position allows for relaxation of the abdominal muscles and thus easier examination of the abdominal area. This position may also be used for vaginal or rectal examination. This position may also be used to test reflexes. The gown is open in the front and

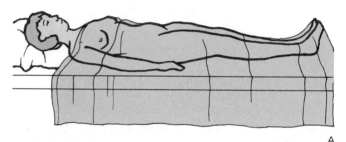

A

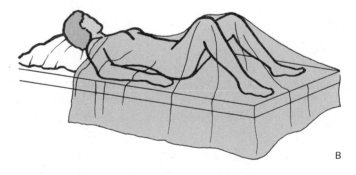

B

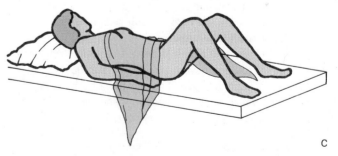

C

FIGURE 16–17 Examination positions: (a). Horizontal recumbent. (b). Dorsal recumbent. (c). Dorsal recumbent with diamond drape

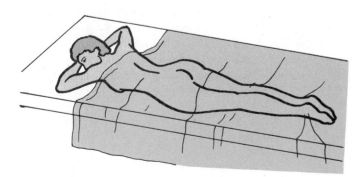

FIGURE 16–18 Prone position

Instruct the patient about the need for a specific position for the examination to be performed. This information should be included with the instructions on preparing for the examination. The patient must understand that the physician needs to examine certain parts of the body or perform certain procedures and tests, and the patient must be positioned in the most accessible manner.

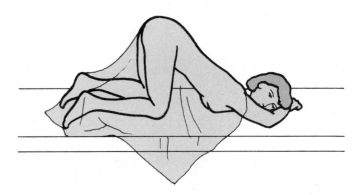

FIGURE 16–20   Knee-chest position

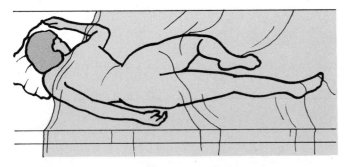

FIGURE 16–19   Sims' position

a drape sheet of cloth or paper is used to cover the patient. The **prone** position is used for examination of the back or spine, with the gown open in the back, Figure 16–18, page 487.

The Sims' position is used in examination and treatment of the rectal area, for enemas, rectal temperature, and sigmoidoscopy, Figure 16–19. This position may also be used for pelvic examinations. This is also called the lateral position.

The knee-chest position is used for rectal examination and specifically for sigmoidoscopy examination, Figure 16–20. When properly done this position helps straighten out the sharp curve in the sigmoid colon and makes it

---

     P R O C E D U R E

Assist Patient to Horizontal Recumbent Position

TERMINAL PERFORMANCE OBJECTIVE: In a simulated situation, using an appropriately prepared examining table and drape, the student will assist the patient to assume the horizontal recumbent position while providing for safety and privacy according to standards identified in the procedure sheet.

1. Check examination room for cleanliness. **Key Point: Always have clean paper on table and a clean pillow cover or clean towel over pillow.**
2. Identify patient. **Key Point: Call patient by name and check chart to avoid error.**
3. Give clear instructions to patient regarding amount of clothing to be removed and where it is to be placed.
4. Instruct patient on use of gown—to be open in front.
5. Assist patient if help is needed. Otherwise respect privacy and modesty of patient by leaving room while patient changes.
6. Instruct patient to sit on side of table.

7. Instruct patient to lie flat on table with legs together.
8. Pull out end extension on table for leg support if needed.
9. Patient may rest head on small pillow if desired.
10. Instruct patient to cross arms on chest or put them at sides of body. To position for dorsal recumbent, ask patient to put bottoms of both feet flat on table with knees flexed.
11. Drape sheet evenly over patient but leave loose on all sides. For vaginal or rectal examination, drape patient with one corner of sheet over chest, a corner wrapped around each leg, and fourth corner over pubic area. Physician will turn back sheet at pubic area.
12. Assist physician as necessary with examination.
13. Assist patient from table if help is needed when examination is completed. Patients may be dizzy from an abrupt change of position.
14. Clean room and replace supplies.

PROCEDURE

Assist Patient to Prone Position

TERMINAL PERFORMANCE OBJECTIVE: In a simulated situation, using an appropriately prepared examining table and drape, the student will assist the patient to assume the prone position while providing for safety and privacy according to standards identified in the procedure sheet.

1. Check examination room for cleanliness. **Key Point: Always have clean paper on table and a clean cover or clean towel over pillow.**

2. Identify patient. **Key Point: Call patient by name and check chart to avoid error.**

3. Give clear instructions to patient regarding amount of clothing to remove and where it is to be placed.

4. Instruct patient on use of gown—to be open in back. Some offices furnish a modesty gown with a rectangular piece of material to be put on diaper fashion and tied on sides. If so, instruct in use.

5. Assist patient if necessary. Otherwise respect privacy of patient by leaving room while patient undresses.

6. Instruct patient to sit on side of table.

7. Instruct patient to lie flat on table with legs together.

8. Pull out end extension on table for leg support if needed.

9. Cover patient with drape sheet and instruct patient to turn toward you onto stomach, being careful to stay in center of table to avoid a fall. **Key Point: Always instruct patient to turn toward your body to prevent a fall. You can grasp cover drape and keep it smoothly in place as patient turns over.**

10. Instruct patient to turn head to side.

11. Instruct patient to flex arms at elbows with hands at side of head.

12. Drape sheet evenly and loosely on all sides.

13. Assist physician as necessary with examination.

14. Instruct patient to turn on back, being careful to stay in middle of table to avoid fall.

15. Instruct patient to sit up for a moment to regain balance before trying to leave table.

16. Clean room and replace supplies.

---

safer and easier to pass the sigmoidoscope. This position is sometimes called the genupectoral and is used as therapy for postpartum prolapsed uterus. The position is difficult to assume and to maintain for a long period of time. Special care must be taken to keep the patient from falling.

The Fowler's position is used for patients with respiratory or cardiovascular problems, Figure 16–21. The patient who is dyspneic must be in a sitting or semisitting position to breathe comfortably. This position may

be used to examine the trunk of the body (head, neck, and chest area). The position may be semi-Fowler's (partially sitting) or Fowler's (sitting upright). A female patient would be more comfortable in an examination gown opened in front if the sheet covers the chest area on down to the feet.

The lithotomy position is used for vaginal or rectal examination, Figure 16–22, page 491. This position can also be used for examination of the male genital area and for catheterization of a patient.

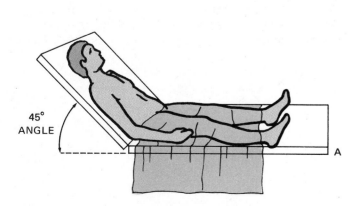
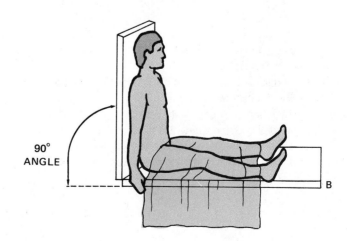

FIGURE 16–21   Fowler's positions: (a). semi: (b). high

Assist Patient to Sims' Position

TERMINAL PERFORMANCE OBJECTIVE: In a simulated situation, using an appropriately prepared examining table and drape, the student will assist the patient to assume the horizontal recumbent position while providing for safety and privacy according to standards identified in the procedure sheet.

1. Check examination room for cleanliness. **Key Point: Always have clean paper on table and a clean pillow cover or clean towel over pillow.**
2. Identify patient. **Key Point: Call patient by name and check chart to avoid error.**
3. Give clear instructions to patient regarding amount of clothing to be removed and where it is to be placed.
4. Instruct patient in use of gown—to be open in back.
5. Assist patient if needed. Otherwise respect privacy and modesty of patient by leaving room while patient undresses.
6. Instruct patient to sit on side of table.
7. Instruct patient to lie on left side. A pillow may be placed under head.
8. Instruct patient to place left arm and shoulder behind body. This places weight of body on chest.
9. Instruct patient to flex right arm with hand toward head in front of body.
10. Instruct patient to flex left leg slightly with buttocks near edge of table being sure patient does not fall.
11. Instruct patient to flex right leg sharply toward chest.
12. Cover patient with a fenestrated drape. If a regular sheet is used, hang drape free from under arms to below knees. Edge will be turned back for procedure.
13. Assist physician as necessary with examination.
14. Instruct patient to turn to back, sit up, and then move from table.
15. Clean and replace supplies.

Assist Patient to Knee-Chest Position

TERMINAL PERFORMANCE OBJECTIVE: In a simulated situation, using an appropriately prepared examining table and drape, the student will assist the patient to assume the knee chest position while providing for safety and privacy, according to standards identified in the procedure sheet.

1. Check examination room for cleanliness.
2. Prepare examination equipment on tray with cover over instruments. Each office will have special equipment, which physician will want you to have ready. Check office procedure manual or make up your own card for each procedure.
3. Identify patient. **Key Point: Call patient by name and check chart to avoid error.**
4. Give clear instructions to patient regarding clothing to be removed and where it is to be placed.
5. Assist patient if needed. Otherwise respect privacy of patient by leaving room while patient undresses.
6. Instruct patient to sit on side of table.
7. Instruct patient to lie down on table.
8. Cover patient with drape.
9. Instruct patient to turn toward you onto stomach, being careful to stay in middle of table.
10. Instruct patient to get on hands and knees.
11. Instruct patient to flex arms and fold under head, bringing chest down to table. If this is too difficult, have patient rest on elbows (genucubital position).
12. Instruct patient to separate knees slightly and keep thighs at right angle to table.
13. A fenestrated drape is usually used, but two small sheets may be draped to meet at rectal area. Diamond drape may also be used.
14. Call physician immediately to complete examination.
15. Assist physician as necessary with examination.
16. Instruct patient to lie flat on stomach and then turn over on back (while staying in middle of table) and sit up before moving from table.
17. Clean room and replace supplies.

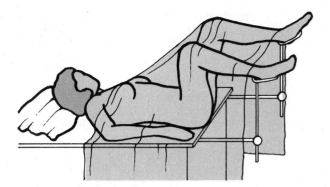

FIGURE 16–22   Lithotomy position

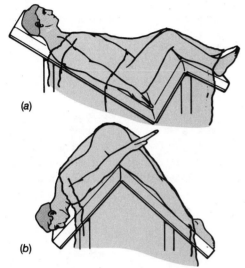

(a)

(b)

FIGURE 16–24   Jackknife position

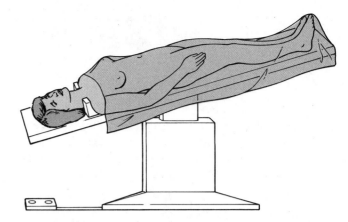

FIGURE 16–23   Trendelenburg position

In the Trendelenburg or shock position the patient is supine with feet elevated slightly, Figure 16–23. This position may easily be accomplished with a power table. This position may be used for postural drainage with the patient turning into various positions. It can be used for a patient with low blood pressure and to displace organs for some abdominal surgical procedures. This position is also useful as a simple test for incompetent valves in persons with varicose veins. After being placed in this position the patient is asked to stand and the physician observes whether the veins fill from above or below.

A special table would be needed for the jackknife position to be comfortable, Figure 16–24. The patient is in a semi-sitting position with the shoulders elevated and the thighs flexed at right angles to the abdomen. This

    P R O C E D U R E

Assist Patient to Semi-Fowler's Position

TERMINAL PERFORMANCE OBJECTIVE: In a simulated situation, using an appropriately prepared examining table and drape, the student will assist the patient to assume the semi-Fowler's position while providing for safety and privacy according to standards identified in the procedure sheet.

1. Check examination room for cleanliness.
2. Identify patient. **Key Point: Call patient by name and check chart to avoid error.**
3. Give clear instructions to patient if clothing is to be removed.
4. Instruct patient on use of gown.
5. Assist patient if needed or leave room while patient undresses.
6. Ask patient to sit at end of table.

7. Raise head of table to desired height for comfort of patient, usually 45-degree angle for semi-Fowler's and completely upright for Fowler's.
8. Ask patient to lean back on rest.
9. Support legs with extension rest at end of table.
10. Drape patient from underarm to below knees.
11. Assist patient as necessary.
12. Ask patient to sit up before lowering head of table. Be sure you understand how to lower head of table. Some tables have a release lever, and it is necessary to support head of table with one hand while releasing lever so that head of table will not fall with a crash.
13. Assist patient from table.
14. Clean room and replace supplies.

P R O C E D U R E

Assist Patient to Lithotomy Position

TERMINAL PERFORMANCE OBJECTIVE: In a simulated situation, using an appropriately prepared examining table and drape, the student will assist the patient to assume the lithotomy position while providing for safety and privacy according to standards identified in the procedure sheet.

1. Check examination room for cleanliness.
2. Assemble necessary equipment.
3. Identify patient. **Key Point: Call patient by name and check chart to avoid error.**
4. Give clear instructions to patient to remove clothing from waist down. If breast examination is also to be performed, ask patient to put on a gown.
5. Assist patient if needed or leave room while patient is undressing.
6. Ask patient to sit at end of table.
7. Instruct patient to lie back on table.
8. Support legs with extension on table. (If no extension, be sure patient moves back on table before lying down.) Newer examination tables allow patient to sit while table is tilted back, leg supports come up under legs, and end of table is lowered, all by use of a foot pedal.

9. Position stirrups as far away from table as possible and adjust height if necessary. If heels are too close to table and buttocks, patient may get leg cramps.
10. Stabilize stirrups so they will remain in position during examination. Some tables are designed so that you must turn a knob at side of table. Some tables have several locking positions for stirrups as they swing outward.
11. Ask patient to move toward end of table while you guide feet into stirrups.
12. Instruct patient to move far enough down so that buttocks are at end of table. **Key Point: Check to see if patient is far enough down by holding hand outside of drape sheet at end of table.**
13. Push in leg rest, position stool for physician, and position light.
14. Assist physician with examination.
15. Ask patient to slide back up on table.
16. Support legs by pulling out extension rest.
17. Instruct patient to sit up before moving from table.
18. Offer tissues to wipe off excess lubricant before dressing.
19. Clean room and replace supplies.

---

position is especially useful for examination and instrumentation of the male urethra.

Complete Chapter 16, Unit 2 in the workbook to help you meet the objectives at the beginning of this unit and therefore achieve competency of this subject matter.

UNIT 3

Preparing Patients for Examinations

OBJECTIVES ....

Upon completion of the unit the student will meet the following terminal performance objectives by verifying knowledge of the facts and principles presented through oral and written communication at a level deemed competent, and will demonstrate the specific behaviors as identified in the terminal performance objectives of the

procedures, observing all aseptic and safety precautions in accordance with health care standards.

1. List the duties that involve the medical assistant in preparing for the complete physical examination (CPE) of a patient.
2. Name the instruments, equipment, and supplies used in the CPE, and state the function of each.
3. Identify each section of the CPE and describe how the physician conducts each part of the examination.
4. Explain the role of the medical assistant in the examination process.
5. List and discuss appropriate patient education for the various parts of the examination.
6. Identify the nine sections of the abdominal cavity and name the visceral organs therein.
7. Define the POMR and SOAP methods of charting patient information.
8. Establish reasons for progress reports.
9. Explain subjective and objective symptoms and give five examples of each.
10. Discuss the seven warning signs of cancer in adults and children.
11. Describe the physical examination schedules for adults and children.

12. Spell and define, using the glossary at the back of the text, all the words to know in this unit.

WORDS TO KNOW ....

acute	inspection
anxiety	L & A
asymmetry	laryngeal
audibility	laxative
auscultation	liaison
baseline	manipulation
bimanual	mensuration
bold	murmur
bruit	objective
caustic	occult
chronic	palpation
coordination	percussion
cytological	pitch
detection	progress report
dimpling	peripheral
douche	physical
duration	prolapse
enema	resonance
evacuate	R/O
explicit	sphincter
exudate	subjective
fasting	subsequent
fistula	symmetry
gait	tentative
glaucoma	tonometer
guaiac	visceral
hernia	void
indigestion	warrant
inguinal	writer
initial	

Assisting with the complete physical examination (CPE), the general physical exam, H & P (history and physical), physical exam (PE), or just plain *physical,* as it is often termed, is not difficult, but complex in that it is a *set* of procedures. The responsibilities of the medical assistant are to prepare the room for the physician and patient, and then the patient for the physician to examine. You may also assist with the exam, or write the findings. In the following pages you will learn this process.

In many facilities, the medical assistant accompanies the physician in the examination room and records the findings while the physician dictates the information as the examination proceeds. The term *writer* is given to the medical assistant who writes what the physician dictates during the exam. One who performs this duty must have sound knowledge in medical terminology, anatomy, and physiology, and of course, good spelling and writing skills. Since the physician bases the diagnosis on these findings, accuracy is vital. Many physicians prefer to write their own findings on plain sheets of lined paper (a common practice is to use a rubber stamp that outlines a

particular exam format), or on specially printed forms in the outlined order of their choice. Still other physicians prefer to dictate the findings of an examination into a recorder for transcription later by the medical assistant.

There is no absolute pattern of examination to follow as long as the examiner is consistent and forms a personal habit so as to be thorough and complete with each patient. The complete examination should include the whole body, from the head to the toes, and front to back, and inside and out. In your career as a medical assistant, you will work with many physicians who may be quite different in their systematic approach to patient care.

Physicians are skilled in a variety of techniques used in evaluating patients in the examination process. In assisting with the H & P, the medical assistant is expected to have a basic knowledge of these procedural terms.

The initial part of the exam is the inspection, in which the physician looks for any abnormalities of speech, skin condition, color, posture, gait, awareness, sensitivity, anxiety, grooming, or general appearance.

Whenever patients come in to the office/clinic for an appointment, whether it is for a checkup or a visit for an illness or injury, it is a perfect opportunity for you to motivate them to practice better health habits. The medical assistant usually has more time than the physician to talk with the patients because many procedures do take time to perform. While you are conducting these matters, you can suggest many different ideas to patients. Often for various reasons, the patient must wait for the physician. Making use of this time for patient education is wise. Sometimes a beginning medical assistant may be at a loss for words with patients and does not know what to talk about with them except for the weather. This may help you learn some appropriate topics to speak with patients about which may benefit them. Table 16–2 out-

TABLE 16–2
The 7 Warning Signs of Cancer

Adults

1. Sore that does not heal
2. Annoying cough or hoarseness
3. Trouble with swallowing or frequent indigestion
4. Unusual bleeding or discharge
5. A thickened area or lump in breast or anywhere on the body
6. A change in a wart or a mole
7. Change in bowel or bladder habits

Children (same as for adults plus the following)

1. The over-all condition seems generally run-down
2. Unexplained stumbling
3. Infant/child cries continually for no apparent reason
4. Any bloody discharge; any spontaneous bleeding or failure to stop bleeding in usual time
5. Anywhere on the body: swelling, lumps, masses, or bumps
6. Change in size and looks of birth marks, moles, etc.
7. Nausea and vomiting for no obvious reason

lines the warning signs of cancer. A few other suggestions for topics to discuss with patients follow.

Palpation is a means of examination by touching with the fingers or hands. Digital (one-finger) palpation is used to examine the anus. **Bimanual** (two-handed) palpation is used in vaginal examinations. Palpation of the breasts is done with the fingertips of both hands.

Percussion is a means of producing sounds by tapping various parts of the body. The physician listens to the sounds to determine the size, density, and location of underlying **visceral** organs. **Pitch,** quality, **duration,** and **resonance** are terms used by physicians when referring to percussion. Direct percussion is termed *immediate* and is done by striking the finger against the patient's body. The type of percussion most often used is *indirect* or *mediate*. With indirect percussion, the examiner's finger is placed on the area and struck with a finger of the other hand.

Auscultation is listening to sounds made by the patient's body. Indirect auscultation is done with the stethoscope to amplify sounds that arise from the lungs, heart, and visceral organs. Sounds heard by this method of examination include **bruits,** murmurs, and rhythms. Direct auscultation is done by placing the ear directly over the area.

Mensuration means measurement. In this part of the examination, the patient's chest and extremities are measured and recorded in centimeters. Usually a standard flexible tape measure is used.

Manipulation is the forceful, passive movement of a joint to determine the range of extension and flexion.

PATIENT EDUCATION

A. To prevent injuries of the face and head:
   1. In working and recreational environments, wear protective head gear: hard hat at work (construction sites), helmet for sports (motorcycle riding, football).
      a. Wear protective face mask/goggles for sports such as football/basketball/wrestling to prevent possible eye injuries.
      b. Use ear plugs to protect the ears from exposure to loud noises that can lead to possible damage to auditory nerves resulting in hearing loss (machinery, band concerts); water when swimming.

B. To protect the skin:
   1. Keep skin clean and soft by using mild soap and water for bathing and a moisturizing lotion as necessary.
      a. Discourage sun worship. Encourage keeping covered in the sun or the use of a sun blocker to prevent damage of ultraviolet rays if one must be in the sun for prolonged periods of time.
      b. Wash hands of (chemical) irritants immediately to prevent caustic burns.

C. To prevent diseases of the respiratory system and other contagious diseases:
   1. Discourage eating, drinking, etc., after others to keep from transmitting viruses and other diseases to others.
   2. Wash hands after handling items in or from public places, which probably have been handled by multitudes of others (money, door knobs, etc.).
   3. Discourage smoking or tobacco use of any kind (post stop smoking pamphlets or meetings for patients to read).
   4. Remind patients of the dangers of drug and alcohol use/abuse (display information about Alcoholics Anonymous meetings).
   5. Encourage exercise/physical fitness programs with the advice of the physician.
   6. Promote proper nutrition and weight control by reminding patients to eat well-balanced meals regularly and help them plan their diets.
   7. Encourage *safe sex* by providing explicit information to teach patients about the dangers of sexually transmitted diseases and AIDS.
   8. Discourage patients from using laxatives and enemas unless specifically ordered by the physician.
   9. Remind patients about immunizations and encourage their compliance.
   10. Encourage patients to read labels for contents of the products they buy and use for their safety.
   11. Remind patients to use seat belts.
   12. Promote regular medical and dental checkups.

In documenting the physical examination, many physicians use the Problem Oriented Medical Record (POMR) method described previously (see Chapter 9, Unit 2). It is sometimes referred to as POS, or problem-oriented system. This system is used for a new patient workup and for patients with serious or chronic illnesses. It is also used to document specific multiple complaints of patients. For acute or single minor complaints, such as a sore throat or a splinter, this system may not be used, for the chief complaint would not warrant such detail. Using this system ensures that pertinent data is recorded in logical order on the patient's chart with each return visit to the physician. Data is recorded under the following headings:

S Subjective findings

O Objective findings

A Assessment of problems

P Plan for treatment

Under subjective findings are those symptoms which the patient feels but which cannot be seen by another. Nausea, joint pain, headache, and abdominal pain are examples of subjective findings. Objective findings are those symptoms that can be seen by another as well as by the patient, such as redness, rash, swelling, watery discharge, or bleeding. It can also include any information concerning the patient that a family member or friend has conveyed to either you or the doctor, and the patient's past health history. Assessment documents measurement of the symptoms. This includes laboratory reports, X rays, vital sign recordings, and other aids to diagnosis.

The tentative diagnosis is made in this section of the patient's chart. The final section of the system outlines the plan of treatment for the patient to follow. This includes referrals, medication, surgery, therapy, exercise, and any further orders to return the patient to better health. Patient education is obviously a great part of this systematic method of record keeping. All action taken in the course of the patient's treatment generates additional information that continually modifies the original data base. Subsequent visits of the patient are recorded in the same manner (SOAP) as was the initial visit on sheets termed *progress notes,* sometimes referred to as *progress reports* or chart notes. Following each entry on the patient's chart should be the signature or initials of the health care provider or the person who performed the procedure.

Preparation of the Examination Room ....

Getting the examination room ready consists of making sure that: the temperature in the room is comfortable; it is clean and tidy; the examination table has a clean covering (either disposable table paper or a cloth sheet); all appropriate instruments, equipment, and supplies are arranged conveniently for use during the examination.

The medical assistant should routinely clean and restock the examination room. Carefully checking the room for necessary items will ensure efficient, expedient patient care. Make sure all equipment is in proper working order and that the room is cleaned following each patient.

These items are displayed and labeled in Figure 16–25 in the order in which they are commonly used for a complete physical examination. You should learn the name and function of each item.

Preparation of the Patient ....

It is a usual practice to schedule the CPE early in the morning because patients are normally required to fast (have nothing by mouth) from midnight on for blood chemistry tests, which are based on a fasting normal range. Other procedures within the examination process are more comfortable if the patient has not eaten before the physical.

When these preliminary tasks have been completed, the medical assistant escorts the patient into the examination room and explains the proceedings, answers any questions, and may begin patient education where appropriate. Triage will have already determined what chief complaints the patient has. You may want to verify what the patient feels is the problem at this point. Make sure that you allow the patient time to use the restroom for comfort during the exam. You should ask the patient to urinate in a specimen cup if he or she did not bring a first morning specimen for you to test (complete

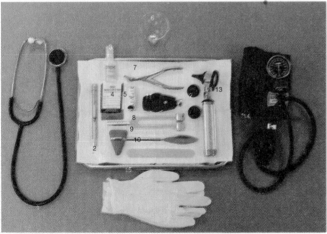

1. stethoscope
2. penlight
3. guaiac/occult blood test developer
4. guaiac/occult blood test
5. flexible tape measure
6. urine specimen container
7. metal nasal speculum
8. tuning fork
9. percussion hammer
10. tongue depressser
11. ophthalmoscope (head)
12. okastic ear/nose speculum
13. otoscope head attached to base handle
14. sphygmomanometer
15. latex gloves

FIGURE 16–25 Instruments and supplies used in the physical examination

instructions for specimen collection are in Chapter 17). Sometimes the physician must delay the examination of the abdominal area because the patient has to **void** or **evacuate** the bowel. Occasionally this is obviously unavoidable even if the patient has already made an elimination. Unnecessary interruptions are annoying besides hindering the patient flow schedule. The success of the physical examination is attributed largely to the preparation of the patient. Until you are sure of yourself in remembering details, it is helpful to keep a checklist in your uniform pocket for handy reference.

The next duty of the medical assistant is to ask the patient to disrobe and put on the examination gown. Explain how by showing the patient, for instance, whether the gown should be open in the front or the back. You should offer assistance with this and show the patient where to store belongings. Pull out the step at the end of the exam table (or provide a portable one) and help the patient up to the exam table. Cover the top of the patient's legs with a drape sheet, which provides both privacy and warmth.

General instructions about the physical may be offered at this point. You may want to tell the patient that some parts of the examination may be uncomfortable, but usually not painful. The patient should be urged to let the physician know of any pain or unusual discomfort during any part of the procedure, and to offer any complaint that has not previously been made known.

Physical Examination Format ....

In reviewing the medical history form in the last chapter (see Figure 15–2), you will notice that the section immediately following, "present illness," has all of the areas outlined for recording the findings of the complete physical examination.

The format of the examination section of this form has been extracted and completed in the following text with an explanation of each of the body areas examined. Hopefully this will help you become familiar with what the doctor does in each section of the physical examination. Even though H & P forms vary in appearance, the contents will basically be the same. In the spaces which say: general appearance, skin, mucous membranes, etc., a brief written description by the examiner is far more helpful for future reference than just writing "normal," or its equivalent N (negative or normal) or simply drawing a straight line which means, no comment.

Notice that the very first part of the physical includes measurement, vital signs, and vision screening, which the medical assistant normally completes. You may want to refer to appropriate units to review these procedures.

The instruments and/or equipment to be used in examining each area of the body are in **bold** print at the beginning of each section where necessary or appropriate. Certainly the patient's chart, pens (one with black ink, and one with red for alerting allergies), and any forms (laboratory request or others) necessary for completion should be at the disposal of the physician and the medical assistant to begin the examination.

(taken from the "in depth" medical history form)

Patient _____ Date _____

PHYSICAL EXAMINATION:

Ht.— recorded in: _____ cm (centimeters) or _____ "
(inches) or _____ ' (feet) and " (inches)

Wt.— recorded in _____ kg (kilograms) or _____ lbs
(pounds)

Temp.— recorded in degrees of _____ Fahrenheit or
_____ Centigrade

Pulse—recorded _____ per minute

Respirations— recorded _____ per minute

Blood Pressure — **stethoscope, sphygmomanometer** —Readings should be taken and recorded from both right and left arms and marked appropriately. It is generally advised that two or more readings be taken, preferably from two different positions (i.e., sitting and standing) and recorded as such.

General Appearance — This generally describes the patient and the state of health, such as "Mr. G. is a spirited, energetic, medium built, well-groomed 34-year-old Hispanic male who has a history of allergies. He has no speech or hearing defects."

Skin — Includes inspection of color (or discoloration), texture, temperature, and assessment of the condition of the hair and nails, as well as lesions, rashes, masses, or swollen areas, scars, wounds, warts, moles, bruises, or any other significant changes the patient reports. •

Eyes — Vision: OD 20/30 OS 20/25 OU 20/30

Ishihara — Record plate numbers that are both seen and not seen by the patient for evaluation or physician may write that patient's color vision is intact for red and green or normal or abnormal after interpreting the results of the test.

Near Vision — Record the number of the line that the patient can read most easily on the Jaeger card. Physician will determine if the patient's near distance acuity is normal or abnormal from test results.

Pupil — Fundus — **ophthalmoscope, tonometer** — The physician uses the ophthalmoscope to look deep into the center of the eye to check the condition of the tiny capillaries behind the retina; if there are no abnormalities there will be what is called a *red reflex,* or a red reflection that fills the pupil as the examiner views the eye. Then testing the pupils for reaction to light is done. During this part of the exam the overhead light is temporarily turned off (by the medical assistant) so that the doctor can watch for pupilary constriction, which if normal will happen right away. The patient is instructed to keep looking straight ahead while this is done in both eyes.

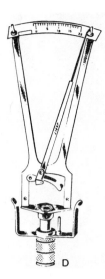

FIGURE 16–26 Schioetz tonometer (Courtesy of J. Jamner Surgical Instruments Inc.)

The examiner looks to see if the patient has eyelashes and brows (or not); checks ocular tension; if the patient exhibits a stare or any ocular protrusion; if the sclera is white; if there is any defect of the cornea or iris; if the pupils are round and equal in size, and if they react to light and accommodation (L & A). At some point during this part of the exam, the examiner will test the patient's **peripheral** vision and the horizontal and vertical fields. These tests are several hand/finger movements made by the doctor, which the patient is instructed to follow while the doctor observes. A test with the tonometer may be done next to detect **glaucoma.** There are several different types of tonometers; a picture of a commonly used one is shown in Figure 16–26. It measures the intraocular pressure by determining the resistance of the eyeball to an indentation made from an applied force. Assistance with this procedure consists of: preparation (by instilling drops to anesthetize the eyes), instruction regarding the procedure, positioning the patient, and handing the instrument to the physician.

Ears — **otoscope, tuning fork** — The examiner inspects the ears for size and for any abnormalities, such as lesions or nodules, or diagonal creasing of the lobe. The otoscope is used to examine the inner ear. Refer to Figure 16–2 for use of the otoscope. The physician traditionally assesses the hearing during examination of the ear with the tuning fork.

Nose — **nasal speculum, penlight (otoscope), alcohol-saturated gauze square** — The physician checks for any outward signs of abnormalities, and then uses a nasal speculum to view the right and left nostril for any lesions, obstructions, **exudate,** tenderness or swelling. A test to check the sense of smell often is done at this point by having the patient close the eyes and identify a common substance such as alcohol.

Oral Mucous Membranes — **penlight, tongue depressor, sterile gauze square, laryngeal mirror, stethoscope** — The physician looks into the oral cavity with a penlight or by using the light of the otoscope (without the ear speculum attached), to check for any unusual condition of the teeth, tongue, throat, and so on. The patient is asked to tilt the head back, hold the mouth open, stick out the tongue, and say, "ahh," while the physician uses the tongue depressor, and/or a gauze square to hold the tongue to the side during the exam of the floor of the mouth. A laryngeal mirror may be used here to check areas difficult to view in the mouth, besides looking down the throat of the patient. It is a good opportunity to remind patients at this point to brush their teeth and use dental floss after eating and have regular dental checkups (especially if there is a noticeable need for dental care). The pharynx and neck are generally examined next by palpation. By auscultation the physician listens to the carotid artery bloodflow for any abnormal sounds. The sound made by the blockage of the carotid artery is referred to as bruit, Figure 16–27.

Chest — **stethoscope** — During this portion of the exam, the patient's gown must be removed to the waist so the physician can inspect the chest for visual signs of abnormality such as lesions, tumors, swelling, skin disorders, etc., as well as observe the patient's breathing. The back is also checked in this manner. The chest is

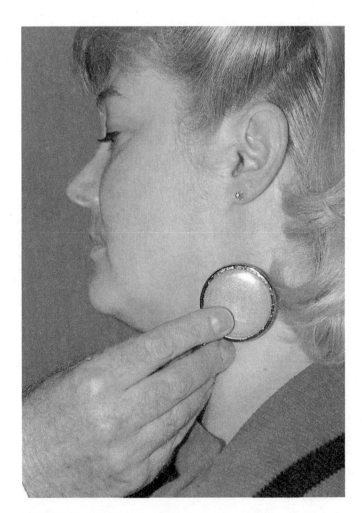

FIGURE 16–27 The doctor performs auscultation of the neck to listen to the blood flow through the carotid artery.

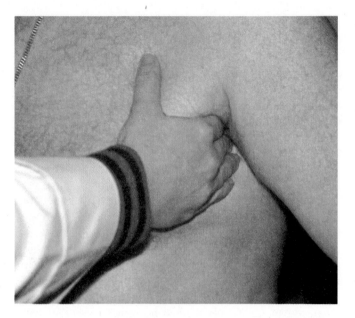

FIGURE 16–28 Palpation of the patient's axillary region by the examiner

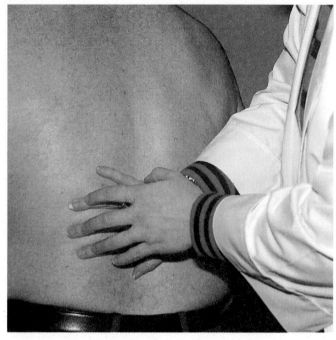

FIGURE 16–29 The examiner uses blunt percussion to examine the kidney.

HOW TO DO BSE

1. Lie down and put a pillow under your right shoulder. Place your right arm behind your head.

2. Use the finger pads of the three middle fingers on your left hand to feel for lumps or thickening. Your finger pads are the top third of each finger.

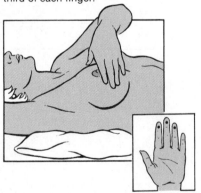

3. Press hard enough to know how your breast feels. If you're not sure how hard to press, ask you health care provider. Or try to copy the way your health care provider uses the finger pads during a breast exam. Learn what your breast feels like most of the time. A firm ridge in the lower curve of each breast is normal.

4. Move around the breast in a set way. You can choose either the circle (A), the up and down (B), or the wedge (C). Do it the same way every time. It will help you to make sure that you've gone over the entire breast area, and to remember how your breast feels each month.

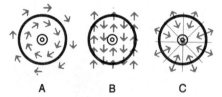

A   B   C

5. Now, examine your left breast using right hand finger pads.

   You might want to check your breasts while standing in front of a mirror right after you do your BSE each month. You might also want to do an extra BSE while you're in the shower. Your soapy hands will glide over the wet skin making it easy to check how your breasts feel.

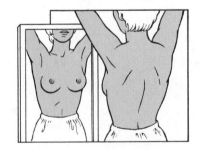

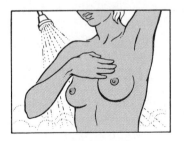

FIGURE 16–30 Breast self-examination (Courtesy of the American Cancer Society)

normally examined next by the physician palpating several areas including the neck and axillary region by using the hands placed against the skin, Figure 16–28. This allows the examiner to feel any nodules, lumps, swelling, or any other abnormal condition of the patient. Percussion is the next means of examination where the doctor taps the fingers over several areas of the chest to evaluate the condition of the underlying structures. Figure 16–29 shows the examiner using blunt percussion to examine the kidney. The stethoscope is used finally in examining the chest to allow the physician to hear the sounds within the chest cavity, including breath sounds in the lungs and the heartbeat. The doctor will ask the patient to breathe through the mouth to make the sounds easier to hear while using the stethoscope.

Breasts — The inspection of the size, shape, symmetry, and position of the breasts and nipples is done first, then palpation while the patient is sitting and then lying down. The examiner looks for abnormalities such as tenderness, discharge from the nipples, swelling or masses, lumps or nodules, dimpling, skin disorders, and any other signs of disease. Routinely patient education should be done at this point in urging breast self-examination after her monthly menstrual period and in scheduling mammograms. An instruction booklet should be provided for the patient to take home, Figure 16–30. Men are also examined for abnormalities of the breasts.

Heart — **stethoscope** — Evidence of heart disease is indicated by many other areas of the body besides the findings from examination of the heart. The examiner visually inspects the chest and then palpates the chest wall to determine the cardiac border. The stethoscope is used to listen to the chambers of the heart to detect different characteristic heart sounds. The physician has the patient move into several positions to achieve maximum audibility, i.e., lying down, sitting up, leaning forward, etc., while the doctor listens for any abnormal sounds, such as a heart murmur.

Lungs — See chest section.

Abdomen — **stethoscope** — Refer to Figure 16–31 for an outlined description of the organs within the nine areas of the abdominal cavity. This will help you to understand the use of the various techniques used by the physician during the examination. For successful exami-

Right Hypochondriac	*Epigastric*	*Left Hypochondriac*
Right lobe of liver	Pyloric end of	Stomach
Gallbladder	stomach	Spleen
Part of duodenum	Duodenum	Tail of pancreas
Hepatic flexure of	Pancreas	Splenic flexure of
colon	Aorta	colon
Part of right kidney	Portion of liver	Upper pole of left
Suprarenal gland		kidney
Right Lumbar	*Umbilical*	*Left Lumbar*
Ascending colon	Omentum	Descending colon
Lower half of	Mesentery	Lower half of left
right kidney	Transverse colon	kidney
Part of duodenum	Lower part of	Parts of jejunum
and jejunum	duodenum	and ileum
	Jejunum and	
	ileum	
Right Inguinal	*Hypogastric*	*Left Inguinal*
Cecum	Ileum	Sigmoid colon
Appendix	Bladder	Left ureter
Lower end of ileum	Pregnant	Left spermatic
Right ureter	uterus	cord in male
Right spermatic		Left ovary in
cord in male		female
Right ovary in		
female		

FIGURE 16–31   The nine sections of the abdominal cavity with underlying visceral organs.

nation of the abdominal cavity, the patient should be lying in the supine position with the head supported by a pillow. The arms should be to the side or folded across the chest. The medical assistant should help the patient into position. You should place a drape sheet over the patient to provide privacy. The physician will inspect the skin (refer to discussion of skin previously), and proceed with the exam usually in this order: inspection, auscultation, palpation, and percussion. The examiner looks for any abnormalities some of which may include hernias, masses, tenderness, or enlargement of organs.

Genitalia — **For both male and female patients, this is an ideal time to stress the importance of using latex condoms during sexual intercourse (vaginal and anal) each and every time.**

Males — **latex gloves, water-soluble lubricant** — (The physician wears latex gloves for this exam.) In general, the doctor inspects the external genitalia for gross **asymmetry,** comparing one side to the other, and checks for any deformities, lesions, swelling or masses, or varicosities, and if the patient has pubic hair or not. Skin temperature is also noted to determine circulation. The penis is examined for lesions, scars, masses, tumors, edema, and discharge. The scrotum is palpated for content and then each side is pressed upward (palpated) while the patient holds his arms over the head and pushes downward with abdominal muscles while the examiner observes for hernias (the patient is instructed to cough during the exam to detect any discomfort with abdominal straining). The physician places a gloved index finger (with water-soluble lubricant) into the rectum to examine the prostate gland and further check the patient internally for **inguinal hernia.** The patient usually stands for the exam; the examiner is seated. Patient education in testicular self-examination (TSE) to **detect** tumors of the testes is appropriate during this portion of the exam, Figure 16–32. Distributing pamphlets is recommended because of the increasing numbers of cases of testicular cancer being reported in young men aged 20 to 35. Early detection may save lives!

Female — **latex gloves, vaginal speculum, water-soluble lubricant, gooseneck lamp, tissues** — Refer to Unit 4 of this chapter for in-depth information regarding the gynecological (GYN) exam. At the time the patient schedules the CPE, she should receive instructions regarding this section of the exam. In general, female patients are advised not to **douche** or engage in sexual intercourse for 24 to 48 hours before the appointment. It is preferred that she make the appointment either before or after the menstrual period (findings may be masked or misinterpreted during this time. Also remind her that routine vaginal douching should be done only by the direction of the physician). This part of the exam is often referred to as a pelvic exam. In general, you may help the patient lie down and then into the lithotomy position by placing your hand at the edge of the exam table and asking the patient to scoot down until she can feel your

These symptoms may be evident with testicular cancer:
— a heavy feeling
— a dragging sensation
— the accumulation of fluid
— breast tenderness

The American Cancer Society recommends that men:
1. begin monthly TSE at 15 years of age;
2. perform careful 3 minute exam following a warm shower or bath when scrotal skin is relaxed;
3. observe for any changes in appearance;
4. manually examine each testis by gently rolling it between fingers and thumbs of both hands to check for any hard lumps or nodules.

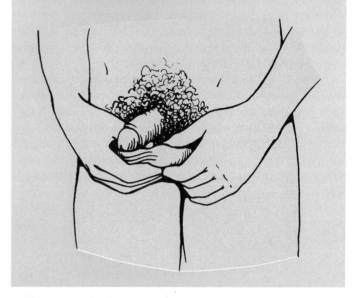

FIGURE 16–32 Testicular self-examination. Men should be advised to be examined by a physician as soon as possible if there are any abnormal findings with TSE.

hand (the buttocks should be just at the edge of the table). Assist the patient in placing the feet in the stirrups and provide a drape for privacy. (The physician wears latex gloves for this exam.) The gooseneck lamp should be placed at the end of the examining table to aid in visual inspection. The physician first inspects the external genitalia for lesions or ulcers, reddening, scratches, edema, inflammation, tumors, cysts or masses, scarring, varicosities, bleeding, or discharge. During this exam, the patient should be instructed to try to relax and breathe slowly and deeply through the mouth. The vaginal speculum is warmed with water before being inserted into the vagina. This part of the exam is for internal inspection and to access vaginal and cervical scrapings, cultures and **cytological** specimens. Using a water-soluble lubricant, a bimanual exam is performed to determine any abnormalities in the female reproductive organs. Offer tissues to the patient following this procedure to remove excess lubricant. Help patient out of stirrups and to a sitting position. Your role in assisting is to hand items to the physician as needed and to offer the patient your support.

Rectum — Male — **latex gloves, water-soluble lubricant, guaiac test paper, tissues** — The patient stands with feet apart and bends over the examination table or is placed in the knee-chest position. The physician, wearing latex gloves and using a water-soluble lubricant, spreads the buttocks and inspects the patient for lesions, fistulas, external hemorrhoids, prolapse, or any other abnormalities. The internal exam determines sphincter control and other abnormalities and is performed as part of the examination of the genitalia (see above). It is followed by a guaiac test for occult blood by the placing of a small amount of stool from the gloved finger on the test paper.

Female — latex gloves, water soluble lubricant, guaiac test paper, tissues — The physician wears latex gloves for this exam. A water-soluble lubricant is used to insert the index finger into the rectum to palpate sphincter control, any fistulas, tumors, hemorrhoids, prolapse, or any other abnormalities. A guaiac test for occult blood is performed by placing a small amount of stool on the test paper from the gloved finger.

Vagina — see above, female genitalia.

Extremities — tape measure — This is a general overall examination of inspection that the physician does during the course of the examination. It begins with the head and neck, and includes evaluation of the patient's gait and posture, the appearance of the back, arms and legs. The examiner also looks for muscle strength, the condition of the patient's circulation, and the range of motion (ROM) of the joints. Sometimes measurements of the chest, arms, and legs are done at this point in the examination with a flexible tape measure and recorded in the patient's chart.

Reflexes — percussion hammer — The patient sits on the exam table with the legs dangling at the side. The patient must be relaxed during these procedures to elicit an involuntary reaction or response (as the absence of such response could mean neuropathy) as the physician strikes the tendon of each extremity. The examiner watches the response of the limb as contraction of the stretched muscle causes the sudden movement. The reflexes tested are biceps, triceps, patellar, Achilles, and plantar, Figure 16–33, page 502.

Lymph nodes — The physician palpates the lymph nodes of the neck, axilla, inguinal, and abdominal areas of the body during the course of the examination to determine if infection is present. Enlargement of these nodes may indicate infection; clustering of nodes may indicate pathology (see Figure 16–28).

In addition to the many examinations already discussed, the physician normally includes many others, such as:

1. *Romberg balance test* — Performed to detect any muscle abnormality. The patient stands with feet together and eyes open; if the balance seems all right, the examiner asks the patient to close the eyes. If there is any muscle abnormality, the patient possibly will fall. You should assist by standing close to

help prevent this from happening.

2. Other tests involve checking for coordination and may include:
   a. The patient sits up and spreads the arms out wide, and touches the fingertip to the nose, first the right and then the left quickly, with eyes open and then closed, Figure 16–34, page 503.
   b. The heel-to-shin test is performed by the patient while lying in the supine position; first the right heel traces the left leg down from the knee, and then the left heel down right leg; may also be done while patient stands.
   c. Alternating motion is a test that may involve tapping the foot or clapping.
   d. The heel-to-toe test of coordination is having the patient touch the right heel to the left great toe, and then the left heel to the right great toe; it can be done while the patient is standing or lying down. The patient is observed and evaluated by the examiner.

Remarks — Physicians note additional observations of important information concerning the patient in this section of the form, i.e., birth mark or scar is noted.

Diagnosis (Diagnoses) — Here the physician makes a decision about the patient's condition based on the health history, symptoms, examination findings, and any other procedures and laboratory tests thought necessary to confirm the decision. The term, R/O or *rule/out,* may be used to indicate that there is not yet conclusive evidence in the decision concerning a patient's condition or in confirming a diagnosis, i.e., R/O gallbladder disease, (awaiting diagnostic X ray studies).

Treatment — This section of the form is where *all* measures for management of the care of the patient are listed, including diet, exercise, physical therapy, medication, surgery, and any others.

Following the completion of the physical examination, the physician will usually leave the patient's chart in the chart holder on the door or in some other designated area for the medical assistant. You should then check the chart for orders to perform any additional procedures for the patient, such as ECG, lab tests, scheduling X rays, or an appointment with a specialist, and so on. After you have finished the procedures, you should write your initials after each one signifying that you completed the orders.

Always be sure to help the patient down from the examination table. Often after sitting there for some time, especially if the (elderly) patient has been lying down, one can become dizzy or lightheaded, and there is the possibility of a fall, which you could prevent. You may also offer the courtesy of assisting them in getting dressed when appropriate, again, with the elderly. Answer any questions they may have about the follow-up appointment or further studies. Always let the patient know how long to expect to wait for reports

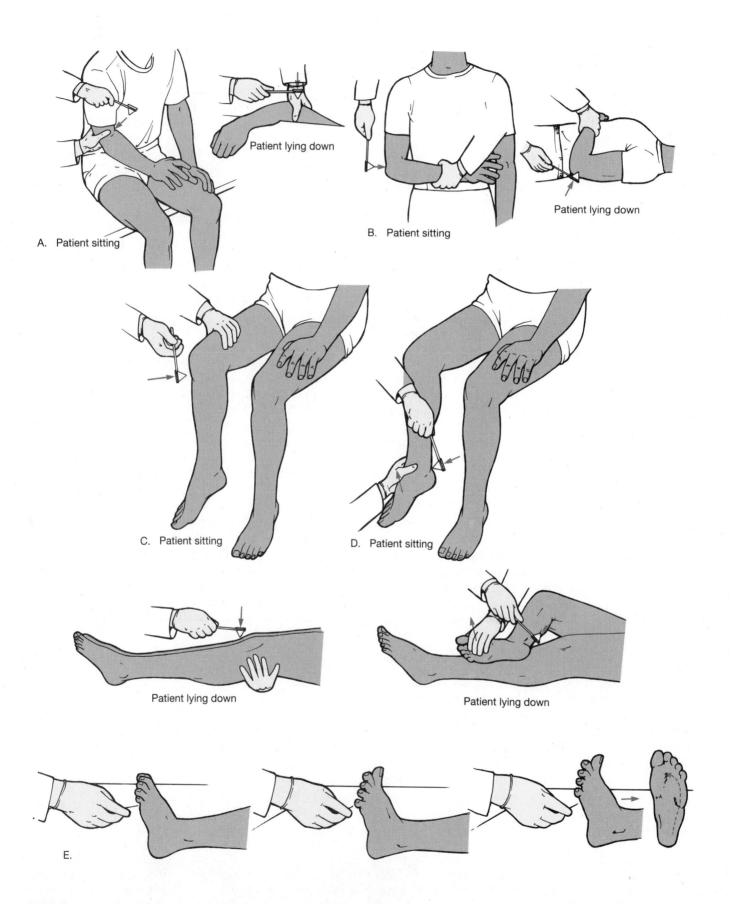

FIGURE 16–33 Percussion hammer is used by physician to test (a) biceps, (b) triceps, (c) patellar, (d) Achilles, (e) plantar reflexes.

A. Patient sitting

Patient lying down

B. Patient sitting

Patient lying down

C. Patient sitting

D. Patient sitting

Patient lying down

Patient lying down

E.

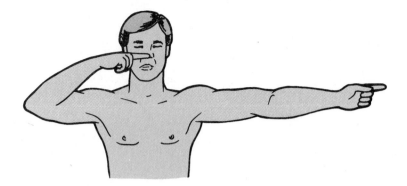

FIGURE 16–34 The physician observes the patient as the finger is touched to the nose to determine normal coordination.

from lab, radiology, or other diagnostic procedures. Tell them when to call and with whom to speak when they phone for the report. It is a common practice to give the patient an appointment a week to 10 days after the physical for a report of the findings; others mail a report, Figure 16–35. Still others phone the patient or have the patient phone the office at a specific day and time. Whatever the policy where you are employed, you must realize that the patient is usually very concerned about what the physician will find and waiting makes the anxiety far worse. Letting patients know about their health status as soon as possible in a professional manner will be appreciated. Filing reports and phoning patients are also duties of the clinical medical assistant.

Patients may ask how often they need to have a physical or a checkup as they call it. You may use Table 16–3 as a guide in giving advice to adult patients about examination and specialty procedures routinely performed on patients. Some physicians recommend annual physicals for their patients, others every 2 to 3

TABLE 16–3
Physical Examination Schedule

Procedure	Age
Electrocardiogram	PRN with baseline established at 40 if not before, thereafter as indicated
Eye exam	Tonometry and funduscopy at 40, then every 4 years
H & P	Every 3 years between ages 20–30 Annually after 40
Mammogram	Baseline at 35, then annually
PAP test pelvic	Begin age 20 (or whenever female becomes sexually active), annually thereafter
Pulmonary function tests	PRN for high-risk patients, chronic obstructive pulmonary disease and smokers
Sigmoidoscopy	2 consecutive at 50, every 3–5 years thereafter
Rectal exam	Begin at 40, then annually
Stool for guaiac	Begin at 40, then annually
Thyroid screening	PRN; baseline at menopause; females every 2 years

This physical exam schedule is meant to serve as a guide. The medical needs of patients will vary as will physicians' recommendations.

From the desk of Dr. H. N. Finklestein

(Today's date)

Dear Mr. G.:

We are pleased to inform you that the results of your physical examination, lab tests, EKG, and Chest x-ray were normal. Your next physical exam should be scheduled within the next 2 - 3 years unless you experience any medical problems. Please feel free to call if you have any further questions or concerns, or if we can be of service to you.

Sincerely,

H.N. Finklestein, M.D.

FIGURE 16–35 Example of report of physical exam.

years unless a specific or chronic medical problem exists. The age of the patient has some consideration in this matter. Pediatric patients should be examined more often than adults and monitored very closely since their growth and development, especially the first year, is so rapid. Initially infants are examined by the physician in the office or clinic at age 3 to 4 weeks. Diet and nutritional concerns are discussed and any laboratory tests or procedures are performed during each of these appointments besides the actual exam. At age 2 months the baby has a checkup and begins the immunization schedule (you will learn about this in detail in Chapter 20). At 4 and 6 months the baby has checkups and continues with the initial series of immunizations. Additional exams and/or immunizations are generally scheduled for the child at ages 9, 12, 15, and 18 months. Even though there are no immunizations needed again until between 4 and 6 years old, children should have annual examinations to detect any diseases or abnormal condition. You will, however, have to check with the physician who employs you, for office policies may vary.

The examinations discussed in this unit are by no means the only ones performed in medical offices and clinics. You will learn many others as you gain experience and knowledge in assisting. To learn other instruments used in medical offices or clinics, refer to the appendix of this text.

Complete Chapter 16, Unit 3 in the workbook to help you meet the objectives at the beginning of this unit and therefore achieve competency of this subject matter.

U N I T   4

Assisting with Special Examinations

OBJECTIVES ....

Upon completion of this unit, the student will meet the following terminal performance objectives by verifying knowledge of the facts and principles presented through oral and written communication at a level deemed competent, and will demonstrate the specific behaviors as identified in the terminal performance objectives of the procedures, observing all aseptic and safety precautions in accordance with health care standards.

1. Instruct a female patient for a Pap test appointment and explain why it is necessary.
2. List and describe the necessary instruments/supplies for a Pap test/pelvic exam.
3. Prepare a female patient for a Pap test/pelvic exam.
4. Demonstrate the proper way to assist with a Pap test/pelvic exam.
5. Prepare the Pap test specimen for laboratory analysis.
6. Explain breast self-examination.
7. Discuss patient education appropriate for females having a pelvic/Pap.
8. Instruct a patient to prepare for a sigmoidoscopy and explain why it is necessary.
9. List and describe the necessary instruments/equipment for a sigmoidoscopy.
10. Explain how to assist with a sigmoidoscopy.
11. Discuss patient education appropriate for patients having a sigmoidoscopy.

12. Demonstrate how to administer an enema.
13. Spell and define, using the glossary at the back of the text, all the words to know in this unit.

WORDS TO KNOW ....

atypical	heartburn
cervical	hormones
constipation	lumen
cytology	maturation
diagnostic	mucosa
disclose	obturator
douche	Papanicolaou
endocervical	occult
endoscope	proctology
enema	sigmoidoscopy
evacuants	suction
evacuate	stool
exfoliated	tarry
feces	trivial
flatulence	tumor
flexible	ulceration
formaldehyde	vaginitis

Many special examinations are performed on patients in various medical practices. Specialties often require additional staff training in assisting with particular procedures.

It is important to stay within your boundaries until such time when you have been properly instructed and evaluated in specific areas.

In this unit, two very common procedures are discussed. One is the Pap test/pelvic examination. In assisting with the CPE (Unit 3), the examination of the vagina and genitalia was described as a part of the total exam; the Pap test is not necessarily done at that time. Frequently women schedule appointments with their general/family practitioners for the Pap test alone, definitely in the specialty of gynecology. One must make the distinction between a *physical* and a *Pap test.* The CPE is a review of systems (ROS) of the total body. The gynecological exam is that of the female reproductive organs only. As a rule, the specialists refer other symptoms or conditions of their patients back to the "family doctor" for treatment.

The sigmoidoscopy is another special diagnostic examination performed in most general or family practices, besides in the specialty practice of internal medicine. Assisting with this procedure requires that you are familiar with the instruments and equipment used by the physician and that you have a sound understanding of the process in giving support to the patient.

With both of these exams it is essential that the patient receive proper preparation before the procedures can be successfully performed. Since the medical assistant is usually responsible for instructing patients, it is important that both verbal and written information is given. In consideration of the patient, the nature of both of these procedures can be embarrassing; having to go through the process only once will be appreciated.

The Pap Test and Hormonal Smears

The **Papanicolaou** technique is a cytologic screening test to detect cancer of the cervix. This method of detection was developed by an American physician, George N. Papanicolaou, in 1883. This simple smear technique can also be used to screen tissue from other parts of the body for **atypical cytology** as the form in Figure 16–36 shows ("special cytology"). Female patients usually have the Pap test done routinely either as a part of the CPE with their family doctor or by their gynecologist. Patients who have complaints of severe menstrual pain or discomfort, unusual vaginal discharge, or lower abdominal pain (or any other problems) may have a Pap smear taken during the pelvic examination to rule out gynecological problems. Women should be especially conscientious in scheduling annual Pap tests if they have a family history of uterine or **cervical** cancer.

Some physicians recommend that females over age 35 have a Pap smear done every 6 months. Others feel that in healthy women one every 1 to 3 years is sufficient. The American Cancer Society recommends that females have a Pap test done at least every 3 years, beginning when they

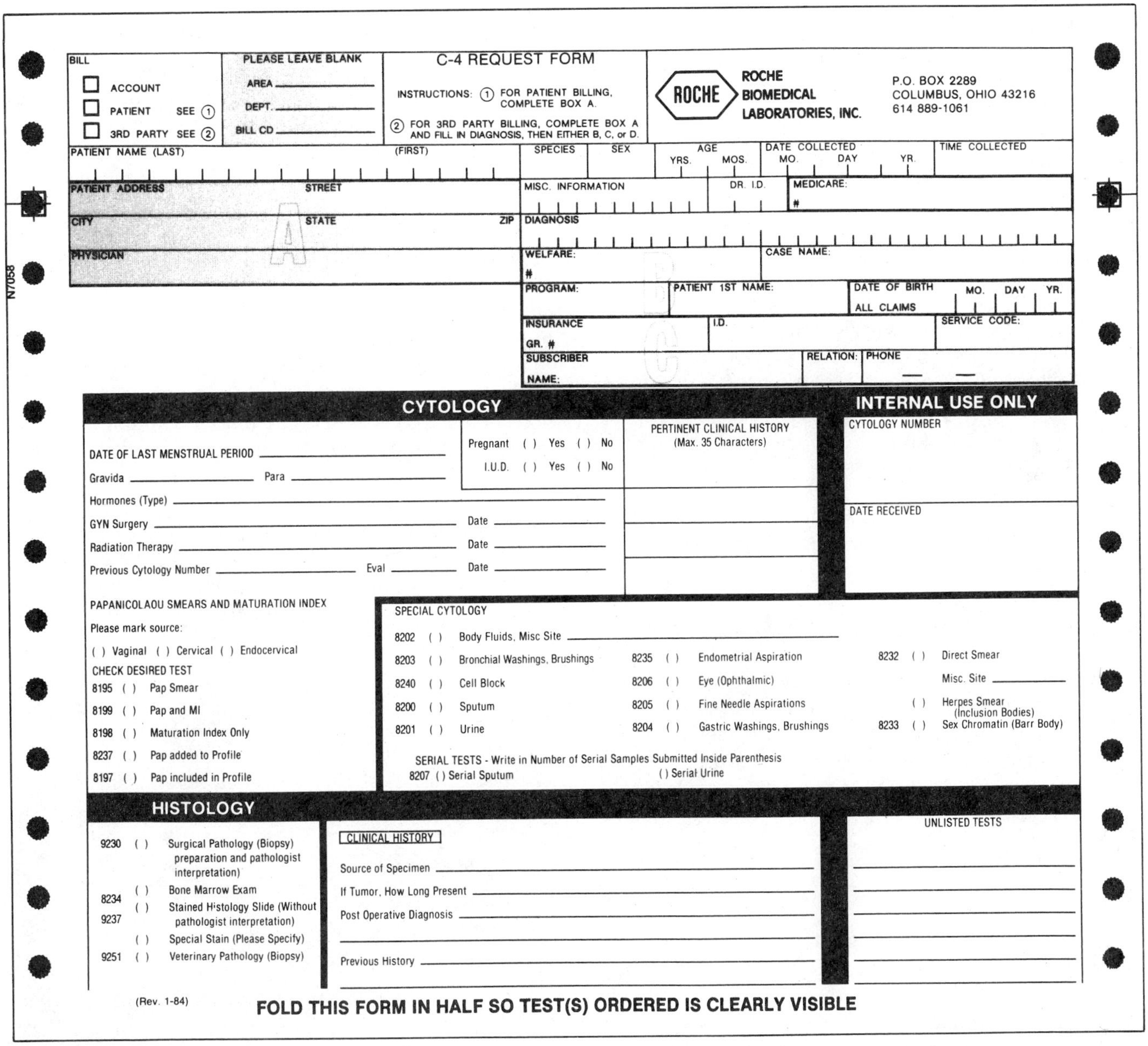

BILL
☐ ACCOUNT
☐ PATIENT SEE ①
☐ 3RD PARTY SEE ②

PLEASE LEAVE BLANK
AREA
DEPT.
BILL CD

C-4 REQUEST FORM
INSTRUCTIONS: ① FOR PATIENT BILLING, COMPLETE BOX A.
② FOR 3RD PARTY BILLING, COMPLETE BOX A AND FILL IN DIAGNOSIS, THEN EITHER B, C, or D.

ROCHE BIOMEDICAL LABORATORIES, INC.
P.O. BOX 2289
COLUMBUS, OHIO 43216
614 889-1061

PATIENT NAME (LAST) (FIRST) SPECIES SEX AGE YRS. MOS. DATE COLLECTED MO. DAY YR. TIME COLLECTED
PATIENT ADDRESS STREET MISC. INFORMATION DR. I.D. MEDICARE: #
CITY STATE ZIP DIAGNOSIS
PHYSICIAN WELFARE: # CASE NAME:
PROGRAM: PATIENT 1ST NAME: DATE OF BIRTH ALL CLAIMS MO. DAY YR.
INSURANCE GR. # I.D. SERVICE CODE:
SUBSCRIBER NAME: RELATION: PHONE

N7058

CYTOLOGY | **INTERNAL USE ONLY**

DATE OF LAST MENSTRUAL PERIOD ______
Gravida ______ Para ______
Pregnant ( ) Yes ( ) No
I.U.D. ( ) Yes ( ) No
PERTINENT CLINICAL HISTORY (Max. 35 Characters)
CYTOLOGY NUMBER
Hormones (Type) ______
GYN Surgery ______ Date ______
Radiation Therapy ______ Date ______
Previous Cytology Number ______ Eval ______ Date ______
DATE RECEIVED

PAPANICOLAOU SMEARS AND MATURATION INDEX
Please mark source:
( ) Vaginal ( ) Cervical ( ) Endocervical
CHECK DESIRED TEST
8195 ( ) Pap Smear
8199 ( ) Pap and MI
8198 ( ) Maturation Index Only
8237 ( ) Pap added to Profile
8197 ( ) Pap included in Profile

SPECIAL CYTOLOGY
8202 ( ) Body Fluids, Misc Site ______
8203 ( ) Bronchial Washings, Brushings
8240 ( ) Cell Block
8200 ( ) Sputum
8201 ( ) Urine
8235 ( ) Endometrial Aspiration
8206 ( ) Eye (Ophthalmic)
8205 ( ) Fine Needle Aspirations
8204 ( ) Gastric Washings, Brushings
8232 ( ) Direct Smear
Misc. Site ______
( ) Herpes Smear (Inclusion Bodies)
8233 ( ) Sex Chromatin (Barr Body)

SERIAL TESTS - Write in Number of Serial Samples Submitted Inside Parenthesis
8207 ( ) Serial Sputum ( ) Serial Urine

HISTOLOGY
9230 ( ) Surgical Pathology (Biopsy) preparation and pathologist interpretation)
8234 ( ) Bone Marrow Exam
9237 ( ) Stained Histology Slide (Without pathologist interpretation)
( ) Special Stain (Please Specify)
9251 ( ) Veterinary Pathology (Biopsy)

CLINICAL HISTORY
Source of Specimen ______
If Tumor, How Long Present ______
Post Operative Diagnosis ______
Previous History ______

UNLISTED TESTS

(Rev. 1-84)

FOLD THIS FORM IN HALF SO TEST(S) ORDERED IS CLEARLY VISIBLE

FIGURE 16–36 Cytology request form (Courtesy of Roche Biomedical Laboratories, Inc.)

When patients come in for their scheduled appointments, here are a few informative topics you might want to discuss with them.

1. Remind the patient at the time she schedules the appointment for a Pap test that she should not douche or engage in sexual intercourse for 24 to 48 hours before the examination. Because the specimen analysis could be misinterpreted during the menstrual flow, the patient should be advised to schedule the test either before or after her period.

2. Explain to female patients that they should *not* douche routinely because it washes away natural protective vaginal secretions that aid in the resistance of possible invading microorganisms. Douching should be done only with the physician's orders.

3. Those female patients who are sexually active should be instructed to use latex condoms when engaging in sexual intercourse for protection against both sexually transmitted diseases and unwanted pregnancies.

4. Educate all females to perform breast self-examination at home routinely after her menstrual period. Pamphlets for distribution can be obtained from the American Cancer Society to help patients with the procedure.

5. Remind all female patients over age 35 to schedule a routine mammography for early detection of breast cancer.

6. Explain to female patients that any of the following symptoms could mean that infection or disease are present and that they should call for an appointment: foul vaginal odor, vaginal discharge that is other than clear, unusual bleeding, vaginal itching or soreness, or any other vaginitis, pain, or discomfort.

7. Advise female patients to refrain from using perfumed toilet articles such as soaps or bubble baths, vaginal sprays and tampons, toilet tissue, or feminine napkins because they may be irritating to the delicate vaginal tissues. Chronic irritation can lead to infection.

engage in sexual intercourse 24 to 48 hours before the scheduled appointment for the same reason.

Prior to bringing the patient into the examination room for the pelvic exam and Pap, the medical assistant should make the necessary preparations. You should wash your hands before you begin. The exam table should have a clean protective covering, either table paper or a cloth sheet. Place a gown and drape sheet on the end of the table for the patient (either cloth or disposable paper). On the Mayo tray near the end of the exam table you should place the instruments and supplies the physician will need to perform the pelvic exam and obtain the Pap smear. In Figure 16–37 the commonly used items for this GYN procedure are displayed. You must learn the names of the instruments and supplies, listed in the following procedure, to efficiently assist the physician. To aid in the inspection part of the pelvic exam, a gooseneck lamp should be placed within reach of the examiner's stool at the end of the table.

Escort the patient to the examination room. Before you continue further preparation of the patient, ask if she needs to empty her bladder and obtain a clean-catch midstream urine specimen if ordered by the physician. Pelvic examinations are uncomfortable for the patients if the bladder is full, besides making the examination difficult for the physician to perform. Examinations that have to be delayed while the patient goes to the rest room disrupt the schedule and are usually unnecessary. Certainly there are exceptions. Some patients may have trouble with bladder control or some other condition that could require frequent trips to the rest room. You should help these patients feel at ease for they will most likely feel embarrassed.

Complete the cytology request form (see Figure 16–36), by making sure that you ask the patient all necessary questions, including complaints she may have and the date of the last menstrual period (LMP, the first day

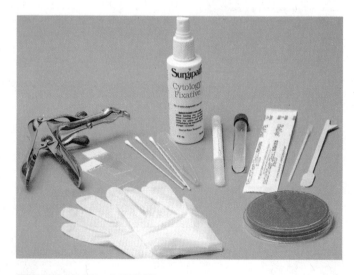

FIGURE 16–37 A GYN/Pap tray setup

become sexually active, or at age 20 if there have been two initial negative Pap test results one year apart. You should check with your employer and advise patients accordingly.

Patients should not douche for 24 to 48 hours prior to the Pap test or the smear may be reported as negative because sloughed-off (exfoliated) cells would have been washed away. The Pap test should not be done during the menstrual flow because red blood cells make the smear difficult to read. Patients should also be advised not to

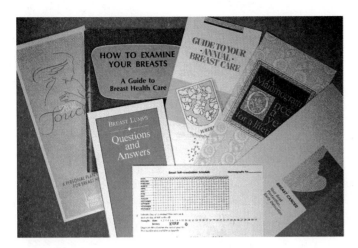

FIGURE 16–38 Breast self-examination pamphlets and schedule

of her last period). Instruct the patient about the procedure, letting her know what to expect, especially if it is the first time for her to have a pelvic exam. Never assume that a patient knows about a procedure whatever her age is. Unfortunately, some health care workers can often be remiss in giving important information to patients. Some patients are both afraid and embarrassed to ask questions because they figure they should already know about procedures. Try to make patients feel comfortable and at ease to help them relax for the exam. You should then instruct the patient to undress completely, where to put her belongings, and how to put on the exam gown (opened in front or back). You should politely offer your assistance. Ask her to leave the door unlocked, or slightly opened, when she is gowned. Allow the patient privacy to change for a couple of minutes. When the patient lets you know she is ready, pull out the foot step at the end of the exam table and help her step up to the exam table and sit at the end. Place the drape sheet over the top of her legs. This will give her privacy and warmth. You should remember to push the foot step back in after the patient has been seated to avoid injury to you or the physician.

Alert the physician that the patient is ready to be examined. (If the patient's appointment is for a Pap alone, or the physician has ordered a pelvic exam only, you should get everything ready, and then get the patient into the lithotomy position just before the doctor goes into the room, otherwise the patient will become uncomfortable and impatient staying in this position for any longer than necessary.) Most physicians prefer that the medical assistant (or nurse) accompany them into the exam room not only to assist with the procedure, but for legal reasons as well.

Because of the importance of early detection of breast cancer, physicians include the breast exam during the patient's annual appointment for the Pap and pelvic (patients should be urged to do breast self-examination

each month following the menstrual period. Giving them a pamphlet of instructions to take with them for this procedure is recommended, Figure 16–38). Explain to the patient that the exam conducted by the physician with the annual Pap test is certainly noteworthy, but insufficient in detecting abnormal breast tissue between visits to the physician. Most women discover a lump or mass in their breasts themselves and report it to the physician. This leads to early detection and treatment. The physician usually listens to the heart and lungs and does a brief general check of the patient first. Then the patient's gown is lowered to the waist while the patient is still sitting up for the inspection part of the breast exam and palpation for lumps and masses. You should then pull the table extension out to support the lower legs and feet and help the patient lie down in assisting the doctor in further palpation for any abnormalities of the breast tissue (often a towel is placed over the chest to provide a sense of privacy for the patient). The abdominal cavity is examined as the examiner palpates the pelvic area. Remind patients to breathe slowly through the mouth to help relax abdominal muscles during the exam.

Following this portion of the exam, you should help the patient into the lithotomy position. Assist her in getting her feet in the stirrups, adjusting them as necessary, and place the drape sheet over her knees. Ask her to scoot down to the end of the table until the buttocks are just at the edge (place your hand at the edge of the table and ask her to keep moving down until she feels the back of your hand). Be careful in assisting patients into positions as the exam tables are usually rather narrow and there *is* the possibility of a patient falling *off* of the table. The gooseneck lamp should be adjusted at the end of the table and the stool

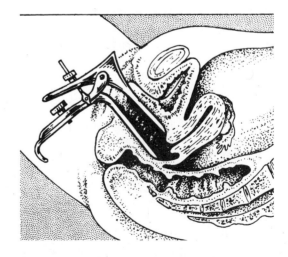

FIGURE 16–39 Lateral view of vaginal speculum in place for inspection and for obtaining specimens. (From Burke, *Human Anatomy & Physiology in Health and Disease*, 3d ed. Copyright 1992, Delmar Publishers Inc.)

comfortably into position for the physician. The medical assistant should put latex gloves on and hand the physician gloves. The vaginal speculum (after running warm water over it) should be handed to the doctor next for use in inspecting the cervix and in obtaining the smear, Figure 16–39, page 507. Hand the physician the spatula to obtain a sample of the vaginal secretions containing the exfoliated cells for analysis. The endocervical brush is used to obtain an endocervical tissue specimen. If the physician requests a Pap and Maturation Index (MI), it means that a hormonal evaluation is necessary in determining the patient's condition. Hold the slides carefully at the frosted end and mark each slide accurately (in pencil) as the physician gives them to you: cervical–C, vaginal–V, endocervical–E. Immediately apply the commercial fixative spray to the slide(s) and put in the container, or place in the jar back to

P R O C E D U R E

Assist with a GYN Examination and Pap Test

PURPOSE: To assist in evaluation of the patient's gynecological condition.

EQUIPMENT: 2 (or more) frosted-end glass slides, Mayo tray, cloth or paper towel, pen and pencil, fixative spray and container to hold slides (or jar with alcohol-ether solution), disposable latex gloves, water-soluble lubricant, vaginal speculum, endocervical brush, vaginal/cervical spatula (Ayer blade), sterile cotton-tipped applicators, tissues, lab request form, rubber band, (cultures and uterine dressing forceps as requested by physician)

TERMINAL PERFORMANCE OBJECTIVE: With all equipment/supplies provided, the instructor role-playing as the physician, and female students role-playing as patients, the students will demonstrate (insofar as feasible) each of the steps required in assisting with the GYN examination and Pap test. The instructor will observe each step. Note that some steps will need to be simulated in the instructional setting.

1. Wash hands; place gown/drape sheet on exam table; cover Mayo tray with towel; assemble all necessary items on tray.
2. Bring patient in and ask for specimen (if ordered) or to empty bladder.
3. Obtain information and complete cytology request form, label slides.
4. Explain: procedure, disrobing, and gowning to patient (assist if needed). Ask her to leave door unlocked when ready.
5. Assist patient onto the exam table and drape.
6. Accompany physician into exam room to assist both the doctor and the patient during the exam.
7. Assist patient into lithotomy position, helping her place her feet in the stirrups (adjust accordingly) and place drape sheet over the knees. (To help her reach the edge of the exam table more easily, ask her to scoot down to the end until she feels the back of your hand.) Place a pillow under her head for comfort.

8. Physician will sit at the end of the exam table on exam stool and adjust the lamp for inspection of vaginal and anal tissues. Hand the physician gloves to put on. You should also put gloves on, run warm water over the vaginal speculum, and hand it and the vaginal spatula to the doctor to obtain Pap smear as you carefully hold the slide by the frosted end. The endocervical brush is used next to obtain a smear from the interior of the cervix. Slides for these specific areas must be marked appropriately: V–vaginal; E–endocervical; and C–cervical for proper analysis to be done at the lab.
9. Immediately apply fixative spray and into place into container, or place in alcohol-ether solution, for transport to lab.
10. The physician performs the bimanual exam after smears have been taken. Assist by placing a small amount of lubricant on the doctor's gloved finger, and handing a fresh glove to the examiner for the rectal exam. Further assistance in obtaining cultures, a biopsy, or any other GYN procedures may be performed at this time. Refer to Figure 16–42 for other instruments that may be used in these procedures that you will assist in handing the physician.
11. Hand tissues to the patient for removal of any residual lubricant. Discard all disposables in biohazardous waste container. If metal speculum was used, place in cool water to soak until it can be properly washed, wrapped, and autoclaved, remove gloves, and wash hands.
12. Help patient sit up, push table extension and stirrups in, and help her down from table when her sense of balance has returned.
13. Instruct patient to dress (give assistance if needed).
14. Advise patient when results will be available and schedule follow-up appointment if indicated.
15. Place specimen(s) in lab pick-up area.
16. Clean and restock exam room to make ready for next patient.

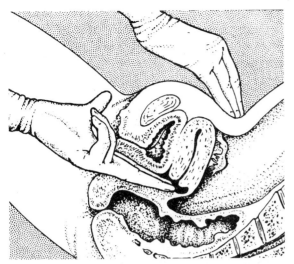

FIGURE 16–40 Bimanual pelvic examination (From Burke, *Human Anatomy & Physiology in Health and Disease*, 3d ed. Copyright 1992, Delmar Publishers Inc.)

back with alcohol-ether solution for transport to the lab. Make sure that you wrap the completed request form around the container and secure with a rubber band.

The bimanual exam is performed following the collection of specimens (Pap smear, cultures, etc.) so that the lubricant will not interfere in the lab analysis. The examiner inserts one finger (with a small amount of water-soluble lubricant) into the vagina, and palpates the pelvic area with the other hand, Figure 16–40. Normally the physician does a rectal examination next. You should hand the doctor another latex glove and lubricant. This is to prevent cross-contamination between the vaginal and rectal tissues. The medical assistant may be asked to write the findings of this examination while the physician conducts the exam alone. Whichever is your role, you will be a valuable assistant to both physician and patient.

When this exam has been completed, offer tissues to the patient to wipe away any residual lubricant. Discard the used tissues in appropriate waste container, remove gloves, and wash hands. Push the stirrups and the extension of the table in and assist the patient in sitting up. After lying down for the exam the patient may either feel faint or dizzy; if she attempts to stand up too quickly she may fall. After she has let you know that she has regained her balance, help her down from the table and ask her to get dressed. Offer assistance to the patient.

REPORT OF CYTOLOGICAL EXAMINATION PAPANICOLAOU TECHNIQUE

Laboratory I.D.
Source of Material
Other Information

Patient Age

Date Received

Patient Name

Physician Name

MATURATION INDEX

Estrogen (0–3+)   Trichomonas   % Superficial
Inflammation (0–3+)   Monilia   % Intermediate
Blood (0–3+)   Erosion Cells   % Parabasal

Class I Negative . . . . .Absence of abnormal or atypical cytology.
Class II Doubtful . . . . .Atypical cytology not suggestive of malignancy.
Class III Suspicious . . . . .Cytology compatible with malignancy or other etiology.
Class IV Highly Suspicious . . . . .Cytology strongly suggestive of malignancy.
Class V Positive . . . . .Cytology practically conclusive of malignancy
Class C . . . . .Insufficient for examination.

REMARKS & RECOMMENDATIONS

screened by

Cytologic
  Classifications for
  the Results of the
  Pap Smear

Class I: Negative, absence of abnormal cells.
Class II: Atypical cytology, but no evidence of malignancy. The atypical cells may be due to inflammation, which causes them to change in character.
Class III: Atypical cytology, suggestive of but not conclusive for malignancy.
Class IV: Abnormal cytology, strongly suggestive of malignancy.
Class V: Abnormal cytology, positive for malignancy

FIGURE 16–41 Cytology report form for Pap test

Remember to advise her when to expect to receive the results of the Pap test and/or other reports in the mail, or when she should call to find out the report(s), Figure 16–41, page 509. Giving these instructions will decidedly reduce unnecessary phone calls to the office. If the physician requests a return appointment for the patient, politely assist her in scheduling it or direct her to the administrative area. As time permits, you may discuss patient education topics either before or after the exam as appropriate to the age and needs of the patient.

The medical assistant should return to the examination room to clean up the exam area. Wear gloves to protect yourself from disease transmission. Discard all disposables in biohazardous and appropriate containers, remove gloves, and wash hands. Restock the supplies as necessary, making the room ready for another patient to be seen. Place the specimen(s) in the proper area for pick-up by the lab representative.

Sigmoidoscopy

Sigmoidoscopy is a diagnostic examination of the interior of the sigmoid colon. It is a useful aid in the diagnosis of cancer of the colon, ulcerations, polyps, tumors, bleeding, and other lower intestinal disorders. The sigmoidoscope is a metal or plastic (disposable) instrument with a light source and a magnifying lens, which permits the mucous membrane of the sigmoid colon to be seen.

The metal and plastic types of scopes are still used to examine patients. Recently, another instrument has been gaining in popularity with physicians. It is a flexible sigmoidoscope, which is shown assembled with items necessary for the procedure to be performed in Figure 16–43. Since it is flexible, it can be inserted much farther into the colon. This instrument makes it possible to view more of the mucous membranes of the intestines.

An obturator is inserted into the sigmoidoscope. The tip of the obturator and scope are lubricated and carefully inserted into the rectum. Then the obturator is removed so that the S shape of the colon can be seen. Patients find this an unpleasant procedure.

As with any examination of the abdominal cavity, you should advise the patient to empty the bladder and evacuate the bowel before the procedure begins. This will make the exam easier for both patient and examiner. During the procedure the patient should be instructed to breathe through the mouth deeply and slowly to relax abdominal muscles. Patients may feel the urge to defecate during any of these colon examinations because of the stretching of the intestinal wall from the instrument passing through and air being introduced with it. If patients use the breathing technique mentioned, this discomfort can be relieved. The procedure should last only a minute or two, especially if patients have followed preparation instructions.

Air is sometimes introduced into the colon (by the examiner's use of the inflation bulb attached to the scope

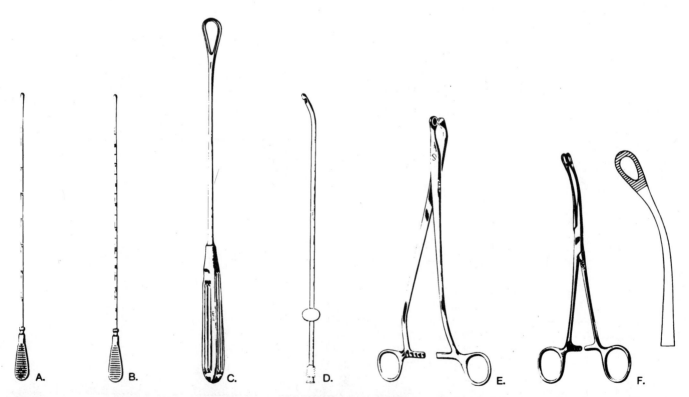

FIGURE 16–42 Additional gynecological instruments used in examinations and procedures: (a). Sims' uterine sound, graduated in inches: (b). Sims' uterine sound, graduated in centimeters: (c). Sims' uterine curette: (d). Randall uterine curette: (e). Toms-Gaylor uterine punch biopsy forceps: (f). Loufe uterine polyp (Courtesy of J. Jamner Surgical Instruments Inc.)

It will most often be the medical assistant who tells the patient how to prepare for the sigmoidoscopy and explains how the test is performed. For successful examination, proper preparation is essential. In addition to having the patient restrict dairy products, raw fruits and vegetables, grains and cereals from their diet, they should be encouraged to drink plenty of clear liquids and eat lightly the day before the scheduled appointment for the sigmoid colon exam. A plain Fleet's enema should be self-administered at home approximately 2 hours before the exam. Physicians may vary the instructions according to the patient's condition. It is best to ask the examiner about the patient before proceeding with instructions. If patients are not completely informed about preparations and the exam is attempted with unsatisfactory results, it will have to be repeated, which is both costly and inconvenient. Satisfactory results are obtained by giving patients both oral and written instructions. This practice will also be helpful in reducing phone calls with trivial questions.

There are occasions, during an appointment for which the patient was "worked in" to the schedules, when the physician feels that the patient's condition warrants the examination of the sigmoid colon. In this case, the physician will order an enema to be given to the patient in the office. A procedure for both assisting with a sigmoidoscopy and administering an enema will follow in this unit.

Some exams, such as diagnostic sigmoidoscopy and X rays, require the use of evacuants by the patient the day before or the morning of the exam. This may present a problem in the patient's personal or employment schedule if instructions are not made clear before the appointment is scheduled. Most patients are fearful of what the diagnostic examination will disclose. Helping them choose a convenient appointment time and explaining the reasons for the preparations they must undergo will usually be appreciated.

When patients come in for rectal or sigmoidoscopy examinations here are a few informative topics that you may discuss with them.

1. Remind them that laxatives and enemas should only be used by direction of the physician.
2. Constipation may be avoided/relieved by including fresh fruits and vegetables, cereals and grains in their diet, drinking plenty of liquids (water), and getting regular exercise.
3. Instruct them that if they have any of the following symptoms persistently it could mean that a disease or an abnormal condition is present and consulting the physician is strongly advised: heartburn or indigestion, nausea and/or vomiting, constipation or diarrhea, excessive gas or bloating, stool that is tarry (black) or other than a normal brown color.
4. Inform patients who are age 40 and over that they should routinely test their stool for occult blood every 2 years for detection of cancer of the colon, or more often if advised by the physician (if family history indicates). All patients over age 50 should test annually.
5. Advise patients to include high-fiber foods in their diets, avoid too much fat (and saturated fats) and cholesterol, and eat red meats very sparingly.
6. Urge patients to eat from a variety of foods (from the food pyramid in Chapter 22) and to eat 4 to 6 small meals rather than 1 or 2 large meals daily to promote better utilization of nutrients and more energy.
7. Suggest to patients that it is better to select snacks and beverages wisely such as: fruits, vegetables and juices over coffee/tea/pop and high-calorie sweets or chips, etc.

with tubing) to distend the wall of the colon for easier placement of the lumen of the endoscope. Patients find this to be uncomfortable and sometimes painful. The physician may need to use a suction pump to remove mucus, blood, or fecal material that is obstructing the view of the colon.

Assistance in handling necessary items to the physician and giving support to the patient are your roles during these exams.

It is certainly not a common procedure to administer an enema to a patient in the medical office or clinic, but is sometimes a necessity in the successful completion of a sigmoidoscopy, other rectal examination, or for other reasons. Even though a patient may have received proper instructions and carried them out before the scheduled appointment, there is no guarantee that the patient achieved success. In the event that the patient comes in for the appointment and is not sufficiently cleaned out for a sigmoidoscopy, the physician may order a cleansing enema so that the exam can be completed. It is generally best to proceed with the planned procedure, even with the delay of the enema. Usually this works out well for patient and staff, for rescheduling presents difficulties for everyone.

Often the patient did follow the list of instructions, but just did not retain the enema solution long enough for it to work. You will more likely be able to encourage the patient to hold the contents of the enema longer. You may want to explain that the longer the contents are held, the more successful the results will be. Otherwise, it may have to be repeated, or the exam rescheduled. Make sure that you use an examination room that is close to the rest room for the patient's convenience when you administer an enema. The enema is a quite simple procedure, one that patients can do at home when advised by the physician. Your patience and understanding are needed here, because most patients are embarrassed to have this done. The procedure that follows will provide the information you need to carry out this duty.

Proper positioning of patients during the exam is important for both the physician's viewing of the rectum and sigmoid colon and the patient's comfort. Proctology tables are designed especially for this procedure. They provide support of the patient's chest and head with the arm resting against the headboard as the table is tilted to the knee-chest position. Those who cannot tolerate this

position are assisted into Sims' position for the exam. Many physicians find this acceptable and it is certainly more comfortable for the patient. You should ask about the physician's preference in patient position since there are many variations.

The physician may wish to view the intestinal mucosa following a normal bowel movement. More often, the patient is instructed to eat a light diet containing plenty of clear liquids and avoiding dairy products for 24 hours before the exam, and to have a plain cleansing enema the morning of, or 2 hours before, the exam. Still other physicians may wish patients to use laxatives

---

PROCEDURE

Assist With Sigmoidoscopy

PURPOSE: To assist in examination of the sigmoid colon to determine its condition.

EQUIPMENT: Disposable latex gloves, water-soluble lubricant, gauze squares, sigmoidoscope, long cotton-tipped swabs, drape sheet (fenestrated–optional), suction machine (container with room temperature water), tissues, (if ordered by physician: biopsy forceps, specimen container for transport to lab, lab request form) pen, patient's chart

TERMINAL PERFORMANCE OBJECTIVE: With all equipment/supplies provided, the instructor role-playing the physician, and students role-playing patients, the student will demonstrate (insofar as feasible) each of the steps required in assisting with the sigmoidoscopy procedure. The instructor will observe each step. Note: some steps will need to be simulated in the instructional setting.

1. Explain procedure to identified patient. Ask patient to empty bladder and bowel.

2. Assemble all needed items on Mayo table near end of examination table. Plug in cord of light source to make sure it works properly, then unplug. (If left on it will be uncomfortably warm for patient and may cause a burn.) **Key Point: If biopsy is scheduled complete lab request form and label specimen container.**

3. Instruct patient to disrobe from waist down and let you know when ready. Assist patient to sit at end of table and cover with drape sheet.

4. Just before physician is ready to begin exam, assist patient into knee-chest or Sims' position, whichever physician prefers.

5. Both medical assistant and physician should wash hands and put on latex gloves.

6. Assist physician by applying about 2 tablespoons of lubricant on gauze square for tip of obturator and tip of

gloved fingers. **Key Point: Physician makes digital examination of anus and rectum prior to insertion of endoscope.**

7. As physician finishes digital exam, plug sigmoidoscope in to light source. Secure air-inflation tubing and have it ready to hand to physician.

8. As physician inserts sigmoidoscope, be ready to hand necessary items as needed. **Key Point: Have suction machine plugged in and suction tip secured for ready use.**

9. If biopsy is taken, hand biopsy forceps to physician and have specimen container open so physician can place tissue in it. **Key Point: Then place cap on container securely and label properly.** Complete lab request form and attach to specimen container with tape or rubber band.

10. Use tissues to clean lubricant and waste from patient's anal area and discard into biohazardous waste container. Assist patient to resting prone position.

11. Clean up area and place used instruments in basin to soak in detergent solution. Remove gloves and wash hands.

12. Assist patient into a sitting position, allowing time for balance to return before you help down from table. Instruct patient to dress (unless patient has an appointment for additional examinations, such as X rays in the same office).

13. For cleaning up the exam table and instruments used you should again wear gloves to prevent disease transmission. A metal scope and the suction tip should be sanitized and prepared for sterilization (autoclaved). Restock the room and make ready for the next patient.

14. Record procedure on patient's chart and initial.

Following sigmoidoscopy, patients should drink plenty of clear liquids to help relieve the usual abdominal discomfort and flatulence. Patients may also find relief in lying in a prone position with a pillow across their midabdominal area to aid in the passage of gas.

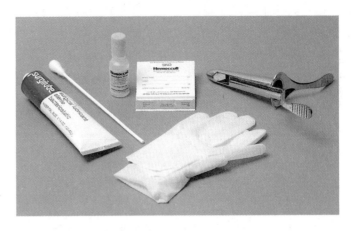

FIGURE 16–44   Rectal examination setup

the day before and an enema the night before and also the morning of the exam. Patients have usually eaten little within the past few days because of their abdominal distress.

In the diagnosis of hemorrhoids, fissures, and ulcerations, the physician usually begins investigative procedures by examining the anus and the interior of the rectum with a proctoscope, Figure 16–44. During the

sigmoidoscopy, the physician may want to take a biopsy of questionable tissue from the sigmoid colon to aid in confirming the diagnosis. It is a good rule to have all possible necessary items available. When the patient has been prepared and the examiner is ready to begin the exam, the medical assistant hands the necessary instruments and supplies to the physician as needed. Remember to advise patients to report any problems, such as bleeding, discharge, swelling, or any other unusual discomfort following any procedure. A biopsy lab request form must be completed and accompany the tissue to the lab. Containers for biopsy specimens have a formaldehyde solution to preserve the tissue until the analysis is done.

There are many other proctological procedures that may need to be performed by the physician for patients in the office setting. Some of the instruments used in these procedures are shown in Figure 16–45. All instruments and items that come in contact with a body cavity must be sterile. One of the duties that the medical assistant is generally responsible for is to make certain that this is so. Autoclaving, which is a method for sterilization of instruments, is discussed in Chapter 19.

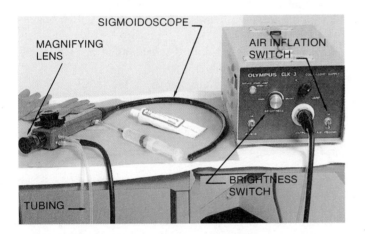

FIGURE 16–43   Parts of the sigmoidoscope are labeled in this photo of the flexible sigmoidoscope setup with suction machine and necessary items for the exam.

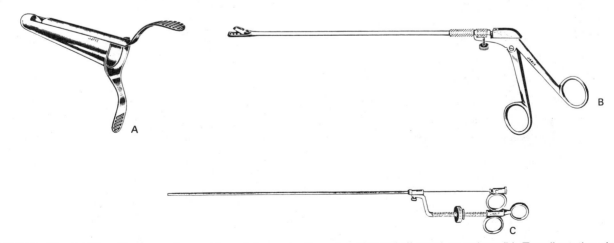

FIGURE 16–45   Additional instruments used in rectal examinations: (a). Brinkerhoff rectal speculum: (b). Turrell rotating shaft rectal biopsy forceps: (c). Norwood rectal snare (Courtesy of J. Jamner Surgical Instruments Inc.)

P R O C E D U R E

Administer Disposable Cleansing Enema

PURPOSE: To stimulate elimination of fecal matter from the lower intestinal tract (and in preparation for diagnostic examinations/tests).

EQUIPMENT: Prepackaged disposable enema (plain Fleet's), water-soluble lubricant, Mayo tray, towel, latex gloves, tissues, drape sheet, pen, patient's chart

TERMINAL PERFORMANCE OBJECTIVE: Provided with an anatomical model of the lower abdominopelvic cavity or a mannequin, and all equipment and supplies required to administer a cleansing enema, the student will first administer the enema to the anatomical model, then the mannequin; in each process the steps of the procedure must be demonstrated in proper order.

1. Explain procedure to patient and instruct to disrobe from the waist down.
2. Provide drape sheet and assist patient on to exam table.
3. Help patient into Sims' position, asking patient to lie on left side and to bring the right knee up to the waist and adjust the drape sheet.
4. Wash hands and put on latex gloves.
5. Remove the protective covering from the tip of the enema container, and apply a small amount of lubricant if necessary (tip *is* prelubricated) to the tip.

6. With one hand separate the buttocks to expose the anus; with the other hold the enema bottle turned upside-down (to eliminate air bubbles), and gently insert the tip between 2 and 4 inches into the rectum, making sure that the tip points in the direction of the patient's navel (remember to advise the patient to breathe deeply and slowly through the mouth to relax the abdominal muscles).
7. Depress the entire contents from the bottle slowly (squeeze from bottom to top of bottle), asking the patient to retain the liquid for as long as possible (at *least* 10 minutes so that the solution may have a chance to work).
8. Withdraw the enema tip slowly and provide patient with tissues. Discard used tissues in biohazardous waste container. Direct patient to rest room as necessary; ask patient to let you check results before flushing and report to physician.
9. Clean up room; discard disposables in appropriate waste containers.
10. Remove gloves and wash hands.
11. Initial chart (signifying that procedure has been completed).

M E D I C A L - L E G A L
E T H I C A L   H I G H L I G H T S

Mrs. Right...

obtains a written contract for third party payment and the written authorization for release of medical information from patients. She respects each patient and keeps information disclosed confidential. She reports suspicious injuries to the proper authorities and sexually transmitted diseases to the health department. She practices safety, assists patients when necessary, and respects their choice of treatment.

Employment outlook: Excellent

Miss Wrong...

forgets frequently to obtain written authorization to release information and contracts for third party payments from patients. She is careless about keeping information confidential. She won't take the time to report suspicious injuries or sexually transmitted diseases because it is too much trouble. She is often careless about safety practices, and shows little respect to patients.

Employment outlook: Poor

Complete Chapter 16, Unit 4 in the workbook to help you meet the objectives at the beginning of this unit and therefore achieve competency of this subject matter.

REFERENCES

A Guide for Eye Inspection and Testing Visual Acuity. National Society for the Prevention of Blindness, Inc., 1991.

Kunz, Jeffrey R. M. and Finkel, Asher J. eds. *The American Medical Association Family Medical Guide.* New York: Random House, 1987.

Morbidity and Mortality Weekly Report (MMWR) 32, no. 1, (January 14, 1983): 1-17.

MMWR Supplement, 36, no. 25 (August 21, 1987).

Mosby's Medical, Nursing, & Allied Health Dictionary. 3d ed. St. Louis: C.V. Mosby Company, 1990.

Ohio Department of Health, 246 N. High St., Columbus, OH 43215; and Columbus Health Department, 181 S. Washington Blvd., Columbus, OH 43215. "Child Daycare Center Communicable Disease Chart." Columbus, February 1986.

Reader's Digest Illustrated Encyclopedic Dictionary. Pleasantville, NY: Reader's Digest Association, Inc., 1987.

Schneidman, Rose; Lambert, Susan; and Wander, Barbara. *Being a Nursing Assistant.* 3d ed. Robert J. Brady, 1982.

Sherman, Jacques L. Jr. and Fields, Sylvia K. *Guide to Patient Evaluation History Taking, Physical Examination, and the Nursing Process.* 5th ed. New York: Medical Examination Publishing Company, Elsevier Science Publishing Co., Inc., 1988.

Simmers, Louise. *Diversified Health Occupations.* 2nd ed. Albany: Delmar, 1988
_____. Nurses Reference Library, Assessment. Springhouse, PA: Springhouse, 1983.

Taber, Clarence W. *Taber's Cyclopedic Medical Dictionary.* 14th ed. Philadelphia: F. A. Davis Co., 1983.

Titmus Optical, Inc. Petersburg, VA, 1985.

U.S. Department of Health and Human Services, Public Health Service Center for Disease Control, Atlanta, GA 30333. "Recommendations for Prevention of HIV Transmission in Health Care Settings." Atlanta, 1987.

Webster's *New World Dictionary, The 100,000 Entry Edition.* New York: Penguin, 1971.

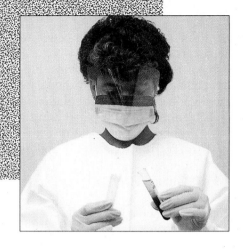

C H A P T E R   1 7

Specimen Collection and Laboratory Procedures

The medical assistant will be responsible for a number of laboratory testing procedures when assisting the physician in the medical office. To be effective in this role, you must know the normal range of various laboratory tests and the proper preparation and procedure for each. An office policy manual for laboratory procedures, as well as one from the laboratory where specimens are sent for analysis, should be kept in a handy place for reference. The knowledgeable medical assistant can make patients feel more at ease about these procedures and elicit more cooperation.

You must follow laboratory instructions exactly in obtaining, preparing, labeling, and sending all specimens for analysis. Accurate typing or printing of all the necessary information on the lab request forms will help to expedite testing and reporting from the laboratory and eliminate unnecessary phone calls. As reports of tests are returned, it will be your responsibility to alert the physician to any abnormal results. This is usually done by circling or underlining the abnormal finding in red ink. As ordered by the physician, you may contact the patient concerning the reports and follow-up procedures.

All lab reports should be filed in the patient's chart as soon as possible after the physician has read them. A special marking, stamp, or the physician's initials on the lab reports will indicate that they are ready to be filed.

Almost every medical practice is equipped with a standard microscope, which is used to examine objects that cannot be seen with the naked eye. The microscope is most helpful in identifying microorganisms in urine and other body fluids and tissues. It is also used in determining blood cell counts. You must develop basic skill in operation and care of the microscope.

Public health officials at the Centers for Disease Control in Atlanta, Georgia, recommend that **all health professionals follow universal precautions.** These "universal blood and body-fluid precautions," or "universal precautions," are required as a means of infection control and should be used consistently for all patients, especially when the health status of the patient is unknown (such as in an emergency situation). Making these universal precautions a *habit* is *vital* for your future health. The precautions recommend:

1. Routine use of appropriate barriers to prevent contact with mucous membranes, blood, or any other body fluid of a patient
2. Routine, proper, thorough handwashing
3. Immediate placing of used sharps and needles in biohazard puncture-proof containers
4. Use of disposables in resuscitation procedures
5. Refraining from direct patient care if you have an exudative skin condition (or other contagious disease)
6. Especially strict adherence to precautions during pregnancy

Many serious diseases can be spread by careless acts. The two most feared are hepatitis B (HBV) and human immunodeficiency virus (HIV), which is the cause of acquired immunodeficiency syndrome (AIDS). Research efforts continue in finding vaccines for AIDS and HIV. There is a vaccine for the prevention of HBV, which all health care providers should have administered if they are exposed to blood or other hazardous body fluids or infectious waste in the course of their duties. If all health care workers follow these precautions to help in the control of contagious diseases, it will set a good example for the public (remember, actions speak louder than words).

Guidelines for Lab Safety ....

1. Proper handwashing before and after any and every procedure, before and after gloving, must become a habit for all health workers for self-protection from disease transmission.(Immediately washing **any** skin surface thoroughly that has been contaminated with any blood or body fluids is vital.)
2. Gloving is always a must when handling *any* blood or body fluid specimens.
3. Cover all scratches, paper cuts, or any breaks in the skin with a bandage after handwashing and before gloving for self-protection against possible contamination.
4. Never eat, drink, chew gum, smoke, or place hands or fingers to mouth or place any item in your mouth (such as a pen or pencil) while working.
5. Wear protective gloves, mask, gown (or apron), and goggles when splashing of any blood or body fluids is possible while you are working, Figure 17–1.

6. Always recap or close bottles, jars, tubes, etc., immediately after desired amounts are obtained to avoid spills, waste, and accidents.
7. Clean up spills immediately to avoid accidents, Figure 17–2. Spilled blood or any body fluids should be flooded with a liquid germicide or bleach solution (a 1:10 ratio) before cleaning up with paper towels (wear latex gloves). Commercial preparations may also be used to solidify liquids, which makes cleanup easier.
8. Record lab test results immediately on charts or in logs to ensure accuracy.
9. Work in a well-lighted, properly ventilated, uncluttered, quiet area for better concentration.
10. Discard all disposable sharp instruments, lancets, syringes and needles (intact) in proper biohazard puncture-proof containers, Figure 17–3 (**never** break needles off, handle after use, or reuse). Place

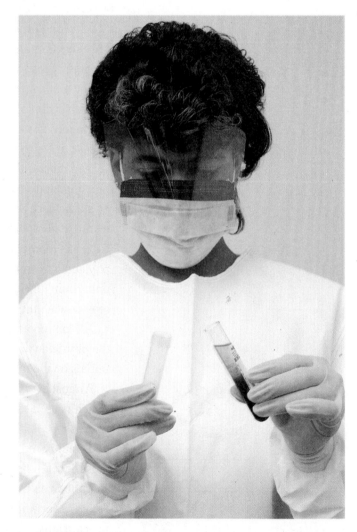

FIGURE 17–1 This medical assistant is wearing protective barriers: latex gloves, gown, face shield and mask—as she prepares to pour serum from a centrifuged blood tube to the transfer tube for laboratory analysis.

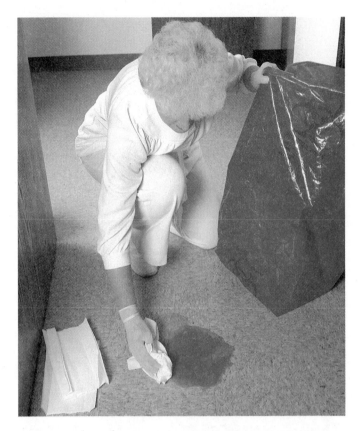

FIGURE 17–2 This medical assistant is wearing latex gloves to clean up a specimen spill. The biohazardous waste bag is used to dispose of the contaminated materials.

reusable metal instruments in a disinfectant solution after rinsing in cold water in preparation for proper cleaning and sterilization.

11. Discard *all* hazardous waste in proper containers, Figure 17–4.

12. Make periodic checks of all electrical appliances and

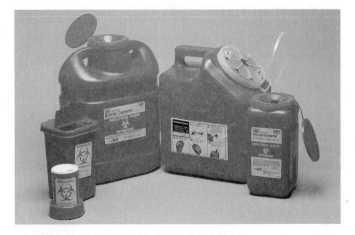

FIGURE 17–3 A few of the various sizes of biohazard puncture-proof containers are displayed (they are a bright red or yellow to alert caution). Biohazardous waste containers should be autoclaved when full and returned to the biohazard agency for proper disposal.

equipment for frayed wires or faulty operation and tag for repair if needed.

13. Make sure that your hands are dry before using any electrical appliances or equipment.

14. Report all accidents to your supervisor or instructor immediately.

15. Clearly post emergency phone numbers near the telephone in the lab (i.e., local fire, police, emergency medical unit, and poison control center), Figure 17–5, page 520.

16. Have available (nearby or in the lab) first aid items (i.e., sterile gauze, bandages, tape, etc.) for emergency use.

17. Post clearly the sign over the functional emergency

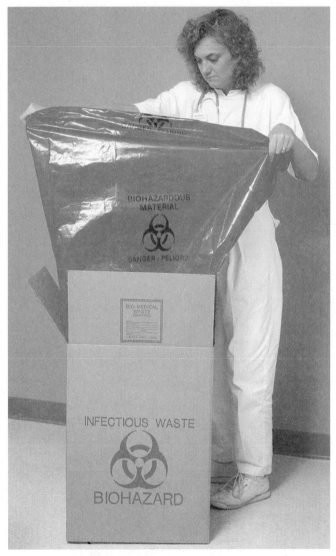

FIGURE 17–4 This medical assistant is placing a sturdy disposable plastic bag marked with the biohazardous waste symbol into a durable cardboard box marked the same for collection of infective waste material. When full, these boxes are picked up by an agency for incineration or for autoclaving before disposal in a public landfill.

FIGURE 17–5 Example of recommended phone numbers to post near each phone for emergency assistance.

eye wash station in the lab, Figure 17–6.

18. Do not wear loose-fitting or bulky clothing or jewelry that could contribute to accidents while working with machines or equipment in the lab or any area in the office or clinic.

19. Use gas or air valves and Bunsen burners with caution. Keep flammable chemicals away from them.

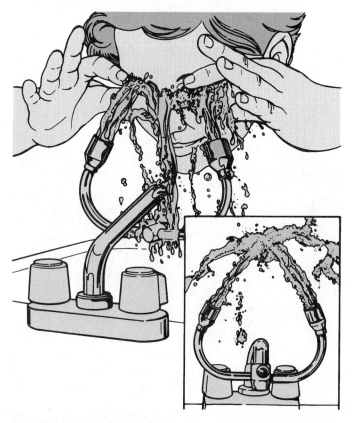

FIGURE 17–6 The emergency eye wash fountain connects to existing plumbing. The two streams of water wash both eyes continuously and simultaneously.

PATIENT EDUCATION

Many patients may be frightened or confused about some of the laboratory procedures requested by the physician to aid in diagnosis. You may perform some of these in the office or clinic setting or send the patient to the lab for tests. If you send patients elsewhere, make sure you give accurate directions on how to get there.

Each test or procedure must be explained clearly and concisely to relieve patients' anxiety. Use language that patients will understand. Most people have little or no knowledge of medical terminology.

Certain lab tests require preparation by patients prior to arrival (i.e., fasting, taking or omitting certain medications, etc.). Be sure to instruct patients in these preparations and have clear, concise, written instructions available. Do not presume that patients know all about a procedure even if they have had the test before. Often new techniques require additional or different instructions for preparation. Medical technology is constantly changing. It is important for health care providers (including medical assistants) to keep abreast of new developments in medicine. Inform patients that some procedures can cause temporary discomfort and how it may be relieved.

Give patients enough time to look over the printed instruction sheet or pamphlet and make certain you answer all of their questions thoroughly before they leave.

20. Use only paper disposable cups for drinking.

21. Designate a "dirty" and a "clean" area in your lab, and enforce this policy.

22. Package broken glass or any sharp unusable item in a sturdy cardboard box or puncture-proof container marked "caution—broken glass" to discard in the proper waste receptacle. (This will protect unsuspecting custodial personnel from injury.)

23. Never lean into work area when working with flame or chemicals (pour at arm's length) to avoid self-injury or accident.

UNIT 1

The Microscope

OBJECTIVES

Upon completion of this unit, the student will meet the following terminal performance objectives by verifying knowledge of the facts and principles presented through oral and written communication at a level deemed competent, and will demonstrate the specific behaviors as

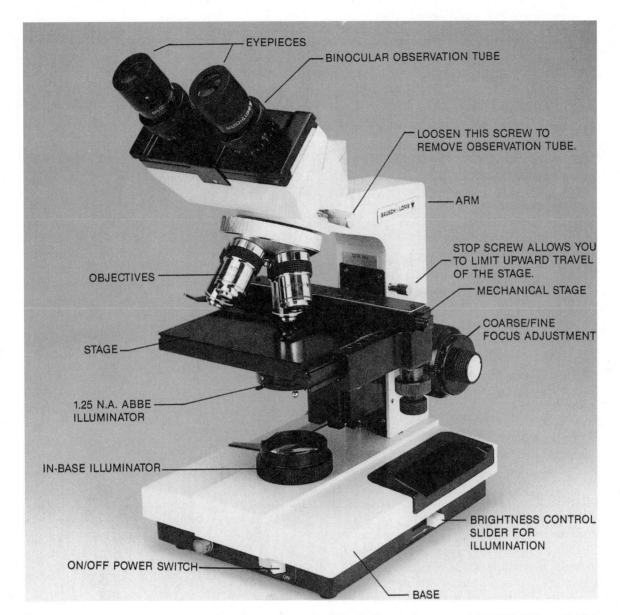

FIGURE 17–7 Parts of the microscope (From Simmers, *Diversified Health Occupations*, copyright 1988, Delmar Publishers Inc.)

identified in the terminal performance objectives of the procedures, observing all aseptic and safety precautions in accordance with health care standards.

1. Identify the parts of the microscope and the purpose of each.
2. Adjust and focus the objectives and state their magnification power.
3. Adjust the light and mirror for proper viewing.
4. Demonstrate how to clean the microscope (lens, stage, mirror).
5. Explain the general purpose of the microscope in the medical office.
6. Demonstrate the proper way to carry a microscope.
7. Spell and define, using the glossary at the back of the text, all the words to know in this unit.

WORDS TO KNOW ....

binocular
compensate
condenser
lpf (low-power field)
magnify
minute

monocular
objective
proficient
specimen
technical

The microscope is an essential piece of equipment in the laboratory of almost every medical practice. It is used to examine and identify **minute** objects that cannot be seen with the naked eye. Microscopes are fine and expensive **technical** instruments that must be handled with great respect. The operation and care manual should be kept handy for reference, because each microscope is

Use Microscope

PURPOSE: To gain skill in the use of the microscope.

EQUIPMENT: Microscope, electrical outlet for light source of microscope, specimen on glass slide with frosted end, cover glass (used usually for wet specimens only), lens cleaning tissues, latex gloves

TERMINAL PERFORMANCE OBJECTIVE: Provided with all necessary equipment/supplies, the student will demonstrate the use of the microscope following the steps in the procedure with the instructor observing each step.

1. Wash hands and put on latex gloves.
2. Assemble necessary equipment.
3. Clean ocular lens with lens cleaning tissues.
4. Plug microscope light source into electrical outlet and turn on light switch at front base of microscope.
5. Place specimen slide on stage with frosted end up, between clips, and secure over opening of stage. Note: Frosted end is used for labeling the specimen in pencil.
6. Watch carefully as you raise substage so that it does not come into direct contact with slide.
7. Turn revolving nosepiece to low-power objective (10X) and begin to focus coarse-adjustment dial until a wide

shaft can be seen.

8. When outline of specimen is in view, turn fine-adjustment dial until specimen can be seen in detail.
9. Adjust substage diaphragm lever or adjust mirror to obtain proper lighting.
10. If sharper detail is needed, carefully turn revolving nosepiece to intermediate-power objective and adjust fine-focus dial.
11. When using oil-immersion lens objective or hpf, oil should be used very sparingly. **Key Point: A cover slide should be used and lens must be cleaned after each use. Adjustment must be made for amount of light needed by adjusting diaphragm lever under stage.**
12. When specimen has been identified turn light off and return all items to proper storage area. **Key Point: Microscope stage should be cleaned as well as any slides that are not disposable.**
13. Remove gloves and wash hands.
14. Results of examination should be recorded or reported to physician as directed.

---

slightly different. The amount of routine maintenance required will vary with the amount of use.

The part of the microscope that supports the eyepiece is called the arm. Figure 17–7, page 521, shows the labeled parts of a binocular microscope. The proper way to carry the microscope is to grasp the arm with one hand and place the other hand under the base, holding it at waist level. The electrical cord for the light source should be loosely wrapped and secured with a twist tie or a rubber band. Wrapping the cord too tightly may cause the enclosed wires to break and lead to a short that could cause an electrical fire. The cord of the microscope should be kept loosely wrapped and out of the work area when not in use. It should always be unplugged by grasping the plug, never by pulling the cord. As with any electrical appliance, all surrounding surfaces and hands should be dry. Wet hands, floors, and so on, can lead to electric shock.

A binocular microscope has two eyepieces. The monocular microscope has only one eyepiece or ocular lens. The eyepiece or ocular lens is in the upper part of the tube of the microscope. The eyepiece contains a lens to magnify what is being seen.

The body tube leads to the revolving nosepiece. Attached to the revolving nosepiece are three (sometimes four) small lenses called objectives, each of which

has a different magnifying power. The shortest has the lowest power. It is called the low-power field, or lpf. On most microscopes, it will magnify the object to be viewed 10 times, or make it 10X larger than when viewed by the naked eye. The low-power field is the lens used to scan the field of interest and to focus in on the specimen. To position each objective, you simply rotate the nosepiece until you hear a click.

For greater detail in viewing the specimen, turn the nosepiece to the next longer objective, the high-power lens. It will magnify the object approximately 40 times, or 40X. The longest objective is the oil-immersion objective. This high-power lens magnifies objects about 100 times, or 100X. Using the fine-focus dial will bring the specimen into good definition.

The stage of the microscope has two clips which hold the specimen slide to be viewed. Just underneath the stage is a substage where a condenser is held that regulates the amount of light directed on the magnified specimen. It has a shutter or diaphragm to control the amount of light desired. The substage may be raised or lowered in focusing on the specimen.

A supply of lens tissue paper should be kept nearby to clean the lenses after each use. Makeup, oil, secretions from the eyes, and dust can make it difficult to see through the lens, besides being a possible means of transmitting disease among office personnel. Eyeglasses are not necessary when performing microscopic work, because the microscope may be focused to compensate for all visual defects except astigmatism.

It will take time and patience to learn how to operate the microscope. The supervision of an experienced operator is essential to becoming proficient in its use and care.

Complete Chapter 17, Unit 1 in the workbook to help you meet the objectives at the beginning of this unit and therefore achieve competency of this subject matter.

U N I T   2

Capillary Blood Tests

OBJECTIVES ....

Upon completion of this unit, the student will meet the following terminal performance objectives by verifying knowledge of the facts and principles presented through oral and written communication at a level deemed competent, and will demonstrate the specific behaviors as identified in the terminal performance objectives of the procedures, observing all aseptic and safety precautions in accordance with health care standards.

1. State the purpose of wearing latex gloves when performing laboratory procedures.
2. List and discuss the regulatory bodies that govern the POL.
3. List and discuss the laboratory practices that yield quality assurance in the POL.
4. Explain the reasons for performing capillary blood tests in the medical office.
5. Perform skin puncture procedures to obtain capillary blood specimens.
6. Complete a health department request form for the PKU test and obtain the blood specimen for it.
7. Obtain hemoglobin and hematocrit levels.
8. Operate a microhematocrit centrifuge.
9. Operated a hemoglobinometer.
10. Perform a blood glucose screening test with glucometer (or color chart on bottle) from reagent strip.
11. Explain the purpose of the GTT (glucose tolerance test).
12. Give instructions and patient education for the preparation of a patient for a GTT.
13. Make calculations of blood cells using the hemocytometer.
14. Perform a red/white blood cell count.
15. Prepare a blood smear for a differential count.
16. List each type of white blood cell and state the function of each.
17. Spell and define, using the glossary at the back of the text, all the words to know in this unit.

WORDS TO KNOW ....

allosteric	metabolism
carbohydrates	neonate
centrifuge	OSHA
CLIA	pallor
differential	percentage
diffuse	phagocytosis
erythropoiesis	phenylalanine
glucose	PKU (phenylketonuria)
HCFA	POL
hematocrit	polycythemia
HHS	puncture
implement	regulatory
insignificant	reticuloendothelial
insulin	stat
laboratory	sterile
lancet	tolerance
meniscus	waiver

Laboratory Classification and Regulation ....

The physician's office laboratory (POL) falls under many regulatory bodies. The complexity of the laboratory tests performed will determine which classification the POL is and under which body it is regulated. Table 17–1, page 524, outlines the three laboratory classifications under the CLIA-88 (Clinical Laboratory Improvement Amendments, 1988).

A Certificate of Waiver allows *only* those tests to be performed in a POL that are on the final list of waivered tests. Waivered tests are those that basically have an insignificant risk to the patient if an error is made in the test results. This means that there would be no significant risk or harm done to the patient. Application for this certificate is obtained from the HHS (Department of Health and Human Services). Laboratory tests on the certificate of waiver list may be billed to Medicare and Medicaid. This certificate must be renewed every 2 years for a moderate fee. Tests performed in the POL must be restricted to this list.

Level I laboratory tests must be performed under more strict regulations. Any abnormal test results that apply to a previously undiagnosed condition of a patient must be referred to a level II lab to be verified.

Regulatory bodies periodically inspect laboratories and medical offices to ensure quality assurance and quality control. Quality assurance in the health care field refers to all evaluative services and the results compared with accepted standards. Quality control implies that operational procedures are used to implement the quality assurance program. To determine these standards many aspects of care are taken into account. First, the cost, place, accessibility, treatment, and benefits of health care are evaluated. The next step is comparing the

TABLE 17–1
Laboratory Classifications

Proposed Certificate of Waiver Tests (Exempt)

Urinalysis by reagent strip or tablet

Microscopic urine sediment

Urine pregnancy tests

Occult blood in stool

Microscopic examination of:

   Pinworm preparation

   Vaginal wet mount preparation

   KOH (Potassium hydroxide) preparation of cutaneous scrapings

   Semen analysis

   Gram stain (of discharge and exudate)

Screen-slide card agglutination test for:

   ASO (antistreptolysin O)

   CRP (C-reactive protein)

   Infectious mononucleosis screening

   Rheumatoid factor screening

   Sickle cell screening (nonelectrophoresis method)

Ovulation tests (visual color test for human luteinizing hormone)

Whole blood clotting time

Glucose reagent strip screening

Spun microhematocrit

Erythrocyte sedimentation rate

Proposed Level I Tests

Cholesterol screen (qualitative and semiqualitative determinations)

Urine cultures for colony counts (excluding identification and susceptibility)

Red and white blood cell counts

Hematocrit

BUN (blood urea nitrogen) uric acid

Glucose

   Creatinine

Direct strep–antigen test

Proposed Level II Tests

All other remaining tests under CPT 80000 series including:

Automated multichannel chemical profiles

Radioimmunoassay procedures

Drug and toxicology procedures

Coagulation studies

These classifications are based on the complexity of the tests and the risks involved in the reporting of an error in the results.

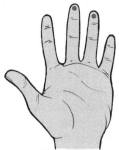
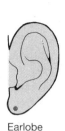
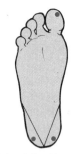

Infant's heel/great toe   Earlobe   Ring/great finger

B.

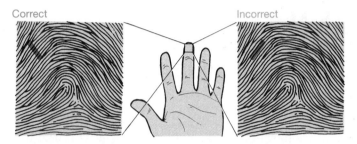

Correct   Incorrect

FIGURE 17–8 (a). These skin puncture sites are recommended because of abundant capillary blood flow for obtaining a specimen. They are also desirable sites for convenience of the patient. (b). Skin punctures should be made across fingerprints, not parallel to them.

findings with standard results. Finally, the appropriate recommendations for improving health care are noted.

Both level I and II laboratories are required to follow quality assurance programs. The purposes of quality assurance programs are to evaluate the quality and effectiveness of health care according to accepted standards and to ensure accuracy and validity in testing procedures. These levels of POLs must also participate in proficiency testing programs for the test procedures that they perform and keep strict records of quality control.

Other bodies that provide regulation inspections of a POL are HCFA (Health Care Financing Administration) and OSHA (Occupational Safety and Health Administration). Private agencies also issue accreditations and/or state licensing for approved operation of the POL. The laboratory may be operated under a provisional certificate, which is issued until the HHS inspects the facility. Certificates must be renewed every 2 years. Inspections may be made, unannounced, anytime. If OSHA, a separate inspecting body from CLIA, finds a POL in noncompliance of regulations during a visit (scheduled or not), a $10,000 fine per item, per employee (per visit) applies.

In the POL, no matter what classification, the following practices should be followed to ensure reliable and accurate data, and to ensure quality health care to patients; quality assurance involves *proper:*

1. Patient identification
2. Patient preparation and specimen collection

3. Specimen processing and transportation
4. Instrumental and technical performance
5. Safety
6. In-service training and education of all health care personnel

All state and federal health and safety regulations and laws apply to the POL according to the three lab classifications. It is important to stay abreast of the current regulations that apply to the facility where you are employed.

Skin Puncture ....

Capillary blood tests are frequently performed in the medical office or clinic because of the small amount of blood required, usually one to a few drops. Because most patients are extremely apprehensive, you must develop skill not only in performing the procedures but in conveying reas-surance to the patient. When skin puncture procedures are done correctly, the patient should feel minimal discomfort. Displaying confidence in carrying out the procedures competently will ensure patient safety and comfort.

Capillaries are minute blood vessels which convey blood from the arterioles to the venules. At this level, blood and oxygen diffuse to the tissues and products of metabolic activity enter the bloodstream. For this reason, capillary blood is an ideal sample for the screening of hematocrit, hemoglobin, blood glucose, and PKU levels and other screening tests that require a very small amount of blood.

Capillary blood is just under the surface of the skin. The most practical sites to use are the ring and great finger, the earlobe, and in infants the heel or great toe, Figure 17–8A & B.

The Autolet is widely used by diabetic (and other) patients in their homes for simple blood tests that require

P R O C E D U R E

Puncture Skin With Sterile Lancet

PURPOSE: to obtain a few drops of capillary blood for screening tests.

EQUIPMENT: Latex gloves, sterile **lancet**, Figure 17–9, page 526, alcohol, cotton balls, gauze squares, Mayo table.

TERMINAL PERFORMANCE OBJECTIVE: Provided with all necessary equipment/supplies, and using other students as patients, the student will demonstrate the skin puncture procedure following all steps to obtain capillary blood for test(s) specified by the physician/instructor. The instructor will observe each step.

1. Identify patient. **Key Point: Call patient by name and check chart to avoid error.**
2. Explain the procedure to the patient.
3. Inspect patient's fingers (or other puncture sites) and select most desirable site.
   Key Points:
   a. **Main sites are ring or great finger, earlobe, infant's lateral areas of heel.**
   b. **Some patients have a preference for a particular site.**
   c. **Earlobe is less sensitive to pain than fingers.**
   d. **Do not use areas that are bruised, calloused, or injured.**
4. Wash hands, put on latex gloves, and assemble needed items on Mayo table.
5. Wipe desired site with an alcohol-saturated cotton ball and let dry. Do not blow the skin to expedite drying; you will contaminate the area with microorganisms from your mouth.

6. Take sterile lancet out of package without contaminating point. **Key Point: Another must be used if point is touched.**
7. Hold patient's finger (or other site) securely between your thumb and great finger. In your other hand hold lancet, pointed downward, with thumb and index or great finger. Puncture site quickly with a firm, steady down-and-up motion to approximately a 2-mm depth. **Key Point: Control entry and exit of lancet in same path to avoid ripping skin.**
8. Discard first drop of blood by blotting away with dry gauze square. First drop may contain traces of alcohol or tissue fluid that would dilute sample and make test inaccurate.
9. Keep applying gentle pressure on either side of puncture site until necessary amount of blood has been obtained. **Key Point: Too much pressure will cause tissue fluid to mix with blood.**
10. Wipe site with alcohol-saturated cotton ball and ask patient to hold dry gauze square over it for a minute or so. **Key Point: Check site to be sure bleeding has stopped. Determine if patient is allergic to adhesive before applying bandage to puncture site (use gauze square and hypoallergenic tape if allergic).**
11. Remove gloves, wash hands, and discard used items in proper receptacle.

Most patients, especially youngsters, are apprehensive about having blood taken. The medical assistant must calmly explain to each patient that screening tests such as a hemoglobin or a blood glucose are performed with a small amount of blood taken from the finger, earlobe, or infant's heel. Let the patient know ahead of time what you are going to do to gain cooperation. You should tell the patient that there will be a little pain or discomfort during the initial skin puncture, but it will not last long. Reassure the patient that this procedure is short-lived and necessary for the physician to assist in making a diagnosis or evaluating the condition. Remember to advise the patient to keep the puncture site clean and dry for 24 hours with a fresh bandage as necessary.

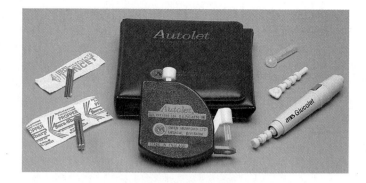

FIGURE 17–9 A variety of sterile lances and devices to use for obtaining capillary blood samples

water. Alcohol tends to toughen the skin if used for extended periods of time.

With strict regulations regarding quality control and quality assurance, it is advisable to keep a log book to record all specimens and the results of the tests performed. The log should include:

1. The date
2. Patient's name
3. Test performed
4. Results of the test
5. Your initials

capillary blood, Figure 17–10A, and 17–10B. You may be given the duty of instructing patients in use of the Autolet. Patients who use this technique daily should simply wash the puncture site thoroughly with soap and

---

   P R O C E D U R E

Puncture Skin With Autolet

PURPOSE: To obtain a few drops of capillary blood for tests.
EQUIPMENT: Autolet, disposable platform (yellow—standard puncture depth of approximately 2 mm, orange—super-puncture depth of approximately 3mm), sterile lancet, alcohol, cotton balls, gauze squares, latex gloves, Mayo table.
TERMINAL PERFORMANCE OBJECTIVE: Provided with all necessary equipment/supplies, and using other students as patients, the student will demonstrate the steps in the procedure for obtaining capillary blood using the Autolet. The instructor will observe each step.

1. Identify patient. **Key Point: Call patient by name and check chart to avoid error.**
2. Explain procedure to patient.
3. Inspect patient's fingers (or other puncture sites) and select most desirable site.
4. Wash hands, put on latex gloves, and assemble all necessary items on Mayo stand.
5. Pull arm of Autolet back to activating button. It holds in place when click is heard.
6. Place sterile lancet securely into socket. Next, place appropriate platform, recessed surface down, into platform slot at base of Autolet.

7. Wipe puncture site with alcohol-saturated cotton ball and let dry.
8. Twist protective covering from tip of sterile lancet and press recessed surface against site firmly so that skin enters opening of platform, Figure 17–10.
9. Hold patient's finger steady with one hand and with other hand press activating button to puncture site with lancet. Rest Autolet on Mayo stand and proceed.
10. Apply gentle pressure to both sides of puncture site with your thumb and great finger. Blot first drop of blood from puncture site with dry gauze square.
11. After a sufficient amount of blood has been obtained for desired test, wipe puncture site with alcohol-saturated cotton ball and ask patient to apply gentle pressure to site with dry gauze square for a minute or so. **Key Point: Check site to be sure bleeding has stopped. Determine if patient is allergic to adhesive before applying bandage to puncture site (use gauze square and hypoallergenic tape if allergic).**
12. Remove gloves, wash hands and discard used items in proper receptacle.

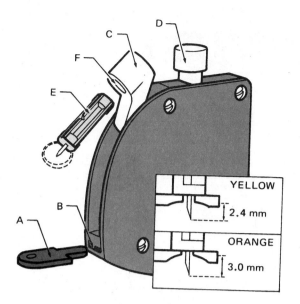

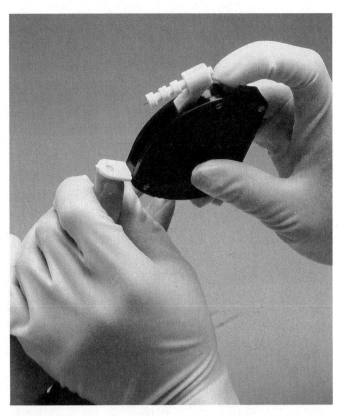

FIGURE 17–10A   Autolet components: (a) platform, (b) platform slot, (c) spring-loaded arm, (d) activating button, (e) lancet, (f) lancet socket

PKU Test

A screening test done with capillary blood from an infant's heel or great toe is the **PKU** (phenylketonuria). Phenylketonuria is a congenital disease due to a defect in

FIGURE 17–10B   Press the recessed surface against the site so that the skin enters the opening of the platform.

P R O C E D U R E

Obtain Blood For PKU Test

PURPOSE: To obtain a blood specimen for determination of PKU (phenylketonuria) level in blood.

EQUIPMENT: PKU health department form, Autolet/sterile lancet, latex gloves, cotton balls, alcohol, gauze squares, round adhesive bandage, patient's chart, pen, stamped envelope addressed to health department

TERMINAL PERFORMANCE OBJECTIVE: Provided with all necessary equipment/supplies, and using other students as patients, the student will demonstrate the steps of the procedure for obtaining a blood specimen for determination of phenylketonuria level in the blood. The instructor will observe each step.

Note: This procedure may be simulated by using a clinical lifelike doll and milk colored with red food coloring for practice.

1. Wash hands, put on latex gloves, and assemble needed items on Mayo table.
2. Identify patient. Ask parents to name patient and check chart to avoid error.
3. Explain procedure to parent and ask for necessary information to complete form. Be sure to write the exact birth weight of the infant on the form and the date and time the test was performed. Ask for their assistance in holding infant still during procedure.
4. Wipe desired site with alcohol-saturated cotton ball and let dry.
5. Take sterile lancet out of the package without contaminating point.
6. Secure infant's great toe/lateral heel with your great finger and thumb and gently apply pressure to produce a large drop of blood. Carefully blot onto one of outlined circles on end of form soaking the test paper from the back of the form. **Key Point: Repeat until each circle has been entirely saturated.**
7. Wipe puncture site with alcohol-saturated cotton ball and apply dry gauze square. Ask parent to hold against puncture site. Then place small round bandage over area.
8. Place completed test form into protective envelope and then into an envelope addressed to health department with physician's return address.
9. Record procedure on patient's chart and initial.
10. Remove gloves, wash hands, discard used items in proper receptacle, and return items to proper storage area.
11. File report in patient's chart when received in return mail after physician has checked the results.

CCO70H1889158Q

ALL INFORMATION MUST BE PRINTED

L-65397

BIRTHDATE: ☐☐ / ☐☐ / ☐☐   TIME: ☐☐ : ☐☐   (USE 24 HOUR TIME ONLY)

BABY'S NAME:
(last, first)

HOSPITAL PROVIDER NUMBER:

HOSPITAL NAME:

MOM'S NAME:
(last, first, initial)

MOM'S ADDRESS:

MOM'S CITY: OHIO   ZIP:

MOM'S RACE: MOM'S AGE: MOM'S SSN: ☐☐☐ - ☐☐ - ☐☐☐☐

MOM'S PHONE: (☐☐☐) ☐☐☐ - ☐☐☐☐   MOM'S COUNTY:

MOM'S ID: BABY'S ID:

SPECIMEN DATE: ☐☐ / ☐☐ / ☐☐   TIME: ☐☐ : ☐☐   (USE 24 HOUR TIME ONLY)

PHYSICIAN NAME:

PHYSICIAN ADDRESS:

CITY: OHIO ZIP:

PHYSICIAN'S PHONE: (☐☐☐) ☐☐☐ - ☐☐☐☐   PHYSICIAN PROVIDER NO: ☐ . ☐☐☐☐☐

ODH ONLY: ☐ SPECIAL:

TEST RESULTS:

☐ SCREENING TEST NORMAL FOR:
   PKU, HOM, GAL, HYPOTHYROIDISM,
   HEMOGLOBINOPATHIES

☐ SCREENING TEST NORMAL FOR:
   PKU, AND HOM ONLY

☐ SCREENING TEST NORMAL:
   ☐ PKU   ☐ HOM   ☐ GAL
   ☐ HYPOTHYROIDISM   ☐ HEMOGLOBINOPATHIES

☐ SCREENING TESTS ABNORMAL:

_____

SEE FOOTNOTE _____ ON BACK

☐ SPECIMEN REJECTED FOR REASON:

BABY SEX: ☐ MALE   ☐ FEMALE
BIRTH WEIGHT: ☐☐☐☐ GRAMS
PREMATURE: ☐ YES   ☐ NO
ANTIBIOTICS: ☐ YES   ☐ NO
TRANSFUSION: ☐ YES   ☐ NO
SPECIMEN: ☐ FIRST   ☐ SECOND
SUBMITTER: ☐ HOSPITAL / BIRTH CENTER
             ☐ PHYSICIAN
             ☐ HEALTH DEPARTMENT
             ☐ OTHER: (name below)

ODH COPY

HEA 2518 _____

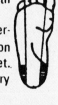

FILL ALL CIRCLES WITH BLOOD
BLOOD MUST SOAK COMPLETELY THROUGH
DO NOT APPLY BLOOD TO THIS SIDE

FIGURE 17–11 (a). PKU blood test form (b). Instructions

the metabolism of the amino acid, phenylalanine. This unmetabolized protein, phenylalanine, accumulates in the bloodstream and can prevent the brain from developing normally. If this condition goes undetected and untreated, the result is mental retardation. This screening is required by law in most states and all Canadian provinces, either by blood test or urinalysis. The blood test requires that a few drops of the infant's blood be soaked through the outlined circles (from the back) of the treated paper attached to the health department form, Figure 17–11. This duplicated form must be completed accurately. Parents usually bring the form with them on the infant's first office visit unless the procedure was performed at the hospital nursery. After completion of the instructions, the form (intact with all copies) should be mailed to the health department. A report of the results of the screening test will be mailed back to the physician to be filed in the infant's chart. This test is limited to newborns (neonates) and their biological parents.

Hemoglobin and Hematocrit ....

Hemoglobin and hematocrit screening tests also require a few drops of capillary blood. Usually the ring or great finger is used in children and adults because these fingers are not so sensitive as the index finger. The thumb is usually too tough-skinned, and the little finger is generally too small and would not yield an adequate amount. The patient's age or preference will help you decide which site to choose.

Hematocrit is a screening test to determine anemia. Anemia is a condition in which there is a lack of circulating red blood cells. Erythrocytes transport oxygen to

INSTRUCTIONS FOR NEWBORN SCREENING SPECIMENS

1. Cleanse infant's heel with alcohol swab.
2. Puncture heel in fleshy lateral or medial posterior portion with sterile disposable lancet. Wipe puncture site with dry sterile swab.
3. Allow large blood droplet to form. Touch blood droplet to center of circle on **ONE SIDE** of filter paper card **ONLY**. Observe reverse side of card and insure that blood has soaked completely through before removing card from infant's heel.
4. Repeat step 3 to fill **ALL FIVE CIRCLES. DO NOT** squeeze heel excessively to obtain blood.
5. Allow card to **AIR DRY** 2 hours at room temperature on a non-absorbent surface. **DO NOT** stack cards together while drying.
6. After blood spots are completely dry, place card in ODH self-addressed laboratory mailing envelope. **MAIL** within **48 HOURS.**

CORRECT   **INCORRECT**

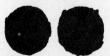   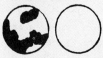

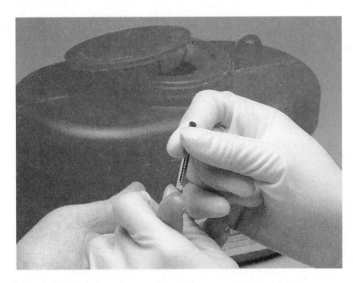

FIGURE 17-12 Skin puncture is made with sterile lancet across fingerprints.

the entire body. When there are not enough of them to supply all of the cells, symptoms of paleness, fatigue, drowsiness, among others, begin to be apparent in patients. Polycythemia may be indicated by an abnormally high reading. Polycythemia is a condition of having an excessive number of erythrocytes. Some of the symptoms are similar to anemia—weakness and fatigue. Redness of the skin (opposite of anemia) and pain of the extremities, often with black and blue spots, is observed in some patients with polycythemia. You should become familiar with all of the symptoms of the diseases for which you perform screening tests so that you may alert the physician to any changes that patients may tell you. Often patients disclose important information to you and then do not say anything to the doctor because they think you have already reported it.

To perform a microhematocrit screening test, you begin by cleansing the skin site with alcohol using a

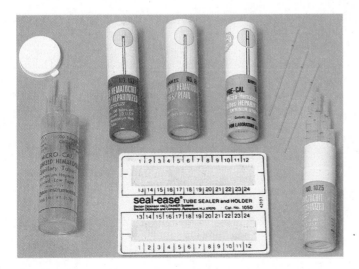

FIGURE 17-13 Microhematocrit tubes

gauze square or cotton ball. A sterile lancet is used to puncture the skin, Figure 17-12. Very small glass tubes, called microhematocrit tubes, are used to collect the blood sample, Figure 17-13. Many of them are marked with a fill line at about the three-quarter point. The tube fills very quickly by capillary action if the puncture site is deep enough, usually about 2 mm. A small amount of clay sealant is carefully placed in one end of the microhematocrit tube to seal the opening so that blood will not leak out. Make sure that there is no trace of red visible around the end of the tube with clay (even a minute hairline path of red will cause *all* of the blood in the tube to spin out during centrifugation).

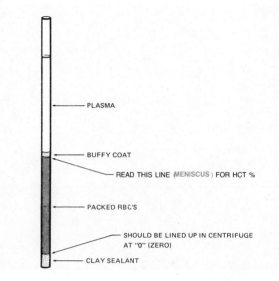

FIGURE 17-14 A labeled hematocrit tube after centrifugation

The tube is then placed in a microhematocrit centrifuge where spinning for approximately 3 minutes will separate the blood components by centrifugal action. The tube after centrifugation has three layers: plasma, a thin yellowish layer called the buffy coat, and packed red blood cells, Figure 17-14. Contained in the buffy coat are the white blood cells and the platelets.

The hematocrit is expressed as the percentage of the total blood volume made up of red blood cells (erythrocytes) or as the volume in cubic centimeters (cc) of erythrocytes packed by centrifugation in 100 cc of blood. The normal hematocrit range for adult males is 40 to 54% and for adult females 37 to 47%.

Figure 17-17, page 534, shows a centrifugal hematology system that analyzes finger-puncture or venous blood samples to provide the following values:

- hematocrit
- platelet count
- total white blood cell count
- total granulocyte count
- percentage granulocytes
- total lymph/mono count
- percentage lymphs/mono

TABLE 17-2

Approximate Relationship Between Hematocrit, Red Cell Count and Hemoglobin in Adults

Hematocrit (%)	For Red Cells of Normal Size—To Be Used for Checking Purposes Only* Red Cell Count (× 1 million per cubic millimeter of blood)	Hemoglobin (in grams per 100 cc)
30	3.4	9.8
31	3.6	10.4
32	3.7	10.7
33	3.8	11.0
34	3.9	11.3
35	4.0	11.6
36	4.1	11.9
37	4.3	12.4
38	4.4	12.8
39	4.5	13.1
40	4.6	13.3
41	4.7	13.6
42	4.8	13.9
43	4.9	14.2
44	5.1	14.8
45	5.2	15.1
46	5.3	15.4
47	5.4	15.7
48	5.5	16.0
49	5.6	16.2
50	5.7	16.5
51	5.9	17.1
52	6.0	17.4
53	6.1	17.7
54	6.2	18.0
55	6.3	18.3
56	6.4	18.6
57	6.6	19.1
58	6.7	19.4
59	6.8	19.7
60	6.9	20.1
61	7.0	20.3

NORMAL HEMATOCRITS	NORMAL RED CELL COUNTS	NORMAL HEMOGLOBINS
Men: Range 40–54%	Men: Range 4,600,000–6,200,000	Men: Range 14.0–18.0 grams
Aver. 47%	Aver. 5,400,000	Aver. 15.8 grams
Women: Range 37–47%	Women: Range 4,200,000–5,400,000	Women: Range 11.5–16.0 grams
Aver. 42%	Aver. 4,800,000	Aver. 13.9 grams

*The relationship shown between hematocrit and red cell count is based on normal cells (which have an average mean corpuscular volume of 0.87). The relationship between hemoglobin and red cell count is based on normal cells (with a mean corpuscular hemoglobin of 29). These relationships do not hold true in cases of microcytic or macrocytic anemias which probably will not be more than 5 to 10% of blood examined by clinical laboratories and blood banks.

Determine Hemocrit (Hct) Using Microhematocrit Centrifuge

PURPOSE: To determine the volume of packed erythrocytes in whole blood.

EQUIPMENT: Autolet/sterile lancet, microhematocrit tube(s), sealing clay, microhematocrit centrifuge, latex gloves, cotton balls, alcohol, patient's chart, pen (if hemoglobin is done by this procedure, conversion chart will also be needed to determine Hb), Table 17–2.

TERMINAL PERFORMANCE OBJECTIVE: Provided with all necessary equipment/supplies, and using other students as patients, the student will demonstrate the steps in the procedure for determining hematocrit (Hct) readings using the microhematocrit centrifuge. The instructor will observe each step.

1. Assemble needed items on Mayo table. **Key Point: Check to see that centrifuge is plugged into electrical outlet.**
2. Identify patient and explain procedure. **Key Point: Call patient by name and check chart to avoid error.**
3. Put on latex gloves.
4. Follow desired skin puncture procedure.
5. Hold microhematocrit tube, as you would hold a pencil or pen, horizontally with opening just by drop of blood that appears at puncture site. To assist flow of blood, which enters tube by capillary action, Figure 17–15(a), page 532, continue holding tube horizontally but tilted slightly downward until blood reaches fill line or three-fourths point. **Key Point: Obtain as many tubes as ordered, usually one or two. Hold tip of gloved finger over Hct tube to keep blood from flowing out.**
6. Wipe outside end of glass tube with gauze square, while still holding it horizontally. Carefully seal *only one end* of the tube by placing it into the clay and turning it until the entire end is solid clay (do not apply too much pressure or the *glass* tube will break), Figure 17–15(b). Only a

very small amount of clay is needed. You may leave the tube standing up in the tray until you are finished tending to the needs of the patient.

7. Have patient hold dry gauze square on puncture site. **Key Point: Check to make sure bleeding has stopped.**
8. Secure sealed end of tube against rubber padding in centrifuge (clay end of tube is always toward you). Balance centrifuge with another tube opposite it. If two or more patients' tubes are placed in centrifuge at same time, make sure that you note numbers of spaces to avoid a mix-up, Figures 17–16(a) and 17–16(b), page 533.
9. Close inside cover carefully over tubes and lock into place by turning dial clockwise. Then close and lock outside cover. **Key Point: Listen for it to click into place.**
10. Turn timer switch to 3–5 minutes. (Most timing switches indicate that you turn past desired time and then back to time you want set.) It will automatically turn off.
11. Wait until centrifuge has completely stopped spinning and unlock covers. (Opening a centrifuge before it stops spinning is most dangerous—centrifugal force pulls objects such as hair, jewelry, loose sleeves of lab coats, etc. into it.) Read results by placing bottom line of packed RBCs (up to buffy coat but not including it) against calibrated chart in centrifuge where tube is resting, Figure 17–16(c) and (d). (There is usually a magnifying glass attached to centrifuge to assist in reading Hct accurately.) Keep cover of centrifuge closed when not in use.
12. Discard used items in proper waste receptacles, remove gloves, and wash hands.
13. Record reading on patient's chart as a percentage, for example, Hct 47%, and your initials.
14. Return items to proper storage areas.

Figure 17–18, page 535, shows the steps in preparing the blood tubes for use in the centrifugal hematology system.

In determining the hemoglobin (Hb) level of the blood, a conversion chart may be used when the hematocrit percentage (Hct %) is known; it may also be used to check the red blood cell count when hemoglobin and hematocrit (H & H) are known, Table 17–2. Hemoglobin is an **allosteric** protein found in erythrocytes, which transports molecular oxygen in the blood. A most reliable and simple way to determine hemoglobin level is with the hemoglobinometer, Figure 17–19, page 536. The normal range of hemoglobin for males is 14 to 18

grams per 100 ml of blood, and for females 12 to 16. Physicians may order an H & H to get a more definite idea of the patient's red cell volume.

Blood Glucose Screening ....

Another capillary blood test performed in most medical practices today is the blood **glucose** screening. It is done with a drop of blood obtained from a skin puncture. A drop of blood is applied directly to a chemically treated reagent strip. After timing (as directed by the manufacturer), the strip is blotted and read by comparing the color of the reagent strip with the color chart on the bottle. A

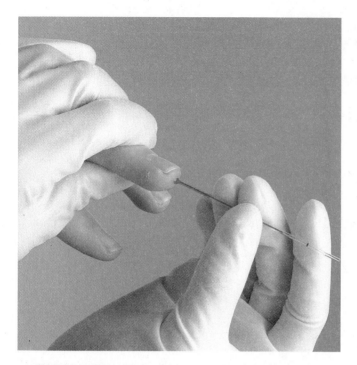

FIGURE 17–15(A) To fill the microhematocrit tube, hold the tip just to the drop of blood.

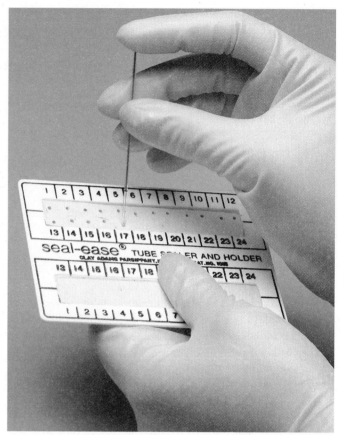

FIGURE 17–15(B) Carefully push glass tube into clay to seal one end before centrifugation.

more accurate reading may be obtained by reading the reacted reagent strip in a glucometer, Figure 17–21, page 536. There are several types, some of which may take a few moments to warm up before they can be used for reliable testing. Unless the machine has an automatic calibration mechanism incorporated within it, you should calibrate the glucose meter and follow directions for use according to the manufacturer's specifications. The operation manual and directions should be kept near the instrument for reference.

The normal fasting blood glucose range is from 80 to 120 mg/100 ml blood. The term *fasting* means that the patient has had nothing to eat or drink for a specific period of time, usually for 8 to 12 hours prior to the test. Fasting means that the patient should not even chew gum, eat mints, smoke, or drink water. Any stimulation of the digestive system may alter the results of the scheduled laboratory test.

GTT—Glucose Tolerance Test ....

The standard glucose tolerance test (GTT) determines a patient's ability to metabolize carbohydrates. This test is used primarily to aid in the diagnosis of diabetes mellitus and hypoglycemia. Usually, the patient is advised to eat a high-carbohydrate diet for 3 days before the scheduled GTT. The night before the procedure, the patient is required to have nothing to eat or drink from midnight on, or to fast for 8–12 hours before the test begins.

Fasting samples of blood and urine are obtained from the patient to begin this procedure. Then the patient is given 100 g of glucose (commercial preparation) orally. A half hour after the patient has consumed the glucose drink, samples of blood and urine are taken. Every hour thereafter, both blood and urine samples are taken for up to 6 hours, or for whatever time period the physician has ordered. Since accuracy is critically important in this test, timing and precise readings of the tests are vital in assessing glucose metabolism.

With today's highly skilled laboratory technicians, you will probably do few blood tests in the medical office. Some offices have their own labs in which laboratory technicians are employed to carry out tests that the medical assistant is not trained to do or is not licensed to do by law. The blood screening tests already mentioned are simple and require a minimal amount of instruction to perform. Proficiency in performing these minor tests will come with practice.

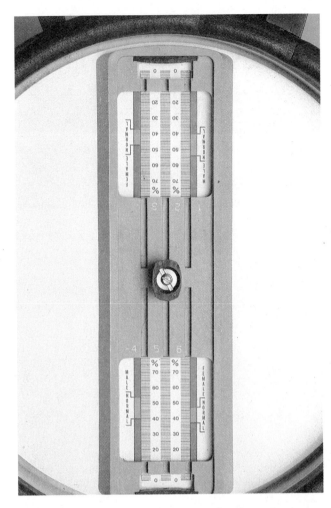

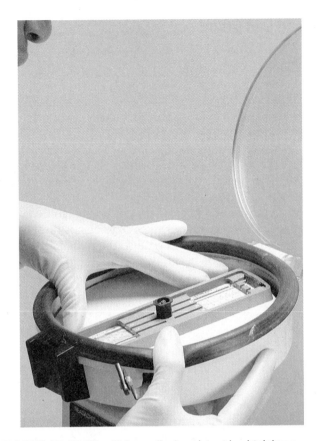

FIGURE 17–16 (C)   This medical assistant is obtaining a hematocrit reading by looking down onto the tube against the values chart within the centrifuge.

FIGURE 17–16 (A)   There are groove slots for up to six microhematocrit tubes to be centrifuged at once. Be sure to note the space number for each patient's hematocrit tube and write it down to avoid a mix-up. The clay sealant tray also has numbers along its side to help you keep track of several patients' specimens.

You may want to use the same number on the tray as in the centrifuge for each patient when there are two or more.

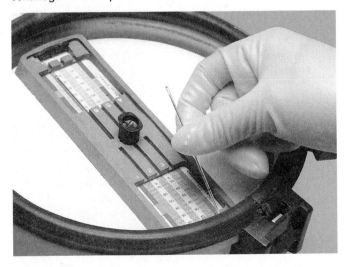

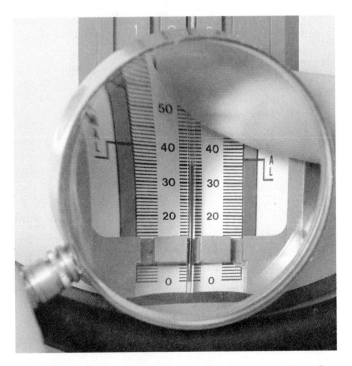

FIGURE 17–16 (D)   After centrifugation the hematocrit reading is obtained by placing the sealed end of the tube against the padding, making sure that the line between the packed red cells and the clay is at "0" (zero). Read the hematocrit at the bottom of the meniscus (the curved line where the red cells and the buffy coat meet). The reading in this photo is 35%.

FIGURE 17–16 (B)   Carefully place sealed end of tube (toward you) against the rubber padding in the microhematocrit centrifuge.

Blood Cell Count

Be sure to determine if it is lawful and within laboratory governing regulations before performing *any* diagnostic laboratory tests. Many of these tests must be performed by only licensed clinical laboratory technicians. These regulations have been made for quality assurance purposes. On occasion the physician wants to know a patient's red or white blood cell count immediately rather than waiting for lab results, to aid in diagnosis. Performing the test right in the office offers convenience to the physician and the patient as well. There are also times when the laboratory service may not be available, such as evenings and weekends when the physician is on call. For these reasons, especially in rural settings where a clinical laboratory may not be readily available, the medical assistant may be asked to perform a red or white blood cell count. Medical offices or clinics may have mechanical devices specifically designed to perform these types

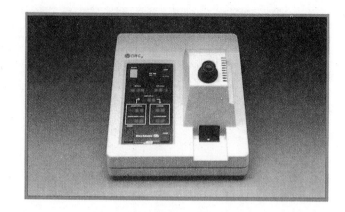

FIGURE 17–17 The QBCII, a centrifugal hematology system (Courtesy of Becton Dickinson and Company)

of blood counts for which in-service training should be provided by your employer, Figure 17–25, page 539.

P R O C E D U R E

Hemoglobin (Hb) Determination Using The Hemoglobinmeter

PURPOSE: Estimating the amount of Hb (iron-carrying protein) in the blood.

EQUIPMENT: Hemoglobinometer, glass chamber slide, hemolysis applicator (plastic or wooden), Autolet/sterile lancet, cotton balls, alcohol, latex gloves, gauze squares, Mayo table, batteries/light bulbs (as needed), patient's chart, pen

TERMINAL PERFORMANCE OBJECTIVE: With all necessary equipment/supplies provided, and using other students as patients, the student will demonstrate the steps required to perform a hemoglobin determination using the hemoglobinometer. The instructor will observe each step.

1. Assemble all needed items on Mayo table, check batteries and light bulb in hemoglobinometer and change if needed.
2. Explain procedure to identified patient.
3. Wash hands and put on latex gloves. Follow the desired skin puncture technique (procedure in this unit).
4. Pull the glass chamber out of the side of the hemoglobinometer and fix the lower part of the slide so that it is slightly offset.
5. Place a large drop of blood directly onto the offset glass chamber surface from the patient's finger (or other puncture site), Figure 17–20(a), page 536. Wipe the patient's finger with an alcohol-saturated cotton ball and give patient a dry gauze square to hold over the puncture site. **Key Point: Check to be sure bleeding has stopped.**
6. Mix the blood on the slide with the hemolysis applicator

to break down the cell membranes to release the hemoglobin. This is seen when the appearance of the blood becomes clear from cloudy and will take up to 45 seconds, Figure 17–20(b).

7. Push the chamber into the clip and place into the slot on the left side of the hemoglobinometer, Figure 17–20(c).
8. Hold the hemoglobinometer in your left hand at eye level, while using your left thumb to turn on the light by depressing the button on the bottom of the instrument. Look into the instrument to see a split green field.
9. Slide the button on the right side of the meter with your right thumb and index finger, while still looking into the meter, until a matching solid green field occurs. Leave the sliding scale on the calibrated line where the solid green field appeared.
10. Read the hemoglobin level at the top calibration scale for it is most frequently used (there are 4 on the scale). It is read in grams of hemoglobin per 100 ml of blood.
11. Wash chamber (and hemolysis applicator if reusable) with a detergent solution, rinse, dry and return to the hemoglobinometer for the next use, wash hands. Discard disposable items in proper receptacle, return items to proper storage area.
12. Remove gloves and wash hands. Place gloves in the proper receptacle.
13. Record the reading in the patient's chart, i.e., 14.5 gm/100 ml, initial.

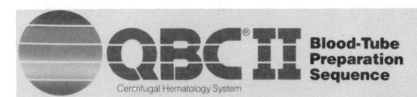

QBC® II Centrifugal Hematology System

Blood-Tube Preparation Sequence

| **Capillary Tube Preparation** Specimen: Finger-puncture blood | **Venous Tube Preparation** Specimen: EDTA-anticoagulated venous blood, well mixed and at room temperature. |

1 From end *nearest* two black lines, fill tube to level between the lines. Roll tube between fingers to mix blood with tube coating. Wipe blood from tube with lint-free cloth.

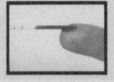

Insert end of tube nearest red lines into Pipetter. Aspirate blood specimen. Wipe blood from tube with lint-free cloth.

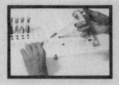

2 Invert slightly and allow blood to flow to other end. Roll tube between fingers AT LEAST 10 TIMES OR FOR AT LEAST 5 SECONDS to mix blood with orange coating.

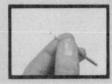

Press distal end of tube into closure. Remove tube from Pipetter. Twist closure to form a leak-tight seal.

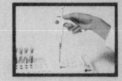

3 Press distal end of tube into closure. Twist closure to form a leak-tight seal.

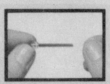

Roll tube between fingers AT LEAST 10 TIMES OR FOR AT LEAST 5 SECONDS to mix blood with tube coatings.

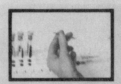

4 Slide tube over float. Gently push until float is inside tube as far as possible. Carefully lift closure end of tube until float is free of tray slot.

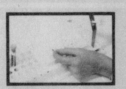

Slide tube over float. Gently push until float is inside tube as far as possible. Carefully lift closure end of tube until float is free of tray slot.

5 Insert open end of tube under flange of rotor nut, then lower tube into rotor slot of centrifuge. Slide closure against outer rim. Balance rotor if necessary, but retain tube identification. Install rotor cover and close lid. Centrifuge for 5 minutes.

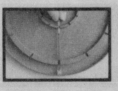

Insert open end of tube under flange of rotor nut, then lower tube into rotor slot of centrifuge. Slide closure against outer rim. Balance rotor if necessary, but retain tube identification. Install rotor cover and close lid. Centrifuge for 5 minutes.

6 Press the "CAP" mode key of the Reader. Insert the QBC Capillary-Blood Tube. Read the 7 interfaces according to instructions on reverse side of this card.

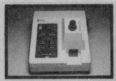

Press the "VEN" mode key of the Reader. Insert the QBC Venous-Blood Tube. Read the 6 interfaces according to instructions on reverse side of this card.

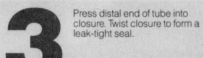

BECTON DICKINSON

Becton Dickinson
Primary Care Diagnostics
One Becton Drive
Franklin Lakes, NJ 07417-1882

© 1988 Becton Dickinson and Company
QBC is a trademark of Becton Dickinson and Company.
Printed in U.S.A.

QBC-7538H 6/88

4270-000-025 Rev A (7/88)

The QBC System is protected by U.S. Patent Numbers: 4,027,660; 4,082,085; 4,077,396; 4,159,896; 4,156,570; 4,091,659; 4,141,654; 4,137,755; 4,181,609; 4,209,226; 4,259,012; 4,190,328; as well as many foreign patents. Other patents pending.

FIGURE 17–18 Blood tube preparation sequence. After preparing the blood tubes, insert them into the QBC II for reading. (Courtesy of Becton Dickinson and Company)

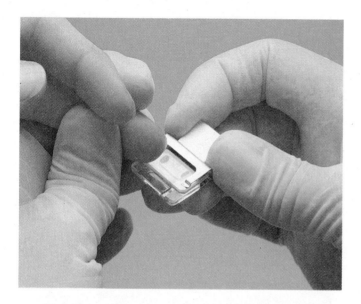

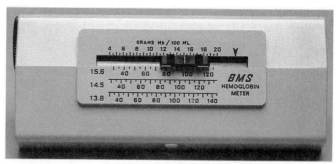

FIGURE 17–19 The hand-held hemoglobinometer

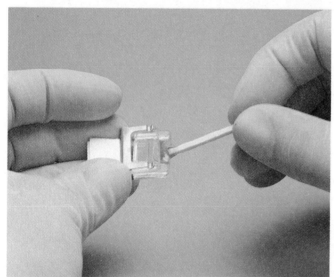

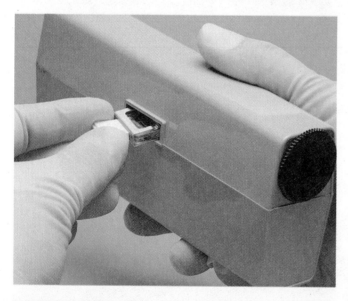

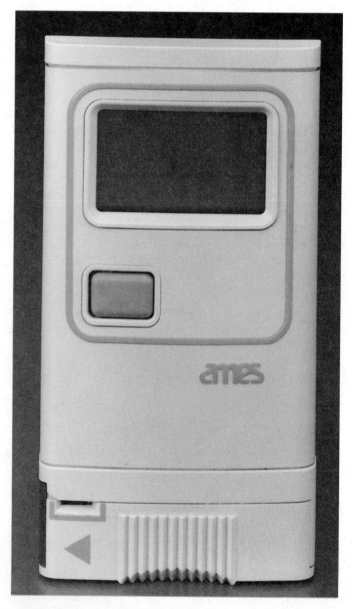

FIGURE 17–20 (A) Place capillary blood on glass chamber.
(B) Mix (hemolyze) blood with hemolysis applicator (wooden stick). **(C)** Push chamber into the clip and place in the slot in the side of the hemoglobinometer.

FIGURE 17–21 The Glucometer III for blood glucose screening tests, (Courtesy of Banyan International Corporation)

ORAL GLUCOSE METABOLISM

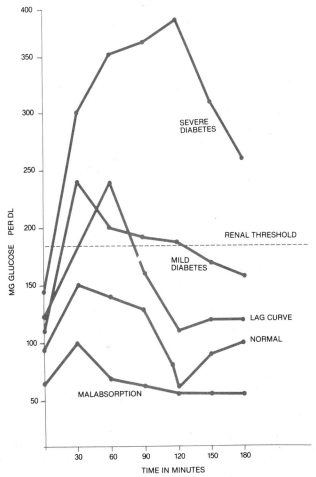

FIGURE 17–22 Graph of 3-hour glucose metabolism

The procedure for a GTT should be carefully explained to patients to gain their full cooperation. Many physicians order a 4-hour GTT. The graph in Figure 17–22 shows glucose metabolism for 3 hours (180 minutes). It is important to instruct patients to take along something to occupy their time (i.e., crossword puzzles, reading or writing materials, sewing) during this long procedure. They should also be told about the possibility of feeling weakness or fainting during the test. Patients must stay at the facility the entire time. Excessive sweating is also a common occurrence that one may experience. These symptoms should be reported to the lab technician or to whoever is administering the test. These reactions are considered normal when the blood glucose level falls as **insulin** is secreted into the blood in reaction to the glucose that has been ingested. Figure 17–23, page 538, shows a laboratory report form for glucose metabolism for a 3-hour GTT.

To do these procedures, you must become proficient in the use of a method of obtaining the blood sample and mixing it with a diluting solution to prepare the blood cells for counting on the hemocytometer. Mouth pipetting is an obsolete procedure on the advice of public

---

   P R O C E D U R E

Screen Blood Sugar (Glucose) Level

PURPOSE: To determine the sugar (glucose) level of the blood.
EQUIPMENT: Autolet/sterile lancet, reagent strips, bottle (for color chart) glucometer, latex gloves, cotton balls, alcohol, gauze squares, watch or clock, facial tissue
TERMINAL PERFORMANCE OBJECTIVE: Provided with all necessary equipment/supplies, and using other students as patients, the student will demonstrate the steps required in the procedure for determining blood glucose levels. The instructor will observe each step.

1. Assemble all needed items on Mayo table. **Key Point: If glucometer is to be used, make sure it has been turned on required time and has been calibrated for accuracy (follow manual of instruction).**
2. Identify patient and explain procedure. **Key Point: Call patient by name and check chart to avoid error. Be sure that patient has been fasting prior to testing.**
3. Wash hands and put latex gloves on.
4. Follow desired skin puncture procedure.
5. Open reagent strip bottle and take one of plastic strips out

without touching chemically treated pads. Re-close bottle.
6. From patient's finger apply large drop of blood so that pad is completely covered.
7. Begin timing *immediately* (stat) for *exactly* the amount of time specified by the manufacturer. Give patient dry gauze square to hold over puncture site after wiping it with alcohol-saturated cotton ball.
8. After the specified time, immediately blot pad firmly and quickly. **Key Point: Follow manufacturer's instruction precisely for timing and blotting.**
9. Immediately place the reagent strip into glucometer meter and close the door. The number displayed is the blood glucose level, Figure 17–24, page 539, OR Hold pad next to color chart of reagent strip bottle to compare color. The closest color match will indicate approximate glucose (sugar) level in blood.
10. Discard all used items in proper receptacle, remove gloves, and wash hands.
11. Record in patient's chart; for example, 98 mg/100 ml of blood. Initial.

DATE	PATIENT		ADDRESS	
☐ GLUCOSE TOLERANCE TEST			_____ HOURS	
TIME	BLOOD SUGAR	URINE SUGAR	ACETONE	PATIENT'S CONDITION (SYMPTOMS)
FASTING	mg/100ml			
½ HR	mg/100ml			
1 HR	mg/100ml			
2 HR	mg/100ml			
3 HR	mg/100ml			
4 HR	mg/100ml			
5 HR	mg/100ml			
6 HR	mg/100ml			
PHYSICIAN		PHONE	TECHNOLOGIST	

FIGURE 17–23 Laboratory report form for glucose tolerance test

health officials because of the danger of disease transmission. Mechanical devices are now used to draw solutions into a pipette as necessary. Figure 17–26, pages 542–543, presents a commonly used method for determining red and white blood cell counts. It is important to make certain which diluting fluid is used for either red or white blood cell counts. The reservoirs are marked, as are the containers they come in, as to which should be used. Practice in performing the procedures for erythrocyte and leukocyte counts is necessary for you to gain expertise in this skill.

Red Blood Cells. A red blood cell (erythrocyte) count is performed when symptoms indicate possible anemia. A decrease in the number of RBCs constitutes a form of anemia. The normal RBC count range for males is 4 to 6 million per cubic millimeter of blood and for females 4 to 5 million.

The function of the RBC is to transport oxygen to and carry carbon dioxide from the cells. It also contributes to the acid-base balance of the blood. If there is an insufficient number of RBCs in the bloodstream, the patient's symptoms will be lack of energy, fatigue, and, in severe cases, shortness of breath (SOB), pounding of the heart, rapid pulse, and **pallor.**

The iron-carrying protein, hemoglobin, gives the RBC its color. Erythrocytes have a biconcave disk shape and no nucleus when mature. They are formed in the red bone marrow of adults (**erythropoiesis**) and in the liver, spleen, and bone marrow of the fetus. The average life span of the RBC is about 120 days. The **reticuloendothelial** system, mostly the liver, bone marrow, and spleen, removes the worn-out red blood cells from the circulatory system.

P R O C E D U R E

Count Erythrocytes (RBCs) Manually

PURPOSE: To estimate the number of RBCs in a blood sample.
EQUIPMENT: Disposable self-filling diluting pipette with a plastic reservoir prefilled with exact amount of diluting solution, hemocytometer with cover glass slide, microscope, hand tally counter, pad and pen, patient's chart, detergent solution, gauze squares, latex gloves, paper towels, Mayo table
TERMINAL PERFORMANCE OBJECTIVE: Provided with all necessary equipment/supplies, the student will demonstrate each of the steps required to perform a manual RBC count. The instructor will observe and check each step.

1. Wash hands and put on latex gloves. Assemble needed items on Mayo table near patient.
2. Explain procedure to identified patient and perform skin puncture to obtain capillary blood sample.
3. Refer to Figure 17–25, and follow directions for filling the Unopette® pipette and reservoir.
4. After you have the hemocytometer charged with the solution, allow the cells to settle for 2–3 minutes on ruled counting chamber.
5. Carefully place slide on stage of microscope, turn light source on, and move nosepiece to select low-power objective. Scan square in ruled area for even distribution of cells. Check other side of slide in the same manner.
6. When an equal distribution of cells has been determined, turn nosepiece to high-power objective and focus on top left square in red counting area, Figure 17–27(A), page 544. Ruling is much smaller than in white blood cell field. Adjust light and fine focus as necessary. Count only cells with a concave, disk-like appearance that are on the top and left lines and within squares. Count in a pattern to avoid recounting cells, Figure 17–27(B). Count cells in all five squares in order from A to E. There are 16 smaller squares in each larger square. Write the number of cells counted in each larger square. Count both sides to be certain of equal distribution of cells.
7. Add total number of cells counted in all five squares (of one side of hemacytometer) and multiply by 10,000 to get the number of RBCs in a cubic millimeter of blood.
8. Record RBC count on patient's chart and initial.
9. Wash hemocytometer with detergent solution, rinse, and dry with paper towels. Return items to proper storage area, discard used disposable items in proper receptacle, remove gloves, and wash hands.

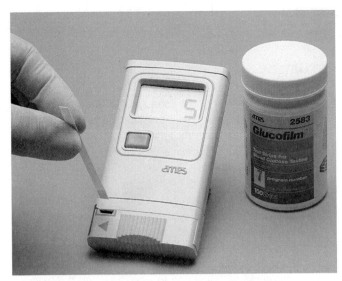

FIGURE 17–24 Insert reagent strip into glucometer and read glucose level after hearing the beep at 22 seconds.

White Blood Cells

A white blood cell (leukocyte) count is done when symptoms indicate possible infection in the body. An increase in WBCs signifies that the process of phagocytosis (WBCs combating infection by engulfing microorganisms or other foreign particles or cells and forming pus) is taking place. The normal leukocyte count for males and females is from 5 to 10 thousand per cubic millimeter of blood. Leukocytes are formed in the bone marrow, lymph nodes, spleen, and the lining of various visceral organs. The chief function of the WBCs is to aid in the body's defense against disease.

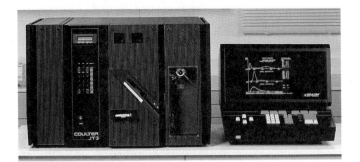

FIGURE 17–25 The COULTER® JT3 Hematology system was designed to meet the needs of the moderate-volume health care facility

Differential Count

One of the most vital tests generally performed with the complete blood count (CBC) is the differential count. This count determines the number and percentage of each of the five different types of white blood cells (leukocytes). Each has a specific function as outlined in Table 17–3, page 541. Preferably the differential count is made from a fresh whole blood specimen. This blood smear is usually sent to a clinical or hospital laboratory where it is stained by a skilled certified laboratory technician who also determines the platelet count. The morphology of the erythrocytes is also noted during this microscopic examination. Figure 17–28, page 544, is a drawing of normal blood cells.

Some laboratories provide an apparatus for slide preparation of blood smears, which will be demonstrated at your request. A blood smear can be obtained from capillary or venous blood by placing a moderate

---

P R O C E D U R E

Count Leukocytes (WBCs) Manually

PURPOSE: To estimate the number of WBCs in a blood sample.

EQUIPMENT: Disposable self-filling diluting pipette with a plastic reservoir prefilled with exact amount of diluting solution, hemocytometer with cover glass slide, microscope, hand tally counter, pad and pen, patient's chart, detergent solution, gauze squares, latex gloves, paper towels, Mayo table

TERMINAL PERFORMANCE OBJECTIVE: Provided with all necessary equipment/supplies, the student will demonstrate each of the steps required to perform a manual WBC count. The instructor will observe and check each step.

1–5. Same as for RBC counts.
  6. When an equal distribution of cells has been determined, leave nosepiece on low-power objective and

focus on top left square in the WBC counting area, Figure 17–27(a), page 544. Count the cells in each of the 16 small squares, counting those on the top and left lines and all cells within the squares. Adjust the fine focus as needed. White blood cells will look like solid dark dots, like periods on this page. Follow the pattern for counting cells as in Figure 17–27(b), page 544. Use the hand tally counter to record the number of cells you see. Count cells in all four large outer squares in order from 1–4. Write the number of cells counted in each of the four large squares.

  7. Add total number of cells in all four squares and multiply by 50 to get the total number of WBCs in a cubic millimeter of blood.

8–9. Same as for RBC counts.

Making A Blood Smear

PURPOSE: To make an adequate blood smear for a *differential* white blood cell count.

EQUIPMENT: Latex gloves, sterile lancet (or skin puncture device with sterile lancet) or CBC (lavender-stoppered) blood collection tube with needle adapter attached, or needle and syringe (for venipuncture procedure), alcohol, cotton balls or gauze squares, fresh clean glass slides with frosted ends, pencil, pen, laboratory request form, patient's chart

TERMINAL PERFORMANCE OBJECTIVE: Provided with all necessary equipment/supplies, the student will demonstrate the steps required to make an adequate blood smear for a differential white blood cell count. The instructor will observe and check each step.

1. Explain procedure to identified patient. Complete laboratory request form. Print patient's name and date on the frosted end of the glass slide with the pencil.
2. Assemble all needed items on Mayo table near patient.
3. Wash hands and put on latex gloves.
4. Perform desired method for obtaining blood specimen (either capillary or venous blood may be used).
5. Place a small drop of blood approximately a quarter inch from the frosted end of the glass slide (the drop of blood should be approximately one-eighth of an inch in diameter), Figure 17–29, page 545. If blood is obtained from the patient's finger, touch the drop of blood carefully to the slide (do not press the blood onto the slide or smudging will occur). If the blood is obtained by needle and syringe, depress plunger to allow a drop of blood to fall onto the end of the glass slide. If the blood is obtained from the needle and adapter, press in on the CBC blood tube attached (within the adapter) to allow a drop of blood to fall onto the glass slide.

6. Hold the corners of the frosted end of the glass slide down on a flat surface with the thumb and index finger of one hand, and with the other hand hold the second glass slide with the thumb and index (or great) finger at a 45 degree angle (if smear is too thick, the angle of spreading should be decreased; too thin, increased). Rest the spreader slide against the first one and move it back carefully into the drop of blood. The blood will follow the edge of the slide evenly across the glass. Move the angled slide toward the frosted end quickly and gently (pressure will hemolyze blood cells). (The second glass slide is used to evenly spread the blood over the first slide thereby distributing the blood cells for the differential white blood cell count.) The smear should have a *feather-edge.* This is the area of the blood smear where the technician examines the cells. If the slide has been prepared properly, the red cells will be in an even monolayer and the white blood cells will be evenly distributed. It should not be too thick or cells are overly crowded, making counting difficult; if too thin it results in an inadequate number of cells to count.
7. Allow the blood smear to air dry, or carefully fan it in the air to expedite drying (blowing on the smear may disturb the cells). Quickly drying the cells helps them keep their shape and avoids reduction in their size.
8. Place blood smear into appropriate container (attach completed lab request form) for transport to laboratory. Generally the slide will accompany a CBC request with a lavender stoppered blood-filled tube.
9. Remove latex gloves and wash hands. Discard all waste in appropriate containers.
10. Initial procedure in patient's chart.

---

drop of blood on a glass slide (frosted side up) and labeling it with pencil. A second glass slide is used to distribute the blood cells evenly over three-fourths of the slide, ending in a feathered tip. Practice is necessary in developing skill and proficiency in making good blood smears.

The procedure for making a blood smear for the purpose of a differential count includes directions regarding various methods of obtaining blood specimens.

Complete Chapter 17, Unit 2 in the workbook to help you meet the objectives at the beginning of this unit and therefore achieve competency of this subject matter.

UNIT 3
Venous Blood Tests

OBJECTIVES

Upon completion of this unit, the student will meet the following terminal performance objectives by verifying knowledge of the facts and principles presented through oral and written communication at a level deemed competent, and will demonstrate the specific behaviors as

TABLE 17–3
Categories of White Blood Cells and Their Functions

White Cell Type	Percent in Normal WBC	Function
Granulocytes		
Neutrophils		Phagocytosis and killing of bacteria; release of pyrogen that produces fever
Segmented	56	
Band	3	
Eosinophils	2.7	Phagocytosis of antigen-antibody complexes; killing of parasites
Basophils	0.3	Release of chemical mediators of immediate hypersensitivity
Lymphocytes	34	
B lymphocytes		Humoral immunity; production of specific antibodies against viruses, bacteria, and other proteins
T lymphocytes		Cell-mediated immunity including delayed hypersensitivity and graft rejection; regulation of immune response
Monocytes	4	Phagocytosis of microorganisms and cell debris; cooperation in immune response

identified in the terminal performance objectives of the procedures, observing all aseptic and safety precautions in accordance with health care standards.

1. Prepare blood specimens to be sent to an outside laboratory.
2. Perform a venipuncture by either the sterile needle and syringe method or the vacuum method.
3. Explain how to obtain serum from whole blood.
4. Determine an erythrocyte sedimentation rate (ESR).
5. List the different colors used to code blood specimen tubes and what they stand for.
6. Spell and define, using the glossary at the back of the text, all the words to know in this unit.

WORDS TO KNOW ....

elasticity	heparin	sedimentation
gauge	legible	tourniquet
hematoma	oxygenate	venipuncture
hemolysis	prothrombin	venous

Venous means pertaining to the veins. As veins return blood to the heart and lungs to be **oxygenated** and recirculated, they carry the waste products of the body. Venous blood tests permit measurement of the kind and amount of those waste products.

Venipuncture ....

When more than a few drops of blood are required to perform tests, a venipuncture is performed. **Venipuncture** is the surgical puncture of a vein.

Usually the patient is seated in a chair with the arm supported for the venipuncture procedure. In the event that a patient does faint from this position, the needle must be withdrawn, the **tourniquet** removed, and a bandage held over the puncture site first. Then the patient must be helped carefully to the floor. Spirits of ammonia may be used to help revive the patient. The physician should check the patient before you proceed further. Patients who say they feel faint should put their head down between their knees. Usually this will help within a few minutes and the procedure can be accomplished with no further interruptions. Often following a complete physical examination, the patient may still be lying on the examination table. This makes an ideal work area for the medical assistant and the position for the patient is most comfortable. In case the patient feels faint there is no worry of accidental falling when the patient is lying down. The law regarding venipuncture varies from state to state. Usually the physician is aware of it and will not ask you to perform the procedure unless it is lawful.

PATIENT EDUCATION

Explaining the procedure and making the patient comfortable will be of great importance. If the patient shows any signs of apprehension, ask the patient to lie down and try to relax. This eliminates the possibility of a patient falling as the result of fainting during the procedure. Some patients experience a queasy (nauseated) feeling, so it is a good idea to keep an emesis basin nearby. Displaying competency and efficiency in carrying out the procedure will gain the patient's confidence and cooperation.

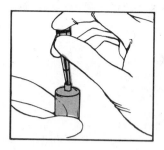

1. Puncture diaphragm

Using the protective shield on the capillary pipette, puncture the diaphragm of the reservoir as follows:

a. Place reservoir on a flat surface. Grasping reservoir in one hand, take pipette assembly in other hand. Push tip of pipette shield firmly through diaphragm in neck of reservoir, then remove.

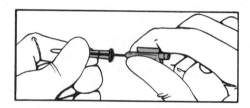

b. Remove shield from pipette assembly with a twist.

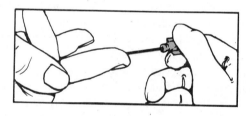

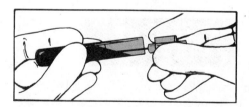

2. Add sample

Fill capillary with sample and transfer to reservoir as follows:

a. Holding pipette *almost* horizontally, touch tip of pipette to sample. (See alternate methods in illustrations above.) Pipette will fill by capillary action. Filling is complete and will stop automatically when sample reaches end of capillary bore in neck of pipette.

b. Wipe excess sample from outside of capillary pipette, making certain that no sample is removed from capillary bore.

c. Squeeze reservoir slightly to force out some air. Do not expel any liquid. Maintain pressure on reservoir.

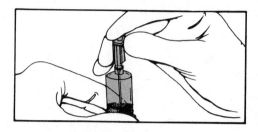

d. Cover opening of overflow chamber with index finger and seat pipette *securely* in reservoir neck.

e. Release pressure on reservoir. Then remove finger from pipette opening. Negative pressure will draw blood into diluent.

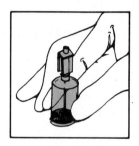

f. Squeeze reservoir *gently* two or three times to rinse capillary bore, forcing diluent into, *but not out of,* overflow chamber, releasing pressure each time to return mixture to reservoir.

CAUTION: If reservoir is squeezed too hard, some of the specimen may be expelled through the top of the overflow chamber.

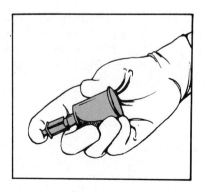

g. Place index finger over upper opening and gently invert several times to thoroughly mix sample with diluent.

3. Count cells (option 1)

Mix diluted blood thoroughly by inverting reservoir (see 2g) to resuspend cells immediately prior to actual count.

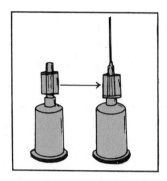

a. Convert to dropper assembly by withdrawing pipette from reservoir and reseating securely in reverse position.

b. Invert reservoir, gently squeeze sides and discard first three or four drops.

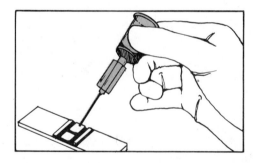

c. Carefully charge hemacytometer with diluted blood by gently squeezing sides of reservoir to expel contents until chamber is properly filled.

OR

3. Transfer contents (option 2)

Transfer thoroughly mixed contents of each reservoir to appropriately labeled test tubes or corresponding cuvettes as follows:

a. Convert reservoir to dropper assembly by withdrawing pipette and reseating securely in reverse position as shown above.

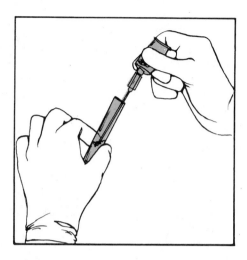

b. Place capillary tip into appropriately labeled test tube or cuvette which will accommodate 5.0 ml of reagent and squeeze reservoir to expel entire contents.

OR

3. Store diluted specimen (option 3)

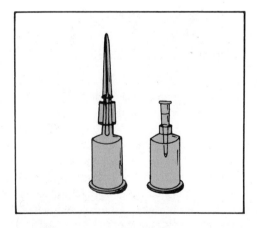

Cover overflow chamber with capillary shield or remove capillary and insert tip of shield firmly into reservoir opening. (Note time for which diluted specimen remains stable for each test.)

FIGURE 17–26 Procedure for using the Unopette® system to collect and prepare blood specimens for hematology and chemistry studies. Each unit of the system consists of a disposable diluting pipette and a plastic reservoir containing a premeasured volume of reagent for diluting. (Courtesy of Becton Dickinson VACUTAINER Systems)

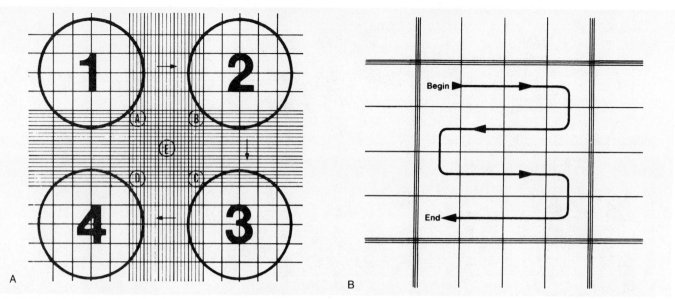

FIGURE 17–27 Counting blood cells. (a). The ruled counting area on the surface of the counting chamber (hemocytometer), white blood cells are counted in the four large outside corner squares (labeled 1, 2, 3, and 4) and red blood cells are counted in the five smaller squares (labeled A, B, C, D, and E) contained in the middle square. (b). Pattern for counting cells

The area of choice for venipuncture is most often the inner arm at the bend of the elbow, Figure 17–30. The veins in this area are the median basilic and the median cephalic (commonly referred to as antecubital veins). A means of promoting better palpation and sometimes visual position of the veins is a tourniquet. Tourniquets are available in many materials. Soft, flat vinyl/rubber tubing is probably most popular. It is also economical. It comes in widths of 1 to 2 inches and can be cut into any length desired, usually from 12 to 16 inches. Thinner

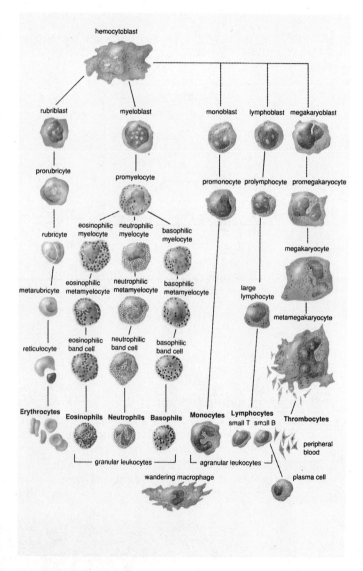

FIGURE 17–28 Blood cells and platelets

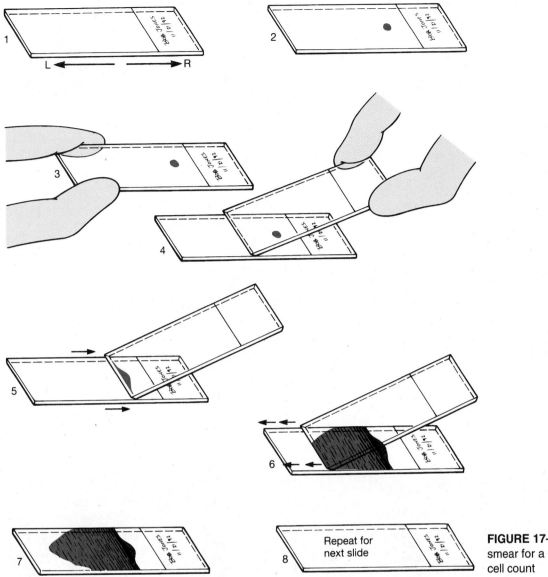

FIGURE 17–29 Making a blood smear for a differential white blood cell count

vinyl or rubber tubing is also popular, but it tends to pinch the skin. Tubing is easily washed with a detergent solution and quickly cleaned with alcohol and a cotton ball. Velcro tourniquets are cloth strips, approximately $1\frac{1}{2}$ to 2 inches wide. They are not so easily cleaned and are not elasticized so cannot be used on patients with larger than average arms.

The tourniquet is placed on the patient's upper arm, about inches above the elbow. Before applying the tourniquet it is a good idea to check both arms of the patient or simply ask which arm is better for this procedure. Many patients have had the procedure performed and know that one arm is better. Some patients will have a preferred arm because of their work or planned activities. Some patients are extremely difficult to obtain blood from. It may be necessary in these cases to draw the sample from a vein on the back of the hand. These veins are small and the procedure is painful. The tourniquet should be applied just above the wrist in this case. Venipuncture must always be done carefully to avoid

causing a hematoma (collection of blood just under the skin). Gentle pressure applied immediately on withdrawing the needle will help avoid this problem.

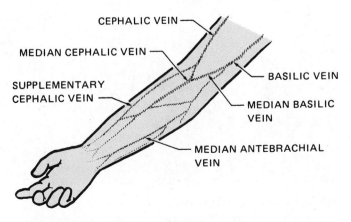

FIGURE 17–30 The veins of the arm. The median cephalic vein is most often used for venipuncture.

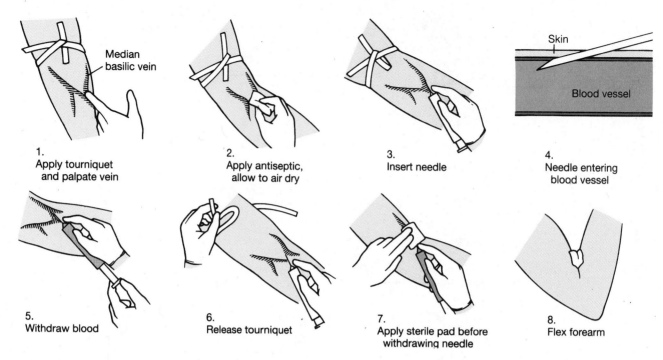

1.
Apply tourniquet and palpate vein

Median basilic vein

2.
Apply antiseptic, allow to air dry

3.
Insert needle

4.
Needle entering blood vessel

Skin

Blood vessel

5.
Withdraw blood

6.
Release tourniquet

7.
Apply sterile pad before withdrawing needle

8.
Flex forearm

FIGURE 17–31 Collecting a venous blood specimen by needle and syringe method

Use a cotton ball saturated with alcohol to swab the entire area. The alcohol will help make the skin more sensitive to your touch. Slowly move your fingertip across the patient's arm at the bend of the elbow. Veins have elasticity and will give somewhat when depressed. Feeling the subtle spring-back movement will help you find a suitable vein for the procedure. Having the patient clench the fist will help make the veins stand out, to the touch if not to the sight.

There are two methods of performing this procedure: (1) the syringe/sterile needle method, and (2) the vacuum

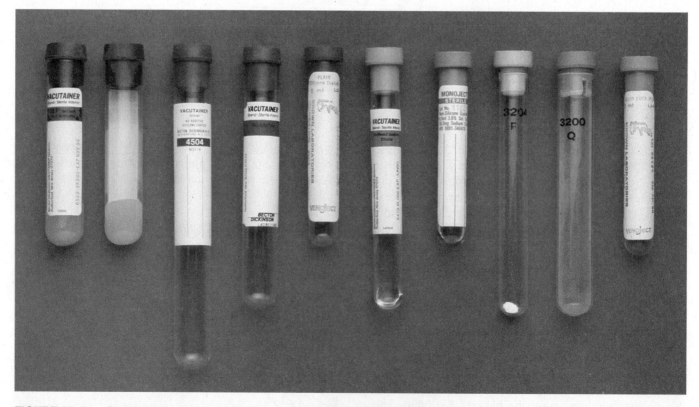

FIGURE 17–32 Blood collection tubes (from left to right): red/gray for whole blood with gel for serum separation; red for whole or clotted blood specimens; lavender for whole blood tests (contains anticoagulant); blue for whole blood for coagulation tests (contains anticoagulant); gray for whole blood for glucose tests (contains anticoagulant)

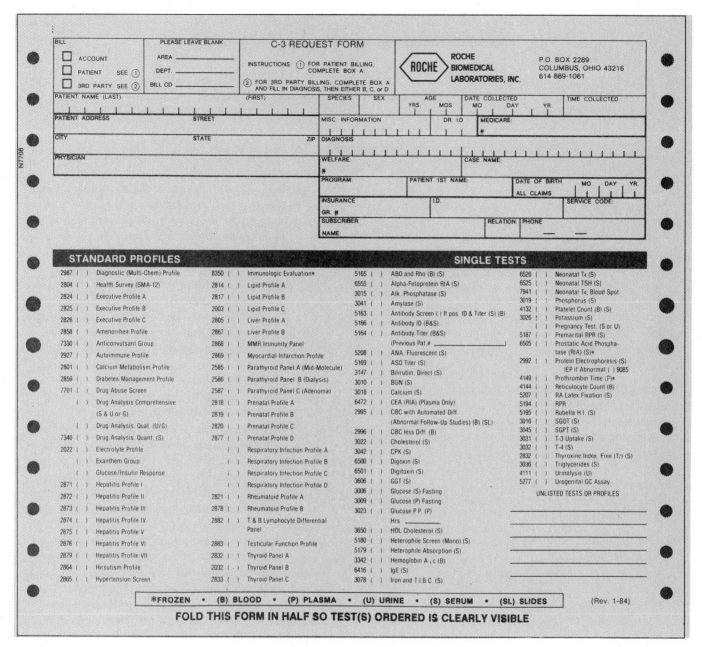

FIGURE 17–33 Laboratory request form for hematology

tube/sterile needle method. Sterile technique must be used because a foreign object is introduced directly into the vein.

A 20–21-gauge needle is usually used. The gauge must be large enough to allow blood to flow through the needle without causing hemolysis (breakdown of blood cells).

The needle and syringe method is always used when very small veins are involved because it is less damaging to the tissues than the vacuum method, Figure 17–31. The size of the syringe will vary according to the amount of blood needed. Usually a 20 to 30-cc syringe is used when drawing several tubes, each 5 to 15 ml.

The vacuum method is probably the most popular because it is so convenient. Blood specimens enter directly into the tubes for the desired tests rather than having to be transferred. It is vital that the correct tubes be used, however.

Specimen test tubes are color coded for the various hematology departments in the lab, Figure 17–32. Red-stoppered tubes come in sizes ranging from 3 to 15 ml. They are used to collect whole blood that is allowed to clot so that the serum can be drawn off by centrifugation. The serum can be drawn out by a disposable pipette and deposited into a transfer tube, which is labeled for the particular test to be done. There are other methods to easily transfer serum from the centrifuged tube. The most efficient way is to use the red/gray stoppered tube, which has a gel in the bottom. During centrifugation, the gel liquifies and travels to the center of the tube separat-

Obtain Venous Blood With Sterile Needle And Syringe

PURPOSE: To obtain venous blood specimens when the amount needed is more than a few drops.

EQUIPMENT: Sterile needle (20–21 G, 1–1$\frac{1}{2}$ inch length), adequate size syringe for specimen tubes, pen, patient's chart, alcohol, latex gloves, cotton balls, tourniquet, lab request form, rubber band, gauze squares, adhesive bandage, spirits of ammonia, emesis basin, and biohazardous waste container should be within reach

Note: A utility bucket is a convenient way to carry all necessary items for venipuncture procedures. It should be stocked with lab request forms, specimen tubes, cotton balls, alcohol dispenser, syringes, sterile needles, sharps container, latex gloves, tourniquet, frosted end slides, adapter for vacuum tube method, pen and pencil, rubber bands, gauze squares, spirits of ammonia, and bandages. This handy carrier may be set next to the patient. It should be restocked daily during routine checking of supplies.

TERMINAL PERFORMANCE OBJECTIVE: Provided with all necessary equipment/supplies, and using a training arm model, the student will demonstrate the steps necessary for obtaining venous blood using the sterile needle and syringe method. The instructor will observe each step. Note: The instructor will determine the student's skill in the performance of this procedure on other students/patients. Use the picture guide in Figure 17–31, page 546, to help you with this procedure.

1. Wash hands, put on latex gloves, and assemble all needed items on Mayo table next to patient: **Key Point: Label all required specimen tubes and complete lab request form.**

2. Identify patient. **Key Point: Call patient by name and check chart to avoid error.**

3. Explain procedure to patient and ask if there is a preferred venipuncture site. If patient has no preference, visually check both arms and select a vein which can be palpated (felt) easily with your fingertip after application of alcohol. **Key Point: Ask patient to lie down if there is any sign of apprehension. Most commonly, patient will be sitting down with arm extended and supported on arm rest of chair or on a table. Providing a comfortable position will relax the patient and elicit better cooperation.**

4. Secure needle onto syringe by holding needle guard in one hand and turning syringe barrel clockwise. Push plunger of syringe all the way in to release any air from barrel. **Key Point: Loosen needle guard but keep it over tip of needle to protect it from contamination and set aside.**

5. Apply tourniquet to patient's upper arm, about 3 inches above bend in elbow. Bring ends of tourniquet up evenly and cross them. Switch, so that you are holding an end in each hand comfortably. Stretch end in your right hand to apply gentle pressure over area of arm while you hold other end against patient's arm. Tuck excess of stretched end under section which is held against arm so that there is nothing in way of puncture site. **Key Point: Proceed quickly, as tourniquet may not be left on any longer than 1 minute. If tourniquet is applied too tightly it will prevent blood flow and patient will be most uncomfortable.**

6. Clean site with lightly alcohol-saturated cotton ball and let air dry. **Key Point: Blowing on site to dry it will contaminate tissue.** Ask patient to make a fist and hold it until you say to release it. This will assist further in making vein stand up. Take off needle guard and, with bevel of needle up, insert needle tip into vein with a quick and steady motion, following path of vein at approximately 15-degree angle. Holding skin at site to stretch it slightly will help keep vein from moving as puncture takes place. **Key Point: Needle should be inserted no more than 1/4 to 1/2 inch or it may pass through vein.**

7. Hold barrel of syringe in one hand and with other hand pull plunger back slowly and steadily until barrel is filled with amount of blood needed to fill specimen tubes.

8. Ask patient to release clenched fist. Release tourniquet by quickly pulling up on end of portion which is tucked in. Pull needle out in same path as it was inserted and place gauze square over site as needle is withdrawn. **Key Point: Ask patient to bend arm slightly to help stop bleeding.**

9. Quickly fill required specimen tubes by inserting needle into rubber-stoppered end. Vacuum tubes fill easily because vacuum draws blood in. Forcing blood into tubes by pushing plunger of syringe will cause hemolysis. If tubes are not vacuum type, gently push plunger of syringe to fill tubes. **Key Point: Specimen tubes must be filled quickly, for clotting will begin within minutes in barrel of syringe. Blood smears should be made at this time if needed.**

10. Gently mix blood in tubes that contain an anticoagulant in a figure-eight motion. Stand red-stoppered tubes vertically to clot so that serum can be drawn after centrifugation. **Key Point: Do not shake or mix blood in red-stoppered tubes or hemolysis will occur.**

11. Deposit needle and syringe intact in sharps biohazardous waste container. Wrap labeled specimen tubes together with lab request form and secure with rubber band. **Key Point: Keep near centrifuge so that serum-only transfer tube(s) may be added when completed.**

12. Attend to patient's needs; apply bandage over puncture site.

13. Discard disposables in proper receptacle and return items to proper storage area. Remove gloves and wash hands.

14. Record procedure on patient's chart and initial.

ing the red cells from the serum. You can then carefully pour the serum into a transfer tube and label for analysis. Another method is to place a slender rubber-tipped tube down carefully into the centrifuged tube (pushing the tube down forcefully will result in hemolysis) just to the meniscus of the packed red cells. The screened filtered opening at the rubber end of the inner tube allows the serum to fill the tube leaving the red cells at the bottom. You pour off the serum into a transfer tube and label for analysis. Lavender-stoppered tubes, or CBC tubes, are usually 5 or 10 ml. They are also used to collect whole blood specimens but they contain an anticoagulant so that tests which require whole blood may be performed. Gray-stoppered tubes are used in blood glucose tests and are usually 5 ml. They contain a different anticoagulant from the CBC tubes. Blue-stoppered tubes (sometimes green) are most often 5 ml and are used to collect specimens for testing prothrombin time, blood gases, and pH. The anticoagulant is different from the glucose tube or the CBC tube and is called heparin. Tests drawn in the blue tubes should be performed within 2 hours for accurate results. Blood should be drawn into the tubes in the order that they have been discussed if tubes for various tests have been ordered.

Blood in specimen tubes that contain an anticoagulant must be mixed immediately in a figure-eight motion 8 to 10 times. Gentle mixing will prevent hemolysis. The tubes with the red stoppers must be allowed to stand vertically and undisturbed for at least 20 to 30 minutes to allow clotting to occur. The tube(s) must then be properly balanced in a centrifuge and spun for 20 to 30 minutes. The serum, which is a clear, light yellow liquid, is then carefully drawn off with a pipette (usually disposable ones provided by the laboratory) or by using one of the methods discussed earlier. Refer back to Figure 17–1, page 518, to see the serum separated from the centrifuged red blood in the tube the medical assistant is holding and preparing to pour into the transfer tube.

Blood collection tubes and supplies must be checked for the expiration date, and if out of date, not used. This is in compliance with quality control and quality assurance regulations. A log book must be kept of all specimens collected and sent for analysis. The log book must contain the following information:

1. Date collected
2. Patient's full name, address, and phone number
3. Date sent to lab
4. Test requested
5. Date results received
6. Test results

Saf-T Clik Shielded Blood Needle Adapter

Instructions For Use
PREPARATION

1. Before attaching needle, push ends of Saf-T Click® together to insure outer sleeve is seated.

2. Open needle cartridge. Twist to break the tamperproof seal. Remove cartridge cap to expose rear needle with threaded hub. Do not remove front needle cover. Use up to 1½″ blood collection needle.

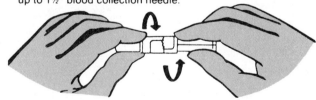

3. Attach needle to Safety Adapter. Screw needle into Safety Adapter until firmly seated.

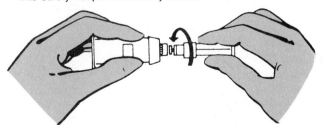

AFTER VENIPUNCTURE

4. When sampling is complete, grasp the Safety Adapter's outer sheath sliding it forward over the exposed contaminated needle until a distinctive "CLICK" is heard. "LOCKED, LOCKED" is visible when Adapter is locked. The contaminated needle is now safely covered.

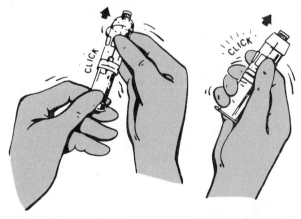

Two Handed Technique   One Handed Technique

5. Discard the Safety Adapter/Contaminated Needle Assembly according to hospital procedures. Do not reuse needle/Safety Adapter.

FIGURE 17–34   Instructions for using the Saf-T Clik® shielded blood needle adapter (Courtesy Ryan Medical, Inc.)

PROCEDURE

Obtain Venous Blood With Vacuum Tube

PURPOSE: To obtain venous blood specimens when the amount needed is more than a few drops.

EQUIPMENT: Multiple sample sterile needles (20–21 G, 1–1$\frac{1}{2}$ inch length), plastic adapter (the Saf-T Click shielded blood needle adapter is recommended for safety), labeled specimen tubes (vacuum), alcohol, latex gloves, sharps container, cotton balls, gauze squares, tourniquet, lab request forms, rubber bands, pen, patient's chart, bandages, biohazardous waste container

TERMINAL PERFORMANCE OBJECTIVE: Provided with all necessary equipment/supplies, and using a training arm model, the student will demonstrate the steps necessary for obtaining venous blood using the vacuum tube method. The instructor will observe each step. Note: The instructor will determine the student's skill in the performance of this procedure on other students/patients.

1–2. Same as for needle and syringe.

3. Secure needle onto adapter by screwing grooved end of needle into grooved tip of adapter, holding needle guard and turning adapter in clockwise motion. Set aside.

4. (Same as for needle and syringe.)

5. Clean site with lightly alcohol-saturated cotton ball and let air dry. (Blowing on site to dry it will contaminate skin.) Push rubber-stoppered end of vacuum tube into adapter until needle is inserted just into rubber to hold tube in place, Figure 17–36. Ask patient to make a fist and hold it. This will assist further in making vein stand up. Take off needle guard and, with bevel of needle up, insert tip of needle into vein with a quick and steady motion, following path of vein at approximately a 15-degree angle. **Key Point: Holding skin at site to stretch it slightly will help keep vein from moving as puncture takes place. Needle should be inserted no more than $\frac{1}{4}$ to $\frac{1}{2}$ inch or it may pass through vein.**

6. Hold adapter with one hand and with other hand place your index and great fingers on either side of protruding edges of adapter. Push vacuum tube completely into adapter with your thumb, allowing needle to puncture rubber stopper. Blood will flow into tube by vacuum force if other end of needle is in vein properly. When tube is filled, pull it out of adapter by holding it between your thumb and great finger and pushing against adapter with your index finger. **Key Point: Fill required number of tubes for tests ordered by physician. Begin with red, then gray, lavender-blue, in that order. Remember to mix blood with anticoagulant gently by figure-eight motion.**

7. Ask patient to release clenched fist. Release tourniquet by quickly pulling up on end of portion which is tucked in. Pull needle out of vein in path of insertion and place gauze square over site as needle is withdrawn. Ask patient to bend arm slightly to help stop bleeding and apply gentle pressure. **Key Point: If a blood smear is needed for a differential, turn CBC (lavender) tube (still attached to adapter) upside down and gently press tube down to release drop of blood onto glass slide.** Make blood smear, or as many as have been ordered, label frosted end with pencil, air dry quickly and send with other specimens.

8. Set red tubes vertically to clot so that serum can be obtained by centrifugation for serum-only tests.

9. Same as steps 10–14 for needle and syringe, except for disposing of needle from plastic adapter carefully into biohazardous waste/sharps container. If Saf-T Click is used, dispose of the entire locked unit in the biohazardous waste/sharps container. Table 17–4 lists laboratory normal value ranges of commonly performed venous blood test results.

Often specimens are sent by mail or shipped to out of town or out of state to laboratories for analysis, Figure 17–33, page 547. The federal government requires that specimens are shipped/transported in securely closed, watertight containers. Blood tubes should be enclosed in a second durable watertight container. Then specimens should be wrapped in layers of paper towels to absorb any possible breakage or leakage during transportation. The doubly secured specimens are then placed in a shipping container of fiberboard, wood, or heavy cardboard with a label stating it is biohazardous. It is then ready for safe transport to the reference laboratory. A second label should read: in case of breakage send to this address: Centers for Disease Control, Attention: Biohazards Control Office, 1600 Clifton Road, Atlanta, GA 30333.

Figure 17–34, page 549, shows instructions for use of the Saf-T Clik shielded blood needle adapter. It was designed to protect the phlebotomist from accidental needle injury, thereby reducing possible disease transmission. This adapter may be used with all standard blood collection needles and does not change the procedure for venipuncture. After its use, the phlebotomist simply slides the protective sheath forward until the "click" is heard and the needle is safely covered and

TABLE 17–4
Normal Values of Commonly Performed Laboratory Tests

Chemistry

Total cholesterol	130–200 mg/dl
HDL cholesterol	45–65 mg/dl
LDL cholesterol	90–130 mg/dl
Glucose	80–120 mg/dl
Triglyceride	40–150 mg/dl
Creatinine	0.7–1.4 mg/dl
Uric acid	3.5–7.5 mg/dl
BUN	8–20 mg/dl
Sodium	132–142 mEq/L
Potassium	4–5 mEq/L
Chloride	98–106 mEq/L
CO_2	25–32 mEq/L

Hematology

White blood cell count	5.000–10,000/mm3
Red blood cell count	3.5–5.5 x 10/mm3
Hemoglobin	12–16 g/dl
Hematocrit	35.5–49%
Sedimentation rate	0–10 mm/hr
Platelet count	150,000–350,000/mm3
Coagulation	
Prothrombin time	11–13 sec

locked so that there is no danger of injury to the phlebotomist or patient. Figure 17–35 is an actual photo of Saf-T Click shielded blood needle adapter covered and locked after use. It is completely disposable and must be discarded in the biohazardous waster receptacle.

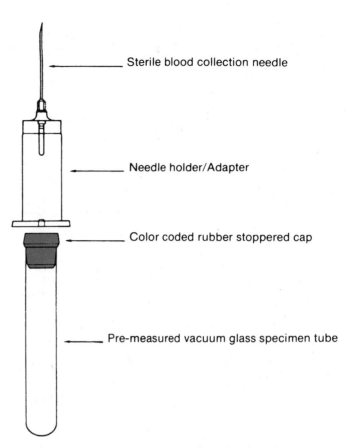

FIGURE 17–36 The VACUTAINER system for venous blood collection

- Sterile blood collection needle
- Needle holder/Adapter
- Color coded rubber stoppered cap
- Pre-measured vacuum glass specimen tube

Erythrocyte Sedimentation Rate

The erythrocyte sedimentation rate is also known as the ESR, the sed rate, and the SR. It is the rate at which red blood cells settle in a particular calibrated tube within a given amount of time, usually 1 hour. Some physicians are interested in 15-minute readings in addition to the standard 1-hour reading. The purpose of the test is to

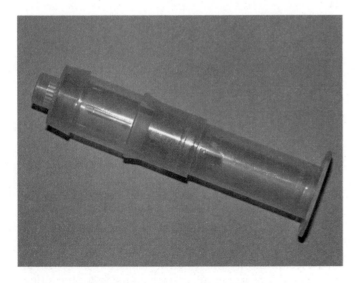

FIGURE 17–35 The Saf-T Clik® adapter locked after use (Courtesy of Ryan Medical, Inc.)

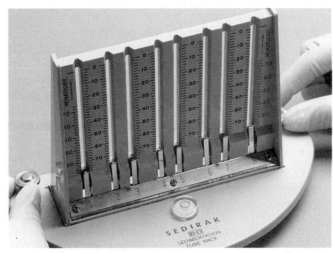

FIGURE 17–37 The sedimentation tube rack must be level for accurate reading of the ESR tube.

Complete An ESR Using The Wintrobe Method

PURPOSE: To determine the rate at which the red blood cells (erythrocytes) fall in a given amount of time (usually 1 hour). Sometimes, additionally, physicians request recorded readings at 15-minute intervals up to 1 hour.

EQUIPMENT: (Disposable) calibrated glass ESR tube-Wintrobe method, rubber bulb (to use with long tapered glass pipette), or plastic disposable pipette, tube holder with level, fresh blood specimen from CBC tube, timer or timepiece, latex gloves, pen, patient's chart, paper towels, detergent solution in long basin to wash pipette and bulb if used. Figure 17–37, page 551, shows the medical assistant adjusting the dials on either side of the tube rack to make it stand level.

TERMINAL PERFORMANCE OBJECTIVE: Provided with all necessary equipment/supplies, the student will demonstrate all required steps to complete the procedure for an ESR. The instructor will observe each step.

1. Assemble needed items on level counter space. Wash hands and put on latex gloves.
2. Carefully set tube into leveled stand. **Key Point: If more than one ESR is being done, mark slot number down next to patient's name on note pad near stand and time it was set.**

3. Carefully fit rubber bulb onto large end of glass pipette if used. Depress bulb end of pipette and place tip of pipette into bottom of blood-filled specimen tube. Slowly fill the pipette with blood by letting up on depressed bulb. Place tip of blood-filled pipette to the very bottom of calibrated sed rate tube carefully without touching sides.
4. Slowly press bulb and fill Wintrobe tube to precisely the 0 line, keeping tip of pipette below meniscus, Figure 17–38.
5. Immediately set timer for 1 hour, or write down exact time that you set tube in stand and check reading in exactly 1 hour.
6. Discard disposables, wash and return other items to proper storage area, remove gloves, and wash hands.
7. Read Wintrobe tube at calibrated line where red cells and plasma separate, Figure 17–39. **Key Point: If meniscus of plasma is above 0 line (2 lines are allowed) add 1 or 2 to reading, depending on line that meniscus is closest to when time is up. Normal range for ESR, Wintrobe method is males, 0 to 6.5, females 0 to 15 mm/hr.**
8. Record on patient's chart; for example, ESR 29 mm/hr. (Wintrobe) and initial.

---

determine the degree of inflammation in the body. When inflammation is present, red cells become heavier than normal. The ESR may be performed in the medical office or clinic. Whole blood is required, and the usual procedure is to draw blood into a lavender-stoppered tube that contains an anticoagulant. The test should be performed within 2 hours of being drawn for accurate results. The erythrocyte sedimentation rate is useful in the diagnosis and evaluation of diseases of the respiratory tract, and in cancer, arthritic, and Collagen's patients. It may also be used in determining the extent of dehydration in burn victims. Sed rates are performed with several different types of calibrated cylindrical tubes. The most common methods and their normal ranges are:

	Males	Females
Culter	0–8	0–10 mm/hour
Wintrobe	0–6.5	0–15 mm/hour
Westergren	0–15	0–20 mm/hour

The normal rate at which red blood cells fall is 1 mm every 5 minutes. Since the readings vary according to which method is used, it is essential that the method be recorded with the results on the patient's chart. Females

tend to have higher readings than males, especially during menstruation and in pregnancy.

Complete Chapter 17, Unit 3 in the workbook to help you meet the objectives at the beginning of this unit and therefore achieve competency of this subject matter.

U N I T   4

Urine, Sputum, and Stool Specimens

OBJECTIVES ....

Upon completion of this unit, the student will meet the following terminal performance objectives by verifying knowledge of the facts and principles presented through oral and written communication at a level deemed competent, and will demonstrate the specific behaviors as identified in the terminal performance objectives of the procedures, observing all aseptic and safety precautions in accordance with health care standards.

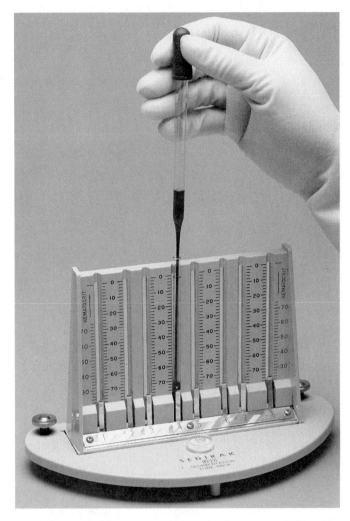

FIGURE 17–38 Fill the calibrated tube from the solid blood-filled pipette, keeping the tip just below the meniscus to precisely the 0 (zero) line.

1. Explain the methods of urine collection: clean-catch midstream, catheterization, infant collection, random.
2. Perform routine urinalysis: physical, chemical, and microscopic examination.
3. Instruct patients in collection of urine, sputum, and stool for analysis.
4. Obtain a catheterization urine specimen from a female patient.
5. Determine specific gravity of urine using a urinometer.
6. Describe the reagent strips used in chemical urinalysis.
7. Describe the proper storage of urine specimens until analysis can be performed and the reasons for it.
8. Complete a lab request form.
9. Record the results of a urinalysis on the patient's chart.
10. Discuss patient education regarding respiratory, digestive, and urinary systems.
11. Discuss the collection process of specimens sent for drug and/or alcohol analysis.
12. Spell and define, using the glossary at the back of the text, all the words to know in this unit.

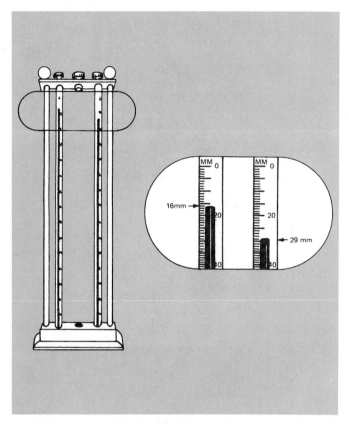

FIGURE 17–39 Reading a Wintrobe tube: the tube on the left reads 16mm/hr, on the right 29 mm/hr.

WORDS TO KNOW ....

amber	physical
cancer	quantity not sufficient
caustic	(QNS)
chemical	random
clarity	renal threshold
crenated	supernatant
dextrose	turbidity
feces	urinalysis
last menstrual period	urinary tract infection
(LMP)	(UTI)
laxative	urination
occult	

In addition to obtaining blood specimens and preparing them for laboratory tests, the medical assistant will probably be responsible for collecting specimens of other body fluids from patients or instructing the patients to do so. The specimens that you must obtain and prepare for analysis most often are urine, sputum, and stool. The same standard information (the patient's name, age, sex, etc.) should accompany each specimen on the appropriate laboratory request form. In addition, specimens must be obtained and sent to the lab in the proper containers to avoid misunderstanding by lab personnel.

PHYSICAL EXAMINATION:

Appearance __CLEAR, STRAW-COLORED__

pH __4.5 TO 7.5__   Specific Gravity __1.010 TO 1.025__

CHEMICAL ANALYSIS:

Albumin (protein) __NONE TO TRACE__   Urobilinogen __NEG.__

Sugar (glucose, dextrose) __NONE__   Porphyrins __NEG.__

Ketones (acetone) __NONE__   PKU __NEG.__

Bilirubin __NONE__   Occult Blood __NEG.__

MICROSCOPIC EXAMINATION:

Cells: Epithelial __FEW__

          WBC's __0 TO 4__

          RBC's __FEW TO OCCASIONAL__

Casts: Hyaline __NEG.__

          Epithelial __NEG.__

          Blood __NEG.__

Crystals: __FEW__

Other: __NEG.__

FIGURE 17–40   Lab report shows normal values for a routine urinalysis.

Most specimens should be refrigerated if there is a delay in transporting them to the laboratory. Many specimen containers already have a preservative added to prevent deterioration so that refrigeration is not necessary. A laboratory procedure manual should be kept at hand for reference on how to prepare specimens.

Urine Specimens ....

Urinalysis is probably the most frequently performed test in the medical office. Examination of urine consists of three major areas of testing: physical, chemical, and microscopic, Figure 17–40.

Specimens for urinalysis are usually collected in plastic disposable containers, Figure 17–41. The time that the urine specimen was obtained should be noted on the container with the patient's name, the date, and the test to be performed on the specimen. Ideally, urinalysis should be performed within 2 hours of collection to avoid bacterial growth and the decomposition of cells. If there is a delay, the specimen should be refrigerated.

The first morning urination is the most concentrated and therefore most often the choice for accurate test results. In addition, patients usually have little difficulty in obtaining random urine specimens upon request in the medical office. Random refers to nonscheduled and/or no preparation required. Most physicians prefer

that the specimen be a midstream sample. Partial voiding before catching the specimen will clear the urethra of any sloughed off cells, bacteria, mucus, or other debris that could interfere with accurate test results. Patients

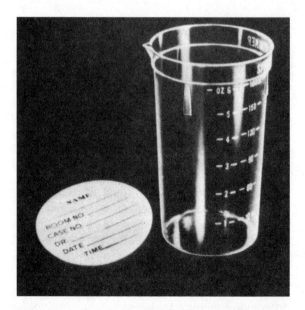

FIGURE 17–41   Urine specimen cup with identification label. (From Caldwell & Hegner, *Health Care Assistant*, 5th ed. Copyright 1989, Delmar Publishers Inc.)

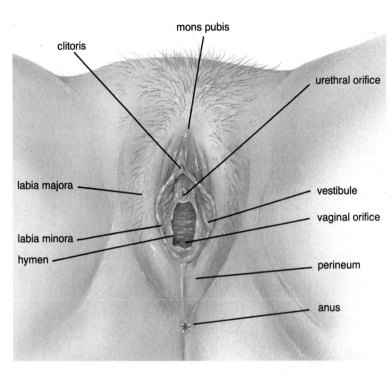

FIGURE 17–43 External female genitalia (From Caldwell & Hegner, Nursing Assistant, 6th ed. Copyright 1992, Delmar Publishers Inc.)

should be instructed to wash the genital area with soap and water, rinse well, wipe the genitals with several antiseptic-soaked cotton balls (usually zephrin chloride is used), begin to void into the toilet, and after a few seconds catch about 3 ounces in the urine container.

The 24-Hour Urine Specimen

On occasion, a 24-hour urine specimen will be called for. Usually a written laboratory order will be given to the patient, and instruction will be given by the laboratory technician, but you may be given this responsibility. Printed instruction sheets are most helpful in this procedure. The patient is given a large container with a preservative already added. This container will hold all of the urine the patient voids in a 24-hour period and must be refrigerated throughout this time. The patient must keep a record of the date and exact time that the collection begins, which should be at the second urination of the day. Then every time the patient voids, day and night, for the next 24 hours, the patient should urinate into a clean smaller container and add the urine to the larger container. The last specimen included in the test period is the first urination of the next morning. When completed, the specimen should be taken to the laboratory as soon as possible, and kept cool during transporting with ice in a portable cooler. Again, it is necessary to check the lab manual for directions in preparing specimens because some 24-hour urine samples should not have the preservative added.

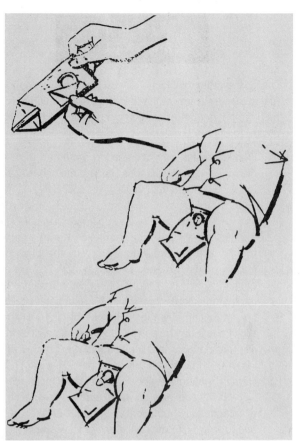

FIGURE 17–42 Pediatric urine collection unit in place: (a). Female (b). male

Pediatric urine collection bags fit over the genital area of either sex and are secured with adhesive, Figure 17–42. The infant's skin should be washed and dried thoroughly before application if the bag is to stay in place. You may have to instruct the parent in the procedure so that it can be done at home. It may be necessary to transfer the urine into a regular specimen container for transporting. You should advise the parent to label the specimen with the baby's name and the date and time of the urine collection.

The lab report will be given to the physician within a few days depending on the type of tests performed. As with any lab test, the patient will be anxious to know the results and should be notified as soon as possible.

Catheterization. You may be asked to either perform or assist with the procedure of urinary bladder catheterization, the introduction of a catheter (tube) through the urethra into the bladder for withdrawal of urine.

There are basically three reasons for catheterizing patients:

1. to obtain a sterile urine specimen for analysis
2. for relief of urinary retention
3. to instill medication into the bladder, after the bladder is emptied

During the patient's office visit you may have an opportunity to discuss a few of the following areas which may help the patient better understand proper health habits in regard to urinary problems.

1. Remind patients to avoid using perfumed toilet articles (i.e., tissue, tampons, soaps, etc.) that are irritating to delicate vaginal tissues.
2. Advise patients to void when they feel the urge because delay can cause bladder stress and irritation.
3. Instruct female patients to practice Kegel exercises to increase the sphincter control of the bladder to improve urine retention. This exercise is done by pushing down with the lower pelvic muscles (as in forcing urination), counting to 10, and then squeezing back counting down to 1. Repeating this routine several times a day helps to strengthen muscle control.
4. Remind patients that they should drink plenty of fluids, avoiding caffeine drinks.
5. Remind patients (especially females) that taking a shower instead of a tub bath reduces the possibility of infection. (Bubble baths should be taken rarely because they irritate delicate vaginal tissues.)
6. Advise female patients that wearing pants that are too tight, as well as nylon underwear, may be irritating to delicate vaginal tissues. Cotton is recommended because it breathes, allowing heat and moisture to escape.

This procedure is not performed routinely. In most cases, it is done by a urologist, a physician who specializes in diseases of the urinary system. However, some physicians in obstetrics-gynecology and general and family practice may delegate this duty to the medical assistant to aid in the diagnosis of the patient. Generally, the physician will order a culture and sensitivity analysis of the urine obtained from catheterization. This is done to determine what microorganism is present and what medication will be effective in treatment. You must be authorized by the physician to perform the procedure. The physician generally will have you observe several catheterizations to become familiar with the procedure. After you have demonstrated the skill under the direct supervision of the physician, you will be released to perform catheterizations alone. If any doubt or problem occurs during the catheterization procedure, the physician should be notified immediately.

Generally, physicians will catheterize male patients for it is a more difficult procedure and sometimes painful. Assistance in assembling the necessary items

and helping the physician during the procedure may be the medical assistant's role.

Sterile technique must be maintained throughout the procedure. Contamination of any of the items during the procedure is possible, and these should be discarded and another sterile item used to continue the procedure. Carelessness may result in severe bladder infection or injury to the patient. You should follow the procedure for putting on sterile gloves given later in the text.

French catheters are used in performing simple catheterizations. The Foley catheter is used when the catheter will remain in the urinary bladder. Sterile, disposable catheterization kits are available that contain all necessary items to perform the procedure. Some have only the catheter tube, which attaches to the sterile specimen container directly. This is convenient for obtaining a sterile urine specimen. Other items must be assembled to properly carry out the procedure.

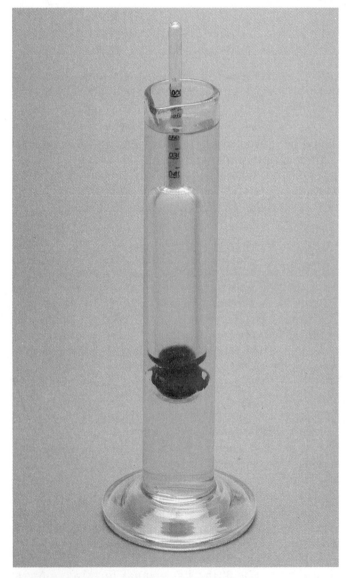

FIGURE 17–44 The reading for specific gravity is done immediately at the meniscus when spinning stops.

Catheterize Urinary Bladder

PURPOSE: To obtain a sterile urine specimen from the urinary bladder for laboratory analysis.

EQUIPMENT: Sterile tray covered with sterile towel, sterile gloves, sterile towels, sterile specimen container with lid, sterile basin to catch excess urine, sterile catheter (French type, sizes 12–16), sterile cotton balls, sterile medicine cup, sterile 4 x 4 inch gauze squares, sterile forceps, sterile plastic sheet, antiseptic solution, sterile lubricant, sterile gloves, gooseneck lamp, Mayo table

TERMINAL PERFORMANCE OBJECTIVE: With all equipment/supplies provided, and using a training model or mannequin in lieu of a patient, the student will demonstrate the steps required to perform a urinary bladder catheterization. The instructor will observe each step. Note: To prevent injury/disease transmission/embarrassment, this procedure should not be practiced before other students. Simulation should be made by the instructor if models are not available.

1. Place catheter kit on Mayo table next to examination table and explain procedure to identified patient. Adjust position of lamp and turn on.

2. Ask patient to lie back on table and assist her into dorsal recumbent position with her feet in stirrups. **Key Point: Drape patient with sheet and expose external genitalia only.**

3. Pull out footrest. Open outer wrapping of sterile kit. Place sterile towel between patient's knees, touching only corners. Then place sterile plastic sheet under patient's buttocks in same way. **Key Point: Kit may now be placed on footrest between patient's legs within reach during procedure.** Ask patient to keep her knees apart.

4. Wash and dry hands and put on sterile gloves, being careful not to contaminate your gloved hands. Pour antiseptic solution over cotton balls in medicine cup. Open urine specimen container and keep on sterile field. Apply sterile lubricant to one of gauze squares.

5. With left hand spread labia and wipe genitalia once with each of three antiseptic-soaked cotton balls (front-to-back motion) and discard onto Mayo table, using right hand. Keep left hand in place and do not touch sterile items with it as it is now contaminated. Place tip of catheter in lubricant and other end of catheter tube into basin.

6. Holding catheter tube about 4 inches from lubricated tip with your right thumb and index finger, insert tip gently into urinary meatus (located below clitoris and above vaginal opening) about 2 to 3 inches, Figure 17–43, page 555. Patient should be instructed to breathe slowly and deeply to relax abdominal muscles and tissues so that procedure is not painful. Tell patient that feeling uncomfortable will last only a few minutes until tube is withdrawn. Procedure should not be painful to the patient. Any unusual complaints should be brought to physician's attention immediately.

7. After insertion of tip of catheter, urine flow should begin immediately into basin. Flow may be stopped by closing metal clamp attached to tubing. Position other end of tube into specimen container and release clamp to collect urine specimen. Allow remainder of urine from bladder to flow into basin.

8. Withdraw catheter tube gently when urine flow stops and dry area with sterile gauze squares or cotton balls. Secure lid onto urine specimen container and set aside. Turn lamp off and return it to usual position. Remove all items from footrest.

9. Discard gloves and other disposable items and place any reusable items in basin to soak in cold water until you have time to wash and sterilize them. Wash hands. Label specimen for analysis and complete request form if sending to outside lab.

10. Assist patient in either sitting up or relaxing in a horizontal recumbent position.

11. Assist patient from table to dress (assist further if needed), and clean off examining table. Remember to wear gloves whenever handling any items soiled with blood or any body fluids. After you have completed the procedure you should discard gloves before you assist the patient from the table. For cleaning up soiled items you must reglove.

12. Record procedure and measured amount of urine (in both basin and specimen container) on patient's chart and initial. Include information about physical properties of urine, rate of flow, and any abnormal or significant observations.

Physical Urinalysis

Physical properties of urine include the appearance (color), specific gravity, **turbidity** (**clarity**), and color. Standard color descriptors are light straw, straw, dark straw, light **amber**, amber, and dark amber. Clarity is described as clear, slightly cloudy, cloudy, and very cloudy. Specific gravity indicates the concentration of urine. It is measured with a glass urinometer and calibrated float, Figure 17–44. The weight of substances

Determine Specific Gravity Using Urinometer

PURPOSE: To determine the specific gravity of urine.
EQUIPMENT: Clean dry glass urinometer and float, fresh urine specimen, tongue depressor, and disposable gloves
TERMINAL PERFORMANCE OBJECTIVE: Provided with the necessary equipment/supplies, the student will demonstrate the steps of the procedure for determining specific gravity of urine. The instructor will observe each step.

1. Wash hands, put on gloves, and assemble all needed items on level counter.
2. Mix urine well with tongue depressor and fill glass container about three-fourths full. **Key Point: If there is not enough urine to complete the specific gravity test write QNS (quantity not sufficient).**

3. Hold the slender, clear end of the float between your thumb and index finger and place the larger end into the glass container holding the urine.
4. Roll the tip of the float quickly between your thumb and index finger.
5. Watch the spinning action at eye level and read the measurement immediately when it stops.
6. Record the reading on the patient's chart.
7. Discard urine and tongue depressor. Wash, rinse, and dry urinometer and float. Remove gloves and wash hands. **Key Point: The float should be kept dry and handled carefully because the bottom may easily be cracked.**

contained in urine is assessed by comparing the specific gravity of urine with that of distilled water, which is 1.000. The specific gravity of urine is normally form 1.010 to 1.025. Lighter colored urine usually has a lower specific gravity, and darker urine a higher one.

The color of urine can be affected by disease, some medications, and food. Urine with a strong ammonia-like odor may be alkaline from a high concentration of bacteria. Urine with a high glucose level (glycosuria) may have a fruit-sweet odor. Glycosuria is caused by a high glucose level in the blood, which spills into the urine when the renal threshold is reached.

Blood in the urine (*hematuria*) may give the specimen a red or rusty color. However, foods with strong color, such as beets, also produce redness in the urine and stool. Patients should be advised that this is only temporary and told not to worry. If medication is known to cause urinary discoloration, the patient should be told in advance to avoid undue stress.

Chemical Urinalysis

Any urine specimen that has been refrigerated should be returned to room temperature before testing.

Reagent strips are convenient and relatively inexpensive diagnostic tests which reveal the presence of abnormal substances in the urine. The reagent strips provide both qualitative and quantitative assessment. Qualitatively, they reveal the presence of an abnormal substance; quantitatively, they determine how much of the substance is present. The substances include sugar (glucose), protein (albumin), ketone (acetone), bilirubin, urobilinogen, blood, nitrite, *p*H, leukocytes, and specific gravity. The treated paper end of the reagent strip reacts chemically with the urine, and if a sufficient amount of a substance is

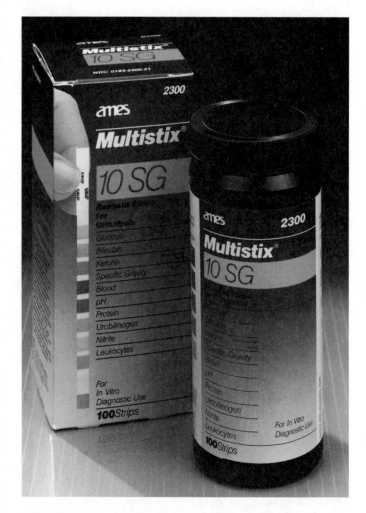

FIGURE 17–45 Multistix® reagent strips for urinalysis (Courtesy of Miles Inc. Diagnostics Division)

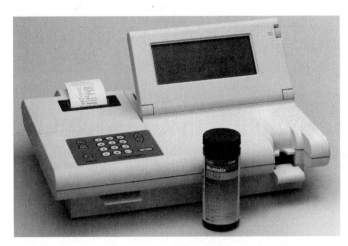

FIGURE 17–46 This urine chemistry analyzer provides quick and accurate test results. (Courtesy of Miles Inc. Diagnostics Division)

present in the urine, the strip changes color. The strip is then compared to the color chart on the bottle.

Fresh urine specimens should be used, and exact tim-ing of the tests is vital. Adequate lighting is also impor-tant to view the colors of the reagent strips and the changes that may occur. If there is no reaction (no change in color), the results are recorded as negative.

Care must be taken to protect the reagent strips from exposure to light, heat, and moisture. Reagent strip bot-tles must be capped immediately after use and stored in a dry, cool area (but not refrigerated). The strips are bot-tled in light-resistant glass with a moisture-absorbent agent included. They must not be used after the expira-tion date on the bottle.

Many companies manufacture urine tests. One test that is commonly used because of its wide range is the Multistix 10 SG reagent strip test (Ames Co.), Figure 17–45. Each reagent strip bottle has a package insert with instructions, which should be precisely followed.

The Multistix 10 SG is also used in the Clinitek 100 urine chemistry analyzer, Figure 17–46. This instrument provides standardized readings of reflectance photome-try on a screen (with abnormal results highlighted) as well as a printed record for the patient's file.

 P R O C E D U R E

Test Urine With Multistix 10 SG

PURPOSE: To detect *p*H, protein, glucose, ketones, blood, bilirubin, urobilinogen, leukocytes, and specific gravity in urine.

EQUIPMENT: Multistix 10 SG reagent strips, fresh urine spec-imen, disposable gloves, watch or other timepiece, tongue depressor, patient's chart, pen, adequate lighting to read color chart on reagent bottle (for accurate test results, use before expiration date on the bottle)

TERMINAL PERFORMANCE OBJECTIVE: Provided with all nec-essary equipment/supplies, the student will demonstrate the steps required to perform the procedure for using Multistix 10 SG. The instructor will observe each step.

1. Wash hands, put on gloves, and assemble all needed items on cleared counter.
2. Stir urine with tongue depressor to evenly distribute constituents throughout specimen.
3. Remove cap from bottle and take out one reagent strip without touching test paper end. Place cap securely back on bottle. **Key Point: Study times given on bot-tle for reading each test section.**
4. Dip test paper end of reagent strip into urine specimen, then quickly remove it by touching edge against inside of container to allow excess urine to run off. **Key Point: If strip is too saturated treated test paper chemicals will run together and make results inaccurate.**
5. Place reagent strip next to color chart on bottle by hold-ing bottom of bottle in left hand and strip by right thumb and index finger. Read results by comparing color of reacted reagent strips to color chart on bottle. Place bottle on its side and hold at bottom with left hand. Hold reagent strip in right hand with thumb and index finger and line up with color chart on bottle. Read test results from bottom to top in order of smaller to larger timings. Proper timing is essential for accurate results. Wash hands.
6. Begin timing tests immediately. For example:
   - 2 minutes—leukocytes
   - 60 seconds—nitrite
   - 60 seconds—urobilinogen
   - 60 seconds—protein (albumin)
   - 60 seconds—pH
   - 50 seconds—blood
   - 45 seconds—specific gravity
   - 40 seconds—ketone
   - 30 seconds—bilirubin
   - 30 seconds—glucose (quantitative)
   - 10 seconds—glucose (qualitative)
7. Discard used reagent strip and other disposables and return Multistix 10 SG to proper storage area. Remove gloves and discard in proper receptacle. Wash hands.
8. Record results as indicated for each section on patient's chart, with name of test, and initial.

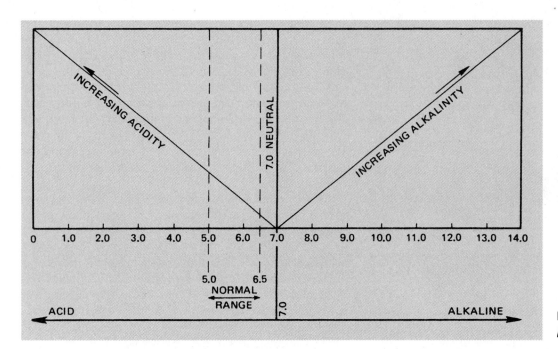

FIGURE 17–47 Scale of pH for urine

The pH range for normal urine is from 5.0 to 7.0, Figure 17–47. Above 7.0 is considered alkaline, and below 5.0 is acid. If a urine specimen has a pH over 7, it probably contains a great number of bacteria, which make the urine alkaline. This will destroy the urinary casts that are formed in the kidney. Urinary casts are important in the diagnosis of a patient's condition.

Diseases of the kidney and urinary tract infections (UTI) produce protein (albumin) in the urine that is not normally present. A patient with a trace or reading of 1+ or more of protein on a random specimen will probably

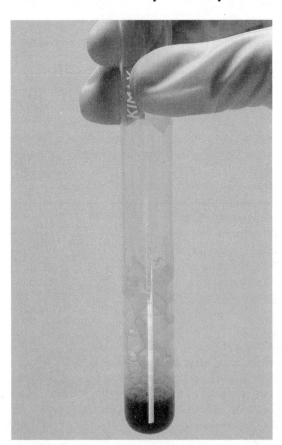

FIGURE 17–48 Carefully hold test tube at the top to avoid possibly being burned from boiling caused by chemical reaction of Clinitest tablet with solution.

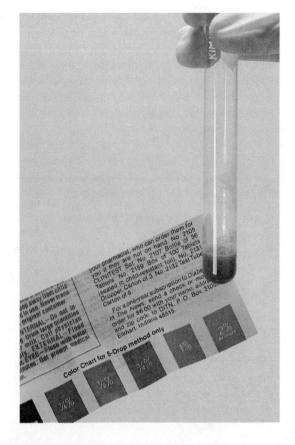

FIGURE 17–49 Compare reaction color with chart 15 seconds after boiling stops after gently swirling to mix solution.

Determine Glucose Content Of Urine With Clinitest Tablet

PURPOSE: To determine the glucose content of urine.

EQUIPMENT: Clinitest tablets with color chart for test result (must be used before expiration date to ensure accurate results), glass test eyedropper, fresh urine specimen, disposable gloves, small container of water, test tube rack, tongue depressor, watch or timepiece, proper lighting

TERMINAL PERFORMANCE OBJECTIVE: Provided with all necessary equipment/supplies, the student will demonstrate the steps in the procedure for using Clinitest tablets. The instructor will observe each step.

1. Wash hands, put on gloves, and assemble needed items on adequate counter space.
2. Stir urine with tongue depressor and fill dropper halfway with urine.
3. Hold test tube near top between thumb and index finger and with other hand release 5 drops of urine into test tube.
4. Rinse dropper and fill halfway with water. Release 10 drops of water into test tube and mix gently.
5. Set test tube in rack and open bottle. Take one Clinitest tablet out by shaking it into cap from bottle without touching it. Drop tablet from cap directly into test tube with mixed urine and water. **Key Point: Moisture on hands may react with tablet and cause a burn. Recap bottle.**
6. Watch reaction, Figure 17–48. As soon as boiling stops, allow exactly 15 seconds before carefully grasping test tube at top, gently tilting it back and forth and swirling contents, and then comparing color of mixture in bottom of test tube with closest color on chart, Figure 17–49. Results are determined in percentage of milligrams per deciliter.
7. Rinse test tube in cool water. Wash with detergent, rinse and dry test tube and dropper, and return items to proper storage. Discard disposable items. Remove disposable gloves and discard in proper receptacle. Wash hands.
8. Record reading on patient's chart.

---

be asked to have a first morning sample checked to see if the protein is in the concentrated urine.

Ketone (acetone) bodies are not normally present in the urine. They are the result of fat metabolized in the digestive tract. Their presence could indicate severe diabetes mellitus, starvation, a high-fat diet, or body wasting. A highly concentrated amount of ketones is called ketonuria. Many patients who have been fasting before coming in to the medical office for blood and urine tests may show a high ketone urine level, which is usually insignificant.

Bilirubin (bile) is an orange or yellowish pigment which is a product of degenerated RBCs that release hemoglobin in the liver. This waste product is normally excreted through the intestines. In patients who have liver damage or disease, bilirubin will appear in the urine, often before they develop symptoms and appear jaundiced.

Urobilinogen is bilirubin that has been converted in the intestines by coli bacteria. This chemical reaction gives feces its brown color. Urobilinogen is excreted through the intestines normally. Large amounts are produced when the heart, spleen, and liver are diseased or dysfunctioning.

Blood in the urine is termed hematuria. Presence of blood in the urine indicates damage of the kidney from injury or from disorders and diseases of the urinary tract. Blood is found normally in the urine specimens of menstruating females. If the specimen is necessary immediately for a diagnosis, a catheterized specimen may be required.

Nitrite is present in urine that contains microorganisms. The action of the invading bacteria converts nitrates in the normally sterile urine to nitrite. Urine which has been left unrefrigerated may contain nitrite due to the action of bacteria present in an alkaline urine. This is why urinalysis should be done as soon as possible after collection.

Phenistix is a reagent strip that detects the presence of phenylketonuria (PKU) in infants. This test may be done like the others by dipping the reagent strip into a fresh urine specimen and timing the reaction.

Glucose (sugar, **dextrose**) is not normally present in the urine, but it may spill out from the kidney when the bloodstream is saturated. Female patients may have a high glucose level during pregnancy and postpartum. Further tests should then be performed to determine the cause. Glucose in the urine may indicate presence of the disease diabetes mellitus. Some patients have a low renal threshold, which may explain the presence of glucose in the urine. Patients with a high glucose level are usually asked for several specimens from different times of the day, with blood tests. The results are evaluated by the physician with other findings from the patient's history before a final diagnosis is made.

Another reliable way to determine the amount of glucose in the urine is with the Clinitest tablet. Instructions for use are enclosed with each kit and may be used by diabetic patients in daily monitoring of their glucose level at home. Bottles which contain Clinitest tablets are light-resistant and should be kept in a dry, cool storage area to ensure accurate test results. As with all medications and

PROCEDURE

Obtain Urine Sediment For Microscopic Examination

PURPOSE: To obtain urine sediment to determine microscopic contents of urine.

EQUIPMENT: Fresh urine specimen, disposable gloves, two glass test tubes, centrifuge, frosted-end glass slides with cover glass, tapered pipette, patient's chart, pen, pencil, tongue depressor, microscope with light source, urine sediment chart, timer or timepiece

TERMINAL PERFORMANCE OBJECTIVE: Provided with all necessary equipment/supplies, the student will demonstrate all steps required in the procedure for obtaining urine sediment. The instructor will observe each step.

1. Wash hands, put on gloves, and assemble all needed items on cleared counter surface near centrifuge.
2. Stir urine specimen with tongue depressor and pour equal amounts (approximately 10 cc) into each of two test tubes or use plain water in one of test tubes.
3. To balance centrifuge, place test tubes on opposite sides. Urine should be spun at 1,500 revolutions per minute for 3 to 5 minutes. **Key Point: Set timer or write down time.**
4. When centrifuge has completely stopped, lift out tube containing urine specimen and carefully pour off urine **(supernatant).**
5. There will still be a few drops of urine in the bottom of test tube with sediment. **Key point: Gently tap bottom of tube on counter or against your palm to mix urine and sediment together.**
6. Obtain a drop or two of urine sediment with a tapered pipette and place it on a clean frosted-end glass slide.
7. Place a cover slip over specimen, allow it to settle, and place on stage of microscope.

   Unless you are highly experienced in this area, the physician will conduct the examination from this point

on. Consult with your employer as to the office policy in this matter before proceeding with the examination.

8. View slide under low-power objective first. Scan for casts and epithelial cells, Figure 17–50. **Key Point: Use dim light.**
9. Change to high-powered objective to view structures such as blood, bacteria, and crystal cells. At least 10 different fields should be viewed. Turn light off when finished. **Key Point: Heat from light will dry out slide and destroy specimen.**
10. Record microscopic observations on patient's chart. Casts and epithelial cells are counted as few, moderate, or many; for example:

    blood casts—few/lpf

    epithelial cells—many/lpf

    Red and white blood cells and bacteria are counted by number seen under microscope using high-power objective or by terms, occasional or loaded (to describe too many to count); for example:

    WBCs—loaded/hpf

    bacteria—occ/hpf

    Red blood cells which are shrunken, or **crenated,** will appear smaller than average and will have a jagged surface.
11. Rinse glass items, wash in detergent solution if not disposable, rinse well, and dry on paper towels. Test tubes may be placed bottom up to drain on paper towels. Return items to proper storage area. Remove disposable gloves and discard in the proper receptacle. Wash hands.

---

chemical preparations, Clinitest should be kept out of the hands of children. These tablets should not come in contact with skin, or a *caustic* reaction with the skin's moisture will result in a burn. Patients who use Clinitest, or other home test kits, keep a record of the results and either phone the medical office or bring the report in to be filed in their chart.

Pregnancy tests are often performed with urine specimens. Female patients usually bring a urine specimen into the medical office in their own containers. They should be instructed to wash, rinse, and dry these carefully before using.

The ideal urine specimen for pregnancy testing is obtained from the first morning urination, which contains

the greatest concentration of chorionic gonadotropin, the hormone on which most pregnancy tests are based. For certain biological pregnancy tests, animals are used. If this type of test is to be performed, the patient should be instructed to discontinue medications or the test results may be inaccurate.

If pregnancy tests are performed in the medical office, the package insert instructions should be followed exactly. Most are simple and easy to complete. Pregnancy tests performed in the medical office take only a few minutes and patients may want to wait for the results. If the test is positive (meaning that pregnancy is evident), the patient may have several questions and may wish to consult further with the

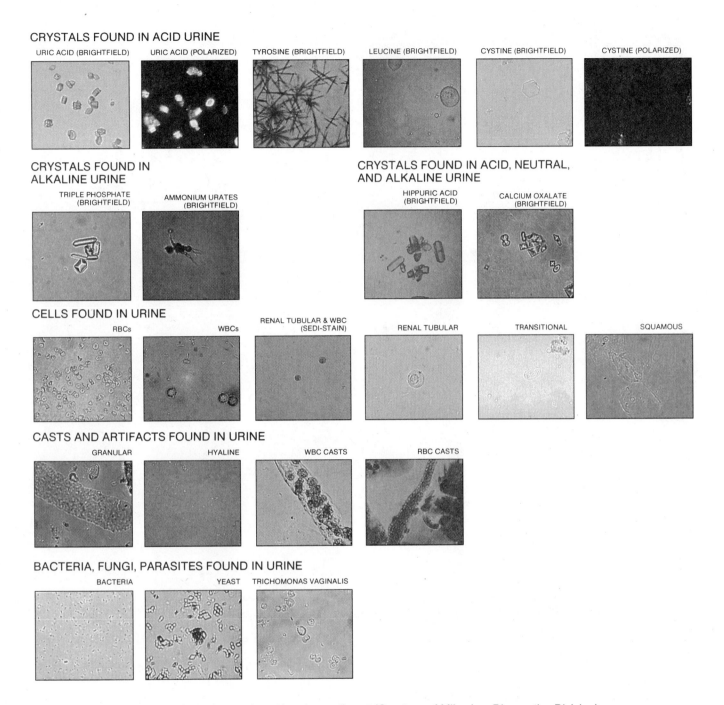

CRYSTALS FOUND IN ACID URINE

URIC ACID (BRIGHTFIELD) | URIC ACID (POLARIZED) | TYROSINE (BRIGHTFIELD) | LEUCINE (BRIGHTFIELD) | CYSTINE (BRIGHTFIELD) | CYSTINE (POLARIZED)

CRYSTALS FOUND IN ALKALINE URINE

TRIPLE PHOSPHATE (BRIGHTFIELD) | AMMONIUM URATES (BRIGHTFIELD)

CRYSTALS FOUND IN ACID, NEUTRAL, AND ALKALINE URINE

HIPPURIC ACID (BRIGHTFIELD) | CALCIUM OXALATE (BRIGHTFIELD)

CELLS FOUND IN URINE

RBCs | WBCs | RENAL TUBULAR & WBC (SEDI-STAIN) | RENAL TUBULAR | TRANSITIONAL | SQUAMOUS

CASTS AND ARTIFACTS FOUND IN URINE

GRANULAR | HYALINE | WBC CASTS | RBC CASTS

BACTERIA, FUNGI, PARASITES FOUND IN URINE

BACTERIA | YEAST | TRICHOMONAS VAGINALIS

FIGURE 17–50 Crystals, cells, and casts found in urine sediment (Courtesy of Miles Inc. Diagnostics Division)

physician. Routine scheduling of an appointment is advised.

Patients are usually advised to bring a urine specimen for a pregnancy test no earlier than 10 days after the first missed menstrual period. Refrigeration is necessary if the specimen cannot be taken directly to the laboratory. The laboratory request form and patient's chart should contain the age of the patient and the date of the last menstrual period (LMP) along with the standard information requested.

Collection of Specimens for Substance Analysis

You may be given the responsibility of collecting specimens for drug (chemical) and alcohol analysis. You must be sure to explain the procedure thoroughly before you have the patient complete and sign the consent/release form for the blood or urine test (or both). The form will state that the purpose of the test is to screen for the presence of drugs, alcohol, and chemical substances. The signature of the patient on this form gives authorization

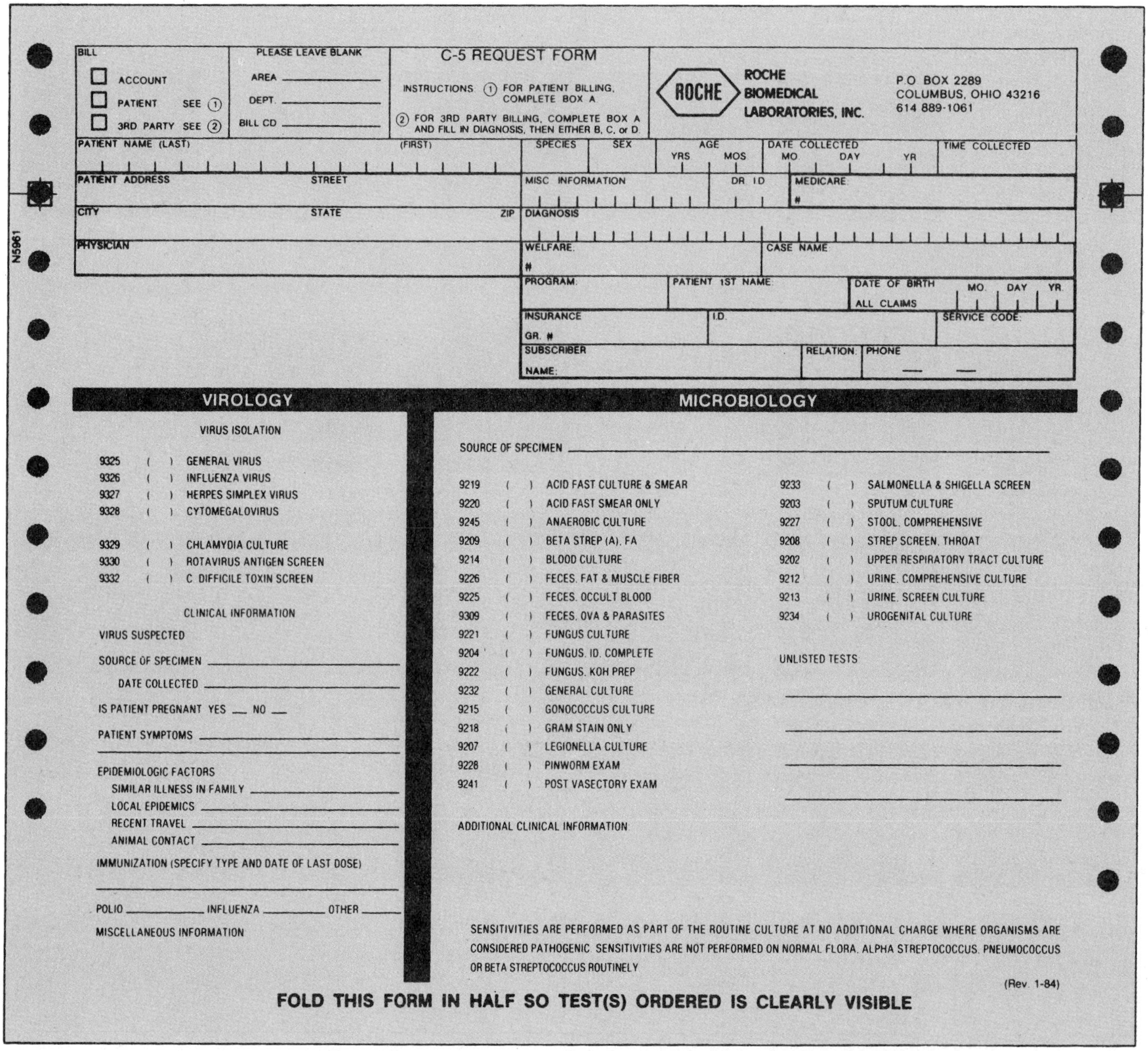

BILL

☐ ACCOUNT
☐ PATIENT SEE (1)
☐ 3RD PARTY SEE (2)

PLEASE LEAVE BLANK
AREA ____
DEPT. ____
BILL CD ____

C-5 REQUEST FORM

INSTRUCTIONS (1) FOR PATIENT BILLING, COMPLETE BOX A
(2) FOR 3RD PARTY BILLING, COMPLETE BOX A AND FILL IN DIAGNOSIS, THEN EITHER B, C, or D.

ROCHE BIOMEDICAL LABORATORIES, INC.
P.O. BOX 2289
COLUMBUS, OHIO 43216
614 889-1061

PATIENT NAME (LAST) (FIRST) | SPECIES | SEX | AGE YRS MOS | DATE COLLECTED MO DAY YR | TIME COLLECTED
PATIENT ADDRESS STREET | MISC INFORMATION | DR I.D. | MEDICARE #
CITY STATE ZIP | DIAGNOSIS
PHYSICIAN | WELFARE # | CASE NAME
PROGRAM | PATIENT 1ST NAME | DATE OF BIRTH ALL CLAIMS MO. DAY YR.
INSURANCE GR. # | I.D. | SERVICE CODE
SUBSCRIBER NAME | RELATION | PHONE

VIROLOGY

VIRUS ISOLATION

9325 ( ) GENERAL VIRUS
9326 ( ) INFLUENZA VIRUS
9327 ( ) HERPES SIMPLEX VIRUS
9328 ( ) CYTOMEGALOVIRUS

9329 ( ) CHLAMYDIA CULTURE
9330 ( ) ROTAVIRUS ANTIGEN SCREEN
9332 ( ) C. DIFFICILE TOXIN SCREEN

CLINICAL INFORMATION

VIRUS SUSPECTED
SOURCE OF SPECIMEN ____
DATE COLLECTED ____
IS PATIENT PREGNANT YES __ NO __
PATIENT SYMPTOMS ____
EPIDEMIOLOGIC FACTORS
SIMILAR ILLNESS IN FAMILY ____
LOCAL EPIDEMICS ____
RECENT TRAVEL ____
ANIMAL CONTACT ____
IMMUNIZATION (SPECIFY TYPE AND DATE OF LAST DOSE)
POLIO ____ INFLUENZA ____ OTHER ____
MISCELLANEOUS INFORMATION

MICROBIOLOGY

SOURCE OF SPECIMEN ____

9219 ( ) ACID FAST CULTURE & SMEAR
9220 ( ) ACID FAST SMEAR ONLY
9245 ( ) ANAEROBIC CULTURE
9209 ( ) BETA STREP (A), FA
9214 ( ) BLOOD CULTURE
9226 ( ) FECES, FAT & MUSCLE FIBER
9225 ( ) FECES, OCCULT BLOOD
9309 ( ) FECES, OVA & PARASITES
9221 ( ) FUNGUS CULTURE
9204 ( ) FUNGUS, ID, COMPLETE
9222 ( ) FUNGUS, KOH PREP
9232 ( ) GENERAL CULTURE
9215 ( ) GONOCOCCUS CULTURE
9218 ( ) GRAM STAIN ONLY
9207 ( ) LEGIONELLA CULTURE
9228 ( ) PINWORM EXAM
9241 ( ) POST VASECTORY EXAM

9233 ( ) SALMONELLA & SHIGELLA SCREEN
9203 ( ) SPUTUM CULTURE
9227 ( ) STOOL, COMPREHENSIVE
9208 ( ) STREP SCREEN, THROAT
9202 ( ) UPPER RESPIRATORY TRACT CULTURE
9212 ( ) URINE, COMPREHENSIVE CULTURE
9213 ( ) URINE, SCREEN CULTURE
9234 ( ) UROGENITAL CULTURE

UNLISTED TESTS

ADDITIONAL CLINICAL INFORMATION

SENSITIVITIES ARE PERFORMED AS PART OF THE ROUTINE CULTURE AT NO ADDITIONAL CHARGE WHERE ORGANISMS ARE CONSIDERED PATHOGENIC. SENSITIVITIES ARE NOT PERFORMED ON NORMAL FLORA, ALPHA STREPTOCOCCUS, PNEUMOCOCCUS OR BETA STREPTOCOCCUS ROUTINELY

(Rev. 1-84)

FOLD THIS FORM IN HALF SO TEST(S) ORDERED IS CLEARLY VISIBLE

N5961

FIGURE 17–51 Laboratory request form for study in determining different types of microorganisms.

for you to collect the specimen(s) for this purpose, prepare it for transport to the laboratory for analysis, and release the results to the agency (employer) where it was requested. Generally this information is an employment requirement. It can also be required for legal reasons. These specimens should be collected very carefully. The consent form and the test request form must accompany the specimens to the laboratory. Information regarding the samples includes:

1. Purpose of the test
2. Number of specimens
3. Comments about: (urine) color, temperature, *p*H and specific gravity
4. Collector's name
5. Site of collection/date/time

The signature of the collector then verifies that the sealed specimen sent is the same one that was received from the patient (at the site) whose name is on the request and consent forms. This multiple (five) copy form is color-coded for routing purposes. Copies are given to:

1. Medical review officer
2. Laboratory
3. Patient
4. Collector
5. Employer

CYTOLOGY-PAP TECHNIQUE			DIAGNOSTIC INFORMATION (Please complete this section)

FIGURE 17–52 Cytology request form

Patients should be informed that all medications, drugs, and alcohol which have been consumed within the last 30 days prior to the test will be revealed by the testing process. OTC (over-the-counter) medications are included. Explain that concealing information is certainly not advised because it would only make a possible problem situation worse for them. A section on the form allows the patient to list all substances consumed in the last month. Patients should be advised to be specific and state what was taken and how much. Ask patients to think about this before completing the form so that they can remember exactly to complete the form accurately.

Discarding specimens may present a problem, with odor caused by the bacterial growth. Pouring urine specimens down the sink is a common practice, but it should be done carefully. Running cold water for a few seconds will flush the trap under the sink. Routine daily use of a few tablespoons of baking soda will keep the drain clean and help eliminate odors.

Sputum Specimens ....

Sputum specimens are sent to the laboratory for analysis of the secretions from the patient's lower respiratory tract. The patient is instructed to obtain the specimen from deeply coughing up the secretions from the bronchial tubes, the trachea, and the lungs into a sterile specimen container. Saliva and mucus from the mouth and nasal passages are not the desired secretions for the sputum analysis and interfere with the test results. The physician may wish to induce coughing in some patients to obtain the specimen in the medical office. Otherwise the patient should be instructed to collect the secretions at home. The patient must understand that the most productive cough will probably occur in the morning soon after waking. This specimen will be the most concentrated. Explain why it is important to follow directions in obtaining a sputum specimen, and that the physician needs accurate information to make a diagnosis. Instruct the patient that this procedure will help identify certain organisms that might not be diagnosed otherwise. Be sure to answer all questions about the process of obtaining the specimen.

The sterile specimen cup (usually a disposable cardboard or plastic container) should be prelabeled with the patient's name and other standard information. The patient should be instructed to fill in the time and date of the specimen and transport it to the medical office as soon as possible. The container should be no more than half full and securely sealed. If it will be more than an hour until the specimen is received by the lab, it should be refrigerated.

PATIENT EDUCATION

When you are giving instructions to patients concerning the collection of sputum specimens, you may also want to advise them about health habits regarding the respiratory tract. Some of the areas you may want to remind them of are listed.

1. Advise patients not to smoke; give advice about stop-smoking programs.
2. Instruct patients to drink plenty of fluids, especially if they have a respiratory ailment.
3. Remind patients to help diminish transmission of viruses and other germs by using disposable paper products at home when a family member is sick.
4. Advise patients to wash hands often, especially when they are infected or when another family member is sick.
5. Urge them to take all the prescribed medication, as directed, for infections to avoid a recurrence of the illness.
6. Advise patients to get proper rest and diet to help them regain strength and resistance to disease.

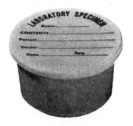

FIGURE 17–53 Laboratory stool specimen container with identification lid ᵃFrom Caldwell & Hegner, *Health Care Assistant*, 5th ed. Copyright 1989, Delmar Publishers Inc.)

Some sputum specimens require collection of secretions of the patient's productive coughing episodes over a period of 24 hours or up to 72 hours. In this case, the secretions will be placed in a larger container and must be refrigerated and appropriately labeled. The appropriate laboratory request form, Figure 17–51, page 564, must be completed with important information regarding the specimen and the patient and accompany the specimen to the lab for proper analysis.

The sputum specimen is analyzed for fungal infections, tuberculosis, and pneumonia. **Cancer** is detected from sputum by the Papanicolaou stain. This test requires a special request form identifying the source of the specimen, Figure 17–52, page 565. This specimen should be sent in the appropriate container with a 95% alcohol solution.

Stool Specimens

Stool specimens (feces) are probably the most difficult to instruct patients to obtain. There is a certain amount of embarrassment for both the patient and the medical assistant in regard to this procedure. Nevertheless, it is an extremely important specimen. Microbial organisms, ova, and **occult** (otherwise invisible and/or hidden) blood may be determined from careful examination of the fecal material.

Patients are instructed to obtain the stool specimen at home, usually within a few days of the request. For the patient who has a daily bowel movement, this will be no problem. For patients who have difficulty with daily elimination, it may take a few days. Patients should use **laxatives** only by order of the physician. Straining during a bowel movement may cause hemorrhoids and is never recommended. You may suggest that the patient drink plenty of fluids to help avoid constipation.

A very small amount of stool is required for laboratory tests. The patient is usually advised to use a tongue depressor or similar stick that can be disposed of to get a sample of stool (the size of a half dollar) from the toilet after a bowel movement. Female patients should be careful not to contaminate the specimen with urine or blood. The stool should be placed in a container which has been labeled with the date and time of collection, Figure 17–53. If the specimen cannot be taken directly to the lab or brought to the medical office, it must be refrigerated to prevent bacterial growth.

Complete Chapter 17, Unit 4 in the workbook to help you meet the objectives at the beginning of this unit and therefore achieve competency of this subject matter.

UNIT 5

Bacterial Smears and Cultures

OBJECTIVES

Upon completion of this unit, the student will meet the following terminal performance objectives by verifying knowledge of the facts and principles presented through oral and written communication at a level deemed competent, and will demonstrate the specific behaviors as identified in the terminal performance objectives of the procedures, observing all aseptic and safety precautions in accordance with health care standards.

1. Obtain a smear for bacteriological examination.
2. Heat-fix a smear for staining.
3. Explain the reason for heat-fixing specimens.
4. Complete a Gram stain.
5. List common diseases caused by gram-positive and gram-negative bacteria.
6. Obtain a throat culture and streak an agar plate.
7. Describe growth media for cultures.
8. Label specimens for analysis.
9. Record information concerning specimens on the patient's chart.
10. Spell and define, using the glossary at the back of the text, all the words to know in this unit.

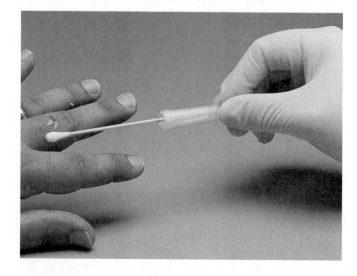

FIGURE 17–54 Use a sterile swab to obtain a specimen from a wound.

Instruct Patient To Collect Sputum Specimen

PURPOSE: To instruct patients in collection of an adequate sputum specimen for laboratory analysis.

EQUIPMENT: Sputum specimen container/lid, label, pen, patient's chart, lab request form, note pad, rubber band, printed instruction sheet (optional)

TERMINAL PERFORMANCE OBJECTIVE: Provided with all necessary equipment/supplies, and using other students as patients, the students will demonstrate the steps of the procedure for instructing a patient in the collection of a sputum specimen for analysis. The instructor will observe each step.

1. Assemble items next to patient.
2. Write patient's name on specimen cup label and complete lab request form.
3. Explain physician's orders to identified patient. Give printed instructions or write out if you feel patient has a difficult time understanding you.
4. Instruct patient to remove lid from sterile specimen container and to expel secretions from a first morning coughing episode into the center of cup, being careful not to touch inside of cup. Container should not be more than half full.
5. Instruct patient not to allow tears, sweat, mucus from nose and/or mouth, or any other substance to enter cup. **Key Point: Secretions must be coughed up (expectorated) from lower respiratory tract (lungs, bronchial tubes, and trachea) or test will not be acceptable.**
6. When secretions have been obtained and cup sealed with its cover, patient should write time and date that it was obtained on label and lab request form and bring it to lab or medical office as soon as possible. **Key Point: If patient cannot bring specimen in within 2 hours after collection, it should be refrigerated.**
7. Secure completed lab request form to specimen container with a rubber band or tape. Send to lab. **Key Point: If patient prepares specimen at home, show patient how to do this.**
8. Record that instruction was given to patient in sputum collecting and initial.

WORDS TO KNOW ·····································

agar
exudate
gram-negative

gram-positive
microscopic

The possibility of disease transmission is extremely high in handling any type of specimen, especially those of patients suspected of having infections. Proper hand-washing and sterile technique must be used at all times to break the cycle of the infection. Eating, drinking, chewing gum, smoking, and any other hand-to-mouth gesture should be avoided to prevent possible self-contamination. Any items used must be carefully washed or properly disposed of to prevent others from becoming infected. Disposable items are almost exclusively used in medical practice today for this reason.

Bacteriological Smear ·····························

Identification of microorganisms that cause disease is accomplished by obtaining a smear or a culture from the area of the body that appears to be infected. To make a smear, a sample of the exudate (drainage) is taken from the throat, mouth, ear, eye, nose, vagina, anus, the surface of the skin or from within a wound by introducing a sterile cotton swab into the area, Figure 17–54. The swab is then rolled over two-thirds of a frosted-end slide, Figure 17–55. The smear is air dried

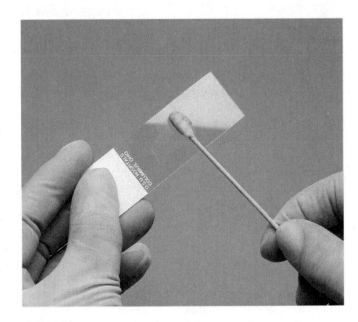

FIGURE 17–55 Rolling the specimen onto the glass slide from left to right covering two-thirds of the area

P R O C E D U R E

Instruct Patient To Collect Stool Specimen

PURPOSE: To instruct patients to obtain an adequate stool specimen for laboratory analysis.

EQUIPMENT: Specimen container with lid, lab request form, pen, patient's chart, label, rubber band, printed instructions (optional) tongue depressors, note pad

TERMINAL PERFORMANCE OBJECTIVE: With all necessary equipment/supplies, and using other students as patients, the student will demonstrate the steps of the procedure for instructing a patient in collecting an adequate stool specimen for laboratory analysis. The instructor will observe each step.

1. Assemble items next to patient.
2. Write identifying information on request form and label (usually cover) and affix to specimen cup.
3. Identify patient and explain physician's orders. Give

printed instructions or write out if necessary.

4. Instruct patient to obtain a small amount of stool (about a tablespoon) from next bowel movement, within next few days. Explain that nothing else should be placed in cup besides stool (no tissue paper, urine, etc.). Patients may defecate onto a paper plate and obtain a small specimen from plate, which is then discarded. Or they may use a tongue depressor to obtain specimen from toilet bowl.
5. Instruct patient to place specimen in cup, secure cover tightly, and write date and time specimen was obtained on cover of cup; then bring specimen to lab or medical office with request form as soon as possible. **Key Point: Specimen should be refrigerated if it cannot be received by lab within 2 hours to prevent bacterial growth.**

at room temperature and then *heat-fixed,* or passed through a flame, Figure 17–56. This seals the specimen to the glass so that it won't wash off during the staining process.

After preparation of a bacteriological smear, determination of the microorganism causing the infection must be made by the physician. Your role is that of obtaining and preparing the smear.

P R O C E D U R E

Prepare Bacteriological Smear

PURPOSE: To adhere a specimen to a glass slide for examination under the microscope.

EQUIPMENT: Specimen (on labeled cotton swab), disposable gloves, clean frosted-end glass slide, forceps, bunsen burner, matches, slide staining rack, pencil, pen, patient's chart (if sent to outside lab: slide holder, lab request form, rubber band or tape)

TERMINAL PERFORMANCE OBJECTIVE: With all necessary equipment/supplies provided, the student will demonstrate the steps of the procedure for preparing a bacteriological smear for microscopic analysis. The instructor will observe each step.

1. Wash hands and put on disposable gloves. Assemble all needed items on counter space. Pencil patient's name on frosted end of glass slide. **Key Point: Complete lab request form, including source of specimen, and wash hands.**
2. Prepare as many smears of specimen as ordered by

physician by rolling cotton swab evenly over two-thirds of glass slide, holding slide with thumb and great finger.

3. Light bunsen burner or other source for flame and adjust to a blue flame. (Blue flame is hottest.)
4. Hold frosted part of slide with your thumb and index finger or with forceps and pass specimen portion of slide through blue part of flame, smear side up, slowly (taking about 2 seconds) two or three times. This is called heat-fixing. **Key Point: Excessive heating will destroy specimen.** Turn bunsen burner or other source for flame off.
5. Place heat-fixed smear on staining rack to cool for staining procedure or place on stage of microscope for observation by physician.
6. Discard used disposables and return other items to proper storage area. Remove disposable gloves and discard in the proper receptacle. Wash hands.
7. Record procedure on patient's chart and initial.

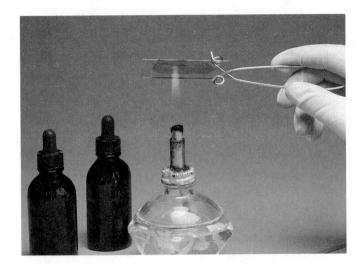

FIGURE 17–56   Heat-fixing the specimen onto the glass slide

Culturing

Culturing is a means of isolating a disease-causing microorganism for identification. It takes far longer than a bacteriological smear but is still a relatively simple procedure. A specimen is obtained and placed in a culture medium, which contains nutrients comparable to human tissue to encourage growth of microorganisms. The medium is agar, a gelatinlike substance, mixed with sheep's blood.

Explain to the patient that a throat culture is necessary to identify certain organisms. Be sure to tell the

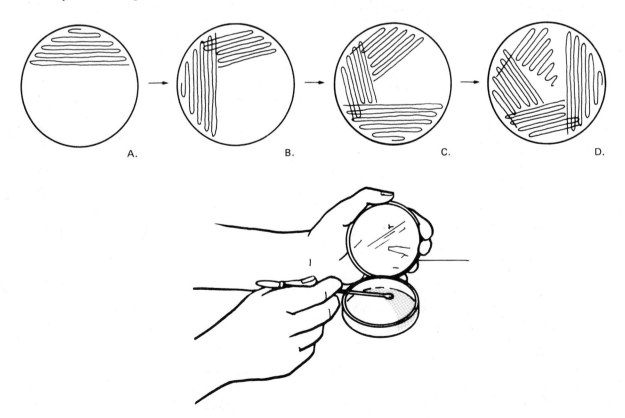

A.   B.   C.   D.

FIGURE 17–57   Pattern for smearing a plate (From Simmers, *Diversified Health Occupations*, copyright 1988, Delmar Publishers Inc.)

PROCEDURE

Obtain A Throat Culture

PURPOSE: To isolate a disease-causing organism to determine effective treatment of the patient.

EQUIPMENT: Culture plate (Petri dish), sterile cotton swabs, sterile tongue depressor, disposable gloves, pen, patient's chart, pen-light (optional), wax crayon or label for culture plate (if sent to outside lab, request form and label for culture plate, clear tape, tissues)

TERMINAL PERFORMANCE OBJECTIVE: Provided with all necessary equipment/supplies, and using a life-like clinical doll infant/small child under close supervision, or other students as patients, the student will demonstrate the steps required to perform the procedure for obtaining a throat culture. The instructor will observe each step.

1. Assemble needed items near identified patient. Label culture plate and complete request form if required. Wash hands and put on gloves.

2. Identify patient. **Key Point: Call patient by name and check chart to avoid error.**

3. Explain procedure to patient and assist patient to comfortable position. Sitting is usual position for adults. **Key Point: It may be easier to work with children if they are lying down. Assistance may be necessary with unruly small patients.**

    Note: If you must obtain a throat culture without assistance from a small child/infant, it may prove easier if you sit with child on your lap. Place child's right arm under your left arm. Hold child's left wrist with your left hand and cradle head between your left wrist and left shoulder. This will free your right hand to obtain specimen. Gently touch throat of child with back of your left thumb to encourage mouth to open. With your right hand, hold swab securely, quickly insert it and swab back of throat with a rolling motion. (Insert swab at corner of mouth behind teeth to prevent child from biting

it.) Use flexible swabs (wooden stick swabs may break if bitten and splintering is a danger when working with small children or infants). Touch only back of throat.

4. Open sterile swab and ask patient to open mouth as wide as possible. Quickly examine with light source.

5. Depress tongue with sterile tongue depressor held in one hand. Hold sterile swab in other. Ask patient to say "ah" to assist depression of tongue (this also prevents patient from feeling gag reflex by diverting attention). Quickly insert swab into back of throat and roll over at least two areas, touching areas with obvious exudate.

6. Remove swab and depressor from patient's mouth. Some physicians order a nasopharyngeal culture (NPC) in which a specimen is obtained from the nasal passages and throat. This is accomplished by inserting a sterile swab into nasal cavities (one for each nostril) and applying each to culture plate, or into a transport media if sent to a lab, Figure 17–58. Attend to patient, offer tissues. Tearing may result from procedure.

7. Immediately apply specimen to agar of Petri dish, smearing it as shown in Figure 17–59 or place swab into container for transportation to lab. Tape request form securely.

8. Place identification label on bottom of Petri dish or write patient's name, date, time, and source on bottom with wax crayon. Secure cover with clear tape.

9. Discard all disposable items in proper receptacle. Remove gloves and dispose of them in the proper receptacle. Wash hands. Place culture in incubator bottom up to prevent moisture, which is released from growth of microorganisms, from accumulating on cover and drowning microorganisms, Figure 17–60.

10. Remove gloves and wash hands.

11. Record procedure on patient's chart and initial.

patient that there might some momentary discomfort in obtaining the specimen, and answer all questions about the process of obtaining the specimen. The specimen is taken directly from the affected area of the patient with a sterile swab and distributed over the agar in a Petri dish of clear plastic using the pattern shown in Figure 17–57, page 569. Many cultures are streaked with a fine wire loop (pictured in the foreground of Figure 17–56, page 569), which is sterilized by flame to prevent cross-contamination when distributing the specimen. The culture plate is then placed in an incubator for 24 to 48 hours to provide the proper temperature for bacterial growth. Many physicians in pediatrics, general, and

family practice obtain, incubate, and read their own cultures, not only for the patient's convenience, but for their own.

The Petri dish must be properly labeled for identification purposes. This includes the patient's name, the date and time the specimen was taken, and the source of the specimen. This information should be written on the bottom of the Petri dish with a wax crayon or label.

Petri plates and other types of transport media for culturing specimens should be prepared according to the outside laboratory's directions. The culture media are disposable and should be discarded in securely tied biohazardous plastic bags in the proper receptacle.

As you obtain throat cultures from patients you may want to give them some helpful advice concerning their condition. Generally when a person has a sore throat it is associated with other respiratory symptoms as well. The following suggestions may provide some relief from discomfort and help them toward better health.

1. Advise patients to drink plenty of liquids (fruit juices) and to eat sensibly from the basic food groups.
2. Urge patients to get extra rest and dress comfortably (according to the weather/temperature outside).
3. Suggest use of gargles or throat lozenges (or both) to relieve painful sore throat.
4. Remind them to avoid tobacco/smoking.
5. Instruct them to cough/sneeze into tissue and discard into proper waste container wherever they are to prevent the spread of germs.
6. Remind them not to eat or drink after others and to use disposables at home when there is illness.

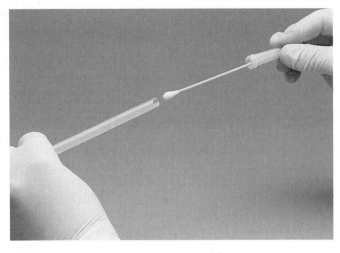

FIGURE 17–58 Place swab with specimen into transport container with culture media for laboratory analysis.

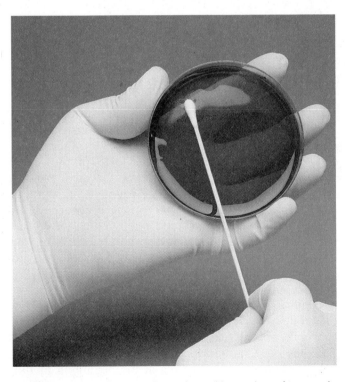

FIGURE 17–59 Smear culture plate with specimen from swab.

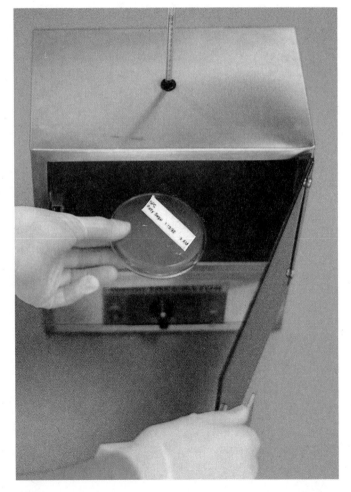

FIGURE 17–60 Place the culture plate in the incubator agar side up.

Prepare Gram Stain

PURPOSE: To stain a heat-fixed bacteriological smear for microscopic identification.

EQUIPMENT: Heat-fixed slide (frosted end labeled), slide rack and tray, crystal (or gentian) violet dye, water wash bottle, forceps, Gram's iodine, alcohol (or acetone), Safranin solution (or dilute fuchsin), timer or timepiece, immersion oil, microscope with light source, pen, patient's chart, pencil, cover glass slides, eye-droppers, paper towels; disposable gloves and plastic apron (optional)

TERMINAL PERFORMANCE OBJECTIVE: Provided with all necessary equipment/supplies, the student will demonstrate the steps in the procedure for preparing a Gram stain. The instructor will observe each step.

1. Assemble all needed items on counter and wash hands. **Key Point: If apron and disposable gloves are to be used, put them on now.**

2. Place heat-fixed slide on staining rack, specimen side up, over tray. **Key Point: All solutions should be recapped immediately after each use to avoid accidents.**

3. Open crystal violet (gentian) dye and fill dropper. Apply over entire specimen area of the slide and time for 60 seconds, Figure 17–62.

4. Hold frosted end of slide with forceps or thumb and index finger and tip slide to allow stain to run off into tray. Wash slide with water, letting flow begin at top and run down.

5. Place slide flat on rack. Fill dropper with Gram's iodine and apply over entire specimen. Tilt slide to allow iodine to run off into tray. Refill dropper with Gram's iodine and leave on for 60 seconds.

6. Wash slide with water, tilting to direct runoff into tray, and replace flat on rack.

7. Apply alcohol (or acetone) with dropper for a few seconds until purple color in excess runoff is gone.

8. Tilt slide and wash with water immediately. Return flat to rack.

9. Apply Safranin solution with dropper to counterstain specimen and wash off with water immediately.

10. Hold slide by frosted end and wipe excess solutions from back. Tap side of slide onto paper towel to help remove excess liquid. Allow slide to air dry. **Key Point: Slide may be blotted between paper towels, but be careful not to rub slide or specimen may be destroyed.**

11. Apply small drop of immersion oil to specimen and place on microscope stage to view under oil-immersion objective. Turn light on to view and off when finished. **Key Point: Cover slide may be used to help preserve specimen for future viewing.**

12. Discard disposables, wash used items, and return items to proper storage. Wash hands.

13. Record procedure and results on patient's chart and initial.

Gram Staining

The purpose of Gram staining is to make heat-fixed bacteria visible for **microscopic** identification, Figure 17–61. The two most common divisions of bacteria are **gram-positive** and **gram-negative.** The infectious diseases most commonly caused by these bacteria are:

- *Gram-positive bacteria:* botulism, diphtheria, lobar pneumonia, rheumatic fever, streptococcal sore throat, tetanus

- *Gram-negative bacteria:* bacillary dysentery, cholera, gonorrhea, meningitis, pertussis, plague, typhoid fever

Bacteria have certain characteristic formations and are identified by their size and shape. Cocci appear in clusters. Staphylococci form grapelike clusters. Bacteria that form pairs are called diplococci. Those that form chains are streptococci. Bacteria with capsule-like coverings are called spore-forming.

Gram-positive bacteria take a violet (purple) color from the Gram stain procedure. Gram-negative bacteria take a red or pink color from the counterstain. Without the staining process the bacteria are colorless. In preparing the slide, you should avoid getting the crystal (or gentian) violet dye on the hands, clothing, or counter as it is difficult (sometimes impossible) to remove. Alcohol and acetone are helpful in removing the dye in some cases.

Refer to Table 17–5, page 574, for examples of how different bacteria stain the particular color of purple (positive) or pink (negative).

Complete Chapter 17, Unit 5 in the workbook to help you meet the objectives at the beginning of this unit and therefore achieve competency of this subject matter.

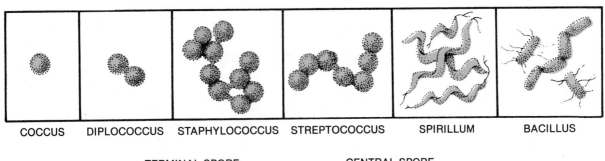

COCCUS DIPLOCOCCUS STAPHYLOCOCCUS STREPTOCOCCUS SPIRILLUM BACILLUS

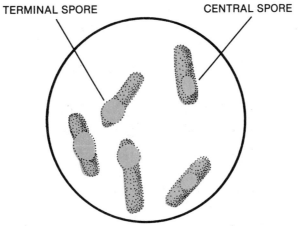

TERMINAL SPORE CENTRAL SPORE

BACILLI WITH CENTRAL AND TERMINAL SPORES

FIGURE 17–61 Shapes of bacteria

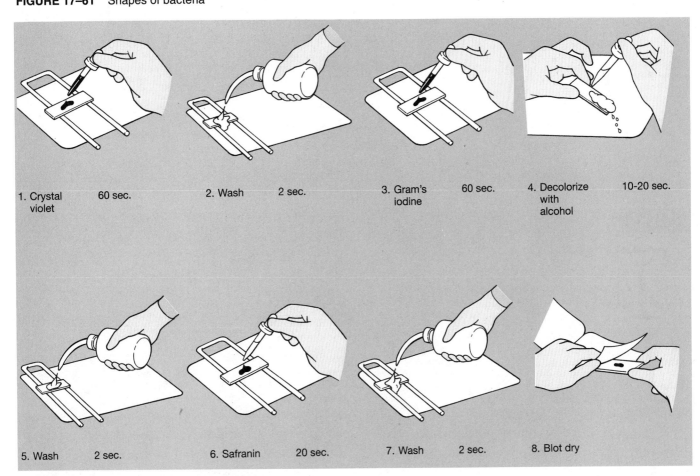

1. Crystal violet 60 sec.

2. Wash 2 sec.

3. Gram's iodine 60 sec.

4. Decolorize with alcohol 10-20 sec.

5. Wash 2 sec.

6. Safranin 20 sec.

7. Wash 2 sec.

8. Blot dry

FIGURE 17–62 Gram staining procedure

TABLE 17–5

Some Important Pathogenic Bacteria and Their Reaction to the Gram Stain (From Fong and Ferris, *Microbiology for Health Careers,* 4th ed. Albany: Delmar, 1987.)

Gram-Positive Reaction (+) (Reaction of Purple Stain)		Gram-Negative Reaction (–) (Loss of Purple Stain)		Gram-Variable Reaction (+/–)	
Bacterium	Disease It Causes	Bacterium	Disease It Causes	Bacterium	Disease It Causes
Bacillus anthracis	Anthrax	*Bordetella pertussis*	Whooping cough	Mycobacterium leprae	Leprosy
Clostridium botulinum	Botulism (food poisoning)	*Brucella abortus* (bovine strain)	Infectious abortion in cattle and undulant fever in man	Mycobacterium tuberculosis	Tuberculosis
Clostridum perfringens	Gas gangrene, wound infection	*Brucella melitensis* (goat strain)			
Clostridium tetani	Tetanus (lockjaw)	*Brudella suis* (porcine strain)			
Corynebacterium diphtheriae	Diphtheria	Esherichia coli	Urinary infections		
Staphylococcus aureus	Carbuncles, furunculosis (boils), pneumonia, septicemia	*Haemophilus influenzae*	Meningitis, pneumonia		
Streptococcus pyogenes	Erysipelas, rheumatic fever, scarlet fever, septicemia, strep throat, tonsilitis	*Neisseria gonorrhoeae*	Gonorrhea		
		Neisseria meningitidis	Nasopharyngitis, meningitis		
Streptococcus pneumoniae	Pneumonia	*Pseudomonas aeruginosa*	Respiratory and urogenital infections		
		Rickettsia rickettsii	Rocky mountain spotted fever		
		Salmonella paratyphi	Food poisoning, paratyphoid fever		
		Salmonella typhi	Typhoid fever		
		Shigella dysenteriae	Dysentery		
		Treponema pallidum	Syphilis		
		Vibrio cholerae	Cholera		
		Yersinia pestis	Plague		

MEDICAL-LEGAL ETHICAL HIGHLIGHTS

Ms. Right...
enters laboratory specimens in the log book as they are received. She efficiently follows up by reporting the results as soon as possible. She is ever mindful of universal precautions and respects the privacy of patients keeping all records confidential.

Promotion outlook: Excellent

Miss Wrong...
is careless in recording laboratory specimens in the log book. She is also negligent in following universal precautions. Results are not reported in a timely fashion because she misplaces them, thereby jeopardizing confidentiality and privacy of patient information.

Promotion outlook: Poor

REFERENCES

Fong, Elizabeth, and Ferris, Elvira. *Microbiology for Health Careers,* 4th Ed. Albany: Delmar, 1987.

Garza, Diana, and Becan-McBride. *Phlebotomy Handbook.* 2d ed. East Norwalk, CT: Appleton and Lange, 1989.

Miller, Benjamin F., and Keane, Claire Brackman. *Encyclopedia and Dictionary of Medicine and Allied Health,* 3d ed. Philadelphia: W.B. Saunders, 1983.

Mosby's Medical & Nursing Dictionary, 3d ed. St. Louis: C.V. Mosby, 1990.

Nurse's Ready Reference Diagnostic Tests. Springhouse, PA: Springhouse, 1991.

Raphael, Stanley S. Lynch's Medical Laboratory Technology. 3d ed. Windsor, Ontario: W.B. Saunders, 1976.

Taber, Clarence W. *Taber's Cyclopedic Medical Dictionary.* 14th ed. Philadelphia: F.A. Davis, 1983.

Ware, Barbara E. *CLIA '88 Physician's Office Laboratory, Are You Ready?* June 1991.

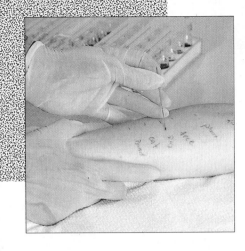

CHAPTER 18

Diagnostic Tests, X Rays, and Procedures

Diagnostic tests, X rays, and procedures will be discussed in this chapter. The medical assistant has a multiple role in these diagnostic aids. You will be responsible for instructing and preparing patients for procedures, tests, and X rays. In some cases, you will either carry out the test(s) or procedure(s), or assist the physician. After completion, you will alert the physician of the results, and from the order of the doctor notify the patient, and then file the report of the results in the patient's chart.

Often as a part of the CPE the physician may order certain tests or other procedures, i.e., chest X ray, mammography, intravenous pyelegram, etc. If these diagnostic tests are performed on site, the results may often be determined while the patient is still present. If referrals must be made for diagnostic tests, etc., patients may be asked to return within a week to 10 days for a final report of the findings. This gives the medical assistant and the physician time to gather reports in the patient's chart for review and evaluation. You may want to advise patients to bring a list of their concerns with them so they won't forget to ask necessary questions. This practice may reduce the number of phone consultations required.

U N I T   1

Diagnostic Tests

OBJECTIVES ···

Upon completion of this unit, the student will meet the following terminal performance objectives by verifying knowledge of the facts and principles presented through oral and written communication at a level deemed competent, and will demonstrate the specific behaviors as identified in the terminal performance objectives of the procedures, observing all aseptic and safety precautions in accordance with health care standards.

1. Describe scratch, patch, and intradermal skin tests, state their purpose; and perform each test under supervision.
2. Describe the schedule and instructions for administering allergy injections.
3. Discuss patient education concerning allergies and treatment.
4. Spell and define, using the glossary at the back of the text, all the words to know in this unit.

adrenalin

adverse

anaphylactic

antibody

antigen

contact dermatitis

desensitizing

eosinophil

epinephrine

extract

histamine

hypersensitive

immune

interpret

obsolete

systemic

venom

wheal

Skin Tests ....

Three procedures are commonly used to determine allergic reactions in patients. They are the scratch, intradermal, and patch tests. The physician determines the diagnosis by evaluating the results of the tests along with the patient's medical history, physical exam, and other laboratory tests. The medical assistant may assist the physician in performing these tests or may perform them by order of the physician. Tests should always be performed under the direct supervision of the physician.

Three tests involve introducing an antigen directly into the patient's skin to induce a reaction. If the reaction is negative (normal) there will be no change in the appearance of the skin following testing. A normal immune reaction occurs in the body when an antigen and antibody unite and the foreign substance is excreted by the body.

A positive allergic reaction to a test is shown by a raised area on the skin, much like a mosquito bite, called a wheal (hive). This is due to interaction of the antigen and antibody, which releases histamine and is termed a hypersensitive reaction. Histamine is naturally produced by the body to attach itself to certain cells to cause dilation of blood vessels and contraction of smooth muscles. Most cells release histamine during allergic reactions. As a part of the normal inflammatory response of the body, histamine protects tissue against injury (the scratch test) and it is the reason that redness and a wheal are produced. The inflammatory response of the body is specific in that it is the whole body's defense against infection, chemicals, or other physical factors.

Besides histamine, researchers are still finding that other chemicals are released during the allergic response. Millions of people have allergies to a variety of substances including certain foods, pollens, dust, drugs (medications), chemicals, venom of stinging insects, animal dander, molds, pollutants, and other allergens. Reaction to these substances ranges from slight to severe. Severe reactions can be life-threatening. A life-threatening reaction must be counteracted with an injection of adrenalin immediately to prevent anaphylactic shock. Symptoms of anaphylactic shock initially include intense anxiety, weakness, sweating, and shortness of breath.

Symptoms may continue to include hypotension, shock, arrhythmia, respiratory congestion, laryngeal edema, nausea, and diarrhea.

Those who have known allergies to the venom of stinging insects, for example, or to certain foods that produce intense life-threatening allergic reactions are instructed to carry an anaphylactic shock kit with them at all times. The kit contains a self-injecting dose of adrenalin for emergency use.

Treatment for many allergy patients consists of an allergy immunotherapy program. Over a considerable period of time, this therapy gradually provides immunization against the substance that the person is allergic to. Increasing amounts of the allergen are injected as long as the patient can tolerate each dose. Treatment generally takes a few years. It is usually effective in reducing symptoms of most allergies. Often patients bring their serum from the allergy specialist to the family doctor's office or clinic for administration. All allergy serum should be refrigerated unless otherwise specified. These desensitizing injections of allergy serum (which patients refer to as "allergy shots") should always be administered under the direct supervision of a physician because anaphylactic shock can occur within seconds even in unsuspecting individuals. Following any injection, the patient must be observed for 20 minutes for possible reaction. Any reaction or unusual symptom must be reported to the physician and noted on the patient's chart, as well as on the schedule sheet accompanying the allergy serum. An example of this schedule is shown in Figure 18–1.

Since patients generally continue this therapy once a week (or even more frequently) over a few years, it is wise to change the injection sites frequently. A practical method of keeping a record of where the allergy serum is injected each time is by alternating arms and

Patient's Name   Lot Number of Serum
Account Number   Expiration Date

INSTRUCTIONS FOR ADMINISTRATION

—Preparations should always be made for physician to treat anaphylaxis should it occur.

—Patients who are being treated with beta-blocker medications should not be given allergy serum.

—Use 27G 1/2" needle.

—Administer 3/8" to 1/2" into subcutaneous tissue between deltoid and biceps muscle (but not into the muscle).

—Aspirate plunger of syringe to ensure needle is not in a blood vessel.

—Reschedule patient for injection if s/he is feverish or is wheezing.

—Observe patient for possible reaction for 20 minutes following injection.

—Administer cold packs on site if local redness, itching, or wheal develops—alert physician for administration of antihistamine PRN.

—If a systemic or general reaction occurs, such as hives, sneezing or wheezing, alert physician for dosage and administration of epinephrine (subcutaneous).

—**Contact allergist for rescheduling instructions if systemic reaction occurs.**

SCHEDULE

Administer allergy serum injections every _____ days. If no adverse reaction occurs, resume scheduled dose. If adverse local reaction occurs, resume schedule with the last well-tolerated dose. Proceed with the following schedule until maximum dose is reached and well-tolerated. Then repeat maximum dose tolerated until vial is empty.

Dose	Date Administered	Adverse Reaction
0.10 cc	month/day/year	type of reaction
0.15 cc	initials of one who	if any (note the
0.20 cc	administered the	severity and
0.30 cc	injection	symptoms of
0.40 cc	and which arm	the patient)
0.50 cc	was injected	
*0.50 cc	Rt or L	

*Reorder before last dose is administered. Allow 2 weeks for delivery.

FIGURE 18–1   Example of schedule and instructions for allergy serum injections

numbering the injection sites. This pattern allows up to 18 injection sites and then it can be repeated. This may help in preventing tissue damage from recurring frequent injections of the same area. Keep track of the pattern on the schedule that comes with the allergy serum, or in the patient's chart by recording which arm, the number of the injection site, and of course, the date and your initials.

Figure 18–2, page 580, shows an illustration of (a) a suggested clockwise pattern and (b) charting method. Refer to Chapter 20 for the procedure for administering injections.

The size of the wheal is interpreted by the physician after a timed 20 to 30 minute period. Wheals are measured in centimeters by using a tape measure or by comparison, Figure 18–3, page 580. A trained skin tester may observe the reaction and make an interpretation by inspection alone.

Extracts of substances that are commonly the cause of allergy in patients are manufactured in applicator bottles. These should be refrigerated and the expiration date noted for accurate test results. Many of the skin testing extracts vary in strength from one company to another. Since specific allergens may also differ geographically, skin tests are sometimes unreliable. Standardization would be helpful, but new methods are being researched, and skin testing may one day become an obsolete procedure.

Scratch Test

Desirable sites for the scratch test are the arms and the back, depending on the number of tests to be performed and, in some cases, the preference of the patient. Small children are easier to restrain if they are lying face down while the test is being administered. The area to be tested should be comfortably accessible to both patient and physician or assistant. The patient must stay in the same position for at least 20 minutes, so comfort is essential for compliance.

The tests should be numbered in a pattern with washable ink on the surface of the skin. Explain to the patient that there will be some discomfort when administering either the scratch test or the intradermal test, but it will not last long. Instruct the patient to inform you of any itching or swelling at the site of injection. Advise the patient to avoid scratching the area for accurate interpretation following the prescribed timing of the test(s). Several extracts may be applied to the patient's skin in rows from evenly spaced applicators that have been dipped into various bottles of allergen substances. The applicator provides a small drop of the substance on the skin in preparation for the scratch test. Figure 18–4 shows a medical assistant applying seven different extracts on the patient's skin. Usually the skin is prepared with alcohol and allowed to air-dry. Alcohol may also be used to remove the ink after the test is completed. A sterile needle or lancet is used to tear the surface of the skin in a scratch of about $\frac{1}{8}$ inch or less to allow a drop of the antigen to enter the epidermis, Figure 18–5. Some test materials are packaged in sealed glass capillary tubes, the contents of which are shaken onto the skin after the tube is snapped. Only a small drop should be used. Otherwise, antigens may run together, and test results will be inaccurate. The scratches should be from $1\frac{1}{2}$ to 2 inches apart, allowing possible reactions to spread without interfering with each other. A control is used for comparison in inter-

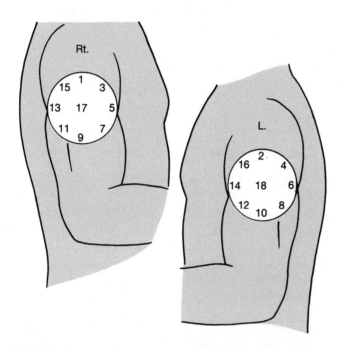

FIGURE 18–2 (a) This alternating pattern of injection allows 18 sites to help prevent possible tissue damage. Repeat as needed.

Progress Notes		
Patient's Name		
Date		
Page		
4-16-92	0.10 cc	Rt arm #1 jy
4-24-92	0.15 cc	L arm #2 jy
5-1-92	0.20 cc	Rt arm #3 jy
5-8-92	0.30 cc	L arm #4 jy

FIGURE 18–2 (b) Example of charting allergy serum injections on patient's chart.

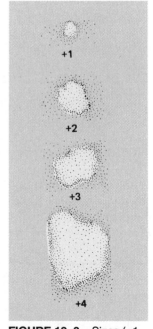

FIGURE 18–3 Sizes (+1 to +4) of wheals in reactions to skin test

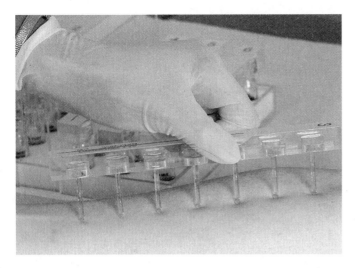

FIGURE 18–4   Placing allergy extract solutions on the skin with the multiple applicator

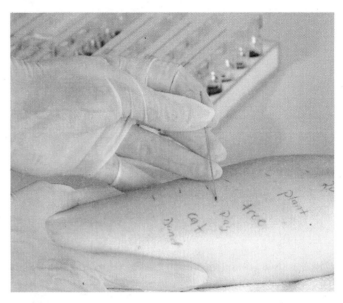

FIGURE 18–5   Each extract is labeled with ink for identification. The medical assistant uses a sterile lancet to scratch the skin, allowing the extract to enter the epidermis.

preting the results. This is a nonallergy-producing plain base fluid.

Reactions usually occur within the first 20 minutes (Itching at the test site may be relieved by application of cold or ice packs), Figure 18–6, page 582. Many physicians wish to recheck the test sites in 24 hours for delayed reactions. If the physician's interpretation of the

skin tests is consistent with the patient's history and physical examination findings, more advanced studies will not be necessary. It is not advisable to perform intradermal tests on patients who have had positive scratch tests.

    P R O C E D U R E

Perform a Scratch Test

PURPOSE: To determine an allergy-causing substance.
EQUIPMENT: Sterile needle(s) or lancet(s), allergen (extract), cotton balls, alcohol, pen, patient's chart, timer or timepiece, control, and disposable gloves
TERMINAL PERFORMANCE OBJECTIVE: Provided with all necessary instruments/supplies and a suitable simulated skin surface (such as an orange), the student will demonstrate each of the steps required in the scratch test procedure. Each step will be observed by the instructor.

1. Assemble all needed items near patient on Mayo table, wash hands, and put on gloves.
2. Explain procedure to identified patient as you prepare test site with alcohol-saturated cotton ball. Sites most commonly used are upper arm and back. **Key Point: Help patient find comfortable position.**
3. Apply small drop of extracts onto site and continue until all extracts are applied.
4. Mark site(s) with initial abbreviation or number of extract in pen if more than one test is to be administered. Leave about $1\frac{1}{2}$–2 inches between test sites.

5. Remove sterile needle or lancet from package without contaminating it. Make $\frac{1}{8}$-inch scratch in surface of skin.
6. Begin timing 20-minute period.
7. As soon as 20-minute time period is up, check each site after cleansing with alcohol-saturated cotton ball. Be careful not to wipe off the identification of the extract until after interpretation of reaction has been made by tester/physician. Wash hands.
8. Compare reaction of site with package insert drawings or measure in centimeters. **Key Point: Cold packs or ice bag may be applied to site to relieve itching.** (Note: It should be noted that this step cannot be realistically carried out when a simulated surface is used. However, until the new medical assistant gains experience on the job, the physician will probably make this comparison personally.)
9. Discard disposables in proper receptacle, return items to proper storage area, remove gloves, and wash hands.
10. Record test results on patient's chart.

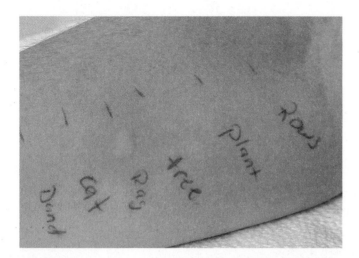

FIGURE 18–6 After timing skin tests for 20 minutes, note reaction on patient's chart. Pictured is a +3 wheal reaction to ragweed.

Intradermal Test

The intradermal test, thought to be more accurate, is often performed if the scratch test is negative or unclear. Although the solutions used for intradermal tests are about 100 times more dilute than those used for scratch tests, they are still potentially dangerous. Severe reactions may occur, however, with either method. Generally the diluted solutions used prevent systemic reactions. Intradermal test sites are performed at spaced intervals on the forearm, Figure 18–7, or scapular area. In the event of a severe adverse reaction, a tourniquet can be applied proximal to the site when the arm is used. The intradermal test can also be referred to as the *subcutaneous test*. Serum or vaccine is sometimes used in intradermal testing. If the initial test is negative, it is often repeated with a stronger solution. Usually the reaction time is 15 to 30 minutes. Epinephrine should be administered about an inch above the site by order of the physician if severe reaction occurs.

In performing an intradermal test, a fine-gauge needle (usually 26 G and $\frac{3}{8}$ to $\frac{5}{8}$ inch long) is used. The antigen is

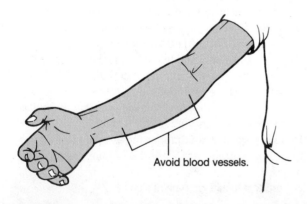

Avoid blood vessels.

FIGURE 18–7 The forearm is the most common area for up to 14 sites for intradermal skin tests.

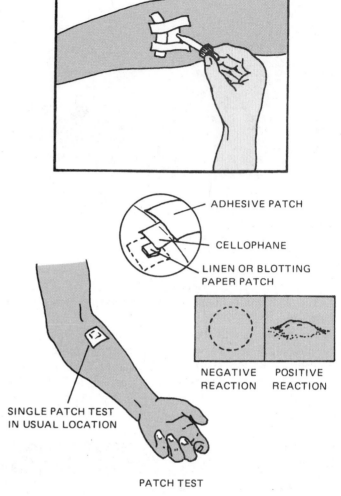

ADHESIVE PATCH

CELLOPHANE

LINEN OR BLOTTING PAPER PATCH

NEGATIVE REACTION   POSITIVE REACTION

SINGLE PATCH TEST IN USUAL LOCATION

PATCH TEST

FIGURE 18–8 Patch test application. Instruct patient to keep patch dry and in place until results are read by physician.

introduced into the dermal layer of the skin in minute dosages of 0.01 to 0.02 cc by sterile technique. The area will appear as a small blister from the fluid raising the skin. The reaction period is up to 30 minutes and the interpretation of the results is the same as in the scratch tests. Some antigens such as fungi and bacteria produce delayed reactions from 24 to 48 hours after administration.

Intradermal tests are sometimes used by physicians to determine medication sensitivity or immunization needs. Follow the procedure for intradermal injections in Chapter 20.

Patch Test

The patch test is done to determine the cause of contact dermatitis. A patch consisting of a gauze square saturated with the suspected allergy-causing substance is placed on the surface of the skin and secured with nonallergenic tape, Figure 18–8. The arm is the usual site of choice for convenience. The results are read after a 24-hour and then a 48-hour time period. A control is

Apply a Patch Test

PURPOSE: To determine the causative substance of suspected contact dermatitis.

EQUIPMENT: Commercially prepared paper with suspected substance or gauze saturated with substance, alcohol, cotton balls, gauze squares, nonallergenic tape, pen, patient's chart

TERMINAL PERFORMANCE OBJECTIVE: After practicing with water in lieu of the suspected substance, students will be provided with all necessary supplies, including the suspected substance; using another student as a patient, the student will demonstrate each of the steps required in carrying out the skin patch test, including the 48-hour recheck. The instructor will observe each step.

1. Assemble items next to patient on Mayo table, wash hands, and put on gloves.
2. Explain procedure while assisting identified patient to comfortable sitting position.
3. Clean test site with alcohol-saturated cotton ball and let air dry.
4. Apply suspected substance to test site and secure with nonallergenic tape. **Key Point: Usually it is placed near unaffected area in patients with contact dermatitis.** Remove gloves and wash hands.
5. Record date, time, substance, and area tested on patient's chart. Initial.
6. Schedule patient to return in 48 hours.
7. Instruct patient to keep area clean and dry until return appointment.
8. Remove patch; read results and record.

---

thought necessary and should be placed on the arm near the patch if the substance of the patch test is not a known skin irritant. Redness or swelling of the area indicates a reaction and its interpretation is based on grading as for scratch and intradermal tests.

PATIENT EDUCATION

During the allergy patient's visit, especially if recently diagnosed as such, giving the patient advice concerning the condition and the prevention of further problems will be well received. The following are a few suggestions for discussion with patients who have allergies.

1. Urge patients to follow the allergy serum desensitizing schedule closely to help build up immunity to the substance to which they are allergic.
2. Advise them to avoid what they are allergic to if at all possible.
3. Instruct patients to read all labels carefully (household products, clothing, consumable products, etc.) to identify possible allergens.
4. Urge them to develop and practice good health habits, such as sensible well-balanced diet, proper rest and exercise.
5. Advise them to take only prescribed medication and to avoid OTC medications unless advised by the physician.
6. If patients have a known severe reaction to a particular substance, remind them to carry their kit with them at all times.

Nasal Smear

A helpful aid for years in the diagnosis of allergies has been a smear done with nasal secretions to observe the eosinophil count. If there are many and they are clumped together, there is a strong indication of allergy. This is a simple means of screening for an allergy and is usually the first step in the testing program.

Complete Chapter 18, Unit 1 in the workbook to help you meet the objectives at the beginning of this unit and therefore achieve competency of this subject matter.

UNIT 2

Cardiology Procedures

OBJECTIVES ....

Upon completion of this unit, the student will meet the following terminal performance objectives by verifying knowledge of the facts and principles presented through oral and written communication at a level deemed competent, and will demonstrate the specific behaviors as identified in the terminal performance objectives of the procedures, observing all aseptic and safety precautions in accordance with health care standards.

1. Explain the reasons for performing an ECG.
2. Describe the electrical conduction system of the heart.
3. Describe the reason for mounting an ECG tracing.
4. Apply limb and chest electrodes properly.
5. Perform a routine 12-lead ECG.
6. Define *artifacts* and list their causes on an ECG.

7. State the purpose of a Holter monitor and explain the procedure to a patient.
8. Demonstrate the procedure for proper hook-up of a Holter monitor.
9. State the purpose of defibrillation.
10. Describe cardiac stress testing and discuss the proper placement of the electrodes.
11. State the purpose of cardiac stress testing.
12. Discuss patient education regarding the heart.
13. Spell and define, using the glossary at the back of the text, all the words to know in this unit.

WORDS TO KNOW ....

amplifier	interpretive
arrhythmia	interval
artifacts	limbs
atrial depolarization	mechanical
augmented	multichannel
cardiology	precordial
computerized	Purkinje
countershock	reliable
current	repolarization
defibrillator	sedentary
electrocardiogram	segment
electrocardiograph	simultaneous
electrode	somatic
electrolyte	standardization
galvanometer	stylus
Holter monitor	trace
impulse	treadmill
interference	voltage
intermittent	

In family and general practice, internal medicine, and **cardiology,** a procedure frequently used in the diagnosis of heart disease and dysfunction is the **electrocardio-**

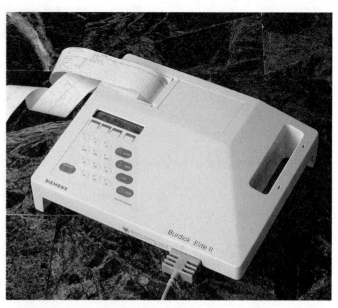

FIGURE 18–10   The portable single channel Burdick Elite II (Courtesy of Siemens Burdick, Inc.)

gram. This procedure is painless and safe, and patients should be told so to eliminate apprehension.

You will obtain the electrocardiogram (recording) (EKG/ECG) by operating the **electrocardiograph** (machine). Figures 18–9 through 18–11 show three widely used models of ECGs.

Through a process of electrical transmission, this machine **traces impulses** of the heart on paper to create a permanent record of its activity.

All muscle movement produces electrical impulses. The ECG is a recording of the electrical impulses of the heart muscle. To accomplish this, **electrodes,** some of which are shown in Figure 18–12 (a, b, and c), and in Figure 18–13, the various types of **electrolyte** are pictured for use with metal electrodes, are placed on the patient's **limbs** and chest, which pick up the electrical

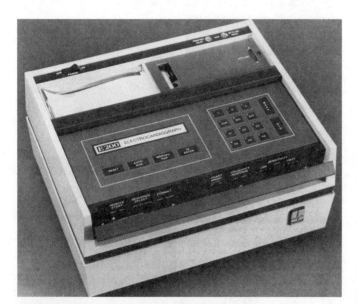

FIGURE 18–9   The portable E200 electrocardiograph (Courtesy of Siemens Burdick, Inc.)

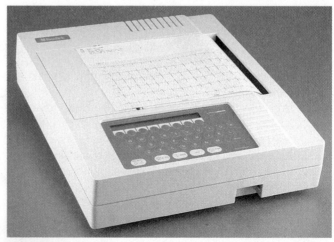

FIGURE 18–11   The multichannel Burdick E350 (Courtesy Siemens Burdick, Inc.)

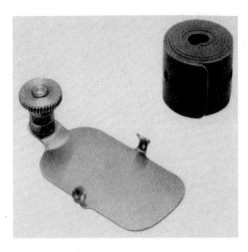

FIGURE 18–12 (a). Limb electrode and strap.(Courtesy of Siemens Burdick, Inc.)

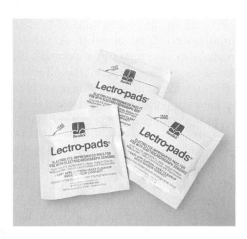

FIGURE 18–13 (a). Presaturated electrolyte pads. (Courtesy of Siemens Burdick, Inc.)

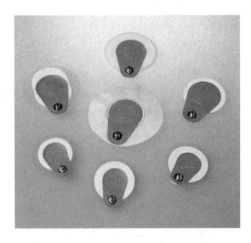

FIGURE 18–12 (b). Blue Max electrodes. (Courtesy of Siemens Burdick, Inc.)

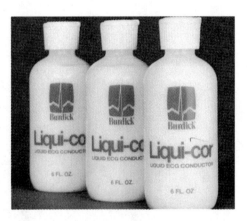

FIGURE 18–13 (b). Electrolyte lotion. (Courtesy of Siemens Burdick, Inc.)

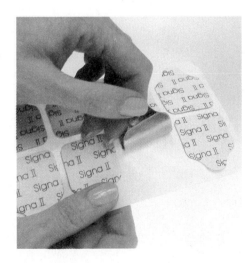

FIGURE 18–12 (c). Signa II disposable sensors (Courtesy of Siemens Burdick, Inc.)

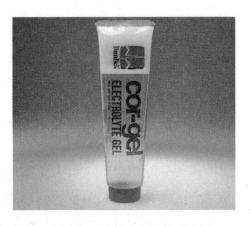

FIGURE 18–13 (c). Electrolyte used with defibrillator. (Courtesy of Siemens Burdick, Inc.)

current produced by the contractions of the heart. These minute impulses are transmitted to the electrocardiograph by metal tips (or clips) of the patient cable (wires) attached to the electrodes. Figure 18–14 displays Astro-Clips sometimes referred to as the "universal clip" because they can be used with most types of electrodes. The current enters the electrocardiograph through the wires to reach the amplifier, which enlarges the impulses. They are transformed into mechanical motion by the galvanometer. The stylus produces a printed representation on ECG paper. ECG paper is made for the different types of machines, standard, single, and multichannel, Figure 18–15. As the heated stylus moves against the tracing paper, the impulses given off by the heart are recorded. The tracing paper should be handled carefully to protect it from being accidentally marked. Dot matrix paper makes tracings easy to read and copy because they are clear and legible.

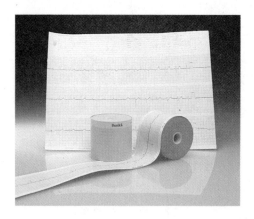

FIGURE 18–15   (a). ECG blush coat paper. (Courtesy of Siemens Burdick, Inc.)

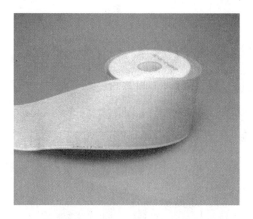

FIGURE 18–15   (b). Single channel paper. (Courtesy of Siemens Burdick, Inc.)

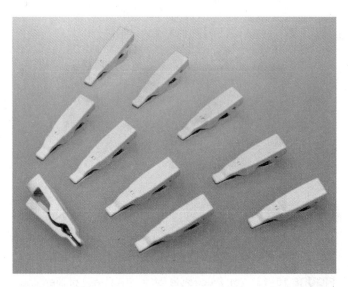

FIGURE 18–14   Astro clips. (Courtesy of Siemens Burdick, Inc.)

Some ECGs are mounted onto permanent folders for filing, Figure 18–16. The ECG trimmer is a handy tool for cutting the ECG tracings in preparation for mounting, Figure 18–17.

The ECG is interpreted by the physician, usually the one who ordered the procedure. Some physicians prefer to have a cardiologist interpret the ECG and send the results in the form of a written report with a copy of the tracing. The physician will read the ECG and compare the measurement, rate, rhythm, duration of the electrical waves, intervals, and segments with known normal ECG readings.

Path of Electrical Impulses ....

The heart is a four-chambered pump that produces minute electrical current by muscular contraction, Figure 18–18. An electrical impulse originates in the modified myocardial tissue of the SA (sinoatrial) node, causing

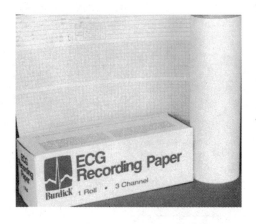

FIGURE 18–15   (c). Multichannel paper. (Courtesy of Siemens Burdick, Inc.)

the atria to contract, Figure 18–19. This contraction is the beginning of atrial depolarization, which is the first part of the cardiac cycle. The first impulse as recorded on the graph paper is termed the P wave. The impulse

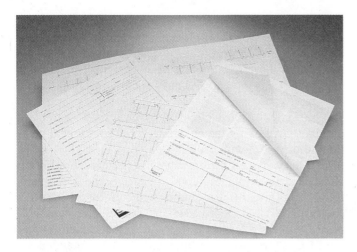

FIGURE 18–16 Various types of mounts for ECG tracing paper for patient's permanent record. (Courtesy of Siemens Burdick, Inc.)

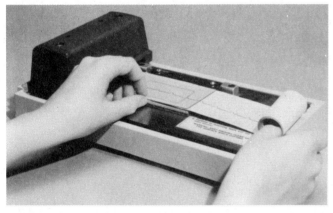

FIGURE 18–17 ECG trimmers used to process tracings for mounting (Courtesy of Siemens Burdick, Inc.)

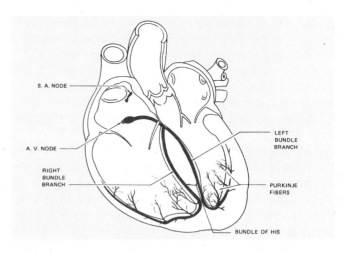

FIGURE 18–18 Anatomy of the heart

continues through the heart tissue to the AV (atrioventricular) node, to the bundle of His, and spreads to the Purkinje fibers. These fibers cause the muscles of the ventricles to contract and produce the QRS complex of waves on the ECG paper. The T wave on the graph paper follows, representing the repolarization of the ventricles, or the time of recovery before another contraction.

Routine Electrocardiograph Leads ....

The routine ECG consists of 12 leads, or recordings of the electrical activity of the heart from different angles. The first three leads are called standard or bipolar leads and are labeled with Roman numerals I, II, and III. These leads are obtained by placing limb electrodes on the

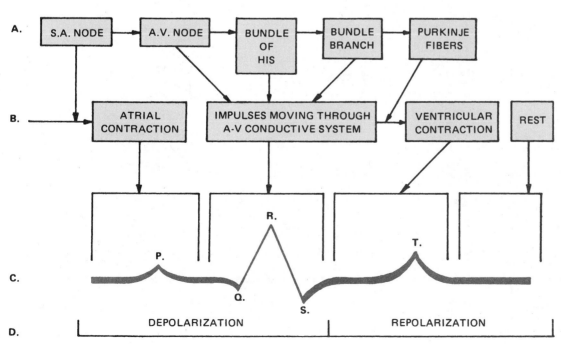

FIGURE 18–19 Diagrammatic representation of cardiac impulses on ECG tracing: (a). Course of electrical impulses. (b). Cardiac muscle reaction to impulses. (c). ECG tracing of impulse waves. (d). Phases of cardiac cycle (Courtesy of Siemens Burdick, Inc.)

fleshy part of the upper outer arms and the inner lower calves, Figure 18–20. Lead I records the electrical voltage difference between the right arm and left arm. Lead II records the difference between the right arm and left leg. Lead III records the voltage difference between the left arm and left leg, Figure 18–21.

The augmented leads are the next three in the standard 12-lead ECG. They are aVR, aVL, and aVF. aVR is the recording of the heart's voltage difference between the right arm electrode and a central point between the left arm and the left leg (augmented voltage right arm). aVL is the recording of the heart's voltage difference between the left arm electrode and a central point between the right arm and the left leg (augmented voltage left arm). aVF is the recording of the heart's voltage difference between the left leg electrode and a central

point between the right arm and left arm (augmented voltage left leg or foot). The term augmented means to become larger. Since these three leads are produced by such small impulses, the amplifier of the ECG machine augments their size sufficiently for recording them on the graph paper.

The six standard chest or precordial leads are obtained by moving the electrode to the anatomical positions shown in Figure 18–22.

The lead selector switch must be set for each different chest lead to obtain the correct code. Some electrocardiographs have an automatic lead marker to identify each of the 12 standard leads as the selector switch is turned. Others require the operator to mark each lead of the ECG. A standard marking code is recommended for use either with the manual or automatic method. Some

LEAD ARRANGEMENT AND CODING

STANDARD LIMB LEADS

LEAD MARKING CODE	LEAD	ELECTRODES CONNECTED	COLOR CODE			
					BODY	INSERT
•	LEAD 1	LA and RA	RL		GREEN	LT. GREEN
	LEAD 2	LL and RA	LL		RED	LT. RED
	LEAD 3	LL and LA	RA		WHITE	LT. GRAY
			LA		BLACK	LT. GRAY

AUGMENTED LIMB LEADS

LEAD MARKING CODE	LEAD	ELECTRODES CONNECTED	COLOR CODE			
					BODY	INSERT
••	aVR	RA and (LA-LL)	RL		GREEN	LT. GREEN
	aVL	LA and (RA-LL)	LL		RED	LT. RED
	aVF	LL and (RA-LA)	RA		WHITE	LT. GRAY
			LA		BLACK	LT. GRAY

CHEST LEADS

LEAD MARKING CODE	LEAD	ELECTRODES CONNECTED	COLOR CODE		
				BODY	INSERT
•••	V₁	V₁ and (LA-RA-LL)	V₁	BROWN	RED
	V₂	V₂ and (LA-RA-LL)	V₂	BROWN	YELLOW
	V₃	V₃ and (LA-RA-LL)	V₃	BROWN	LT. GREEN
••••	V₄	V₄ and (LA-RA-LL)	V₄	BROWN	LT. BLUE
	V₅	V₅ and (LA-RA-LL)	V₅	BROWN	ORANGE
	V₆	V₆ and (LA-RA-LL)	V₆	BROWN	VIOLET

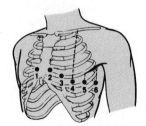

V1 Fourth intercostal space at right margin of sternum
V2 Fourth intercostal space at left margin of sternum
V3 Midway between position 2 and position 4
V4 Fifth intercostal space at junction of left midclavicular line
V5 At horizontal level of position 4 at left anterior axillary line
V6 At horizontal level of position 4 at left midaxillary line

FIGURE 18–20 Proper placement of electrodes for the standard routing 12-lead ECG and lead marking codes. (Courtesy of Siemens Burdick, Inc.)

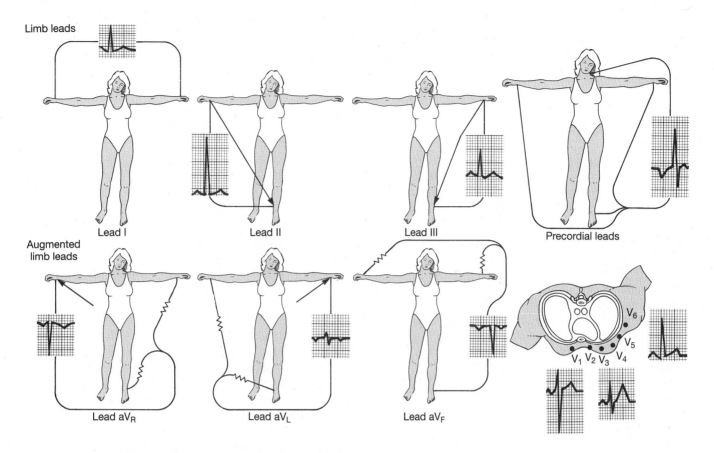

FIGURE 18–21   Voltage difference between leads (Courtesy of Siemens Burdick, Inc.)

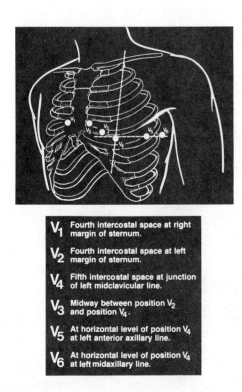

V₁	Fourth intercostal space at right margin of sternum.
V₂	Fourth intercostal space at left margin of sternum.
V₄	Fifth intercostal space at junction of left midclavicular line.
V₃	Midway between position V₂ and position V₄.
V₅	At horizontal level of position V₄ at left anterior axillary line.
V₆	At horizontal level of position V₄ at left midaxillary line.

FIGURE 18–22   Recommended positions for precordial ECG leads (Courtesy of Siemens Burdick, Inc.)

physicians prefer other codes. It is best to follow the policy where you are employed.

Interference

As with any procedure, a full explanation must be given to the patient to gain cooperation. Providing privacy and adequate draping of the patient during the procedure will ease patient apprehension and avoid chills. The patient must be relaxed for a good tracing to be obtained, as any movement of the patient may cause **interference** on the tracing. Shivering from nervousness or cold can produce muscle voltage artifacts for example. This additional activity is called **somatic** tremor. Arm electrodes should be placed close to the shoulders of the upper outer arms to decrease the possibility of muscle voltage **artifacts,** Figure 18–23, page 591.

Other artifacts which may appear on the ECG, called AC interference, are caused by electrical activity. The latest models of electrocardiographs have sensitive filtering devices that eliminate most of the interference, but it is still recommended that a room with a minimum of electrical wiring be used for the ECG procedure. All power cords should be kept away from the patient, and the patient table should be away

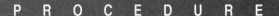
Obtain a Standard 12-Lead ECG (EKG)

PURPOSE: To obtain a graphic representation of the electrical activity of the patient's heart

EQUIPMENT: Electrocardiograph, ECG paper, four metal limb electrodes and straps, [or disposable pregelled adhesive electrodes as appropriate for use with patient cable of ECG machine—lead wires with snaps, clips, or tips (use chest strap if necessary) to attach to electrodes], patient cable, electrolyte (pads, cream, or gel), chest strap, treatment table, pillow, drape sheet, tissues, paper towels, ECG mount, footstool, tongue depressor, patient's chart, pen, disposable razor

TERMINAL PERFORMANCE OBJECTIVE: Provided with an electrocardiograph and all essential equipment/supplies and using other students as patients, the student will demonstrate each of the steps required in obtaining a standard 12-lead ECG reading/recording. The instructor will observe each step. Note: The specified disrobing may be simulated.

1. Plug in ECG machine to outlet away from known electrical interference. Plug in patient cable wire to machine. Assemble electrodes and attach to straps. Apply electrolyte pads and set aside. Turn machine on. Wash hands.

2. Ask patient to disrobe from waist up and remove clothing from lower legs. Provide privacy and show patient where to put belongings. Explain procedure.

3. Assist identified patient onto treatment table and cover with drape sheet. Ask patient to lie down. Pull leg rest out. Adjust pillow under patient's head for comfort.

4. Apply chest strap by placing hard plastic end under left side of patient and weighted end against right side of patient's chest. Recover chest with drape sheet.

5. Place arm electrodes (with electrolyte) on fleshy outer area of upper arm with connectors pointing toward shoulders. Straps should be moved one space tighter than relaxed. Leg electrodes (applied with electrolyte) should be placed on fleshy inner area of lower leg near calf, connectors pointing toward upper body. If gel or cream is used, use a small amount, the size of a dime, and spread with tongue depressor. If disposable electrodes are used, use tongue depressor or gauze square to rub sites vigorously to increase circulation and promote better contact of the electrodes.

6. Connect lead wire tips to appropriate electrodes by screwing tightly in place all pointing down, or by snapping or clipping electrodes securely in place. **Key Point: Power cord should be pointing away from patient.**

7. Place chest electrode (electrolyte side up) under chest strap and secure until needed, or attach all 6 pregelled disposable adhesive chest electrodes V1 through V6 (shaving dense chest hair as necessary for placement of electrodes), Figure 18–27.

8. Turn lead selector switch to STD and adjust stylus to center of graph paper.

9. Move record switch to 25-mm/second position and run for a few seconds to adjust centering of stylus. Make standardization mark 2 mm wide and 10 mm height. Then turn off, or with computerized electrocardiograph (single and multichannel), press "auto" and run the 12-lead ECG; and proceed to appropriate instructions for steps #13 though #17.

10. Turn lead selector switch to lead I and run 8 to 12 inches of tracing. Proceed in same manner for leads II and III. Run 4 to 6 inches each of leads aVR, aVL, and aVF. **Key Point: Lead selector switch should be allowed a second or two to pause between leads to allow for adjustment.**

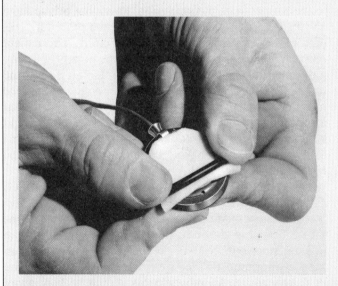

FIGURE 18–27 (a). Chest lead electrode held in place with chest strap. (Courtesy of Siemens Burdick, Inc.)

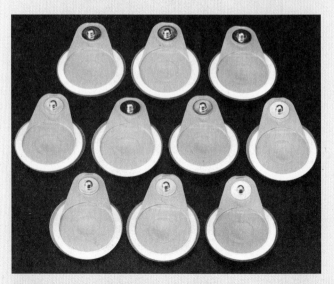

FIGURE 18–27 (b). Adhesive pregelled disposable electrodes (Courtesy of Siemens Burdick, Inc.)

This permits steadier centering of tracing. Standardization should appear at beginning of each lead if requested by physician; otherwise at beginning of tracing and whenever sensitivity switch is changed to either reduce or enlarge size of cardiac cycles. **Key Point: Each lead should be marked accordingly either manually or automatically by the machine.**

11. Turn lead selector switch either to V of V1 depending on machine you are using. Place chest electrode in proper position and standardize. Run 4 to 6 inches of recording. Turn switch to AMP OFF when changing electrode positions to keep stylus from moving about. Move chest electrode to V2 for second chest lead and run 4 to 6 inches of recording, then to V3, and so on. **Key Point: Turn the run switch to AMP off after each of the chest or precordial leads. Allow stylus to adjust to next lead by pausing a few seconds so that centering is certain and standardize as instructed. Mark each lead.**

12. Turn lead selector switch back to STD slowly, one lead at a time to avoid stripping gears of dial. Run recording out until baseline only appears and turn machine off.

13. Tear off tracing from machine. **Key Point: Immediately mark it with patient's name, age, day's date, and your initials.** Roll or loosely overlap tracing back and forth, secure with paper clip carefully, and set aside.

14. Remove tips of lead wires from limb electrodes by unscrewing ends. Remove chest electrode and strap and limb straps and electrodes from patient. Clean sites with a warm wet paper towel and dry. Discard used towels in proper receptacle.

15. Assist patient to sitting position and then down from table when ready. Assist patient in dressing if necessary.

16. Change table paper and pillow cover and discard used disposables. Wash hands.

17. Placing tracing in patient's chart, initial ECG order, and place in appropriate area for physician to read. Or, mount tracing on desired form and place in patient's chart for physician to review. **Key Point: Record any unusual findings or observations on patient's chart.**

from the wall to eliminate the possibility of electrical interference from the wall. The patient must be properly connected with the electrodes and properly grounded. Using good technique will also reduce AC

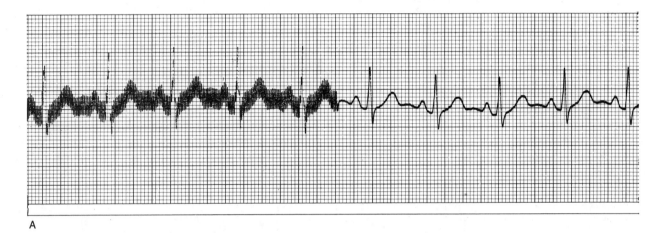

A

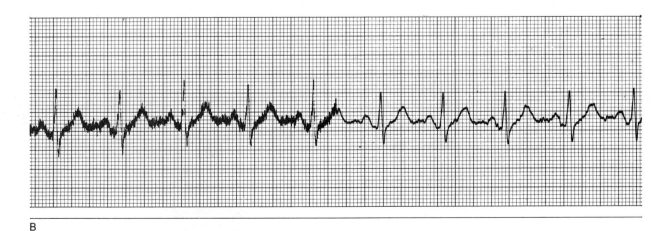

B

FIGURE 18–23 ECG interference: (a). Somatic tremor, or involuntary muscle movement. (b). AC (alternating current) (Courtesy of Siemens Burdick, Inc.)

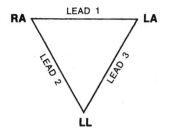

LOCATION OF SOURCE OF ARTIFACTS

Leads 1, 2, and 3 can be helpful in locating the source of interference. Refer to the triangle. Notice that each limb electrode is involved in recording two of the three leads. This means that if an artifact is observed in two leads but not in the third, the artifact is probably caused by a condition at or near the electrode that is common to the two leads. Examples: tremor on leads 1 and 3 and not on lead 2 indicates that the left arm is the probable source since it is common to leads 1 and 3. Similarly, a large amount of AC interference appearing in leads 1 and 2 and a smaller amount in lead 3, would most likely indicate that the AC source is near the right arm. If interference problems cannot be readily solved, contact your Burdick dealer or The Burdick Corporation for the name of your nearest Burdick field representative. They have equipment to help you find the interference source and can offer suggestions to eliminate or reduce the problem.

FIGURE 18–24 Sources of artifacts from leads (Courtesy of Siemens Burdick, Inc.)

interference. The sources of artifacts from different leads is shown in Figure 18–24.

Wandering baseline can be caused by corroded or improperly applied electrodes or by an unequal amount of electrolyte on the electrodes. Another cause is improperly cleaned skin. Oils, creams, and lotions should be removed from the patient's skin with alcohol or the conduction of electrical impulses will be impaired. Interrupted baseline is caused by an electrode becoming separated from the wire or by a broken lead wire. Follow manufacturer's instructions for repairing the electrocardiograph.

To further ensure a good ECG the operator must use clean electrodes. Metal electrodes should be cleaned with a mild detergent solution after each use and with scouring powder and a cloth as needed. The rubber straps should also be washed with a mild detergent solution after each use. A proper amount of electrolyte must be used with each electrode to provide maximum electrical conduction. Individual packets of pretreated disposable pads are available for convenience.

Many offices and clinics still use a standard electrocardiograph with the metal electrodes and limb straps. All of the computerized channel ECG machines require the disposable electrodes and electrolyte pads. These are widely used because of their convenience. Because they are obviously more expensive, you should use them wisely and avoid unnecessary waste.

Standardization

The standardization of the ECG is necessary to enable a physician to judge deviations from the standard. The usual standardization mark is 2 mm wide and 10 mm high. This mark should begin each lead to provide a reliable reading. If the tracing is too large, the sensitivity button should be turned down to $\frac{1}{2}$ to produce a standardization mark 5 mm high and 2 mm wide. If the tracing is too small, the sensitivity button can be turned up to 2 making the impulse 20 mm high and 2 mm wide. You must pay close attention to the tracing as it is being run to make adjustments as needed. Figure 18–25, shows the standardization marking from and electrocardiograph with the sensitivity dial set at $\frac{1}{2}$, 1, and 2.

The stylus should be centered in the middle of the paper. The baseline will allow you to observe the centering and make adjustments as necessary. The temperature of the stylus can be adjusted to control the thickness of the line.

The tracing paper is normally run at a speed of 25 mm per second. If the ECG cycles are too close together, the speed can be changed to 50 mm per second, Figure 18–26. This adjustment should be noted in pen on the tracing.

The physician may order a standard 12-lead ECG with a rhythm strip. This simply means that you should record a long strip, usually 12 inches, or for a period of seconds

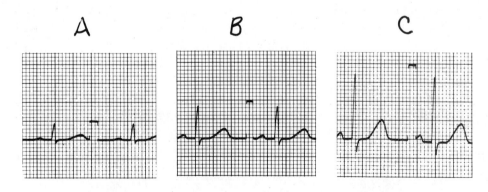

A   B   C

FIGURE 18-25 Standardization markings with sensitivity dial set on (a) 1/2, (b) 1, (c) 2. (Courtesy of Siemens Burdick, Inc.)

(generally 30, or however long the physician orders for the rhythm strip) of lead II in addition to the standard tracing. This gives the physician a better look at the rhythm of the heartbeat and how often an irregularity occurs.

Any obvious abnormality should be brought to the physician's attention immediately if the patient is experiencing pain or discomfort at the time it is observed.

The ECG is an extremely important procedure. Every detail must be performed accurately.

It is extremely important that the patient be relaxed and comfortable during the ECG procedure. Reassure the patient by answering any questions. Explain that the machine does not "put electricity" into the body. Your calm, efficient manner will help the patient relax.

The computerized electrocardiographs have many timesaving features. They have simultaneous 12-lead interpretive analysis. Date are not only printed out, but also stored in its memory. The entire ECG tracing is generated in about 1 minute. There is no time involved in mounting. A manual mode provides additional leads, such as the rhythm strip of lead II which may be run from 10 seconds to however long the physician requests. These machines are relatively light weight and can be easily moved if necessary.

The ECG can detect damage from previous heart attacks, enlargement of the heart muscle, disturbances in the rhythm, and other abnormal conditions. It is usually recommended for patients between the ages of 35

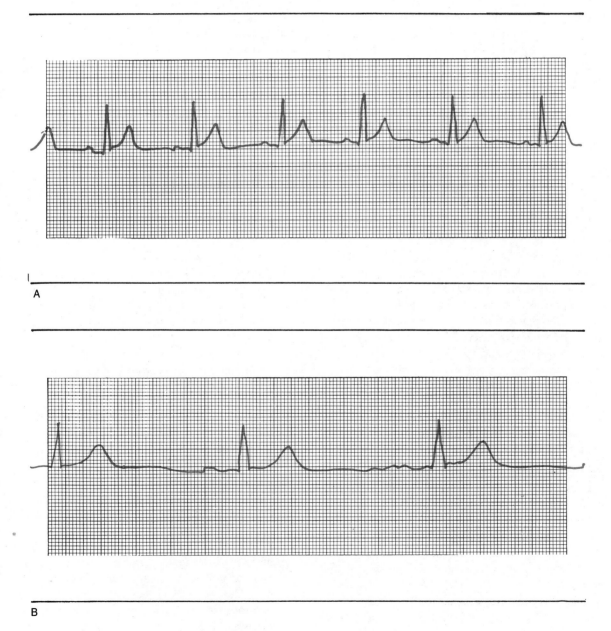

FIGURE 18–26 ECG paper: lead II run at 25 mm/sec (a) and lead II run at 50 mm/sec (b). Lead II is also known as a rhythm strip.

and 40 to establish a base reading. Physicians may then refer to this ECG in the event of later problems. Most often an ECG is performed along with the routine annual physical examination every 5 to 10 years after a baseline normal reading has been established. Some physicians prefer to have a tracing more often, even annually, for patients who have a history of hypertension, are smokers, are obese, or have a high serumcholesterol level. Another factor in heart problems is a sedentary life-style, which is usually accompanied by obesity.

Stress Tests

ECG stress tests are done by some physicians on a routine basis for patients with a high risk of developing heart disease. They are more often done in a limited manner for patients interested in starting a strenuous exercise program or those who continue to have heart pain even after a routine ECG has been read as normal. Figure 18–28, illustrates the BaseLine prep kit and instructions for cardiac stress testing. The stress test ECG is done while a patient is exercising either on a bicycle or treadmill under careful supervision. Figure

18–29, page 596 shows a physician reading the computerized printout of a stress test in progress. The medical assistant monitors the patient's blood pressure while he exercises on the treadmill. The purpose of this test is to detect the unknown cause of the patient's heart trouble. Even with ECGs and other diagnostic tests the physician cannot predict future heart attacks.

Holter Monitoring

Patients who have normal routine ECGs but still have intermittent or irregular chest pain or discomfort, are often tested over a period of 24 hours or more by a device known as a Holter monitor. This method of recording the electrical activities of a patient's heart for a period of time is also referred to as an ambulatory (walking) or "24-hour ECG." The ECG electrodes are attached to the patient's chest wall. A portable cassette recorder (monitor) is attached to a belt worn around the patient's waist. Figure 18–30, page 596, shows the anatomical placement of electrodes. During the prescribed period of time, usually 24 hours, the patient's heart action is recorded. The patient is asked to keep a diary of all activities and note any pain or discomfort

---

P R O C E D U R E

Holter Monitoring

PURPOSE: To detect chest pain and cardiac arrhythmias; to evaluate chest pain and cardiac status following pacemaker implantation or after an acute myocardial infarction; and to determine correlation of symptoms and activity.

EQUIPMENT: Disposable razor/shaving cream, alcohol and swabs, pregelled adhesive electrodes, lead wires, appropriate batteries/recorder, standard ECG, diary for patient, belt for recorder, nonallergenic tape to secure electrodes PRN, drape sheet, patient's chart, pen

TERMINAL PERFORMANCE OBJECTIVE: With all equipment and supplies provided, the student will demonstrate the steps of the procedure for hooking up a patient for the Holter monitor. The instructor will observe each step.

1. Explain procedure to identified patient. Ask patient to remove clothing from the waist up (provide a drape sheet). Assist patient to sit at the end of the examination table.
2. Wash hands and assemble equipment and supplies on Mayo table near patient.
3. Test Holter for proper working order and replace with new batteries.
4. Use shaving cream and razor to remove chest hair if necessary. Rinse and dry electrode sites and clean

with alcohol swabs.

5. Rub each site vigorously with gauze square and apply electrodes and lead wires carefully, making sure there is good skin contact. Use extra tape to secure electrodes and wires. Refer to Figures 18–30 and 18–31, page 596.
6. Place the belt around the patient's waist and advise patient in care of recorder and precautions (refer to text). Assist patient in dressing to help avoid disturbing wires and electrodes. Remind patient not to take a tub bath or shower during 24-hour period.
7. Instruct patient to go about routine daily activities, but to be sure to note in diary any symptoms or problems experienced, (time it occurred and how long it lasted).
8. Record date and time that monitor began on patient's chart and in the patient's diary, and initial.
9. Give patient diary to take with him/her and a return appointment time.
10. When patient comes in for appointment the next day, assist in disrobing; remove electrodes and wires, clean electrode sites, and place cassette from recorder in computerized ECG for printout of tracing. Place diary and recording of ECG in patient's chart for evaluation by physician and initial.

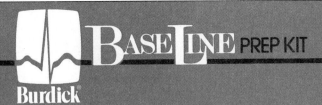

BASELINE PREP KIT

Burdick

INSTRUCTIONS FOR USE

Special Note: Proper skin preparation is a critical step in obtaining the best Base Line results.

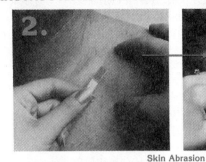

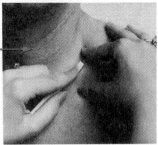

1.

Site Preparation
☐ To free skin from all body oils, cleanse **each** sensor placement site with alcohol swabstick.

2.

Skin Abrasion
☐ Place the Burdick Skin Rasp between thumb and index finger with the rough portion against the skin.

☐ Using moderate pressure, stroke each Blue Max sensor site (gel area only) two or three times.

3. Blue Max Sensor Placement
☐ Remove protective backing from Blue Max Sensor.

☐ Pointing the blue snap tab toward the lower center of the abdomen, place the gel portion of the sensor over the prepared site.

☐ Pressing on the foam ring of sensor **only**, secure sensor to the skin.

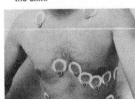

* RA: Right Arm (RA) Sensor should be placed to the extreme right while still remaining on the clavical bone.
* LA: Left Arm (LA) Sensor should be placed to the extreme left while still remaining on the clavical bone.
* RL: Right Leg (RL) Sensor should be placed on the lower portion of the right rib cage.
* LL: Left Leg (LL) Sensor should be placed on the lower portion of the left rib cage.
* V1: Fourth intercostal space at right margin of sternum.
* V2: Fourth intercostal space at left margin of sternum.
* V4: Fifth intercostal space at junction of left mid-clavicular line.
* V3: Midway between V2 and V4.
* V5: At horizontal level of V4 at left anterior axillary line.
* V6: At horizontal level of V4 at left mid-axillary line.

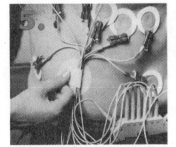

4.

E.C.G. Cable Connection to Blue Max Sensor
☐ Apply cable lead by lifting sensor offset tab and pinching cable and sensor snap button together.

5.

Burdick Cable Restraint Placement/Cable Bundling
☐ Remove protective paper from the inner circle, then from the outer circle of the adhesive area.

☐ Adhere the Burdick Cable Restraint over the lower abdomen with the tab pointing either to the right or left.

☐ Remove the protective paper from the Cable Restraint Tab.

☐ Taking up all the slack in the lead cables, bundle over the Cable Restraint Tab center.

☐ Fold tab over cables and press firmly, holding cables in place.

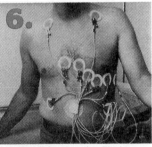

6.

Securing Cable Junction Block
☐ Secure cable junction block to belt/harness.

7. PROCEED WITH STRESS TEST.

©1988 Burdick Corporation, 915 North Plum Grove Road, Suite C, Schaumburg, IL 60173 (312) 882-4550

FIGURE 18–28 BaseLine prep kit instructions for stress testing (Courtesy of Siemens Burdick, Inc.)

experienced during this monitoring. Figure 18–31, shows the medical assistant giving instructions to the patient about recording any problems. The patient is instructed to press the "event button" when any cardiac symptoms are experienced. At the end of the test period, the patient returns to have the electrodes and monitor removed. The cassette is then placed in a computerized analyzer for a permanent printout of the results (or sent to a laboratory for interpretation). Evaluation of the 24-hour tracing reveals any cardiac **arrhythmias,** chest pain, and effectiveness of cardiac medications, and correlates any symptoms with the patient's activity at the time it occurred. You should instruct patients to carry on with all routine daily activities during this test. Advise patients to take a "sponge bath" and not to get into a tub or shower while conducting this monitoring heart test. Ask patients to avoid using electric blankets or being around metal detectors, magnets, and high-voltage areas because these might interfere with the recording. This method of monitoring is also used in evaluating the status of recovering cardiac patients. Another version of this test permits the patient to activate the recording device only when experiencing symptoms. This patient-activated monitor can be worn for several days.

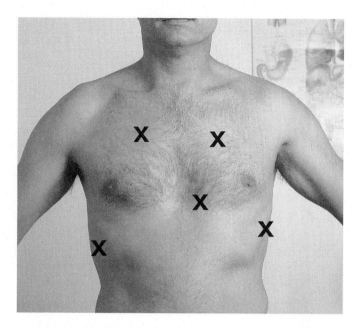

FIGURE 18–30 Anatomical placement of chest electrodes for Holter monitoring.

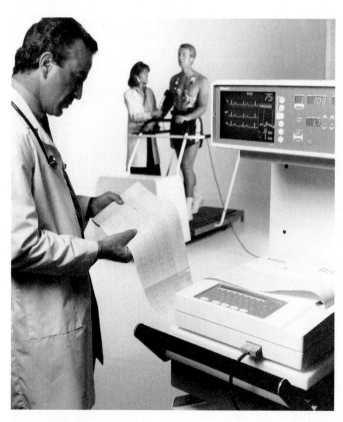

FIGURE 18–29 The EXTOL 350 ST Stress system (Courtesy of Siemens Burdick, Inc.)

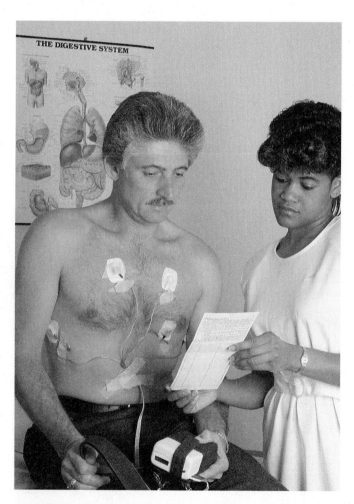

FIGURE 18–31 The medical assistant shows the patient the diary and gives instructions regarding the Holter monitor before securing it around his waist.

During the time you spend with patients in performing electrocardiographic testing and its instruction, you will have ample opportunity to give patients some of the following suggestions.

1. Remind them to eat a low-fat, low-cholesterol diet, and keep their salt/sodium intake at a minimum.
2. Advise them to get proper rest and exercise and keep their weight at an acceptable level.
3. Instruct cardiac patients to take their prescribed medication regularly and to report any problems they may experience to the physician immediately.
4. Remind them to keep their scheduled appointments and make a list of questions for the doctor to review with them at that time.
5. Advise them not to take OTC medications.
6. Urge them not to use tobacco and to avoid alcoholic beverages.

Many medical offices, clinics, and emergency centers are equipped with a defibrillator, Figure 18–32. These units are designed to provide countershock by a trained individual to convert cardiac arrhythmias into regular sinus rhythm. Part of your routine duties may be to check this, and other equipment and supplies, to ensure that they are in proper working order and that everything is ready in case of a cardiac emergency. Employers offer in-service training periodically to all employees in assisting with emergency procedures. All employees should

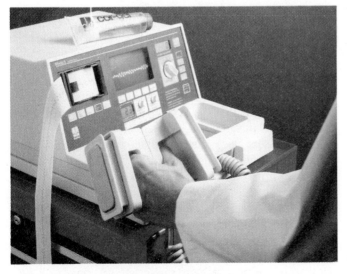

FIGURE 18–32 The Medic IV defibrillator and Cor-gel (electrolyte gel) (Courtesy of Siemens Burdick, Inc.)

have current CPR cardiopulmonary resuscitation (CPR) certification.

Complete chapter 18, Unit 2 in the workbook to help you meet the objectives at the beginning of this unit and therefore achieve competency of this subject matter.

UNIT 3

Diagnostic Procedures

OBJECTIVES ··

Upon completion of this unit, the student will meet the following terminal performance objectives by verifying knowledge of the facts and principles presented through oral and written communication at a level deemed competent, and will demonstrate the specific behaviors as identified in the terminal performance objectives of the procedures, observing all aseptic and safety precautions in accordance with health care standards.

1. Describe a spirometry test and state the purpose of it.
2. Instruct a patient about the spirometer and demonstrate how to use it.
3. Explain what magnetic resonance imaging (MRI) is.
4. List reasons for contraindication of the MRI.
5. Describe ultrasound and state the purpose of it.
6. Explain the patient preparation for ultrasound procedures.
7. Explain the reason for a Hemoccult sensa test and the procedure to be followed.
8. Perform and interpret a Hemoccult sensa slide test.
9. Discuss patient education concerning the procedures in this unit.
10. Spell and define, using the glossary at the back of this text, all the words to know in this unit.

WORDS TO KNOW ··

claustrophobia	occult
diaphanography	oscilloscope
echocardiography	reagent
echoes	resonance
electromagnetic	sonogram
guaiac	sophisticated
imaging	spirometer
implants	thermography
magnetic	transducer
maturity	transillumination
noninvasive	ultrasonic scanning

Vital Capacity Tests

Vital capacity is defined as the greatest volume of air that can be expelled during a complete, slow, unforced expiration following a maximum inspiration. Vital capacity should equal inspiratory capacity plus expiratory reserve. Vital capacity is usually reported in both absolute values and statistically derived values based on the age, sex, and height of the patient. The statistical value is reported as a percentage.

Several devices are used to measure the capacity of the lungs. Many physicians prefer to use the hand-held spirometer, which comes with vital capacity charts.

Vital capacity testing is performed to evaluate patients who are suspected to have pulmonary insufficiency. The spirometer is an instrument used to test the capacity of the lungs. Vital capacity testing aids in the diagnosis of and degree of functional or obstructive abnormalities. It also helps the physician find the cause of dyspnea and evaluate the effectiveness of medication and therapy.

When scheduling patients for these tests of vital capacity, it is important to advise them to eat lightly and not to smoke for at least 6 hours before the appointment. Patients should refrain from routine treatment, and medication should not be taken until after the test is completed.

In preparing to perform this diagnostic procedure, instruct the patient regarding the necessary steps and demonstrate the use of the spirometer. Routine procedures, such as, height, weight, and vital signs should be taken and recorded on the patient's chart. Showing the patient how to hold the instrument and what is expected will yield a more accurate test result. Disposable mouthpieces are used to prevent disease transmission. Most spirometers are computerized and have a printout of the results within minutes of administering the test. You should type in the patient's name, age, height, race and sex, account number, and any other information if applicable, before you start the test.

Figure 18–33 pictures the medical assistant coaching a patient through the procedure. A clip is placed on the patient's nose to force the expired air out of the lungs directly into the mouthpiece (make sure patient's mouth is sealed around the mouthpiece) and into the spirometer. Instruct the patient to stand up straight and to take in a slow deep breath. Coach the patient to expel all the air from the lungs quickly until s/he cannot exhale any more, within approximately 15 seconds. Give the patient a couple of practice runs before beginning the official test because it is an awkward procedure for most people. Follow each of the expirations with a few seconds of resting for the patient. Watch for signs of stress, dizziness, coughing, or other problems the patient may have during the test. Generally 3 to 5 expirations are tested. The results are analyzed by the computerized instrument and the diagnostic data are printed for evaluation by the

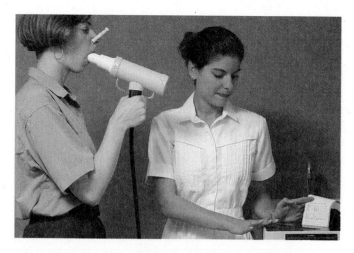

FIGURE 18–33 The medical assistant operates the computerized spirometer while the patient blows exhaled air from the lungs into the disposable mouthpiece.

physician. Test results below 80% are usually considered abnormal. This spirometry reading is placed in the patient's chart, along with a notation of any symptoms or problems the patient may have had during the test, and your initials. Spirometry tests should not be performed when the patient has been diagnosed with angina, acute coronary insufficiency, or recent myocardial infarction. Allow the patient to sit and relax to wait for consultation with physician. Instruct the patient to resume medication and therapy routine as directed by the physician.

You may be instructed to schedule patients for further pulmonary function studies to be performed by a pulmonary and thoracic specialist. More sophisticated equipment may be necessary to evaluate a patient's condition.

Sonographic Studies

Sonograms are records obtained by ultrasonic scanning. Ultrasonography is a technique in which internal structures are made visible by recording the reflections, or echoes, of ultrasonic sound waves directed into the tissues. These high-frequency sound waves are conducted through the use of a transducer (a hand-held instrument resembling a microphone). While the transducer is held against the body area to be tested, it sends sound waves through the skin to various organs. As the echoes are sent back, the transducer picks them up and changes them into electrical energy. This energy is transmitted into an image on a monitor, or printed out on paper in wavy lines. The picture formed on the screen represents a cross section of the organ. Photos of these images are taken for permanent records. The physician interprets these images to aid in the diagnosis and treatment of the patient. Echocardiography is a technique used to examine the heart: echoes are converted into electrical impulses, which create a picture of the tissues being examined on an oscilloscope.

> (1) ABDOMINAL ULTRASOUND: Take nothing by mouth after midnight. No breakfast on the morning of the examination.
>
> (2) PELVIC ULTRASOUND: Drink 24–30 ounces of fluid 1 hour before the examination. Do not urinate after drinking the fluid.
>
> (3) FETAL ULTRASOUND: Drink 24–30 ounces of fluid 1 hour before the examination. Do not urinate after drinking the fluid.

FIGURE 18–34 Preparation for ultrasound

Ultrasonography is useful in examination of the abdominopelvic cavity to locate aneurysms of the aorta and other blood vessel abnormalities. The size and shape of internal organs can also be determined with ultrasound. It can be of value in the identification of cysts and tumors of the eye and in the detection of pelvic masses and obstructions of the urinary tract. In obstetrics and gynecology, where the radiation of X ray examinations is avoided, ultrasound is useful in the diagnosis of multiple pregnancies and in determining the size, maturity, and position of the fetus. Patient preparation may vary but usually the patient is instructed to drink a large amount of water, up to a quart. This will distend the bladder and help to push the uterus into place as well as increase the conduction of the sound waves. Sonograms are not useful in viewing the lungs, for echoes are not created by structures containing air.

When scheduling patients for this type of study, you should give them a few important instructions. They should avoid eating foods that produce gas and drink plenty of fluids (specific amounts are required for certain tests) as mentioned earlier, for example, in determining the size of the fetus, Figure 18–34. Explain to the patient that s/he will be asked to lie down on an examination table and that the procedure lasts approximately 45 minutes to an hour. It is an accurate and painless diagnostic tool. A gel or lotion is used to produce better sound wave conduction and to allow the transducer to glide more easily across the skin.

Besides being a diagnostic procedure, ultrasound is used in the treatment of diseased or injured muscle tissue. Sound waves vibrate into the tissues producing heat, which helps to relieve inflammation and pain. It also increases circulation, which speeds up healing of injured muscle tissues. Another common use of ultrasound is in dentistry. Sound vibrations make it possible for tartar to be painlessly removed from the teeth.

Specific in-service training is necessary before using this instrument because the patient can be burned if precautions are not followed precisely.

Other uses are being discovered as research continues in this field. Other methods besides ultrasound and x rays are used to detect masses and cysts in the body. One is called **thermography.** As the name implies, thermography is a measurement of the "heat" patterns given off by the skin. This method is sometimes used to detect masses and cysts in breast tissue. Changes in the images produced are usually suggestive of a problem with breast tissue. A "hot spot" pattern may detect a breast mass. When this is the case, mammography is the next step in determining the diagnosis.

Another method to detect breast tissue masses and cysts is the **diaphanography.** A bright light, or **transillumination,** is shown through the breast tissue. This means of examination can show a difference between a solid tumor and a cyst in breast tissue. However, very small cancers are not detected by this method, and again, mammography is the next diagnostic test to determine the patient's condition.

MRI—Magnetic Resonance Imaging ....

A technique to view the structures inside the human body is called MRI, **magnetic resonance imaging.** This method allows physicians to examine a particular area of the body without exposing the patient to X rays or surgery. This **noninvasive** procedure, which may range from 30 to 60 minutes, requires that the patient lie on a padded table that is moved into a tunnel-like structure, Figure 18–35.

There is no advance patient preparation required for this examination. The MRI procedure becomes an *invasive* procedure only when an intravenous contrast media is administered to the patient under certain conditions. This *contrast enhanced* technique is done during the last series of images of the examination to detect certain pathologies. The patient may resume normal activity following the procedure. There are no known harmful effects to the patient from this imaging technique.

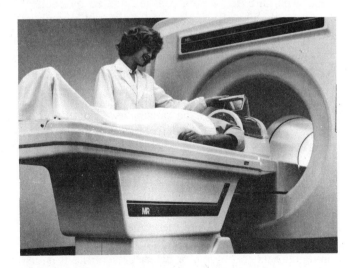

FIGURE 18–35 Magnetic resonance imaging (MRI System) (Courtesy of GE Medical Systems)

The magnetic resonance machine scans all planes of a body structure to produce an image processed by a computer, without moving the patient, Figure 18–36. Radio signals are sent from the scanner that are influenced by strong magnetic fields to which the body responds. Figure 18–37 shows an image of the lumbar spine in the sagittal plane. Note the herniated disc and the clarity of the image. The MRI has reduced a great number of diagnostic exploratory surgeries. It is most useful in helping to diagnose brain and nervous system disorders, cardiovascular disease, cancer, and diseases of the visceral organs. MRI is also used to help monitor the effectiveness of treatment. Since the MRI uses a strong electromagnetic field, it is extremely important that any metal objects be removed before the procedure is performed. The technician will request that the patient remove all metallic objects including jewelry, hairpins, and nonpermanent dentures before being placed in the tunnel for the MRI. Patients should be interviewed thoroughly regarding their health history. Inform the patient that at the facility where the MRI will be performed, they will generally be asked to sign a consent form prior to the procedure. Female patients should refrain from even wearing mascara since tiny metallic flakes may be present in it. During the procedure, these minute pieces of metal may become hot and burn the patient.

During the process the many repetitive noises sound like clanging and banging, humming, and whirring. This is just the sound of the electromagnetic field. There are no sensations of pain and no known side effects. The patient must be still and relax for the test to be properly completed. The technician observes the patient during the entire time. Patients may speak to the technician by the use of a microphone inside the tunnel.

The MRI procedure is contraindicated in patients who have pacemakers, metallic implants, are in the first trimester of pregnancy, are severely claustrophobic, or obese. The claustrophobia can be handled by counseling and/or the use of a sedative administered by a physician before the procedure is begun.

Hemoccult® Sensa® Tests ....

Hemoccult sensa is the trademark for a guaiac reagent strip test used to detect the presence of occult blood, Figure 18–38. The test may detect bleeding in the digestive tract that is otherwise not detectable. It is a diagnostic aid in the detection of cancer of the colon. Hemoccult sensa tests are usually given routinely to patients aged 40 and over following a complete physical exam or if the patient's symptoms indicate their use. Hemoccult sensa slides are recommended for both men and women who have a personal or family history of colorectal cancer, polyps, or ulcerative colitis. It is also advised as a screening for people who have a personal

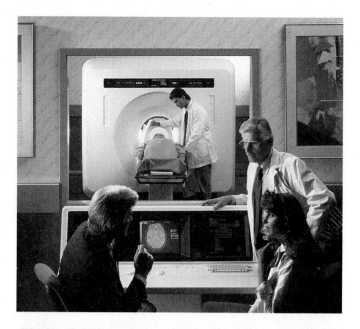

FIGURE 18–36 Magnetic resonance imaging system. The scan is shown on the computer screen on the console in the foreground. (Courtesy of GE Medical Systems)

history of inflammatory bowel disease. Bleeding may be caused by peptic ulcers, hemorrhoids, polyps, and other conditions of the bowel tract. It can also be an early symptom of cancer of the colon. This test was designed to help detect hidden blood in the stool early enough for corrective measures to be taken. Since cancer of the colon is one of the leading cancer killers in the United States, it makes sense to follow the simple, easy-to-use screening test that could help save one's life. Instruct patients how to collect specimens at home and to return them in the double-layered, leak-proof

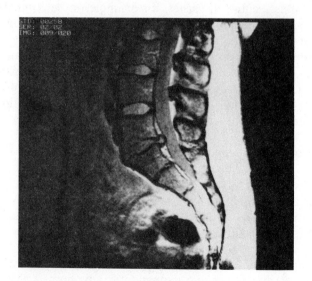

FIGURE 18–37 MRI scan showing a herniated disc in the lumbar spine (Courtesy of GE Medical Systems)

PROCEDURE
HEMOCCULT® SLIDES

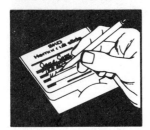

Identification
Write, or have patient write his name, age, address, phone number, and date specimen was collected in space provided on front of each slide.

Preparation

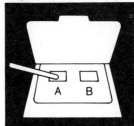

1. Collect small stool sample on one end of applicator.
2. Apply thin smear inside box A.
3. Reuse applicator to obtain second sample from different part of stool. Apply thin smear inside box B.
4. Close cover. Return slide to physician.
CAUTION: Protect from heat.

Development of Test

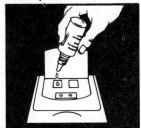

1. Open flap in back of slide and apply two drops of Hemoccult® Developer to guaiac paper directly over each smear.
2. Read results within 60 seconds.
ANY TRACE OF BLUE ON OR AT THE EDGE OF THE SMEAR IS POSITIVE FOR OCCULT BLOOD.

Development of Performance Monitors®

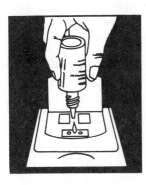

1. Apply ONE DROP ONLY of Hemoccult® Developer between the positive and negative Performance Monitors®.
2. Read results within 30 seconds.
A BLUE COLOR WILL APPEAR IN THE POSITIVE PERFORMANCE MONITOR®, AND NO BLUE WILL APPEAR IN THE NEGATIVE PERFORMANCE MONITOR®, IF THE SLIDES AND DEVELOPER ARE FUNCTIONAL.

IMPORTANT NOTE: Follow the procedure exactly as outlined above and on the preceding page. Always develop the test, read the results, interpret them and make a decision as to whether the fecal specimen is positive or negative for occult blood BEFORE you develop the Performance Monitors®. Do not apply Developer to Performance Monitors® before interpreting test results. Any blue originating from the Performance Monitors® should be ignored in the reading of the specimen test results.

READING AND INTERPRETATION OF THE HEMOCCULT® TEST
the world's leading test for fecal occult blood

Negative Smears*

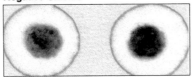

Sample report: negative
No detectable blue on or at the edge of the smears indicates the test is negative for occult blood.
(See **LIMITATIONS OF PROCEDURE**.)

Negative and Positive Smears*

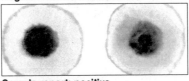

Positive Smears*

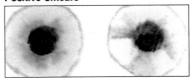

Sample report: positive
Any trace of blue on or at the edge of one or more of the smears indicates the test is positive for occult blood.

FIGURE 18–38 Hemoccult® Sensa® test (Courtesy of SmithKline Diagnostics, Inc.)

mailing envelope as soon as possible; otherwise people have a tendency to forget.

The Hemoccult sensa test is easy to complete. It requires proper lighting to compare the color change of the reagent paper to the control. Two drops of developer are applied to each stool smear, A and B, and one drop to the control area. If the test area turns blue as compared to the positive control, then the Hemoccult sensa is reported as positive. Further studies will then be ordered by the physician to determine where in the colon the bleeding is occurring.

Intestinal bleeding may be intermittent (not all the time). Giving the patient three slides with smears of two sections of stool for each increases the detection of the

Perform a Hemocult Sensa Test

PROCEDURE: To determine the presence of occult blood in the stool.

EQUIPMENT: Hemoccult sensa slide(s) prepared by patient, developer, timer or timepiece, patient's chart, pen

TERMINAL PERFORMANCE OBJECTIVE: Provided with all necessary equipment/supplies and using samples obtained from own stool, the student will demonstrate each step in the Hemoccult sensa testing procedure.

1. Wash hands and assemble items needed for testing on counter.
2. Open test side of Hemoccult sensa paper slide.
3. Remove cap from bottle of developer.
4. Place two drops of developer on each of the sections of reagent paper slide: A, B.

5. Immediately begin timing 60 seconds. **Key Point: At 30 seconds watch closely for any change of color which may be developing. Read within 60 seconds.**
6. Compare test with control color and read results.
7. Place one drop of developer between positive and negative control. Read within 10 seconds.
8. Record test results on patient's chart as either positive or negative. **Key Point: Positive reading means that there is occult blood in the stool. Negative means that no occult blood is present. If first slide is negative and second and third are positive, record as:**
Hemoccult sensa slides: 1. neg
                                     2. pos
                                     3. pos

PATIENT EDUCATION

The patient is advised to avoid eating red meat and foods known to cause digestive tract distress for 48 hours prior to the test and until the specimens are collected. Patients should also avoid processed meats and liver and all raw fruits and vegetables. Instruct patients not to take iron supplements, or vitamin C (in excess of 250 mg a day), aspirin, or other nonsteroidal anti-inflammatory medications for a week before and during collection of specimens. Advise patients to eat well-cooked pork, fish, and poultry; cooked fruits and vegetables; and high-fiber foods such as breads and cereals. Smears of three consecutive bowel movements are requested for testing. The patient should complete the information label on each of the paper Hemoccult sensa slides, filling in the time and date that the samples were obtained. The test kit contains a flushable paper sheet to cover the water in the toilet. (Advise the patient to flush the toilet prior to placing this tissue on top of the water.) This will allow the stool to fall onto the tissue making it easier to obtain the specimens. Remind the patient that the stool samples should be taken from two separate sections with the wooden stick. The sticks should be disposed of in a plastic bag in a waste receptacle, not the toilet.

presence of blood in the bowel tract. Ask patients to follow instructions printed on the envelope carefully.

Complete Chapter 18, Unit 3 in the workbook to help you meet the objectives at the beginning of this unit and therefore achieve competency of this subject matter.

UNIT 4
Diagnostic X ray Examinations

OBJECTIVES ·······································

Upon completion of this unit, the student will meet the following terminal performance objectives by verifying knowledge of the facts and principles presented through oral and written communication at a level deemed competent, and will demonstrate the specific behaviors as identified in the terminal performance objectives of the procedures, observing all aseptic and safety precautions in accordance with health care standards.

1. Instruct patients in preparation for radiological studies.
2. Discuss the importance of diet in preparation of X rays.
3. Explain why pregnant women should not have X rays.
4. Discuss X rays that require no preparation.
5. Discuss the importance of patient education in scheduling a mammography.
6. Spell and define, using the glossary at the back of the text, all the words to know in this unit.

WORDS TO KNOW

absorb	fluoroscope
artifact	iodine
compression	IVP
conjunction	KUB
contract	lesion
contrast	mammography
CTAT	planes
cystoscope	radiation
diagnostic	radioactive
distends	radiograph
electromagnetic radiation	radiologist
electron	radiopaque
enema	residual barium
evacuants	retrograde
evacuate	roentgen
flatus	therapeutic
flexible	

Radiological Studies

Radiological studies are made by the use of X rays (roentgen rays), which are high-energy electromagnetic radiation produced by the collision of a beam of electrons with a metal target in an X ray tube. An X ray photograph is taken of the requested part of the patient's body and a permanent film picture is made. Patients must follow preparation instructions for certain radiological studies. Bone studies do not require preparation and are performed to aid in the diagnosis of tumors, fractures, and other disorders and diseases. Chest X rays do not normally need advanced preparation. Therapeutic X rays are used in the treatment of cancer. Following are the most commonly ordered radiological studies for which you may be responsible in scheduling and preparing patients.

Gallbladder—Cholecystogram

The gallbladder stores bile that is produced in the liver to break down fat in the digestive process. When the gallbladder malfunctions, the patient experiences abdominal discomfort (nausea) and pain. The cholecystogram enables the physician to diagnose the cause of the patient's distress.

In preparation for this study of the gallbladder, the patient must follow a prescribed diet and take prescribed medication (a contrast medium) to make the gallbladder visible on the X ray film, Figure 18–39. Generally the day before the exam, the patient is advised to avoid drinking alcoholic and carbonated beverages because these drinks may produce flatus (gas). Unless otherwise specified by the physician, you should remind patients to take their regularly prescribed medication(s).

1. Two days prior to exam, starting at 6 P.M. take 1 tablet of Oragrafin every 5 minutes until 6 tablets have been taken.
2. On day prior to exam, repeat step 1.
3. Day prior to exam, take 4 oz of Neoloid or 3 Dulcolax 5 mg tablets from 2–4 P.M.
4. Evening before exam, eat a fatfree meal—dry toast, tea, fruit, jello.
5. Nothing by mouth after midnight.
6. No breakfast.

FIGURE 18–39 Preparation for gallbladder series

Upper GI Series—Barium Swallow

For this study the patient must drink the chalky tasting contrast medium during the examination while the radiologist observes the flow of the substance directly by means of a fluoroscope. The contrast medium is a mixture of barium and water, usually flavored to increase palatability. Radiologic films are taken for a permanent record of the upper digestive tract. During the study the

PATIENT EDUCATION

Undergoing radiological studies can be frightening to some patients. Assure the patient that the studies are done in a controlled environment. Always provide clear and concise oral *and* written instructions for examinations that require advance preparation. Be sure that the patient understands the necessary preparations. Answer all questions. Emphasize the importance of being on time for the radiological appointment to avoid unnecessary delays, since some examinations are very long.

If the patient is not familiar with the facility where the X ray studies are scheduled, give specific instructions (and a map) of how to get there and where to park. Patients appreciate this courtesy. Often, this information is printed on the appointment/information sheet the facility provides to medical offices and clinics for referral appointments.

It is of vital importance that you advise all female patients who are of childbearing age to inform you if they are pregnant, or could possibly be, if X rays are considered as a part of the assessment of their condition. X rays are contraindicated in pregnant females, especially in the first trimester because radiation is damaging to the fetus. During triage you should always ask females for the date of the last menstrual period (LMP) for documentation in their chart. This will help in preventing any misunderstanding concerning a possible pregnancy. Other diagnostic exams can be performed that are safe for the fetus during this time as necessary.

Most patients with gallbladder trouble already know they should avoid fatty foods. The usual preparation for a cholecystogram is a nonfatty evening meal the night before the scheduled appointment. Foods which are permitted are fresh fruits and vegetables, lean meat (broiled), toast, bread, jelly, and coffee or tea. Fatty foods will cause the gallbladder to **contract** and empty the contrast medium, which the patient usually takes following the evening meal.

The medication is usually in pill form, with directions to swallow 1 tablet every 5 minutes with a minimum amount of water until all are consumed. Repeating this a second night is necessary to define the gallbladder sufficiently. This takes approximately half an hour. Spreading the consumption of the contrast medium out over this period of time allows the gallbladder to **absorb** the substance. The patient is instructed to eat or drink nothing after midnight the night before the cholecystogram is performed. In addition to these preparations, many physicians request an **enema** or laxative or both to help remove fecal material and gas which could cause shadows, blockages, or other **artifacts**.

Often when the series of **radiographs** is completed, patients are told to return after a meal containing fats to observe radiographs that show how the gallbladder functions during digestion of fats.

Preparation requires that the patient eat a light evening meal and then only clear liquids, Figure 18–40. The patient should have nothing to eat or drink from midnight until after the X ray series the next day. Prescribed medications are allowed, taken with water. Dairy products, carbonated beverages, and alcohol are not permitted. The digestive tract should be clear of all foods to avoid blockage of or shadows on the anatomical structures to be observed.

Constipation may result from the barium and patients should be advised to drink plenty of clear liquids to help relieve it. You should also mention that their stool may appear lighter than usual from the white barium and that this should not be a cause for concern. Laxatives are ordered only by the physician. Patients should phone the medical office if any problem arises.

ESOPHAGUS, UPPER GI SERIES

1. Nothing by mouth after midnight.
2. No breakfast.

IF SMALL BOWEL

1. Day prior to exam—Take 4 oz. of Neoloid or 3 Dulcolax 5 mg tablets from 2–4 P.M.
2. Nothing by mouth after midnight.
3. No breakfast.

FIGURE 18–40   Preparation for upper GI series

patient is positioned so that different angles of the digestive organs can be seen.

The physician observes the functioning of the esophagus, stomach, duodenum, and small intestine as the barium passes. Such disorders or diseases as hiatal hernias, peptic or duodenal ulcers, and tumors may be diagnosed as a result of the upper GI series.

Lower GI Series—Barium Enema

In this examination, barium sulfate is the contrast medium. It is introduced into the colon by an enema tube, and the radiologist observes the flow into the lower bowel. Many physicians order a barium enema with air-contrast. This procedure **distends** the barium-filled colon with air to make the structures more visible by fluoroscopy. Permanent radiographs are taken periodically during the procedure. This study is helpful in diagnosing diseases of the colon, tumors, and **lesions.**

The barium enema procedure generally takes several minutes and produces discomfort and some pain. Patients should be told to breathe through the mouth slowly and deeply to help relax the abdominal muscles.

A strong urge to defecate is normal and patients often cannot resist the urge. After several films have been taken the patient generally is allowed to use the toilet. Then the study of the lower bowel is completed.

Patients should be encouraged to drink plenty of liquids for the next few days to help evacuate the **residual barium** sulfate in the lower colon.

Intravenous Pyelogram

In studies of the genitourinary system, the intravenous pyelogram (**IVP**) requires that the patient prepare with laxatives, enemas, and fasting, Figure 18–42. The IVP consists of an intravenous injection of **iodine,** the contrast medium, to define the structures of the urinary system. A **retrograde** pyelogram is a study of the urinary tract done by inserting a sterile catheter into the urinary meatus, through the bladder, and up into the ureters. The

Patients must prepare for this study by precisely following instructions, usually beginning the day before the appointment. The instructions generally include laxatives and enemas to clear the bowel of fecal matter and gas. The patient should eat lightly, avoid dairy products, and drink plenty of clear liquids to encourage more comfortable evacuation. Patients should have nothing to eat or drink past midnight the night before the X ray, Figure 18–41. On the day of the appointment, the patient should have an enema 2 hours before the scheduled appointment.

BARIUM ENEMA OR COLON EXAMINATION.

a. Beginning the morning of the day before the examination, change to an all liquid diet*, as outlined below. Do not take any more solid food until after the examinations.

b. At 12:30 PM., or 1/2 hour after lunch on the day before the examination, drink entire contents of a bottle of Citrate of Magnesia (10 oz.).

c. At 1:00 PM., drink one glass of fluid.

d. At 3:00 PM., take 2 Dulcolax tablets with a large glass of water.

e. At 4:00 PM., drink one large glass of fluid.

f. At 5:00 PM., or as close as possible, liquid dinner.

g. At 6:00 PM., drink one large glass of fluid.

h. Bedtime—drink one large glass of fluid.

i. You may have one cup of coffee, tea, or water on the morning of the examination.

*ALL LIQUID DIET
You may have any of the following: Coffee, tea, carbonated beverages, clear gelatin desserts, strained fruit juice, bouillon, clear broths, tomato juice. Do not drink milk of any kind.

Please call office if you have any questions regarding above instructions.

FIGURE 18–41 Preparation for barium enema

radiopaque contrast medium then flows upward into the kidneys. This diagnostic test is usually done in conjunction with cystoscopy. Patients should have iodine-sensitivity tests prior to the examination to determine the possibility of an allergic reaction. A voiding cystogram may be ordered in conjunction with an IVP. In this case the contrast medium is injected into the bladder by catheter and no special patient preparation is needed.

ALL LIQUID DIET

You may have any of the following: coffee, tea, carbonated beverages, sherbet, clear gelatin desserts, strained fruit juice, bouillon, clear broths, tomato juice. Do not drink milk of any kind.

1. Day prior to exam—4 oz. of Neoloid or 3 Dulcolax 5 mg tablets from 2–4 P.M.
2. Liquids only after midnight.

FIGURE 18–42 Preparation for intravenous pyelogram (IVP)

KUB

The KUB (kidneys, ureters, bladder) is an X ray of the patient's abdomen, sometimes termed "flat plate of abdomen," Figure 18–43. This requires no patient preparation and is used in the diagnosis of urinary system diseases and disorders. It may also be useful in determining the position of an intrauterine device (IUD) or in locating foreign bodies in the digestive tract. In some cases surgery is indicated to remove an object which may block the normal digestive flow, but many small objects are easily passed with solid foods, especially in young

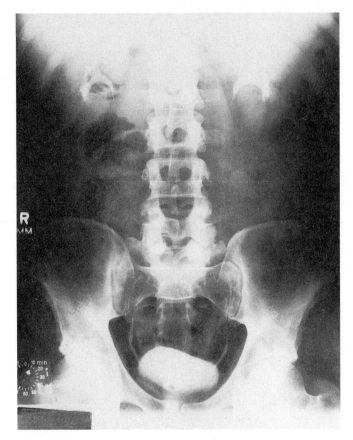

FIGURE 18–43 Radiological Xray of kidneys, ureters, and bladder (KUB); no patient preparation is necessary.

The medical assistant should schedule the mammography during the first week following the patient's menstrual cycle, since the breasts must be compressed firmly during the procedure to obtain a satisfactory image for diagnostic purposes, Figure 18–45. During this time the patient would experience less discomfort. Since this procedure is often very uncomfortable and even sometimes painful in many women, there are other suggestions that may be helpful in reducing the discomfort. For instance, it is advisable to tell patients to omit caffeine from their diets for 7–10 days prior to this examination to reduce the possible effects of swelling and soreness that caffeine often produces. Compression of the breasts during this procedure requires less radiation to be used. It also allows a much clearer picture to be taken of the breast tissue. Following this exam, some areas of the breast(s) may sometimes become temporarily discolored. However, it does not damage the breast tissue and should not be alarming. At the advice of the physician, a mild analgesic may be taken to relieve any discomfort or aching that may be experienced by the patient.

Explaining these details to the patient and requesting their cooperation with the radiology technician during this procedure will be most helpful in obtaining a quality mammogram for diagnostic study by the physician. It is also important to let the patient know when the results will be available so they will not have to contend with unnecessary worry. Remind patients again of the importance of breast self-examinations on a continuing basis. The mammography is not a substitute for this important means of detection.

To ensure the best results for your mammogram, please follow these procedures prior to your appointment:

    a. BE SURE TO NOTIFY OUR PERSONNEL IF YOU ARE PREGNANT.

    b. Please shower or bathe as close to your appointment time as possible.

    c. Do not use deodorants, powders, perfumes, and etc. on the breast or underarm areas.

    d. You will only have to undress to the waist, so wear an easily removable top such as a blouse.

FIGURE 18–44 Instructions for mammography

children whose internal structures are more flexible. The physician ultimately makes this decision in patient care.

Mammography

Mammography aids in the diagnosis of breast masses, some of which may be as small as 1 cm in size or less. Women who practice self-examinations regularly each month and find lumps in breast tissue early have a much better cure rate if a malignancy is found. Breast self-examination (see chapter 16, Unit 3) and regular examinations by the physician should be strongly reinforced to female patients in addition to their scheduled mammography. The American Cancer Society recommends a baseline mammography between the ages of 35 to 39 for all women; between ages 40 and 49 every 1 to 2 years; and, over age 50 every year. At any time a lump is found, patients should be advised to see the physician at once for examination. This procedure requires the patient to move into various positions so that different angles of the breast tissue may be X rayed. The X ray pictures are called mammograms. Patients are usually advised to wear slacks or a skirt for ease in preparation for the procedure, Figure 18–44, since it is necessary to undress to the waist for the examination. The only preparation required is that the patient wash the chest and underarms and rinse and dry thoroughly. No deodorants or powders are to be used the day of the mammography because the film on the skin from these substances could interfere with the radiograph. As a courtesy to patients, you should remind them to take soap, deodorant, and a fresh blouse with them.

Body Scans

Rapid scanning of single-tissue planes is performed by a process that generates images of the tissue in "slices" about 1 cm thick. This method of radiology is called the CAT (computerized axial tomography) scan or CTAT (computerized transaxial tomography). These procedures can be performed in seconds and aid in diagnosis of diseases and disorders of the breast or other internal organs.

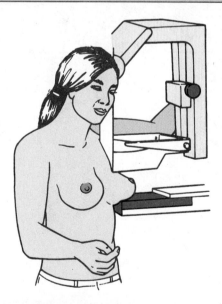

FIGURE 18–45 Breasts compressed by plates during mammography

The branch of medicine that uses radionuclides in the diagnosis and treatment of disease is nuclear medicine. Almost any organ of the body may be viewed and recorded by having the patient ingest, or be injected with, radioactive material.

Uptake studies refer to procedures in which patients ingest a radioactive substance under careful supervision and return within 24 hours to have the amount of radioactive substance in a particular organ measured. The radioactive thyroid uptake determines the function of the thyroid gland, for example. Tumors of the thyroid may also be determined by this method. In female patients pregnancy should be determined prior to the radioactive thyroid uptake, for it is seriously damaging to the fetus, especially within the first trimester of pregnancy.

Complete Chapter 18, Unit 4 in the workbook to help you meet the objectives at the beginning of this unit and therefore achieve competency of this subject matter.

MEDICAL-LEGAL ETHICAL HIGHLIGHTS

Mr. Right...

documents procedures and their results following their completion and initials. He completes follow-up reports of results in an efficient manner and shows respect for the confidentiality of patient information. He always remembers to advise patients of risks or precautions concerning procedures including X ray precautions regarding pregnancy.

Employment advancement: Excellent

Ms. Wrong...

documents procedures and results when she remembers to do it, just as she often forgets to send out follow-up reports. She is careless about leaving patient records out for anyone to see, which violates patients' confidentiality and privacy. She occasionally remembers to advise patients about risks and precautions concerning procedures before they are performed. She usually remembers to tell pregnant women about the dangers of X rays to the fetus.

Employment outlook: Poor

REFERENCES

Diagnostic Tests, Nurse's Ready Reference, Springhouse PA: Springhouse Corporation, 1990.

Mosby's Medical, Nursing, and Allied Health Dictionary, 3d ed. St. Louis: C.V. Mosby, 1990.

Siemens Burdick, Inc., Schaumburg, Illinois 60173

Wendt-Bristol Diagnostic Center, 1550 Kenny Road, Columbus OH.

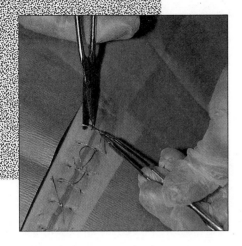

C H A P T E R   1 9

Minor Surgical Procedures

As a clinical medical assistant, you may assist with a variety of sterile procedures. Maintaining medical asepsis is vital to prevent the transmission of diseases *before, during,* and *following* any of the invasive surgical procedures performed in the medical office/clinic. In compliance with the universal precautions, proper barriers, such as latex gloves, gown, face mask/shield, must be worn to protect the health care staff from possible contamination while performing these procedures. All disposable waste must be placed in a plastic biohazardous bag and discarded properly to prevent disease transmission.

Setup for various procedures may vary slightly according to the physician's preference. However, sterile technique will always remain the same for any invasive procedure. The basic information for assisting both the physician and patient is covered in this chapter.

OBJECTIVES ....

Upon completion of this unit, the student will meet the following terminal performance objectives by verifying knowledge of the facts and principles presented through oral and written communication at a level deemed competent, and will demonstrate the specific behaviors as identified in the terminal performance objectives of the procedures, observing all aseptic and safety precautions in accordance with health care standards.

1. Explain scheduling, preop and postop instructions of patients for minor office surgery.
2. Discuss the importance of obtaining the consent form for the surgical procedure.
3. Demonstrate skin preparation procedure for surgical site.
4. Prepare treatment room and minor surgical tray setup.
5. Discuss various procedures that require sterile technique.
6. Demonstrate procedure for assisting with minor surgery.
7. Demonstrate how to put on and remove sterile gloves properly.
8. Discuss proper care of surgical instruments.
9. Demonstrate proper way to remove sutures.
10. Discuss important information that should be recorded on patient's chart.
11. Spell and define, using the glossary at the back of the text, all the words to know in this chapter.

anesthesia
anesthesiologist
anesthetic
antiseptic
appropriate
authorize
biopsy
coagulation
contaminate
cryosurgery
dominant
electrocautery
electrocoagulation
expiration
fenestrated

hemophilia
histology
hypoallergenic
incision and drainage
   (I & D)
invasive
microbial
polyp
postoperative (postop)
preoperative (preop)
schedule
stress
suture
taut
wart

The medical assistant is usually responsible for scheduling minor office surgery. Surgery may include removal of a sebaceous cyst, wart, or foreign object; circumcision; vasectomy; skin biopsy; incision and drainage (I & D); out-patient dilation and curretage; (D & C) or insertion of an IUD.

You must be mindful of the amount of time required for each type of surgical procedure you schedule. Advise patients as you make their appointments how long they should plan to be on the day of their minor surgery. Depending on the type of procedure being performed, patients may need to make arrangements for someone to bring them for the appointment and take them home. Occasionally patients do not feel well enough following a surgical procedure to drive or travel alone and should have some assistance for at least a few hours. Because it is unpredictable how an individual patient may react to even a minor surgical procedure, it is best to advise *all* patients to arrange for assistance to ensure their safety and well-being. You should also advise them about possibly taking appropriate time off from work or arranging for home care, depending on the procedure scheduled.

You must first be sure that the patient understands the procedure and the instructions regarding preoperative (preop) and postoperative (postop) care. Most medical facilities have printed instructions for patients. This eliminates any misunderstandings, and patients feel more at ease knowing they can refer to it. Patients should be advised of the appropriate clothing to be worn on the day of the surgery. Loose-fitting clothing, or clothing easy to put on and take off, and not their "Sunday best" should be suggested as appropriate for the anatomical area of surgery. It is a good practice to phone the patient the day prior to the appointment, not only to reassure the patient and answer any questions but to confirm the physician's schedule.

The day before the scheduled surgery, you should get all the necessary surgical instruments and supplies ready.

All surgical instruments must be properly labeled and autoclaved. Most of the instruments will already have been sterilized, as they should be done after each use. The basic setup for most minor surgical procedures includes the following sterile items: scalpel handle and blades, hemostats (straight or curved), needles holder, needles and suture material (catgut or silk), suture scissors, thumb forceps, probe, gauze squares, sponges, vial of anesthetic medication, syringes, needles, towels, and bandages. Some of these supplies may be wrapped and sterilized together. Items that need to be added are dropped onto the sterile field after the wrap has been carefully unfolded on the Mayo table by sterile technique. Autoclaved items remain sterile if they have been properly processed and have been protected from moisture for 30 days. Packages should be checked before use for any tears or other signs of tampering to ensure sterility.

Most items used today are disposable and come already sterile in the manufacturer's packaging. You must make sure that the package has not been torn or punctured to ensure sterility. The sterilization of the product is guaranteed only to a certain date marked on the package, and this date must be checked.

A variety of minor invasive surgical procedures are performed in the medical office and each requires several instruments. Figure 19–1 shows an example of a surgical instrument tray setup and supplies commonly used in minor office procedures. You must become familiar with the physician's preference for particular items and the way they are to be arranged for use. Until you are certain about the details of a particular procedure, you may want to keep a notebook handy for reference.

When the patient arrives for the surgery the consent form, an example of which is shown in Figure 19–2, must

---

PATIENT EDUCATION

Preop

In scheduling, advise patient of:
1. Approximate length of time for procedure
2. Appropriate clothing to wear at appointment
3. Amount of time to fast as instructed by physician
4. Arranging for someone to accompany him/her
5. Anticipated time to take off work or arranging for home care.

When patient arrives for appointment
1. Provide written instructions regarding the surgical procedure and follow-up care
2. Explain surgical consent form and obtain patient's signature
3. Answer any questions concerning procedure
4. Ascertain if the patient has any allergies to any medications, including topical preparations, and adhesive tapes.

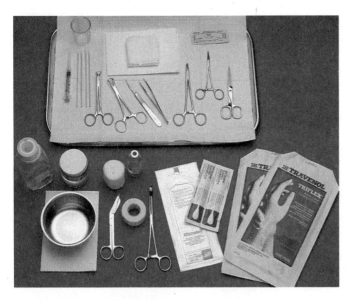

FIGURE 19–1 An example of a surgical setup tray.

first be explained to the patient and completed. You should allow the patient time to ask any questions about the procedure and answer them adequately. The patient's signature must be on the consent form and filed in the chart. If the patient is a minor, or incompetent, the person authorized to give consent must sign for the patient following an explanation of the procedure and answering any questions. The Patient's vital signs should be taken and any complaints or problems should be recorded on the patient's chart. The patient should then empty the bladder before being positioned and draped for the procedure.

Most procedures are performed under local anesthesia. A physician always administers the anesthetic. Large group practices may have a qualified anesthesiologist on staff. A careful medical history must be taken from the patient to determine possible allergic reactions. This helps avoid complications during and after the procedure.

If the patient discloses a family history of hemophilia, a serious blood clotting disease, or is himself a hemophiliac you should bring it to the physician's attention immediately. This information should be

---

CONSENT TO OPERATE

Date _____ Time _____ A.M. P.M.

1. I authorize the performance upon _____
   of the following operation _____
   to be performed under the direction of Dr. _____.
2. The following have been explained to me by Dr. _____.
   A. The nature of the operation _____
   _____
   _____
   _____

   B. The purpose of the operation _____
   _____

   C. The possible alternative methods of treatment _____
   _____

   D. The possible consequences of the operation _____

   E. The risks involved _____
   _____

   F. The possibility of complications _____
   _____

3. I have been advised of the serious nature of the operation and have been advised that if I desire a further and more detailed explanation of any of the foregoing or further information about the possible risks or complications of the above listed operation it will be given to me.
4. I do not request a further and more detailed listing and explanation of any of the items listed in paragraph 2.

   Signed _____
   (Patient or person authorized
   to consent for patient)

Witness _____

FIGURE 19–2 Surgical consent form

Prepare Skin For Minor Surgery

PURPOSE: To remove hair from surgery site to prevent infection and to clean the skin and apply antiseptic solution to reduce microbial growth.

EQUIPMENT: Small basin, 4 x 4 inch gauze squares (sponges), safety razor and blades, scissors, antiseptic soap solution, emesis basin, gooseneck lamp, sterile drape sheet or towels (or **fenestrated** drape sheet), sterile gloves, Mayo table, sterile forceps and container, sterile water for irrigation, Figure 19–4

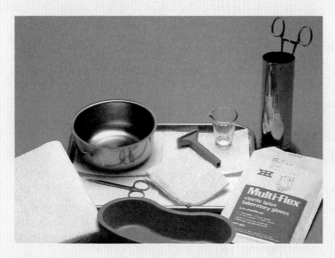

FIGURE 19–4   Example of skin prep tray

TERMINAL PERFORMANCE OBJECTIVE: Provided with all necessary equipment and supplies and other students to act as patients, the student will demonstrate each of the steps required in the skin-prep procedure. Note: in the instructional setting, preparing the forearm may be sufficient; moreover, the shaving process may be demonstrated by using a razor with no blade.

1. Wash and glove hands, and assemble all needed items.
2. Identify patient. Call patient by name and check chart to avoid error.
3. Explain procedure to patient. Ask patient to remove necessary clothing. Assist patient if necessary. Explain where patient should put belongings.
4. Assist patient into proper position on treatment table and drape with sheet or light bath blanket as directed by physician.
5. Position Mayo table over patient near surgical site. Adjust gooseneck lamp to light area to be shaved.
6. Place gauze squares in soapy solution and use one at a time to soap area to be shaved. After use discard each into emesis basin, Figure 19–5 (a) & (b).

7. If skin-prep site is covered by scalp hair, beard, or pubic hair, use scissors to clip hair in preparation for shaving. Use caution when clipping hair with scissors and in shaving with razor to avoid both self-injury and harm to the patient. If reusable razor is the method, very carefully place new razor blade in razor to prevent self-injury. Shave hair by placing razor against skin at about a 30-degree angle, Figure 19–6. Hold skin **taut** for easier shaving. Shave in direction hair grows. Wipe soap and hair from razor with tissue. Swish razor through soapy water, shake excess water from it, and shave next area.
8. Remove all soap and hair from area by wetting sterile gauze square with sterile water. Dry area with sterile gauze squares.

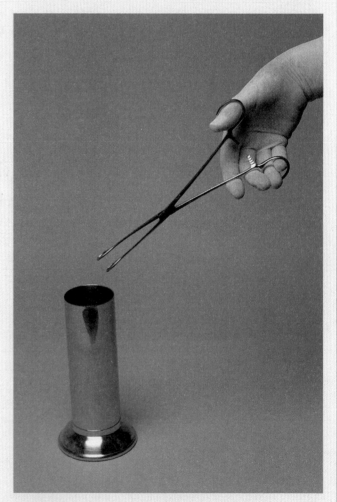

FIGURE 19–5 (A)   Remove transfer forceps from container without touching sides.

9. Apply antiseptic solution to surgery site with gauze square held by transfer forceps. **Key Point: Begin**

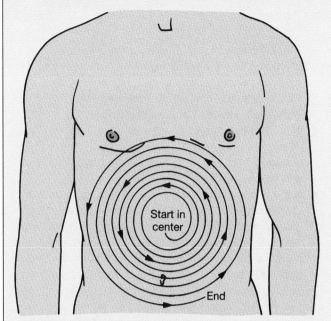

FIGURE 19–5 (B) Apply all solutions in this pattern to the skin. Prepping the skin with antiseptic solution should begin at the center of the incision site and proceed outward in one continuous circular motion as shown.

application in center of site and move outward in a circular motion, see Figure 19–5.

10. Cover sterile area with sterile drape sheet or towel until physician is ready to begin. **Key Point: Instruct patient not to touch sterile field (both sterile field of surgical site and instrument tray setup).**

11. Discard disposable items and return other items to proper storage area. Remove gloves and wash hands.

12. Attend to patient's comfort. Patients are usually apprehensive about even most minor surgical procedures. Reassurance at this time is most important.

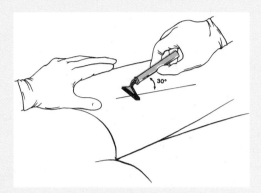

FIGURE 19–6 Angle of shaving surgery site

---

marked in red ink on the patient's chart. Hemophilia is a sex-linked hereditary trait that occurs mostly in males. Patients who have this diagnosis must have surgery of any type *only* at a completely equipped, well-staffed medical-surgical hospital for their safety and well-being.

In procedures requiring that a biopsy be taken for analysis, careful labeling and handling of the specimen is vital. The laboratory provides a formalin solution container for preservation of the tissue specimen. This container is sterile and the specimen must be placed directly in the solution with sterile transfer forceps. A completed lab request form must accompany the specimen for analysis.

In certain surgical procedures, such as in removing warts or polyps, an electrocautery device may be used. Often this is used to control bleeding of the surgical site by electrocoagulation. Controlled high-frequency current is applied by the physician to the surgical area to coagulate the blood to close the incision. If the reusable tips are preferred by the physician for surgical procedures, they must be autoclaved to prevent possible cross-contamination. Disposable tips are available. Figure 19–3 illustrates a Hyfrecator.

Another method used in removing skin tags, warts, and other skin disorders and growths, is by cryosurgery.

Often certain gynecological treatments and surgical procedures are performed with this instrument. This process uses subfreezing temperature to destroy/remove tissue.

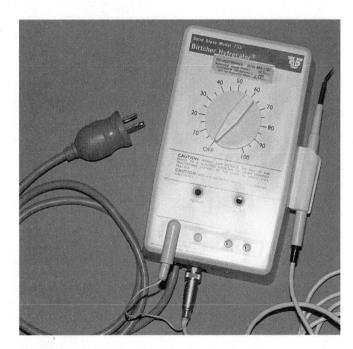

FIGURE 19–3 Hyfrecator (electrocautery unit).

Put On Sterile Gloves

PURPOSE: To protect both patient and medical assistant from contamination.

EQUIPMENT: Package of sterile latex gloves of proper size

TERMINAL PERFORMANCE OBJECTIVE: After practicing with clean gloves, each student will be provided with a package of sterile latex gloves; standing in front of a clean, clear counter surface, each student will then demonstrate the correct method of putting on sterile gloves. The instructor will observe each step.

1. Remove wristwatch, rings, and other jewelry of hands and wrists and perform surgical scrub using nail brush. Thoroughly dry hands with sterile towels. **Key Point: Hands are now clean but unsterile.**

2. Tear seal and open package of sterile gloves as you would open a book. Place on clean counter surface with cuff end toward your body. **Key Point: Do not touch inside of package.**

3. Grasp glove for your **dominant** hand by fold of cuff with finger and thumb of your nondominant hand, Figure 19–7(a). Insert dominant hand, carefully pulling glove on with other hand, keeping cuff turned back. **Key Point: Dominant hand is now gloved and sterile, Figure 19–7(b).**

4. Place gloved fingers under cuff of other glove and insert nondominant hand, Figure 19–7(c). Put glove on by pulling on inside fold of cuff, Figure 19–7(d). Avoid touching thumb of dominant hand to outside cuff of other glove where it has been contaminated.

5. Now both hands are gloved and sterile. Place fingers under cuffs to smooth gloves over wrists and smooth out fingers for better fit. **Key Point: Check for tears and holes.**

6. Keep hands above waist level. Do not touch anything other than items in sterile field or you will **contaminate** gloved hand and must reglove with another sterile pair.

7. Remove gloves by pulling glove off dominant hand with thumb and fingers, Figure 19–7(e). Hold outside cuff and pull glove off inside out. Slip ungloved hand into palm of gloved hand and slip glove off inside out, Figure 19–7(f). Most sterile gloves are disposable. If not, place them in appropriate container until you can sanitize them. **Key Point: Be careful not to touch contaminated side of gloves when removing.**

8. Wash hands.

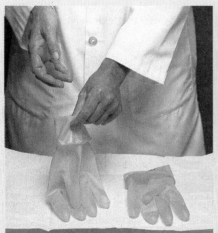
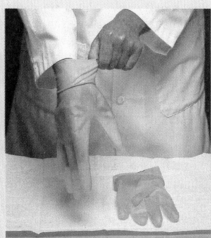
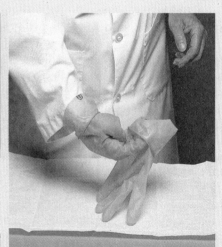

FIGURE 19–7 (a). Pick up glove for dominant hand with thumb and index finger of nondominant hand by cuff. (b). Carefully pull glove onto dominant hand, keeping cuff turned down (touch only the cuff). (c). With dominant hand gloved, pick up other glove by fingers under cuff.

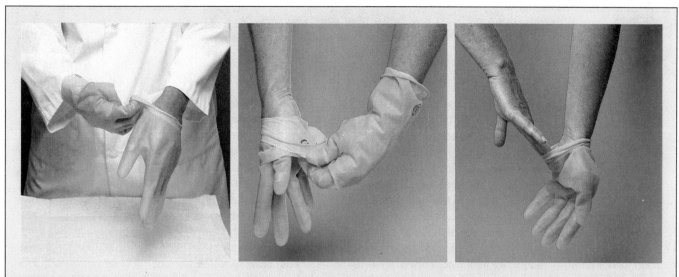

FIGURE 19–7 (d). Pull glove onto nondominant hand by placing fingers under cuff. (e). Pull glove off of dominant hand with thumb and fingers holding outside of cuff. (f). Place ungloved fingers between glove and hand (at palm) and pull off (do not touch outside of contaminated glove) inside out.

Generally the substances used are solid carbon dioxide or liquid nitrogen. It is sometimes referred to as cold cautery.

Skin Preparation

Preparation of the area of skin that will be affected by the surgical procedure is called skin prep. Because body hair encourages microbial accumulation, it is usually shaved. The skin cannot be completely sterilized or the cells would be destroyed, but an antiseptic is used to reduce microbial growth.

Many physicians still prefer the use of a stainless steel razor with disposable blades, but there are also disposable skin-prep kits that contain all the necessary items for this procedure. If a reusable razor is preferred for hair removal in preparation for the surgery site, it must be autoclaved to prevent possible disease transmission. A new blade must be used for each patient. To protect yourself and the patient from possible disease transmission, you should wear latex gloves during the skin-prep procedure. Practice in the procedure for this skill is necessary to become proficient.

You must be extremely careful to avoid nicking the patient's skin. Microorganisms can enter the body through a break in the skin and an infection could develop from carelessness. If this should happen, the physician must be notified immediately.

Sterile Gloves

If the physician wishes you to assist directly with the surgical procedure, sterile gloves must be worn. Dressing changes should also be performed wearing sterile gloves to protect both yourself and the patient. In addition, you may assist with lacerations resulting from injury, needle biopsies, and the insertion of IUDs. All of these procedures require sterile technique.

A thorough surgical scrub should be performed for 6 minutes. If it has been within 48 hours since last surgical scrub was performed, 3 minutes is sufficient.

Assisting with Procedures

Assisting with surgical procedures requires basic knowledge in several areas. The medical assistant should learn anatomy and physiology, medical terminology, and the names and uses of the instruments used in minor office procedures. You should also develop skills in human relations. With experience, you will become more sensitive and aware of the patient's needs. The more knowledge you acquire about procedures and the items necessary to perform them, the more perceptive you will be in assisting the physician.

The following procedures in assisting with minor surgical procedures and suture and skin staple removals are valuable skills that require self-discipline and personal integrity. Keeping a sterile field is of monumental importance for the well-being of the patient. It is also of utmost importance for medical-legal reasons. If sterile technique is not practiced, and infection can result. Patients are very much aware of their rights. You must respect the medical profession and the patient in practicing these skills to the very best of your ability.

Assist With Minor Surgery

PURPOSE: To assist physician in the performance of a surgical procedure and to provide support for the patient.

EQUIPMENT: Basic setup, sterile: needle and syringe, needle holder, appropriate suture, scalpel handle and blade, thumb forceps, surgical scissors, hemostats, retractor, 2 or 3 pairs of latex gloves, gauze squares, cotton-tipped applicators, alcohol pad, fenestrated sheet or towels, towel clamps, bandages; bandage scissors, tape, ordered anesthetic, antiseptic (small glass container for antiseptic solution), plastic biohazardous waste bag (and waste receptacle), patient's chart, pen, histology request form for laboratory analysis if biopsy is indicated, Mayo tray table

TERMINAL PERFORMANCE OBJECTIVE: Provided with all necessary equipment/supplies, the instructor role-playing as physician, and the students role-playing as patients, the student will demonstrate (insofar as possible) each of the steps required in assisting with minor surgery. The instructor will observe each step. Note: Some steps will need to be simulated in the instructional setting.

1. Wash hands.
2. Assemble appropriate equipment/supplies on counter or table near Mayo tray. Position Mayo tray table next to treatment table and check expiration dates of sterile items.
3. Bring scheduled patient into treatment room. Advise patient to empty bladder. When patient returns, take vital signs and record. Explain procedure to patient and obtain signature on consent form. If biopsy is to be taken, complete lab request form for histology analysis.
4. Instruct patient to disrobe as necessary for procedure and advise where to place belongings. Assist patient if needed. Allow privacy and ask patient to let you know when ready for positioning.
5. Assist patient to treatment table and into desired position for surgery. Perform skin-prep procedure. Give patient support and understanding and answer any questions at this time. Drape patient appropriately.
6. Place sterile towel on Mayo tray by holding the underneath sides of it (the top side must be untouched). Put sterile latex gloves on. Open all sterile items (as ordered by physician for scheduled surgery) carefully by holding them at the tabs; drop them onto the sterile field without touching them. Place instruments and other sterile items in the order that they will be used in the procedure. Do not reach, cough, sneeze, wave, talk, or cross over the sterile field or it will become contaminated. Carefully cover with a sterile towel until physician is ready to begin. Remove gloves and wash hands.
7. When physician is ready to begin the surgical procedure, remove the sterile towel from the prepared sterile setup. Assist physician by handing sterile gloves, use alcohol

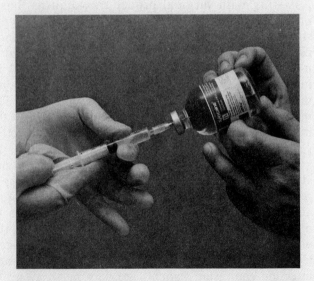

FIGURE 19–8 Hold the anesthetic solution in a convenient position so the physician can fill the syringe without contamination. (From Simmers, *Diversified Health Occupations,* 2d ed. Copyright 1988, Delmar Publishers Inc.)

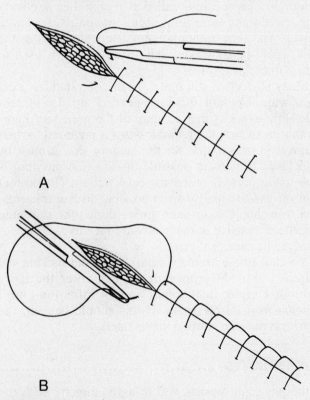

A

B

FIGURE 19–9 Two examples of suturing techniques: interrupted (individual) sutures (a) and continuous sutures (b).

prep to wipe the top of the anesthetic vial, and hold it for physician to draw out the amount needed, Figure 19–8.

8. If you are to assist with surgical procedure, wash hands and put on sterile gloves. Hand instruments and other sterile items to physician as needed, mop excessive blood with gauze sponges PRN, open specimen container labeled for biopsy to be placed into by physician. You may assist the physician in suturing the incision by clipping each individual suture after the knot is tied by the physician, Figure 19–9. You should perform any other assistance as directed by physician during the procedure PRN. If additional sterile items are needed during the procedure, open the package and hand to physician for removal, or drop onto the center of the sterile field. Table 19–1 describes various surgical instruments used in minor office procedures (see

TABLE 19–1
Instruments Used in Minor Office Surgical Procedures

Figure Number	Category: Description	Use
	Operating Scissors:	
A	*Deaver* $5\frac{1}{2}$" (14 cm) straight, sharp-sharp	Cut tissue and suture
B	*Sistrunk* $5\frac{1}{2}$" (14 cm) slightly curved	Same
C	*Deaver* $5\frac{1}{2}$" (14 cm) straight, sharp-blunt and curved, sharp-blunt	Same
	Bandage Scissors:	
D	*Lester* $5\frac{1}{2}$" (14 cm) sidecurved	Cut dressings, tape
E	*Knowles finger* $5\frac{1}{2}$" (14 cm)	Same
F	*Spencer suture* $3\frac{1}{2}$" (8.75 cm)	Cut suture
G	*Littauer stitch* $5\frac{1}{2}$" (14 cm)	Same
	Petit-Point Hemostats:	
H	*Mosquito* $4\frac{3}{4}$" straight-curved	Grasp tissue to hold, clamp, or pull out of the way
I	*Mosquito* $3\frac{1}{2}$" straight-curved	Same
	Towel Forceps:	
J	*Backhaus* (clip) $3\frac{1}{2}$" (8.75 cm)	Grasp towels, dressing; hold drape towels in place (use caution—will puncture skin)
K	*Jones* (clip) 3"	Same
L	*Knife Handle #3* 5" (12.5 cm) holds blades 10, 12, 15	Accept blades
M	*Blades*	Cut tissue
	Sponge-Holding Forceps:	
N	*Foersfer* 7" (18 cm) straight smooth jaws or serrated	Pick up and hold dressings
	Needle Holders:	
O	*Brown* $5\frac{1}{4}$" (13.5 cm)	Grasp suture needle
P	*Collier* 5" (13 cm)	Same
	Dressing and Tissue Forceps:	
Q	*Thumb* 4" (10 cm) serrated	Pick up dressings, delicate tissue
R	*Tissue* $4\frac{1}{2}$" (11 cm) 1 x 2 teeth	Grasp tissue securely for control during dissection or suturing
S	*Adson* serrated, extra delicate, 0.8 mm-wide tip	Pick up delicate tissue
T	*Semken dressing* $4\frac{3}{4}$" (12 cm) serrated	Pick up dressings
U	*Cushing* $7\frac{1}{4}$" (18.5 cm) serrated handle, scraper end, bayonet, 1 × 2 teeth	Close skin
V	*Plain splinter* $3\frac{1}{2}$" (8.75 cm)	Remove splinters
W	*Judd-Allis tissue* 6" (15 cm)	Grasp tissue

Appendix pages 741 and 742 for illustrations).

9. When surgery is completed, assist in (or perform) cleaning and bandaging the surgery site, remove gloves, and wash hands. Tend to the patient by helping into sitting position to regain balance, and when stable, from the table. Assist in dressing if necessary. Give patient education regarding return visit, care of surgery site, and any other orders from physician. Ask patient if allergic to adhesive, if so use hypoallergenic tape to secure bandage.

10. Put on gloves to clean up treatment table, discard disposable items in biohazardous bag, place instruments in detergent solution to soak after rinsing with cold water, remove gloves and wash hands, restock room.

Assisting with surgical procedures requires you to become efficient in completing many details. Of primary concern is patient education in both preoperative and postoperative care. Many physicians prefer to perform minor surgical procedures first on the day's schedule. The doctor may require that patients fast for a certain period of time before the procedure. Fasting lessens the possibility of nausea and vomiting, which some patients may experience during and following any type of surgery. It is best to check with the doctor regarding preference in preop instructions.

PATIENT EDUCATION

Usual care of patient:
1. Keep site clean and dry
2. Place no stress on the area
3. Drink plenty of fluids
4. Get proper rest
5. Eat a sensible well-balanced diet
6. Return for follow-up appointment.

Patients should report to the physician any of the following:
1. Unusual pain, burning, or other uncomfortable sensation
2. Swelling, redness, or other discoloration
3. Bleeding or other discharge
4. Fever above 100°F (37.7°C)
5. Nausea and vomiting
6. Any other problem or symptom.

Following suture removal patients should be advised to:
1. Keep the site dry for at least 24 hours
2. Cover the area to keep it clean
3. Apply supportive bandaging PRN
4. Report any sign of infection immediately to physician.

Often patients are apprehensive about even the most minor surgical procedure. You must display confidence, concern, and understanding to each individual about the particular procedure. Allow enough time following the explanation of the procedure for the person to think about what was said. Offer to answer questions of patients even if they do not ask.

Make sure that return appointment visits are confirmed and reminder cards are given to patients before they leave the office. Phoning patients the next day is an excellent way to follow-up and reassures them that you and the physician are genuinely concerned about their progress. It will also bring to the physician's attention any problems that could be eliminated early. If patients do have complaints, it is best to have the physician check the problem as soon as possible.

Advise patients about symptoms that may occur following the surgery and to report them immediately to the physician.

Follow-up visits are essential so that assessment of progress can be made by the physician and for the removal of sutures. In general, you should advise all patients who have had any minor surgical procedure to limit their activity for at least a couple of weeks, or however long the physician has ordered according to the procedure performed.

Specific instructions such as soaking or applying topical medications will be given by the physician for certain individual cases. Physicians generally instruct patients (or teach you how to instruct patients) about packing or special bandaging procedures, such as with ingrown toenail removals. Physicians may prescribe an analgesic for minor pain and discomfort the patient may experience following the procedure.

Patients usually see the family/general practitioner for suture removal following laceration repair from an injury or from a diagnostic procedure such as heart catheterization. You may have this duty to perform. It is vital that you check the emergency room report regarding the number of sutures put in, so you can be sure to remove all of them. Check the report also for a tetanus booster and record on the patient's chart to bring the immunization

Remove Sutures

PURPOSE: To remove suture(s) from healing laceration/incision.

EQUIPMENT: Sterile: thumb forceps, sutures removal scissors (or staple extractor), gauze squares, latex gloves, cotton-tipped applicators, butterfly or steristrip closures; antiseptic solution, hydrogen peroxide, basin with warm soapy water, bandages, tape, towels, biohazardous waste bag, bandage scissors, patient's chart, pen

TERMINAL PERFORMANCE OBJECTIVE: Provided with all necessary equipment and supplies, and using a mannequin/model as the patient, the student will demonstrate the steps required to remove sutures. The instructor will observe each step. Simulation should be made by the instructor.

1. Wash hands and move Mayo table next to treatment table, or where patient will be during the procedure.
2. Assemble all necessary items on Mayo table tray, Figure 19–10.

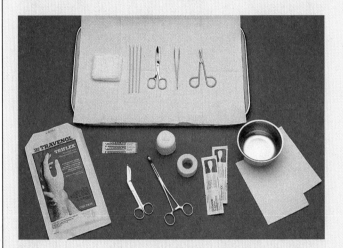

FIGURE 19–10 Example of a suture removal tray setup

3. Bring scheduled patient to treatment room. Ask patient about healing condition of incision/laceration, take vital signs, and record on patient's chart. (If sutures resulted from a laceration injury, ask appropriate questions regarding where, when, tetanus booster, (file ER report in chart) etc., and record.
4. Ask patient to remove appropriate clothing for inspec-

tion of healing incision (offer help PRN).
5. Assist patient to treatment table and into required position and drape appropriately. Explain procedure and answer any questions.
6. Put gloves on and remove bandage. Clean incision with antiseptic solution using cotton-tipped applicators. If bandage has stuck to the incision (record condition of site on chart: excessive blood, or drainage), apply gauze squares that have been soaked with the soapy warm water solution, *or* hydrogen peroxide, to the area for a few minutes to loosen bandage from sutures and scab (pulling off a stuck bandage may reopen the wound, and/or pull sutures out) as this will make removing the bandage much easier. Advise physician that the incision site is ready to be checked.
7. After physician orders suture removal, open sterile package containing the necessary instruments on the Mayo tray and proceed. Grasp the knot of the suture material with thumb forceps and gently, but firmly, pull up making just enough space to place the suture removal scissors to clip the suture as close to the skin as possible, Figure 19–11, page 620. Pull the suture with the forceps (back) toward the healing incision so that no stress is put on it. (Pulling the suture away from the site could possibly pull the incision open). **Key Point: Do not pull suture that has been on the surface of the skin (exposed to the outside) through the path of the suture being removed or infection may develop.** Continue in this manner until all sutures are removed.
8. Apply antiseptic solution to site and allow to air dry. Apply steristips or butterfly, closure if necessary for support during healing process, and bandage. Ask if patient is allergic to adhesive, if so use hypoallergenic tape to secure bandage, (ask also about allergies to topical preparations such as povidone-iodine mixture, or any medications).
9. Remove gloves and wash hands.
10. Instruct patient to keep the bandage clean and dry for 24 to 48 hours, or as directed by physician. Advise patient to avoid undue stress for appropriate amount of time for the anatomical area. Give patient education regarding home care and follow-up appointment if ordered by physician.

11. Record on progress notes in patient's chart: (1) anatomical area of incision/laceration; (2) condition of site; (3) number of sutures removed; (4) type of antiseptic applied; (5) support closures applied; (6) type of bandage applied, and your initials. Be sure to include the ER report if sent from facility where injury was treated, and record tetanus booster if applicable.

Note: If skin staples (or clips) are to be removed, the physician will usually perform the procedure. However, you may be instructed to do so. Basically, skin staples are removed in the following manner: Follow Steps 1 though 7 above and proceed to:

Place the sterile staple extractor under staple (one at a time) and squeeze handles of extractor completely closed, Figure 19–12. (Explain to patient that a tugging sensation may be felt.) Lift staple away from skin and place in biohazardous waste bag. Continue process until all are removed. Resume procedure above with Step 8.

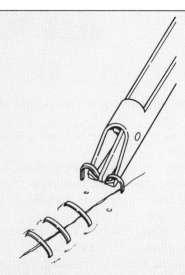

FIGURE 19–12 Removal of a staple. Staple extractor reforms the staple (clip). Then the staple is lifted from the incision.

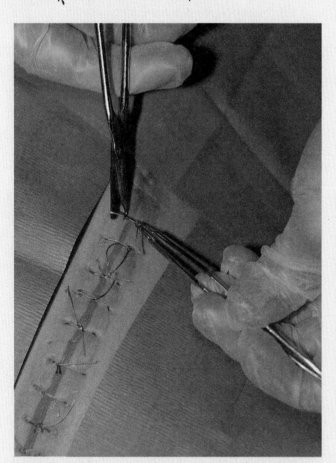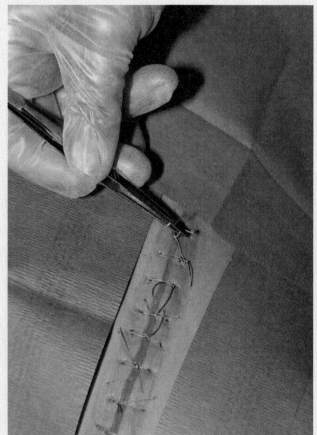

FIGURE 19–11 Suture removal. (a). Grasp suture knot with thumb forceps, and place the curved tip of the suture removal scissors just next to the skin under the suture and clip. (b). Gently pull the suture knot up and toward the incision with thumb forceps to remove (pulling the suture away from the incision may reopen it).

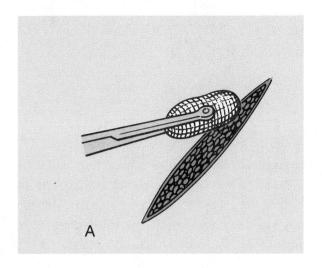

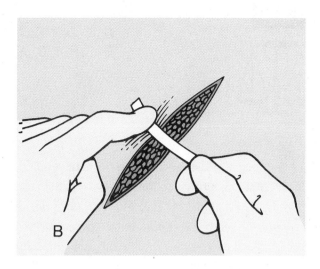

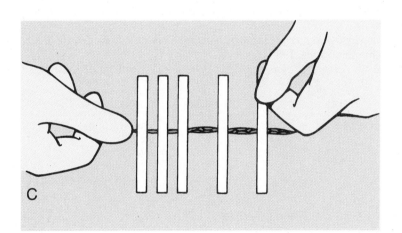

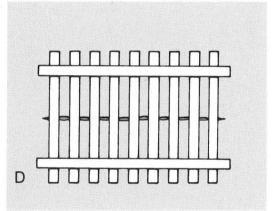

FIGURE 19–13 (a). Use transfer forceps with sterile gauze to apply antiseptic. (b). Apply steristrip closure to center of incision. (c). Apply closures to each side for evenness. (d). Apply closures parallel to incision for support.

record up to date. Before you remove the sutures, check the number of days that the physician who put them in recommended, and ask your physician-employer to inspect the healing wound. Physicians generally order additional closure materials to cover healing incisions/ lacerations following suture removal, Figure 19–13. This procedure gives support to the wound and offers the patient more flexibility. Additionally, physicians advise using an Ace bandage to offer more protection and support of surgical areas of the extremities, especially for pediatric and physically active patients. Application of an Ace wrap increases circulation of the area, which hastens the healing process.

Until you are confident in assisting with various office surgeries, it is suggested that you keep a notebook or file cards to help you learn the instruments and steps required for each procedure.

Complete Chapter 19 in the workbook to help you meet the objectives at the beginning of this chapter and therefore achieve competency of this subject matter.

MEDICAL-LEGAL
ETHICAL HIGHLIGHTS

Ms. Right...

explains the procedure to the patient prior to obtaining written consent from the patient for any procedures that involve risk. She provides printed information about the procedure for the patient to take home. If a third party is responsible for payment, she obtains a written contract.

Employment advancement: Excellent

Miss Wrong...

often forgets to obtain written consent form and third party contract for procedures involving risk. She tells the patient about the procedure and says not to worry about anything, that everything will be all right. She never gives out printed information because she can never remember where she put it.

Employment advancement: Poor

REFERENCES

J. Jamner Surgical Instruments, Inc., 1991, 9 Skyline Drive, Hawthorne, New York 10532.

Mosby's Dictionary of Medical, Nursing and Allied Health, 3d ed. St. Louis: C. V. Mosby, 1990.

Procedures, The Nurse's Reference Library, Nursing 83 Books, Springhouse, PA: Intermed Communications, 1983.

Taber, Clarence W. *Taber's Cyclopedic Medical Dictionary,* 14th ed. Philadelphia: F. A. Davis, 1983.

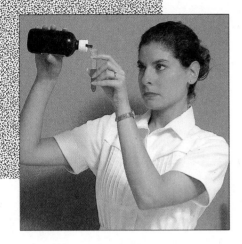

C H A P T E R 2 0

Assisting with Medications

A dministering medications is one of the most sensitive and important duties that the medical assistant will perform.

You must first become familiar with the medications which are most frequently given to patients. Knowing the properties of the medications will help in answering patients' questions and recognizing common side effects that patients may exhibit. The *Physicians' Desk Reference*, or PDR, and the *Physicians' Desk Reference for Nonprescription Drugs* will become valuable resources. Because these resources are frequently referred to, they should be kept in a central accessible place for use by all members of the health care team. You should also become familiar with the many terms and abbreviations used in administering medications. Some of the most common ones are included in this chapter and in the Appendix.

The laws may vary from state to state in regard to your administering medications. You should check with your employer about this matter. Some physicians prefer always to administer medications to patients themselves, thereby lessening this possible medical-legal concern.

A review of basic math skills will be helpful in preparing medications. The areas in which to practice are: addition, subtraction, multiplication, division, fractions, decimals, percentages, and ratio–proportion. Refer to Table 20–5, page 632, for examples of these math problems. Accuracy and care must always be taken in assisting with and administering medications to patients.

U N I T 1

Prescription and Nonprescription Medications

OBJECTIVES ···

Upon completion of this unit, the student will meet the following terminal performance objectives by verifying knowledge of the facts and principles presented through oral and written communication at a level deemed competent, and will demonstrate the specific behaviors as

Throughout this chapter you should be mindful of all medical-legal/ethical implications. Listed below are a few important reminders.

1. Secure medications or prescription pads in locked storage.
2. Report theft of medications or prescription pads to authorities.
3. Dispose of expired medications properly.
4. Obtain and file written consent from patients for experimental drugs.
5. Give printed information about and obtain written consent for immunizations.
6. Record medication refills on patient's chart.
7. Keep narcotics records accurate and up to date.
8. Keep physician's narcotics registration current and on file.

identified in the terminal performance objectives of the procedures, observing all aseptic and safety precautions in accordance with health care standards.

1. Demonstrate how to use PDRs for both prescription and nonprescription medications.
2. Explain how to properly phone in prescriptions to a pharmacist.
3. Demonstrate how to write a prescription as ordered by the physician.
4. Discuss the drugs that are under federal regulation according to category, or Schedules I through V.
5. Define abbreviations commonly used in regard to medications.
6. Demonstrate how to record medications properly on the patient's chart.
7. Explain how to categorize medications used in the medical office.
8. Discuss medical/legal/ethical concerns regarding medications.
9. Spell and define, using the glossary at the back of the text, all the words to know in this unit.

WORDS TO KNOW ....

accuracy	OTC
administer	PDR
Drug Enforcement	pharmaceutical
Administration (DEA)	pharmacology
dispense	prescribe
expertise	prescription
facility	reference
license	resource
narcotic	vial

Commonly Prescribed Medications ....

Because of the nature of each type of medical practice, certain medications will be more commonly prescribed than others. It is a good idea to keep a list of these medications handy with the most often questioned information. This list should include the usual dosage and possible side effects. The entire staff should become knowledgeable about these medications.

The list in Table 20–1 is meant as an introduction. The common names of some of the drugs are listed. Consulting a **PDR** or other resource for complete information is suggested.

PATIENT EDUCATION

Many patients are very anxious about receiving medication, whether by mouth or by injection. Careful and complete explanation of the procedure and the need for medications is essential in calming the patient. The patient must understand when and how to take prescribed medications to receive the full benefits of these medications. Some medications are to be taken before meals or after meals, with certain fluids or excluding certain fluids, and in the presence or absence of certain foods or other medications. Carefully explained verbal and written instructions are essential for the patient's compliance. The patient must understand that the medication dosage cannot be changed without first consulting the physician.

TABLE 20–1
Selected Drug Classifications

CLASSIFICATION	ACTION	EXAMPLES
Analgesic	An agent that relieves pain without causing loss of consciousness	acetaminophen (Tylenol) aspirin ibuprofen (Advil, Motrin)
Anesthetic	An agent that produces a lack of feeling. May be local or general depending on the type and how administered.	morphine, lidocaine HCL (Xylocaine) procaine HCL (Novocaine)
Antacid	An agent that neutralizes acid.	Amphojel, Gelusil, Mylanta, Aludrox, Milk of Magnesia
Antianxiety	An agent that relieves anxiety and muscle tension.	benzodiazepines: diazepam (Valium) and chlordiazepoxide HCL (Librium)
Antiarrhythmic	An agent that controls cardiac arrhythmias.	lidocaine HCL (Xylocaine) propranolol HCL (Inderal)
Antibiotic	An agent that is destructive to or inhibits growth of microorganisms.	penicillins (Pentids, Duracillin, Polycillin, Pipracil, Augmentin) cephalosporins (Reflin, Mandol, Rocephin)
Anticholinergic	An agent that blocks parasympathetic nerve impulses.	atropine, scopolamine, trihexyphenidyl HCL (Artane)
Anticoagulant	An agent that prevents or delays blood clotting.	heparin sodium, Dicumarol, warfarin sodium (Coumadin)
Anticonvulsant	An agent that prevents or relieves convulsions.	carbamazepine (Tegretol) phenytoin (Dilantin) ethosuximide (Zarotin)
Antidepressant	An agent that prevents or relieves the symptoms of depression.	ethosuximide (Zarotin), monoamine oxidase (MAO) inhibitors: isocarboxazid (Marplan), phenelzine sulfate (Nardil), amitriptyline HCL (Elavil), imipramine HCL (Tofranil)
Antidiarrheal	An agent that prevents or relieves diarrhea.	Lomotil, Pepto-Bismol, Kaopectate
Antidote	An agent that counteracts poisons and their effect.	naloxone (Narcan)
Antiemetic	An agent that prevents or relieves nausea and vomiting.	Tigan, Dramamine, Phenergan, Reglan, Marinol
Antihistamine	An agent that acts to counteract histamine.	Dimetane, Benadryl, Seldane
Antihypertensive	An agent that prevents or controls high blood pressure.	methyldopa (Aldomet) clonidine HCL (Catapres) metoprolol tartrate (Lopressor)
Anti-inflammatory	An agent that counteracts inflammation.	naproxen (Naprosyn), aspirin, ibuprofen (Advil, Motrin)
Antimanic	An agent used for the treatment of the manic episode of manic-depressive disorder.	lithium
Antineoplastic	An agent that kills or destroys malignant cells.	busulfan (Myleran) cyclophosphamide (Cytoxan)
Antipyretic	An agent that reduces fever.	aspirin, acetaminophen (Tylenol)
Antitussive	An agent that prevents or relieves cough.	codeine, dextromethorphan
Bronchodilator	An agent that dilates the bronchi.	isoproterenol HCL (Isuprel) albuterol (Proventil)
Contraceptive	Any device, method, or agent that prevents conception.	Enovid-E 21, Ortho-Novum 10/11-21; 10/11-28 Triphasil-21
Decongestant	An agent that reduces nasal congestion and/or swelling.	oxymetazoline (Afrin) epinephrine HCL (Adrenalin) phenylephrine HCL (Neo-Synephrine) pseudoephedrine HCL (Sudafed)
Diuretic	An agent that increases the excretion of urine.	chlorothiazide (Diuril) furosemide (Lasix) Mannitol (Osmitrol)
Expectorant	An agent that facilitates removal of secretion from bronchopulmonary mucous membrane.	guaifenesin (Robitussin)
Hemostatic	An agent that controls or stops bleeding.	Humafac, Amicar, vitamin K

TABLE 20–1
Selected Drug Classifications (continued)

CLASSIFICATION	ACTION	EXAMPLES
Hypnotic	An agent that produces sleep or hypnosis.	secobarbital (Seconal); chloral hydrate ethchlorvynol (Placidyl)
Hypoglycemic	An agent that lowers blood glucose level.	insulin; chlorpropamide (Diabinese)
Laxative	An agent that loosens and promotes normal bowel eliminations.	Metamucil powder, Dulcolax
Muscle relaxant	An agent that produces relaxation of skeletal muscle.	Robaxin, Norflex, Paraflex, Skelaxin, Valium
Sedative	An agent that produces a calming effect without causing sleep.	amobarbital (Amytal) butabarbital sodium (Buticaps) phenobarbital
Tranquilizer	An agent that reduces mental tension and anxiety.	Thorazine, Mellaril, Haldol
Vasodilator	An agent that produces relaxation of blood vessels; lowers blood pressure.	isorbide dinitrate (Isordil) nitroglycerine
Vasopressor	An agent that produces contraction of muscles of capillaries and arteries; elevates blood pressure.	metaraminol (Aramine) norepinephrine (Levophed)

(From Rice, *Principles of Pharmacology for Medical Associates,* copyright 1989, Albany, NY; Delmar Publishers. Used with permission)

Pharmaceutical References ....

The PDR is a valuable resource that the medical assistant should keep handy in the medical office. The purpose of the PDR is to provide accurate, reliable, and current information about all prescribed medications and related products. You may need to consult the PDR for the proper spelling, strength, or other information concerning medications, which are not given frequently, to assist the physician in accurately prescribing medications.

One of your responsibilities may be to order the current edition of the PDR so that the practice may keep abreast of the newest pharmaceuticals approved by the Food and Drug Administration (FDA). This reference book is published annually. A supplement with the latest information is sent to subscribers quarterly. There are nine sections:

1. Manufacturers' index (white)
2. Product name index (pink)
3. Product classification index (blue)
4. Generic and chemical name index (yellow)
5. Medications in color and actual size for identification assistance
6. Product information section (white, alphabetically)
7. Diagnostic product information (green)
8. Listings of poison control centers
9. Guide to management of drug overdose

Guidelines for using the PDR:

1. The pink section alphabetically lists the brand of (if described) generic names of medicines and products. The manufacturer of the product appears next with either one or two page numbers. The first page number refers you to the picture section for identification of the product and the next page number is for the information about the product in the white section.
2. The yellow section alphabetically lists the generic or chemical names of the products with the manufacturer listed beside it and the pages on which information may be obtained.
3. The blue section contains products in alphabetical order according to their classification.
4. The green section contains current information about diagnostic products also listed in alphabetical order.

Note: The medical assistant should become familiar with the PDR's contents page with each new edition to become proficient in assisting the physician with needed information. The *Physicians' Desk Reference for Nonprescription Drugs* is also another valuable resource that can be of great assistance in identifying over-the-counter (OTC) medicines that patients use for self-medication. The format of this reference book is almost identical to the PDR for prescription products. A section on patient education material and support groups is also included, besides diagnostic home use products.

Getting familiar with the arrangement of both PDRs will prove its worth very quickly when a difficult situation is encountered in the medical practice.

Many other sources of information about pharmacology are used by physicians. Most offices have more than one reference for this purpose. *The National Formulary,* the *Pharmacopoeia of the United States of America* (USP), and the *Pharmacopoeia Internationalis* are three.

Writing Prescriptions ....

A prescription is a written order for a particular medication or treatment for a particular patient by a licensed physician. It is a legal document. Most prescriptions are hand written by the physician, especially those for narcotics. However, some physicians delegate the task of

FIGURE 20–1

DEA NUMBER (MAY BE PRINTED)   TELEPHONE NUMBER

PHYSICIAN'S NAME
ADDRESS ZIP

PATIENT'S NAME _____ DATE _____

ADDRESS _____

Rx

Sig:

Refill _____ Times

Please label ( )

PHYSICIAN'S SIGNATURE

DEA NUMBER (MAY BE PRINTED)   TELEPHONE NUMBER

PHYSICIAN'S NAME, ADDRESS, ZIP

PATIENT'S NAME _____ Date _____

ADDRESS _____

Sig:	LABEL MEDICATION	mg/cc	Quantity	Refills
Rx 1.				
Rx 2.				
Rx 3.				
Rx 4.				
Rx 5.				

PHYSICIAN'S SIGNATURE

FIGURE 20–1 Sample prescription blanks for single medication (a) and multiple medications (b)

writing the information on the prescription blank to the medical assistant. The physician will then check the prescription and sign it. Any medication that is **prescribed** must be recorded on the patient's chart. Figure 20–1 shows examples of prescription blanks. When the physician prescribes only one medication for a patient, the single medication prescription pad is used. Physicians use the multiple medication prescription pads for those patients whose condition requires several medications to be prescribed at a time. This eliminates having to write in the patient's name, date, etc., on each single prescription order. It also saves the doctor from having to sign each individual sheet.

The prescription should contain the:

- Date
- Patient's full legal name and complete address
- Rx symbol (means recipe, or "take thou")
- Name of drug and amount
- Pharmacist's instructions
- Patient's instructions
- Signature of physician
- Physician's full name, address, and phone number
- Physician's DEA number

This standard information helps the pharmacist fill the prescription. It is much easier for pharmacists today to fill

Form DEA (Jun 1990) – 224　　OMB No. 1117-0014

APPLICATION FOR REGISTRATION
UNDER
CONTROLLED SUBSTANCES ACT OF 1970

Please PRINT or TYPE all entries.

No registration may be issued unless a completed application form has been received (21 CFR 1301.21).

NAME

PROPOSED BUSINESS ADDRESS

CITY　　STATE　　ZIP CODE

RETAIN Copy 3. Mail Orig. and 1 copy with FEE to:

UNITED STATES DEPARTMENT OF JUSTICE
DRUG ENFORCEMENT ADMINISTRATION
CENTRAL STATION
P. O. Box 28083
WASHINGTON, D.C. 20038 - 8083
For INFORMATION, Call: (202) 307 7255

See "Privacy Act" Information on reverse

THIS BLOCK FOR DEA USE ONLY

REGISTRATION CLASSIFICATION: Submit Check or Money Order Payable to the **DRUG ENFORCEMENT ADMINISTRATION** in the Amount of **$ 60.00** (3 year registration period)

● **FEE MUST ACCOMPANY APPLICATION**

1. BUSINESS ACTIVITY: *(Check ☑ ONE only)*

A ☐ RETAIL PHARMACY　B ☐ HOSPITAL/CLINIC　C ☐ PRACTITIONER *(Specify Medical Degree, e.g., DDS, DO, DVM, MD, etc.)*　D ☐ TEACHING INSTITUTION *(Instructional purposes only)*

2. SCHEDULES: *(Check ☑ all applicable schedules in which you intend to handle controlled substances. See Schedules on Reverse of Instruction Sheet.)*

SCHEDULE II NARCOTIC ☐　SCHEDULE II NONNARCOTIC ☐　SCHEDULE III NARCOTIC ☐　SCHEDULE III NONNARCOTIC ☐　SCHEDULE IV ☐　SCHEDULE V ☐

3. ☐ CHECK HERE IF YOU REQUIRE ORDER FORMS.

4. **ALL APPLICANTS MUST ANSWER THE FOLLOWING:**

(a) Are you currently authorized to prescribe, distribute, dispense, conduct research, or otherwise handle the controlled substances in the schedules for which you are applying, under the laws of the **State** or jurisdiction in which you are operating or propose to operate?

☐ YES - **State** License No. ____________
☐ Not Applicable　☐ Pending

☐ YES - **State** Controlled Substance No. ____________
☐ Not Applicable　☐ Pending

(b) Has the applicant ever been convicted of a crime in connection with controlled substances under State or Federal law, or ever surrendered or had a Federal controlled substance registration revoked, suspended, restricted or denied, or ever had a State professional license or controlled substance registration revoked, suspended, denied, restricted or placed on probation?　☐ YES　☐ NO

(c) If the applicant is a corporation (other than a corporation whose stock is owned and traded by the public), association, partnership, or pharmacy, has any officer, partner, stockholder or proprietor been convicted of a crime in connection with controlled substances under State or Federal law, or ever surrendered or had a Federal controlled substance registration revoked, suspended, restricted or denied, or ever had a State professional license or controlled substance registration revoked, suspended, denied, restricted or placed on probation?　☐ YES　☐ NO　☐ NOT APPLICABLE

IF THE ANSWER TO QUESTIONS 4(b) or (c) is YES, include a statement using the space provided on the **REVERSE** of this part.

● *ATTACH CHECK HERE* ●

Print or Type Name Here - Sign Below　　Applicant's Business Phone No.

SIGN HERE ▶　*Signature of applicant or authorized individual*　　*Date*

Title (If the applicant is a corporation, institution, or other entity, enter the TITLE of the person signing on behalf of the applicant ((e.g., President, Dean, Procurement Officer, etc....))

5. CERTIFICATION FOR FEE EXEMPTION

☐ CHECK THIS BLOCK IF INDIVIDUAL NAMED HEREON IS A FEDERAL, STATE, OR LOCAL OFFICIAL.

The Undersigned hereby certifies that the applicant herein is an officer or employee of a Federal, State or local agency who, in the course of such employment, is authorized to obtain, dispense, or prescribe controlled substances or is authorized to conduct research, instructional activity or chemical analysis with controlled substances, and is exempt from the payment of this application fee.

Signature of Certifying Official　　*Date*

Print or Type Name

Print or Type Title

Name of Institution or Agency

WARNING: SECTION 843(a)(4) OF TITLE 21, UNITED STATES CODE, STATES THAT ANY PERSON WHO KNOWINGLY OR INTENTIONALLY FURNISHES FALSE OR FRAUDULENT INFORMATION IN THIS APPLICATION IS SUBJECT TO IMPRISONMENT FOR NOT MORE THAN FOUR YEARS, A FINE OF NOT MORE THAN $30,000.00 OR BOTH.

Mail the Original and 1 copy with FEE to the above address. Retain 3rd copy for your records.

FIGURE 20–2 Example of a DEA physican registration form.

TABLE 20-2

Schedules of Controlled Substances

DRUG CATEGORY	POTENTIAL FOR ABUSE (ADDICTION)	MEDICAL USE	POTENTIAL FOR DEPENDENCE	EXAMPLE
Schedule I	High	—Unaccepted —Limited to research	High	Heroin, LSD, marijuana, peyote
Schedule II	High	—Accepted —Tightly restricted	Severe psychic or physical	Amphetamines, morphine
Schedule III	Less than I or II Low to moderate	Current	High psychological	Certain opioids, barbiturates and some depressants
Schedule IV	Low	Acceptable	Limited physical and psychological	Phenobarbital propoxyphene
Schedule V	Low	Acceptable	Limited physical and psychological	Small amounts of codeine in cough preparations and analgesics

prescriptions because of prepared and prepackaged medications. Although it is rare, however, some medications must still be prepared by the licensed pharmacist from the directions on the prescription. When phoning in prescriptions, you must give the pharmacist all the information that the prescription contains. To ensure accuracy, you should ask the pharmacist to repeat the information. This practice will help avoid dangerous misunderstandings.

When patients have their prescriptions filled by a pharmacist, the container often has an instruction label on it. Pharmacists frequently use one or more of these labels to alert the patient of special instructions or warnings regarding a particular medication ordered by the doctor. Warning labels are made in a variety of bright colors to attract attention to their messages, Figure 20–3.

All physicians who prescribe, dispense, or administer medications in the United States must register with the U.S. Department of Justice, Drug Enforcement Administration (DEA), under the Controlled Substances Act of 1970. A form must be filled out, with the physician's state license number and signature, and accompanied by a standard fee, Figure 20–2. If the physician moves the medical practice, this change of address must be reported in writing to the nearest DEA field office. Registration must be renewed every 3 years. The certificate must be filed at the registered location and be available for inspection by officials on request. If the physician practices medicine in one or more locations, as long as it is within the same state, individual registration must be filed for each address only if controlled substances are administered or dispensed at each place. If prescriptions only are written at other locations, registration needs to be filed with the DEA just for the primary location. Physicians must be in compliance with these requirements of the 1984 Diversion Control Amendments to administer, dispense, or prescribe any

controlled substance. A current printed schedule of controlled substances is enclosed with the application and this should also be kept on file. Table 20–2 lists the drugs that are under federal control according to their

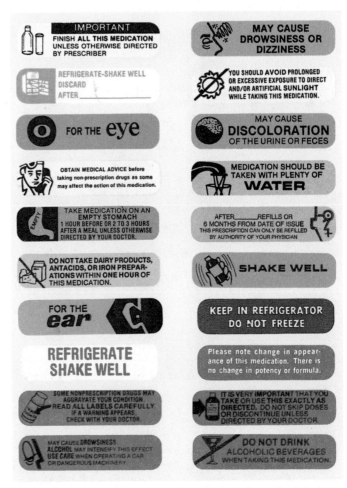

FIGURE 20–3 Examples of instructions and warning labels for prescription medications.

TABLE 20–3

Abbreviations and symbols commonly used in administering medications

Abbreviation	Meaning	Abbreviation	Meaning
@	at	hs	bedtime, hour of sleep
āā	of each	IM	intramuscular
ac	before meals	inj	injection
ad	up to	IV	intravenous
AD	right ear	k	potassium
adde	add, let it be added	kg	kilogram
ad lib	as much as needed, as desired	m	minim
agit	shake, stir	M	mix
agNo$_2$	silver nitrate	mcgm	microgram
alt dieb	alternate days	M et f pil	mix and make into pill
alt hor	alternate hour	M et f pulv	mix and make into powder
alt noc	alternate nights	M et sig	mix and label
am	morning	mg, mgm	milligram
ante	before	ml	milliliter
aq	water	noct	night
aq bull	boiling water	non rep	do not repeat
aq com	tap water, common water	NPO	nothing by mouth
aq dist	distilled water	o h	every hour
aq ferv	hot water	o m	every morning
aq frig	cold water	OS	left eye
aq susp	water suspension	OD	right eye
AS	left ear	OU	in each eye, both eyes
AU	in each ear, both ears	oz, ℥	ounce
Ba	barium	pc	after meals
bid	twice a day	pil	pill
/c, c̄	with	po	by mouth
cap(s)	capsule(s)	prn, PRN	as necessary, whenever necessary
cc	cubic centimeter	pt	patient
comp	compound	pulv	powder
contra	against	qd	every day
coq	boil	qh	every hour
DC, Disc	discontinue	q (2,3,4) h	every (2,3,4) hours
dil	dilute	qid	four times a day
div	to be divided	qns	quantity not sufficient
dos	doses	qod	every other day
dr, ʒ	dram	qs	quantity sufficient
EENT	eye, ear, nose and throat	rep	let it be repeated
elix	elixir	Rx, ℞	take, recipe
emul	emulsion	/s, s̄	one-half
et	and	sat	saturated
ext	extract	sc, sub cu, SC, Subc	subcutaneous (under the skin)
f, ft	make, let there be made	Sig, Sig, S	write on label, give directions
Fe	iron	sol	solution
fl	fluid	ss, s̄s̄	one-half
G	gauge	stat, STAT	immediately
garg	gargle	suppos	suppository
GI	gastrointestinal	syr	syrup
Gm, gm	gram	T, tbsp	tablespoon
gr	grain	tab	tablet
gt	drop	tid	three times a day
gtt	drops	tr, tinct	tincture
GU	genitourinary	tsp	teaspoon
guttat	drop by drop	u	unit
h	hour	ung	ointment
H$_2$O$_2$	hydrogen peroxide		

TABLE 20–4
Commonly used weights and measures

UNITS OF VOLUME				UNITS OF WEIGHT			
1	liter	= 1000	milliliter	1	gram	= 1000	milligrams
0.001	liter	= 1	milliliter	0.001	gram	= 1	milligram
	or			1	kilogram	= 1000	grams
	1		cubic centimeter	0.001	kilogram	= 1	gram

Commonly used metric measurements

VOLUME			WEIGHT		
0.1	liter	= 1 deciliter	0.1	gram	= 1 decigram
0.01	liter	= 1 centimeter	0.01	gram	= 1 centigram
0.001	liter	= 1 milliliter	0.001	gram	= 1 milligram
10.0	liter	= dekaliter	10.0	grams	= 1 dekagram
100.0	liters	= 1 hectoliter	100.0	grams	= 1 hectogram
1000.0	liters	= 1 kiloliter	1000.0	grams	= 1 kilogram

Metric units, divisions, and multiples

VOLUME EQUIVALENTS		WEIGHT EQUIVALENTS	
Metric	Apothecaries'	Metric	Apothecaries'
1 milliliter	= 15 or 16 minims	0.06 gram or 60 milligrams	= 1 grain
4 milliliters	= 1 dram	1 gram or 1000 milligrams	= 15 grains
30 milliliters	= 1 ounce	500 milligrams	= $7\frac{1}{2}$ grains
500 milliliters	= 1 pint	4 grams	= 1 dram
1000 milliliters	= 1 quart	30 grams	= 1 ounce

Equivalency chart for volumes and weights

VOLUME	WEIGHT
60 minims = 1 (fluids) dram	60 grains = 1 dram
8 drams = 1 (fluids) ounce	8 drams = 1 ounce
16 drams = 1 pint	12 ounces = 1 pound
2 pints = 1 quart	

Apothecary measurements

actual or potential level for abuse or addiction in five categories or schedules.

Since there is no medical use for any of the drugs in Schedule I, prescriptions are prohibited. Drugs in Schedule II must have a written or typed prescription order with the physician's personal signature and DEA registry number. These medications may not be refilled. If a genuine emergency situation arises, the doctor may phone in a limited amount of medication to the pharmacist for the patient. A written, signed prescription order must be presented to the pharmacist within 72 hours for the controlled substance in compliance with DEA regulations. In Schedule III of controlled substances, medications may be ordered by phone or written prescription to the pharmacist. Five refills may be ordered within a 6-month period. Schedule V medications are subject to state and local regulations. A written prescription for these medicines is not necessarily required.

TABLE 20–5
REVIEW EXAMPLES OF MATH PROBLEMS

Addition

```
  876
  493
+ 521
 1890
```

Subtraction

```
  691          581
-  98        -  98
  593          483
```

Multiplication

```
    437
 x   25
   2185
   874
 102925
```

To Prove
Divide your
answer by
437

```
         25
437)10925
    874
   2185
   2185
```

Division

```
     56.80
70)3976.00
   350
   476
   420
   560
   560
```

To Prove
Multiply
your answer
by 70

```
   56.80
 x   70
3976.00
```

Decimals

Addition	Subtraction	Multiplication	Division
87.43	796.37	394.75	272.52$\frac{1}{5}$
+ 39.57	− 55.62	x 68.29	35)9538.27
127.00	740.75	3552.75	70
		7895	2538.27
		315800	2450.00
		236850	088.27
		26957.4775	70
			18.27
			17.5
			.77
			7

Fractions $\frac{\text{numerator}}{\text{denominator}}$

Addition
$$\frac{2}{5} + \frac{4}{5} = \frac{6}{5} = 1\frac{1}{5}$$

$$\frac{1}{5} = \frac{3}{15}$$
$$+ \frac{1}{3} = \frac{5}{15}$$
$$\frac{8}{15}$$

$$1\frac{7}{8} = 1\frac{35}{40}$$
$$+ 7\frac{7}{10} = 9\frac{28}{40}$$
$$10\frac{63}{40} = 11\frac{23}{40}$$

Subtraction $\frac{3}{5} - \frac{1}{3} = \frac{9}{15} - \frac{5}{15} = \frac{4}{15}$

$$3\frac{7}{16} - 2\frac{1}{8} = 3\frac{14}{32} - 2\frac{4}{32} = 1\frac{10}{32} = 1\frac{5}{16}$$

Multiplication $\frac{2}{5} \times \frac{7}{16} = \frac{1}{5} \times \frac{7}{8} = \frac{7}{40}$

$$\frac{1}{5} \times \frac{7}{10} = \frac{1}{5} \times \frac{7}{10} = \frac{7}{50}$$

Division $\frac{1}{12} \div \frac{2}{3} = \frac{1}{12} \times \frac{3}{2} = \frac{1}{8}$

$$1\frac{1}{4} \div 3 = \frac{5}{4} \times \frac{1}{3} = \frac{5}{12}$$

Percentages To find out what percent (%) one number is to another, use the number following the word "of" as a denominator and make a fraction. Divide the numerator by the denominator, for example:

25 is what percent of 35?

$$\frac{25}{35} = \frac{5}{7} = \quad .70 \quad =70\%$$
```
        7)5.00
          4 9
            10
```

Ratio Ratios show how one quantity relates to another and are separated by a colon (:), for example:

$20 : 100 = \frac{20}{100} = .20$ parts or 20%

Proportion A set of two equal ratios is a proportion. In the equation a double colon (::) separates each of the equal ratios, for example:

To mix a cleaning solution knowing the correct portions for a small amount you can find out how much baking soda to use to make a larger amount, using x for the unknown amount.

$\frac{1}{2}$ cup baking soda : 16 oz. water :: x amount of baking soda : 32 oz. water

$$\frac{1}{2} : 16 :: x : 32$$
$$.5 : 16 :: x : 32$$
$$16x = 32 \times .5$$
$$16x = 16$$
$$x = 1 \text{ cup baking soda}$$

Recording Medications

You will be expected to read and record many types of medications. Memorizing the commonly used abbreviations and symbols given in Table 20–3, page 630, will prepare you to carry out this responsibility. Another useful reference is the list of equivalent weights and measures given in Table 20–4, page 631. These will be needed in ordering medications. An extended list of these is given in the Appendix.

Basic math skills should be among your many areas of expertise. These skills may mean monetary savings to your employer, because there are competitive prices for everything, including medical supplies and medications. When ordering injectables, for instance, you may find that a multiple-dose vial is more economical for the needs of the practice than a single-dose vial. Determining what is cost effective for the practice and shopping for the best values will make you an asset to the practice. Table 20–5 provides examples of the common math problems you may encounter in determining costs, dosages, and other mathematical calculations in the medical setting.

Pharmaceutical representatives will undoubtedly visit the medical facility from time to time, bringing detailed information concerning prices and the newest products. These representatives are always willing to answer questions. Many of these companies offer support in the area of education for members of the American Association of Medical Assistants.

Storing Medications

In storing medication, "a place for everything and everything in its place" is the rule. Many necessary forms, prescription blanks, and records must be kept. Commonly used medications must be rotated according to their expiration dates. The most practical way to store medications is to categorize them by their classification as in Table 20–1, page 625. Medications may also be stored alphabetically. Labeling shelves increases efficiency, as do pull-out shelves.

Complete Chapter 20, Unit 1 in the workbook to help you meet the objectives at the beginning of this unit and therefore achieve competency of this subject matter.

UNIT 2

Methods for Administering Medications

OBJECTIVES

Upon completion of this unit, the student will meet the following terminal performance objectives by verifying knowledge of the facts and principles presented through oral and written communication at a level deemed competent, and will demonstrate the specific behaviors as identified in the terminal performance objectives of the procedures, observing all aseptic and safety precautions in accordance with health care standards.

1. List and describe the various methods of medications.
2. Demonstrate how to instruct patients in the method of medication ordered by the physician.
3. Explain how to apply a transdermal patch medication properly.
4. Discuss precautions in applying a transdermal patch medication.
5. Identify each time and explain the importance of checking medications prior to administration.
6. Discuss patient education to females regarding vaginal medications.
7. List considerations regarding drug action in the body.
8. Spell out and define, using the glossary at the back of the text, all the words to know in this unit.

WORDS TO KNOW

BSA (body surface area)	parenteral
buccal	salve
douche	sublingual
infusion	suppository
interaction	tolerance
nomogram	topical
ointment	transdermal

Administering Medication

There are many methods of medicating patients, and even though you may not administer every type, you should know something about each one. You will also assist in the preparation of different types of medications for patients and in the instruction of patients in specific directions for taking medications. The methods of administering medications are: oral, including sublingual and buccal; by inhalation; topical, including transdermal; vaginal; rectal and urethral; and by injection.

When administering any medication to a patient you should follow a standard format checklist to make certain that you are accurate and efficient. Develop the habit of using the checklist that follows to help you to achieve this standard of quality patient care. Before you administer the medication always be sure that you have the correct:

1. Patient
2. Medication
3. Dose/amount
4. Route/method
5. Technique
6. Time/schedule

It is common practice, and sound advice, when giving any medications to follow these precautions:

- Compare the medication order to the container when taking the container from storage
- Compare the medication order to the container when preparing the medication
- Compare the medication order to the container before administering the medication
- Compare the medication order to the container when returning the container to storage

This practice ensures accuracy in giving any medication.

If there is ever a chance that a medication was given in error, the necessary action must be taken immediately. Admitting such a mistake is not a pleasant experience, but it is necessary for the well-being of the patient. Reporting the error to the physician at once is essential.

Properly instructing the patient about how a medication should be taken is extremely important. If the patient does not understand the directions or the need for carrying out the physician's orders, then the medication will be virtually useless and may be dangerous, as the patient may not take it, or may take it incorrectly. Patients who are given medication that may induce drowsiness should be made aware of the dangers of driving or operating machinery while taking the medication. Even though the physician may give these instructions to patients, you should make sure the information is clearly understood before the patient leaves the office. You should be mindful of recording all medications given to patients, including sample packages. On the patient's chart, record the name of the medication, the strength, directions for use, and how many dispensed. Writing the directions for use for the patient will eliminate possible confusion for the patient. Package inserts enclosed with all medication contain the necessary information. This same information is found in the PDR. If there is any further question, the PDR should be consulted.

It may seem unlikely that one would make a mistake and administer a medication to a patient in error. However, care must be taken in identifying the patient for whom the medication is intended before it is administered or this could be possible. Many offices and clinics care for so many patients in the course of the daily schedule, with multiple family members being seen in the same treatment room for example, that if particular attention is not given, an error could result.

Reading the label of the ordered medication and the amount or dose when you obtain it from storage, as you prepare it, just before you administer it, and finally again, after you have administered it, will safeguard you from committing an error. If an error is made, necessary steps must be taken immediately in reporting it to the doctor for emergency care to be given if necessary.

The route or method of administering medication is equally important. Carefully reading the order provides instruction in how the physician wants the medication to be administered, i.e., topical—applying a cream or other preparation to the skin; by injection—intramuscular, subcutaneous, intradermal; transdermal—skin patch; or orally—buccal or sublingual. All of these are certainly very different.

Technique refers to how the method is administered, i.e., skill in giving the different types of injections; the manner in which you apply a topical preparation; or the way in which you administer an inhalation treatment to a patient.

Attention must be given to time and schedule in administering medicines. For example, immunizations must be given within a certain time frame for maximum effectiveness in the immunity process of the patient. What time a medication is administered is also important to the well-being of the patient. For instance, some medicines should not be taken when the stomach is full, and some should not be taken when the stomach is empty. Checking the time the patient has eaten last is important. Time also should remind you to check the expiration date of the medication to be sure of its quality strength.

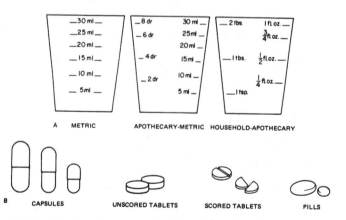

FIGURE 20–4 Means of administering oral medication: (a). Medicine cups. (b). Capsules, tablets (unscored and scored), and pills

PROCEDURE

Obtain and Administer Oral Medication

PURPOSE: To obtain the ordered oral medication and administer it to the patient.

EQUIPMENT: Ordered oral medication (for practice, any tiny candies), medicine cup (disposable), disposable paper cup filled with water, medicine tray

TERMINAL PERFORMANCE OBJECTIVE: Provided with all necessary equipment/supplies, and using other students as patients, the student will demonstrate the steps required to obtain the ordered oral medication and administer it to the patient. The instructor will observe each step.

1. Obtain medication from storage area and read label carefully, comparing it to order. **Key Point: Work in a well-lighted area and avoid distractions.**
2. Calculate dosage if necessary and wash hands.
3. Take bottle cap off and place inside up on counter. **Key Point: Do not touch inside of bottle or cap or it will be contaminated.** Read label of medication container.
4. If pill or capsule form, pour desired amount into cap. Then pour medication into medicine cup. If liquid medicine, pour directly into medicine cup to calibrated line of ordered amount. **Key Point: Hold measuring cup at eye level with thumbnail placed at desired amount, Figure 20–5.** Syrup or liquid medications may also be given in disposable plastic measuring spoons. Liquids should be poured from the opposite side of the bottle's label to prevent the contents from dripping and discoloring the label.
5. Place medication container on tray and ordered dose in medicine cup. Place cup of water on tray for patient to take with medicine. Read label of container again.
6. Take medication tray to patient and confirm identification. Explain procedure.
7. Give patient medication and offer cup of water. Observe patient taking medicine and report any reaction or problem to physician.
8. Discard disposables and return medication container and tray to proper storage area. **Key Point: Read label of medication container again.**
9. Record information on patient's chart and initial.

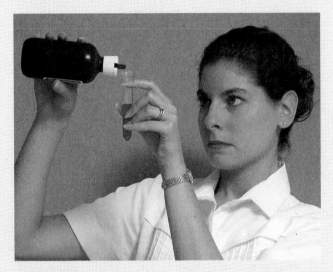

FIGURE 20–5 Pour liquids at eye level with thumbnail held at point of amount needed.

Most oral medications are intended for absorption in the small intestine. The remaining methods are **parenteral,** or intended for absorption outside the digestive system.

Oral Administration

One of the most common methods of administering medications is the oral method. These medicines are in the form of pills, tablets, capsules, lozenges, syrups, sprays, and other liquids, which are swallowed, Figure 20–4. These medications are usually given to patients as prescriptions, although they may be administered in the office. For example, an analgesic may be given to a patient while in the office for relief of pain. Sabin (immunization against polio) is given orally to infants and children in the medical office by the physicians or the medical assistant. Medicine which is given or sold to patients to be taken home is said to be dispensed.

Oral medications have many advantages. An obvious one is their convenience. If a patient exhibits an intolerance or an adverse reaction to an oral medication, the remedy may be to just discontinue the medicine. The reaction to a single oral dose would certainly be much less dangerous than if the medication were given by injection. They are also easily stored and are economical for the medical practice and the patient.

Sublingual and Buccal. This sublingual method of administering medication involves placing the medication, usually tiny tablets, under the tongue. This introduces the medication immediately into the bloodstream. An example is nitroglycerine, for patients who suffer from angina. Tiny tablets are also administered by the buccal method, or placed in the mouth between the gum and the cheek. The medication is then absorbed through the mucous membranes. Patients should avoid eating, drinking, or chewing while the medication is in place. Instruct patients how to use these medications properly because sublingual and buccal medications should not be swallowed whole or their intended action would be delayed and ineffective.

Inhalation Administration

Medications given to patients by the inhalation method are in the form of gases, sprays, fluids, or powders to be mixed with liquid and used with equipment that will produce a mist or vapor. These are breathed into the respiratory tract. The patient usually self-administers the medication at home. After being instructed properly, the patient should feel comfortable in doing so. Manufacturers prepare instruction material on the proper use and care of their equipment. You should keep a file of these for the most commonly prescribed medications.

A form of inhalation medication that should be kept in every medical practice is oxygen. Although it isn't given often in most practices, it should be available for emergency use. Many companies offer instruction in the use and care of such equipment. They also offer various home oxygen treatment programs for patients who need this treatment daily. Setting aside a time when this service could benefit the entire medical staff would be advantageous.

Topical Administration

Topical medications are used in treating diseases or disorders of the skin by application to the skin in some form. They come in sprays, lotions, creams, **ointments,** paints, **salves,** wet dressings, and adhesive patches.

Topical medications must be applied as instructed for maximum effect. For example a patient should apply a medication to reduce itching with gentle single strokes. If the medication is rubbed into the skin vigorously, the itching will increase from the heat produced from the friction, which increases the circulation.

The patch type of medication, commonly called the *transdermal patch,* is a convenient method of choice for medicating patients for many medical conditions. It is painless, and ensures patient compliance. The patch is placed on the skin according to the directions of the pharmaceutical company. It then releases minute dosages of the desired medicine into the patient's tissues, which carry it into the circulatory system. The patient receives timed-release treatment without worrying about when to take medication. Patients return as scheduled or as indicated to have the patch changed or removed. The effectiveness of the medication is then evaluated. Patients are also instructed to apply the transdermal patch themselves. When applying the transdermal patch, one must be extremely careful when handling it to avoid getting

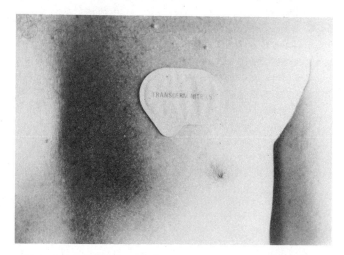

FIGURE 20–6 (B) When applied to the skin, Transderm-Nitro® delivers nitroglycerin at a constant and predetermined rate through the skin directly into the bloodstream. One patch gives 24-hour protection against the pain of angina pectoris due to coronary artery disease. (Courtesy of CIBA-GEIGY)

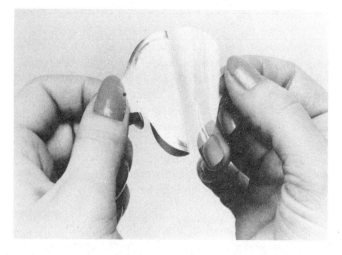

FIGURE 20–6 (A) The Transderm-Nitro® skin patch is applied once a day. It helps prevent the pain of angina by delivering a steady level of nitroglycerin to the body. The patch provides medication without interfering in a patient's daily activities. (Courtesy of CIBA-GEIGY)

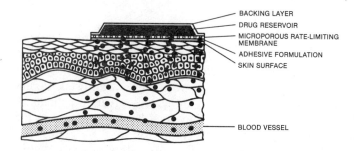

FIGURE 20–6 (C) The Transderm-Nitro® is a multilayer unit. It consists of a backing layer, a reservoir of nitroglycerin, a rate-controlling membrane, and an adhesive layer which has a priming dose of nitroglycerin. (Courtesy of CIBA-GEIGY)

CAUTIONS

If your physician has prescribed ''under-the-tongue'' nitroglycerin tablets in addition to Nitro-Dur II, you should sit down before taking the ''under-the-tongue'' tablet. If dizziness should occur, notify your physician. This may be an indication that the ''under-the-tongue'' tablet dosage needs to be reduced.

POSSIBLE SIDE EFFECTS

The most common side effect experienced by people taking nitroglycerin is headache. Your physician may tell you to take a mild analgesic to relieve the headache.

Some people may experience dizziness. This is due to a slight decrease in blood pressure, which is usually experienced when a person changes position, from lying flat to sitting upright or from sitting to standing. If this occurs, sit down until the dizziness stops, then notify your physician. He may wish to reduce your Nitro-Dur II dosage.

In some people, nitroglycerin preparations may cause the skin to feel flushed or the heart to beat faster. If this should occur, notify your physician; again, he may wish to change your Nitro-Dur II dosage.

Nitro-Dur II is a unique drug that depends on direct contact with the skin to work. For this reason, the skin should be reasonably hair-free, clean and dry.

INSTRUCTIONS FOR USE
PLACEMENT AREA

☐ Select a reasonably hair-free application site. **Avoid** extremities below the knee or elbow, skin folds, scar tissue, burned or irritated areas.

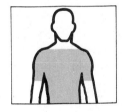

APPLICATION

☐ Wash hands before applying.

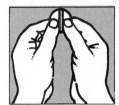

☐ Hold the unit with brown lines facing you, in an up and down position.

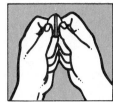

☐ Bend the sides of unit away from you.

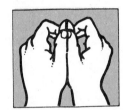

☐ Then bend the sides toward you, until the clear plastic backing ''snaps'' down the middle.

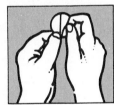

☐ Peel off both halves of the clear plastic.

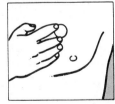

☐ Apply the sticky side of the unit to the selected body site.

☐ Wash hands to remove any drug.

☐ It is important to use a different application site every day.

REMOVAL

☐ Gently lift unit and slowly peel away from skin.
☐ Wash skin area with soap and water. Towel dry. Wash hands.

SKIN CARE

1. After you remove Nitro-Dur II, your skin may feel warm and appear red. This is normal. The redness will disappear in a short time. If the area feels dry, you may apply a soothing lotion.
2. Any redness or rash that does not disappear should be called to your physician's attention.

OTHER INFORMATION

1. Allow Nitro-Dur II to stay in place for 24 hours unless otherwise instructed by your physician.
2. Showering is permitted with Nitro-Dur II in place.
3. Apply your Nitro-Dur II the same time every day, preferably before going to bed. This allows it to adhere firmly to your skin while you are sleeping, when body movement is minimal.
4. Nitro-Dur II should be kept out of reach of children and pets.
5. Store at controlled room temperature—15-30° C (59-86° F). Do not refrigerate.
6. Nitro-Dur II is boxed so that you have a 30-day supply. Be sure to check your supply periodically. Before it runs low, you should visit your pharmacist for a refill or ask your physician to renew your Nitro-Dur II prescription.
7. It is important that you do not miss a day of your Nitro-Dur II therapy. If your schedule needs to be changed, your physician will give you specific instructions.
8. Nitro-Dur II has been prescribed for you. Do not give your medication to anyone else.
9. Nitro-Dur II is for prevention of angina; not for treatment of an acute anginal attack.
10. Notify physician if angina attacks change for the worse.

If you have any questions about Nitro-Dur II, ask your physician or pharmacist.

FIGURE 20–7 Transdermal infusion system for the administration of nitroglycerin (Courtesy of Key Pharmaceuticals)

the medication on the fingers. A priming dose of medication is in the adhesive edge of the patch. The medication intended for the patient can also be absorbed by the person who applies it. If one is not careful to wash the hands with soap and water immediately after application of the transdermal medicating patch, the effects could be undesirable or even dangerous to the one who applied it. Traces could also be transferred to another person, which could also present problems. Wearing disposable gloves when applying transdermal patches is a suggested practice, especially when a potential adverse reaction is possible for the person who applies the patch.

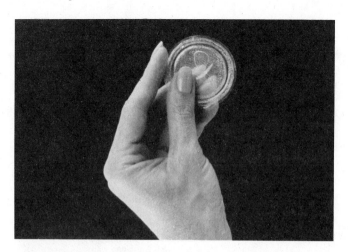

FIGURE 20–8 (A) Estraderm®, a low-dose estrogen skin patch. Less than 2 inches in diameter, the wafer-thin patch contains 17-ß estradiol, which is identical to the estrogen produced naturally before menopause. The patch releases small amounts of medication at a relatively constant and controlled rate through the skin directly into the bloodstream. It relieves menopausal symptoms such as hot flashes, night sweats, and vaginal dryness. The patch is worn on a dry, non-oily part of the trunk of the body. (Courtesy of CIBA-GEIGY)

1. A SEALED BACKING THAT HOLDS THE DRUG IN THE SYSTEM.
2. A RESERVOIR CONTAINING ESTRADIOL.
3. A MEMBRANE THAT CONTROLS THE RELEASE OF ESTRADIOL.
4. A NON-ALLERGENIC ADHESIVE THAT KEEPS THE PATCH ON THE SKIN.
5. A PROTECTIVE PEEL STRIP.

FIGURE 20–8 (B) The Estraderm® skin patch is a multilayered unit. (Courtesy of CIBA-GEIGY)

Several commonly prescribed medications are available as transdermal systems. Figure 20–6, page 636, shows the once-a-day Transderm-Nitro® patch to help control the pain of angina. The instructions for use of another transdermal nitroglycerin infusing system are shown in Figure 20–7, page 637. Figure 20–8 shows a skin patch containing a low dosage of estradiol, a form of the hormone estrogen. The medication is used to relieve menopausal symptoms such as hot flashes, night sweats, and vaginal dryness. Figure 20–9 shows the instructions for the use of a transdermal system of administering scopolamine for the prevention of nausea and vomiting due to motion sickness. You should remind patients that medications to prevent motion sickness should be taken or applied anywhere from 30 minutes to 4 hours before travel for effectiveness.

Transdermal patches containing time-released amounts of nicotine have become popular as a means of quitting the cigarette habit. These are intended to curb the craving for smoking. Patients may obtain a prescription for the patches, which supply decreasing doses of nicotine over a 3-month period. The patch is changed every 24 hours. They are relatively expensive, but the initial expense is a sound investment in the long run for good health.

Vaginal Administration

Vaginal medications are applied as creams, **suppositories,** tablets, **douches,** foams, ointments, tampons, sprays, and salves, Figure 20–10.

PATIENT EDUCATION

You must make sure the patient understands the proper method of self-administration of vaginal medications, because many women are embarrassed about asking. For example, many women may not know that vaginal medications should be used during the menstrual flow, as this is an ideal time for growth of microorganisms.

Vaginal medications may seem undesirable because they tend to be messy. Since most vaginal medications are ordered for use at bedtime, better patient compliance is gained. You may also advise patients to use disposable panty liners or, with the advice of the physician, to insert a tampon to hold the medication in the vaginal canal.

Stress to female patients the importance of completing the prescribed treatment plan which the doctor has ordered. Often patients stop using a medication after a few doses or a few days because the symptoms seem to clear up. Unless all of the prescribed medication is used, the condition or problem could return. Many self-medications are available for women with gynecological symptoms. You should urge patients to seek advice from the physician if their complaints do not improve with the use of these OTC products as they may have a serious condition.

You may also want to instruct female patients in good personal hygiene. Advertising has made women believe that they should be clean "inside and out." But frequent douching or bathing with perfumed soaps or other toilet articles may leave the body open to infection by washing the natural body secretions away or irritating the delicate vaginal tissues. Patients should be made aware that vaginal sprays and douches are really not necessary. Daily showering or bathing should be sufficient. Excessive odor and vaginal discharge are symptoms of infection and should be brought to the attention of the physician.

How to Use Transderm Scōp

Transderm Scōp may be kept at room temperature until you are ready to use it.

1. Plan to apply one Transderm Scōp disc at least 4 hours before you need it. **Wear only one disc at any time.**
2. Select a hairless area of skin behind one ear, taking care to avoid any cuts or irritations. Wipe the area with a clean, dry tissue.
3. Peel the package open and remove the disc (Figure 1).
4. Remove the clear plastic six-sided backing from the round system. Try not to touch the adhesive surface on the disc with your hands (Figure 2).
5. Firmly apply the adhesive surface (metallic side) to the dry area of skin behind the ear so that the tan-colored side is showing (Figure 3). Make good contact, especially around the edge. Once you have placed the disc behind your ear, do not move it for as long as you want to use it (up to 3 days).
6. *Important:* **After the disc is in place, be sure to wash your hands thoroughly with soap and water to remove any scopolamine. If this drug were to contact your eyes, it could cause temporary blurring of vision and dilation (widening) of the pupils**

(the dark circles in the center of your eyes). This is not serious, and your pupils should return to normal.
7. Remove the disc after 3 days and throw it away. (You may remove it sooner if you are no longer concerned about motion sickness.) After removing the disc, be sure to wash your hands and the area behind your ear thoroughly with soap and water.
8. If you wish to control nausea for longer than 3 days, *remove* the first disc after 3 days and place a new one *behind the other ear,* repeating instructions 2 to 7.
9. Keep the disc dry, if possible, to prevent it from falling off. Limited contact with water, however, as in bathing or swimming, will not affect the system. In the unlikely event that the disc falls off, throw it away and put a new one behind the other ear.

This leaflet presents a summary of information about Transderm Scōp. If you would like more information or if you have any questions, ask your doctor or pharmacist. A more technical leaflet is available, written for your doctor. If you would like to read the leaflet, ask your pharmacist to show you a copy. You may need the help of your doctor or pharmacist to understand some of the information.

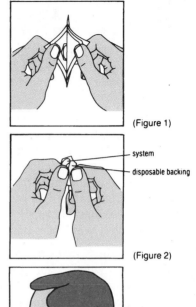

(Figure 1)

system

disposable backing

(Figure 2)

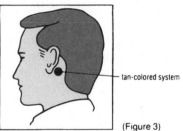

tan-colored system

(Figure 3)

FIGURE 20–9 Transderm® Scōp is a prescription transdermal system that administers scopolamine for the prevention of nausea and vomiting associated with motion sickness. The disc is placed behind the ear several hours before traveling and prevents symptoms for up to 3 days. (Courtesy of CIBA-GEIGY)

Considerations of Drug Action ....

Several considerations may affect how the body responds to a drug. These are age, weight, and body surface area (BSA), method of administration, tolerance, allergies, time, and interaction. Pediatric and geriatric patients, and some individuals, usually require a smaller dose than an average adult. To achieve a specific blood level of a medication, the dosage must be calculated according to the patient's weight. Special medications, such as chemotherapy drugs, are determined by the

BSA, which is derived by plotting the patient's height and weight on a **nomogram.** The different methods of administering medications and the rate at which the body uses them varies. Medications given by injection are circulated in the bloodstream rapidly; transdermal patch infusion systems deliver small amounts of medication in a sustained time-release manner; oral medicines take considerable time before they are absorbed by the small intestines, and so on for each of the methods. If a patient has to take a particular medication for a long period of time, a tolerance may develop. An increase in the amount, or a change in medicine, may be necessary for the desired effect to take place. An allergy to a medication may occur at any time in an individual. Careful attention must be given to the medical history and to the patient's responses during the interview. Further, the medical assistant must be alert to notice any notations in red ink signifying allergies. Many patients take several medications daily. Helping the patient determine what to take medicine with and when to take it will encourage the desired result.

Complete Chapter 20, Unit 2 in the workbook to help you meet the objectives at the beginning of this unit and therefore achieve competency of this subject matter.

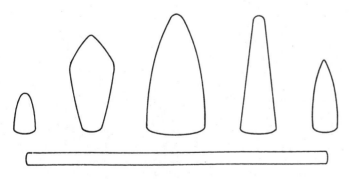

FIGURE 20–10 Suppositories: urethral, vaginal, and rectal

U N I T   3

Injections and Immunizations

OBJECTIVES

Upon completion of this unit the student will meet the following terminal performance objectives by verifying knowledge of the facts and principles presented through oral and written communication at a level deemed competent, and will demonstrate the specific behaviors as identified in the terminal performance objectives of the procedures, observing all aseptic and safety precautions in accordance with health care standards.

1. Correctly identify the parts of a syringe and needle.
2. Name the tissue layers and sites of injection for intradermal, intramuscular, and subcutaneous injections.
3. Demonstrate how to administer intradermal, intramuscular, and subcutaneous injections properly.
4. Demonstrate how to reassure an apprehensive patient in preparation for an injection.
5. Demonstrate how to recap a needle properly after filling a syringe from a vial or an ampule.
6. Demonstrate the proper way to discard a used needle and syringe.
7. List and explain the immunization schedule for normal infants and children and adults.
8. Explain the importance of informing patients, or the responsible party for a minor, verbally and in writing, of both the benefits and the risks of immunizations before they are administered.
9. Discuss the importance of patient education regarding medications.
10. Demonstrate how to instruct patients in self-administration of insulin injections.
11. Identify the various sites for administering insulin injections.
12. Spell and define, using the glossary at the back of the text, all the words to know in this unit.

WORDS TO KNOW

ampule	haemophilus	measles
antitoxin	hepatitis B	paroxysmal
attenuated	HIB/Hib	stage
anaphylactic	immunization	pertussis
booster	incubation	photophobia
catarrhal stage	influenza	polio
cholera	insulin	retardation
debridement	intradermal	rubella
decline stage	intramuscular	rubeola
diphtheria	intravenous	risk
disciplinary	lethal	series
epiglottis	mumps	sensitivity
flu	meningitis	subcutaneous
tetanus	trimester	vial
toxin	typhoid	Z-tract
toxoid	vaccine	

Injections

You will be helping to prepare and possibly to administer medications in the form of injections. Since this method of medication introduces the substance directly into the tissues, where it quickly enters the patient's bloodstream, extreme caution must be practiced. The proper technique must be learned under supervision. Latex gloves should be worn to administer an injection. Medication should only be given to patients when a physician is available nearby should the patient exhibit any adverse reaction. There is always a possibility of anaphylactic shock. Refer to Chapter 18, Unit 1 for symptoms of anaphylactic shock. In the event that this situation occurs, the physician should be notified to administer the immediate treatment of injecting epinephrine just above the initial injection site. Following the injection into the muscle or subcutaneous tissue, the area should be massaged. This is to aid in speeding the distribution of the epinephrine into the circulatory system as fast as possible. You should keep taking the patient's vital signs until the patient is stable. Provisions should always be made for emergency situations. Even though the patient's past history reveals no sensitivity to a particular drug, there is no guarantee of what the next dose may do.

The term *hypodermic* simply means under the skin. You must become familiar with the parts of the syringe and needle as well as proficient in handling them. Figure 20–11 pictures a needle and syringe with labeled parts. Practice with different types of syringes and needles; filling the syringe with varying amounts of sterile water from a vial and ampule will give you confidence. Use an orange to practice inserting different needle lengths at different angles of injection, Figure 20–12. This should

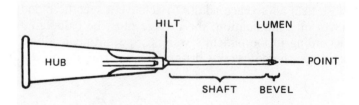
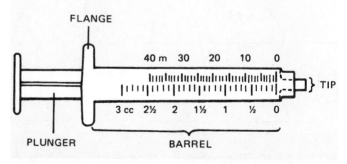

FIGURE 20–11   A hypodermic needle and 3-cc syringe

General Guidelines for Teaching Patients about Medications

The following are general considerations patients need to know about taking prescribed medication:

1. Take only the medicine that has been prescribed by the physician for you.
2. Never share your medicine with anyone else, not even family members.
3. Take your prescribed medication when and only as directed, not more or less, to maintain proper blood level for its desired effect in your treatment.
4. Keep *all* medicines (or any chemicals) out of the reach of children.
5. Phone the physician's office immediately if you experience any reaction (regardless of how minor) to any medication or immunization.
6. Report any OTC (over-the-counter) or home remedy medication that you are taking to the physician.
7. Eat a well-balanced diet and include plenty of fluids while taking your medication. (Avoid foods/beverages that you have been instructed to stay away from because they may interfere with the action of the medicine).
8. Refrain from alcoholic beverages or any other drugs (both OTC and home remedy-type) that are not prescribed by the physician while you are taking prescribed medication to avoid dangerous side effects.
9. Women should report to the physician if they are pregnant, plan to become pregnant, or are nursing mothers before taking any medication.
10. Never save some of your prescription for a later date (i.e., antibiotics, take only as directed).
11. Throw old medicines away—flush down the toilet—after they are 6 months old.
12. Direct questions that patients have regarding diet, activity, dosage, or any concern about their medications to the physician's attention immediately.
13. To avoid confusion and gain compliance, explain to patients that generic products and brand name products are the same.
14. Caution patients about taking medications that could cause them to become sleepy, interfere with their concentration, or affect their ability to operate machinery or drive.

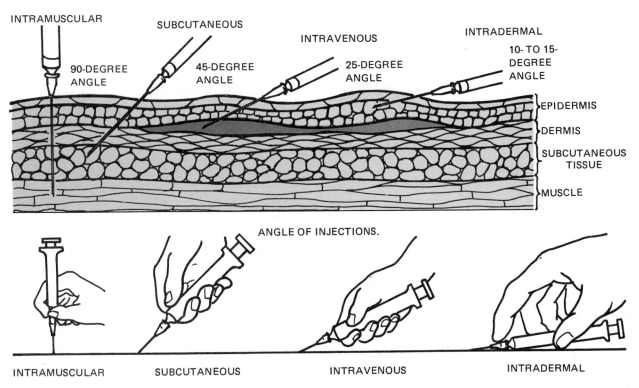

ANGLE OF INSERTION FOR PARENTERAL INJECTIONS.

ANGLE OF INJECTIONS.

FIGURE 20–12 Angle of injections

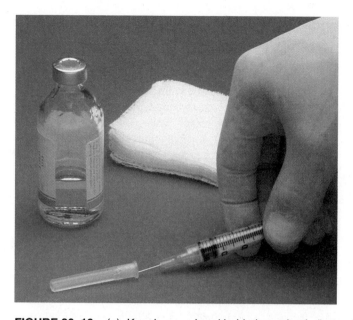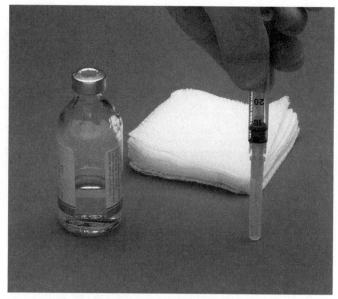

FIGURE 20–13 (a). Keeping one hand behind your back, "scoop" the cap onto the needle carefully so it does not become contaminated. (b). Secure the cap onto the hub of the syringe by pressing the tip against a hard surface.

be done under supervision for instruction, practice, evaluation, and/or correction in developing proper technique. While becoming proficient in handling the syringe and needle confidently, and thereafter, one must use caution to avoid dangerous needle sticks. It is recommended that to prevent injuries needles *never* be recapped. Used needles and syringes should be discarded intact in the biohazardous sharps waste container. Even though you are strongly urged to never recap needles, in reality it may be necessary in certain circumstances to do so. For your safety you should recap a needle by placing your nondominant hand behind your back, and holding the syringe and needle intact "scoop" the cap onto the needle, Figure 20–13. Keeping your other hand behind you will lessen the chance of being tempted to use it to recap the needle, the point at which most needle sticks occur. Some needle and syringe units have a shield that locks into place over the used needle to prevent injury to the user.

Injectible medications also come in single-dose, prefilled, disposable sterile syringes and cartridges. This method guarantees an accurate dosage and is also convenient and time-saving. The single-dose units are assembled by inserting the cartridge into a reusable injector as illustrated in Figure 20–14.

In injecting medications, technique is extremely important. If injections are given carelessly, injury to the nerves, blood vessels, and tissues can occur, as can infection. These can lead to legal action. When proper technique is used, however, giving medications by injection can be a minimally painful experience for the patient.

You can help relieve the patient's anxiety by explaining the procedure. Being honest with patients is most important. In the case of children's immunizations, for example, it is far better to explain that the injection will hurt for a minute, than to say it won't. You may give the child a simplified explanation of the disease for which the immuniza-

tion is meant. This may help the child understand how it is really better in the long run to hurt for a minute rather than suffer the dreaded disease. If the child shows extreme apprehension, it is advisable to have assistance in restraining the child before proceeding with the injection. Instructing parents in how they can explain injections to their children can be helpful. Many parents use injections as **disciplinary** threats. This is not an acceptable practice. It not only creates anxiety for the child but makes the work of the health care team more difficult. Some pharmaceutical companies provide badges of courage or other awards to pediatric patients who display bravery in receiving their immunization injections. This gives the child a sense of pride in good behavior and makes future visits much easier for all concerned.

Authorization forms should be in order before immunizations are administered to minors. You should allow sufficient time for parents (or those responsible for the child) to read the information regarding the vaccine and have all questions answered before obtaining the authorization signature. This form must be filed in the patient's chart.

The site to be injected should be free from restricting clothing. Patients should be asked to remove these items of clothing while the medication is being prepared.

Follow correct gloving procedure before you begin to administer the injection. Proper preparation of the skin at the site of injection is necessary before and after injecting the medication, since microorganisms can enter the body through a break in the skin. Alcohol is the antiseptic usually used, because it is least irritating to the skin and is economical.

Proper disposal of used needles and syringes is also of vital importance in preventing possible accidents to the medical and custodial staff of the **facility** and avoiding transmission of disease. Nondisposable needles and syringes must be properly sanitized and autoclaved

TUBEX® Injector

NOTE: The TUBEX® Injector is reusable: do not discard.
DIRECTIONS FOR USE:

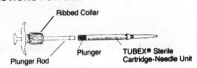

Ribbed Collar
Plunger Rod
Plunger
TUBEX® Sterile Cartridge-Needle Unit

To load a TUBEX® Sterile Cartridge-Needle Unit into the TUBEX® Injector

CLOSE   OPEN

1. Turn the ribbed collar to the "OPEN" position until it stops.

2. Hold the Injector with the open end up and fully insert the TUBEX® Sterile Cartridge-Needle Unit.

CLOSE

Firmly tighten the ribbed collar in the direction of the "CLOSE" arrow.

3. Thread the plunger rod into the plunger of the TUBEX® Sterile Cartridge-Needle Unit until slight resistance is felt.

The Injector is now ready for use in the usual manner.

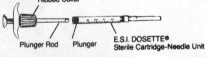

Ribbed Collar
Plunger Rod   Plunger
E.S.I. DOSETTE® Sterile Cartridge-Needle Unit

To load an E.S.I. DOSETTE® Sterile Cartridge-Needle Unit into the TUBEX® Injector

CLOSE   OPEN

1. Turn the ribbed collar to the "OPEN" position until it stops.

2. Hold the Injector with the open end up and fully insert the E.S.I. DOSETTE® Sterile Cartridge-Needle Unit.

CLOSE

Firmly tighten the ribbed collar in the direction of the "CLOSE" arrow.

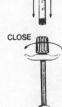

3. Thread the plunger rod into the plunger of the E.S.I. DOSETTE® Sterile Cartridge-Needle Unit until slight resistance is felt.

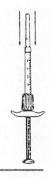

4. Engage the needle-cap assembly by pulling the cap down over the silver cartridge hub. The needle is fully engaged when the silver hub is completely covered.

The Injector is now ready for use in the usual manner.

To administer
Method of administration is the same as with conventional syringe. Remove needle cover by grasping it securely; twist and pull. Introduce needle into patient, aspirate by pulling back slightly on the plunger, and inject.

To remove the empty TUBEX® or DOSETTE® Cartridge-Needle Unit and dispose into a vertical needle disposal container

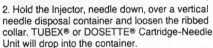

1. Do not recap the needle. Disengage the plunger rod.

2. Hold the Injector, needle down, over a vertical needle disposal container and loosen the ribbed collar. TUBEX® or DOSETTE® Cartridge-Needle Unit will drop into the container.

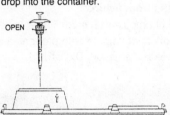
OPEN

3. Discard the needle cover.

To remove the empty TUBEX® or DOSETTE® Cartridge-Needle Unit and dispose into a horizontal (mailbox) needle disposal container

1. Do not recap the needle. Disengage the plunger rod.

2. Open the horizontal (mailbox) needle disposal container. Insert TUBEX® or DOSETTE® Cartridge-Needle Unit, needle pointing down, halfway into container. Close the container lid on cartridge. Loosen ribbed collar; TUBEX® or DOSETTE® Cartridge-Needle Unit will drop into the container.

3. Discard the needle cover.

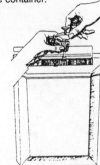

The TUBEX® Injector is reusable and should not be discarded.

Used TUBEX® or DOSETTE® Cartridge-Needle Units should not be employed for successive injections or as multiple-dose containers. They are intended to be used only once and discarded.

NOTE: Any graduated markings on TUBEX® or DOSETTE® Sterile Cartridge-Needle Units are to be used only as a guide in mixing, withdrawing, or administering measured doses.

Wyeth-Ayerst does not recommend and will not accept responsibility for the use of any cartridge-needle units other than TUBEX® or E.S.I. DOSETTE® Cartridge-Needle Units in the TUBEX® Injector.

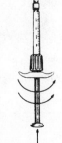

FIGURE 20–14   Directions for using the TUBEX "Hands-Off" injector. Note that latex gloves should be worn when administering any injection. (Courtesy of Wyeth-Ayerst Laboratories)

Withdraw Medication from Ampule

PURPOSE: To withdraw an ordered amount of medication into a syringe from an ampule.

EQUIPMENT: Ampule of medication (sterile water for injection), medication tray, sterile gauze square, sterile needle and syringe

TERMINAL PERFORMANCE OBJECTIVE: Provided with all necessary equipment/supplies, the student will demonstrate each of the steps required to withdraw medication (sterile water for instructional purposes) from an ampule; the procedure will be repeated three times, each time withdrawing a specific quantity of fluid as predetermined by the instructor.

1. Place sterile gauze square over middle of ampule and hold between thumb and index finger of one hand, Figure 20–15. **Key Point: Sterile gauze will keep any fragments of glass from flying.**
2. Flick pointed end of ampule with index finger to release medication into bottom of ampule before opening.
3. Grasp tip of ampule and snap off. Discard tip.

4. Make sure that syringe and needle are secured by turning barrel to right while holding needle guard. Remove guard.
5. Expel air from syringe by pushing down on plunger. Insert tip of needle into solution while holding ampule in upright position. **Key Point: Do not touch rim of ampule to maintain sterile technique.**
6. Draw back plunger quickly and steadily to fill syringe with medication, Figure 20–16. **Key Point: Keep needle point below meniscus level of liquid to avoid air bubbles entering syringe.** (Note: If air bubbles do enter, turn syringe pointing up and gently tap the barrel to free the bubbles to the top. Gently push plunger up to release the air bubbles.)
7. Replace needle guard by gently scooping it onto the needle to maintain sterility and safety. Place filled syringe on medication tray.
8. Discard ampule and gauze in proper receptacle.

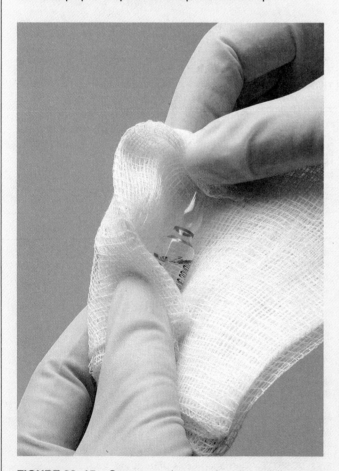

FIGURE 20–15   Snap open the ampule using sterile gauze for protection from possible flying glass fragments.

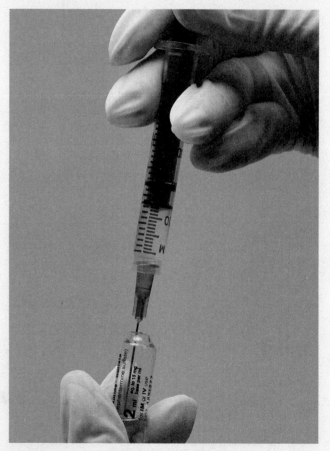

FIGURE 20–16   Keep needle point below meniscus of the liquid with ampule upright.

Withdraw Medication from Vial

PURPOSE: To withdraw an ordered amount of medication into a syringe from a vial.

EQUIPMENT: Multiple- and single-dose vials (sterile water for injection), alcohol-saturated cotton ball, sterile needle and syringe, medication tray

TERMINAL PERFORMANCE OBJECTIVE: Provided with all necessary equipment/supplies, the student will demonstrate each of the steps required in withdrawing medication (sterile water for instructional purposes) from multiple- and single-dose vials; the procedure will be repeated three times, each time withdrawing a specific quantity of fluid as predetermined by the instructor.

1. Calculate dosage if required and wash hands.
2. Use alcohol-saturated cotton ball to clean rubber-topped vial.
3. Secure needle onto syringe by holding needle guard and turning barrel of syringe to right.
4. Remove needle guard and pull back on plunger to fill syringe with same amount of air as medication that has been ordered. **Key Point: This prevents vacuum from forming in vial and thus makes it easier to withdraw solution.**
5. Hold syringe by barrel between thumb and fingers and with other hand hold vial upside down, Figure 20–17. Insert needle into rubber top and push plunger in, expelling air into vial.
6. Pull back on plunger so desired amount of medication will flow into syringe, keeping needle below level of solution to avoid air bubbles. Air takes up space where medication should be and dosage would not be correct if air remained. To release air bubbles if they appear, flick barrel of syringe with finger in quick, hard motion. They will be released into hub of syringe. Push plunger carefully to make sure they are out of needle. Invert vial and syringe before withdrawing needle from vial.
7. Let go of plunger. Hold barrel of syringe and pull needle out of vial, keeping syringe in vertical position. Check

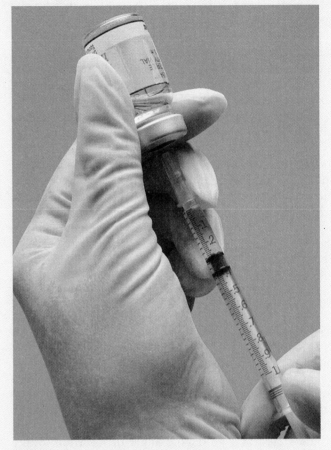

FIGURE 20–17 Hold the vial upside down at eye level and insert needle into the rubber-topped vial.

for air bubbles. Replace needle guard by carefully scooping it onto the needle to keep sterile and for safety.
8. Keep medication with loaded syringe on medication tray to ensure proper identification. Place alcohol-saturated cotton ball with syringe to administer medication.

---

before using again. Disposable syringes and needles should be used only once and discarded properly. Keep the needle guard on the needle until just before you are ready to administer the injection (again, this is a situation where recapping a needle may be necessary. Remember to scoop the cap onto the needle; do not use your other hand or you risk a needle stick, besides risking contamination of the needle before it is to be used for injecting the patient.) Afterward dispose of the entire syringe and needle intact in the biohazardous sharps container according to universal precautions recommenda-

tions. *Do not recap.* Remove latex gloves before handwashing.

Before you can become proficient in injecting medications, you must first learn to withdraw medications into the syringe accurately. Medications for injection are available in single-dose and multiple-dose ampules or vials.

Intradermal Injections

Intradermal injections are used in allergy and tuberculin testing. The intradermal injection is administered just under the surface of the skin with a fine-gauge needle, 26G or 27G. The needle is generally $\frac{3}{8}$ to $\frac{5}{8}$ inch in length, and the angle of the insertion into the skin 10 to 15 degrees, Figure 20–18. The sites for this type of injection are usually the anterior forearm and the mid back area. Proper positioning of patients is vital for the accuracy of results as well as for the patient's comfort. Intradermal injections themselves go very quickly, but the patient must be observed for 20 minutes or more after the administration. Make sure the patient's forearm is supported on the treatment table while sitting comfortably, or have the patient lie on the treatment table.

A small wheal should develop at the site of injection to give evidence that the medication is in the dermal layer of the skin. Very small amounts of medication, from 0.01 to 0.05 cc, are administered by this method. The patient should be watched carefully and any reaction reported to the physician at once. The speed of the reaction and the size of the wheal should be recorded. Most allergy testing is done under the direct supervision of the physician. In the event of a hypersensitive reaction, a preparation of epinephrine may be injected by order of the physician.

Subcutaneous Injections

Subcutaneous injections are used to administer small doses of medication, usually not more than 2.0 cc. The injection is most often given in the upper outer part of the arm (deltoid area), abdominal area, or upper thigh (midvastus lateralis area), Figure 20–20, page 648. The length of the needle ranges from $\frac{1}{2}$ to $\frac{5}{8}$ inch and the gauge from 25G to 27G. Subcutaneous injections are administered at a 45-degree angle of insertion. Many medications, including allergy injections, insulin, and immunizations are administered by the subcutaneous method. Refer to Chapter 18, Unit 1 for specific details in giving allergy injections. The patient should be asked to sit or lie on the treatment table for safety.

Intramuscular Injections

As the name suggests, **intramuscular** injections are made into muscle tissue. The most common sites for this method of injection are the deltoid (upper outer arm), gluteus medius (upper outer portion of the hip), ventrogluteal (lateral outside portion of the hip), and vastus lateralis (midportion of the thigh), Figures 20–21 and 20–22, page 649. Proper positioning of patients is important. For injections in the deltoid area, the patient should be sitting. If the site is the gluteus muscle, ask the patient to lie in prone position on the treatment table with the toes pointed inward, or to lean over the treatment table and stand on the non-injection-site leg. This will allow the muscle to relax and make the procedure much easier. For injection of the vastus lateralis site, the patient may be sitting or lying in the horizontal recumbent position.

The site of injection must be recorded so that injection sites can be rotated. This practice is necessary when patients receive injections routinely, to reduce the possibility of muscle tissue damage.

In the administration of IM injections, the needle is from 1 to 3 inches in length or longer, for it must penetrate many layers of tissue. The angle of injection is 90 degrees. IM injections are indicated when large doses of medication or irritating substances must be given. Dosage may vary from 0.5 to 3.0 ml. Medications given by IM method are absorbed quickly by the rich blood supply of the muscle tissue.

The gauge of the needle ranges between 18G and 23G to accommodate the density of the substance. In giving injections intramuscularly to pediatric patients, the gauge and length of the needle may be smaller.

For injecting substances that may be irritating or cause discoloration of the subcutaneous tissues, the **Z-tract** IM method is used. Tissue is displaced by holding it to the side of the injection site. Following injection of the medication, the tissue is moved back over the site blocking any residual substance. Using this technique prevents the irritating medication from following the path of the needle and leaking out into the tissues. After Z-tract IM administration, the injection site

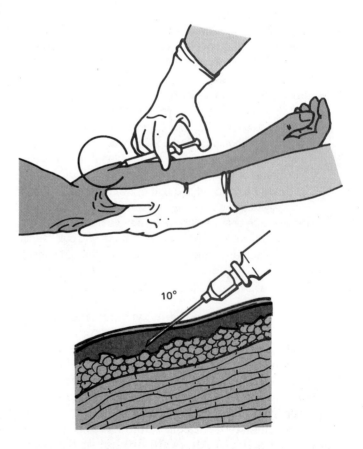

FIGURE 20–18   Intradermal injection

Administer Intradermal Injection

PURPOSE: To inject liquid solutions of 0.01 cc and 0.05 cc into the dermal layer of tissue for allergy and immunity testing of patients.

EQUIPMENT: Medication (sterile water for injection in vial/ampule), cotton balls, adhesive bandage (or hypoallergenic tape), sterile needle and syringe (needle is usually $\frac{3}{8}$ to $\frac{5}{8}$ inch length and 25G to 27G), medication tray, alcohol, patient's chart, pen, latex gloves

TERMINAL PERFORMANCE OBJECTIVE: Provided with all necessary equipment/supplies, the student will demonstrate each of the steps required in administering an intradermal injection; three injections will be administered to a latex training arm with the instructor observing each step. The dosage amount will be determined by the instructor each time.

1. Wash and glove hands and prepare syringe with ordered amount of medication. Replace needle guard by carefully scooping it onto the needle. **Key Point: Read label or medication and compare with order.**
2. Place medication tray near patient. Compare medication order with patient's chart, identify patient, and explain procedure.
3. Use alcohol-saturated cotton ball to clean injection site. **Key Point: Allow alcohol to air dry. Blowing on site to dry it out will cause contamination.**
4. Remove needle guard. Hold patient's skin taut between thumb and fingers to steady area to be injected. With other hand insert needle at a 10- to 15-degree angle of insertion and slowly expel medication from syringe by depressing plunger. **Key Point: Bevel of needle should be up to allow medication to accumulate in dermal layer of skin. Substance will cause a wheal to develop, distending skin.**
5. Remove needle quickly by angle of insertion and wipe site with alcohol-saturated cotton ball. **Key Point: Do not massage injection site.**

6. Observe patient and time reaction. Give patient instructions as ordered and answer questions. Determine if patient is allergic to adhesive before applying a bandage. Hypoallergenic tape is recommended.

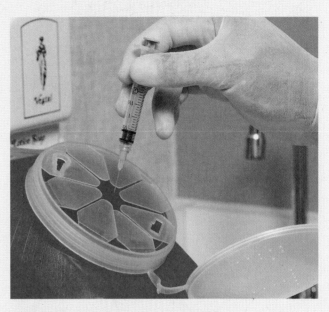

FIGURE 20–19 Discard entire used syringe and needle intact into sharps biohazardous container to prevent dangerous needle sticks.

7. Discard disposable items. (Place entire syringe and needle intact in the biohazardous sharps container according to universal precautions recommendations, Figure 20–19.) Wash and sterilize reusable items, remove gloves, and wash hands. Return medication and tray to proper storage area.
8. Record information and initial.

should *not* be massaged for this action would encourage the irritating substance to circulate into the subcutaneous tissues.

Intravenous Injections

The intravenous, or IV, method of injection is used by the physician usually in an emergency situation. You are not qualified to administer medications by this method but may prepare medications to be given intravenously. IV medications have an immediate effect on the patient for they are introduced directly into the bloodstream.

Needles are 1 to $1\frac{1}{2}$ inches in length and are usually 20G to 21G. Intravenous preparations vary in amount from a few ml to much larger doses, which are given by IV drip. The items needed are: needle and syringe, medication, tourniquet, alcohol-saturated cotton balls, adhesive bandage, and IV stand if necessary.

Usually you will draw up medication in the syringe for an intravenous injection. After filling the syringe, be sure to carefully recap the needle by the scoop method to avoid contaminating the needle. You then place the vial or ampule on the medication tray so that the physician can check to be certain it is correct. You may be asked to

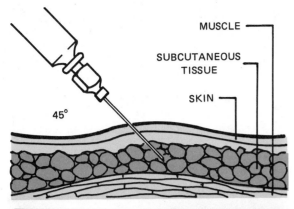

MUSCLE

SUBCUTANEOUS
TISSUE

SKIN

45°

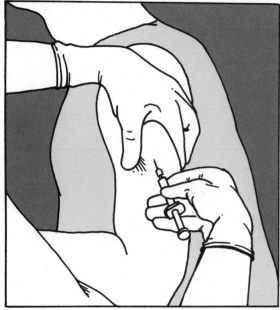

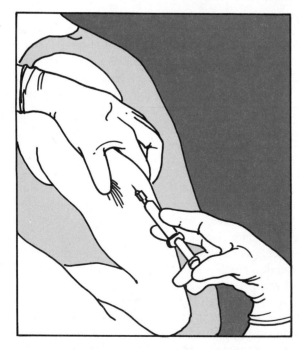

FIGURE 20–20 Subcutaneous injection

stay with the patient while waiting for the emergency squad or ambulance to transport the patient to the hospital. Observing the patient for signs of distress and reactions to the administered medication is an important responsibility. The physician must be notified immediately of any complications. All information should be recorded on the patient's chart.

The medical assistant is often the one who will give instruction to the diabetic patient in the technique of self-administration of daily **insulin** injections. You may be of great help in demonstrating the proper method of filling a syringe, preparing the injection site, and acquiring skill in injecting the insulin. Figure 20–23, pages 650–651, shows a step-by-step self-injection outline for the patient who needs daily insulin injection. Generally, the physician teaches the patient initially about diet, dosage, and the different types of insulin. You may be delegated to do follow-up patient education in this area. Since the insulin-dependent diabetic patient must administer this injection at home to him/herself at least once each day, you should instruct the patient to follow a pattern of rotation of injection sites, an example of which is shown in Figure 20–24, page 652. Explain to the patient to number each area of the body that is injected each time in the boxes in an alternating rotation

PATIENT EDUCATION

It is vitally important that all patients are instructed properly in safety regarding storage, use, and disposal of used syringes and needles. The medical assistant must stress that all of these materials must be kept safely out of reach of children. The potential danger of used and discarded needles must be stressed to avoid possible accidents. Remind patients not to remove the needle from the barrel of the syringe after use. Provide patients with sharps containers. Advise patients to keep these containers in a safe place at home and to return them to their medical facility when they return so the medical assistant can dispose of them properly. Having patients follow this safety procedure will help avoid unnecessary punctures to the skin. This is an especially important precaution for diabetics, who are prone to develop infections from such punctures.

It is also of vital importance to remind the diabetic patient to record daily blood glucose levels and ketone test results as well as the dosage amount of insulin. Impress on the patient how important it is to bring this record to the next appointment for the physician to review. This daily information, along with an interview, examination, and laboratory findings, helps the physician to make adjustments as necessary in the treatment plan for each patient.

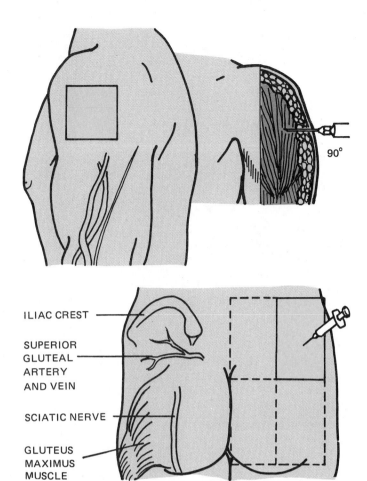

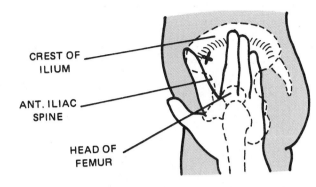

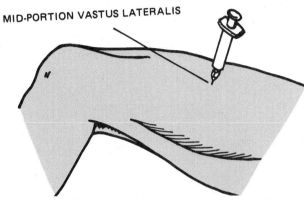

FIGURE 20–22   IM sites, ventrogluteal and vastus lateralis

FIGURE 20–21   IM sites, deltoid and gluteus medius

pattern. This method offers the patient the means to develop his/her own personal schedule. Printed patient education material for patients is available from most pharmaceutical companies to help patients gain an understanding of their diabetes. You may also want to

TABLE 20–6
Immunization Schedule of Normal Infants and Children

AGE	VACCINE(S)
2 months	DTP-1, Hib Haemophilus influenza - type B (diphtheria, tetanus **toxoid** and pertussis vaccines) OPV-1 (oral, attenuated poliovirus vaccine)
4 months	DTP-2, Hib OPV-2
6 months	DTP-3, Hib
15 months	MMR 1 (measles, mumps, rubella)
18 months	DTP-4, Hib OPV-3 (completes primary series)
4–6 years	DTP-5, MMR 2 OPV-4
14–16 years	Td (adult tetanus and diphtheria toxoid) (should be repeated every 10 years)

ADULT IMMUNIZATIONS	
Td	every 10 years (more often if severe/dirty injury or laceration)
Pneumovax	Once administered at age 60–65
Influenza A and B	Annually, age 65 and over
Hepatitis B	One series of 3 injections

Preparing and Injecting the Dose of Insulin

Preparing the Dose of Insulin

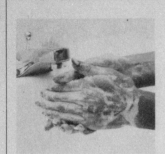

1

Wash your hands.

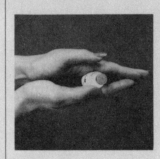

2

Gently roll the insulin bottle several times to mix the insulin. Be sure it is completely mixed. Do not shake bottle. Flip off the colored protective cap on the bottle, but **do not** remove the rubber stopper.

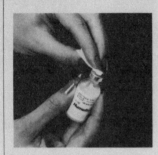

3

Wipe top of bottle with alcohol swab.

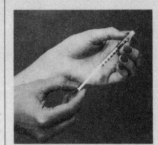

4

Remove the needle cover. Draw air into the syringe by pulling back on the plunger. The amount of air should be equal to your insulin dose.

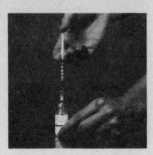

5

Put the needle through rubber top of insulin bottle. Push plunger in. The air injected into the bottle will allow insulin to be easily withdrawn into syringe.

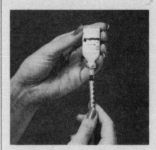

6

Turn bottle and syringe upside down in one hand. Be sure tip of needle is in insulin. Your other hand will be free to move the plunger. Draw back on plunger slowly to draw the correct dose of insulin into syringe.

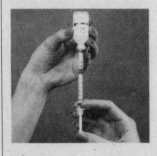

7

Check for air bubbles. The air is harmless, but too large an air bubble will reduce the insulin dose. To remove air bubbles, push insulin back into the bottle and measure your correct dose of insulin.

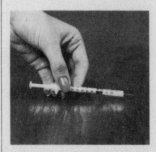

8

Double-check your dose. Remove needle from bottle. Cover needle with guard or lay syringe down so that needle does not touch anything.

Lilly

60-HI-2018-4   PRINTED IN USA   600781-108640   OCTOBER 1986   © 1986 ELI LILLY AND COMPANY

FIGURE 20–23   Instructions for self-administration of insulin (Courtesy of Eli Lilly and Company)

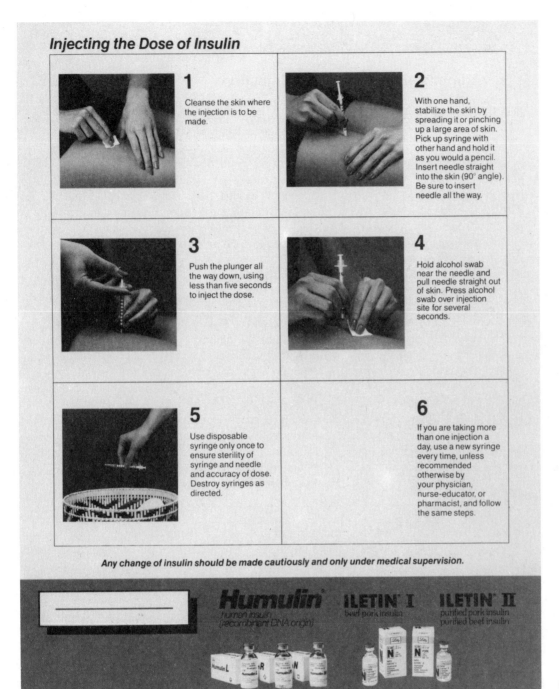

Injecting the Dose of Insulin

1 Cleanse the skin where the injection is to be made.

2 With one hand, stabilize the skin by spreading it or pinching up a large area of skin. Pick up syringe with other hand and hold it as you would a pencil. Insert needle straight into the skin (90° angle). Be sure to insert needle all the way.

3 Push the plunger all the way down, using less than five seconds to inject the dose.

4 Hold alcohol swab near the needle and pull needle straight out of skin. Press alcohol swab over injection site for several seconds.

5 Use disposable syringe only once to ensure sterility of syringe and needle and accuracy of dose. Destroy syringes as directed.

6 If you are taking more than one injection a day, use a new syringe every time, unless recommended otherwise by your physician, nurse-educator, or pharmacist, and follow the same steps.

Any change of insulin should be made cautiously and only under medical supervision.

Humulin human insulin (recombinant DNA origin)

ILETIN I beef pork insulin

ILETIN II purified pork insulin purified beef insulin

FIGURE 20–23
(Continued)

refer patients to educational programs held at local hospitals or through the American Diabetes Association.

Immunizations

Our immune system acts in response immediately on invasion of disease-causing microorganisms. If the exposure to the disease is slight and our susceptibility is low, our immune response may defend us from coming down with the disease itself. However, if we are susceptible to the disease, meaning our resistance is low, we come down with the disease, experience the symptoms, and are sick. Antibodies are produced to protect us, making us resistant, from further attacks of the specific pathogen that has made us sick. For instance, if one gets mumps, the body produces antibodies to destroy the mumps-causing organisms. After recovery from this illness, antibodies against mumps will protect one from coming down with it again. This is a process which is called *natural immunity.*

Artificial immunity is produced by administering **immunizations** or **vaccines** made from the dead or harmless infectious agents that trigger the immune response in the body to manufacture antibodies against

PROCEDURE

Administer Subcutaneous Injection

PURPOSE: To inject aqueous solutions of 0.5 to 2.0 cc into the subcutaneous tissue.

EQUIPMENT: Medication (sterile water for injection in vial/ampule), alcohol, cotton balls, adhesive bandage (hypoallergenic tape), sterile needle and syringe (needle is usually $\frac{1}{2}$ to $\frac{5}{8}$ inch, 25G), latex gloves

TERMINAL PERFORMANCE OBJECTIVE: Provided with all necessary equipment/supplies, the student will demonstrate each of the steps required in administering a subcutaneous injection; three injections will be administered to a latex training arm with the instructor observing each step. The dosage amount will be determined by the instructor each time.

1. Compare orders with medication and wash and glove hands. Prepare syringe and place on medication tray.
2. Compare medication order with patient's chart, identify patient, explain procedure, and ask patient to remove necessary clothing.
3. Use alcohol-saturated cotton ball to clean injection site. Remove needle guard.
4. Hold patient's skin taut between thumb and fingers of one hand and with other hand hold syringe securely.
5. Insert needle (bevel down) at a 45-degree angle with a steady penetration. Let go of patient's skin.

6. With one hand hold barrel of syringe while pulling back on plunger slightly with other hand to make sure a blood vessel has not been penetrated. If no blood appears in syringe, proceed by slowly pushing down on plunger to expel medication into tissues. If blood appears in syringe, pull needle out carefully at angle of entry. Discard medication, syringe, and needle. Replace with new syringe and medication.
7. Pull needle out at angle of insertion and wipe injection site with alcohol-saturated cotton ball. Replace with dry one and gently massage area to help distribute medication into tissues.
8. Observe patient for possible reaction and report to physician if so. Desensitizing allergy injections may take 15 to 20 minutes to cause a reaction. Instruct patient to wait for a full 20 minutes in case of a possible reaction. Answer questions. Determine if patient is allergic to adhesive before applying a bandage. Hypoallergenic tape is recommended.
9. Discard used disposable items. (Place entire syringe and needle in sharps container.) Wash and sterilize reusable items, remove gloves, and wash hands. Return medication and tray to proper storage area.
10. Record information and initial.

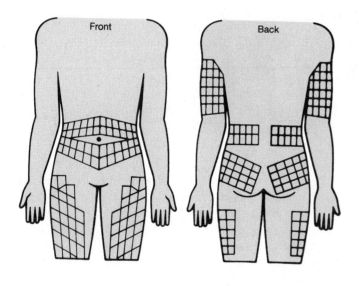

FIGURE 20–24 Selection and rotation of insulin injection sites

the particular disease-causing agent. Occasionally, one has a slight reaction during this process by experiencing mild symptoms of the disease or having a slight fever. In this process one becomes immune (resistant) to the disease. The immunization schedule, Table 20–6, page 649, is the recommendation of public health officials in the United States against the usual childhood diseases (UCHD) and suggested vaccines for adults (especially high-**risk** patients). Immunization schedules may vary in other countries for infants, children, and adults. You should make sure before administering any immunization that the patient does not have an active illness or fever. If this is the case the vaccine should be rescheduled when the patient is well. Check also the patient's health/medical history to be sure the patient has no past history of convulsions or allergies of any kind. If an allergy is known, bring it to the attention of the physician *before* the vaccine is administered. You may want to look the immunization up in a medications reference book for contraindications, precautions, and warnings. It is strongly advised that the parent/patient be made aware of the benefits and risks of all vaccines. Sufficient time should be given to the responsible person to read printed material after a verbal explanation is given regarding the vaccine(s). An opportunity must be provided for any questions of the parent/patient to be answered by the doctor before administration of immunization(s). When more than one dose of a vaccine is necessary to reach adequate immunization against a particular disease, such as the DPT injections, it is referred to as a primary "series." Each of these should be given with at least 6 to 8 weeks between each dose within a reasonable period of time. The primary series requires a booster for the immunization to be most effective and complete. In years past, these diseases were dreadful illnesses, which often caused death and affected children and adults. In the following text is a brief description of each of the diseases, the symptoms, the method of transmission, incubation period, and its treatment. This is to help you in answering questions about the diseases in the immunization schedule when patients ask "why" they need to have the vaccine. Certainly a few seconds/minutes (or even hours) of discomfort are well worth the minor suffering to gain protection from a potentially fatal disease.

The anatomy and physiology section of this text (Chapter 13) provides information regarding pneumonia and influenza, which are diseases affecting the respiratory system. A brief description follows.

Influenza. Commonly referred to as "the flu," influenza is a disease caused by a myxovirus that affects the respiratory tract. It is spread by direct contact, by droplet infection from the vapor of coughing and sneezing from an infected person, and by indirect contact from handling soiled items (such as used tissues) of the patient. The incubation period is between 1 and 4 days. Symptoms include sudden onset of fever, chills, sore throat, cough, muscle aches and pains, general malaise, and weakness. Treatment for the flu consists of bed rest, increased intake of fluids, antipyretics, and mild analgesics. Immunization against some strains of influenza is recommended for high-risk patients, such as the elderly, those with chronic illness, respiratory distress, or other conditions that warrant protection from infectious disease.

Pneumonia. This is an acute inflammation of the lungs. Eighty-five percent of pneumonia cases are caused by the *pneumococcus* bacterium. Pneumonia may also be caused by other bacteria, as well as by a virus, rickettsiae, and fungi. The pneumococcus bacterium disease (pneumonitis) is spread by droplet infection and direct contact with an infected person. The incubation period is

P R O C E D U R E

Administer Intramuscular Injection

PURPOSE: To inject large amounts of medication, 0.5 cc to 3.0 cc, and oil-base substances or irritating solutions which are more easily tolerated in the muscle tissue.

EQUIPMENT: Medication (sterile water for injection in vial/ampule), cotton balls, alcohol, adhesive bandage (or hypoallergenic tape), sterile needle and syringe (needle usually is 1 to 3 inches length, 18G to 23G), medication tray, patient's chart, pen, latex gloves

TERMINAL PERFORMANCE OBJECTIVE: Provided with all necessary equipment/supplies, the student will demonstrate each of the steps required in administering an intramuscular injection; three injections will be administered to a latex training arm with the instructor observing each step. The dosage amount will be determined by the instructor each time.

1. Wash and glove hands and prepare syringe with ordered amount of medication. Replace needle guard. Place medication on tray. **Key Point: Read label of medication and compare with order.**

2. Compare medication order with patient's chart. Identify patient and explain procedure. Ask patient to remove necessary clothing.

3. Use alcohol-saturated cotton ball to clean injection site. Remove needle guard. **Key Point: Allow alcohol to dry.**

4. Secure a large area of skin (to accommodate large amount of medication) between thumb and fingers of one hand. With other hand, grasp syringe midway as you would a dart and hold over site at 90-degree angle. Insert needle quickly with firm and steady action. **Key Point: Avoid force when injection to keep bruising to a minimum.** Pull back plunger to make sure a blood vessel has not been penetrated. If no blood is seen in barrel of syringe, proceed by pushing down on plunger and expelling medication into muscle. If blood appears in syringe barrel, pull needle out quickly at angle of insertion. Discard syringe, needle, and medication and begin again with new syringe and medication.

5. Pull needle out at angle of insertion carefully and quickly. Wipe injection site with alcohol-saturated cotton ball and gently massage area to help distribute medication.

6. Observe patient for any reaction and report to physician if needed. Determine if patient is allergic to adhesive before applying a bandage. Hypoallergenic tape is recommended.

7. Discard disposable items. (Place entire syringe and needle in sharps container.) Wash and sterilize reusable items, remove gloves, and wash hands. Return medication and tray to proper storage area.

8. Record information and initial.

Administer Intramuscular Injection by Z-Tract Method

PURPOSE: To inject irritating substances deep into the muscle layer of tissue. These irritating substances would cause tissue discoloration and irritation if given in the subcutaneous tissues from leakage in following the path of the needle when administered. The site of injection is in the gluteal muscle of the buttocks (upper outer quadrant; for some medications the deltoid muscle may be used). Dose is from 0.5 cc to 3.0 cc.

EQUIPMENT: Medication (sterile water for injection in vial/ampule), cotton balls, alcohol, adhesive bandage (or hypoallergenic tape), sterile needle and syringe (needle usually is 2 to 3 inches, 19G to 21 G), sterile gauze square, medication tray, patient's chart, pen, latex gloves

TERMINAL PERFORMANCE OBJECTIVE: Provided with all necessary equipment/supplies, the student will demonstrate each of the steps required in administering a Z-tract intramuscular injection using a clinical mannequin; three injections will be administered with the instructor observing each step. The dosage will be determined by the instructor.

1–3. Same as for intramuscular injection.

4. Use sterile gauze square to securely hold patient's skin at injection site to one side to displace skin/tissues until injection is completed. Insert needle into gluteal muscle of buttocks at a 90-degree angle, holding syringe as you would a dart. First and second fingers may be used to aspirate while thumb and ring finger hold syringe near needle end. If no blood is seen in barrel of syringe, proceed by expelling medication into muscle. Wait a few seconds before removing needle. If blood is seen in barrel of syringe, pull needle out quickly at angle of insertion, expel blood, replace needle, and begin again. **Key Point: Read package insert of medication carefully. There may be additional instructions for certain medications.** Some Z-tract injection instructions suggest that 0.5 cc of air be in syringe to follow medication to prevent leakage from needle track.

5. Pull needle out at angle of insertion and let go of skin quickly so that displaced tissue will cover needle track and prevent it from leaking into surrounding subcutaneous tissues. Cover injection site with alcohol-saturated cotton ball and hold in place for a few seconds. **Key Point: Do not massage area for this could cause tissue irritation and discoloration.**

6–8. Same as for intramuscular injection.

---

only a few hours after exposure to the bacteria. The symptoms are abrupt in onset and include severe chills, high fever, headache, chest pain, dyspnea, rapid pulse, cyanosis, and cough with blood-stained sputum. Bed rest, increased fluid intake, analgesics, antipyretics, and in many cases oxygen, are necessary for successful treatment of the patient. Pneumovax is a vaccine to protect high-risk patients from contracting the disease.

Haemophilus influenza Type B. Hemophilus or **haemophilus,** also known as **Hib** and **HIB,** is a disease caused by a small gram-negative, nonmotile parasitic bacterium that leads to severe destructive inflammation of the larynx, trachea, and bronchi. The disease is transmitted by droplet airborne infection. Incubation is from 1 to 3 days. The symptoms are sudden onset of fever, sore throat, cough, muscle aches, weakness, and general malaise. General care is bed rest, increased fluid intake, antipyretics, antibiotics, and analgesics as necessary. Because this particular disease affects infants and small children, immunization is recommended to this population. Each year this illness attacks 1 in every 200 infants in the United States; the most at-risk group is between the ages of 6 months and 5 years. With the rise in popularity of day care centers, immunization against the Hib bacterium is a most sensible way to prevent this often resistant-to-antibiotic disease from spreading through the very young population in the United States. Complications of this childhood disease include **meningitis,** which could result in damage to the nervous system, or in mental **retardation; epiglottitis,** could cause a child to choke to death if immediate treatment is not given; and joint infections, and forms of crippling arthritis. The Hib vaccine is administered in a series of 3 subcutaneous or intramuscular injections at ages 2, 4, and 6 months, see Table 20–6. A booster is given at age 18 months.

The MMR vaccine protects children from 3 childhood diseases.

Measles, Mumps, and Rubella. **Measles** is medically termed **rubeola.** It is also referred to as "old-fashioned," and 10-day measles. It is spread by direct contact, droplet infection, and by indirect contact from infected items of a patient. It has a 10- to 21-day incubation period. In the prodromal stage (earliest) the patient exhibits fever, malaise, runny nose, cough, sometimes conjunctivitis, and progresses with loss of appetite, **photophobia,** sore throat, and eventually Koplik's spots (the red skin rash). The cause is the rubeola virus, which is an acute and highly contagious viral disease involving the respiratory tract. Complications of measles can result in deafness, brain damage, and pneumonia. Treatment for measles is bed rest, increased fluid intake, antipyretics, antibiotics, cough medicine, and calamine lotion. the patient should be kept in isolation to prevent transmission to other. Quiet activity is suggested for the patient during recovery time, usually a few days.

Mumps is an acute contagious febrile disease that causes inflammation of the parotid and salivary glands. Parotitis is transmitted by droplet infection or direct contact with an infected person. The usual incubation period is from 14 to 28 days. Symptoms include chills and fever, headache, and pain below and in front of the ear(s) for 5 to 7 days' duration. Another symptom is pain between the ear and the angle of the jaw with drinking or eating acidic substances. Bed rest and a soft diet, including increased fluid intake, is recommended. Application of cold packs to control swelling of the glands of the neck, and in males, of the testicles in orchitis, is advised.

Rubella, also called German measles or 3-day measles, is an acute contagious viral disease characterized by an upper respiratory infection. If a female acquires rubella during the first trimester of pregnancy, fetal abnormalities may result. You should remind female patients in childbearing years of this concern and to be tested for a rubella antibody titer, and/or to be vaccinated before becoming pregnant. *Females should not be vaccinated during pregnancy.* Be sure to determine this before administering the vaccine. Rubella is transmitted by droplet infection and by direct contact. The incubation period is from 12 to 23 days. Symptoms include slight fever, sore throat, drowsiness and malaise, swollen glands and lymph nodes, arthralgia, and a diffuse fine red rash, Figure 20–25. Treatment is bed rest, liquids, antipyretics, and sponge baths. Complications of rubella can result in blindness, deafness, brain damage, heart defects, enlarged liver, and bone malformation.

Diphtheria. This acute infectious disease is caused by *Corynebacterium diphtheriae,* which is a gram-positive, nonmotile, nonspore-forming, club-shaped bacillus. Diphtheria diagnosis is confirmed by throat culture. Transmission is by direct and indirect contact. The incubation period is between 2 and 5 days. Symptoms include headache, malaise, fever, and sore throat with a yellowish white or gray membrane. Treatment consists of adequate liquids and a soft diet, antibiotics, bed rest, and in some cases a tracheostomy. The Schick test is an interdermal injection of a minute amount of the diphtheria toxin used to determine the degree of immunity to the disease. Little or no reaction indicates immunity (the presence of antibodies).

Pertussis. Whooping cough, or pertussis is an acute infectious disease characterized by respiratory drainage, then a peculiar paroxysmal cough, which ends in a whooping inspiration (sounds like a shrill trumpeting cry; the name comes from the whooping crane that makes this sound). This disease is most common in children under 4 years of age, although it can affect children of all ages if they have not been immunized against it. Pertussis is caused by the small, nonmotile, gram-negative bacillus *Bordetella pertussis.* It is transmitted by direct and indirect contact. The incubation period is from 7 to 14 days. Symptoms of whooping cough include: in the catarrhal stage—an increase in leukocyte count marked by lymphocytosis, respiratory drainage, sneezing, slight fever, dry cough, irritability, loss of appetite; in the paroxysmal stage—violent cough with whooping inspiration sounds, forceful vomiting that can evoke hemorrhaging from various portions of the body from the straining; and in the decline stage—decline in coughing and return of appetite. A trace cough may last for several months to 2 years.

Tetanus. This acute, potentially fatal, infectious disease affects the central nervous system. Tetanus was commonly

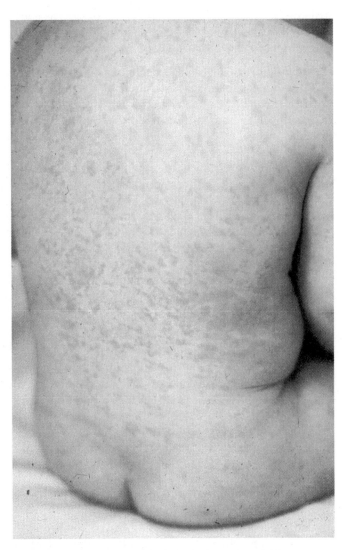

FIGURE 20–25 Eleven-month-old infant with rubella (postnatal). This infant has a typical discrete macupapular erythematous rash indistinguishable from that seen in other viral illnesses.

referred to as "lockjaw." Motor nerves transmit impulses from the infected central nervous system to muscle. It is caused by the bacillus *Clostridum tetani,* the **toxin** of which is one of the most **lethal** poisons known. The bacillus is found in superficial layers of the soil. It is a normal inhabitant of the intestinal tracts of horses and cows. Tetanus affects only wounds that contain dead tissue, transmitted commonly in puncture wounds, abrasions, lacerations, and burns. There is a short incubation period of 3 to 21 days, and a longer one of 4 to 5 weeks. The symptoms of tetanus are stiffness of the jaw, esophageal muscles, and sometimes neck muscles. Progressing rigidity follows soon with fixed jaw (thus lockjaw), altered voice, fever, painful spasms of all body muscles, irritability, and headache. Immediate cleaning of the wound and **debridement** are necessary initially in treatment. Maintaining an airway is vital as well as administering **antitoxin.** Additionally, treatment consists of sedation, controlling muscle spasms, maintaining fluid balance, penicillin G, tracheostomy, and oxygen as necessary. The patient must be in a quiet room to prevent the triggering of muscle spasms.

Hepatitis B. This is a highly contagious, potentially fatal, form of viral hepatitis. It is caused by the **hepatitis B** virus (HBV). It has been known as "serum hepatitis." Hepatitis B is transmitted by contaminated serum in blood transfusions or by using contaminated needles or instruments. It has an incubation period of 14 to 50 days. The symptoms are slow at onset with fever, malaise, loss of appetite, nausea, and vomiting, progressing to include jaundice, weakness, dark urine, and whitish stool. Bed rest and a forced-fluid diet are recommended. Alcohol and fats should be eliminated from the patient's diet. The hepatitis B vaccine is urged for all who may be at risk, especially *all health care workers.* It is though to be in widespread proportions everywhere and immunization is strongly urged to protect the country's population and to prevent a massive epidemic.

Other vaccines. All of the immunizations mentioned thus far are vaccines administered by injection. As with any parenteral administration of medications, it is important to instruct the patient to relax as much as possible during the procedure. Tense or tight muscles around the site of injection will make not only the procedure itself an unpleasant experience, but will have an after-effect of unnecessary soreness of the area. Becoming proficient in technique, besides developing a good rapport and educating the patients you serve, is fundamental.

A vaccine administered orally is the **polio** immunization. It is kept frozen until just before it is to be administered. It should never be refrozen. As you can see in the immunization schedule, this vaccine is administered to infants and young children. It is made from the pathogenic microorganisms and is **attenuated,** which makes it

less virulent. The disease it protects against is known as infantile paralysis, or poliomyelitis, which is the acute infection and inflammation of the gray matter of the spinal cord caused by the polio virus. As the name suggest, children are more susceptible than adults. It is transmitted by the oral-fecal route. Incubation is usually from 7 to 12 days (and can be from 5 to 35). The symptoms begin with fever, malaise, headache, nausea and vomiting, slight abdominal discomfort, and general paralysis (if respiratory muscles are involved it is likely to be fatal). Treatment consists of relieving symptoms, bed rest, mild analgesics, sedatives as necessary, fluid and salt balance, laxatives or enemas as necessary to relieve constipation, oxygen, respirator, and tracheostomy if necessary. Physical and occupational therapy are needed as the patient recovers.

Remind patients to protect themselves and their families against all of these diseases to prevent the return of epidemics. There are other diseases, such as **cholera** and **typhoid,** for which there are vaccines to prevent

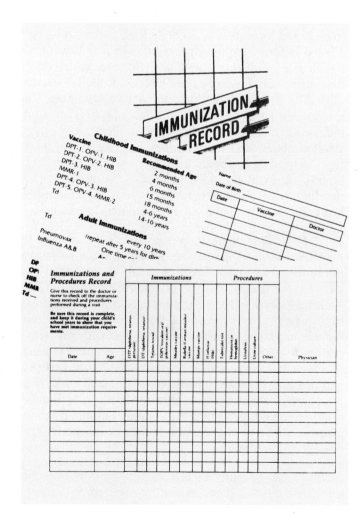

FIGURE 20–26 Immunization schedule and records

dangerous epidemics that have the potential to wipe out entire populations. Many underdeveloped countries have such situations even today. Immunizations other than what appears in the schedule in Table 20–6 are not recommended on a routine basis in most Western countries. Health officials advise immunizations as determined necessary. Travel to some countries requires immunizations against particular diseases before entry is permitted. To provide up-to-date immunization information by country, computer data bases have been established. One such program containing health information for travelers on over 200 countries is available from Immunization Alert, Storrs, Connecticut. Current information may also be obtained at local and state health departments. You should provide the patient with a card or booklet to accurately record each immunization, the month, day and year for each, Figure 20–26, as well as recording each vaccine on the patient's chart. Any reaction, no matter how slight, must also be recorded on the patient's chart. Remind patients to make appointments and carry the immunization record (or a copy) with them at all times.

Because of the continuing research and advances in the production of vaccinations against many infectious diseases, these illnesses are rarely experienced in developed countries, except in severely poverty-stricken areas. Unfortunately, however, third world nations are still constantly fighting a losing battle against communicable diseases. Deaths from them are staggering in number. This is mainly due to inadequate education, poor living conditions, and lack of funding for vaccines.

Complete Chapter 20, Unit 3 in the workbook to help you meet the objectives at the beginning of this unit and therefore to achieve competency of this subject matter.

MEDICAL-LEGAL ETHICAL HIGHLIGHTS

Mrs. Right...

makes sure that all prescription pads are secured at all times to prevent theft. She keeps accurate records of narcotics and reminds the physician about keeping current narcotics registration. In the event of theft of any medication or prescription pad, she reports it immediately to the proper authorities. When patients agree to take experimental drugs, she obtains written consent. She disposes of all expired medicines properly. She explains about immunizations to patients and obtains written consent from them. She remembers to record medication refills on the patients' records.

Promotion outlook: Excellent

Ms. Wrong...

never concerns herself about securing prescription pads, and therefore, wouldn't even know if one were missing. She pays no attention to recording refills of prescriptions on the patient records, saying that the patient should tell the doctor that they got more medicine when they come in for the next appointment. Her haphazard narcotics records and the physician's narcotics registration forms are always misplaced so she doesn't know if they are accurate or current. She rarely obtains a written consent form from patients for experimental drugs or for immunizations. She pays no attention to expiration dates on medicines she prepares or puts away.

Promotion outlook: None

REFERENCES

American Medical Association Family Medical Guide, rev. ed. New York: Random House, 1987.

Code of Federal Regulations and Drugs 21, 1990.

Erickson, Belle. *Nurse's Clinical Guide Dosage Calculations.* Springhouse, PA: Springhouse Corporation, 1991.

Mead Johnson, Nutritional Division Distributors of b-CAPSA I Vaccine (Haemophilus b Polysaccharide Vaccine). Praxis Biologics, Inc., Rochester, N.Y. Write for booklet.

Miller, Benjamin F., and Keane, Claire Brackman. *Encyclopedia and Dictionary of Medicine, Nursing and Allied Health,* 3d ed. Philadelphia: W. B. Saunders, 1983.

Morbidity and Mortality Weekly Report (MMWR), 32, no. 1 (January 14, 1983).

Mosby's Medical, Nursing, & Allied Health Dictionary, 3d ed. St. Louis: C. V. Mosby Co., 1990.

Physician's Desk Reference. Oradell, NJ: Medical Economics, updated annually.

Physician's Desk Reference for Nonprescription Drugs. Oradell, NJ: Medical Economics, updated annually.

Physician's Manual. U.S. Department of Justice, DEA, revised 1990.

Taber, Clarence W. *Taber's Cyclopedia Medical Dictionary*, 14th ed. Philadelphia: F.A. Davis, 1983.

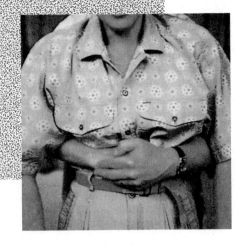

Medical Emergencies

The emergency situations a medical assistant is most likely to encounter will depend on the employer's practice. However, if an accident occurs near a physician's office the victim may appear in your waiting room with an injury which does not fall within your practice area. You must know how to evaluate the situation and respond in the manner expected from a member of a health care team. This chapter will present guidelines for preventing accidents and describe emergency procedures and first aid care of accident victims.

U N I T   1

Safety in the Medical Office

OBJECTIVES

Upon completion of this unit, the student will meet the following terminal performance objectives by verifying knowledge of the facts and principles presented through oral and written communication at a level deemed competent.

1. Identify potential office hazards.
2. List steps to take in accident-proofing an office.
3. Describe methods of fire prevention in the office.
4. Explain why fire/earthquake/severe weather drills are needed.
5. Discuss steps of an evacuation procedure and include the manner in which it should be carried out.
6. Explain where a fire extinguisher should be affixed and why.
7. Spell and define, using the glossary at the back of the text, all the words to know in this unit.

WORDS TO KNOW

accessible	drill
ambulate	extinguisher
conceal	evacuation
concise	procurement
crisis	volatile
disaster	

Reports of injuries reveal that a large percentage occur in the home. A medical office may also present dangers for employees and patients. As described in Chapter 6, you should do a daily check of the waiting room to be sure all electrical wires, furniture, and carpet are in good repair. No throw rugs should be on the floor.

All medications should be in a locked cupboard or in drawers not easily **accessible** to patients. Spills of any kind should be cleaned up immediately. Any medications dropped must be located and destroyed. File drawers and cupboard doors should be closed when not in use to avoid both head injuries and falls from tripping over them. All equipment cords should be **concealed** where people will be moving about. No prescription blanks should be left where they could be forged and used illegally for drug **procurement**.

A very young child should never be left unattended. Patients who are ill are sometimes unsteady when they attempt to **ambulate**; always assist these patients as needed. Never leave ill or elderly patients unattended on an examination table.

Learn to give clear, **concise** instructions to patients. When you position the patient for examinations your instructions are important in obtaining the desired results and in maintaining the safety of the patient moving about on the table.

Be sure office staff knows when the autoclave is in operation so that burns will not result from touching the machine.

Computers need to be situated so that glare is not present on the screen. Employees using computers or word processors should rest the eyes by looking away from the screen at regular intervals.

If chemicals are kept in the office for laboratory work, care must be taken to store them properly. Some chemicals become **volatile** when kept beyond the expiration date, so these dates need to be carefully monitored.

Fire prevention is of utmost importance for the safety of everyone. There are rare exceptions to the "no smoking" regulations in medical and public facilities. Even though this is true, there is still a possibility of the danger of a match, lighter, or cigarette dropped into furniture, a planter, or trash container by someone looking for an ashtray. Some facilities provide ashtrays just outside the entrance for this very reason. However, you should keep an eye on it for people tend to use this ashtray as a trash disposal as well. This can become a prime setting for a fire to start. Ashtrays should be emptied often and the contents (possibly smoldering smoking materials) flushed down the toilet.

Fire **extinguishers** should be affixed on a wall closest to the lab or kitchen area where the potential for a fire is the greatest. It should be checked periodically by the fire department for effectiveness. Each employee should be instructed in the proper use of it in case of fire.

Electrical outlets which do not work should be checked by an electrician, as a defective outlet may cause a fire. Frayed wires of any electrical appliance or office equipment must not be used until repaired. Do not attempt to tape or fix a frayed wire for the danger of fire or shock to you and others is too great. Coffee pots boil dry and can burn, as can boiling water sterilizers. Some office procedure manuals require that all electrical appliances be unplugged each night.

The office should have an established policy so that all employees know what to do in the event of a fire or severe weather warning, such as a tornado alert. Natural **disasters** are certainly unpredictable and can claim many

lives if necessary steps are not taken immediately. **Evacuation** from a building of all persons is necessary in cases of fire, possible explosions, or other similar dangers. Exit signs should be clearly posted. All stairways and hallways should be free from clutter to allow safe passage. In an earthquake (and in a tornado), however, it is advisable for persons to take shelter in a door frame or under a sturdy structure and *not* go outside. For example, in areas of the country where earthquakes are known to occur, children in school settings are taught to immediately get under their desks for shelter from falling objects. Going outside may result in being struck by objects, electrical power lines, and falling trees and buildings. Electrical power is usually disrupted during such a situation or severe storm. Never use an elevator in any threatening situation because the power could be cut off at any time and those in the elevator could be trapped or killed. Some medical facilities, such as hospitals, clinics, and group practices, have emergency generators for just these types of situations.

Routine **drills** psychologically prepare you for sensible and safe actions should an emergency situation occur. A practical time to review drill procedures is at staff meetings or during orientation of a new employee. Studies have shown that those who are prepared have a greater chance of surviving a **crisis** than those who did not know what to do or how to act. Keeping a calm and commanding attitude and acting in an efficient manner helps to reduce panic in a stressful situation. This will allow others to follow your example in leading them to safety. It is not practical to decide at the time of such an emergency what to instruct your patients and the employees to do. Each member of the health care team should have specific tasks to accomplish in such emergencies. Complete Chapter 21, Unit 1 in the workbook to help you meet the objectives at the beginning of this unit and therefore achieve competency of this subject matter.

UNIT 2

Medical Office Emergency Procedures

OBJECTIVES ....

Upon completion of this unit, the student will meet the following terminal performance objectives by verifying knowledge of the facts and principles presented through oral and written communication at a level deemed competent, and will demonstrate the specific behaviors as identified in the terminal performance objectives of the

procedures, observing all aseptic and safety precautions in accordance with health care standards.

1. Describe the universal emergency medical identification system.
2. Assemble and maintain an emergency tray of appropriate drugs and equipment.
3. Describe the symptoms and first aid for:

   ■ bee, wasp, and hornet stings
   ■ bites, animal and human
   ■ burns
   ■ convulsions
   ■ diabetic coma and insulin shock
   ■ dislocations
   ■ fainting
   ■ foreign bodies
   ■ fractures
   ■ heart attack
   ■ heat and cold exposure
   ■ hemorrhage
   ■ poisoning
   ■ respiratory emergencies
   ■ shock
   ■ sprains and strains
   ■ stroke
   ■ wounds

4. List symptoms of substance abuse (drugs and alcohol).
5. List methods of obtaining local emergency services.
6. Discuss the purpose of applying heat and cold packs.
7. Discuss the importance of following universal precautions in caring for injuries.
8. Spell and define, using the glossary at the back of the text, all the words to know in this unit.

WORDS TO KNOW ·····························

activate	diaphoresis	perfusion
antihistamine	emetic	prophylactic
aspiration	exogenous	psychopathic
cessation	flushed	rotate
complicated	forge	shock
confront	incision	superficial
convulsion	ingest	syncope
delirium tremens	molten	universal

A medical emergency is any situation in which an individual suddenly becomes ill or has an injury in circumstances calling for swift and decided action. You should first identify the person if at all possible and determine who to contact as next of kin. If the patient is conscious you should try to obtain information regarding the illness or injury. If the patient is unconscious you should check for a universal emergency medical identification symbol, Figure 21–1. This symbol, designed by the American Medical Association, is worn like a dog

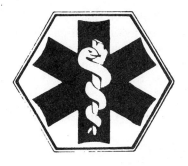

FIGURE 21–1   Universal emergency medical identification symbol

tag around the neck, wrist, or ankle. If you find this symbol, you should check for an identification card, which will tell you the health problem the patient has, Figure 21–2. You should encourage patients who have serious heart conditions, diabetes, allergies, or a laryngectomy to wear such a symbol.

As part of your preparation for an emergency, you and your employer should list the supplies and equipment that would be necessary to handle an emergency that could come under your care. Then set aside a place in the office where these items will always be ready for use. All employees in the office should know where the items are and how they are to be used. You should have a supply of sterile dressings, bandage material, and adhesive tape; easily activated hot and cold packs; disposable syringe and needle units with adrenaline, narcotics, and antihistamines. Adrenaline (epinephrine) is available in cartridge units ready for use. Other supplies include: Ipecac, an effective emetic; tubes of glucose for use in diabetic patients suffering from a severe hypoglycemic reaction; and an oxygen tank with a mask. Oxygen tanks should be routinely checked on a monthly basis to determine how much oxygen is still available. If the amount is insufficient during an emergency, an unfortunate situation could result. Only disposable face masks and tubing should be used for each patient. They should be used only once and discarded in the proper

EMERGENCY
I am a laryngectomee (no vocal cords).
I breathe through an opening in the neck, not through the nose or mouth.
If artificial respiration is necessary:
1. Keep neck opening clear of all matter.
2. Don't twist head sidewise.
3. Apply oxygen only to neck opening.
4. Don't throw water on head.
5. Mouth-to-opening breathing is effective.

FIGURE 21–2   Emergency medical identification card

receptacle. Any supplies used should be replaced immediately. A backup supply must be available at all times. Rotate the supplies so that you use older supplies first, and be careful to check dates on medications to be sure they have not expired.

First Aid for Sudden Illness and Injuries ....

Bee, Wasp, and Hornet Stings

Bees, wasps, and hornets cause deaths every year. If the victim of a sting is not sensitive to the sting, the result may only be a painful swelling with redness and itching. When several stings are received at one time, the victim may become quite ill. The patient may develop severe hives or edema of all tissues.

When a patient is severely allergic to stings, they can cause acute illness with shortness of breath. The patient may become restless, complain of headache, or have mottled blueness of the skin. In the cases where shortness of breath is not apparent, the victim may appear to be in shock and have severe nausea, vomiting, and blood may be evident in diarrhea. The severely allergic patient should always have a special emergency kit close at hand when there is any possibility of a sting. Refer to Chapter 18 for discussion about anaphylactic shock and stings. If there is evidence of anaphylactic shock, epinephrine should be given as a life-saving measure.

A honeybee leaves the stinger in the skin, and it should be immediately removed by scraping it out carefully with a sharp object. Never grasp the stinger with your fingers or a tweezers, as that would inject more of the venom. Wasps, hornets, and yellow jackets retain their stingers and can sting repeatedly.

Bites

An animal bite may tear skin and cause a bruise. The bite is dangerous because of the possibility of infection and rabies. The animal should be held for observation for at least 15 days to see if it is rabid. The bite must be reported to the police or local health authorities, who will examine the animal for rabies. The wound should be thoroughly cleansed with an antiseptic soap and rinsed well. The area should be bandaged and immobilized, and the victim should be examined by a physician as soon as possible. The decision must be made regarding the use of antirabies serum. If the skin is broken and the animal cannot be tested, antirabies serum should be used. When the animal can be observed for 15 days and is found to be free of rabies, no serum is necessary.

There is also concern regarding human bites because of AIDS and hepatitis B. The only way AIDS could be transmitted in this manner is if the bite breaks the skin and the person doing the biting has bleeding gums. It is still necessary to cleanse the wound thoroughly, cover with a sterile bandage, and have a physician examine the

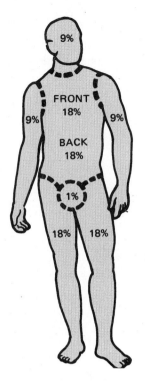

FIGURE 21–3 (A) Diagram for use in calculating the extent of burns or other injuries for an adult

area. Patients who have sustained such a bite from another person should be advised to have a series of three injections to be immunized against hepatitis B.

Burns

The severity of a burn is determined by the amount of skin surface and the layer of skin involved, Figures 21–3 (a) and (b) and 21–4. Any amount involving 15% of the total body surface (TBS) is considered a serious or critical burn. Burns occur as a result of radiation from the sun or a heat lamp, or contact with electricity, chemicals, or heat. A first-degree burn is a superficial injury resulting in reddening of the skin and severe pain. A sunburn or contact with boiling water or steam may cause this type of burn. It will heal without special treatment.

Treating the area with cold water or ice packs should stop the pain and may even keep the burn from progressing into deeper tissue layers. The application of butter or ointments will hold the burn in and cause more pain as well as being a problem to remove. In treatment of burns a physician may use an antiseptic ointment, which can easily be washed off.

A second-degree burn, which affects 30% of the TBS of an adult (20% of TBS of a child), involves both reddening and blistering because the burn extends into deeper layers of skin. The leakage of plasma and electrolytes from the capillaries damaged by the burn into the surrounding tissues raises up the epidermis to form blisters. Patients should be cautioned to refrain from breaking blisters as this opens up the area to infection. Blisters will heal more quickly if they are opened by a

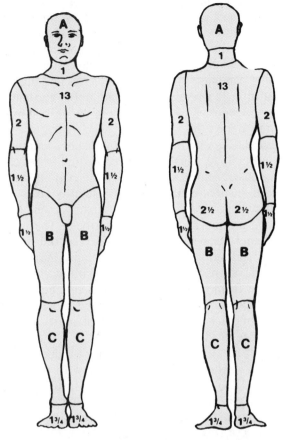

Relative percentages of areas affected by growth

	At birth	1 yr	5 yr	10 yr	15 yr	Adult
A: Half of head	9½%	8½%	6½%	5½%	4½%	3½%
B: Half of thigh	2¾%	3¼%	4%	4¼%	4½%	4¾%
C: Half of leg	2½%	2½%	2¾%	3%	3¼%	3½%

FIGURE 21–3 (B) Lund and Browder chart for estimating the extent of burns. Because this chart takes proportional age-size differences into account, it can be used for infants and children, as well as for adults. (Adapted with permission from *Surgery, Gynecology, & Obstetrics* 79:352, 1944)

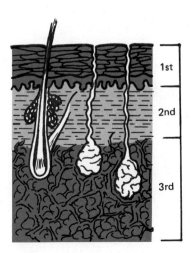

FIGURE 21–4 Layers of skin in relation to degree of burn

physician, who would first paint the area with an anti-septic and then open them with a sterilized needle. The area should then be covered with a sterile gauze pad bandaged in place. First aid for a second-degree burn would involve treatment for shock, removal of any jewelry as edema may be severe, as much fluid as the patient can take, and covering the burn area with a sterile dressing. A victim of severe sunburn would be encouraged to soak in a tub of cold water and take large amounts of fluid. Pain medication as advised by the physician, may be taken to ease painful burns. Some medications increase the danger of exposure to the sun. It is important to warn patients of this potential problem. Pharmacists generally place a warning label on the patient's prescription bottle.

Third-degree burns involve the epidermis, dermis, and subcutaneous tissues and require surgical care. They affect 10% to 15% of the TBS. The patient should receive immediate treatment for shock. No first aid can be given to the burn area except for clothing burned to the tissue should be removed only under sterile conditions in surgery by the physician. Cover the area with a sterile dressing.

Some physicians use the term fourth-degree burn for burns involving all the layers of skin, muscle, and even bone. This can result from an industrial injury such as contact with molten metal. The intense heat of a burning building or a chemical fire could cause this type of burn.

An electrical burn may result from contact with electrical power lines or lightning. The circuit breaker should be cut off and the electric power company should be called immediately. In the case of an electrical burn, the primary aid is to remove the victim from the contact with the power source. This can best be done by the use of a wooden stick or cloth or special heavy gloves used to pull the victim away from the electrical power source. The rescuer could also be injured if contact is made with the electrical source. Depending on the total voltage that the victim has come in contact with, the articles used to free the victim can still conduct electricity. There should be immediate care for shock and cardiopulmonary resuscitation (CPR) if breathing or pulse is absent.

Chemical burns are treated by removing any clothing from the area and then flooding the area with water for at least 15 minutes. The one exception to the rule of immediate flooding with water is a carbolic acid burn, which should be flooded first with alcohol and then with water. A dry chemical should be brushed off carefully before flushing the patient's skin because some chemicals, such as lime, are activated by water. These burns should all be covered with a sterile dressing after thorough washing with water. A chemical burn of the eye should be flooded with water continuously for at least 20 minutes. A physician should always examine and treat eye burns immediately. Any other acid burn to the skin should be flushed with water for at least 5 minutes.

Convulsions

Convulsions may occur when the patient has high body temperature, head injuries, brain disease, or brain disorders such as epilepsy. A convulsion is a severe involuntary contraction of muscles that causes the patient first to become rigid and then to have uncontrollable movements. The patient becomes unconscious and may be injured during the seizure. The face and lips may become cyanotic, and the patient may stop breathing. The patient may also lose bladder and bowel control and bite the tongue. When the convulsion has stopped the patient may be confused and complain of headache.

During the convulsion do not restrain movement. You should move objects that might cause injury. If possible, put a padded tongue depressor or soft object between the teeth to prevent biting the tongue. However, do not force any object between the patient's teeth or it could cause vomiting, **aspiration,** or spasm of the larynx. Keep the head turned to the side to prevent choking from profuse salivation. Never attempt to force the mouth open or pour water over the face. Allow the patient to rest or sleep after the seizure is over. Artificial respiration should be given if necessary. Emotional support should be given as the patient regains composure because this situation can cause the person to feel awkward.

Diabetic Coma and Insulin Shock

Diabetic patients may present emergency situations by going into diabetic coma or insulin shock, Table 21–1. A diabetic coma is caused by an increased amount of sugar in the blood. This may be caused by eating sweets or failing to take insulin. The patient may complain of confusion, dizziness, weakness, or nausea. Vomiting may occur. Respiration may be rapid and deep. The skin may be dry and **flushed.** The patient's breath has a sweet or fruity odor, which may be evident some distance away. The patient can lapse into unconsciousness and die from this condition if not treated immediately. The patient should be transported by ambulance to the nearest hospital for immediate care.

Insulin shock may occur from an excess amount of insulin in the body. This can happen if food is not eaten regularly in measured amounts, if the patient vomits after taking insulin, or if too much insulin is taken. The patient may have muscle weakness, anxiety, mental confusion, and a rapid and irregular heartbeat. The patient may be hungry and have **diaphoresis.** The skin will be cold, pale, and moist. The patient may lapse into a coma and may develop convulsions. The patient should be given some form of sugar. Sweetened orange juice or tubes of glucose are often used. The sugar should control the shock but if it does not the patient must be transported at once to a hospital.

You must be alert to the possibility of diabetic coma or shock in a known diabetic patient with the above symptoms. If the patient can talk, ask if insulin or food has been taken. This will give you a better idea of the need for treatment of coma or shock. If you do not know the diagnosis, it is safer to give a spoon of sugar, because insulin shock can cause brain damage, which is not reversible. Recent studies indicate that by placing a very small amount of sugar under the tongue of an unconscious person it may be absorbed rapidly in the blood stream.

TABLE 21–1
Causes and symptoms of diabetic coma and insulin shock

DIABETIC COMA OR ACIDOSIS	INSULIN SHOCK OR REACTION
Causes	
Too little insulin	Too much insulin or oral hypoglycemic drug
Too much to eat	Too little to eat
Infections, fever	An unusual amount of exercise
Emotional stress	
Symptoms	
Skin: Dry and flushed	Moist and pale
Behavior: Drowsy	Often excited
Mouth: Dry	Drooling
Thirst: Intense	Absent
Hunger: Absent	Present
Vomiting: Common	Usually absent
Respiration: Exaggerated, air hungry	Normal or shallow
Breath: Fruity odor of acetone	Usually normal
Pulse: Weak and rapid	Full and bounding (gives patient feeling of heart pounding)
Vision: Dim	Diplopia (double)
First aid: Keep patient warm	If conscious, give patient sugar or any food containing sugar (fruit juice, candy, crackers, etc.)
Obtain medical help immediately.	Obtain medical help immediately.

Dislocations

At least half of all dislocations involve the shoulder, but dislocations are possible of any freely moving joint. When a bone end slips out of the socket or when the capsule surrounding a joint is stretched or torn, a dislocation is likely to occur. There is usually severe pain and obvious deformity of the joint area. There may be loss of function of the affected limb. There is also noticeable swelling. Dislocations are best treated by a physician. The only first aid measure is to immobilize the dislocation during the trip to the medical office or hospital. Treat all sprains, strains, and dislocations as if a fracture. Splint the injured limb in the position in which you find it to avoid additional injury to the accident victim.

Fainting

A temporarily diminished supply of blood to the brain may cause fainting. The medical term for fainting is **syncope.** A patient who feels faint should lower the head between the legs or lie down with feet elevated to improve the blood circulation to the head. The patient who is about to faint may be pale, perspiring, have cold clammy skin, and complain of dizziness or nausea. Another term or slang phrase you may hear to describe the strange color which some patients turn before they get sick and vomit or pass out is "turning green." An emesis basin should be handy in case the patient vomits. Each examination room should be supplied with aromatic spirits of ammonia capsules, which can easily be broken and used to arouse the patient. These should not be held directly under the nose but passed back and forth about 6 inches under the nose. The patient should be kept in a reclining position until fully recovered and then may be given sips of water. The patient should regain consciousness within 5 minutes from a simple fainting episode. If not, the physician should check the patient. You should keep checking the patient's vital signs to determine that the patient is stabilized before allowing the patient to leave. Realize that in this situation, too, the patient needs emotional support.

Foreign Bodies

Foreign bodies are substances or objects which become lodged in any part of the human body where they do not belong. It is fairly common for a speck of dirt, soot from a fire, or an eyelash to lodge in the eye, for example. Always wash your hands before touching the eyes. A foreign body under the lower lid can usually be seen easily and can be removed with a bit of cotton or a fold of tissue moistened with sterile water. If a foreign body is under the upper lid, it may be possible to remove it by pulling the upper lid over the lower lid. If this procedure is not successful it may be necessary to grasp the eyelashes and carefully turn back the upper lid over a cotton swab,

Figure 21–5. When the object is located it may be removed with a folded piece of sterile gauze moistened with sterile water. Any object lodged on the cornea should be removed by a physician. A sterile compress should be placed over both eyes to keep the eye from moving until a physician can examine it. A sterile eye irrigation solution should be kept on hand for just this type of emergency. Use it to continuously flush the affected eye for 20 minutes to prevent further tissue damage, or to remove a foreign substance (such as dust). Refer to Chapter 16 for the procedure regarding eye irrigation.

First aid for an object lodged in the ear consists of placing several drops of warm olive oil, mineral oil, or baby oil into the ear, pulling back on the earlobe to straighten the external canal, while the head is leaning toward the uninjured side, Figure 21–6, page 666. Then let the oil run out and see if the object will come out with it. Never try to dig an object out of the ear; damage can be done to the eardrum. If first aid measures are not successful, a physician should examine the patient.

You may get a call from a parent who is frightened because a child has swallowed a small object. It is best for the physician to perform a fluoroscopic examination to see if the object is in the stomach. If the object is not sharp it will probably pass on through the intestinal tract and be eliminated in normal fashion.

Splinters can generally be removed with a needle if at home or with a splinter thumb forceps in the office, Figure 21–7, page 666. The skin should be washed with soap and water. The needle should be held over a flame until it is thoroughly heated and then cooled before making a slit

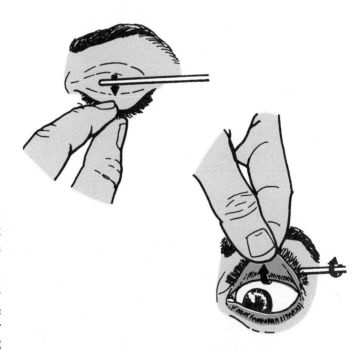

FIGURE 21–5 Removing a foreign object from the upper eyelid by turning the eyelid back over a cotton-tipped swab or the stem of a wooden kitchen match

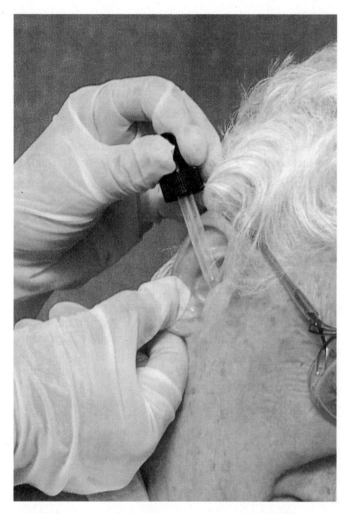

FIGURE 21–6 After the patient's head is tipped to the side, insert eardrops by pulling back on the earlobe so as to straighten the external canal.

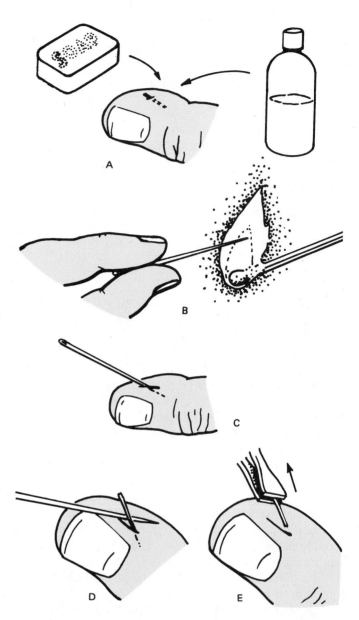

FIGURE 21–7 Removing a splinter. (a). Clean area around splinter. (b). Heat needle in flame and let it cool. (c). Cut the skin over the splinter. (d). Lift the splinter partially out. (e). Remove the splinter with tweezers.

over the splinter. The splinter forceps should be wrapped and sterilized in the autoclave. Lift the end of the exposed splinter with the needle and remove by grasping with a pair of tweezers. If a splinter or thorn is under a fingernail it is best to have a physician remove it. After the splinter or thorn is removed the area should again be washed with soap and water and covered with a Band-Aid.

One of the hazards of fishing or of being around individuals who are casting for fish is that of hooks becoming embedded in fingers, backs, scalps, or any part of the anatomy that is exposed. It is best for a physician to use a local anesthetic for such removal. If you do not have a physician near at hand, you should push the barb through the flesh and then cut it off with a pair of nipper pliers, Figure 21–8. After this is done you can back out the remainder of the hook. The other possibility is to cut off the shank of the hook and pull out the barbed end. After the hook is removed, the area should be carefully cleaned and a dry dressing applied. If the removal is done away from the office, the patient should be seen by a physician for a tetanus toxoid booster or tetanus anti-

serum as needed. The physician may also prescribe an antibiotic.

Fractures

Fractures are breaks in bone caused by trauma or bone disease. In a *closed* or *simple fracture* there is no open wound. In an *open* or *compound fracture* there is an open wound. First aid for an open fracture is to control bleeding and to splint without moving the bone ends. The patient may also need to be treated for shock. You should check the PMS (pulse, and motor and sensory reflexes). Capillary refill of the distal area to all fracture sites on an injured limb will be impaired. To ensure good

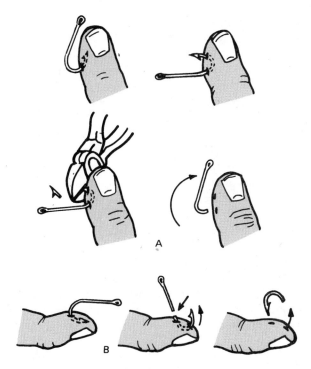

FIGURE 21–8 Removing a fish hook by cutting the barb (a) and cutting the shank (b)

perfusion and nonimpaired neurologic function, treatment must be administered as soon as possible. A fracture can be diagnosed only by an X ray unless bone ends can be seen in an open wound or severe deformity is present. A physician is the only person who should attempt to straighten, or reduce, a fracture.

In addition to the fractures described in Chapter 13, Unit 5, you may have patients with extracapsular fractures, where the bone is broken just outside the joint; intracapsular fractures, where the bone is broken inside the joint; fracture dislocations, where the break is **complicated** by the end of the bone being out of the joint; pathologic fractures, or breaks at the site of a bone tumor or bone disease; longitudinal fractures, where the break is parallel with the bone; transverse fractures, where the break runs across the bone; and oblique fractures, where the break slants across the bone.

Heart Attack

When you are **confronted** with a patient who is complaining of severe chest pain, it is extremely important for the physician to diagnose whether the patient is suffering from a heart attack or indigestion. Other terms for a heart attack are coronary thrombosis, coronary occlusion, and myocardial infarction. The cause is usually a blockage of one or more of the coronary arteries. The patient may also complain of pain radiating down one or both arms and a tightness of the chest or pain radiating into the left shoulder and jaw (mandible). The pulse is usually rapid and weak. The patient may be perspiring profusely, have cyanotic lips and fingernails, and may be anxious and agitated.

Never allow such a patient to walk or carry objects such as a heavy purse or coat. If you have a wheelchair, help the patient into the chair. In the absence of a wheelchair, use any chair with rollers to move the patient to an examination room. Most cardiac patients prefer to have the head elevated.

The physician may want you to administer oxygen or prepare an injection for the patient. If the patient has a medication such as nitroglycerine, it should be given immediately. The patient should be quickly but calmly transported to a hospital if the physician is not in the office. If the physician is in, he or she will want an electrocardiogram done immediately, so you should loosen clothing and connect the ECG at once. Treat for shock by maintaining body heat. If the patient should stop breathing, start artificial respiration, and if there is no pulse, start CPR. These procedures will be discussed under respiratory emergencies. Always have the emergency tray with IV equipment ready for the physician.

Heat and Cold Exposure

Excessive heat is especially critical for elderly patients and you should recognize the differences between heatstroke and heat exhaustion. The patient suffering from heatstroke will have a red, dry face. The skin will be hot and dry and the temperature may be very high. The pulse will be strong, and respirations may be loud and difficult. The pupils of the eyes will be dilated but equal. The patient may have muscle tenseness or even convulsions. Treatment is bed rest with head elevated and the use of cold packs. The patient may be given normal saline infusion to force fluids.

In heat exhaustion the face is pale, cool, and moist. The skin is cool and clammy with profuse perspiration. There may be slight temperature elevation. The pulse is weak and rapid, and the respirations are quiet and shallow. The muscles may be tense. The pupils of the eyes are normal. The patient should be put in recumbent position with head lowered and warmth maintained for treatment of shock. If the patient is conscious, salt tablets may be given along with fruit juices in large amounts. If the patient is unconscious, an IV isotonic saline solution may be required.

The patient who is exposed to high temperatures for a long period of time in industry or at home may suffer from heat cramps. These patients may have diaphoresis and should drink large amounts of water. The problem is that they lose a large amount of body salt. The patient will complain of severe muscle cramps of the abdomen and legs and may also complain of faintness, dizziness, and exhaustion. First aid is designed to replace salt by taking salt tablets or drinking a solution of one teaspoon of table salt in a quart of water. If there is a problem with nausea when the patient uses salt tablets or table salt, a coated salt tablet may be given, or the patient may be encouraged to drink cool water with the salt tablets. Ice water should not be taken.

Exposure to freezing temperatures will often result in frostbite. The body parts most often damaged by cold are the hands, feet, ears, and nose. Symptoms that might indicate damaged tissue are a tingling sensation with numbness followed by pain and redness of the skin. If exposure is continued, the patient may complain of burning and itching. Sensation may be completely lost. The first aid required is to warm the part as quickly as possible by placing it in water with a temperature of 103° to 107° (39° to 41°C). This will help to reduce tissue damage. Never rub frostbite because this will cause tissue damage. Hot tea or coffee will help because they are both a stimulus and dilate blood vessels to increase circulation. The patient should not be allowed to smoke because the effect is to constrict blood vessels and decrease circulation.

Hemorrhage

It is important to understand what the different sources of bleeding are to determine the seriousness of hemorrhage. Arterial bleeding will produce bright red blood in spurts. If the ruptured artery is a large branch, death can occur in 3 minutes or less. Bleeding from a vein will produce a steady flow of dark red blood. It is important to control this bleeding quickly because of the danger of an air bubble getting into the bloodstream and causing a blockage in the heart. Any bleeding from capillary damage will produce a steady ooze from the wound area. This type of bleeding will often clot without first aid measures being taken.

Internal bleeding causes symptoms you should be able to recognize. They are similar to those of shock. The patient may have a rapid weak pulse, shallow breathing, cold clammy skin, dilated pupils, dizziness, faintness, thirst, restlessness, and a feeling of anxiety. Internal hemorrhage might need to be controlled by surgery. The patient must be kept in a recumbent position with strictly limited movement until the physician takes over care.

Internal bleeding may be difficult to detect unless it leads to external signs. The patient who coughs up bright red blood may have a lung hemorrhage. Vomiting bright red blood could mean the patient has an ulcer that has started bleeding. If the patient is coughing up what looks like coffee grounds it could indicate chronic slow bleeding into the stomach. If the patient notices coal-black stools there is probably a loss of blood in the intestines. If the patient has rectal hemorrhage it is likely to be from a lesion in the lower colon. A patient with severe abdominal pain from trauma may have a ruptured internal organ such as a kidney, liver, or spleen.

Epistaxis (nosebleed) may be the result of excessively dry air over a prolonged period of time, hypertension, injury, or simply blowing the nose too hard. First aid for epistaxis is to elevate the head and pinch the nostrils closed for at least 6 minutes. Keep the patient in a sitting position with the head tilted forward so that the blood trickling down the throat will not be aspirated. The use of a cold compress over the nasal area or on the back of the neck may be helpful. A piece of gauze may be placed between the lips and gums with pressure against this area for several minutes. Specially treated gauze is best to use for nasal packing because cotton is difficult to remove. A physician should be consulted if bleeding is not easily controlled. Sometimes the addition of humidity to the air will relieve the patient who has recurrent epistaxis.

If a pregnant patient experiences vaginal bleeding, you need to determine the kind of flow. If there is gushing blood, the patient should lie down immediately with feet elevated and an emergency squad should be called. If there has been discharge of clots or tissue substance, this should be taken to the hospital for analysis. Your employer will let you know how these emergencies should be handled.

Poisoning

Poison is not only **ingested,** it is absorbed, inhaled, injected, and produced by bites and stings.

If you get a call regarding a possible ingestion of poison, you should always ask what was taken, how much was taken, and the time it was taken. You should know the location and the telephone number of the local Poison Control Center so that you can direct callers to the best source of help. If an antidote is on the label of the poison, the patient should be given the antidote only after approval or order of the Poison Control Center or the physician. It is usually safe to dilute the poison with water or milk. If the substance is one which should be removed after diluting you may use Ipecac or large amounts of warm water or activated charcoal to induce vomiting. The area at the back of the tongue known as the gag reflex may be touched to cause vomiting also. If table salt is available you may add a small amount to warm water to induce vomiting. The patient should not be encouraged to vomit if a strong alkali, acid, or petroleum product has been ingested.

For poisoning from plants such as mushrooms or from bacterial-contaminated shellfish, the emergency treatment is to keep the patient as quiet as possible and induce vomiting.

Poisoning by inhalation may be caused by the use of cleaning fluids and sprays in a poorly ventilated area. Carbon monoxide poisoning may be caused by a faulty exhaust system in an automobile. First aid for inhalation poisoning is pulmonary resuscitation and immediate care in a hospital.

Poisoning by injection is usually the result of drug abuse. The patient may exhibit symptoms from confusion to excitement to hallucinations to convulsions. These patients need hospitalization for proper treatment.

Patients who are sensitive to insect stings may suffer anaphylactic shock and die if proper measures are not taken. They may show a decrease in blood pressure and difficulty breathing (dyspnea). They should be kept quiet and medical help obtained at once. The stinger should be brushed off. Any attempt to squeeze the stinger will inject more poison into the skin.

Many patients suffer from contact with poison ivy, poison sumac, and poison oak. A person who is sensitive to these poisons may not need to touch the plant but merely to pet a dog or cat which has come in contact with it. The patient will complain of reddening of the skin and blister formation that itches and is easily spread to other portions of the body. The physician may need to prescribe antihistamines (for relief of severe itching) and ointments (effective in clearing up the inflammation).

Respiratory Emergencies

One of the most common medical emergencies is an obstructed airway. The obstruction must be cleared away immediately as brain damage may result in 4 minutes from lack of oxygen. A person who is choking signals by placing the hand at the throat, Figure 21–9. Such an individual may make no sound but simply fall from the chair if nothing is done.

The method used to relieve an obstructed airway is a manual thrust, or subdiaphragmatic abdominal thrust also known as the Heimlich maneuver. You should stand behind the victim and reach around the waist. Clench one hand to make a fist and grasp your fist with the other hand. Place the thumb side of the fist against the midline of the victim's abdomen between the waist and the rib cage, Figure 21–10. Thrust fist inward and upward six to ten times in a quick, firm movement to move air out of the

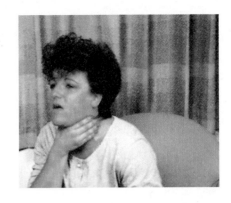

FIGURE 21–9 Universal distress signal for choking (From Caldwell & Hegner, *Health Care Assistant*, 5th ed. Copyright 1989, Delmar Publishers Inc.)

lungs and with enough force to dislodge the obstruction. A chest thrust may be used if the victim is pregnant or has a problem with exogenous obesity. Chest thrusts are exerted downward. The abdominal thrust may be performed on an unconscious victim by sitting astride the victim's thighs. The heel of one hand is placed on the midline of the breastbone (sternum). The second hand is placed on top of the first, and the thrust is inward and upward. A choking victim who is alone may use the abdominal thrust with the fist or may thrust against a chair back or any hard object of adequate height.

If the thrusts have dislodged the obstruction but not expelled it from the victim's mouth, then the finger sweep is performed. Open the victim's mouth by tilting the head back (do not use the former head tilt; use the modified jaw thrust) with one hand and moving the jaw forward to lift the tongue away from the back of the throat. Insert the index finger of the first hand along the side of the cheek and sweep deeply into the mouth in a

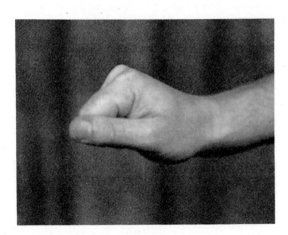

FIGURE 21–10 Hand placement for abdominal thrust (From Simmers, *Diversified Health Occupations*, 2d ed. Copyright 1988, Delmar Publishers Inc.)

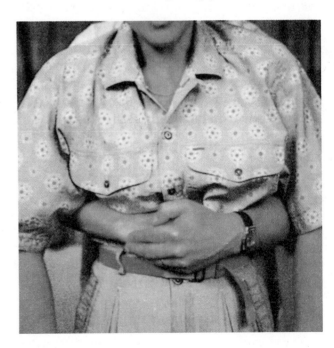

P R O C E D U R E

Give Mouth-to-Mouth Resuscitation

TERMINAL PERFORMANCE OBJECTIVE: In a simulated situation, using a training manikin, the student will demonstrate that he/she has learned the procedure in the course taught by a certified instructor by explaining each step as it is being demonstrated with 100% accuracy. Remember that you must follow universal precautions even in emergency situations when you may come into contact with blood or body fluids.

1. Position victim on back and use finger sweep of mouth to remove any foreign material.
   Key Points:
   a. **This may be accomplished with your finger alone or with a gauze sponge if these are available.**
   b. **This procedure is necessary to clear mouth area for mouth-to-mouth contact.**
2. Use modified jaw thrust, thereby moving tongue from back of throat. **Key Point: This opens victim's airway and determines whether victim is breathing independently. Continue with procedure if there are no breath sounds.**
3. Pinch victim's nostrils together with your fingers of one hand while leaving other hand on forehead to keep head tilted. **Key Point: This prevents escape of air through nose.**
4. Take a deep breath and then seal your mouth over victim's and breathe two times into the victim's mouth. Refill your lungs after each breath. This forces air into lungs for oxygen and carbon dioxide exchange. Breathe at a rate of 1 to $1\frac{1}{2}$ seconds for each breath.
   Key Points:
   a. **If mouth is injured, hold it shut and blow into nose.**
   b. **With small child, place your mouth over mouth and nose and blow into both, adjusting the force of your breaths to the size of the child.**
5. Turn your head to one side and listen for return of air. **Key Point: Watch chest for movement.**
6. Repeat this cycle of blowing and listening with approximately 12 breaths per minute for adults and 20 for children until breathing is fully restored or another medical helper takes over or physician is in charge. **Key Point: Number of breaths correspond to average number of breaths per minute for adults and children.**

hooking action. Be careful not to push an obstruction deeper into the throat. If it is possible to dislodge an obstruction, be sure to remove it from the mouth. If dentures are worn it is helpful to remove them. If the patient has vomited it is extremely important to turn the patient on the side and jut the jaw to keep an open airway and prevent inspiration of material into the lungs.

A patient suffering from severe edema of the vocal cords as a result of an allergic reaction to food or stings of bees or wasps must be hospitalized as quickly as possible.

The victim of a drowning must receive artificial respiration immediately. This can be given before the patient is taken from the water if there is help to support the patient while mouth to mouth resuscitation is given. Any surviving drowning victim needs to be hospitalized for follow-up of delayed reactions which are apt to occur. Poisoning by toxic gases such as carbon monoxide or suffocation may also require immediate artificial respiration.

The patient suffering from an asthma attack might have severe difficulty breathing. The physician must determine the treatment needed but you can be helpful in attempting to calm the patient. Remove the patient to a clean air environment. Emotional upset may start a severe asthmatic attack.

Some medications will cause a slowing or cessation of breathing. Electric shock may cause respiratory paralysis. The victim must be moved away from the source of the electricity and then be given artificial respiration and CPR if necessary.

All medical assistants should take a standard first aid course and a course in CPR. The following procedures are for review purposes only and should not be used as the primary means of learning these skills.

CPR must be learned by taking a course from a certified instructor. Procedures are constantly being refined and the procedure you learn should be the one you practice. There is currently a recommendation that a one-way valve face piece be used in a health care environment as a guard against AIDS. If that is not possible, the mouth-to-nose method is recommended. According to the American Heart Association, two-man CPR is no longer used or taught to basic emergency care providers. The exception to the teaching or the practice of two-man CPR is to persons in an advanced training program.

The CPR procedure has some variations when used for a child or infant. Infants are generally considered to be under 1 year of age and children ages 1 to 8. Adult procedure would be used for anyone over 8.

Shock may be associated with many different kinds of injuries and is a serious depressor of vital body functions. Symptoms include a rapid, thready, weak pulse; shallow, rapid respirations; dilated pupils; ashen

P R O C E D U R E

Give Cardiopulmonary Resuscitation

TERMINAL PERFORMANCE OBJECTIVE: In a simulated situation, using a training manikin (Figure 21–11), the student will demonstrate that he/she has learned the procedure in the course taught by a certified instructor by explaining each step as it is being demonstrated with 100% accuracy. Remember that you must follow universal precautions even in emergency situations when you may come into contact with blood or body fluids.

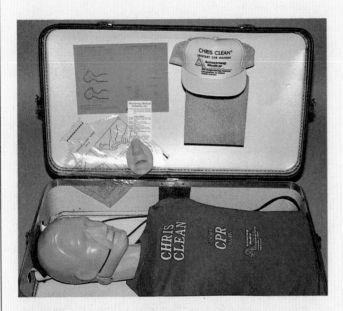

FIGURE 21–11   Cris clean CPR training manikins with disposable parts

1. Position manikin on back on blanket on floor.
   Key Points:
   a. Victim must always be in recumbent position on firm surface (floor or ground).
   b. Never practice this procedure on a person.
2. Gently shake victim and ask "Are you OK?" Call for help. **Key Point: This should always be done so that you will not forget with a real patient.**
3. Place one hand on forehead to tilt head back and use the other hand to lift chin, Figure 21–12. **Key Point: This opens airway.**
4. Check for breathing by putting your ear close to victim's nose and mouth and watch chest for rise and fall. **Key Point: Check for 3 to 5 seconds.**
5. If victim is not breathing, keep airway open, pinch nose, seal your mouth over victim's, and breathe twice into victim's mouth. Refill your lungs after each breath.
   Key Points:
   a. Watch chest for evidence that air is entering lungs.
   b. Request that someone get help if victim is not breathing.
6. Check for carotid pulse by placing your index and middle fingers into natural groove at side of neck. Take at least 5 to 10 seconds to locate pulse. **Key Point: Check carefully as pulse will probably be weak.**
7. If victim has a pulse, continue mouth-to-mouth respirations at rate of one breath every 5 seconds (12 times per minute). **Key Point: Correct timing can be obtained by counting one, one thousand; two, one**

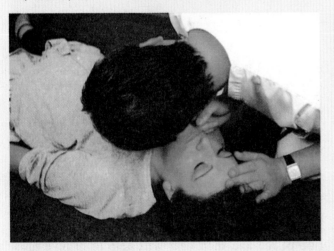

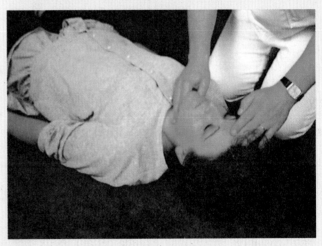

FIGURE 21–12   Basic CPR for adults: (a). After opening the airway, look, listen, and feel for breathing; if the victim is not breathing, give two slow, full breaths. (b). Palpate the carotid pulse for at least five seconds to determine whether or not the heart is beating. (c, page 672). Use smooth, even motions to compress the chest straight down, about 1 to 2 inches in an adult. (From Simmers, *Diversified Health Occupations*, 2d ed. Copyright 1989, Delmar Publishers Inc.)

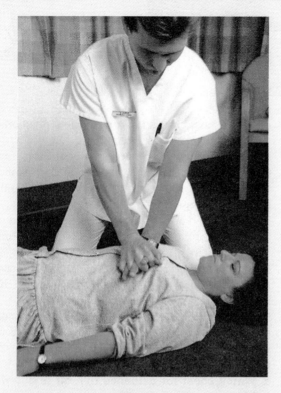

thousand; three, one thousand; four, one thousand; and breathe. Go to Step 16.

8. If victim does not have a pulse, chest compression must be started. Locate lower margin of victim's rib cage and follow it to notch where ribs meet sternum in center of chest.

9. Place index finger on lower end of sternum.

10. Heel of hand closest to head is then placed on lower sternum next to index finger of first hand.

11. Place heel of hand which located notch over hand on sternum and lock fingers. Hold fingers high, away from body.

12. Rise on your knees so your shoulders are directly over hands on victim's sternum. Lock your elbows and keep arms straight.

13. Use a smooth, even motion to push straight down on chest and compress about 1 to 2 inches for a count of 15 compressions. A count of one and, two and, three and, etc. will help you obtain correct rate. (The rate of compressions is 80 to 100 times per minute.)

14. After administering 15 compressions, give victim two mouth-to-mouth respirations or ventilations **Key Point: Do this without moving from your position beside body.**

15. Repeat 4 cycles of compressions and respirations before pausing to check for breathing and presence of carotid pulse.
    Key Points:
    a. **If no pulse is felt, resume compressions and respirations.**
    b. **check every few minutes or when second rescuer arrives.**

16. You must not discontinue CPR unless victim recovers, someone takes over for you, a physician pronounces victim dead, or you become so exhausted that you cannot continue.

17. Use alcohol or Zephiran to clean manikin. It is recommended that manikins with disposable mouthpieces and air bags are used in training for CPR, as shown in Figure 21–11, page 671, to prevent disease transmission. For those manikins that have no disposable parts, they must be carefully and faithfully cleaned after each use with a clean gauze pad soaked in a liquid chlorine bleach and water solution, or with rubbing alcohol. The soaked gauze pad should remain on the area for at least 30 seconds and then wiped clean. It should be dried with a clean gauze pad.

color; and cool clammy skin. All of these result from decreased blood volume, as there is diminished cardiac output and the blood pressure drops. It is possible for shock to cause death even when the injury causing the shock is not life-threatening. First aid measures include placing the patient in recumbent position with feet elevated unless there is a head injury, in which case the patient is kept flat. If the patient has difficulty breathing or has a chest injury, the head and shoulders should be elevated. It is best to place a blanket under and over the patient to maintain body warmth but not to overheat.

Anaphylactic shock is an acute allergic reaction to a foreign substance, which may include certain foods, bee stings, or injections of therapeutic or prophylactic substances. The patient will have severe difficulty breathing, blueness of the skin, and may have convulsions. The emergency supplies of epinephrine and oxygen should be immediately available for use by the physician or by the medical assistant under the direction of the physician. No patient should be given an allergy injection and then be allowed to leave the office immediately as anaphylactic shock may result from these injections. Patients may also have severe reactions to penicillin.

Sprains and Strains

Strains are the result of overuse of a muscle or group of muscles. They may be caused by improper lifting or by slipping while moving a heavy object. First aid is to rest the injured muscles in a comfortable position. Application of ice and then heat will help to relieve muscle strain. The physician may prescribe an analgesic or muscle relaxant.

Sprains are injuries to ligaments surrounding a joint. They are usually the result of twisting the joint and are sometimes so severe that a fracture may also occur.

Give Cardiopulmonary Resuscitation to Infants and Children

TERMINAL PERFORMANCE OBJECTIVE: In a simulated situation, using a training manikin, the student will demonstrate that he/she has learned the procedure in the course as taught by a certified instructor by explaining each step as it is being demonstrated with 100% accuracy. Remember that you must follow universal precautions even in emergency situations when you may come into contact with blood or body fluids.

1. Gently shake infant or child or tap bottom of foot to check for consciousness. Place infant or child on back on firm surface. **Key Point: Send someone for help if there is no response.**

2. Tip victim's head back and lift chin to open airway, Figure 21–13. **Key Point: Be careful not to tip head too far back as this can cause obstruction of airway in infant.**

3. Listen and watch for breathing. Place ear by mouth to listen. Also feel for breath on cheek and watch chest for breathing.

4. If no breathing is observed, give 2 slow breaths, 1 to 1 seconds each.
   Key Points:
   a. **For infants, cover nose and mouth with your mouth and breathe gently.**
   b. **For a child, cover mouth and pinch nostrils and carefully give two slow breaths.**

5. For a child, check carotid pulse as for an adult. For an infant, check pulse over brachial artery by putting your middle fingertips on inside of upper arm halfway between elbow and shoulder. At the same time, keep airway open. **Key Point: Child's pulse should be checked at brachial artery for no longer than 10 seconds.**

6. If pulse is present, continue giving an infant one breath every 3 seconds and a child one ventilation every 4 seconds. Go to Step 8.

7. If no pulse is present, start cardiac compression. For an infant, use two fingers to compress middle of sternum to 1 inch at rate of 100 per minute. For a child use adult hand position, but use only the heel of one hand. Compress 1 to $1\frac{1}{2}$ inches at rate of 80 to 100 times per minute. Give one breath for every 5 compressions.
   Key Points:
   a. **Be sure infant or child is on a firm surface or is being supported in back while administering compressions.**
   b. **Correct rate for infants could be counted as one, two, three, four, five, breathe.**
   c. **Correct rate for child would be one and two and three and four and five and breathe.**

8. Do 10 cycles of compression and breath, and then check for breathing and pulse. **Key Point: Do not take more than 5 seconds for this check.**

9. If no pulse, give one breath and continue cycle until help arrives.

10. Clean manikin at end of practice according to manufacturer's instructions.

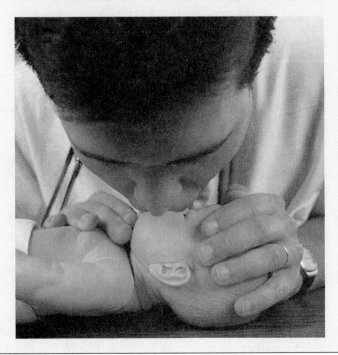

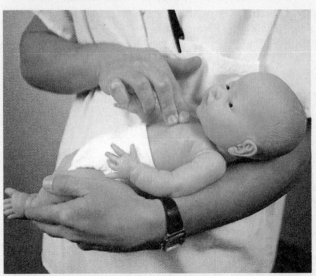

FIGURE 21–13 Basic CPR for infants (From Caldwell & Hegner, Health Care Assistant, 5th ed. Copyright 1989, Delmar Publishers Inc.)

Treatment is to elevate the sprained area and apply ice for the first 24 hours. The ice should be applied as soon as possible after the injury takes place. An elastic bandage is helpful but should not be put on too tightly. Temporary support may be given to an ankle by use of a cravat bandage, which may be applied over the shoe. (Note: a cravat is a folded, triangular bandage.)

Applying Heat and Cold Treatments. In the treatment of injuries often physicians order the application of a heat or cold pack, Figure 21–14. The physician will give specific instructions concerning the length of time and where to apply the treatment.

Many offices and clinics today use disposable heat and cold packs because of their convenience. These plastic packs contain chemicals that are activated by either squeezing the bag and mixing the contents to produce cold, or by bending a metal disc to initiate heat. Many of these disposable packs are reusable by boiling or freezing them, which is of further convenience to the patient. With either of these packs it is recommended that the pack be placed in a cloth covering or a cloth or disposable towel be placed next to the area to protect the skin. If the physician requests moist heat or cold treatment, you should use a clean moist cloth towel between the plastic pack and the skin. Moisture better facilitates conduction of cold to tissues. Moist heat is less likely to cause burns of the skin or dry it. It also provides deeper penetration to tissues. Unless otherwise ordered by the physician, the pack should be left in place for 20 minutes at a time. The maximum is 30 minutes. Generally the standard instruction is on 20 minutes and off 10. This may be repeated to increase circulation, but constant hot or cold is never advised.

Application of cold decreases local circulation temporarily, bacterial growth, and body temperature. It also is a temporary anesthetic, relieves inflammation, helps control bleeding, and reduces swelling. The average temperature is between 50° and 80°F (10° to 26.7°C). Cold applications are used in burns, sprains, strains, and bruises and in the initial treatment of injuries to the eye.

Heat applications are used to increase tissue temperature, circulation, and rate of healing. When heat is applied to an injured area, pain decreases. The average temperature is between 105° and 120°F (40.6° to 49°C). Heat treatments are used to relieve congestion in deep muscle layers and visceral organs and muscle spasms.

Stroke

For a patient with a cerebrovascular accident (CVA), you should loosen the clothing and be sure the patient is positioned so as not to choke on excess saliva. The common terms for a CVA are stroke, apoplexy, or cerebral thrombosis. A CVA is the result of a ruptured blood vessel in the brain. A CVA can also be caused by an occlusion of a blood vessel. The patient may have a light stroke with very little damage or an immediate paralysis in the form of sagging muscles on one side of the face or inability to use an arm or leg. One entire side of the body may be paralyzed. The patient may complain of numbness. The pupils of the eyes may be unequal in size. There may be mental confusion, slurred speech, nausea, vomiting, or difficulty in breathing and swallowing. Avoid any unnecessary movement of the patient. Keep in mind that the patient who appears to be unconscious or unable to speak may be able to hear what is being said.

Wounds

You should be able to recognize and treat many types of wounds. Abrasions involve a scrape of the epidermis with dots of blood and possibly the presence of foreign material such as dirt or gravel. First aid is to carefully clean the area with soap and water, apply an antiseptic solution or ointment, and cover with a dressing. If the abrasion resulted from contact with rusty metal or an unusually dirty object, a tetanus toxoid or antitoxin may be required.

A wound caused by a sharp object that leaves a clean cut is called an incision and may need sutures to close. Some people prefer to use tape for closure rather than sutures. The area must be carefully cleaned with soap and water, and an antiseptic may be applied before covering with a sterile dressing. A laceration is a tearing of body tissue and is more difficult to clean and suture properly. Special care must be taken to avoid infection. In the first aid care of an incision or laceration, the first concern must be control of bleeding. This is accomplished with direct pressure to the wound area and elevation of the wound area, Figure 21–15. If direct pressure is not effective, indirect pressure on the appropriate pressure point should be used, Figure 21–16. A puncture wound is one made with a pointed object such

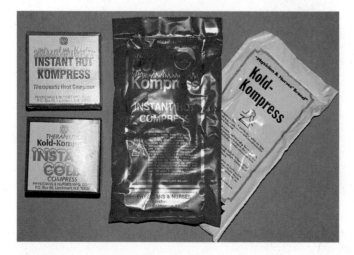

FIGURE 21–14 Examples of heat and cold disposable packs before activating chemicals

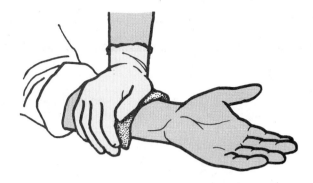

FIGURE 21–15 Direct pressure

as an icepick, knife, or nail. First aid is to clean the wound area and if necessary enlarge the hole with a probe to allow for irrigation with antiseptic solutions. A puncture wound may be the result of an animal bite or human bite. It is usually possible to identify the type of bite by looking at the shape of the wound. For example, a snake bite would show a two-fang wound; it generally would be treated with a tourniquet tight enough to prevent venous return. Ice packs might also be used to prevent absorption of venom. Treatment must be given at once. A human bite is identified by the shape of the denture and needs to be carefully cleaned. An animal bite may result in a laceration. Any bite, human or animal, that breaks the skin should be seen by a physician. It is also important to report animal bites to the health department authorities so that the animal can be confined and checked for rabies. The bite should be cleaned thoroughly by washing with soap and water and dressed. If the animal shows evidence of rabies, a full 14 days of vaccine injections is necessary to protect the patient. A gunshot wound entrance will be a small deep puncture site with evidence in some cases of powder burns. This type of wound needs to be treated by a physician. First aid would be to keep the patient in shock position and carefully monitor vital signs while taking measures to control hemorrhage. Gunshot or stab wounds must be reported to the police. The location of either of these wounds would dictate the first aid measures to be taken. If a lung puncture is suspected, do not remove the object; sent the patient immediately to an emergency facility.

Substance Abuse

Drug dependency is an increasing problem that will often create emergency situations. You need to know the symptoms associated with the various substances abused so that appropriate questions may be asked in taking a history from family members, Table 21–2, pages 676–679.

The authorities are greatly concerned about marijuana use because it is often contaminated by addition of other substances. It may also be a stepping stone to more serious substance abuse. The effects of marijuana are swings

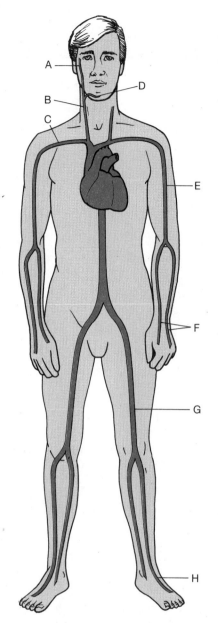

FIGURE 21–16 Pressure points: temporal artery (A), carotid artery (B), subclavian artery (C), facial artery (D), brachial artery (E), radial artery (F), femoral artery (G), dorsalis pedis (H)

from an unreasonable feeling of well-being, to disorientation in time, confusion, and irritability. The individual may lose the ability to accomplish anything requiring effort or concentration. Chronic asthma and bronchitis may also result.

The LSD user is described as experiencing sudden changes in the physical sense, and more acute sensory impressions. These individuals sometimes seem to be happy and sad at the same time. The effects are not always the same, and users describe "good trips" and "bad trips." These individuals may lose all sense of proportion and judgment and fancy themselves as having unusual powers. The user of LSD may develop strong **psychopathic** tendencies.

TABLE 21–2
Commonly abused substances

DRUG	PRESCRIPTION (BRAND NAME)	MEDICAL USE	HOW ADMINISTERED	STREET NAME
LSD	None	None	Orally, injection	Acid, cubes, purple haze
Psilocybin, psilocin	None	None	Orally (ingested in natural form)	Magic mushrooms
Inhalants: Gasoline, airplane glue, paint thinner, dry-cleaning solution	None	None	Sniffed inhaled	
Nitrous oxide (N₂O)	Nitrous oxide	Anesthetic in dentistry	Inhaled	Laughing gas, whippets
Nitrites: Amyl, butyl	Amyl nitrite	Vasodilator	Inhaled, sniffed	Poppers, locker room, rush, snappers
Marijuana, hashish	None	None	Orally, smoked	Pot, grass, reefer, weed, Columbian, hash, hash oil, joint, sinsemilla
Tranquilizers	Librium, valium, tranxene	Antianxiety, muscle relaxant, sedation	Orally	
Narcotics	Percodan	Analgesic	Orally, injection	
	Codeine	Analgesic	Orally, injection	School boy
	Heroin	None	Injection sniffed	Dreamer, junk, horse, smack
	Morphine	Analgesic	Injection, smoked	

The chronic cocaine abuser may have elevated blood pressure, rapid pulse, dilated pupils, and may be nervous and apprehensive.

Amphetamines are powerful central nervous system stimulants and require a prescription for purchase, but there is considerable black market production of lookalikes. The illegal user of this type of drug develops a dependence and requires larger and larger amounts to obtain the desired "high." Abuse of this drug may cause hallucinations severe enough to require hospitalization. Large doses make patients irritable and may create difficulty in speaking clearly. Amphetamines also affect blood pressure and respirations, and cause arrhythmia of the heart. The pupils may be dilated, and excess sweating, headache, and diarrhea may be experienced.

Barbiturates are also addictive. They lower blood pressure and respiratory rate and the patient may suffer from mental disorientation, slurred speech, and staggering gait. An overdose of a barbiturate may cause death. The sudden withdrawal of barbiturates may cause nausea, delirium, convulsions, and death.

Alcohol dependence may result in emergency situations because of accidents in which alcoholics are involved. Alcohol acts as a depressant on the central nervous system and becomes addictive. The patient may develop grand mal epilepsy or **delirium tremens** when alcohol is withdrawn.

You must be aware of the problems of narcotic addiction. It is important to keep any narcotic supply in the office locked in a cabinet at all times. Physicians are

TABLE 21–2
Commonly abused substances

LENGTH OF EFFECTS (HRS)	POSSIBLE SYMPTOMS OF USE	HAZARDS OF LONG-TERM USE/OVERDOSE	SYMPTOMS OF WITHDRAWAL
Variable	Dilated pupils, illusions, mood swings, hallucinations, poor perception of time and distance	Breaks from reality, emotional breakdown, flashback	Not reported
Variable	Poor motor coordination, impaired vision, poor memory and thought processes, abusive and violent behavior	High risk of sudden death; weight loss; and damage to brain, liver, and bone marrow	
	Lightheaded feeling	Death by anoxia, muscle weakness, neuropathy	
Seconds to minutes	Slowed thought process, headache	Anemia, death by anoxia	
2–4	Euphoria, increase in appetite, short-term memory loss, disorientation, loss of interest and motivation, neglect of appearance	Lung damage, possible reproductive system damage, loss of motivation, damage to immune system and heart, interference with psychological maturation, impaired memory perception, psychological dependence	Insomnia, hyperactivity, and decreased appetite reported in some individuals
4–8	Drowsiness, confusion, slurred speech, impaired judgment, drunken behavior without odor of alcohol, constricted pupils	Nausea, addiction with severe withdrawal symptoms, loss of appetite, death from overdose, shallow respiration, cold and clammy skin, dilated pupils, weak and rapid pulse, coma	Anxiety, insomnia, tremors, delirium, convulsions, possible death
3–6	Nausea, drowsiness, respiratory depression, constricted pupils, lethargy, euphoria	Addiction with severe from overdose, loss of appetite	Watery eyes, runny nose, loss of appetite yawning, irritability panic, chills, sweating, cramps, nausea
3–6			
3–6	Needle marks		
3–6			

careful to regulate the narcotics prescribed for a patient but patients may see more than one physician for the purpose of obtaining narcotic prescriptions. You should be certain prescription pads are not left where they can be stolen and the name of the physician forged. It is also important to keep syringes and needles where patients cannot easily obtain them. You should be able to recognize chronic narcotic abusers. Some might have scars over veins used for injecting substances such as heroin or crack cocaine. The addict may attempt to cover up pin-point pupils by wearing dark glasses. These individuals may have ulcerated areas at the injection sites and also frequently suffer from hepatitis from use of dirty needles. To prevent being unnecessarily exposed, you should always remember to use universal precautions when caring for all patients, especially when the risk of AIDS and hepatitis B is so great.

Emergency Services ....

You should be able to contact the service that will be able to give the most help in an emergency. Contact the fire and police departments before you need them to find out what help is available and the quickest way to obtain that help. Find out what information must be reported in an emergency. The list of emergency numbers should be posted by every phone in the office and on a card on the emergency supply tray. All office staff should be aware of this information. The card kept on the tray can be handed

TABLE 21–2
Commonly abused substances

DRUG	PRESCRIPTION (BRAND NAME)	MEDICAL USE	HOW ADMINISTERED	STREET NAME
Hallucinogens (drugs that alter one's perception of reality)	PCP (Phencyclidine)		Orally, smoked inhaled, snorted, injection	Angel dust, killer weed, supergrass, hog, PeaCe Pill
	Sernylan	Veterinary anesthetic		
Mescaline	None	None	Orally, injection	Mesc, cactus
Alcohol	Ethanol	None	Swallowed in liquid form	Booze, hooch, brew
Depressants (drugs that depress the CNS)				
Chloral hydrate	Notec, somnos	Hypnotic	Orally	Downer
Barbiturates	Butisal, nembutal, phenobarbital, seconal, secobarbital	Anesthetic, anticonvulsant, sedation, sleep	Orally, injection	Barbs, downers, yellow jackets, red devils, blue devils
Glutehimide	Doriden	Sedation, sleep	Orally	
Methaqualone	Parest, quaalude, somnafac	Sedation, sleep	Orally	
Stimulants (drugs that stimulate the CNS)	Cocaine	Local anesthetic	Injection, sniffed, smoked, or snorted, orally	Coke, crack, rock, snow, toot, white lady
Amphetamines	Dextroamphetamine Biphetamine Benzedrine	Hyperkinesis, narcolepsy, weight control	Orally, injection	Speed, uppers, pep, pills, meth, bennies, dexies, black beauties,
Phenmatrazine	Preludin	Weight control	Orally	lid poppers
Methylphenidate	Ritalin, cylert, didrex	Hyperkinesis	Orally	
Nicotine		None	Smoked (snuff or chew)	Coffin nail, smoke, butt

TABLE 21–2
Commonly abused substances

LENGTH OF EFFECTS (HRS)	POSSIBLE SYMPTOMS OF USE	HAZARDS OF LONG-TERM USE/OVERDOSE	SYMPTOMS OF WITHDRAWAL
Variable	Slurred speech, blurred vision, confusion, aggression, uncoordination, agitation, needle marks	Anxiety, depression, impaired memory and perception, death from accidents/overdose	Not reported
	Illusions and hallucinations, poor perception of time and distance	Longer, more intense trip episodes, psychosis	
Hours—depends on amount consumed	Impaired muscle coordination, and judgment	Heart and liver damage, death from overdose, death from auto accidents, addiction	Weakness, sweating, hyperreflexia, delirium tremens
5–8	Drowsiness, confusion, slurred speech, impaired judgment, drunken behavior without odor of alcohol, constricted pupils	Nausea, addiction with severe withdrawal symptoms, loss of appetite, death from overdose, shallow respiration, cold and clammy skin, dilated pupils, weak and rapid pulse, coma	Anxiety, insomnia, tremors, delirium, convulsions, possible death
1–16	Needle marks		
4–8			
4–8			
2	Restlessness, anxiety, intense short-term euphoria followed by dysphoria, dilated pupils, increased pulse rate and blood pressure, insomnia, loss of appetite	Intense psychological dependence, sleeplessness and anxiety, lung and nasal passage damage, death from overdose	Apathy, long periods of sleep, irritability, depression, disorientation
2–4	Excess activity, mood swings, irritability, nervousness, needle marks, dilated pupils, increased pulse rate and blood pressure,	Loss of appetite, hallucinations, paranoia, convulsions, coma, agitation, increase in body temperature, death from overdose	Apathy, long periods of sleep, irritability, depression, disorientation
2–4	insomnia, loss of appetite		
2–4			
Variable	Smell of tobacco, stained teeth and fingers, high carbon monoxide levels	Cancers of the lung, throat, mouth, esophagus, heart disease, emphysema, irritation/diseases of the GI and urinary tract; frequent URI, "smoker's cough"	Irritability, insomnia, nervousness

to a family member to call for help while you administer first aid to the patient or assist the physician in this care.

If all emergency care fails and the patient should die in the office and the physician is not there at the time, the medics may be called to pronounce the patient deceased. Arrange, if possible, for the body to be removed from the office through a back door and not the waiting room. The police must be notified, and usually they notify the coroner who will pick up the body for postmortem examination. A copy of the death certificate should be filed in the deceased patient's chart. It is important to find out what the procedure is in the area where you are working. The local statutes dictate the procedure to be followed.

Complete Chapter 21, Unit 2 in the workbook to help you meet the objectives at the beginning of this unit and therefore achieve competency of this subject matter.

UNIT 3

First Aid Care of Accidents and Injuries

OBJECTIVES

Upon completion of this unit, the student will meet the following terminal performance objectives by verifying knowledge of the facts and principles presented through oral and written communication at a level deemed competent, and will demonstrate the specific behaviors as identified in the terminal performance objectives of the procedures, observing all aseptic and safety precautions in accordance with health care standards.

1. Demonstrate the proper method of cleaning a wound.
2. Demonstrate application of dressing and recurrent turn bandages.
3. Demonstrate application of dressing and open spiral bandage.
4. Demonstrate application of dressing and closed spiral bandage.
5. Demonstrate application of dressing and figure-eight bandage to the hand.
6. Demonstrate application of cravat bandage to the head.
7. Demonstrate application of triangular bandage to the head.
8. Demonstrate application of sling.
9. Demonstrate application of tube gauze.
10. Demonstrate fitting and instruction in use of crutches.
11. Demonstrate fitting and instruction in use of cane.
12. Demonstrate instruction in use of walker.
13. Demonstrate movement of patient from wheelchair to and from examination table.
14. Spell and define, using the glossary at the back of the text, all the words to know in this unit.

 ## P R O C E D U R E

Clean Wound Areas

TERMINAL PERFORMANCE OBJECTIVE: Provided with all necessary equipment and supplies, and using other students as patients, the student will demonstrate the steps in this procedure for cleansing wounds. The instructor will observe each step. Remember that you must follow universal precautions even in emergency situations when you may come into contact with blood or body fluids.

1. Assemble basin, mild detergent with warm water, sterile gauze sponges, sterilized sponge forceps, and latex gloves.
2. Wash your hands thoroughly with soap and water. Put on gloves.
3. Grasp several gauze sponges with sponge forceps.
4. Dip into warm detergent water.
5. Wash wound and wound area to remove microorganisms and any foreign matter.
   Key Points:
   a. **Be careful not to injure patient further with instrument. Wash wound area with sponges only.**

   b. **Work from inner to outer area 2 to 3 inches around wound as you would for surgical prep. This will prevent bringing microorganisms from surrounding skin into open wound.**
6. Rinse thoroughly with clean tap water. **Key Point: This can best be done under warm running water. The physician may order sterile water for irrigation to rinse the wound.**
7. Blot wound dry with sterile gauze.
8. Cover with dry sterile dressing and bandage in place.
9. Advise patient to call physician immediately if evidence of infection should develop. **Key Point: Patient should be told to watch for redness, swelling, and sensation of pain or fever. Typed instructions should be given patient for follow-up care.**
10. Clean up work area. Place all blood-stained materials in the biohazardous waste bag and into proper receptacle for safe disposal.
11. Remove gloves and wash hands.

PROCEDURE

Prepare Basic Suture Setup

TERMINAL PERFORMANCE OBJECTIVE: Provided with all necessary equipment and supplies, the student will demonstrate all steps required in the basic suture setup procedure. The instructor will observe each step. Remember that you must follow universal precautions even in emergency situations when you may come into contact with blood or body fluids.

1. Wash your hands.
2. Assemble local anesthetic as directed by physician, sterile dressings and bandages, tape, and appropriate drape.
3. On a sterile towel, assemble sterile gloves, syringe and needle, hemostats, scissors, sponges, suture and needle holder, and forceps.
   Key Points:
   a. **Your office procedure manual should list items your employer wants ready.**
   b. **As you gain experience, you should also have your own reference cards to help you remember wishes of your employer in regard to various procedures.**
4. You may be instructed to bandage area when suturing is completed.
   Key Points:
   a. **Always hold dressing material by edges which will not touch wound.**
   b. **In bandaging, be careful to make bandage snug enough to hold dressing in place but not so tight that circulation is impaired or patient is uncomfortable.**
5. You are usually expected to give patient instructions for follow-up care. **Key Point: Have follow-up instructions in printed form as patients are often so upset because of trauma that they do not comprehend what you tell them.**
6. Make an appointment for suture removal.
7. Clean up work area.

WORDS TO KNOW ....

axilla   friction   recurrent

Human skin cannot be sterilized, but the microorganisms that may be harmful can be washed off with soap and water using **friction** at the skin surface. The procedure of cleaning a wound is usually the responsibility of the medical assistant. If bleeding has been severe, no attempt should be made to clean the area because the patient will need medical care. A pressure bandage should be applied securely and the patient taken for emergency medical care immediately. If the office/clinic

---

PROCEDURE

Apply Bandage in Recurrent Turn to Finger

TERMINAL PERFORMANCE OBJECTIVE: Provided all necessary equipment and supplies and using other students as patients, the student will demonstrate the steps in the procedure for recurrent turn. The instructor will observe each step. Remember that you must follow universal precautions even in emergency situations when you may come into contact with blood or body fluids.

This procedure will show you how to bandage after the wound area has been covered so there should be no possibility of coming into contact with blood or body fluids.

1. Wash hands.
2. Assemble supplies: dressing, scissors, bandage, antiseptic or medication as ordered.
3. Carefully open dressing by grasping edge and place over injury area.
4. Secure dressing with bandage of gauze, which is started at the proximal end of the finger on the palm side and then directly over the finger to the proximal end on the back of the hand and repeated several times.
5. Hold recurrent turns in place with spiral turns.
6. Secure by tying off at proximal end of finger. The tying off may be accomplished by using a figure-eight turn:
   a. From the finger take the end of the bandage diagonally across the back of the hand to the wrist.
   b. Circle the wrist once or twice.
   c. From the opposite side of the wrist, continue back to finger and loop.
   d. Repeat the figure eight several times and tie off at wrist, or tape in place.
7. Clean up area.

policy is to treat such emergencies, you should notify the appropriate staff and follow the procedure quickly to prepare for treatment of the patient. When the wound does not bleed excessively and does not involve tissues below the skin, the area should be thoroughly cleaned.

If a wound is superficial and will heal well with simple cleaning and protection from contamination, there is no need for sutures. Some clean cuts may be closed with adhesive steristrips or butterfly closures. You will be responsible for having suture setup packets sterilized and ready for use when the physician needs them. The emergency patient who needs suturing may come to the office with a pressure dressing in place to control hemorrhage. You should wait for instructions from the physician before removing a pressure dressing. You may question the patient or a relative to find out what caused the wound and how large and deep it is. You should also inquire about the most recent tetanus immunization booster and record the

information on the patient's chart. The physician will write the orders for the necessary immunization(s) the patient may need. You should not proceed with any medication or injection until the order has been written by the physician.

An injury to fingers or toes or an amputation can be effectively bandaged with the use of a non-stick dressing over the wound area which is held in place with **recurrent** turns, Figure 21–17.

An injury on the arms or legs will require a dressing to be held in place with an open or closed spiral bandage, Figure 21–18.

A wound on the palm or back of the hand may be protected with a dressing and a figure-eight bandage to hold the dressing in place.

When a dressing is needed for the forehead, ears, or eyes, a cravat may be used to hold the dressing in place. A cravat can be made from a triangular bandage, Figure 21–21.

P R O C E D U R E

Apply Bandage in Open or Closed Spiral

TERMINAL PERFORMANCE OBJECTIVE: Provided all necessary equipment and supplies and using other students as patients, the student will demonstrate the steps in the procedure for application of open and closed spiral bandage. The instructor will observe each step. Remember that you must follow universal precautions even in emergency situations when you may come into contact with blood or body fluids.

This procedure will show you how to bandage after the wound area has been covered so there should be no possibility of coming into contact with blood or body fluids.

1. Wash hands.
2. Assemble needed supplies.
3. Carefully open dressing, touching only edge, and place over wound area.
4. Anchor bandage by placing end of bandage on bias at starting point.
5. Encircle part, allowing corner of bandage end to protrude.
6. Turn down protruding tip of bandage.
7. Encircle part again.
8. Continue to encircle area to be covered with spiral turns spaced so that they do not overlap.
   OR
   Form closed spiral by continuing to encircle with overlapping spiral turns until all open spaces are covered.
9. Complete bandage by tying off or taping in place
   Key Points:
   a. **Tape should be long enough to hold bandage snugly in place.**
   b. **Tape should be applied to run in opposite direc-**

tion from body movement.
   c. **Tearing adhesive tape is made easier by holding edge between thumbnails and forefingers and using a quick rotary direction of hands in opposite directions, Figure 21–19.**
10. Clean up work area.

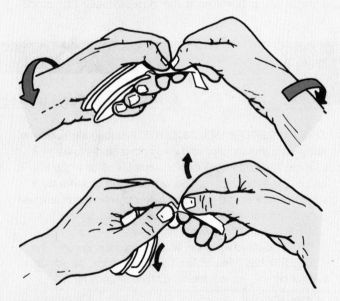

FIGURE 21–19 Tearing adhesive tape is much simpler when holding the edge of the strip between the thumbnails and forefingers and using a quick rotary motion of the hands in opposite directions.

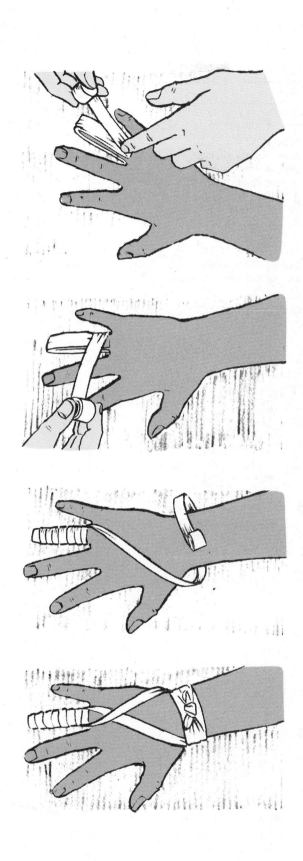

FIGURE 21–17 Recurrent turn on finger (From Simmers, *Diversified Health Occupations*, copyright 1988, Delmar Publishers Inc.)

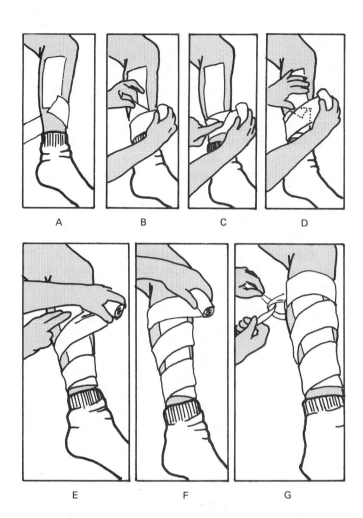

FIGURE 21–18 Application of bandage in open spiral

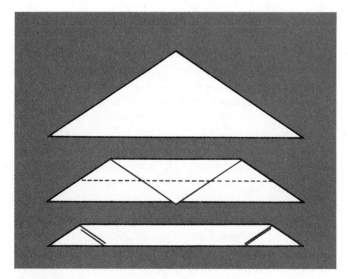

FIGURE 21–21 Folding a triangular bandage to make a cravat bandage (Adapted from Simmers, *Diversified Health Occupations*, copyright 1988, Delmar Publishers Inc.)

PROCEDURE

Apply Figure-Eight Bandage to Hand and Wrist

TERMINAL PERFORMANCE OBJECTIVE: Provided all necessary equipment and supplies and using other students as patients, the student will demonstrate the steps in the procedure for applying a figure-eight bandage to hand and wrist. The instructor will observe each step. Remember that you must follow universal precautions even in emergency situations when you may come into contact with blood or body fluids.

This procedure will show you how to bandage after the wound area has been covered so there should be no possibility of coming into contact with blood or body fluids.

1. Wash hands.
2. Assemble needed supplies.
3. Apply dressing, taking care not to touch any part which will touch wound area.
4. Anchor bandage with one or two turns around palm of hand.
5. Roll gauze diagonally across front of wrist and in figure-8 pattern around the hand as many times as necessary, Figure 21–20.

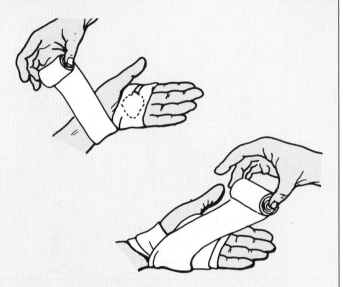

FIGURE 21–20 Figure-eight bandage

6. Tie off at wrist.
7. Clean up work area.

PROCEDURE

Apply Cravat Bandage to Forehead, Ear, or Eyes

TERMINAL PERFORMANCE OBJECTIVE: Provided all necessary equipment and supplies and using other students as patients, the student will demonstrate the steps in the procedure for applying a cravat bandage to the head. The instructor will observe each step. Remember that you must follow universal precautions even in emergency situations when you may come into contact with blood or body fluids.

This procedure will show you how to bandage after the wound area has been covered so there should be no possibility of coming into contact with blood or body fluids.

1. Wash hands.
2. Assemble needed supplies.
3. Carefully place dressing over wound taking care not to touch area which will be over wound.
4. Place center of cravat over dressing, Figure 21–22.

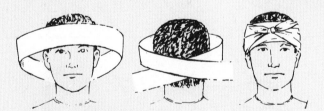

FIGURE 21–22 Applying a cravat bandage to the head (Adapted from Simmers, *Diversified Health Occupations*, copyright 1988, Delmar Publishers Inc.)

5. Take ends around to opposite side of head and cross them. Do not tie.
6. Bring ends back to starting point and tie them.
7. Clean up work area.

A bandage that is particularly useful in keeping a dressing in place over a large head wound or a burn is the triangular bandage.

A sling is often used to support an arm after a fracture or injury to the shoulder or arm. It is important to learn the correct way to put a sling on a patient and to practice with the patient standing, sitting, and lying down. Care must be taken to elevate the hand properly. You must also be sure that the sling is tied to one side and never over the spine where a knot is extremely uncomfortable.

Triangular bandages may be made from muslin or purchased in individual packages. Some physicians like to use a print material for children. The standard adult sling is about 55 inches across the base and 36 to 40 inches along the sides.

The easiest and probably the quickest way to bandage arms, legs, fingers, and toes is with a tubular gauze bandage, Figure 21–25. This is accomplished with the use of a cylindrical cage applicator. The amount of gauze you expect to use is stretched over the applicator and placed over the extremity.

It is often necessary for a patient to walk with crutches to give a foot, ankle, knee, or leg injury an opportunity to heal. It is important for the crutches to

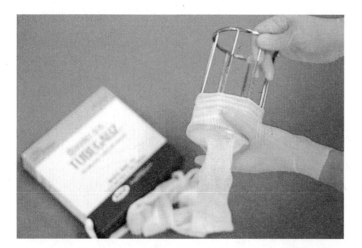

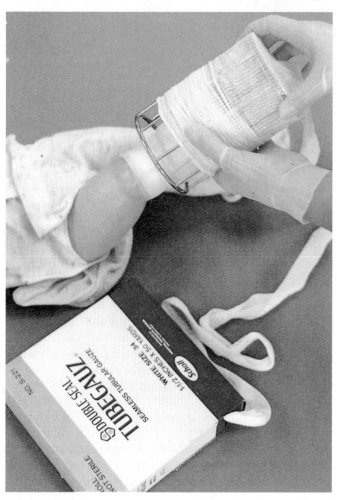

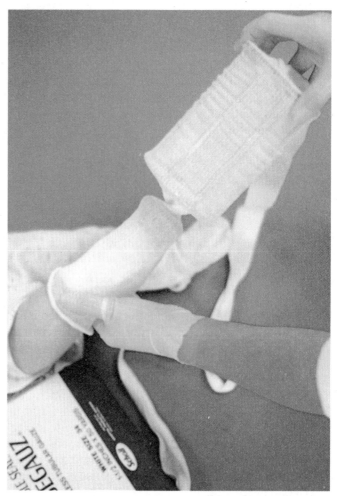

FIGURE 21–25 a). Push tube-gauze onto cylinder and allow for excessive amount. (b). Place cylinder with tube-gauze over injured extremity carefully. (c). Hold end of tube-gauze gently above injury and pull cylinder away from extremity, twisting the gauze. Repeat applications as desired for protection of wound.

PROCEDURE

Apply Triangular Bandage to Scalp

TERMINAL PERFORMANCE OBJECTIVE: Provided all necessary equipment and supplies and using other students as patients, the student will demonstrate the steps in the procedure for applying a triangular bandage to the scalp. The instructor will observe each step. Remember that you must follow universal precautions even in emergency situations when you may come into contact with blood or body fluids.

This procedure will show you how to bandage after the wound area has been covered so there should be no possibility of coming into contact with blood or body fluids.

1. Wash hands.
2. Assemble needed supplies.
3. Carefully place dressing over wound area without touching body of dressing.
4. Fold a hem about two inches wide along base, Figure 21–23.
5. With hem on outside, place bandage on head so that middle of base is on forehead close to eyebrows and point hangs down back.
6. Bring two ends around head above ears and cross them just below bump at back of head.
7. Draw ends snugly around head and tie them in center of forehead.
8. Steady head with one hand and with other draw point down firmly behind to hold compress securely against head. Grasp point and tuck it in to area where bandage ends cross.
9. Clean up work area.

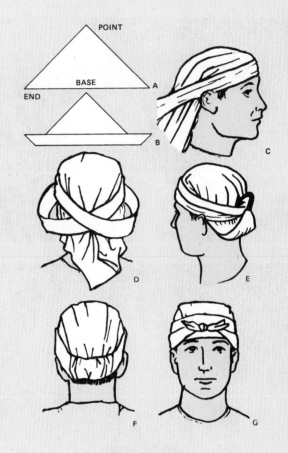

FIGURE 21–23 Applying a triangular bandage to the scalp

be adjusted to the correct height. This is accomplished by holding the crutches up to the side of the patient and adjusting them so that the underarm pad is 2 to 3 inches below the axilla. The handhold should be adjusted so that the hands fit comfortably with the arms extended. The axillary pad and handhold should be foam padded for comfort. The patient should be instructed to stand on the uninjured foot while swinging the injured leg forward as the crutches are moved forward. The weight of the body should be on the hands and never on the axillary area since it can cause nerve damage.

The patient who needs only a cane for support should have one that is the proper length to fit comfortably in the hand with the arm hanging naturally at the side. Many canes are adjustable; if not, they must be fitted to the correct length. Canes come in a variety of materials and types. An elderly patient usually has less trouble with a quad-base cane. The patient should carry the cane on the strong or uninjured side. The cane should swing forward with the injured extremity. Part of the weight is carried by the cane being firmly placed on the floor simultaneously with the injured extremity.

Apply Arm Sling

TERMINAL PERFORMANCE OBJECTIVE: Provided all necessary equipment and supplies and using other students as patients, the student will demonstrate the steps in the procedure for applying an arm sling. The instructor will observe each step.

1. Wash hands.
2. Place one end of bandage over shoulder on uninjured side and let other end hang down over chest, Figure 21–24.
3. Pull point behind elbow of injured arm.
4. Pull end of bandage which is hanging down up around injured arm and over shoulder. Elevate hand 4 to 5 inches above elbow. Tie ends together at side of neck (never over spine).

5. Bring point of bandage at elbow over front of sling and pin to sling with safety pin.

   Key Points:

   a. **If pin is not available, twist point until it is snug against elbow and tie a single knot.**
   b. **Be sure ends of fingers extend slightly beyond edge of sling so you may observe fingers for circulation.**

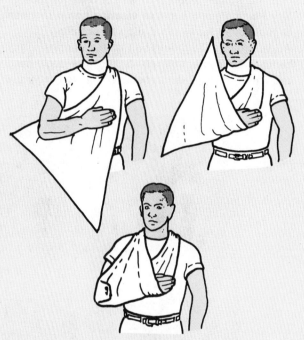

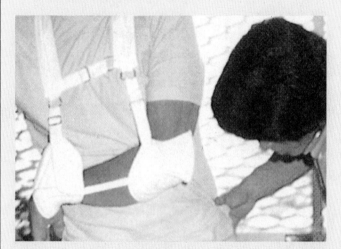

FIGURE 21–24 (a). Buckle type of arm sling for support. (b). Applying an arm sling

A walker is useful for patients who because of age or physical condition cannot safely use crutches. The walker may be adjusted to proper height for the patient. The patient must be cautioned not to step too closely to the walker as it is then difficult to stay balanced. The patient should move the walker forward and then step into the walker while leaning slightly forward on the walker.

When a patient comes to your office in a wheelchair, you need to know how to help that patient from the wheelchair to the examination table and back again.

If you have had to put a patient onto an examination table from a wheelchair, you will need to return that patient to a wheelchair to leave the office.

All of the procedures in this chapter need to be practiced many times so that you feel comfortable and confident when the need arises to use them.

Complete Chapter 21, Unit 3 in the workbook to help you meet the objectives at the beginning of this unit and therefore achieve competency of this subject matter.

Instruct Patient in Use of Crutches

TERMINAL PERFORMANCE OBJECTIVE: Provided with all necessary equipment and supplies, and using other students as patients, the student will demonstrate the steps of this procedure to instruct a patient in using crutches. The instructor will observe each step.

1. Identify patient and physician's orders.
2. Assemble equipment. Make sure crutches are intact (hand pads and rubber tips), and stable.
3. Stabilize patient upright near wall or chair for support. **Key Point: Patient must be wearing nonskid shoes or foot coverings to avoid slipping or falling.**
4. Adjust crutches to patient so that the handles of the crutches are comfortable with a 30-degree angle bend of the elbows with 2 inches between the area under the

arm and the top of the crutches.
Key Points:
a. **Explain to the patient to support his/her weight at the handle and not under the arm, and to take small steps slowly to avoid getting off balance and possibly falling.**
b. **Instruct patient to stand on his or her good foot while swinging the injured leg forward with crutches.**

Crutches should be placed approximately 4 to 5 inches in front and 4 to 5 inches to the side of the patient's heels.

Use Figure 21–26 to show the ordered gait to walk safely with crutches.

5. Record and initial on patient's chart.

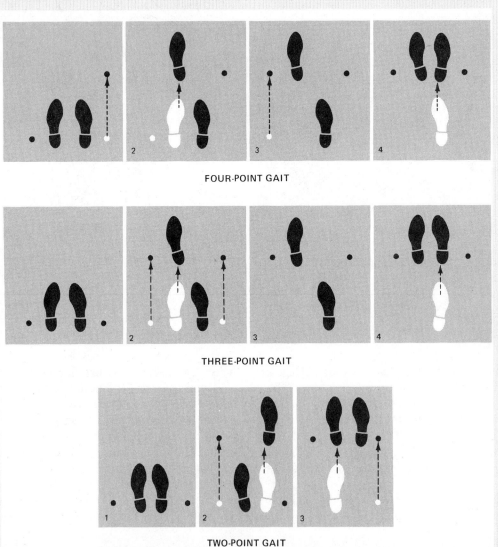

FOUR-POINT GAIT

THREE-POINT GAIT

TWO-POINT GAIT

FIGURE 21–26 (a). Four-point gait. (b). Three-point gait. (c). Two-point gait. (From Simmers, *Diversified Health Occupations*, copyright 1988, Delmar Publishers Inc.)

Instruct Patient in Use of Cane

TERMINAL PERFORMANCE OBJECTIVE: Provided with all necessary equipment and supplies, and using other students as patients, the student will demonstrate the steps of this procedure for instructing a patient in the use of a cane. The instructor will observe each step.

1. Identify patient and physician's orders.
2. Assemble equipment. Check cane for intact rubber tip. **Key Point: Patient must be wearing nonskid shoes or foot coverings to avoid slipping or falling.**
3. Adjust height of cane so that patient's elbow is flexed comfortably at approximately a 25- to 30-degree angle, and that the handle of the cane is positioned just below hip level of the uninjured or strong side.
4. Demonstrate to the patient the gait ordered to safely ambulate by:
   a. moving the cane and injured extremity forward simultaneously,
   b. then moving the strong/uninjured extremity forward. **Key Point: Observe patient and be alert to assist patient and rescue in case of fall.**
5. Explain to patient how to go up stairs:
   a. Move the uninjured extremity up first.
   b. Then move injured extremity up. Remind patient to use cane for support.
6. Explain to patient how to go down stairs:
   a. Move uninjured extremity down first.
   b. Then move injured extremity down. Remind patient to use cane for support.
7. Instruct patient to take small, slow steps to prevent getting off balance or falling to the side. **Key Point: Answer questions of patient and give emotional support.**
8. Record and initial on patient's chart.

Instruct Patient in Use of Walker

TERMINAL PERFORMANCE OBJECTIVE: Provided with all necessary equipment and supplies, and using other students as patients, the student will demonstrate the steps in the procedure to instruct a patient in the use of a walker.

1. Identify patient and physician's orders.
2. Assemble equipment. Check walker for rubber tips, pads at handles, and stability.
3. Stabilize patient upright near wall or chair for support. **Key Point: Patient must be wearing nonskid shoes or foot coverings to avoid slipping or falling.**
4. The height of the walker should be adjusted so that the handles are at the patient's hip level, and the bend of the patient's elbows is at a comfortable 25- to 30-degree angle.
5. Position the walker with the patient inside it.
6. Instruct patient to pick up the walker and move it slightly forward and walk into it.
   Key Points:
   a. **Instruct patient to keep all four feet of walker on the floor.**
   b. **Explain to patient not to slide the walker or it could slip and cause a fall.**
   c. **Instruct patient not to step too close to walker as doing so may cause loss of balance.**
   d. **Observe patient and be ready to assist in case of possible fall.**
7. Record and initial on patient's chart.

Assist Patient From Wheelchair to Examining Table

TERMINAL PERFORMANCE OBJECTIVE: Provided necessary equipment and using other students as patients, the student will demonstrate the steps in the procedure for assisting patient from wheelchair to examination table. The instructor will observe each step.

1. Unlock wheels of chair and wheel patient to examination room area. **Key Point: Wheelchairs should always be locked in position when sitting still to prevent unexpected movement. This is accomplished by flipping brake on each wheel.**
2. Position chair as near as possible to place you want patient to sit on table.
3. Lower table to chair level. **Key Point: If this cannot be done, position footstool beside table.**
4. Lock wheels on chair.
5. Fold footrests back. **Key Point: If necessary, assist patient in moving feet.**
6. Stand directly in front of patient with feet slightly apart to give a good base.
7. Bend knees and have patient place hands on your shoulders while you place your hands under patient's armpits to assist patient to standing position. **Key Point: Pause in this position for a moment before next step.**

8. Maintaining position of hands pivot or side step to position in front of table, Figure 21–27.
9. Place one foot slightly behind you for support and help patient to sitting position on table.
10. If patient still needs support, place one hand around back of patient. Help patient raise legs to table by placing free arm under legs and lifting them as patient turns. **Key Point: If patient needs to remove clothing get someone to help you. One person balances patient while other removes necessary clothing.**
11. Place pillow under head of patient and cover with drape. **Key Point: Never leave a very ill patient alone on a table. There is danger of a fall.**
12. Unlock chair wheels and move chair out of way of physician.

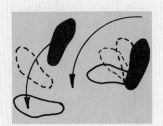

FIGURE 21–27 Position of the feet when assisting patient from wheel chair onto examination table

---

Assist Patient From Examining Table to Wheelchair

TERMINAL PERFORMANCE OBJECTIVE: Provided necessary equipment and using other students as patients, the student will demonstrate the steps in the procedure of assisting the patient from examination table to wheelchair. The instructor will observe each step.

1. Reposition chair and lock wheels.
2. Assist patient to sitting position on table. **Key Point: Support back if necessary. Lift legs of patient as patient is turned until feet dangle over edge of table.**

3. Ask patient to put hands on your shoulders. Support patient on sides below armpits. **Key Point: Have stepstool in place if table is not lowered to chair height.**
4. Support patient into standing position.
5. Side step or pivot patient to position in front of chair. **Key Point: Assist patient in putting on robe or clothing if necessary.**
6. Have patient reach back to arms of chair as you help in lowering patient into chair.
7. Adjust footrests.
8. Unlock wheels and return patient to waiting room.

Mr. Right...

has taken first aid and CPR courses and remains current in certification so he can administer emergency assistance when needed. He keeps the emergency phone numbers updated by each phone in the office. He makes a routine check of the office daily for safety hazards and deals with problems immediately. He makes sure that all exits are free of obstacles and marked clearly. He also makes sure that emergency evacuation routes are visible for the general public.

Promotion outlook: Excellent

Ms. Wrong...

doesn't want to renew her certification in CPR or first aid because she doesn't have time. She takes the list of emergency phone numbers with her from phone to phone and frequently misplaces them. Once in a while she looks over the office to see if there are any safety hazards and if the emergency evacuation instructions are still on the wall by the exit, which is blocked with the delivery of supplies from yesterday.

Promotion outlook: Termination

R E F E R E N C E S

American Red Cross, *Adult CPR,* 1988.

Mosby's Medical, Nursing, and Allied Health Dictionary, 3d ed. St. Louis: C.V. Mosby, 1990.

The Nurse's Reference Library, Procedures, Nursing 83 Books, Springhouse, PA: Intermed Communications, 1983.

Simmers, Louise. *Diversified Health Occupations,* 2d ed. Albany, NY: Delmar Publishers, 1988.

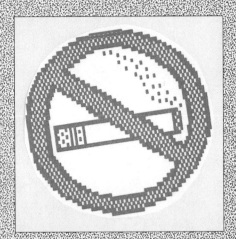

Desired Behavior and Employability Skills

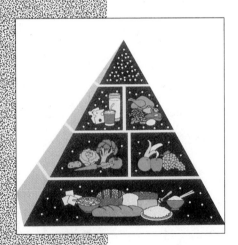

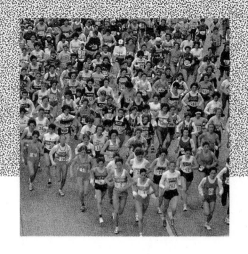

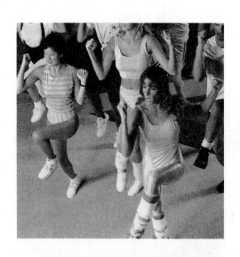

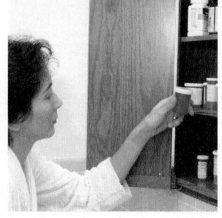

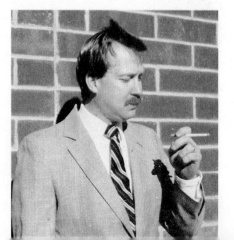

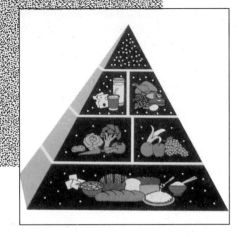

CHAPTER 22

Personal Behaviors Influencing Health

As you gain experience in the field, it will soon become apparent that patients have a tendency to depend on you for advice. The physician prescribes a treatment plan for the patient to follow and usually discusses it with the patient. Almost always the patient's next step is to ask you to explain the details. Therefore, you must have a complete understanding of the policies of the health care facility. Personal opinions should be restrained. This chapter concerns the significance of diet, exercise, and weight control and the way personal behavior influences health. The use of habit-forming substances and treatment and support groups will be discussed. These areas are vitally important to you personally, as well as to the patients you will serve.

U N I T   1

Nutrition, Exercise, and Weight Control

OBJECTIVES ·······································

Upon completion of this unit, the student will meet the following terminal performance objectives by verifying knowledge of the facts and principles presented through oral and written communication at a level deemed competent.

1. Explain the significance of diet and exercise to health.
2. Name and discuss the six food groups of the food pyramid.
3. Name the fat-soluble vitamins.
4. Name the water-soluble vitamins.
5. Name the essential minerals.
6. Discuss ways to encourage patient compliance in weight control.
7. Discuss the importance of sleep and a positive outlook

PATIENT EDUCATION

You will notice that this chapter primarily concerns educating the patient on staying well. When educating the patient about the importance of a good diet and proper exercise, you must be supportive and empathetic. If you can gain the patient's confidence, you will be in a better position to help the patient attain certain goals. Whether the patient is dieting, exercising, or working to stop smoking, encourage realistic goals. Offer praise whenever possible no matter how small the accomplishments.

in regard to health.

8. List guidelines for promoting good health.
9. Demonstrate range-of-motion exercises.
10. Demonstrate flexibility exercises.
11. Spell and define, using the glossary at the back of the text, all of the words to know in this unit.

With today's attention to physical fitness, the medical assistant must be well informed to answer the countless inquiries patients make concerning diet and exercise programs. The physician will decide what is best for each patient after all data from the medical history, examination, laboratory findings, and other pertinent information have been evaluated. It is up to you to reinforce the physician's orders and help patients adapt those orders to their particular life-styles.

As you begin to practice skills in communicating information to patients regarding treatment plans and their overall health, it is important for you to have a basic understanding of the meaning of health. Health is defined by the World Health Organization as a state of complete physical and mental or social well-being. Health is not merely the absence of disease or infirmity. All things conducive to good health are referred to as healthful. Healthful living habits are essential for one to maintain being in good physical condition or in staying physically fit. Fitness, therefore, refers to being in good

---

DO:
— exercise regularly
— eat a sensible, well-balanced diet
  include high-fiber, low-fat, cereal and grain foods
— practice health and safety rules at home and work
— include spiritual/emotional nurturing

DON'T:
— smoke or use tobacco
— drink alcohol in excess
— expose skin to sun for prolonged periods
— use drugs or medications unless prescribed for a specific purpose
— overeat or gain too much weight
— expose yourself to unnecessary X rays

FIGURE 22–1 Guidelines for good health

---

physical condition or being healthy. There are simple guidelines that can help to keep us in good health, increase vitality, and may even increase life expectancy. Figure 22–1 outlines the suggestions advised for the general population. Those who are in the health care professions are urged to set a good example to those patients for whom we are models.

Nutrition ....

Patient education in proper nutrition is one of your many responsibilities. Nutrition is defined as the sum of the processes involved in taking in, assimilating, and utilizing nutriments. This includes the processes by which the body uses food for energy, maintenance, and growth.

The Food Guide Pyramid

The food guide pyramid was introduced in the spring of 1992 by the United States Department of Agriculture. This pyramid concept replaces the "food wheel" and the old basic four food groups that have been used since 1946. The pyramid is divided into 6 sections; the foods listed in the largest sections are those foods that should be consumed in the greatest quantities. Notice that at the top of the triangle, for example, are fats, oils, and sweets; this indicates that foods such as butter, salad oil, candy, and other sweets should be used sparingly. Explaining the food pyramid to patients will encourage healthful eating habits. Eating sensibly makes people feel better and more energetic. When people feel well they have a more positive outlook on life. It is a good idea to post the food guide pyramid shown in Table 22–1 near the scale or on the wall of the examination room. An attractive poster is an even better way to suggest good eating habits. Figure 22–2 illustrates an example of a colorful poster to catch the eye of patients to give them a visual reminder of healthy food choices. You may want to place a note regarding the "other" foods that have only slight nutritional value (fats, oils, and sweets) next to the poster. This reminder may help patients realize the importance of avoiding large amounts of the foods found at the top of the pyramid. Some patients have never been educated in this area of importance. Many pharmaceutical companies offer complimentary instructional materials.

Vitamins and Minerals

Vitamins are organic substances found in foods that are essential to good health and growth. Vitamins are called micronutrients. As the name implies, only a trace quantity is required for enzymatic reaction in the body. If the body does not receive adequate vitamins or does not absorb them sufficiently, deficiency diseases may result. The major ones are rickets, scurvy, and beriberi. Rickets is the result of a deficiency in vitamin D, scurvy, of vitamin C or ascorbic acid, and beriberi, of vitamin B or thiamine.

TABLE 22–1
The Food Guide Pyramid

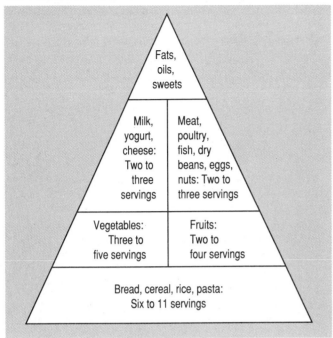

Vitamins A, D, E, and K are fat-soluble vitamins. Vitamin C and the B complex vitamins are water-soluble.

With a well-balanced diet, there is little likelihood of vitamin-deficiency diseases. Prepared foods display a list of their nutritional values on their labels for consumer information. Vitamins are added to many foods because of their loss in preparation. Patients will be advised by the physician if a vitamin or mineral supplement is necessary.

Minerals are naturally occurring nonorganic, homogeneous, solid substances. Thirteen are said to be essential to good health. They are supplied by a variety of meats and vegetables. Minerals found to be missing most often from the diet are calcium, iron, and iodine. Metabolic disturbances can be caused by insufficient amounts of zinc, copper, magnesium, and potassium.

The principal micronutrients are listed in Tables 22–2 and 22–3, pages 698–702. Careful study of these charts will give you an understanding of the food sources, the function of each in the body's growth and repair, the effects of deficiency and toxicity, and the dosages recommended for daily intake.

Several servings of fiber-rich foods (fruits, vegetables, peas and beans, whole grain cereals) should be included in the daily diet to promote a healthy digestive tract and prevent constipation. Notice that the sections of the food pyramid that list these nutrients are more than half the size of the entire pyramid to show their importance. Encourage patients to modify cooking techniques by using less fats, oils, and sugars (smallest portion of pyramid) and by baking, broiling, boiling, roasting, grilling,

poaching, or steaming meats and other foods instead of frying. These modified cooking practices can also help to reduce the amount of calories, cholesterol, sodium, and sugar, as well as saturated and total fat, from the diet. Review the information in Chapter 13 regarding the immune system and foods that aid the body in defense against disease.

Supplements

When patients suffer from loss or lack of appetite or they cannot tolerate a normal diet, it may be necessary for the physician to prescribe a protein-vitamin-mineral food supplement. These food supplements come in the form of a powder or liquid for oral or tube feeding as required by the patient's condition. Patients who might need this type of treatment are the chronically ill, postoperative, underweight, anemic, and anorexic. This treatment should be conducted only under the supervision of a physician. Remind patients to take these supplements regularly as directed for their intended affect.

Weight Control

A good weight-control program should contain foods from the food guide pyramid to be nutritionally sound. Eating should be an enjoyable, relaxing experience. But in our fast-food society, people tend to eat more food, with more calories, more often. A calorie is a unit of heat, and all food substances have caloric value, Table 22–4, pages 703–704. All of the body's processes burn calories to provide energy and sustain life. If you overeat regularly, the unused calories are stored as fat. If you reduce calorie intake, the fat will be used by the body for

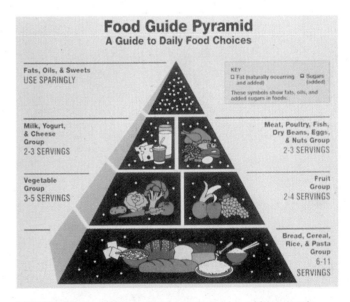

FIGURE 22–2 The four food groups and nutritious meals prepared using foods from each group (From *How to Eat for Good Health*, courtesy of NATIONAL DAIRY COUNCIL®)

TABLE 22–2
Recommended daily dietary allowances of vitamins and minerals

	AGE (YEARS)	WEIGHT kg	lb	HEIGHT cm	in	PROTEIN (g)	VITAMIN A (µg RE)†	VITAMIN D (µg)‡	VITAMIN E (mg α TE)§
Infants	0.0–0.5	6	13	60	24	kg x 2.2	420	10	3
	0.5–1.0	9	20	71	28	kg x 2.0	400	10	4
Children	1–3	13	29	90	35	23	400	10	5
	4–6	20	44	112	44	30	500	10	6
	7–10	28	62	132	52	34	700	10	7
Males	11–14	45	99	157	62	45	1000	10	8
	15–18	66	145	176	69	56	1000	10	10
	19–22	70	154	177	70	56	1000	7.5	10
	23–50	70	154	178	70	56	1000	5	10
	51+	70	154	178	70	56	1000	5	10
Females	11–14	46	101	157	62	46	800	10	8
	15–18	55	120	163	64	46	800	10	8
	19–22	55	120	163	64	44	800	7.5	8
	23-50	55	120	163	64	44	800	5	8
	51+	55	120	163	64	44	800	5	8
Pregnant						+30	+200	+5	+2
Lactating						+20	+400	+5	+3

WATER-SOLUBLE VITAMINS

VITAMIN C (mg)	THIAMINE (mg)	RIBOFLAVIN (mg)	NIACIN (mg NE)	VITAMIN B$_6$ (mg)	FOLACINE (µg)	VITAMIN B$_{12}$ (µg)
35	0.3	0.4	6	0.3	30	0.5**
35	0.5	0.6	8	0.6	45	1.5
45	0.7	0.8	9	0.9	100	2.0
45	0.9	1.0	11	1.3	200	2.5
45	1.2	1.4	16	1.6	300	3.0
50	1.4	1.6	18	1.8	400	3.0
60	1.4	1.7	18	2.0	400	3.0
60	1.5	1.7	19	2.2	400	3.0
60	1.4	1.6	18	2.2	400	3.0
60	1.2	1.4	16	2.2	400	3.0
50	1.1	1.3	15	1.8	400	3.0
60	1.1	1.3	14	2.0	400	3.0
60	1.1	1.3	14	2.0	400	3.0
60	1.0	1.2	13	2.0	400	3.0
60	1.0	1.2	13	2.0	400	3.0
+20	+0.4	–0.3	+2	+0.6	+400	+1.0
+40	+0.5	–0.5	+5	+0.5	+100	+1.0

TABLE 22–2

Recommended daily dietary allowances of vitamins and minerals (continued)

| | | MINERALS | | | |
CALCIUM (mg)	PHOSPHORUS (mg)	MAGNESIUM (mg)	IRON (mg)	ZINC (mg)	IODINE (µg)
360	240	50	10	3	40
540	360	70	15	5	50
800	800	150	15	10	70
800	800	200	10	10	90
800	800	250	10	10	120
1200	1200	350	18	15	150
1200	1200	400	18	15	150
800	800	350	10	15	150
800	800	350	10	15	150
800	800	350	10	15	150
1200	1200	300	18	15	150
1200	1200	300	18	15	150
800	800	300	18	15	150
800	800	300	18	15	150
800	800	300	10	15	150
+400	+400	−150	††	−5	+25
+400	+400	−150	††	+10	+50

energy and you will begin to shed the extra weight. You should make patients aware that they should eat their meals slowly because it takes approximately 20 minutes for the brain to realize that the stomach is full. Those who follow this practice in a relaxed atmosphere eat *less* and digest their food better. It is now recommended that eating several (5 to 6) small meals daily not only allows for better utilization of nutrients by the body for more energy, but is much easier on the digestive tract. This practice also helps in weight control.

A variety of magazines, books, and businesses offer weight-control plans that promise success for each individual. Over-the-counter drugs promise miraculous weight loss in a matter of weeks. You can be influential in helping patients avoid possible health hazards by warning them of the danger in these quick-weight-loss programs. Many people do lose weight in a short time, but they gain it right back as soon as the program ends. Others do permanent damage to their health.

One respected and worthwhile weight-loss program is Weight Watchers. Most people who have reached their weight-loss goals through this program have maintained a satisfactory weight because they have learned how to change their eating habits. Many support groups offer similar programs. Positive reinforcement is one of the keys to their success. Many physicians realize the frustration of trying to reduce and suggest these support groups to patients. You may want to encourage patients who are trying to follow a diet by suggesting low-calorie recipes or cooking techniques. Showing genuine interest in patients' needs will help them reach their goals.

Therapeutic Diets

Therapeutic diets are used in the treatment of patients with a specific disease or disorder. So that patients will comply with treatment, these special diets must be presented in a workable manner. The patient's life-style and background must be taken into consideration and certain adjustments made on the part of the patient. For the patient to give full cooperation, you must explain acceptable reasons for changes in diets. This area of patient education is vitally important and may take a considerable amount of time. Some physicians refer patients with special dietary needs to a Registered Dietician (RD). Dieticians work closely with other health care team members in therapeutic diet planning.

Exercise

In addition to a well-balanced diet, adequate exercise and sufficient rest are essential to good health. Special diets and exercise programs must be approved for individuals by the physician, who will determine the patient's needs and tolerance from careful examination and medical history. This is done to safeguard the patient from overexertion and stress.

TABLE 22–3

Principal micronutrients

MICRONUTRIENT	PRINCIPAL SOURCES	FUNCTIONS	EFFECTS OF DEFICIENCY AND TOXICITY	USUAL THERAPEUTIC DOSAGE
Vitamin A	Fish liver oils, liver, egg yolk, butter, cream, vitamin A-fortified margarine, green leafy or yellow vegetables	Photoceptor mechanism of retina; integrity of epithelia; lysosome stability, glycoprotein synthesis	*Deficiency:* Night blindness, perifollicular hyperkeratosis, xerophthalmia; keratomalacia *Toxicity:* Headache; peeling of skin, hepatosplenomegaly, bone thickening	10,000–20,000 µg (30,000–60,000 IU/day)
Vitamin D	Fortified milk is main dietary source, fish liver oils, butter, egg yolk, liver, ultraviolet irradiation	Calcium and phosphorus absorption, resorption, mineralization, and collagen maturation of bone; tubular reabsorption of phosphorus (?)	*Deficiency:* Rickets (tetany sometimes associated); osteomalacia *Toxicity:* Anorexia; renal failure; metastatic calcification	*Primary Deficiency* 10–40 µg (1400–1600 IU)/day *Metabolic Deficiency* 1–2 µg/day 1.25–(OH)$_2$D$_3$ or 1α–(OH)D$_3$
Vitamin E group	Vegetable oil, wheat germ, leafy vegetables, egg yolk, margarine, legumes	Intracellular antioxidant; stability of biologic membranes	*Deficiency:* RBC hemolysis, creatinuria; ceroid deposition in muscle	30–100 mg/day
Vitamin K (activity) Vitamin K$_1$ (phytonadione) Vitamin K$_2$ (menaquinone)	Leafy vegetables, pork, liver, vegetable oils, intestinal flora after newborn period	Prothrombin formation; normal blood coagulation	*Deficiency:* Hemorrhage from deficient prothrombin *Toxicity:* Kernicterus	In situations conductive to neonatal hemorrhage, 2–5 mg during labor or daily for 1 wk prior; or 1–2 mg to newborn
Essential fatty acids (linoleic, arachidonic acids)	Vegetable seed oils (corn, sunflower, safflower); margarines blended with vegetable oils	Synthesis of prostaglandins, membrane structure	Growth cessation, dermatosis	Up to 10 g/day
Thiamine (vitamin B$_1$)	Dried yeast; whole grains; meat (especially pork, liver), enriched cereal products, nuts; legumes; potatoes	Carbohydrate metabolism, central and peripheral nerve cell function, myocardial function	Beriberi; infantile and adult (peripheral neuropathy, cardiac failure; Wernicke-Korsakoff syndrome)	30–100 mg/day
Riboflavin (vitamin B$_2$)	Milk, cheese, liver, meat, eggs, enriched cereal products	Many aspects of energy and protein metabolism integrity of mucous membranes	Cheilosis; angular stomatitis; corneal vascularization; amblyopia, sebaceous dermatosis	10–30 mg/day
Niacin (nicotinic acid, niacinamide)	Dried yeast, liver, meat, fish, legumes, whole-grain enriched cereal products	Oxidation-reduction reactions, carbohydrate metabolism	Pellagra (dermatosis, glossitis, GI and CNS dysfunction)	Niacinamide 100–1000 mg/day
Vitamin B$_6$ group (pyridoxine)	Dried yeast, liver, organ meats, whole-grain cereals, fish, legumes	Many aspects of nitrogen metabolism, e.g., transaminations, porphyrin and heme synthesis, tryptophan conversion to niacin. Linoleic acid metabolism	Convulsions in infancy, anemias; neuropathy; seborrhea-like skin lesions Dependency states	25–100 mg/day
Folic acid	Fresh green leafy vegetables, fruit, organ meats, liver, dried yeast	Maturation of RBCs; synthesis of purines and pyrimidines	Pancytoperia; megaloblastosis (especially pregnancy, infancy, malabsorption)	1 mg/day

TABLE 22–3
Principal micronutrients (continued)

MICRONUTRIENT	PRINCIPAL SOURCES	FUNCTIONS	EFFECTS OF DEFICIENCY AND TOXICITY	USUAL THERAPEUTIC DOSAGE
Vitamin B$_{12}$ (cobalamins)	Liver, meats (especially beef, pork, organ meats); eggs; milk & milk products	Maturation of RBCs; neural function; DNA synthesis, related to folate coenzymes; methionine and acetate synthesis	Pernicious anemia; fish tapeworm & vegan anemias; some psychiatric syndromes, nutritional amblyopia Dependency states	In pernicious anemia 50µg/day IM first 2 wk, 100 µg twice/wk next 2 mo, thereafter 100 µg/mo
Biotin	Liver, kidney, egg yolk, yeast, cauliflower, nuts, legumes	Carboxylation and decarboxylation of oxalocetic acid; amino acid and fatty acid metabolism	Dermatitis, glossitis Dependency states	150–300 µg/day
Vitamin C (ascorbic acid)	Citrus fruits, tomatoes, potatoes, cabbage, green peppers	Essential to osteoid tissue; collagen formation; vascular function; tissue respiration and wound healing	Scurvy (hemorrhages, loose teeth, gingivitis)	100–1000 mg/day
Sodium	Wide distribution—beef, pork, sardines, cheese, green olives, corn bread, potato chips, sauerkraut	Acid-base balance; osmotic pressure; pH of blood; muscle contractility; nerve transmission; sodium pumps	*Deficiency:* Hyponatremia *Toxicity:* Hypernatremia; confusion, coma	
Potassium	Wide distribution—whole and skim milk, bananas, prunes, raisins	Muscle activity, nerve transmission, intracellular acid-base balance and water retention	*Deficiency:* Hypokalemia; paralysis, cardiac disturbances *Toxicity:* Hyperkalemia; paralysis, cardiac disturbances	
Calcium	Milk and milk products, meat, fish, eggs, cereal products, beans, fruits, vegetables	Bone and tooth formation; blood coagulation; neuromuscular irritability; muscle contractility; myocardial conduction	*Deficiency:* Hypocalcemia and tetany; neuromuscular hyperexcitability *Toxicity:* Hypercalcemia; GI atony, renal failure; psychosis	10–30 ml 10% calcium gluconate soln IV in 24 h
Phosphorus	Milk, cheese, meat, poultry, fish, cereals, nuts, legumes	Bone and tooth formation, acid-base balance, component of nucleic acids, energy production	*Deficiency:* Irritability; weakness; blood cell disorders; GI tract and renal dysfunction *Toxicity:* Hyperphosphatemia in renal failure	Potassium acid and di-basic phosphate parenteral 600 mg (18.8 mEq)/day
Magnesium	Green leaves, nuts, cereal grains, seafoods	Bone and tooth formation; nerve conduction; muscle contraction; enzyme activation	*Deficiency:* Hypomagnesemia; neuromuscular irritability *Toxicity:* Hypermagnesemia; hypotension, respiratory failure, cardiac disturbances	2–4 ml 50% magnesium sulfate soln/day IM
Iron	Wide distribution (except dairy products)—soybean flour, beef, kidney, liver, beans, clams, peaches Much unavailable (<20% absorbed)	Hemoglobin, myoglobin formation, enzymes	*Deficiency:* Anemia; dysphagia; koilonychia; enteropathy *Toxicity:* Hemochromatosis: cirrhosis; diabetes mellitus; skin pigmentation	Ferrous sulfate or gluconate 300 mg orally t.i.d.

TABLE 22–3
Principal micronutrients (continued)

MICRONUTRIENT	PRINCIPAL SOURCES	FUNCTIONS	EFFECTS OF DEFICIENCY AND TOXICITY	USUAL THERAPEUTIC DOSAGE
Iodine	Seafoods, iodized salt, dairy products Water variable	Thyroxine (T_4) and triiodothyronine (T_3) formation and energy control mechanisms	*Deficiency:* Simple (colloid, endemic) goiter; cretinism; deaf-mutism *Toxicity:* Occasional myxedema	150 µg iodine/day as potassium iodide added to salt 1:10–40,000 ppm
Fluorine	Wide distribution—tea, coffee Fluoridation of water supplies with sodium fluoride 1.0–2.0 ppm	Bone and tooth formation	*Deficiency:* Predisposition to dental caries; osteoporosis (?) *Toxicity:* Fluorosis, mottling, pitting of permanent teeth; exostoses of spine	Sodium fluoride 1.1–2.2 mg/day orally
Zinc	Wide distribution—vegetable sources Much unavailable	Component of enzymes and insulin; wound healing; growth	*Deficiency:* Growth retardation; hypogonadism; hypogeusia; in cirrhosis; acrodermatitis enteropathica	30–150 mg zinc sulfate/day orally
Copper	Wide distribution—organ meat, oysters, nuts, dried legumes, whole-grain cereals	Enzyme component	*Deficiency:* Anemia in malnourished children; Menkes' kinky hair syndrome *Toxicity:* Hepatolenticular degeneration; some biliary cirrhosis (?)	0.3 mg/kg/day copper sulfate, orally
Cobalt	Green leafy vegetables	Part of vitamin B_{12} molecule	*Deficiency:* Anemia in children (?) *Toxicity:* Beer-drinker's cardiomyopathy	20–30 mg/day cobaltous chloride, orally
Chromium	Wide distribution—brewer's yeast	Part of glucose tolerance factor (GTF)	*Deficiency:* Impaired glucose tolerance in malnourished children; some diabetics (?)	

Exercise is defined as physical exertion for improvement of health or correction of physical deformity. The safest form of exercise, and one almost everyone can participate in, is walking, but so many different exercise programs are available that people can choose according to their individual needs and goals. A combination of proper diet and proper exercise brings satisfying results in overall good health.

All of the behaviors which influence health are influenced by one's mental (or social) health and vice versa. A positive outlook is most helpful in coping with life in general. (Refer back to Chapter 5.) Learning coping and problem-solving skills can help us deal with the everyday stress and the occasional crisis of routine living. Getting sufficient rest is also necessary for good health. Individuals vary in the number of hours of sleep they require. An "average" number is between 6 and 8 hours in a 24-hour period. Sleep is the natural way for the body to rest and restore itself. Adequate rest equips us with strength to handle various daily situations. People who have trouble sleeping (insomnia) may have either serious physical or emotional (psychological) problems that should be brought to the attention of the physician. Each individual should find outlets to release tension and participate in activities that bring enjoyment and enrichment to his/her life. It is additionally important to practice the virtue of patience and maintain a sense of humor, for it has been said that laughter is the best medicine.

Regular exercise improves circulation and muscle tone and relieves tension. People who have followed an exercise routine regularly report that they experience a better outlook on life, have more energy, and feel healthier. The degree of exertion in any exercise routine

TABLE 22–4
Calorie chart

FOOD AND MEASURES	APPROXIMATE CALORIES	FOOD AND MEASURES	APPROXIMATE CALORIES	FOOD AND MEASURES	APPROXIMATE CALORIES
Apple, baked, 1 large and 2 tbs. sugar	200	Cocoa, half milk, half-water, 1 cup	150	Mushrooms, 10 large	10
fresh, 1 large	100	Cod steak, 1 piece, $3\frac{1}{2}$ by 2 by 1 in.	100	Noodles, cooked, $\frac{3}{4}$ cup	75
Asparagus, fresh or canned, 5 stalks, 5 in. long	15	Cola soft drinks, 6-oz. bottle	75	Oatmeal, cooked, $\frac{3}{4}$ cup	110
Avocado, $\frac{1}{2}$ 4-in. pear	265	Collards, $\frac{1}{2}$ cup, cooked	50	Oil, corn, cottonseed, olive, peanut, 1 tbs.	100
Bacon, 2–3 long slices, cooked	100	Corn, $\frac{1}{2}$ cup	70	Olives, green 6 medium	50
Banana, 1 medium, 6 in. long	90	Corn flakes, 1 cup	80	ripe, 4–5 medium	50
Beans, lima, fresh or canned, $\frac{1}{2}$ cup	100	Cracker, graham, 1 square	35	Onions, 3–4 medium	100
green or yellow, fresh or canned, $\frac{1}{2}$ cup	25	saltine, 2-in. square	15	Orange, 1 medium	80
canned with pork, $\frac{1}{2}$ cup	175	Cream, light, 2 tbs.	65	juice, 1 cup	125
Beef (cooked), corned, 1 slice 4 by $1\frac{1}{2}$ in. by 1 in.	100	heavy, 2 tbs.	120	Parsnip, 7 in. long	100
hamburger, 3 oz.	300	whipped, 3 tbs.	100	Peach, fresh, 1 medium	50
round, lean, 1 medium slice (2 oz.)	125	Custard, $\frac{1}{2}$ cup	130	canned in syrup, 2 lg. halves, 3 tbs. juice	100
sirloin lean, 1 average slice (3 oz.)	250	Eggs, medium	75	Peanut butter, 1 tbs.	100
tongue, 2 oz.	125	Eggplant, 3 slices, 4 in. diam., $\frac{1}{2}$ in. thick, raw	50	Peanuts, shelled, 10	50
Beets, fresh or canned, 2, 2-in. in diam.	50	Flour, 1 tbs., unsifted	35	Pear, fresh, 1 medium	50
Bread, corn (1 egg), 1 2-in. square	120	Frankfurter	125	canned in syrup, 3 halves, 3 tbs. juice	100
rye, 1 slice, $\frac{1}{2}$ in. thick	70–75	Gelatin, fruit flavored, ready to serve, $\frac{1}{2}$ cup	85	Peas, canned, $\frac{1}{2}$ cup	65
white, enriched, 1 slice, average	75	Grapefruit juice, unsweetened, 1 cup	100	fresh, shelled, $\frac{3}{4}$ cup	100
whole wheat, 100%, 1 slice average	75	Grape juice, $\frac{1}{2}$ cup	80	Pepper, green 1 medium	20
Broccoli, 3 stalks, $5\frac{1}{2}$ in. long	100	Griddle cake, 4 in. diam.	75	Pie, apple, 3-in. sector	200
Brussels sprouts, 6 sprouts, $1\frac{1}{2}$ in. diam.	50	Halibut, 1 piece, 3 by $1\frac{3}{8}$ by 1 in.	100	mincemeat, 3-in. sector	300
Butter, 1 tbs.	95	Ham, lean, 1 slice, $4\frac{1}{4}$ by 4 by $\frac{1}{2}$ in.	265	Pineapple, fresh, 1 slice, $\frac{3}{4}$ in. thick	50
Cabbage, cooked, $\frac{1}{2}$ cup	40	Hominy grits, cooked, $\frac{3}{4}$ cup	100	canned, unsweetened, 1 slice, $\frac{1}{2}$ in. thick, 1 tbs. juice	50
raw, 1 cup	25	Ice cream, $\frac{1}{2}$ cup	200	juice, unsweetened, 1 cup	135
Cake, angel, $\frac{1}{10}$ large cake choc, or vanilla, with icing	155	Ice cream soda, fountain size	325	Pork chop, lean, 1 medium	200
2 by $1\frac{1}{2}$ by 2 in.	200	Jellies and jams, 1 rounded tbs.	100	Potato chips, 8–10 large	100
cupcake (med.), choc. icing	250	Lamb, roast, 1 slice, $3\frac{1}{2}$ by $4\frac{1}{2}$ by $\frac{1}{8}$ in.	100	Potato salad with mayonnaise, $\frac{1}{2}$ cup	200
Cantaloupe, $\frac{1}{2}$ $5\frac{1}{2}$-in. melon	50	Lettuce, 2 large leaves	5	Potatoes, mashed, $\frac{1}{2}$ cup	100
Carrot, 4 in. long	25	Liver, 1 slice, 3 by 3 by $\frac{1}{2}$ in.	100	sweet, $\frac{1}{2}$ medium	100
Cauliflower, $\frac{1}{4}$ of head, $4\frac{1}{2}$ in. in diam.	25	Liverwurst, 2 oz.	130	white, 1 medium	100
Celery, 2 stalks	15	Macaroni, cooked, $\frac{3}{4}$ cup	100	Prunes, dried, 4 medium	100
Cheese, American cheddar, 1 cube $1\frac{1}{8}$ in. square	110	Maple syrup, 1 tbs.	70	Pumpkin, $\frac{1}{2}$ cup	50
cottage, 5 tbs.	100	Margarine, 1 tbs.	100	Raisins, $\frac{1}{4}$ cup	90
cream, 2 tbs.	100	Milk, buttermilk, 1 cup	85	Rice, cooked, $\frac{3}{4}$ cup	100
Chicken, $\frac{1}{2}$ med. broiler	270	condensed, $1\frac{1}{2}$ tbs.	100	Rutabagas, $\frac{1}{2}$ cup	30
Chocolate, milk, sweetened, 1 oz.	140	evaporated, $\frac{1}{2}$ cup	160	Salad dressing, French, 1 tbs.	90
malted milk, fountain size	460	skin, 1 cup	85	mayonnaise, 1 tbs.	100
syrup, $\frac{1}{4}$ cup	200	whole, 1 cup	170	Salmon, canned, $\frac{1}{2}$ cup	100
		yogurt, plain, 1 cup	120–160	Sauerkraut, $\frac{1}{2}$ cup	15

TABLE 22–4
Calorie chart (continued)

FOOD AND MEASURES	APPROXIMATE CALORIES	FOOD AND MEASURES	APPROXIMATE CALORIES	FOOD AND MEASURES	APPROXIMATE CALORIES
Soup, condensed, 11 oz. can, mushroom	360	Tapioca, uncooked, 1 tbs.	50	Alcoholic Beverages	
		Tomato juice, 1 cup	60	beer, 8 oz.	120
tomato	230	Tomatoes, canned, $\frac{1}{2}$ cup	25	gin, $1\frac{1}{2}$ oz.	120
vegetable	200	fresh, 1 medium	30	rum, $1\frac{1}{2}$ oz.	150
Spaghetti, cooked, $\frac{3}{4}$ cup	100	Tuna fish, canned, $\frac{1}{4}$ cup, drained	100	whiskey, $1\frac{1}{2}$ oz.	150
Spinach, cooked, $\frac{1}{2}$ cup	20	Turnip, 1, $1\frac{3}{4}$ in. diam.	25	Wines	
Squash,				champagne, 4 oz.	120
summer, cooked, $\frac{1}{2}$ cup	20	Veal roast, 1 slice, 3 by $3\frac{3}{4}$ by $1\frac{1}{2}$ in.	120	port, 1 oz.	50
winter, cooked, $\frac{1}{2}$ cup	50	Waffle, 6 in. in diam.	250	sherry, 1 oz.	40
Sugar, brown, 1 tbs.	50	Wheat flakes, $\frac{3}{4}$ cup	100	table, red or white, 4 oz.	95
granulated, 1 tbs.	50				

will vary with individuals and the physician's advice should be taken.

For patients who cannot engage in strenuous exercise, walking and ROM (range-of-motion exercises) are suggested to improve circulation and promote muscle tone, Figure 22–3. These movements help to move each joint through its full range. Patients who have arthritis, bursitis, and other disabilities can be helped by these exercises. Flexibility exercises increase muscle tone and flexibility of the muscles and also relieve tension, Figure 22–4, page 707. You should be familiar with these so that you can teach them to patients.

Complete Chapter 22, Unit 1 in the workbook to help you meet the objectives at the beginning of this unit and therefore achieve competency of this subject matter.

U N I T   2

Use of Habit-Forming Substances

OBJECTIVES

Upon completion of this unit, the student will meet the following terminal performance objectives by verifying knowledge of the facts and principles presented through oral and written communication at a level deemed competent.

1. List the most commonly abused major groups of drugs and give an example of each.
2. Explain the effects of the most commonly abused substances.
3. Describe the difference between an alcohol-dependent drinker and alcoholic.
4. Describe research into the causes of alcoholism.
5. Describe ways you can be influential in assisting drug addicts and alcoholics toward rehabilitation.
6. Describe the action that tar, nicotine, and carbon monoxide have on the body.
7. List ways a person can stop smoking.
8. List diseases in which smokers have a higher probability rate.
9. Discuss the effects of secondhand smoke.
10. Discuss the stages of drug/alcohol abuse.
11. List signs of drug/alcohol abuse.
12. List organizations and facilities that assist in the rehabilitation of drug addicts and alcoholics.
13. Spell and define, using the glossary at the back of the text, all of the words to know in this unit.

WORDS TO KNOW

acetylcholine	depressant
addiction	detrimental
advantageous	euphoria
Al-Anon	hallucinogen
Al-Ateen	narcolepsy
alcoholic	nicotine
Alcoholics Anonymous	norepinephrine
amphetamine	proclivity
barbiturate	psychedelics
bizarre	stimulant
carbon monoxide	synergism
carboxyhemoglobin	tar
carcinogen	traumatic
cholinergic	veritable

A habit is a pattern of behavior that is acquired over a period of time by repetition. Habits can be either advantageous or disadvantageous depending on the effects

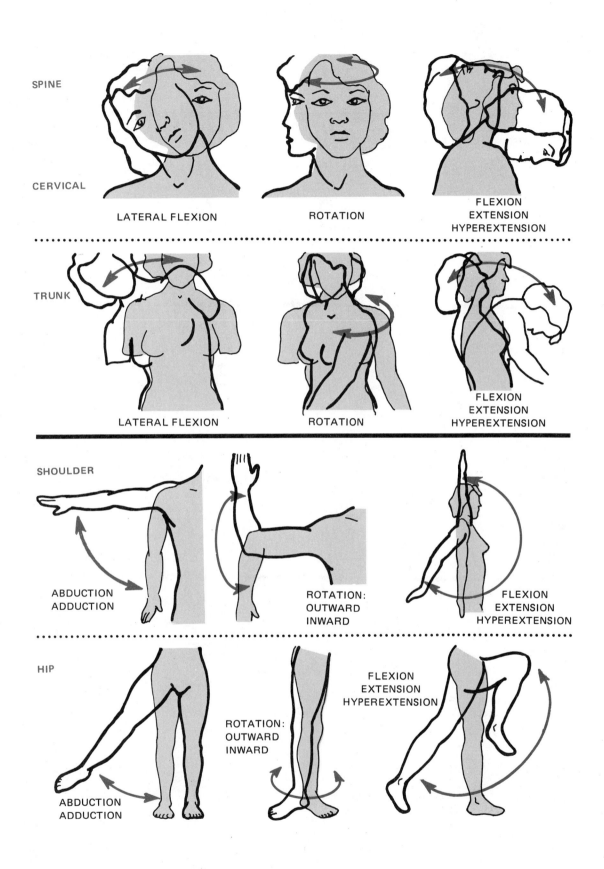

SPINE

CERVICAL

LATERAL FLEXION

ROTATION

FLEXION
EXTENSION
HYPEREXTENSION

TRUNK

LATERAL FLEXION

ROTATION

FLEXION
EXTENSION
HYPEREXTENSION

SHOULDER

ABDUCTION
ADDUCTION

ROTATION:
OUTWARD
INWARD

FLEXION
EXTENSION
HYPEREXTENSION

HIP

ABDUCTION
ADDUCTION

ROTATION:
OUTWARD
INWARD

FLEXION
EXTENSION
HYPEREXTENSION

FIGURE 22–3 Range-of-motion (ROM) exercises

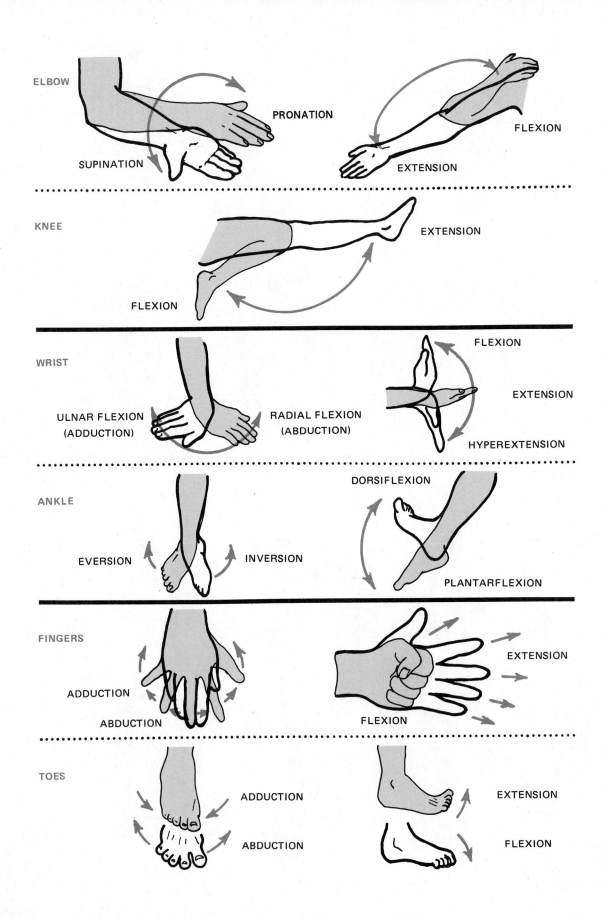

FIGURE 22–3 (Continued)

These exercises are designed to increase the flexibility of the low back extensor ranges and to strengthen the low back flexor muscles. They are to be performed slowly, starting with ten repetitions for each exercise, and increasing gradually to as many as forty or fifty repetitions. These are best performed on a firm, flat surface.

1. Purpose: To strengthen abdominals. Patient lies on back, with hips and knees bent.

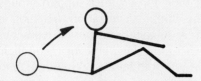

A) Come to sitting position:

    a) Reaching hands past the knees
    b) With arms folded across chest
    c) With hands clasped behind head

2. Purpose: To strengthen hip muscles. Patient lies on back, with hips and knees bent.

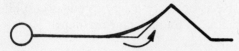

A) Roll the pelvis backwards, flattening the low back curve, pinching the buttocks together, raising the tailbone slightly upwards.

3. Purpose: To stretch the lower back muscles. Patient lies on back, with hips and knees bent.

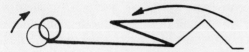

A) Stretch the back by pulling the knees to the chest as close as possible. Curve the back by also ducking the head forward.

4. Purpose: To stretch the lower back and hamstring muscles. Patient sits upright with legs straight.

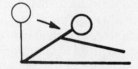

A) Keeping the knees straight, bend the head toward the knees to stretch the lower back and hips.

5. Purpose: To stretch the hip flexor muscles. Patient stands erect.

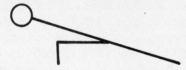

A) Place one foot forward. Lean forward on that leg, keeping the other leg straight, the body bent forward so that a good stretch is felt along the front of the hip and thigh.

6. Purpose: To stretch the lower back and to strengthen the upper leg muscles. Patient stands erect.

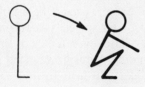

A) Squat down as far as possible and stand up again. Keep feet flat on the floor and curve the back to keep the balance and to stretch the lower back and hip muscles.

FIGURE 22–4 Flexibility exercises

they have. Many of our habits are so much a part of us that we do not even realize they exist. Changing a behavior that has become a habit is difficult. It takes a great deal of patience and encouragement to repattern personal activities. Teaching good health habits to patients is an important duty of the medical assistant. The entire medical staff must strive to set a good example, for example is the best teacher.

In times of stress one may be temporarily inclined to relieve anxiety or depression by using chemical substances. Even individuals under the supervision of a physician may become dependent. Other persons turn to chemical substances to experiment with the feelings they produce. Often this is a response to peer pressure, which can be strong indeed. Regardless of why persons turn to chemical substances, they need to know that dependency and abuse can follow and that the stakes can be very high.

Unfortunately, the influence of advertising has been to encourage chemical substance use by promoting fast relief, quick weight-loss, instant sleep and wakefulness, and a variety of other "feel-good" promises from the makers of chemical products. Although a substance may well relieve symptoms temporarily, the cause of the problem will still exist. If undetermined or undetected physical or emotional problems are not diagnosed and treated, they may balloon into more complex problems which are, of course, only worsened by the abuse of chemical substances. You can play an important part in recognizing potential chemical abusers and helping them take steps toward treatment.

Alcohol

Still the nation's number-one drug problem, alcohol is responsible for the destruction of many lives. Its use is commonly accepted by society and to a great degree encouraged. Most persons who drink alcoholic beverages do so moderately, probably because its effects have been learned from either first-hand observation or educational programs. The responsible social drinker can take alcohol or leave it alone.

On the other hand, a person who is dependent on alcohol has a difficult time doing without a drink. An alcohol-dependent drinker will say that cutting down is not a problem, but is then unable to do so. Daily use of alcohol becomes a need and usually leads to increasingly compulsive drinking. Patients who indicate this during conversation or in giving a medical history may be indirectly asking for help with their problem. Privately disclosing this information to the physician may lead to a treatment or counseling program, which may prevent the patient from becoming an alcoholic. An alcoholic is a drinker who has become totally dependent on alcohol. All areas of the alcoholic's life are affected by it. It is the number-one priority, and control over drinking is nonexistent. More often than not, the occurrence of a tragedy is the reason the alcoholic seeks treatment, either by court order or sometimes voluntarily in an effort to put a productive life back together.

Alcoholism is now recognized as a disease, as serious as cancer or diabetes, which can be treated. It is a major health problem and recognized as such by the American Medical Association, American Osteopathic Association, and American Bar Association. Excessive long-term use of alcohol can reduce resistance to infections and eventually lead to cirrhosis of the liver. It can also add complications to other diseases and conditions. In effect, alcohol works to dissolve all tissues with which it comes in contact.

Research efforts continue in the search for the causes of the disease. Many theories have been offered but none are yet definitive. Current efforts are concentrating on brain chemistry, hereditary traits, and cultural influences. While certain ethnic groups show a proclivity toward alcoholism, others are virtually free of the disease. Studies in these areas suggest almost evolutionary relationships between habits, value systems, and brain chemistry. Many scientists feel that a combination of factors contribute to alcoholism.

Treatment

Alcoholics Anonymous is a well-known support group for the alcoholic, who must admit to being an alcoholic and be willing to start leading a productive life once again. AA was founded in the mid 1930s to help those who were looked on by society as hopeless degenerates. The program has become extremely successful over the years and has directly and indirectly helped millions to reorder their lives. Other support groups have branched from this initial organization. Al-Anon and Al-Ateen are for family members or close friends of the alcoholic to help them understand and cope with their loved ones' illness. Many companies maintain alcoholism assistance and rehabilitation programs for employees who are problem drinkers. It has been realized by employers that this practice is not only a service but is cost-effective as an alternative to training new personnel.

Drugs

(Refer to Table 21–2, pages 676–679) There was a time when we thought of drugs only in connection with a trip to the drugstore to have a prescription filled, perhaps staying long enough to enjoy something at the soda fountain. Today the meaning has changed, and the term evokes the image of illicit chemical substances available on the street. Most of these are impure, diluted, and extremely addictive, as well as expensive.

Throughout civilized history people have had a desire to soothe the anxieties of life and obtain temporary relief from troubles. But our society, as a whole, is today more than ever before looking for instant gratification. Over-the-counter drugs are practically beyond number. It is a mind-boggling experience to look over a well-stocked drug shelf in a retail store and consider all the substances that can allegedly provide "fast and temporary" relief. In this age of fast food, instant car washes, one-hour dry cleaning, and express lanes, the art of patience has seemingly been lost. Our society has become accepting of drug use as a part of life, even a *way* of life, despite the physical and emotional damage, reflected in the high numbers of drug-related deaths from overdose and accident.

The threat of nuclear war, unemployment, an uncertain economy, and a fast-paced life-style make it difficult for many to deal with the challenges of everyday living. For some people the only way to cope with problems is by resorting to mood-altering drugs. But these drugs alter not only one's mood, but also one's perception of reality, and they are dangerous not only to the user but to others as well. The euphoric state they produce exists only in the user's mind.

The reality of drugs in society and the seriousness of their abuse are not going to disappear. A veritable smorgasbord of legal and illegal drugs remains widely available and probably always will be. Educating the public to their dangers seems to be the only hope.

You could be most influential in helping someone, a patient or a family member of a patient, recognize the signs of drug abuse so that intervention may be possible. You should always be supportive and understanding. Avoid being judgmental, sarcastic, or accusatory with patients or others seeking your help. The indications of drug abuse are outlined in Figure 22–5.

There are four basic stages of alcohol and drug abuse. In the first stage, one may show no visible signs in outward behavior. Unfortunately, society has taken somewhat an attitude of acceptance in the use of alcohol and drugs, especially in youth. Experimental use is considered normal, and abuse often goes unnoticed until the second stage has begun. In the second stage, use is more frequent and the habit starts. Frequently signs may include a change in the type of friends one associates with and a decline in motivation and performance at school and work. Stage three shows a marked change in one's mood when domestic problems are common. The abuser may exhibit signs of depression and possibly talk of or attempt suicide. The person affected by abuse has an intense preoccupation to seek drugs for daily use. The fourth and last stage requires that the abuser take the drug in increasing amounts just to feel OK. Outward signs of stage four include coughing, frequent sore throats, weight loss, and fatigue. The person may also overdose and have blackouts. To maintain the habit, the person may have begun a life of crime. Deterioration of relationships and family is most evident. Obviously the sooner help is initiated the better in dealing with this situation. Stay firm in your attitudes, explanations, and efforts in seeking help for one who requests it.

The most commonly misused major groups of drugs and medicines in the United States are depressants, hallucinogens, narcotics, and stimulants. The state of addiction stems from periodic or chronic intoxication; that is, from repeated use. The abuser or addict has an overriding desire for the euphoric effect of the substance and will find a means of obtaining it to fulfill that desire. Because of increasing physiological tolerance of the drug, the user gradually must increase the dosage to maintain the desired effects. The user may also mix two

or more drugs, including alcohol. This practice, referred to as synergism, greatly enhances the intoxicating qualities of each drug into a combined new effect, which can be quite erratic and unpredictable. Though the user may realize the damaging effects of the substance, dependence can become so great that it is quite impossible to stop using the drug without outside intervention and assistance.

Rarely does the drug abuser begin by taking medicine to relieve pain, but more typically to avoid a confrontation with emotional or psychological problems. Hence the addiction is psychological as well as physical. These problems are only made more complex with the addition of mood-altering chemicals.

Depressants

Barbiturates, such as Butisol sodium, Donnatal, and Nembutal, to name a few, are used in the treatment of patients who need sedation or for the relief of anxiety. They are also used to induce sleep, and thus are frequently referred to as sleeping pills. They are also known as downers. They vary in strength and action but function by depressing the activity of the central nervous system. This affects the heart rate, respiration, blood pressure, and temperature. Tolerance to the drug is acquired after frequent use over a relatively short period of time. Psychological effects are similar to those of alcohol and when used with alcohol the danger to the user is great. A person under the influence of barbiturates appears to be intoxicated.

Immediate medical attention must be given in the case of overdose or death is imminent. For a victim who is still awake, the first step is to induce vomiting.

Hallucinogens

Hallucinogens are also referred to as psychedelics or sometimes as "mind-expanding" chemicals. Some of the most commonly used street drugs of this type are LSD, or acid, mescaline, and PCP (angel dust). These chemical substances give the user a distorted look at reality. "Taking a trip" refers to the visual hallucinations seen on those short chemical vacations. However, the images may be horrific, and "coming down" may be traumatic. Even though dependence does not seem to occur, the danger of hallucinogens is in the bizarre behavior that may result, which can cause accidental death to the user and others. In addition, some users experience undesirable "flashbacks" from some hallucinogens, or effects long after the drug was taken.

Marijuana can have hallucinogenic effects on the user. The effects of marijuana are varied and it can be classified in other drug categories as well. It is also referred to as dope, grass, mary jane, pot, reefer, smoke, and weed. It is one of the oldest and probably most widely used drugs next to alcohol, and it has become more socially

---

INDICATIONS OF DRUG/ALCOHOL ABUSE

- Abrupt change in mood/attitudes
- Sharp decline in attendance/performance at school/work
- Resistance to discipline/rules at home/school
- Deterioration in relationships
- Sudden unusual temper outbursts
- Increased frequency in borrowing money
- Stealing from others at home, school, or work
- Increased intense secrecy about actions and belongings
- Associating with new friends

FIGURE 22–5   Warning signs of possible drug or alcohol abuse

acceptable today than ever before. When mixed with other drugs it becomes more powerful and dangerous. Marijuana stimulates the central nervous system and produces a euphoric effect. It also distorts the perception of time and reality and can give rise to feelings of paranoia.

Marijuana may have **detrimental** effects on the respiratory and reproductive systems, and these are being studied. Use in treating nausea in patients undergoing chemotherapy for cancer and use in treating glaucoma have prompted further investigation into potential medical applications.

There is ongoing debate regarding legalization of marijuana. Those who choose to use marijuana are likely to continue whether it is legal or not. There are reports of third-grade youngsters who have already smoked marijuana. Early usage frequently leads to later use of more dangerous drugs.

Narcotics

A narcotic is a drug that produces insensibility or stupor. Legally, the term refers to habit-forming drugs such as opiates: cocaine, heroin, meperidine, and morphine. The lesser narcotics are paregoric, which is used in the treatment of diarrhea and abdominal pain, and codeine, which is a pain reliever. These substances can be obtained legally by a physician's prescription. However, federal, state and local laws prohibit the sale of narcotics for other than medical purposes. These medications are extremely potent and highly addictive. The possibility of overdose is great. Since many physicians store these medications in their offices or clinics, great care must be taken to ensure their security. You have a tremendous responsibility in keeping accurate records of these drugs.

Stimulants

The medical uses for stimulants are few. They are used in the treatment of **narcolepsy,** some cases of mental depression and alcoholism, chronic rigidity following encephalitis, and in some cases of obesity. The central nervous system is stimulated by **amphetamines,** which are referred to as uppers or speed. Abusers take speed in pill form to stay awake, to feel more energetic, or to lose weight. Some abusers inject the drug directly into their veins for a faster, more intense reaction. Others "snort" or sniff it to obtain the effects.

Cocaine was used as a local anesthetic many years ago, but today it is rarely used for medical purposes. Its illegal use is nearly epidemic. Songs have been written about it, and fashionable people use it in combination with other drugs for pleasure. Its effects are short-lived, usually about 12 minutes, and the user must constantly increase the dosage to reach the desired state. It is a stimulant that leaves the user depressed after it wears off. Most cocaine addicts must use other drugs to keep them going. The drug leads to frequent upper respiratory

and gastrointestinal problems. A nasty side effect suffered by many heavy "snorters" is destruction of the nasal passages. It is an extremely dangerous and expensive addiction.

Heavy use of any stimulant results in physical and psychological dependence. Few deaths are reported from abuse of stimulants, but many result from mixing them with other drugs. Physical ailments and emotional problems are the most evident effects of abusing stimulants.

Over-the-counter diet aids are popular stimulants, which are also abused. Their dangers arise when mixed with other drugs or alcohol. Pregnant women and patients with heart disease or hypertension must be particularly discouraged from using stimulants except under the direct supervision of a physician. This advice should be given to anyone in the use of any stimulant.

Probably the most abused stimulant is caffeine, found in coffee, tea, chocolate, and many cola drinks. Caffeine stimulates the central nervous system and also acts as a diuretic. Moderation is advised in its use. Coffee "jitters," for instance, cause one to feel out of sorts and nervous. Abuse can result in many related physical and emotional problems.

Treatment

Comprehensive rehabilitation programs to assist drug abusers are available in a variety of facilities, private and public.

Federal government facilities are located in Fort Worth, Texas, and Lexington, Kentucky. These are Public Health Service hospitals that offer treatment to addicts who volunteer for the program of rehabilitation.

Community hospitals and mental health centers provide these services as well. Staffed by psychiatrists, psychologists, counselors, and social workers, treatment centers give the addict the opportunity to receive therapy that can help in getting to the root of the problems leading to the addiction. Support from the health care team is necessary to assist in the return of the addict to a productive and meaningful life. Finally, Alcoholics Anonymous attracts many drug as well as alcohol abusers to its program.

Smoking ....

According to recent government studies, the risk of premature death due to smoking cigarettes is now the same for men and women. The saying, "You've come a long way baby," is unfortunately true. Nicotine dependence, for those smokers who use 20 (or more) cigarettes per day, is responsible for decreasing life expectancy by one-half. There are over 2,000 substances that have been identified in tobacco smoke. Of these, the three poisons in tobacco smoke that do the most harm are **tar, nicotine,** and **carbon monoxide**.

Tar is the thick, sticky, dark brown or black substance that is carried in inhaling the smoke and deposited in the lungs. Tar is a **carcinogen,** which means that it is capable of producing cancer in tissues with which it comes in contact. Nicotine is believed to be the addictive drug that is absorbed in the lungs and first stimulates and then depresses the nervous system. The stimulation is caused by the release of **norepinephrine** and because nicotine acts similarly like **acetylcholine. Cholinergic** nerves are stimulated by nicotine; and because nerve activity is blocked, depression results. Respiration rate is increased with stimulation of nerve receptors in the carotid arteries to supply more oxygen to the brain. The cardiovascular system is also stimulated with the release of norepinephrine, which causes an increase in blood flow to the heart and a rise in heart rate and blood pressure.

Nicotine seems to inhibit hunger, raises blood sugar levels slightly, and deadens taste buds in smokers.

Carbon monoxide produces still other dangerous effects. Red blood cells pick up carbon monoxide where it binds together to form **carboxyhemoglobin.** This could be the reason why smokers easily become short of breath with even moderate activity. Smokers have approximately 10% of their blood supply in the form of carboxyhemoglobin, which cannot carry oxygen. This is also a factor in the cause of heart attacks and lower birth weight and survival rate of babies of smoking mothers.

In addition, smokers are more at risk to have cancer of the lungs, larynx, lip, esophagus, and urinary bladder; chronic sinusitis and bronchitis; emphysema; URIs; cardiovascular diseases (CAD and ASHD); and peptic ulcers.

Even though these facts have been proven and efforts to discourage smoking in recent years have increased, men and women continue to smoke. The nicotine addiction is difficult for many to overcome. The key to success in the elimination of the smoking habit is first of all becoming thoroughly educated on the facts about smoking. Realizing the health hazards as well as the cost of this habit can be helpful to a smoker in making the decision to stop. Encourage patients, co-workers, family, and friends to consider attending a stop-smoking seminar. Post this information in the waiting room and on the employee's bulletin board. Reward those you know who have stopped smoking by giving them praise and recognition.

Some ways to help the smokers you know to get on the right track to stop their smoking habit are as follows:

1. Keep track of when and why you smoke for at least 2 weeks.
2. Compare a list of reasons why you should and should not stop.
3. Practice not smoking for a period of time (begin with an hour, a morning, a day, etc.)
4. Decide a target date when you are going to give up smoking.
5. Learn deep breathing relaxation exercises and use at least twice a day when tension becomes apparent.

Simply take a deep breath slowly and release slowly, thinking consciously of relaxing. Continue for 5 minutes unless you become dizzy.
6. Find a substitute to replace holding the cigarette.
7. Use nonsugar gums, mints, and mouth sprays to avoid overeating and to help curb the nicotine craving. (Transdermal nicotine patches available by prescription only may help patients break the habit successfully.)
8. Drink plenty of water and eat sensibly. Pay special attention to caloric intake for the first 4 to 8 weeks.
9. Include exercise to relieve tension and restlessness that comes with trying to overcome addiction.
10. Reward yourself with something special with the money saved from not buying cigarettes.

Involuntary smoking and *passive smoking* are terms describing secondhand smoke from active tobacco smokers. It is also called sidestream smoke. Both sidestream and mainstream smoke cause damage to the cells that line the heart and blood vessels. The buildup is a cause of atherosclerosis. Studies have shown that the platelets in the blood of smokers are more likely to clump together abnormally, which can lead to blood clots and the risk of a heart attack. Those exposed to secondhand smoke are not only at higher risk of heart disease and cancer, as are active smokers, they also are more likely to have respiratory illnesses often. Children who are exposed to passive smoke from parents may have poor development and reduced lung function, besides the diseases and disorders already mentioned. Those with chronic respiratory problems are obviously at greatest risk from passive smoke and these individuals certainly should keep from contact to prevent further irritation and difficulty with breathing.

Remind those who smoke to at least think about stopping. Advise them to refrain from smoking around others, especially children and those with respiratory distress. Smoke-free areas should be encouraged, respected, and applauded by those especially in the health care fields. Figure 22–6 illustrates a commonly posted sign requesting "No Smoking."

In patient education pursuits, make sure that you make them aware that tobacco contains poisons that could be fatal to toddlers if swallowed. All smoking materials should be kept out of the reach of children. Remember,

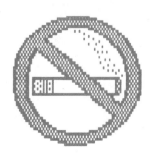

FIGURE 22–6 This common symbol is displayed in most public places with the notation "Thank you for not smoking."

the U.S. Surgeon General's report applies to everyone. **Warning:** The Surgeon General has determined that cigarette smoking is dangerous to your health.

Complete Chapter 22, Unit 2 in the workbook to help you meet the objectives at the beginning of this unit and therefore achieve competency of this subject matter.

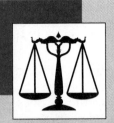

MEDICAL-LEGAL ETHICAL HIGHLIGHTS

Mrs. Right...
keeps the patient education material updated and replenished as necessary. She posts information about meetings and support groups on the bulletin board regularly to keep patients currently informed. She makes an effort to keep attractive displays about nutritional news and advice for patients.

Employment advancement: Excellent

Ms. Wrong...
is lazy and doesn't provide any patient education materials. She says that it's not her job.

Employment advancement: None (Probable termination)

REFERENCES

American Cancer Society. *Eating Smart.* 1989.

American Dietetic Association. *Staying Healthy—A Guide for Elder Americans.* 1990.

Kunz, Jeffrey, R.M., ed. *The American Medical Association Family Medical Guide.* New York: Random House, 1987.

Milliken, Mary Elizabeth. *Understanding Human Behavior,* 4th ed. Albany: Delmar, 1987.

Physicians' Desk Reference. Oradell, NJ: Medical Economics, updated annually.

Taber, Clarence W. *Taber's Cyclopedic Medical Dictionary,* 14th ed. Philadelphia: F.A. Davis, 1981.

United States Department of Health and Human Services, Alcohol, Drug Abuse, and Mental Health Administration. *Saying No.* Rockville, MD, 1981.

United States Department of Health and Human Services. *Diet, Nutrition, and Cancer Prevention.* Washington, D.C., 1987.

United States Department of Health and Human Services. *What You Can Do About Drug Use in America.* Publication No. (ADM) 90-1572. Washington, D.C., 1990.

United States Department of Justice, Drug Enforcement Administration. *Drugs of Abuse.* Washington, D.C., 1989.

Webster's New World Dictionary, 100,000 Entry Edition. New York: Penguin, 1971.

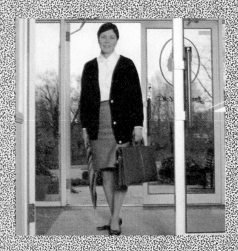

SECTION VI

A Final Note

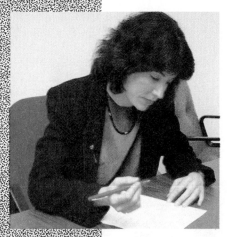

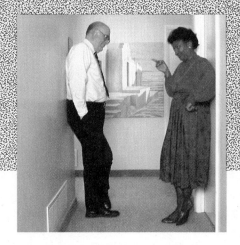

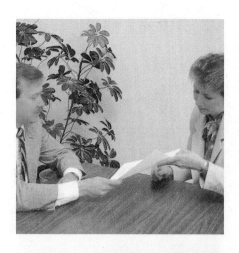

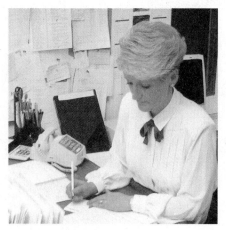

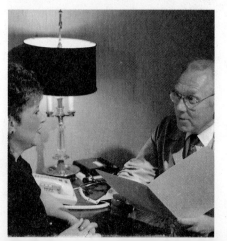

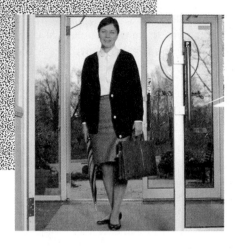

CHAPTER 23

Presenting Yourself For Employment

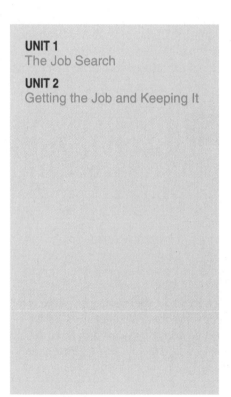

UNIT 1
The Job Search

UNIT 2
Getting the Job and Keeping It

A vast array of jobs require either administrative or clinical skills or a combination of both. Physicians in private practice usually have an average of three employees. In group practice, there may be from five to as many as forty or more, depending on the number of physicians and the size of the facility.

In seeking employment, you must be aware of the different opportunities and decide which area of medical assisting you would prefer. Many medical assistants prefer general or family practice because of its variety and challenge; others enjoy the specialty fields with their new developments and rapid change. There are still many health care facilities whose job descriptions specify particular duties, such as medical secretary, office nurse, or receptionist. The generally trained medical assistant should be able to perform the dual role of administrative and clinical assistant and will therefore be a valuable asset to any medical practice.

This chapter will discuss the steps involved in seeking employment in the health care field as well as presenting ideas for being a valuable employee. These job acquisition skills will be useful in other employment fields as well. Showing a genuine interest in others and the desire to work are the first steps in the job search.

UNIT 1

The Job Search

Upon completion of this unit, the student will meet the following terminal performance objectives by verifying knowledge of the facts and principles presented through oral and written communication at a level deemed competent, and will demonstrate the specific behaviors as identified in the terminal performance objectives of the procedures.

1. Prepare a neat, accurate, and well-organized resumé.
2. Discuss information contained in a resumé and the purpose of each style of resumé.
3. Write a cover letter to accompany a resumé.
4. Reply to a classified ad in the newspaper.
5. Explain employment agency services.
6. List three contacts to assist you in your job search.
7. Define the common abbreviations used in the newspaper "Help Wanted" section.
8. Spell and define, using the glossary at the back of the text, all the words to know in this unit.

WORDS TO KNOW ···

aspirations	functional
attribute	ingenuity
chronological	negotiable
classified	resumé
dual	targeted
elaborate	transcript

The job search begins with the desire to work. A medical assistant with skills in communication and medical office procedures should discover excellent opportunities for employment.

The Resumé

One of the first steps in presenting yourself for employment is to develop a personal resumé. A resumé is an outlined summary of your abilities and experience. It should be complete, accurate, and neatly organized. The resumé will describe to prospective employers your educational background, previous work experience, professional affiliations, community service, personal inter- ests, honors, employment objectives, and whatever else you feel is important for them to know. It need not contain personal information about your marital status, race, religion, age, or any other facts that may be used to discriminate against you illegally. The purpose of the resumé is to inform the prospective employer of how well you measure up to the position for which you are applying.

There are several styles of resumés. You may arrange the information in a variety of ways. Some popular styles include: a traditional format in **chronological** order, a listing of your career objective, in a **functional** plan, or in a **targeted** layout. Figure 23–1 (A) through (E) shows an example of each type. Each of these designs is attractive and easy to read. The *traditional (chronological) approach* shows the reader your background information in an organized fashion. It is a good way to highlight your abilities when you are just beginning the job search. The *career objective* style shows your obvious career choice to the reader and is followed by your abilities and qualifications. It is also a frequently chosen style for the novice. A *chronologically arranged* resumé, page 718, shows the prospective employer your

---

P R O C E D U R E

Prepare a Resumé

PURPOSE: To document information concerning education, experience, and abilities for employment consideration.

Items needed: Paper, pen, dictionary, thesaurus, telephone book, typewriter/word processor

1. Write your complete legal name, address, and phone number. This information may be arranged flush left or centered at the top of the page.
   Refer to Figure 23–1 for the particular style of resumé that is appropriate for you and/or your needs. Use reference materials listed above for accuracy, expression, and correct spelling in composing your resumé.
2. Briefly state your qualifications/abilities, and list the position desired next to the heading of: Job Objective or Job Target.
3. List your educational background, beginning with the most recent or present date. You may note that you will furnish **transcripts**/certificates on request at the bottom of the resumé.
4. List all pertinent employment experience, beginning with the most recent or present date. Include the dates of employment, employer's name, address, and the position you held with a brief description of your responsibilities according to the style of resumé you have selected.
5. List memberships/affiliations in professional organiza- tions. These may be arranged alphabetically or ranked by order of importance.
6. List community service, including volunteer programs and activities as may be appropriate. This is optional.
7. List outside interests briefly as appropriate. This is optional.
8. List references on a separate sheet of paper. State on the bottom of the resumé that references will be furnished on request. You should have at least three references (persons *not* related to you) and no more than five. Permission should be obtained from these persons *before* they are listed.
9. Type the completed resumé on a sheet of bond paper, or use the word processor to enter your information. Underscore (underline) headings for clarity and attractiveness. Check the finished copy for errors (use spell-check program on word processor). Ask a reliable person to proofread your resumé. Have a number of copies printed on quality paper for distribution (off-white, beige, or ivory white are preferred colors).
10. Revise and update your resumé to document additional employment experience, educational achievements, certificates, awards, and personal development. Items of lesser importance should be deleted as more important accomplishments are added.

Sandy Lynn Beach, CMA
4030 Newbank Road
Wheelersburg, Ohio 45794
(614) 555-1212
Qualifications: Certified Medical Assistant
Desired Position: Clinical Medical Assistant
Education:
    1992 to date: Attending evening courses in Nursing, Southern Ohio Technical College, Lucasville, Ohio
                   AAMA National Certification 1990
    1986–87:   Certificate, Ohio Valley Training Academy, Wellston, Ohio. Major: Medical Assisting
    1984:   Diploma, Portsmouth East High School, Portsmouth, Ohio. Major: General Business
EMPLOYMENT EXPERIENCE:
    1990 to date: Administrative Medical Assistant to Wilber Roth, M.D., Rolling Hills, Ohio
    1987–90:   Admissions Clerk, Green Meadows Community Hospital, Green Meadows, Ohio
    1984–87:   Cashier, Garden Inn Restaurant, Hilldale, Ohio
PROFESSIONAL ASSOCIATIONS:
    American Association of Medical Assistants
    Ohio State Society of Medical Assistants
    Scioto County Chapter of Medical Assistants
COMMUNITY SERVICE:
    Red Cross Volunteer
    Big Sisters Association Volunteer
Interests: aerobics, camping, knitting, music, reading
References, transcripts and certificates, furnished upon request.

FIGURE 23–1   Sample Resumés   **A**. Traditional (chronological order) format

Jody C. Lawrence
270 Huxley Road
Avondale, Ohio 41234
(614) 555-1212
CAREER OBJECTIVE
    To establish a career as a Medical Assistant in a professional medical practice in both administrative and
    clinical capacities; To become a Certified Medical Assistant.
EDUCATION
    Independence High School, Major: Business; plan to receive diploma this June
    Southfield Vocational Center, Program Specialty; Medical Assisting; plan to receive vocational certificate
    this June
EXPERIENCE
    Avondale Civic Center; part-time secretary, 29 East Main Street, Avondale, Ohio 41234
    Southfield Family Practice; externship as Student Medical Assistant, 589 Garfield Avenue, Suite 212,
    Southfield, Ohio 41239
ACTIVITIES/HONORS
    Cheerleader, all four years, Independence High School
    Class Secretary, Senior year, Independence High School
    Health Fair Committee, Junior and Senior years, Southfield Vocational Center Honor Roll, all four years
    Vocational Industrial Clubs of America, Class Club Treasurer, Senior year, Southfield Vocational Center
SKILLS
    Typing—65 WPM, transcribing, operating: calculator, IBM computer
    Basic clinical laboratory procedures; CPR
INTERESTS
    Cooking, dancing, poetry, swimming, softball

FIGURE 23–1 B.   "Career objective" style

Sharon R. Beach
4270 Hilldale Drive
Fernridge, CA 95061
(406) 555-1122

Employment Experience

1989–Present	Fernridge Family Health Center
	Clinical Medical Assistant
	Provide patient education regarding therapeutic diets; assist with minor office surgery; perform ECGs and Holter monitors; phlebotomy and routine diagnostic tests.
1986–1989	Brownsville General Hospital
	Phlebotomist/ECG Technician
1985–1986	Ronald L. Botkin, D.O.—General Practice
	Administrative and Clinical Medical Assistant
	Completed medical insurance claim forms; office correspondence; transcription; basic clinical assisting.

Professional Affiliations/Achievements

1985 to Present	Member American Association of Medical Assistants
1990 to Present	CPR Certification
1990	Certified Medical Assistant Certificate

Education

1988	B.A. Degree; Nutrition, Brownsville University
1985	Medical Assistant Program Certificate, Baldwin Community College

FIGURE 23–1 C. Example of chronological resumé

employment history in dated order from present (or most recent) back to the beginning of your work experience. You should highlight the responsibilities of each position. Your present job duties should be emphasized. This will show the employer your strengths. The *functional type resumé* draws attention to the most important areas of your achievements and strengths. You may arrange the information to highlight your abilities but not necessarily in dated order of your employment experience. A *targeted resumé,* page 720, is used for a precise field of employment. It shows the employer your expertise in a particular area. This type of resumé is directed to a specific job title. One that is basic but complete and properly arranged will attract an employer's attention. One that is flashy, too lengthy, or too wordy may well be discarded. A one-page resumé is a preferred length. It should be well-organized and grammatically correct. You should always have someone proofread your resumé because often our own mistakes go unnoticed. Spelling must be correct. There is no need for being **elaborate** in style. A simple typed or printed resumé on quality paper will make the information stand out, which is the sole purpose of it. Describing your objectives clearly will direct the employer's attention to your qualifications for employment. Noting your **aspirations** will give the interviewer some insight as to your long-term goals and your level of ambition. Although the main purpose of the resumé is to communicate your abilities to an employer, it also may spur interest in getting an interview for a specific position. Preparation of a resumé requires you to

systematically list experiences that show your valuable **attributes.** Awards and special certificates should be listed along with the reasons for which they were given. These will interest an employer and may be the deciding factor when the final hiring decision is made.

In composing your resumé you should be aware that some items are optional. Realizing that employers are people too will help you decide about including personal information. This section of your resumé can convey your genuine caring for others and good citizenship in your community. Interests and community service are not required, but often communicate a human touch to the reader. Often the employer can relate to the community service organization you have listed (or one similar). It is possible that you may be selected for an interview over others who are just as qualified because you have communicated to the reader that you are a well-rounded person. Employers are often interested in what you do with the other hours of your day besides work. A person who has a balance in life is usually happier, healthier, and more productive and full of life in general.

The Cover Letter

After you have perfected your resumé, you should do the same in composing a cover letter to send with it. It must state *why* you should be hired for the desired position. The cover letter should be addressed to the person who decides who is interviewed and hired. Finding out the name of the office manager or supervisor may be done

Sharon R. Beach
4270 Hilldale Drive
Fernridge, CA 95061
(406) 555-1122

Communication skills:
- Providing patient education regarding therapeutic diets
- Sending referral, follow-up, and other correspondence
- Scheduling appointments

Administrative skills:
- Completing medical insurance claim forms
- Transcribing medical histories and progress notes
- Date entry of patient information

Clinical Skills:
- Phlebotomy and basic diagnostic laboratory tests
- Electrocardiogram and Holter monitor
- CPR and first aid
- Sterile technique and assisting with minor surgery

Employment Experience:

1989–Present	Fernridge Family Health Center
	Clinical Medical Assistant
	Provide patient education regarding therapeutic diets; assist with minor office surgery; perform ECGs and Holter monitors; phlebotomy and routine diagnostic tests
1986–1989	Brownsville General Hospital
	Phlebotomist/ECG technician
1985–1986	Ronald L. Botkin, D.O.—General Practice
	Administrative and Clinical Medical Assistant
	Completed medical insurance claim forms; office correspondence; transcription; basic clinical assisting

Education:

1985	Baldwin Community College
	Medical Assistant Program
1988	Brownsville University
	B.A. Degree; Nutrition

FIGURE 23–1 D. Functional resumé

by making a simple phone call and asking (be sure to get the correct spelling). Personalizing the letter will gain more attention than will the standard form letter. Let the employer know that your skills and qualifications will be an asset. Make the letter simple and direct to convey what makes you special for the job. Be sure to request an interview and make it clear when and how you can be reached for an appointment to be made. Figure 23–2, page 721, gives sample cover letters.

Both cover letter and resumé must be error free. Employers eliminate numerous resumés by pitching those with spelling or grammatical errors and tears or smudges, or those that are too wordy or unorganized.

Classified Advertisements ....

You may send your resumé to a prospective employer in response to a **classified** ad in the local newspaper. A classified ad is a request for qualified applicants to send information about themselves to a prospective employer. The employer may then request an interview with those who meet the requirements for the position instead of interviewing all persons who may wish to apply. This method of screening saves time for the employer and makes the resumé a most important means of communication. Figure 23–3, page 722, shows abbreviations commonly used in classified advertisements.

In responding to a classified ad, it is customary to write a cover letter to accompany your resumé. This cover letter expresses your desire to be interviewed for the position and describes briefly who you are and what you have to offer.

Public Employment Services ....

All states offer assistance in locating jobs through the state employment service. Local offices of this agency will have job openings on file, including, possibly, the one you are looking for. You simply walk in, fill out the general forms, wait your turn, and then have a conference with an employment counselor. If there are listings which call for your kind of experience and training, you will have immediate leads to begin checking. If no appropriate listings are currently on file, the employment counselor will place your name on file and notify you when listings do materialize. Because this agency is supported by tax dollars, there is no fee for the service.

Private Employment Agencies ....

Private employment agencies offer similar services. A cover letter and resumé should be sent to the agency explaining your area of expertise and desired employment. Many agencies specialize in the medical field and can give efficient service in locating openings in medical assisting. Many potential jobs are "fee paid," meaning that the employer pays the agency's fee. In general, you should avoid positions which require you to pay the fee. This is too often a means of taking advantage of employees. The decision is obviously yours. You may be definitely interested in a particular position for which you have to pay the fee. Carefully weighing the advantages and disadvantages will help you decide if the cost is worth it to you in the long run. A substantial pay increase is an obvious advantage. If you have been waiting for a certain position to open for a relatively long period of time, or the position is unique and rarely provides an opening, it may well be a wise choice to secure it by paying a fee. Often arrangements may be made for the fee to be paid in installments. Fees for finding employment positions are generally based on a percentage of the annual wages of an employee.

Other Contacts ....

A resumé with a cover letter requesting an interview may be sent to many medical offices or health care facilities even if there is no position available. If you ardently wish to be employed in a particular facility, making it known may spark an interest in you as a prospective employee should there be an opening. Introducing yourself through correspondence and specifying your interest in employment should a position become available can be very productive. Employers may keep your letter and resumé on file for as long as a year and respond as the need arises.

Sharon R. Beach
4270 Hilldale Drive
Fernridge, CA 95061
(406) 555-1122
Job Target: Clinical Medical Assistant
Abilities:
 • Communication skills—patient education
 • CPR and first aid
 • Phlebotomy
 • Basic clinical laboratory skills
 • Electrocardiography
Achievements:
 • Certified Medical Assistant
 • Bachelor's degree in Nutrition
 • CPR certification
Employment Experience:
1989–Present   Fernridge Family Health Center
                Clinical Medical Assistant
1986–1989   Brownsville General Hospital
                Phlebotomist/ECG Technician
1985–1986   Ronald L. Botkin, D.O.—General Practice
                Administrative and Clinical Medical Assistant
Professional Affiliations:
 •   Member—American Association of Medical Assistants
Education:
1985   Baldwin Community College
1988   Brownsville University

FIGURE 23–1 E. Example of targeted resumé

Date

Karla Baker, CMA-A
Office Manager
Hilldale Medical Center
Hilldale, Ohio 45102

Dear Ms. Baker:
My training in medical assisting at Ohio Valley Training Academy has provided me with skills in both administrative and clinical areas. I am very interested in securing a position in your health care facility as a **dual** Medical Assistant. I am nationally certified as my enclosed resumé states.

Please let me know if you wish an appointment for an interview. I can be reached at home on Tuesday and Thursday afternoons and every evening at 555-8131.

Thank you for your consideration.

Sincerely,

Sandy Lynn Beach, CMA

FIGURE 23–2 Sample cover letter for a resumé

4270 Hilldale Drive
Fernridge, CA 95061
(406) 555-1122
March 4, 1992

Ms. Doreen Castle
Office Manager
Hopkin's Medical Clinic
739 Mountainview Way
Great Valley, CA 95068

Dear Ms. Castle:
I read your ad in the local paper about the opening for a full-time clinical medical assistant at Hopkin's Medical Clinic. I feel that my training and experience would make me a worthy candidate for this position. As you will see from my resumé, I am a Certified Medical Assistant and have a bachelor's degree in Nutrition.

In addition, my experience in patient education regarding therapeutic diets has helped me to sharpen my communication skills. I also have excellent clinical skills and am current in CPR certification.

I would like to meet with you for an interview at your earliest convenience. Please call me at the number listed above to schedule an appointment. I can be reached at home every evening and on Wednesday afternoons.

Yours truly,

(Miss) Sharon R. Beach, CMA

FIGURE 23–2 Sample cover letter B.

APPT—Appointment	MED—Medical
ASST—Assistant	MGR—Manager
BGN or BEG—Beginning	MOS—Months
COL—College	NEC—Necessary
DEPT—Department	NEG—**Negotiable**
EDUC—Education	OFC—Office
EOE—Equal Opportunity Employer	PD—Paid
EXP—Experience	POS—Position(s)
F—Female	PT—Part Time
FB—*Fringe Benefits*	REF—References
FT—Full Time	REQ—Required
GRAD—Graduate	SAL—Salary
H—Handicapped	SEC—Secretary
HS—High School	T—Temporary
HR—Hour	TRANSP—Transportation
HRS—Hours	WPM—Words per minute
IMMED—Immediate	WK—Week
INT—Interview	WKENDS—Weekends
LIC—License	W/—With
M—Male	Yrs—Years

FIGURE 23–3 Abbreviations used in the "Help Wanted" section of the newspaper

Additional information about job opportunities may be obtained at the public library. Many services, periodicals, and books deal with occupational information, and library personnel can be very helpful. Membership in professional associations is quite helpful in the job search, too. Not only may an association's publications include classified ads, but personal contact with other members at meetings may provide invaluable information about job openings. Participation in community service groups can put you in touch with yet another network of persons who may have information about job openings. Finally, you should not overlook your friends and acquaintances; the job one of them happens to mention in conversation could turn out to be just the one you have been waiting for. If you have a sincere desire to be employed, a job can be found. However, as most people have realized from time to time, it may take patience, persistence, and **ingenuity.**

Complete Chapter 23, Unit 1 in the workbook to help you meet the objectives at the beginning of this unit and therefore achieve competency of this subject matter.

U N I T   2

Getting the Job and Keeping It

OBJECTIVES ....

Upon completion of this unit, the student will meet the following terminal performance objectives by verifying knowledge of the facts and principles presented through oral and written communication at a level deemed competent.

1. Complete a job application form.
2. Discuss the importance of appearance when interviewing and/or applying for a job.
3. State the purpose of a job interview.
4. Explain the importance of promptness and courtesy in a job interview.
5. Explain the reasons for sending a follow-up letter after an interview.
6. Write a follow-up letter.
7. List the qualities employers regard as most important in employees.
8. Discuss "dos" and "don'ts" in interviewing and/or applying for a job.
9. List the most important qualities necessary for job advancement.
10. Discuss each of the 15 commonly asked questions on a job interview.
11. Discuss questions that applicants may ask on a job interview.
12. Spell and define, using the glossary at the back of the text, all of the words to know in this unit.

WORDS TO KNOW ....

apprise	demeanor
arbitrary	fringe
competent	negate
contemporary	reiterate

Application Forms ....

Filling out an application for employment may be your next step. These forms may range from the simple to the complex. Figure 23–4 shows an example of an application form that asks for a minimal amount of information. Often the information is the same as what is contained on your resumé. Remember to take a copy of your resumé with you to help you fill out the job application. Some applications are extremely lengthy (several pages). It may be best if this type is taken home to complete as it may take a considerable amount of time. It is not considered

EMPLOYMENT APPLICATION FORM

PERSONAL

NAME _____ DATE_____

| (LAST) | (FIRST) | (MI) |

ADDRESS—STREET   CITY   STATE   ZIP

PHONE NUMBER   SOCIAL SECURITY NUMBER

POSITION DESIRED:

EXPECTED SALARY OR HOURLY WAGE:

EDUCATION

	NAME OF SCHOOL	ADDRESS	DATE(S)	DEGREE/CERTIFICATE
HIGH SCHOOL				
VOCATIONAL/TECHNICAL				
COLLEGE				
OTHER				

WORK EXPERIENCE—Give present position (or last position held first).

JOB TITLE:	EMPLOYER	ADDRESS	DATES
DUTIES PERFORMED:			
JOB TITLE:	EMPLOYER	ADDRESS	DATES
DUTIES PERFORMED:			

REFERENCES—LIST THREE PERSONS (OTHER THAN RELATIVES) WHO HAVE KNOWN YOU FOR AT LEAST 2 YEARS

NAME/TITLE	ADDRESS	TELEPHONE NUMBER

FIGURE 23–4   Example of an employment application

proper to ask for a phone directory or any other reference when applying for a job. You are supposed to show that you are prepared. In filling out an application for employment, you must be accurate and honest. Being prepared with dates, names, addresses, phone numbers, and other detailed information will expedite completion of the form. You should also be aware of the impression you may give when you apply for employment. Even if you are merely picking up an application to take home to complete, or returning it after you have completed it, your appearance, including your attitude, will certainly be noticed. You should dress for success any time a prospective employer may see you. Other employees will surely notice you and relay the information to the employer, especially if there is a negative impression given.

Because of the professional setting (medical field) for which you are seeking employment, many employers require that the trust of prospective employees is checked. Among the areas of concern are the person's credit rating, police record, and chemical use/abuse. You may be asked to produce these documents or give authorization for the employer to find out about your personal records before you may be considered for hiring.

Since the job application will probably reach the personnel manager's office before you do, it must speak well for you; it must make a good impression on the person who reads it. Applications must be complete, neat, and legible or they will promptly be discarded. Reading and following the instructions on the form is of utmost importance. Most forms begin with directions to print all information requested. Ignoring basic directions of this nature is not the mark of a good candidate for employment. The application form will provide the employer not only with factual information about you but with many other insights as well.

If you take sufficient time and interest in completing the application you will be more likely to be given a personal interview. Additionally, because of the Immigration Reform Act of 1986, employers are required by federal law to ask you for documents that show both your identity and eligibility to work in the United States. Employers will make copies of your documents and return them to you. Further, the Employment Eligibility Verification Form I-9 must be completed and filed in the employee's record along with other important documents. Employers must verify that you are legally entitled to work in the U.S. All applicants and employers must comply with this law. Refer to Chapter 12, Medical Office Management, for more details.

The Interview

An interview is a face-to-face meeting between you and your prospective employer. The day of the scheduled interview you should allow sufficient time to get ready. If you chew gum or smoke cigarettes, leave these at home for this trip. Neither has any place in a job interview.

When applying for a job, your appearance is extremely important. Appearance is an outward indication of who you are. Remember what you learned about nonverbal communication. If you are a sincere, **competent,** and dedicated person, then by all means attend to your appearance accordingly. Nonverbal messages, though silent, can speak loudly.

Most employers expect appropriate attire and some require adherence to a very specific policy concerning mode of dress and general appearance.

If you are interviewing for a clinical position, ask beforehand about what type of dress to wear. Your inquiry will most likely be taken as showing genuine interest. Often employers will want to see you dressed in what you perceive as a "uniform" to see how you will look on the job.

Women who prefer to wear business type attire should dress conservatively in a navy, gray, tan, or brown tailored suit. Bright colors, or jewelry, miniskirts, pants, and frilly outfits are not considered professional attire. Men should also follow this advice and dress conservatively, avoiding outrageous ties, jewelry, and fad clothes. Remember that you should make every effort to make a positive impression with the interviewer concerning yourself and your qualifications, not your ability to show off fashions and accessories. It follows that those interested in employment at a facility should conform to the standards set forth. Following fads in fashion is usually not advisable. Trendy looks are for models for the most part. A medical assistant who is more interested in meeting the requirements of the job than in being the center of attention is more appealing to a personnel manager.

The same rules apply to job interviews that have already been mentioned in terms of the job. Since they are important, they will be **reiterated** once more. All matters concerning personal cleanliness are vital. The following attributes are sure to interfere with or **negate** the possibility of employment: bad breath, dirty or uneven fingernails, dirty or unkempt hair, overpowering aftershave or perfume, unclean teeth, unpleasant or offensive body odor, or untended complexion problems.

The point is this: no matter how well qualified or eager you are, you may not find anyone willing to pay for your services if you fail in certain matters of personal hygiene. Take nothing for granted. Make strict adherence to proper personal grooming a rigid daily rule.

Rushing usually detracts from your appearance and **demeanor.** If the address of the facility is not familiar to you, get directions and plan your time beforehand. (It is a good idea to drive, or have someone take you, a day or two before the scheduled interview to scout out the area to determine the approximate travel time, exact location, parking, bus route, etc. to avoid getting lost or being delayed because of confusion due to construction, etc.) You should arrive about 10 minutes before the appointment. (You may be instructed to arrive up to an hour or more before the interview to complete an application form or to take required preemployment tests.) Arriving too early will make you appear insecure. Being late for almost any reason will make you appear irresponsible and a poor candidate for the position. If you happen to find yourself in this predicament, a telephone call explaining the delay and a sincere apology are in order. Being on time is a sign of reliability, dependability, and conscientiousness.

Introducing yourself with a handshake should initiate a friendly and pleasant conversation. Your manner should tell the interviewer you are happy to be there.

The interview ought to allow sufficient time for each of you to inquire about the other and to discuss the requirements of the position. Often the interviewer will have reviewed your resumé.

You should be prepared to answer questions concerning your career goals and objectives, how you feel about changes, why you decided on this career, your further educational plans, and so on, Figure 23–5. Your answers should be brief, concise, and honest.

In terms of perspective and dimension, the section of the resumé that lists community services is an appealing area to prospective employers. It is an indicator of your concern for others, your involvement, and your enjoyment of working. Many employers will ask what prompted your interest in a particular service area.

Contemporary federal laws are designed to deal with arbitrary discrimination in hiring practices. Toward this end, you should not be asked questions concerning your age, cultural or ethnic background, marital status, or parenthood. Nevertheless, these issues may come up in the course of your interview. You are not required to provide this information if you choose not to. The purpose of the interview is to ascertain the relevance of your experience and character to the job at hand. Should any of these unrelated issues come up, be careful to analyze the context in which they arose (it could be from something you said). In any case, if you are honestly convinced that you have been denied a job because of arbitrary discrimination, be advised that this is illegal, and you have legal recourse.

At some point during the interview, the interviewer may give you a written job description of the position for which you are applying. You will probably be given time to look it over and then asked if you would feel confident about performing the job described. An honest answer is the best. Avoid hedging or bluffing about issues because an experienced interviewer will pick up on your insecurities. Remember that body language tells the rest of the story. If there are one or two duties you have never performed before or one or two pieces of equipment which you know little about, say this but add that you are eager to learn. The employer will appreciate the initiative in your answer. If the job description sounds totally unfamiliar, it is best to say that, too, or if you feel it would be an impossible task. The interviewer will appreciate your openness.

1. What are your qualifications for employment in our facility?
2. Do you have plans for continuing education? If yes, what are your plans?
3. What were your favorite subjects in school and why?
4. Why are you seeking employment with us?
5. What made you decide to enter the medical assisting field?
6. What is your most rewarding experience in life thus far?
7. What are your long-range career goals?
8. What motivates you to do your best?
9. What is the most difficult problem you ever had to deal with? And how did you handle it?
10. What does success mean to you?
11. What relationship should exist between supervisors and those under their supervision?
12. How would you describe yourself?
13. Do you work well under pressure?
14. What are your strengths and weaknesses?
15. What two things are most important to you in a job?

FIGURE 23–5 Fifteen commonly asked questions during interviews

Some positions may have no job description, and the duties involved will be discussed during the interview. Knowing that there are probably as many duties not mentioned as mentioned will give you an idea of the amount of work the job requires.

By the time all of these matters have been dealt with, the interview will be starting to wind down. The interviewer beginning to reach closure will apprise you of this by asking you if you have any further questions. If

1. To see a Job Description
2. About Hours—Work Day Schedule
3. Rate of Pay (if not Discussed by the Close of the Interview)
4. Chances for Advancement or Promotion
5. About Continuing Education—In-Service Programs
6. Fringe Benefits:
    a. Health insurance plan
    b. Dental insurance plan
    c. Eye care
    d. Vacation/time off
    e. Membership dues in AAMA
    f. Profit sharing
    g. Retirement plan
    h. Other
7. Evaluations of Job Performance Periodically

FIGURE 23–6 Questions *you*, the applicant, may ask during an interview

WHEN APPLYING FOR A JOB:	
DO	*DON'T*
ARRIVE ON TIME (10–15 minutes early) SHOW INTEREST—ENTHUSIASM! DISPLAY A POSITIVE ATTITUDE USE COURTESY ACT COMPOSED DRESS APPROPRIATELY KEEP GOOD POSTURE (SIT STILL AND STRAIGHT)	BE LATE! ASK TOO MANY QUESTIONS OR MAKE EXCUSES TALK ABOUT PERSONAL PROBLEMS ACT OVER-CONFIDENT DRUM FINGERS, SWING LEG, TAP FOOT OVERDRESS CHEW GUM/SMOKE

FIGURE 23–7   Reminders in applying for employment

issues of salary, raises, and advancement have not been dealt with previously, this is an appropriate point to mention them. This is also the logical point for you to ask about any other matters you be uncertain about, Figure 23–6, page 725. See Figure 23–7 for the "dos and don'ts" of applying for a job. However, do not drag out this time. Let the interview end smoothly. When it is over, rise and thank the interviewer for his or her time. Firmly shake hands if the interviewer extends a hand, Figure 23–8. Remember to smile and be pleasant and polite as you exit with confidence.

The interviewer may talk to a number of people about a specific job opening in the office. To help the interviewer remember specific facts and traits about each individual, a form such as the one shown in Figure 23–9 may be filled out.

You may be one of many candidates interviewing for a particular job. Therefore, any decision may take some time. Out of courtesy as well as to enhance your image with the interviewer, take the time to compose a follow-

up letter shortly after the interview has taken place. Figure 23–10 offers a sample letter.

What Employers Want Most in Employees .....

The personal investment that you have made with regard to your education and skills training along with all of the effort you have put forth in producing a resumé and interviewing for employment does not stop with being hired. After securing a position, you must continually endeavor to do your best. An employer will expect you to perform with increasing expertise in your position as you continue to gain experience.

Desirable employee qualities that employers generally rank as most important are listed as follows:

1. Communication skills (oral and written)
2. Cooperation
3. Courteousness
4. Dependability
5. Enthusiasm
6. Initiative
7. Interest
8. Math skills
9. Punctuality
10. Reading skills
11. Reliability
12. Responsibility
13. Time management skills

These qualities are fast becoming increasingly more important and are a stark fact in holding a job. Becoming proficient in grammar, including both the written and spoken word, is a must. Speaking in a well-educated manner is necessary to portray a professional image of not only yourself, but of the facility where you are employed. You become a member of a team of medical personnel who reflect each other to the public you serve. Many evening classes, such as a business English course, offer basic review in grammar. Taking the initiative to improve oneself is admirable. Employers recog-

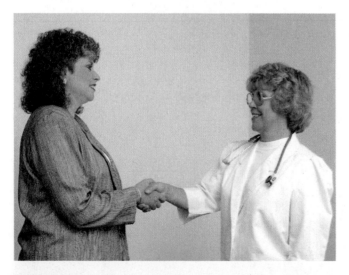

FIGURE 23–8   A firm handshake at the conclusion of the interview conveys courtesy and mutual respect.

INTERVIEW EVALUATION					
Subject	Excellent	Good	Satisfactory	Needs Improvement	Poor
Appearance					
Attitude					
Eye contact					
Self-control					
Voice					
Grammar					
Responses					
Manners					
Resumé					
Comments					
Date					
Employer			Title		
Address			Phone		
Applicant					

FIGURE 23–9 Employers may use a form such as this after an interview to record information about an applicant.

nize these efforts and for those with ambition, rewards will surely follow.

Attendance is most important as schedules must be constantly changed and reassignments made when an employee is absent, especially when it is unexpected. An absent employee affects everyone as work must be divided among other team members. Scheduling personal appointments should be done on your day off or after working hours. If there is an important engagement for which you need time off from your job, you should ask for a meeting with your supervisor to discuss making arrangements for a day off well in advance of the date. Remember that *only when it is absolutely necessary* should you call in sick. If you are not sure about the office policy regarding this issue, you should ask your employer. Employees have a responsibility to report a personal or serious illness to their supervisor as soon as possible. When an emergency involves an accident or acute medical problem, notification of the circumstance will be received with sympathy and concern. Generally employers are most understanding about illness when the reason is genuine. If child care is a problem, and the reason for absence is due to needing someone to care for children, the supervisor should be made aware of the situation. Often supervisors may be helpful in assisting with information that could be a possible solution to the problem. However, repeated occurrences of calling in "sick" just to take a day off will become annoying and

may lead to disciplinary action. Usually offenders are more likely to take off on Mondays and Fridays for long weekends. These are days when schedules are full and all employees are most needed. If one is placed on probation and warned about poor attendance practices and the warnings go unheeded, it could ultimately result in the employee's dismissal.

It is equally important to be on time daily. Being prompt is a valuable personal quality appreciated by both employers and patients. Leaving early is not advised unless absolutely necessary and with permission of the supervisor in advance. When one leaves before the scheduled time it puts an added burden on other team members to finish your job. With each member of the health care team doing what is expected the work will be shared and the group's efficiency will be noticed by your employer. This makes for a harmonious working relationship among employees. You have studied throughout this text about various patient education materials and guidelines for better health. You must have realized by now that you should be practicing what you are expected to teach patients. This can only help you to feel better about yourself, which will be evident to others with whom you come in contact. In good health you will be more productive, energetic, and display better coping skills. All of the qualities important to employers should also be important to you. The secret to success is simple. Strive toward fulfilling the goals you set and do everything in your power to reach them. Your personal satisfaction is surely one goal that will be realized if you follow this plan.

Date

Karla Baker, CMA-A
Office Manager
Hilldale Medical Center
Hilldale, Ohio 45102

Dear Ms. Baker:

Thank you very much for granting me an interview for the Clinical Medical Assistant's position on your staff. The interview was both challenging and stimulating; I found it to be an enjoyable and rewarding experience.

You outlined the duties and responsibilities which come with the position very specifically. This is the type of position for which I have been trained; I feel confident that if I am offered the position, I can handle the responsibilities and become an asset to your staff.

Again, thank you for considering me for this position. I would be most appreciative if you would inform me of your final decision as soon as it is convenient for you.

Sincerely,

Sandy Lynn Beach, CMA

FIGURE 23–10 A follow-up letter

In addition to these qualities, one in particular that the medical assistant must keep in mind is personal appearance. A medical assistant must continually strive to maintain an impeccable appearance; this is essential to ensure job security. Looking your best requires that you compliment your best assets and always keep neat, clean, and attractive to the public eye.

When you obtain employment, you must necessarily dedicate yourself first of all to the task of keeping the job. This is where your work history begins, and it will probably follow you throughout your working life. If the health care field remains your chosen career area and if medical assisting is your point of entry, then you must be determined to become the very best medical assistant you can. Ultimately, your eventual advancement into more responsible medical assisting duties and higher pay will depend largely upon your demonstrated capabilities in performing your administrative and clinical tasks. However, the aforementioned employee qualities will also become significant factors in paving the way for advancement.

Consider this scenario: A physician employs two medical assistants; both are the same age and possess relatively equal administrative and clinical skills. The only differences between the two come down to appearance and attitude. One maintains a considerably nicer appearance than the other, along with a more positive attitude. As the physician's volume of business expands and a promotion and salary increase for one of the positions becomes inevitable, guess which one will likely get the nod from the physician. You do not have to be a genius to figure this one out. In the end, it comes down to common sense.

Employee's name   Job title/position   Date hired

Supervisor   Title   Date of evaluation

Scheduled evaluation/review: ___Initial ___ 3 month ___ 6 month ___ annual ___ *other

*Explain___

Previous review date ___ Rating ___

Comments___

Total days/times: absent ___ Tardy___ Left early___

Rate the following areas of the employee appropriately using the scale from 1 to 10:
1 2 3 4 5 6 7 8 9 10

Job knowledge: very little / limited / adequate / average / good /superior/ outstanding ___

Quality of work: very poor/ fair/ good/ acceptable/ excellent/ superior/ outstanding ___

Quantity of work: inferior/inadequate / does just enough/ average/ superior/outstanding ___

Speed: very slow / below average / average / above average / outstanding ___

Initiative: lacking / needs pushing / adequate / good/ excellent / outstanding ___

Judgement: poor / unreliable / limited / reliable / superior / outstanding ___

Cooperation: very uncooperative / difficult / cooperative / excellent / outstanding ___

Adaptability: poor / slow / satisfactory / good / excellent / superior / outstanding___

Appearance: poor/unprofessional/avg/reluctantly complies with dress code/outstanding ___

Attendance: poor / average / good / excellent / superior / outstanding ___
Total ___

Since last evaluation the employee has:
___Improved ___ made no noticeable change ___ regressed
Recommendation for pay raise: ___Yes ___No
Overall impression:
___unsatisfactory ___ fair ___ satisfactory ___ excellent ___outstanding
Comments of employee's strengths and weaknesses:___

Supervisor's signature___
Employee's signature___

FIGURE 23–11 Example of employee evaluation/review form

The Employee Evaluation/Review ....

Most employers require that employees have regular, routine, or periodic reviews or evaluations regarding their work performance. The time schedule may vary from place to place, but usually the reviews are held initially every 3 months for the first year and then every 6 months thereafter. Some physicians/employers prefer to have annual reviews scheduled unless there is a problem or the employee requests it more often. Evaluations should be regarded in a positive light.

These are generally conducted by the supervisor, the office manager of the facility, and sometimes by the physician-employer. Whoever holds this meeting with the employee offers insightful observations about the person. This is done to point out both positive and negative areas of which the employee may or may not be aware. Most facilities hold regular weekly staff meetings where suggestions, problems, and other important information is discussed. It is vital, however, to have private meetings to discuss personal goals, promotion opportunities, pay increase possibilities, educational pursuits, etc. The review, or evaluation as it is also referred to, is meant for both employer and employee to have just this opportunity. You should use this meeting to your advantage. Let the employer/supervisor know your intentions regarding promotion goals. Ask questions (tactfully) about what has been on your mind (bothering you) regarding policy, dress code, or whatever else you feel is important. You may ask about or schedule your vacation during this meeting. Your supervisor or evaluator may use a form similar to the one shown in Figure 23–11. Usually it will be completed and then offered to you to read. You may be asked to sign it at the bottom indicating that you have read, discussed, and understood the rating on the form. You may request a copy if it is not offered. The original will remain in your employee record and filed with all of the other documents pertaining to your employment. It is a good idea to study the form and heed the rating scale. If you take the review seriously and with an open mind, you will most likely find out some good points and sometimes a couple of not so good things about yourself that you may not have realized before. Try to improve on the not so good things before the next review, i.e., poor attendance, poor grammar, appearance. Showing improvement immediately and continuing on with the improvement will only make good points to remark about on the next review. To the

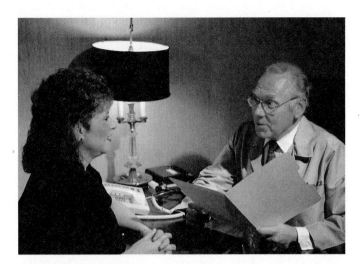

FIGURE 23–12 Employer discussing evaluation review in an open communication

smart individual, a word to the wise should be sufficient. If you show a poor attitude, it will only make matters worse. Remember that the supervisor's job responsibilities require that this evaluation be performed. You should not take the suggestions for improvement or reprimands about poor attendance, for instance, as personal insults. Try to remember the old saying "if the shoe fits, wear it," and consider the source of the remark. If you give the remark a chance to sink in and it doesn't, then possibly there is no just cause for it. Try to remain unaccusing and calm and discuss the problem. Chances are it may be a misunderstanding that can easily be talked out in a matter of seconds. Open dialogue and clear communication works wonders and leads to a better working relationship between you and your employer, Figure 23–12. Many positive results are achieved from reviews for both employee and employer.

Terminating Employment ....

There are many reasons for terminating employment—relocation, advancement to a more responsible position, higher paying jobs, illness, educational pursuits, pregnancy, a change in life-style, etc. There is, however, a major responsibility that an employee has to an employer, that of giving at least a 2-weeks' notice, Figure 23–13. This should be done to give the employer adequate time to fill the position that you will vacate. The notice that you give should be directed to your immediate supervisor, your physician-employer, or other appropriate member of the staff, with carbon copies to whoever else is appropriate for your place of employment. The letter should include the date that will be your last working day. Employers appreciate this considerate gesture, as it allows for a smoother transition of personnel. There is even time for a new person to be hired to work with you so that you may help in the training and explain your job description in more detail.

Date

Marlene Blackstone, CMA-A
Office Manager
Sports Medicine Center
7386 Canyon Road
Anywhere, U.S.A. 10000

Dear Ms. Blackstone:

It is with much regret that I submit this letter as my notice of resignation. My employment over the past five years in Sports Medicine has been a most interesting experience for me. I have learned so much in working with such a fine group of professionals. I am grateful for having had this opportunity.

From the date of this letter I am giving my two week notice; my last day will be (insert date).

Since my husband has taken a new position with his company, we are being transferred out of state. I will miss working with everyone at the center.

My thanks to all of you for making my years of employment at the center something that I can look back on with fond memories.

Sincerely,

Patsy J. Keene, CMA

Date

Maxwell S. Mitchell, M.D.
472 Circle Drive
Anywhere, U.S.A. 10000

Dear Dr. Mitchell:

Please accept this as my letter of resignation. During my employment in your practice I have learned a great deal, and I have greatly enjoyed working for you. However, (at this point the writer may choose to add a sentence or two elaborating on the specific reason for leaving).

My X years of employment with you have been a valuable experience for me; thank you for the opportunity to work and learn.

In accordance with your personnel regulations, this letter is also my two week notice; my last day in the office will be (at least two weeks hence).

Sincerely,

Your name and title or position with your signature

FIGURE 23–13 Letters of resignation

Employment can also be terminated by the employer. This is an unpleasant experience for both employer and employee. The usual cause for termination initiated by the employer is failure to perform job responsibilities. Deficiencies can include being tardy, high absenteeism, failure to get along with coworkers and patients, poor work habits, undependability, dishonesty, poor attitude, and uncooperativeness. On some occasions and in some situations, through employer-employee communication, one may be able to smooth over the conflict and ask if it is possible to change the situation from being fired to accepting a letter of resignation. This is mentioned because misunderstandings *do* happen from time to time. Having a poor work record is something that could follow a person and make it difficult to land another job in the future.

Keeping on your toes can prevent this unwanted dilemma from happening. One should strive to do the best job possible for making a good reference if ever needed.

Summary

Requirements for medical assistant's positions will be as varied as the practice of medicine. The medical assistant may have to be the most versatile member of the health care team. Some physicians still hire medically untrained persons as file clerks, secretaries, receptionists, and the like. More physicians recognize the value of employing trained and experienced medical assistants who have a basic background in the administrative and clinical areas of medical office practice. If you have successfully completed a training program, you have established the basis for a rewarding career.

Employers in medical practice have begun to realize the worth of Certified Medical Assistants. CMAs are usually considered for employment over untrained applicants. Currently, this is true in some states more than in others, but certification may well become a nationwide requirement for employment in medical practice as regulations tighten. Keeping yourself up-to-date by attending continuing education programs, seminars, meetings, and other informative ways will make you a most valued employee. By opting to become a CMA you will demonstrate that you are knowledgeable in basic entry-level skills. Further, you will demonstrate to a prospective employer that you have pride in the profession as well as in your professional skills.

A Final Note

Throughout this chapter much emphasis has been directed toward securing employment. Although it may seem to you that employers ask the impossible as you review their expectations, you must keep in mind that an employee is paid for work performed. Gainful employment is a mutually agreed to contract which is either written or implied. To assist you in gaining a better understanding of why employers have such expectations, you may find it interesting to know how and where they originated.

The concept of the "work ethic" originated from the sixteenth century's Protestant Ethic. During this time period work was considered a sacred task and success in one's work was a sign of divine grace. One was looked down on by society in general if one was thought to have moral flaws such as being lazy, having no ambition, or other undesirable characteristics. Essentially this ideal has not changed. The work ethics of today are basically the same as the original with some minor changes. The word *responsible* can be substituted for sacred. And being a success in one's work is a sign of *ambition, hard work, and perseverance*. These expectations are fair, realistic and sensible. It simply means that one should give an honest day's work for an honest day's wages. Taking the responsibility of providing for oneself financially usually makes most people aware of what is necessary to keep a job. Being a part of the health care team means that you have to be a team player!

Our best wishes for a successful and rewarding career in medical assisting!

Complete Chapter 23, Unit 2 in the workbook to help you meet the objectives at the beginning of this unit and therefore achieve competency of this subject matter.

REFERENCES

Burns, William E. "Jobs for the Future." *Industrial Education*, January 1987.

Hess, Beth B. *Sociology*, 3rd ed. New York: Macmillan, 1988.

Jackson, Tom. *The Perfect Resumé for the '90s*, Doubleday, a division of Bantam Doubleday Dell Publishing Group, Inc., 1990.

Shapiro, Robert J. and Maureen Walsh. "The Great Jobs Mismatch." *U.S. News & World Report*, September 7, 1987.

"Why Me? What Every Applicant Needs To Know about the New Immigration Law," Business & Legal Reports, booklet, 64 Wall Street, Madison, CT 06443-1513, reorder #54i, 1987.

Appendix

Converting Measurements ....

LENGTH	Centimeters	Inches	Feet
1 centimeter	1.000	0.394	0.0328
1 inch	2.54	1.000	0.0833
1 foot	30.48	12.000	1.000
1 yard	91.4	36.00	3.00
1 meter	100.00	39.40	3.28

VOLUMES	Cubic Centimeters	Fluid Drams	Fluid Ounces	Quarts	Liters
1 cubic centimeter	1.00	0.270	0.033	0.0010	0.0010
1 fluid dram	3.70	1.00	0.125	0.0039	0.0037
1 cubic inch	16.39	4.43	0.554	0.0173	0.0163
1 fluid ounce	29.6	8.00	1.000	0.0312	0.0296
1 quart	946.0	255.0	32.00	1.000	0.946
1 liter	1000.0	270.0	33.80	1.056	1.000

WEIGHTS	Grains	Grams	Apothecary Ounces	Pounds
1 grain (gr)	1.000	0.064	0.002	0.0001
1 gram (gm)	15.43	1.000	0.032	0.0022
1 apothecary ounce	480.00	31.1	1.000	0.0685
1 pound	7000.00	454.0	14.58	1.000
1 kilogram	15432.0	1000.00	32.15	2.205

Rules for Converting One System to Another ....

Volumes

Grains to grams—divide by 15
Drams to cubic centimeters—multiply by 4
Ounces to cubic centimeters—multiply by 30
Minims to cubic millimeters—multiply by 63
Minims to cubic centimeters—multiply by 0.06
Cubic millimeters to minims—divide by 63
Cubic centimeters to minims—multiply by 16
Cubic centimeters to fluid ounces—divide by 30
Liters to pints—divide by 2.1

Weights

Milligrams to grains—multiply by 0.0154
Grams to grains—multiply by 15
Grams to drams—multiply by 0.257
Grams to ounces—multiply by 0.0311

Temperature

Multiply centigrade degrees by $\frac{9}{5}$ and add 32
Subtract 32 from the Fahrenheit degrees and multiply by $\frac{5}{9}$

Household Measures and Weights ....

1 teaspoon	$= \frac{1}{6}$ fluid ounce or 1 dram
3 teaspoons	= 1 tablespoon
1 dessert spoon	$= \frac{1}{3}$ fluid ounce or 2 drams
1 tablespoon	$= \frac{1}{2}$ fluid ounce or 3 drams
4 tablespoons	$= 1$ wine glass or $\frac{1}{2}$ gill
16 tablespoons (liq)	= 1 cup
12 tablespoons (dry)	= 1 cup
1 cup	= 8 fluid ounces
1 tumbler or glass	$= 8$ fluid ounces or $\frac{1}{2}$ pint
1 wine glass	= 2 fluid ounces
16 fluid ounces	= 1 pound
4 gills	= 1 pound
1 pint	= 1 pound

Symbols ....

m	minim	s̄	without
ℨ	dram	c̄	with
℥	ounce	–	minus, negative, alkaline reaction
O	pint	+	plus, excess, acid reaction, positive
#	pound, number	×	multiply
℞	recipe, prescription	÷	divide
'	foot, minute	=	equals
"	inch, second	>	greater than

°	degree	<	less than
%	percent	∞	infinity
♂	male	↑	increase
♀	female	↓	decrease

Common Medical Abbreviations ....

a, aa	of each
a.c.	before meals
ad lib	as desired
A & P	anterior and posterior
aq	aqueous, water
BE, ba.en.	barium enema
BlF	black female
bib	drink
b.i.d. BID	twice a day
bm, BM	bowel movement
BlM	black male
BP, B/P	blood pressure
BUN	blood urea nitrogen
c̄	with
C	centigrade
Ca	calcium
CA	carcinoma
cap	capsule
CBC	complete blood count
cc	cubic centimeter
CCU	coronary care unit
CHF	congestive heart failure
cm	cubic centimeter
CNS	central nervous system
CO_2	carbon dioxide
comp	compound
COPD	chronic obstructive pulmonary disease
CPR	cardiopulmonary resuscitation
CSF	cerebrospinal fluid
CVA	cerebrovascular accident
cysto	cystoscopy
D & C	dilatation and curettage
Dil, dil	dilute
DOA	dead on arrival
DPT	diphtheria, pertussis, tetanus
dr.	dram
dx, Dx	diagnosis
ECG	electrocardiogram
EEG	electroencephalogram
EENT	eye, ear, nose, throat
EKG	electrocardiogram
elix	elixir
ER	emergency room
et	and
expl lap	exploratory laporatomy
ext.	extract

F	fahrenheit	OD	overdose
F	female	O.D.	right eye
FBS	fasting blood sugar	OP	outpatient
fl	fluid	OR	operating room
fl. dr.	fluid dram	os	mouth
fl. oz.	fluid ounce	O.S.	left eye
Fx	fracture	O.U.	both eyes
		oz	ounce
GB	gallbladder		
GI	gastrointestinal	Path	pathology
Gm	gram	PBI	protein bound iodine
GP	general practitioner	p.c.	after meals
gr	grain	Peds	pediatrics
gtt Gtt gtts	drop, drops	per	through, by
GU	genitourinary	PID	pelvic inflammatory disease
GYN	gynecology	PKU	phenylketonuria
		PO, p.o.	by mouth
H, h	hour	prn	as desired, needed
HCL	hydrochloric acid	pro time	prothrombin time
Hgb	hemoglobin	Psych	psychiatry
hs	hour of sleep, bedtime	pt	patient, pint
Hx	history	pulv	powder
hypo	hypodermic, under	Px	physical examination
ICU	intensive care unit	q	every
I & D	incision and drainage	qd	every day
IM	intramuscular	q 4 h	every 4 hours
inj	injection	qh	every hour
I & O	intake and output	q.i.d. QID	four times a day
IPPB	intermittent positive pressure breathing	qns	quantity not sufficient
IT	inhalation therapy	qs	quantity sufficient
IUD	intrauterine device	qt	quart
IV	intravenous		
IVP	intravenous pyelogram	R	right
		Ra	radium
k	potassium	RBC	red blood cells
KUB	kidney, ureter, and bladder	REM	rapid eye movement
		rep	let it be repeated
L, lb	pound	R/O	rule out
lat	lateral	ROM	range of motion
liq	liquid	ROS	review of systems
LLQ	left lower quadrant	Rx	prescription, take
LMP	last menstrual period	s̄	without
LUQ	left upper quadrant		
		sig	instructions, directions
m	minim	SOB	short of breath
M	male	sol	solution
mm	millimeter	solv	dissolve
MS	multiple sclerosis	s.o.s.	distress signal
		sp. gr.	specific gravity
NB	newborn	ss	half
no.	number	stat	immediately
noxt.	at night	subq	subcutaneous
NPO	nothing by mouth	syr.	syrup
N & V	nausea and vomiting		
		T	temperature
O	pint	T & A	tonsilectomy and adenoidectomy
OB	obstetrics		

tab	tablet	cramp—spasmus
TIA	transient ischemic attack	
t.i.d.	three times a day	dead—mortuus
tinct.	tincture	deadly—lethalis
TPR	temperature, pulse, respiration	dental—dentalis
TUR	transurethral resection	digestive—pepticus
		disease—morbus
UA	urinalysis	dose—potio
ung.	ointment	
URI	upper respiratory infection	ear—auris
UTI	urinary tract infection	egg—ovum
		entrails—viscera
VD	venereal disease	erotic—amatorius
vin	wine	exhalation—exhalatio
VS	vital signs	expell—expello
		expire—expiro
WBC	white blood cells	external—externus
WF	white female	extract—extractum
WM	white male	eye—oculus; ophthalmos (Gr)
WNL	within normal limits	eyeball—pupula
wt, Wt.	weight	eyelid—palpebra

Selected English, Latin, and Greek Equivalents ....

and—et
arm—brachium; brachion (Gr)
artery—arteria
attachment—adhaesio

back—dorsum
backbone—spina
backward—retro
belly—venter
bend—flexus
bile—billis; chole (Gr)
bladder—vesica
blind—obscurus
blister—pustulo
blood—sanguis; haima, aima (Gr)
blood vessel—vena
body—corpus; soma (Gr)
bone—os; osteon (Gr)
bony—osseus
bowels—intestina, viscera
brain—cerebrum
breach—ruptura
breast—mamma; mastos (Gr)
buttock—gloutos (Gr)

cartilage—cartilago; chondros (Gr)
chest—thorax
choke—strangulo
confinement—puerperium
corn—callus, clavus
cornea—cornu; keras (Gr)
cough—tussio

face—facies
fat—adeps; lipos (Gr)
feel—tactus
fever—febris
finger—digitus
flesh—carnis
foot—pedis; pous (Gr)
forearm—brachium
forehead—frons

gall—bilis
gravel—calculus
gum—gingiva
gut—intestinum

hair—capillus
half—dimidius
hand—manus; cheir (Gr)
harelip—labrum fissum
head—caput; kephale (Gr)
healer—medicus
health—sanitas
hear—audio
heart—cor; kardia (Gr)
heat—calor
heel—calx, talus
hysterics—hysteria

illness—morbus
infant—infas, puerilis
infectious—contagiosus
infirm—debilis
injection—injectio
intellect—intellectus
internal—intestinus

intestine—intestinum; enteron (Gr)
itch—scabies
itching—pruritis

jaw—maxilla
joint—artus; anthron (Gr)

kidney—ren; nephros (Gr)
knee—genu
kneecap—patella

lacerate—lacero
larynx—guttur
lateral—lateralis
leg—tibia
limb—membrum
listen—ausculto
liver—jecur, hepar (Gr)
loin—lapara
looseness—laxitas
lukewarm—tepidus
lung—pulmo, pneumon (Gr)

mad—insanus
male—masculinus
malignant—malignus
maternity—conditio matris
milk—lac
moist—humidus
month—mensis
monthly—menstruus
mouth—os; stoma (Gr)

nail—unguis
navel—umbilicus; omphalos (Gr)
neck—cervis; trachelos (Gr)
nerve—nervus; neuron (Gr)
nipple—papilla
no, none—nullus
nose—nasus; rhis (Gr)
nostril—naris
nourishment—alimentus

ointment—unguentum
orifice—foramen

pain—dolor
patient—patiens
pectoral—pectoralis
pimple—pustula
poison—venenum
powder—pulvis
pregnant—gravida
pubic bone—os pubis
pupil—pupilla

quinsy—angina

rash—exanthema
recover—convalesco
redness—rubor
rib—costa
ringing—tinnitus
rupture—hernia

saliva—sputum
scab—scabies
scalp—pericranium
scaly—squamosus
sciatica—ischias
seed—semen
senile—senilis
sheath—vagina
shin—tibia
short—brevis
shoulder—humerus; omos (Gr)
shoulderblade—scapula
shudder—tremor
side—latus
skin—cutis; derma (Gr)
skull—cranium; kranion (Gr)
sleep—somnus
smell—odoratus
socket—cavum
solution—dilutum
sore—ulcus
spinal—dorsalis, spinalis
spine—spina
spittle—sputum
sprain—luxatio
stomach—stomachus; gaster (Gr)
stone—calculus
sugar—saccharum
swallow—glutio

tail—cauda
taste—gustatus
tear—lacrima
teeth—dentes
testicle—testis; orchis (Gr)
thigh—femur
throat—fauces; pharygx (Gr)
throb—palpito
tongue—lingua; glossa (Gr)
twin—geminus

urine—urina

vagina—vagina; kolpos (Gr)
vein—vena; phleps (Gr)
vertebra—vertevra; spondylos (Gr)
vessel—vas

wash—lavo

water—aqua
wax—cera
weary—lassus
wet—humidus
windpipe—arteria aspera
woman—femina
womb—uterus; hystera (Gr)
worm—vermis
wrist—carpus; karpos (Gr)

yolk—luteum

Prefixes and Suffixes ....

a- an-	without, negative
ab- abs-	away from
ad-	toward
adeno-	gland
aero-	air
-aesthesia	sensation
-algia	pain
ambi-	both
angio-	blood vessel
ano-	anus
ante-	before
anti-	against
arterio-	artery
arthro-	joint
auto-	self
bi-	two, twice
brady-	slow
broncho-	bronchial
cardio-	heart
cata-	down
-cele	tumor, cysts
cent-	hundred
-centesis	puncture
cephal-	head
chole-	gall
chromo-	color
-cide	causing death
circum-	around
-cise	cut
co- com- con-	together
colo-	colon
colpo-	vagina
contra-	against
costo-	rib
cranio-	skull
cysto-	bag, bladder
-cyte -cyto	cell
dacry-	tears
de-	from, down
deca-	ten

deci-	tenth
demi-	half
dent-	teeth
derma-	skin
di-	double
dia	through, between
diplo-	double
dis-	negative, apart
dys-	difficult, painful
ecto-	out, on the outside
-ectomy	cutting out
-emesis	vomiting
-emia	blood
en-	in, into
encephalo-	brain
endo-	within
entero-	intestine
epi-	above, over
-esthesia	sensation
ex- exo-	out
extra-	on the outside
fibro-	connective tissue
fore-	before, in front of
-form	form
-fuge	to drive away
galact- galacto-	milk
gastro-	stomach
-gene -genic	origin, formation
glosso-	tongue
gluco- glyco-	sugar, sweet
-gram	a tracing, record
-graph	machine
-graphy	the process
gyne-	woman
hema- hemato- hemo-	blood
hemi-	half
hepa- hepato-	liver
herni-	rupture
histo-	tissue
homo-	same, similar
hydra- hydro-	water
hyper-	above, increased, over
hypo-	below, under, decreased
hyster-	uterus
-iasis	condition of
ictero-	jaundice
idio-	peculiar to the individual
ileo-	ileum
in-	in, into, not
infra-	beneath
inter-	between
intra- intro-	within

-ism	condition, theory	oophor-	ovary
-itis	inflammation of	ophthalmo-	eye
-ize	to treat by special method	-opia	vision
		orchid-	testicle
karyo-	nucleus, nut	-orrhaphy	to repair a defect
kata- kath-	down	ortho-	straight
kera-	horn, indicates hardness	os-	mouth, bone
-kinesis	motion	-osis	disease, condition of
		oste- osteo-	bone
lact-	milk	-ostomy	to make a mouth, opening
laparo-	abdomen	oto-	ear
-lepsy	seizure, convulsion	-otomy	incision, surgical cutting
leuco- leuko-	white	oxy-	sharp, acid
lipo-	fat		
lith-	a stone	pachy-	thick
-logia -logy	science of, study of	pan-	all, entire
-lysis	disintegration	para-	alongside of
		path- -pathy	disease, suffering
macro-	large, long	ped- (Greek)	child
mal-	bad, poor	ped- (Latin)	foot
-mania	insanity	-penia	too few, lack
mast-	breast	per-	through, excessive
med- medi-	middle	peri-	around
mega-	large, great	pharyng-	throat
-megalia -megaly	large, great, extreme	phelebo-	vein
melan-	black	-phobia	fear
men-	month	-phylaxis	protection
meso-	middle	-plasty	operate to revise
meta-	beyond, over, between, change, transportation	-plegia	a stroke, paralysis
		-pnea	breathing
-meter	measure	pneumo-	air, lungs
metro- metra-	uterus	poly-	many, much
micro-	small	post-	after
mio-	smaller, less	pre-	before
mono-	single, one	pro-	before, in behalf of
multi-	many	procto-	rectum
my- myo-	muscle	proto-	first
myel- myelo-	marrow	pseudo-	false
		psych-	the mind
narco-	sleep	pyelo-	kidney, pelvis
naso-	nose	pyo-	pus
necro-	dead	pyro-	heat
neo-	new		
nephr- nephro-	kidney	re-	back, again
neu- neuro-	nerve	reni- reno-	kidney
niter- nitro-	nitrogen	retro-	backward, behind
non- not-	no	-rhage -rhagia	hemorrhage, flow
nucleo-	a nucleus	-rhaphy	a suturing, stitching
		-rhea	flow
o-	ovum, an egg	rhino-	nose
ob-	against		
oculo-	eye	sacchar-	sugar
-ode -oid	form, shape	sacro-	sacrum
odont-	a tooth	salpingo-	a tube, fallopian tube
oligo-	few	sarco-	flesh
-ology	study of	sclero-	hard, sclera
-oma	a tumor	-sclerosis	dryness, hardness

-scopy	to see	thrombo-	clot
semi-	half	thyro-	thyroid gland
septi-	poison, infection	trans-	across
stomato-	mouth	tri-	three
-stomy	to furnish with a mouth		
sub-	under	uni-	one
super- supra-	above	-uria	urine
syn-	with, together	urino- uro-	urine, urinary organs
tele-	distant, far	vaso-	vessel
tetra-	four	venter- ventro-	abdomen
-therapy	treatment		
-thermy	heat	xanth-	yellow
thio-	sulfur		
thoraco-	chest		

Uniform Care—Stain Removal Chart ....

Treat stains as quickly as possible.

Check fabric labels for care instructions.

Use ENZYME PRESOAKS for protein-based stains such as blood, milk, fruits, grass (Example: "AXION," "BIZ")

Use Prewash spot treatments for greasy stains. (Example: "SPRAY'N WASH," "SHOUT")

Use proper bleach for hard-to-whiten and difficult stains. Examples: Chlorine for whites "CLOROX."

Chlorine will discolor most colors. All purpose bleach for colored "CLOROX 2."

Stain	Method for Washable Fabrics
felt tip pens	Soak in rubbing alcohol at least 30 minutes, preferably overnight. Wash and add bleach.
blood, milk, egg, chocolate, ice cream	Pretest using **enzyme presoak**. Do not use hot, only **cold** water. If presoak is not enough, work in detergent paste. Wash in warm water. Bleach if needed.
butter, grease, oil, margarine, dressings	Prewash with **prewash spot treatment OR** rub detergent paste into stain. Launder.
fruits, juices	Use **enzyme presoak**; bleach if stain still persists **OR** for cherry, peach, pear, plum stains, soak in cool water. For others pour boiling water through stain. Launder.
chewing gum	Place ice cube under gum to harden. Rub off excess with dull knife. If stained, use cleaning fluid.
coffee, tea	Pour boiling water through stretched fabric. Launder in hot water.
cosmetics	Pretreat with detergent paste. Launder in hot water.
grass	Rub detergent paste into stain. Launder in hot water. Use appropriate bleach.
ballpoint ink	Rub white Vaseline into stain. Pretest with detergent paste. Launder using bleach if fabric permits.
mildew	Launder in hot water. Bleach with appropriate bleach.
Scorch, white	Dampen white cloth with hydrogen peroxide and place on stain. Place clean cloth on top. Press.
perspiration	Apply ammonia to wash water for new stain. Use vinegar on old stain. Launder.
shoe polish	Pretreat with detergent paste. Launder.

CONSULT DRY CLEANER FOR ESPECIALLY DIFFICULT STAINS AND CLOTHING LABELED "DRY CLEAN ONLY."

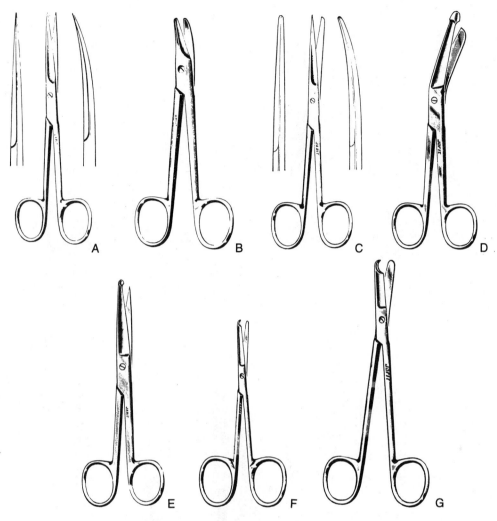

Operating Scissors: (A) Deaver, (B) Sistrunk, (C) Deaver. Bandage scissors: (D) Lester,
(E) Knowles finger, (F) Spencer suture, (G) Littauer stitch
(Courtesy of J. Jamner Surgical Instruments Inc.)

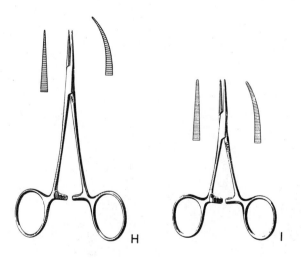

Petit-point hemostats: (H) and (I) mosquito (Courtesy of J. Jamner
Surgical Instruments Inc.)

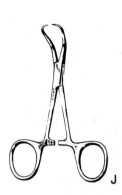

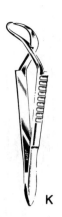

Towel forceps: (J) Backhaus, (K) Jones
(Courtesy of J. Jamner Surgical Instruments Inc.)

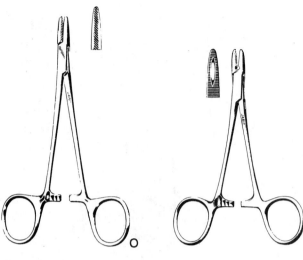

Needle holders: (O) Brown, (P) Collier
(Courtesy of J. Jamner Surgical Instruments Inc.)

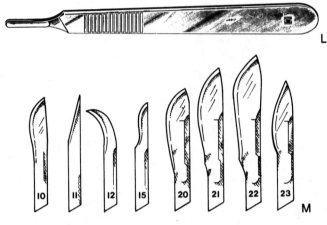

| 10 | 11 | 12 | 15 | 20 | 21 | 22 | 23 |

(L) Knife handle, (M) Blades (Courtesy of J. Jamner
Surgical Instruments Inc.)

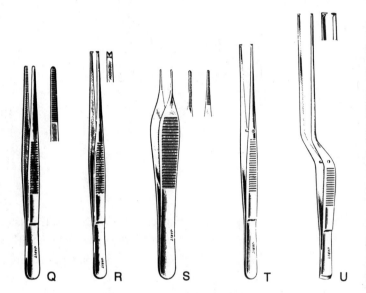

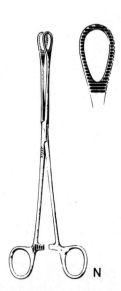

(N) Foerster sponge-holding forceps (Courtesy of
J. Jamner Surgical Instruments Inc.)

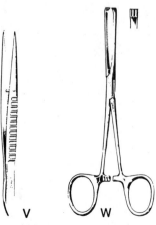

Dressing and tissue forceps: (Q) thumb, (R) tissue, (S) Adson,
(T) Semken dressing, (U) Cushing, (V) plain splinter,
(W) Judd-Allis tissue (Courtesy of J. Jamner
Surgical Instruments Inc.)

Glossary

abandonment—to desert, to give up entirely.

abbess—a mother superior; a woman who is the head of an abbey of nuns.

abdomen—the cavity in the body between the diaphragm and the pelvis.

abdominal—pertaining to the abdomen.

abdominopelvic—pertaining to the anterior body cavity below the diaphragm.

abduct—to move away from the midline.

ablation—a surgical procedure utilizing a resectoscope inserted into the uterus through the cervix.

abnormality—person, thing, or condition that is not normal.

abortion—the termination of pregnancy before the stage of viability; spontaneous or induced.

abrupt—sudden; blunt, curt.

absolute—free as to condition, unlimited in power.

absorb—to suck or swallow up, to drink in.

abstract—a summary of the principal parts of a larger work.

absurd—contrary to sense or reason.

accelerator—increasing action or function.

accessible—capable of being reached.

accommodation—the process of the lens changing shape to permit close vision.

accountant—one who keeps, audits, and inspects the financial records of individuals or businesses.

account history—the past financial record.

accreditation—the assignment of credentials; approval given for meeting established standards.

accumulated—to pile up; collect; gather.

accuracy—correctness, exactness.

acetylcholine—a hormone released at the parasympathetic and skeletal nerve endings.

Achilles tendon—a tendon attaching the gastrocnemius muscle of the leg to the heel.

acidosis—a disturbance of the acid-base balance of the body.

acquaintance—the state of knowing a person or subject.

acquire—to gain by one's own efforts or actions; to get.

acquisition—to acquire; to get by one's own efforts.

acromegaly—a chronic condition characterized by enlargement of bones of the extremities and some bones of the head; thickening of facial soft tissues.

acronym—a word formed from the initial letters of each major word in a term.

action potential—the temporary electrical charge within a cell.

activate—to make active or more active.

acute—sharp, severe. Having a rapid onset, severe symptoms and a short course; not chronic.

addiction—the state of being governed or controlled by a habit, as with alcohol or drugs.

adduct—to draw together toward the midline.

adenitis—inflammation of lymph nodes or a gland.

adequate—equal to the requirement or occasion, sufficient.

adhere—to stick fast, become firmly attached; to be devoted to.

adjustments—changes to fit or bring into harmony.

administer—to manage; to conduct, as in business.

admissions clerk—a person who processes information and forms for a patient who will be entering the health facility.

adrenal—pertaining to the adrenal glands which sit atop each kidney.

adrenaline—an internal secretion derived from the adrenal glands; can be commercially prepared from animal glands; acts as a stimulant.

adrenocorticotrophic hormone (ACTH)—a hormone secreted by the anterior lobe of the pituitary gland.

advantageous—beneficial, profitable.

advocate—one who pleads for or defends a cause or a person.

aerobe—a microorganism which can live and grow only in the presence of oxygen.

afebrile—without fever.

affiliate—to unite, to join or become connected.

agar—a dried mucilaginous substance, or gelatin, extracted from algae, used as a culture medium.

agent—one that acts or has the power or authority to act for another.

aggressive—pushy, assuming the offensive without cause; forceful.

Al-Anon—a support group for family members of alcoholics.

Al-Ateen—a support for teenagers with an alcoholic parent.

albino—a person who lacks pigment in the skin, hair, and eyes, either partial or total; a person with albinoism.

alcoholic—an individual who uses alcohol to excess.

Alcoholics Anonymous—an organization formed to assist alcoholics to refrain from the use of alcohol.

aldosterone—a mineralocorticoid hormone secreted by the adrenal cortex.

alignment—being in proper position.

alimentary canal—the intestinal tract, from the esophagus to the rectum, and accessory organs.

allege—to state positively but not under oath and without proof; to affirm.

allergic rhinitis—inflammation of the nose due to an allergy.

allergist—a physician specializing in the care of patients with allergies.

allergy—an altered or acquired state of sensitivity; abnormal reaction of the body to substances normally harmless.

allosteric—a protein found in erythrocytes that transports oxygen in the blood; hemoglobin.

alopecia—the loss of hair; baldness.

alpha search—look by alphabetical order.

alveoli—microscopic air sacs in the lung.

amber—orange/yellowish color.

amblyopia—lazy eye; a condition characterized by the inward turning of the affected eye.

ambulate—to walk, not be confined to bed.

amniotic—pertaining to the amniotic fluid within the amniotic membrane surrounding the fetus.

amphetamine—a central nervous system stimulant, often referred to as an upper.

amplifier—a device on an electrocardiograph which enlarges the EKG impulses.

ampule—a small glass container that can be sealed and its contents sterilized.

amputate—to cut off, remove a part.

anaerobe—a microorganism having the ability to live without oxygen.

anal—pertaining to the anus or outer rectal opening.

analysis—the examination of anything to determine its makeup; a description of the process or the examination, point by point.

analytical—characterized by a method of analysis, a statement of point-by-point examination.

anaphylaxis—a hypersensitive reaction of the body to a foreign protein or a drug; the term implies symptoms severe enough to produce serious shock, even death.

anatomical—pertaining to the anatomy or structure of an organism.

anatomy—the study of the physical structure of the body and its organs.

anchor—the attachment of a skeletal muscle; the wrapping at the start of a gauze or elastic bandage.

anemia—a deficiency of red blood cells, hemoglobin, or both.

aneroid—operating without a fluid; when used in reference to a sphygmomanometer, measuring by a dial instead of a mercury column.

anesthesia—without sensation, with or without loss of consciousness.

anesthesiology—the study of anesthesia.

anesthetic—an agent which produces insensibility to pain or touch, either generally or locally.

aneurysm—a widening, external dilation due to the pressure of blood on weakened arterial walls.

angina—pain and oppression radiating from the heart to the shoulder and left arm; a feeling of suffocation.

angiography—a radiological study of an artery using a radiopaque medium.

annotating—to provide critical or explanatory notes.

annuity—a sum of money to be received yearly, either in a lump sum or by installments.

anorexia—loss of appetite; with anorexia nervosa, loss of appetite for food not explainable by disease, which may be a part of psychosis.

antagonize—to annoy; to arouse opposition.

antecubital—the inner surface of the arm at the elbow.

anterior—before or in front of.

antibody—a protein substance carried by cells to counteract the effect of an antigen.

antibody-mediated—humoral immunity; when antibodies and complement work together to destroy antigens.

anticoagulant—a substance that prohibits the coagulation of blood.

antigen—any immunizing agent which, when introduced into the body, may produce antibodies.

antihistamine—a class of drugs used to counteract allergic reactions or cold symptoms.

antiseptic—an agent which will prevent the growth or arrest the development of microorganisms.

antitoxin—a protein that defends the body against toxins.

anuria—the absence of urine.

anus—the external opening of the anal canal.

anxiety—a condition of mental uneasiness arising from fear or apprehension.

aorta—the main trunk of the arterial system of the body.

apex—the point, tip, or summit of anything; in reference to the heart, the point of maximum impulse of the heart against the chest wall.

apical—referring to the apex.

apnea—the absence of breathing.

aponeurosis—extension of connective tissue beyond a muscle in round or flattened tendons; a means of insertion or origin of a flat muscle.

appendectomy—the excision of the appendix.

appendicitis—inflammation of the appendix.

appendicular—pertaining to the limbs or things that append (attach) to other parts.

applicable—capable of being applied, suitable.

apprehension—anticipation of something feared, dread; a mental conception.

apprenticeship—a training or learning period; study under the guidance of a skilled, experienced worker.

apprise—to inform.

appropriate—correct, suitable.

aqueous humor—a watery, transparent liquid which circulates between the anterior and posterior chambers of the eye.

arachnoid—a delicate, lacelike membrane covering the central nervous system.

arbitrary—depending on will or whim, self-willed; depending on choice or discretion.

ardently—eagerly, passionately, intensely.

areola—a ringlike coloration about the nipple of the breast.

arrhythmia—without rhythm; irregularity.

arteriography—a radiological study of an artery using a radiopaque medium.

arterioles—small blood vessels connecting arteries with capillaries.

arteriosclerosis—a degeneration and hardening of the walls of arteries.

artery—a blood vessel carrying blood away from the heart, usually filled with oxygenated blood.

arthritis—inflammation of a joint.

articulate—to join together, as in a joint.

artifact—something extraneous to what is being looked for. Activity which causes interference on EKGs.

ascending—referring to that portion of the colon which

ascends from the lower right quadrant to the upper right quadrant of the abdomen.

ascertain—to make certain

asepsis—a condition free of organisms.

aseptic technique—means of performing tasks without contamination by organisms.

asphyxiation—suffocation, loss of consciousness as the result of too little oxygen and too much carbon dioxide.

aspirate—to remove by suction.

assault—a violent attack, either physical or verbal, an unlawful threat to harm another physically, or an unsuccessful attempt to do so.

assess—to determine, to appraise the condition or state.

asset—anything owned that has exchange value, all the entries on a balance sheet that shows the property or resources of a person or business.

asthma—an allergic reaction to a substance resulting in wheezing, shortness of breath, and difficulty in breathing.

astigmatism—blurring of the vision due to an abnormal curvature of the cornea.

asymmetry—lack of same size, shape, and position of parts or organs on opposite sides.

atelectasis—lack of air in the lungs due to the collapse of the alveoli of the lungs.

atherosclerosis—fatty degeneration of the walls of the arteries.

atrial depolarization—the excitement and contraction caused by the SA node at the beginning of the cardiac cycle.

atrioventricular—see **A-V node**

atrium—cardiac auricle; the upper chamber of the heart.

atrophy—wasting away of a muscle.

attenuated—diluted; To reduce virulence of a pathologenic organism.

attribute—quality or characteristic; to give credit for.

audible—loud enough to be hear.

audiometry—testing of the hearing sense.

auditory—pertaining to the sense of hearing; the external canal of the ear.

aural—the ear; temperature measurement using tympanic infrared scanner.

augmented—refers to leads 4, 5, and 6 of the standard 12-lead EKG tracing; these leads are of different voltage.

auscultate—to listen for sounds produced by the body.

authorization—the giving of authority.

autoimmune—a condition wherein the person's antibodies react against their own normal tissues.

autologous—given by oneself.

automation—behavior in an automatic or mechanical fashion.

autonomic—spontaneous; the part of the nervous system concerned with reflex control of bodily functions.

autonomous—self-governing.

autotrophs—microorganisms that feed on inorganic matter.

A-V node—atrioventricular node; the beginning of the Bundle of His in the right auricle/atrium; nerve fibers responsible for the contraction of the ventricles.

axial—pertaining to the spinal column, skull, and rib cage of the skeleton.

axilla—the underarm area, armpit.

axillary—referring to the underarm area.

axon—an extension from a nerve cell.

BSA—see **body surface area**

bacteria—unicellular microorganism concerned with the fermentation and putrefaction of matter; disease-causing agent.

bankruptcy—the state of being bankrupt, being legally declared unable to pay debts.

barbiturate—a sedative or hypnotic drug, also known as a downer.

Bartholin's glands—two small mucous glands, situated one on each side of the vaginal opening at the base of the labia minora.

baseline—the initial information on which additional data is based.

basophil—a granulated white blood cell.

battery—any illegal beating of another person.

benefits—anything that promotes or enhances wellbeing.

benign—non-malignant; not cancerous.

benign hypertrophy—nonmalignant enlargement.

beriberi—a disease resulting from lack of vitamin B, thiamine.

biceps—the muscle of the upper arm which flexes the forearm.

biconvex—the curving out on both sides.

bicuspid—heart valve between the left atrium and left ventricle, also known as the mitral valve.

biennially—happening once in two years.

bile—a secretion of the liver; a greenish-yellow fluid with a bitter taste.

bimanual—two-handed; with both hands.

bimonthly—occurring once in two months.

binocular—pertaining to the use of both eyes; possessing two eyepieces as with a microscope.

biochemistry—a science concerned with the chemistry of plants and animals.

biohazardous—any material that has been in contact with body fluid and is potentially capable of transmitting disease.

biopsy—excision of a small piece of tissue for microscopic examination.

bizarre—odd, unusual, strikingly out of the ordinary.

bladder—a membranous sac or receptacle for a secretion; the gallbladder, urinary bladder.

blood pressure—the amount of force exerted by the heart on the blood as it pumps the blood through the arteries.

body mechanics—the use of appropriate body positioning when moving and lifting objects in order to avoid injury.

body surface area (BSA)—refers to the total surface of the human body.

bolus—a mass of masticated food which is ready to be swallowed.

bookkeeper—one who records the accounts and transactions of a business.

booster—a subsequent injection of immunizing substance to increase or renew immunity.

Bowman's capsule—part of the renal corpuscle; surrounds the glomerulus of the nephron.

brachial—refers to the brachial artery in the arm; the artery used in measuring blood pressure.

bradycardia—slow heart rate.

brain scan—a diagnostic test using a scanner to measure radioisotopes within the brain.

breach—violation of a law, contract, or other agreement.

brochure—a small pamphlet or booklet providing information.

bronchi—the primary divisions of the trachea.

bronchiole—small terminal branches of the bronchi which lack cartilage.

bronchitis—inflammation of the mucous membranes of the bronchial tree.

bruit—an adventitious sound of venous or arterial origin heard on auscultation; usually refers to the sound produced by the mixing of arterial and venous blood at dialysis shunts.

buccal—the mouth; oral cavity.

bulbourethral gland—two small glands, one on each side of the prostate gland, terminating in the urethra by way of a duct.

bunion—a bursa with a callus formation.

bursa—a sac or pouch in connective tissue chiefly around joints.

CAT scan—see **computerized axial tomography**

CLIA—see **Clinical Laboratory Improvement Amendments (1988)**

COPD—see **chronic obstructive pulmonary disease**

calculate—to compute.

calculi—commonly called stones; usually composed of mineral salts.

calibrations—a set of graduated markings to indicate values.

callus—in fractures, refers to the formation of new osseous material around the fracture site.

calorie—a unit for measuring the heat value of food.

calyces—two or more calyx.

calyx—the cuplike division of the kidney pelvis.

cancer—a malignant tumor or growth; specifically the hyperplasia of cells with infiltration and destruction of tissue.

cannula—a tube or sheath enclosing a trocar (triangular bore needle); after insertion the trocar is removed.

capillary—a microscopic blood vessel connecting arterioles and venules.

caption—heading, title, or subtitle.

carbohydrate—an organic combination of carbon, hydrogen, and oxygen as a sugar, a starch, or as cellulose.

carbon dioxide—a gas found in the air, exhaled by all animals; the chemical formula is CO_2.

carbon monoxide—a colorless, odorless, poisonous gas caused by the incomplete combustion of carbon.

carboxyhemoglobin—combined carbon monoxide and hemoglobin in red blood cells.

carbuncle—a staphlococcal infection following furunculosis, characterized by a deep abscess of several follicles with multiple draining points.

carcinoembryonic antigen—a tumor marker which can be detected in the blood when tested.

carcinogenic—cancer causing agents.

carcinogenesis—the malignant transformation of a cell.

carcinoma—a malignant tumor from epithelial tissue.

cardiac—pertaining to the heart.

cardiac sphincter—the muscle which encircles the esophagus where it enters the stomach.

cardinal signs—principal signs: temperature, pulse, respiration, and blood pressure.

cardiologist—a physician specializing in the care of patients with diseases of the heart.

cardiology—the study of the heart and its diseases.

cardiovascular—pertaining to the heart and blood vessels.

carotid—pertaining to the carotid artery.

carpal tunnel syndrome—the symptoms associated with the entrapment of the median nerve within the carpal bones and the transverse ligament at the wrist.

carpals—bones of the wrist.

cartilage—a strong, tough, elastic tissue forming part of the skeletal system; precalcified bone in infants and young children.

cataract—an opacity of the lens of the eye resulting in blindness.

catarrhal—pertaining to inflammation of mucous membranes; causing severe spells of coughing with little or no expectoration.

catastrophic—of great consequence; disastrous.

categorize—to arrange by class or kind; to place like things together.

catheterize—to insert a catheter into a cavity (for example, urinary bladder to remove urine) to remove body fluid.

caudal—pertaining to any taillike structure.

caustic—capable of burning; an agent that will destroy living tissue.

cauterize—to burn with an electrical cautery or chemical substance.

cavities—a hollow space, such as within the body or organs.

cecum—the beginning of the ascending portion of the large intestine which forms a blind pouch at the junction with the small intestine.

celiac disease—dilatation of the small and large intestines.

cell-mediated—direct cellular response to antigens.

cell membrane—the structure which surrounds and encloses a cell.

central—situated at or related to a center.

centrifuge—a machine for the separation of heavier materials from lighter ones through the use of centrifugal force.

centriole—an organelle within the cell.

cerebellum—lower or back brain below the posterior portion of the cerebrum.

cerebral—pertaining to the cerebrum of the brain.

cerebrospinal—referring to the brain and spinal cord.

cerebrospinal fluid—the liquid that circulates within the meninges of the spinal cord and ventricles and meninges of the brain.

cerebrovascular accident—a stroke; hemorrhage in the brain.

cerebrum—the largest part of the brain. It is divided into two hemispheres with four lobes in each hemisphere.

certified—holding a certificate; being certificated; guaranteed in writing.

cerumen—waxlike brown secretion found in the external auditory canal.

cervical—pertaining to the neck portion of the spinal column; also to the entrance into the uterus.

cervix—the entrance into the uterus.

cesarean—surgical removal of an infant from the uterus.

cessation—ceasing or discontinuing.

chaos—a state of complete confusion; disorder.

charting—the recording of data on a record-keeping device.

chemical—pertaining to chemistry.

chemotherapy—the use of chemical agents in the treatment of disease, usually associated with cancer therapy.

Cheyne-Stokes—a breathing pattern characterized by alternating periods of apnea and hyperventilation.

chiropractic—a system of healing based upon the theory that disease results from a lack of normal nerve function; treatment by scientific manipulation and specific adjustment of body structures such as the spinal column.

chiropractor—a health care provider who utilizes

chiropractic methods to treat patients.

chlamydia—a sexually transmitted disease caused by a bacteria that lives as an intracellular parasite.

chloroform—a liquid compound that yields a gas which dulls pain and causes unconsciousness.

cholecystectomy—surgical removal of the gallbladder.

cholelithiasis—stones in the gallbladder.

cholenergic—nerve fibers capable of secreting acetylcholine.

cholera—an acute, specific, infectious disease characterized by diarrhea, painful cramps of muscles, and a tendency to collapse.

chorionic gonadotropin—a hormone detectable in the urine of a pregnant female soon after conception.

choroid—the vascular coat of the eye between the sclera and the retina.

chromosome—structures within the cell's nucleus which store hereditary information.

chronic—continuing a long time, returning; not acute.

chronic obstructive pulmonary disease (COPD)—a syndrome characterized by chronic bronchitis, asthma, and emphysema, or any combination of these conditions, resulting in dyspnea, frequent respiratory infections, and thoracic deformities from attempting to breathe.

chronological—the arrangement of events, dates, etc., in order of occurrence.

chyme—the mixture of partially digested food and digestive secretions found in the stomach and small intestines during digestion of a meal.

cilia—hairlike projections from epithelial cells as in the bronchi.

circulatory—refers to the circulatory system. The process of blood flowing through the vessels to all the cells of the body.

circumcision—surgical removal of the foreskin of the penis.

cirrhosis—an interstitial inflammation with hardening of the tissues of an organ, especially the liver.

civil—pertaining to the rights of private individuals; legal proceedings concerning rights that are not criminal.

clarity—clearness, absence of cloudiness.

classified—arranged in a group or classification according to some system.

claustrophobia—an abnormal fear of being in enclosed or confined places.

clavicle—the collar bone, articulating with the sternum and scapula.

Clinical Laboratory Improvement Amendments (CLIA)—legislation dealing with the operation of a clinical laboratory.

clitoris—an erectile organ located at the anterior junction of the labia minora.

clone—an exact copy.

coagulate—to lessen the fluidity of a liquid substance; to clot or curdle.

coccyx—the tailbone; the last four bones of the spine.

cochlea—the snail-shaped portion of the inner ear.

coitus—sexual intercourse between a man and a woman.

colitis—inflammation of the colon.

collaborate—to work together.

colleague—an associate at work, usually one of similar status.

colon—the large intestine.

colorimeter—an instrument used for measuring the amount of pigments and determining the amount of hemoglobin in the blood.

colostomy—incision of the colon for the purpose of making a more or less permanent opening.

colposcopy—a diagnostic examination to visualize the cervix through a colposcope.

coma—an abnormal deep stupor from which a person can not be aroused by external stimuli.

comminuted—a crushed bone fracture with many fragments.

common bile duct—a duct carrying bile from the hepatic and cystic ducts to the duodenum.

compatible—able to be mixed or taken together without destructive changes (as in blood typing and cross-matching); matching; not opposed to.

compensate—to make amends; be equivalent to.

competent—fit, able, capable.

complement—a group of about twenty inactive enzyme proteins present in the blood.

complexity—the state of being complicated.

compliance—consent; conformity to formal or official requirements.

complicated—not simple, involved; having many parts; not easy to solve.

compound—not simple, composed of two or more parts; with fractures, refers to bone fragments piercing the skin externally.

comprehensive—covering all areas; inclusive.

compression—to exert force against, press.

computerized—to store in a computer; to put in a form a computer can use; to bring computers into use to control an operation.

computerized axial tomography (CAT)—a series of X-ray views of the body used to construct a three-dimensional picture.

conceal—to hide, to keep secret, to withhold, as information.

conceive—to become pregnant; the uniting of the sperm and ovum.

conception—the union of the sperm of a male and the egg of a female; fertilization.

concise—condensed, short.

condenser—part of a microscope substage that regulates the amount of light directed on a specimen.

confidentiality—to be held in confidence; a secret.

confinement—restriction within certain limits.

confirm—to verify or ratify.

conflict—a clash of opinions or interests; a fight or struggle; an inner moral struggle; to come into opposition.

confront—to stand face to face with.

congestive heart failure—a complex condition of inadequate heart action with retention of tissue fluids; may be either right or left side failure, or both.

conjunction—meeting.

conjunctiva—a mucous membrane which lines the eyelids and covers the anterior sclera of the eyeball.

connective—that which connects or binds together; one of the five main tissues of the body.

connotation—something implied or suggested.

consciousness—awareness, full knowledge of what is in one's own mind.

consecutive—following in order, successive.

constipation—a sluggish action of the bowel; usually refers to an excessively firm, hard stool which is difficult to expel, or lack of a bowel movement over a period of time.

constrict—to narrow; to become smaller due to contraction of a sphincter muscle.

contact dermatitis—inflammation and irritation of the skin due to contact with an irritating substance.

contagious—catching; able to be transmitted by contact.

contaminate—to place in contact with microorganisms.

contemporary—happening or existing at the same time; a person living at the same time as another.

context—the part of a written or spoken statement that surrounds a particular word or passage and can clarify its meaning.

contraception—against conception.

contract—to draw together, reduce in size, or shorten.

contractions—the muscle action of the uterus during labor.

contracture—permanent shortening or contraction of a muscle.

contrast—to show difference; in radiology, refers to a radiopaque medium used to outline body organs.

convey—to impart, as an idea; to transfer.

convulsion—attack of involuntary muscular contractions often accompanied with unconsciousness.

coordination—a state of harmonious adjustment or function.

cornea—the transparent extension of the sclera that lies in front of the pupil of the eye.

coronal plane—a line drawn through the side of the body from head to toe, making front and back section.

coronary—referring to the arteries surrounding the heart muscle; also refers to a "heart attack" which involves the coronary arteries.

corpus luteum—the yellow body that develops in the ruptured graafian follicle after the ovum has been discharged.

cortex—the outer portion of the kidney.

corticosteroids—hormones used to treat inflammation.

countershock—(in cardiology) a high intensity, short duration, electric shock applied to the area of the heart, resulting in total cardiac depolarization.

cramp—a spasmodic, painful, contraction of a muscle or muscles.

cranial—pertaining to the cranium or skull.

cranium—the skull; the eight bones of the head enclosing the brain; generally applied to the 28 bones of the head and face.

crenated—notched or scalloped, as the crenated condition of blood corpuscles.

cretinism—a congenital condition due to the lack of the hormone thyroxin.

criminal—of, involving, or having the nature of a crime.

crisis—the turning point of a disease; a very critical period. An emergency situation.

criterion—a standard of criticism or judgment (plural: criteria).

critique—a critical examination of a thing or situation, to determine its nature, worth, or conformity to standards.

Crohn's disease—an inflammation of the GI tract with debilitating symptoms.

cross-match—a blood test used to assure compatibility of the donor to the recipient when transfusing blood.

cryosurgery—the use of a substance at subfreezing temperature to destroy and/or remove tissue.

cryptorchidism—failure of the testicles to descend into the scrotum.

currency—any form of money.

current—happening now; of the present time; the latest information.

Cushing's syndrome—a disorder resulting from the hypersecretion of glucocorticoids from the adrenal cortex.

customarily—by custom, the usual course of action under similar circumstances.

cyanosis—a bluish discoloration of the skin due to lack of oxygen.

cyst—a bladder; any sac containing fluid.

cystic—pertaining to a cyst; of disease, refers to a condition with multiple cysts.

cystic fibrosis—a disease condition of fibrous tumors which have undergone cystic degeneration, accumulating fluid in the interspaces; also known as fibrocystic disease.

cystitis—inflammation of the urinary bladder.

cystoscope—an instrument for examining the interior of the urinary bladder.

cytology—the study of cell life and cell formation.

cytoplasm—cellular matter, not including the nucleus of a cell.

cytotechnologist—a laboratory specialist who prepares and examines tissue cells to study cell formation.

cytotoxic—capable of destroying cells.

D & C—see **dilatation and curettage**

DEA—see **Drug Enforcement Administration**

data—facts from which conclusions can be inferred.

debilitated—weaken; impaired the strength of.

debridement—to clean up or remove, as is done with damaged tissue around a wound.

decline stage—becoming less intense, subsiding. A period of time when the symptoms of disease start to disappear.

dedicated—committed to; set apart for a special use.

deductions—to deduct or subtract; remove, take away.

defamation—to slander, or to attack the reputation of an individual or group.

defecate—to pass stool or move bowels.

defibrillation—to cause fibrillation to end; restore to normal action.

dehydration—withdrawal of water from the tissues naturally or artificially.

delegation—a person or group of persons officially elected or appointed to represent another or others.

delete—to remove, erase.

delirium tremens—a psychic disorder involving hallucinations, both visual and auditory, found in habitual users of alcohol.

deltoid—the muscle of the shoulder.

demeanor—behavior; bearing.

demography—the study of population statistics concerning births, marriage, death and disease as well as many other indicators.

dendrite—an extension from a nerve cell.

denote—to indicate, to mean.

dental assistant—a health care worker employed by a dentist to perform management and clinical functions and provide chairside assistance.

dental hygienist—a licensed health care provider who is trained to X-ray and perform prophylactic treatments on teeth.

dentist—a licensed health provider who cares for the teeth, repairing and replacing as needed.

depict—to represent by a picture; portray.

depleted—consumed, emptied, exhausted.

deposit—to entrust money to a bank or other institution.

deposition—testimony given under oath.

depressant—a drug which causes a slowing down of bodily

function or nerve activity.

depressed—a state of depression, a period of low spirits; referring to a fracture, usually a fracture of the skull where bone fragments are driven (depressed) inward.

deprivation—to be deprived; without; having to do without or unable to use.

dermatitis—an inflammation of the skin, often the result of an irritant.

dermatologist—a physician who specializes in the diseases and disorders of the skin.

dermatology—the study of the skin and its diseases.

dermis—true skin.

descending—refers to the portion of the large intestine from the splenic flexure to the sigmoid.

description—a word picture.

desensitization—the process of making an individual less susceptible to allergens.

detection—find out or discover.

detrimental—harmful, injurious.

devastate—to lay waste, plunder, destroy.

dextrose—a simple sugar, also known as glucose.

diabetes mellitus—a metabolic disease caused by the body's inability to utilize carbohydrates.

diabetic—one afflicted with the condition diabetes.

diagnostic—referring to measures which assist in the recognition of diseases and disorders of the body.

dialysis—removal of the products of urine from the blood by passage of the solutes through a membrane.

diaphanography—a type of transillumination used to examine the breast, using selected wavelengths of light and special imaging equipment.

diaphoresis—profuse sweating.

diaphragm—the muscle of breathing which separates the thorax from the abdomen.

diarrhea—frequent bowel movements, usually liquid or semisolid.

diarthroses—a movable joint; another word for synovial.

diastole—the relaxation phase of the heartbeat; the period of least pressure.

dietician—one who is trained in dietetics, which includes nutrition, and in charge of the diet of an institution.

differential—refers to determining the number of each type of leukocyte in a cubic millimeter of blood.

diffuse—to scatter or spread.

diffusion—a process whereby gas, liquid, or solid molecules distribute themselves evenly through a medium.

digestion—the process by which food is broken down, mechanically and chemically, in the gastrointestinal tract and converted into absorbable forms.

digestive—pertaining to digestion.

digital—pertaining to or resembling a finger or toe, as an examination using a finger or fingers.

dilatation and curettage (D & C)—dilation of the cervix and scraping of the interior lining of the uterus.

dilate—to enlarge, expand in size; to increase the size of an opening.

dimpling—a condition characterized by indentations in the skin.

diphtheria—an acute infectious disease characterized by the formation of a false membrane on any mucous surface, usually in the air passages, interfering with breathing.

diplomate—an advanced status of medical practice.

disability—a legal incapacity.

disaster—an occurrence inflicting widespread destruction and distress.

disciplinary—designed to correct or punish breaches of conduct.

disclose—to uncover, reveal.

discoid—a type of Lupus which is confined to the skin; also called cutaneous.

discrepancy—inconsistencies; variances.

discretion—the use of judgment, prudence.

dislocate—the displacement of a part; usually refers to a bone temporarily out of its normal position in a joint.

dispense—to distribute; to deal out in portions.

displacement—the transfer of emotions about one person or situation to another person or situation.

disposition—the act or manner of putting in a particular order; arrange.

dissect—to cut into separate parts for examination; to separate.

distal—farthest from the center, from the medial line, or from the trunk.

distend—to become inflated, to stretch out.

distinctive—unmistakable, different from anything else.

distort—to misrepresent; to twist out of usual shape.

diverticulitis—inflammation of the diverticula.

diverticulum—a sac or pouch in the walls of a canal or organ, particularly the colon.

doctorate—a postgraduate degree conferred following extensive course work, an individual research project, and the writing of a dissertation; a PhD.

doctrine—the principles of any branch of knowledge; a belief held or taught.

documentary—presenting facts without inserting fictional matter.

dominant—strongest; prevailing, the prime or main.

dorsal—pertaining to the back.

dorsalis pedis—a pulse point palpable on the instep of the foot.

douche—an irrigation of the vagina.

dribbling—uncontrolled leakage of urine from the bladder.

drill—disciplined repetitious exercises as a means of perfecting a skill or procedure.

droplet—a very small drop.

Drug Enforcement Administration (DEA)—a division of the federal government responsible for the enforcement of laws regulating the distribution and sale of drugs.

duodenum—the first segment of the small intestine.

dura mater—the outer membrane covering the brain and spinal cord.

duration—period of time a thing continues.

dwarfism—a condition caused by inadequate growth hormone during childhood.

dysmenorrhea—painful menstruation.

dyspnea—difficult or labored breathing.

dystrophy—progressive atrophy or weakening of a part, such as the muscles.

dysuria—painful urination; difficulty in urination.

ECG/EKG—see **electrocardiogram**

echocardiography—ultrahigh-frequency sound waves directed toward the heart to evaluate function and structure of the organ.

echoes—reflections of sound.

ectopic—in an abnormal position; in pregnancy refers to the

embryo or fetus being outside the uterus.

eczema—a non-contagious skin disease characterized by dry, red, itchy and scaly skin.

edema—a condition of body tissues containing abnormal amounts of fluid, usually intercellular; may be local or general.

effacement—the thinning out of the cervix during labor.

efficiency—the ratio of energy expended to results produced.

ejaculation—the expulsion of seminal fluid from the male urethra.

ejaculatory duct—the duct from the seminal vesicle to the urethra.

elasticity—ability to return to shape after being stretched.

electrocardiogram (EKG, ECG)—a graphic record of the electric currents generated by the heart; a tracing of the heart action.

electrocardiograph—a machine for obtaining a graphic recording of the electrical activity of the heart.

electrocautery—an apparatus used to cauterize tissue with heat from a current of electricity.

electrocoagulation—coagulation of tissue by means of a high-frequency electric current.

electrode—an instrument with a point or a surface which transmits current to the patient's body.

electroencephalogram—a graphic record of the electric currents generated by the brain; a tracing of brain waves.

electrolyte—a substance, which in solution, conducts an electric current.

electromagnet—a soft iron core that temporarily becomes a magnet when an electric current flows through a coil surrounding it.

electromagnetic radiation—rays produced by the collision of a beam of electrons with a metal target in an X-ray tube.

electromyography—the insertion of needles into selected skeletal muscles for the purpose of recording nerve conduction time in relation to muscle contraction.

electron—a minute particle of matter charged with the smallest known amount of negative electricity; opposite of proton.

elements—substances in their simplest form; the basic building blocks of all matter.

elicit—to draw out, to derive by logical process.

eliminate—to remove, get rid of, exclude; also to pass urine from the bladder or stool from the bowel.

elite—choice, superior, select.

ellipses—a mark or series of marks used in writing or printing to indicate an omission, especially of letters or words.

emancipated minor—no longer under the care, custody, or supervision of a parent or guardian.

embolus—a circulating mass in a blood vessel; foreign material which obstructs a blood vessel.

embryo—the initial eight weeks of development after fertilization.

emergency medical technician (EMT)—an individual trained to respond in emergency situations and provide appropriate initial medical treatment.

emesis—to vomit.

emetic—medication that induces vomiting.

empathy—sympathetically trying to identify one's feelings with those of another.

emphysema—a chronic lung disease characterized by overdistention of the alveolar sacs and inability to exchange oxygen and carbon dioxide.

empyema—exudate (pus) within the pleural space of the chest cavity.

enact—to make into law.

encompass—to surround, enclose.

endocardium—the serous membrane lining of the heart.

endocrine—a gland that secretes directly into the blood stream.

endocrinologist—a physician specializing in the diseases and disorders of the endocrine system.

endocrinology—the study of the endocrine or ductless glands of internal secretion.

endocytosis—a cellular process to bring large molecules of material into the cytoplasm of the cell.

endometrium—the mucous membrane lining of the uterus.

endoplasmic reticulum—an organelle within the cytoplasm of a cell.

endorse—to approve, recommend, or sponsor.

endorsement—the act of endorsing; approving.

endoscope—an instrument consisting of a tube and optical system for observing the inside of an organ or cavity.

enema—the instillation of fluid into the rectum and colon.

engorge—to fill with blood to the point of congestion; to devour or engulf.

enhance—to intensify, improve.

entity—a thing having reality.

enucleation—surgical excision of the eyeball.

enumerate—to count separately, name one by one.

enunciate—to speak or pronounce clearly.

enzyme—a complex chemical substance produced by the body, found primarily in the digestive juices, which acts upon food substances to break them down for absorption.

eosinophil—a white blood cell or cellular structure that stains readily with the acid stain eosin; specifically an eosinophilic leukocyte.

epidermis—the outer layer of skin; literally over the true skin.

epididymis—a convoluted tube resting on the surface of the testicle, which carries sperm from the testicle to the vas deferens.

epigastric—pertaining to the area of the abdomen over the stomach.

epiglottis—a cartilagenous lid which closes over the larynx when swallowing.

epilepsy—a chronic disease of the nervous system characterized by convulsions and often unconsciousness.

epinephrine—a hormone produced by the adrenal medulla.

epiphysis—a portion of bone not yet ossified; the cartilagenous ends of the long bones which allow for growth.

episiotomy—an incision in the perineum to avoid tearing during childbirth.

epistaxis—nosebleed; hemorrhage from the nose.

epithelial—pertaining to a type of cell or tissue that forms the skin and mucous membranes of the body.

equity—the value of property beyond the total amount owed on it.

equivalent—equal to in value, size, or effect.

erectile—refers to tissue which is capable of erection, usually due to vasocongestion.

ergonomics—a study of the application of biology and engineering to the relationship between workers and their environment.

erythema—diffuse redness over the skin due to capillary

congestion and dilation of the superficial capillaries.

erythrocyte—a red blood cell (RBC).

erythropoiesis—the formation of red blood corpuscles.

esophagus—a collapsible tube from the pharynx to the stomach through which passes the food and water the body ingests.

essential—necessary; when referring to blood pressure, indicates an elevation without apparent cause.

estrogen—a female hormone produced by the ovaries.

ether—a colorless liquid used to produce unconsciousness and insensibility to pain.

ethical—right, according to the principles of ethics.

etiquette—conventional rules for correct behavior.

euphoria—a feeling of well-being, elation.

eustachian tube—refers to the tube of the middle ear which connects to the pharynx.

evacuate—to empty, especially the bowels.

evacuation—withdrawal, to remove, to make empty.

evaluation—assessment; judgment concerning the worth, quality, significance, or value of a situation, person, or product.

excretion—the process of expelling material from the body.

exemplify—to show by example.

exemption—freed from or not liable for something to which others are subject.

exfoliate—to scale off dead tissue.

exhale—to breathe out.

exocrine—a gland which secretes substances through a duct into the body.

exocytosis—a cellular process which moves materials within the cell to the outside.

exogenous—originating outside an organ or part.

exophthalmia—abnormal protrusion of the eyeball.

expectorate—to spit, to expel mucus or phlegm from the throat or lungs.

expedient—suitable means for achieving or attaining a purpose or end. Of immediate advantage, convenient.

expedite—to hasten.

expend—to spend or use, as with money or energy.

expertise—special knowledge or skill.

expiration—the expulsion of air from the lungs in breathing.

explicit—clearly and definitely expressed; unambiguous; leaving no room for questions.

express—to utter; to make known in words or by action.

extensive—having a wide range.

extensor—the muscle of a muscle team which extends a part, allowing the joint to straighten.

externship—a supervised employment experience in a qualified health care facility as part of the educational curriculum.

extinguish—to put out; put an end to.

extracellular—outside the cell.

extract—a substance distilled or drawn out of another substance.

extremity—refers to the terminal parts of the body—the arms, legs.

exudate—pus; the collection of purulent material in a cavity.

eyewash—a device utilizing water to remove foreign material from the eyes, usually in emergency situations.

facility—a building; in medical situations, a building for the care and treatment of patients.

facultative—able to live under conditions of temperature or oxygen supply which vary; having the capability to adapt to more than one condition, as a facultative anerobe.

fallopian tube—the ovaduct; the passageway for the ova from the ovary to the uterus.

family practice—one which cares for patients of all ages and all conditions not requiring specialization.

fascia—a fibrous membrane covering, supporting, and separating muscles; may also unite the skin with underlying tissue.

fasting—to abstain from food; without food or water.

fatal—causing death.

febrile—pertaining to a fever.

fecal—pertaining to feces.

feces—stool, bowel movement.

femoral—pertaining to the artery that lies adjacent to the femur.

femur—the thigh bone of the leg.

fenestrated—having a window or opening.

fertilization—impregnation of the ovum by the sperm; conception.

fetal—pertaining to a fetus, pregnancy beyond the third month.

fetus—an embryo after eight weeks of gestation.

fibrillation—the quivering of muscle fibers; ineffective, rapid but weak heart action.

fibroid—a tumor made up of fibrous and muscular tissue.

fibula—a long bone in the leg from the knee to the ankle.

filtration—the movement of solutes and water across a semi-permeable membrane as a result of a force such as gravity or blood pressure.

fiscal—of or pertaining to finances in general.

fissure—an ulcer, split, crack, or tear in the tissue.

fistula—an abnormal tubelike passage from a normal cavity or an abscess to a free surface.

flatulence—the existence of flatus or intestinal gas.

flatus—intestinal gas.

flexed—bent, as at a joint.

flexible—easily bent, compliant, yielding to persuasion.

flexor—the muscle of a muscle team that bends a part.

flora—plant life as distinguished from animal life; plant life occurring or adapted for living in a specific environment, as flora in the intestines.

flu—an abbreviation for the word influenza; a respiratory or intestinal infection.

fluoroscope—a device consisting of a fluorescent screen in conjunction with an X-ray tube to make visible shadows of objects interposed between the screen and the tube.

flush—sudden reddish coloration of the skin.

follicle—a small excretory duct or sac or tubular gland; a hair follicle.

folliculitis—a staphlococcal infection of a hair follicle.

foreign—anything which is not normally found in the location; usually refers to dirt, splinters, etc.

foreskin—loose skin covering the end of the penis.

forge—to imitate, especially to counterfeit, as a signature.

formaldehyde—a colorless, pungent gas used in its liquid form to harden tissue for pathological study, or as a germicide, disinfectant, or preservative, according to the strength of the solution.

fovea centralis—a depression in the posterior surface of the retina which is the place of sharpest vision.

fracture—the sudden breaking of a bone.

fraudulent—characterized by cheating and deceit; obtained by dishonest means.

frequency—the need to void urine often, though usually only a small amount at one time.

friction—resistance of one surface to the motion of another surface rubbing over it.

fringe benefits—benefits included in or added to the salary paid, such as health insurance, retirement fund, etc.

frontal—anterior; the forehead bone; refers to the plane drawn through the side of the body from the head to the foot.

functional—practical, working, useful.

fungus—a vegetable, cellular organism that subsists on organic matter, such as bacteria or mold; a disease condition which causes growth of fungal lesions on the surface of the skin.

furuncle—the medical term for a boil.

GYN—see **gynecology**

gait—manner of walking.

gallbladder—a small sac suspended beneath the liver which concentrates and stores bile.

galley proof—printed matter in preliminary form, to be corrected.

galvanometer—an instrument that measures current by electromagnetic action.

gamete—a germ cell; any reproductive body.

ganglion—a mass of nerve tissue which receives and sends out nerve impulses.

gangrene—a form of necrosis; the putrefaction of soft tissue.

gastric—pertaining to the stomach.

gastrocnemius—the large muscle in the calf of the leg.

gastroenterologist—a physician specializing in the care of patients with diseases and disorders of the gastrointestinal tract.

gastroenterology—the study of the stomach and intestines and their diseases.

gastrointestinal (GI)—pertaining to the stomach and intestines.

gastroscopy—examination of the stomach with a gastroscope.

gauge—the size of a needle bore; the smaller the number the larger the needle bore.

gene—a substance within the chromosome that dictates heredity.

generate—to produce, as heat, ideas, power.

generic—general; characteristic of a genus or group.

genetic—pertaining to the genes.

genital herpes—fluid-filled lesions on the external genitalia which are contagious upon direct contact.

genitalia—the external sexual organs.

genucubital—pertaining to the elbows and knees; the knee-elbow position.

genupectoral—pertaining to the knees and the chest; the knee-chest position.

geriatrics—the study and treatment of the diseases of old age.

gerontologist—a physician specializing in the care of the aged.

gigantism—a condition resulting from the overproduction of growth hormone during childhood.

glance—a quick look or view.

glaucoma—a disease of the eye characterized by increased intraocular pressure.

glomerulonephritis—inflammation of the glomerulus of the nephron of the kidney.

glomerulus—the microscopic cluster of capillaries within the Bowman's capsule of the nephron.

glucose—a colorless or yellow, thick, syrupy liquid obtained by the incomplete hydrolysis of starch; a simple sugar.

gluteus maximus—the large muscle of the buttocks.

glycosuria—sugar in the urine.

goiter—an enlargement of the thyroid gland.

golgi apparatus—an organelle within the cytoplasm of a cell.

gonadotrophic—related to stimulation of the gonads.

gonads—the sex glands, the ovaries in the female and the testicles in the male.

gonorrhea—a venereal disease of the reproductive organs which is highly contagious upon direct contact.

graafian follicle—the vesicle in which ova are matured and which releases them when ripened.

graft—a constructed part.

gram-negative—bacteria which take on a pink color with Gram staining process.

gram-positive—bacteria which take on a purple color with Gram staining process.

greenstick—an incomplete fracture, occurring in children.

grillwork—a bar-like device, usually constructed of heavy metal; an open grating for a door or window.

groin—the depression between the thigh and the trunk of the body; the inguinal region.

gross—exclusive of deductions; total; entire.

gross anatomy—refers to the study of those features that can be observed with the naked eye by inspection and dissection.

guaiac—a solution used to test for the presence of occult blood in the stool.

guarantor—a person who makes or gives a guarantee or pledge, often to pay another's debt or obligation in the event of default.

guilds—associations of persons engaged in the same trade or calling for mutual protection.

gynecologist—a physician specializing in the care of diseases and disorders of women, particularly the genital organs.

gynecology (GYN)—the study of diseases of the female, particularly of the organs of reproduction.

HCFA—Health Care Financing Administration.

HHS—Health and Human Services.

HIB/hib—hemophilus influenzae type B.

haemophilus—bacterial strains that grow best in hemoglobin.

hallucinogen—a substance which causes hallucinations.

hamstring—a group of muscles of the posterior thigh.

harassment—continual annoyance; persecution.

hard copy—information printed on a solid surface such as paper instead of displayed on a CRT screen or stored on a disk.

harmonious—having parts combined in a proportionate, orderly, or pleasing arrangement; being peaceable or friendly.

hazardous—dangerous; risky.

health—a state of complete physical and mental or social well-being.

heart block—a condition in which impulses from the S-A node fail to carry over to the A-V node resulting in a slow heart rate and a different rate of contraction between the upper and lower heart chambers.

heartburn—a burning sensation beneath the breastbone, usually associated with indigestion.

hematocrit—an expression of the volume of red blood cells per unit of circulating blood.

hematologist—a physician specializing in the care of patients with disorders and diseases of the blood and blood-forming organs.

hematology—the study of the blood and its diseases.

hematoma—a tumor or swelling which contains blood.

hematuria—blood in the urine.

hemodialysis—a process whereby blood is passed through a thin membrane and exposed to a dialysate solution to remove waste products.

hemoglobin—the combination of a protein and iron pigment in the red blood cells that attracts and carries oxygen in the body.

hemolysis—dissolution; the breaking down of red blood cells.

hemophilia—an hereditary condition, transmitted through sex-linked chromosomes of female carriers; affects males only, causing inability to clot blood.

hemorrhage—abnormal discharge of blood either internally or externally from venous, arterial, or capillary vessels.

hemorrhoidectomy—surgical excision of hemorrhoidal tissue.

hemorrhoids—varicose veins of the anal canal.

hemothorax—blood within the pleural space of the chest cavity.

heparin—a substance formed in the liver which inhibits the coagulation of blood.

hepatic—pertaining to the liver.

hepatitis—inflammation of the liver.

hernia—a projection of a part from its normal location.

herniorrhaphy—the surgical repair of a hernia.

Herpes Simplex—the medical term for fever blister, an acute viral infection of the face, mouth or nose.

Herpes Zoster—the medical term for shingles, an acute viral infection of the dorsal root ganglia.

hesitancy—difficulty in starting a urine stream.

heterosexual—sexual attraction toward the opposite sex.

heterotrophs—microorganisms that feed on organic matter.

hiatus—pertains to a herniation of the stomach through an opening or hiatus.

hiccough—(Also hiccup) a result of the spasmodic closing of the epiglottis and spasm of the diaphragm.

hilum—the recessed area of the kidney where the ureter and blood vessels enter.

hinge—a type of joint.

histamine—a substance normally present in the body.

histologist—(Histotechnologist) a person engaged in the study of the microscopic structure of tissue.

histology—the study of the microscopic structure of tissue.

histoplasmosis—a fungal infection caused by an organism found in bird and bat droppings.

holistic—considering the whole or entire scope of a situation.

Holter monitor—a device that attaches electrodes to a patient's chest for the purpose of obtaining a 24-hour EKG tracing in an accessory tape recorder.

homeostasis—maintenance of a constant or static condition of internal environment.

homosexual—sexual attraction toward the same sex as oneself.

horizontal—not vertical; flat and even; level; parallel to the plane of the horizon.

hormone—a chemical substance secreted by an organ or gland.

hostility—unfriendliness, enmity.

hpf—high-power field; refers to microscope lens.

humble—modest, unassuming.

humerus—the long bone of the upper arm.

humoral—antibody-mediated immunity.

hyaline membrane disease—a condition resulting from incomplete development of the respiratory system in premature infants.

hydrocele—the accumulation of fluid in the scrotum.

hydrochloric acid—a digestive juice found in the stomach.

hygiene—the study of health and observance of health rules.

hymen—a membranous fold partially or completely covering the vaginal opening.

hyperglycemia—increase of blood sugar, as in diabetes.

hyperopia—a defect of vision so that objects can only be seen when they are far away; farsightedness.

hypersensitive—over sensitive; abnormally sensitive to a stimulus of any kind.

hypertension—elevated blood pressure.

hyperthermia—higher than normal temperature.

hyperthyroidism—a condition caused by excessive secretion of the thyroid glands.

hypertonic—having a higher concentration of salt than found in a red blood cell.

hyperventilation—excessive deep and frequent breathing.

hypoallergenic—unlikely to cause an allergic reaction.

hypochondriac—pertaining to the upper outer regions of the abdomen below the thorax; also someone with a morbid fear of disease, resulting in abnormal concern about one's health.

hypogastric—referring to an abdominal area in the middle lower third of the abdomen.

hypoglycemia—deficiency of sugar in the blood.

hypotension—abnormally low blood pressure.

hypothalamus—a structure of the brain between the cerebrum and the midbrain; lies below the thalamus.

hypothermia—below normal body temperature.

hypothyroidism—a condition caused by a marked deficiency of thyroid secretion.

hypotonic—having a lower concentration of salt than found in a red blood cell.

hypoxia—a lack of oxygen.

hysterectomy—surgical removal of the uterus.

hysteroscopy—a procedure utilizing the hysteroscope to view the endometrium of the uterus.

I & D—see **incision and drainage**

IVP—see **intravenous pyelography**

idiopathic—disease without recognizable cause.

ileocecal—the valve between the end of the small intestine and the cecum.

ileostomy—a surgical opening from the ileum onto the abdominal wall.

ileum—the last section of the small intestine.

iliac—the edge or crest of the pelvic bone.

ilium—the hip bone.

illegible—impossible to read.

illicit—improper; unlawful; not sanctioned by custom or law; illegal.

illuminate—to enlighten, throw light on.

imaging—a representation or visual impression produced by a lens, mirror, etc.

immune—protected or exempt from a disease.

immunization—becoming immune or the process of rendering a patient immune.

immunodeficiency—lacking the components necessary to

mount an immune response.

immunoglobulin—a large protein molecule which assists in the immune response.

immunological—pertaining to immunology.

immunosuppressed—a condition wherein the immune system has been overpowered and cannot function adequately.

impacted—refers to a fracture where the broken ends are jammed together.

impaction—a collection of hardened feces in the rectum which cannot be expelled.

impending—to be at hand or about to happen.

implant—something implanted into tissue; a graft; artificial part.

implement—a tool or instrument for doing something; to put into effect.

implication—involvement, bringing into connection.

impotence—inability of a male to obtain or maintain an erection.

impulse—a charge transmitted through certain tissues, especially nerve fibers and muscles, resulting in physiological activity.

inappropriate— not appropriate, out of place.

incinerate—to burn, set afire.

incision—cut.

incision and drainage (I & D)—cutting into for the purpose of providing an exit for material, usually a collection of pus.

inclined—leaning or tending toward.

incomprehensible—beyond belief, not to be grasped by the mind.

incongruous—lacking harmony or agreement.

incontinent—unable to control the bladder or bowel.

incubation—the interval between exposure to infection and the appearance of the first symptom.

incus—the anvil, the middle bone of the three in the middle ear.

indigent—needy, poor, destitute.

indigestion—difficulty in digesting food.

inevitable—unavoidable, destined to occur.

infarct—infiltration of foreign particles; material in a vessel causing coagulation and interference with circulation.

infectious—capable of producing infection; denoting a disease in the body caused by the presence of germs; tending to spread to others.

inferior—below, under.

infertility—inability to achieve conception.

infirmity—illness, disease.

inflict—to strike, to cause punishment.

influenza—an acute illness characterized by fever, pain, coughing, and general upper respiratory symptoms.

infrared—pertaining to those invisible rays just beyond the red end of the visible spectrum which have a penetrating heating effect.

infusion—to instill; introduction of a substance into a vein.

ingest—to eat.

inguinal—referring to the region where the thigh joins the trunk of the body; the groin.

inguinal canal—a passageway in the groin for the spermatic cord in the male.

inguinal hernia—the presence of small intestine in the inguinal canal.

inhale—to breathe in.

initial—the first; beginning; the first letter of each of a person's names.

initiate—to get something started, begin.

inunction—the process of administering drugs through the skin.

inoculating loop—a laboratory instrument used to transfer organisms from one source to another.

inorganic—not living; occurring in nature independently of living things.

inseminate—to impregnate with semen.

insertion—the place where a muscle is attached to the bone that it moves.

insidious—hidden, not apparent.

insignificant—unimportant; petty; of little or no value.

inspect—to examine closely.

inspection—the first part of a physical examination; close observation.

inspiration—to breathe in, inhale.

institute—to originate as a custom.

insufficient—not as much as needed.

insulin—a hormone secreted by the Islands of Langerhans in the pancreas.

intact—unbroken, undamaged.

intangible—that which cannot be touched, easily defined or grasped.

integrity—soundness of character; honesty in particular.

integumentary—the skin; a covering.

intellectualization—to employ reasoning to avoid confrontations or stressful situations.

interaction—to act upon one another.

intercostal—between the ribs.

interference—confusion of desired signals due to undesired signals, as in artifacts on an EKG.

interferon—a lymphokine that helps regulate the activities of macrophages and NK cells.

interleukin—a substance which is a messenger between leukocytes.

intermediate—in the middle.

intermittent—stopping and starting again at intervals.

intermuscular—within the muscle.

interneurons—neurons connecting sensory to motor neurons.

internist—a physician specializing in the care of patients with internal diseases.

internship—a period of time following graduation wherein practice of the profession is performed.

interpersonal—between persons.

interpret—to explain, translate; to determine the meaning.

interval—time between events; space.

intervertebral—between the vertebrae.

intestine—the alimentary canal extending from the pylorus of the stomach to the anus.

intimidate—to make afraid, to frighten.

intracellular—within the cell.

intradermal—within the skin.

intraocular—within the eyeball.

intrauterine device (IUD)—an object inserted into the uterus to prevent pregnancy.

intravenous—to insert into the vein.

intravenous pyelography (IVP)—the insertion of a radiopaque material into the vein for the purpose of X-raying the kidneys and ureters.

intricate—complicated, complex, elaborately interwoven.

intubate—to insert a tube.

intuition—the immediate knowing or learning of something without the conscious use of reasoning.

invasive—diagnostic methods involving entry into living tissue.

inventory—an itemized list of goods in stock.

involuntary—independent of or even contrary to will or choice.

iodine—a nonmetallic element belonging to the halogen group.

iris—the colored, contractible tissue surrounding the pupil of the eye.

irreparable—damaged beyond possibility of repair.

ischemia—temporary and localized anemia due to obstruction of the circulation to a part.

ischium—posterior and inferior portion of the hip bone.

Ishahara—refers to an eye test to determine color vision.

Islet of Langerhans—clusters of cells in the pancreas.

isotonic—having the same concentration of salt as found in a red blood cell.

issue—to send forth; to put into circulation.

Jaeger—a system for measuring near vision acuity.

jaundice—a yellowish discoloration of the sclera and skin due to the presence of bile pigments in the blood.

jejunum—the middle segment of the small intestine, which measures approximately 8 feet in length.

journal—a record of happenings; a diary.

journalizing—entries on the daily log.

judgment—a decision; ability to make the right decisions.

keloid—an overgrowth of new skin tissue; a scar.

keying—pressing a lever or button, as on a typewriter, that is pressed with the finger to operate the machine.

kidney—a bean-shaped organ that excretes urine and is located retroperitoneally, high in the back of the abdominal cavity.

KUB—kidneys, ureters, and bladder; refers to a radiological study.

kyphosis—a convex curvature of the spine; humpback.

L & A—light and accommodation.

labia majora—the two large folds of adipose tissue lying on each side of the vulva of the female; external genitalia.

labia minora—the two mucocutaneous folds of membrane within the labia majora.

laboratory—a room or building in which scientific tests or experiments are conducted.

laboratory technician—a health care worker who performs specialized chemical, microscopic, and bacteriologic tests of blood, tissue, and body fluids.

lacrimal—pertaining to tears; the glands and ducts which secrete and convey tears.

laminectomy—the removal of a portion of the vertebral posterior arch.

lancet—a sharp, pointed instrument used to pierce the skin to obtain a capillary blood sample.

laryngeal—pertaining to the larynx.

laryngectomy—surgical removal of the larynx or voice box.

larynx—the voice box.

lateral—pertaining to the side.

latissimus dorsi—the large muscle of the back.

laxative—a substance which induces the bowels to empty.

ledger—the principal account book of a business establishment, containing the credits and debits.

legible—easy to read, readable.

Legionnaires disease—an acute bronchopneumonia.

leisure—spare or free time, away from the pressure and responsibilities of work.

lens—a part of the eye which bends or refracts images onto the retina.

lesion—an injury or wound; a circumscribed area of pathologically altered tissue.

lethal—deadly; capable of causing death.

leukemia—a disease characterized by a great excess of white blood cells; it exists in a lymphatic and myelogenous form; it is often fatal, especially in adults.

leukocyte—a white blood cell.

liability—anything to which a person is liable, responsible, legally bound.

liaison—intercommunication between two entities.

license—a legal permit to engage in an activity.

licensed practical nurse (LPN)—an individual trained in basic nursing techniques, to provide direct patient care under the supervision of an RN or physician.

ligament—fibrous tissue which connects bone to bone.

ligation—to tie off; the process of binding or tying.

limbs—refers to the arms and legs.

liter—a unit of measure; 1,000 ml or approximately 1 quart.

liver—the largest gland in the body, located in the upper right quadrant of the abdomen beneath the diaphragm.

lithotomy—an examination position wherein the patient lies upon the back with thighs flexed upon the abdomen and legs flexed upon the thighs.

lithotripsy—destruction of stone; stonecrusher.

LMP—last menstrual period.

longevity—a long duration of life; lasting a long time.

longitudinal fissure—the deep cleft between the two hemispheres of the cerebrum.

lordosis—abnormal anterior curvature of the lumbar spine.

lpf—low-power field; refers to microscope lens.

lubb dupp—sounds made by the heart.

lumbar—pertaining to the back, specifically to the five vertebrae above the sacrum.

lumbar puncture—the insertion of a needle between the vertebrae in the lumbar area for the purpose of withdrawing spinal fluid.

lumen—the space within an artery, vein, or capillary; the space within a tube.

lung—the organ of respiration, located within the thoracic cavity.

lupus erythematosus—a chronic autoimmune disease which causes changes in the immune system.

luteinizing—a hormone effect which causes ovulation and progesterone in the female and sperm production and testosterone in the male.

Lyme Disease—a disease caused by a spirochete which is carried by the deer tick.

lymph—a body fluid formed within the tissue spaces and circulated throughout the body.

lymphatic system—a network of transparent vessels carrying lymph fluid throughout the body.

lymphocyte—a type of white blood cell.

lysosomes—an organelle within the cytoplasm of the cell.

MI—see **myocardial infarction**

MRI—see **magnetic resonance imaging**

MUGA—see **multiple-gated acquisition scan**

macule—a discolored spot or patch on the skin neither

elevated nor depressed.

macrophage—a phagocytic cell that destroys antigens.

magnetic—having the properties of a magnet, able to attract.

magnetic resonance imaging (MRI)—a diagnostic test using magnetic waves to visualize internal body structures.

magnify—to make something look larger than it really is.

mailable—an item suitable for mailing.

maintenance—to preserve; the act or work of keeping something in proper condition.

malaise—a feeling of discomfort or uneasiness.

malignant—a cancerous growth; tumor.

malinger—to pretend illness to escape dealing with a situation or obligation.

malleus—the largest of the three bones of the middle ear, also called the hammer.

mammary glands—the breasts.

mammograph—an X-ray of the breast.

management—the act, manner, or practice of managing, handling, or controlling something.

manifestation—act of disclosing; revelation; display.

manipulation therapy—any treatment or procedure involving the use of the hands; movement of a joint to determine its range of extension and flexion; additional manual skills utilized by osteopathic physicians.

marginal—close to the lower limit of acceptability.

marrow—the soft tissue in the hollow of long bones.

masses—a multitude; a large number of people.

mastectomy—surgical removal of a breast.

matrix—a format for establishing a time schedule for appointments.

maturation—refers to a stage of cellular development.

maturity—a state of full development.

measles—a highly contagious disease characterized by the presence of maculopustular eruptions.

mechanical—pertaining to machinery.

medial—pertaining to the middle or midline.

medulla—the inner section of the kidney.

medulla oblongata—enlarged portion of the spinal cord; the lower portion of the brain stem.

melanin—a pigment which gives color to the skin, hair, and eyes.

melanocyte—cells which produce the pigment of the skin, melanin.

membrane—a thin, soft, pliable layer of tissue which lines a tube or cavity or covers an organ or structure.

menarche—the first menstrual period.

Meniere's disease—a disorder of the ear characterized by nausea, vomiting, tinnitus, and hearing loss.

meninges—the membranes covering the brain and spinal cord.

meningitis—inflammation of the meninges of the brain and/or spinal cord.

meniscus—a concave level of fluid in a tube or cylinder.

menopause—the permanent cessation of menstruation.

menorrhagia—excessive menstrual flow, hemorrhage.

menstruate—to periodically discharge bloody fluid from the uterus.

mensuration—the process of measuring.

mercury—a liquid metal used in measurement devices such as thermometers and sphygmomanometers; chemical symbol, Hg.

merit—to deserve reward or praise; excellence.

mesentery—a peritoneal fold connecting the intestine to the posterior abdominal wall.

metabolism—the successive transformations to which a substance is subjected from the time it enters the body to the time it or its decomposition products are excreted, and by which nutrition is accomplished and energy and living substance are provided.

metacarpals—pertaining to the five bones of the hand between the wrist and the phalanges.

metastasis—movement of cancer cells from one part of the body to another.

metatarsals—the five bones of the feet between the instep and the phalanges.

methodical—systematic, following a plan or method.

microbial—related to microbes.

microfiche—a sheet of microfilm capable of accommodating and preserving a considerable number of book pages in reduced form.

microorganism—a microscopic living body not perceivable by the naked eye.

microscopic—visible only with a microscope.

microscopic anatomy—an area of study that deals with features that can be seen only with a microscope.

micturation—the passing of urine.

midbrain—that portion of the brain connecting the pons and the cerebellum.

midline—the middle.

migraine—a severe headache with characteristic symptoms.

minute—a measurement of time equal to 60 seconds; very small, tiny.

misalignment—out of alignment; not straight.

mitochondria—an organelle within the cytoplasm of the cell.

mitosis—the division of a cell.

mitral—the valve in the heart between the chambers of the left side, also known as the bicuspid.

modifies—qualifies or limits the meaning.

molten—melted.

monitor—to oversee or observe.

monoclonal—a laboratory-produced hybrid cell which produces antibodies.

monocular—possessing a single eyepiece as with a microscope.

monocyte—single nucleated cells which leave the blood and enter into tissues to become macrophages.

monotone—all in one tone; speech in an unchanging tone.

mons pubis—a pad of fatty tissue and coarse skin overlying the symphysis pubis in the female.

morphology—a branch of biology dealing with the form and structure of organisms.

motor—refers to the nerves which permit the body to respond to stimuli.

mouth—the oral cavity; can also refer to the opening to organs.

mucosa—pertaining to mucous membrane.

multi-channel—refers to the capability of ECG equipment of processing impulses from multiple leads.

multiple-gated acquisition scan (MUGA)—a diagnostic test to evaluate the condition of the myocardium of the heart.

mumps—an acute contagious disease characterized by inflammation of the parotid gland and other salivary glands.

murmur—a soft blowing or rasping sound heard on auscultation of the heart.

muscle—a type of tissue composed of contractile cells or

fibers which effect movement of the body.

muscle team—a pair of skeletal muscles, one which flexes and one which extends the joint.

muscle tone—a state of muscle contraction in which a portion of the fibers are contracted while others are at rest.

muscular—pertaining to muscles.

musculoskeletal—pertaining to the muscular and skeletal systems.

mutation—a change in an inheritable characteristic; cellular change due to an influence.

myelin—a fatlike substance forming the principal component of the myelin sheath of nerve fibers.

myelography—an X-ray examination of the spinal cord following an injection of a radiopaque material.

myocardial infarction (MI)—blockage of a coronary artery which interrupts the flow of blood to the heart muscle.

myocardium—the muscle layer of the heart.

myometrium—the muscular structure of the uterus.

myopia—a defect in vision so that objects can only be seen when very near; nearsightedness.

myxedema—a condition resulting from the hypofunction of the thyroid gland.

narcolepsy—overwhelming attacks of sleep which the victim cannot inhibit; sleeping sickness.

narcotic—a drug capable of producing sleep and relieving pain or inducing unconsciousness and even death, depending upon the dosage.

nasal—pertaining to the nose.

nausea—an inclination to vomit.

negate—to deny the existence or truth of.

negligent—guilty of neglect; lacking in due care or concern; act of carelessness.

negotiable—capable of being discussed and terms arranged.

neoadjuvant—new attachment process; giving chemotherapy prior to surgery to shrink the tumor before removal.

neonate—a newborn infant.

neoplastic—new abnormal tissue formation; cancer related.

nephrology—the study of the kidney and its diseases.

nephrologist—a physician specializing in the diseases and disorders of the kidney.

nephron—the structural and functional unit of the kidney.

nephrotic syndrome—term applied to renal disease of whatever cause characterized by massive edema, proteinuria, and usually elevation of serum cholesterol and lipids.

nerve—a group of nervous tissues bound together for the purpose of conducting nervous impulses.

net—remaining after all deductions have been made; to clear as profit.

neurilemma—a thin membranous sheath enveloping a nerve fiber.

neurologist—a physician specializing in the diseases and disorders of the nervous system.

neurology—the study of the nervous system and its diseases.

neuron—a nerve cell.

neurosurgery—surgical procedures performed on the nervous system.

neutrophil—a granulated white blood cell.

nicotine—a poisonous alkaloid extracted from tobacco leaves.

nit—the egg of a louse or other parasitic insect.

nocturia—having to void at night.

node—a knot, knob, protuberance, or swelling.

nomenclature—a system of technical or scientific names.

nominal—too small to be considered, or a very small amount.

nomogram—representation by graphs, diagrams, or charts of the relationship between numerical variables.

nonchalant—unconcerned, indifferent.

non compos mentis—general legal term for all forms of mental illness.

non-invasive—a diagnostic method not requiring entry into body tissue.

nonpathogen—an organism which does not produce a disease.

nonspecific urethritis—inflammation of the urethra in males, vaginitis or cervicitis in females, due to bacteria or an allergy to substances used by a sexual partner.

norepinephrine—a hormone secreted by adrenal medulla in response to sympathetic stimulation.

normal saline—a solution with the same salt content as that found within a red blood cell.

nuclear medicine—the branch of medicine which utilizes radionuclides in the diagnosis and treatment of disease.

nucleolus—a structure found within the nucleus of the cell.

nucleus—the vital body in the protoplasm of a cell.

nurse practitioner—an RN with advanced clinical experience and education in a special branch of practice.

nurture—to care for, train, or educate.

nutrition—refers to edible material, food, things that nourish.

nutritionist—a member of the health care team who studies and applies the principles and science of nutrition.

OSHA—Occupational Safety and Health Act.

OTC—see over the counter

objective—the end toward which action is directed; of a disease symptom, perceptible to persons other than the one affected; on a microscope, a lens or series of lenses.

obligate—to bind legally or morally.

observant—quick to notice, watchful.

obsolete—out of use, discarded, no longer useful.

obstetrician—a physician who specializes in the care and treatment of women during pregnancy and childbirth.

obstetrics—the branch of medicine dealing with women during pregnancy, childbirth, and postpartum.

obturator—anything that obstructs or closes a cavity or opening; refers to that internal portion of an examining instrument which facilitates the introduction of the instrument into the body and is then withdrawn permitting visualization of the internal area.

occipital—pertaining to the back part of the head, the posterior lobe of the cerebrum.

occlude—to close up, obstruct.

occult—obscure, hidden.

occupational medicine—diagnosing and treating disease or conditions arising from occupational circumstances.

occupational therapist—a health care worker involved in the use of purposeful activity with individuals who are limited by physical injury or illness, psychosocial dysfunction, developmental or learning disabilities, poverty and cultural differences, or the aging process to maximize independence, prevent disability, and maintain health.

O.D.—oculus dexter, or right eye.

office manager—(Business Office Manager) an individual responsible for the overall operation of the medical office.

ointment—a salve; a fatty, soft substance having antiseptic or healing properties.

olfactory—pertaining to the sense of smell.

oliguria—scanty production of urine.

oncogenes—a gene in a tumor cell.

oncology—the branch of medicine dealing with tumors, usually malignant.

ophthalmologist—a physician specializing in the diseases and disorders of the eye.

ophthalmology—the study of the eye and its diseases.

opportunistic—seizing the opportunity; taking advantage of the situation.

opposition—action against, resistance.

optic—pertaining to the eye or sight.

optic disc—the blind spot where the optic nerve exits from the retina of the eye.

optometrist—a person who measures the eye's refractive power and prescribes correction of visual defects when needed.

oral—pertaining to the mouth.

orbital—refers to the cavity within the skull where the eye is located.

organ—a part of the body constructed of many types of tissue to perform a function.

organ of Corti—terminal acoustic apparatus in the cochlea of the inner ear.

organelles—functional structures within the cytoplasm of a cell.

organic—pertaining to or derived from animal or vegetable forms of life.

origin—the beginning or source of anything; of muscles, the anchor.

orthopedics—the branch of medicine dealing with the structure and function of bones and muscles.

orthopedist—a physician who corrects deformities and treats diseases and disorders of the bones, joints, and spine.

orthopnea—respiratory condition in which breathing is possible only in an erect sitting or standing position.

O.S.—oculus sinister, or left eye; also a mouth or opening.

oscilloscope—an instrument that displays a visual representation of electric variations on the fluorescent screen of a cathode ray tube.

osmosis—the process of diffusion of water or another solvent through a selected permeable membrane.

osseous—bonelike, concerning bones.

osteopathy—any bone disease; also refers to a school of medicine based on the belief that the bony framework of the body largely determines the structural relations of its tissues.

osteoporosis—a condition resulting from a decrease in the amount of calcium stored in the bone.

otitis—inflammation of the ear; can be referenced to the external, middle, or internal ear.

otorhinolaryngologist—a physician specializing in diseases and disorders of the ear, nose, and throat.

otorhinolaryngology—the study of the ear, nose, and larynx and their diseases.

otosclerosis—condition characterized by progressive deafness due to the fixation of the stapes of the middle ear.

O.U.—oculus uterque, or each eye.

ovary—the female gonad which produces hormones causing the secondary sex characteristics to develop and be maintained.

over the counter (OTC)—referring to accessible, nonprescription drugs.

ovulation—the periodic ripening and rupture of a mature graafian follicle and the discharge of the ovum.

ovum—an egg, the female gamete or reproductive cell.

oxalate—a salt of oxalic acid.

oxygen—a colorless, odorless, tasteless gas found in the air; chemical symbol, O_2.

oxygenate—combine or supply with oxygen.

PDR—*Physician's Desk Reference*

PKU—see **phenylketonuria**

POL—physician's office laboratory.

PS—see **postscript**

pacemaker—the S-A node of the heart; also refers to an artificial device which initiates heartbeat.

pallor—lack of color, paleness.

palpate—to feel; to examine by touch.

pancreas—an organ which secretes insulin and pancreatic digestive juice.

pancreatitis—inflammation of the pancreas.

Papanicolaou (Pap) smear—a test to detect cancer cells in the mucus of an organ.

papillae—small protuberances or elevations, such as the taste buds of the tongue.

papillary muscles—muscular attachments to the undersides of the heart valves from the walls of the ventricles, which open the valves during the relaxation phase of the heartbeat.

parabasal—beside, near, an accessory to the base or lower part.

paralytic ileus—paralysis of the intestinal wall with symptoms of acute obstruction.

paramedic—health care providers who provide emergency and supportive medical care. Have additional training beyond EMT status.

parameter—quantity to which an arbitrary value may be given as a convenience in expressing performance or for use in calculations.

parasite—an organism that lives in or on another organism without rendering it any service in return.

parasympathetic—a division of the autonomic nervous system.

parathyroid—small endocrine glands located close to the thyroid gland.

parenteral—other than by mouth.

parietal—a central portion of the cerebrum located on each side of the brain.

paroxysmal—a sudden attack of a disease; fit of acute pain, passion, coughing, or laughter.

patella—the kneecap.

pathogen—any microorganism or substance capable of producing a disease.

pathological—a condition due to a disease.

pathologist—a physician specializing in the interpretation and diagnosis of changes caused by disease in tissues and body fluids.

pathology—the study of the nature and cause of disease.

pathophysiology—the study of mechanisms by which disease occurs, the responses of the body to the disease process, and the effects of both on normal function.

patience—calm in waiting, endurance without complaint.

payee—a person to whom money is paid.

pectoralis major—the principal muscle of the chest wall.

pediatrician—a physician specializing in the diseases and disorders of children.

pediatrics—the branch of medicine dealing with the care of children and their diseases.

pediculosis—the scientific name for lice.

peer—equal; usually refers to someone of similar standing or status.

pelvic—pertaining to the pelvis.

penis—the male external sex organ.

peptic—pertaining to digestion; can also refer to an ulcer of the upper digestive tract.

per capita—for each person.

percentage—rate or proportion of each hundred.

perception—awareness through the senses; the receipt of impressions; consciousness.

percussion—tapping the body lightly but sharply to determine the position, size, and consistency of an underlying structure.

perfusion—passing of a fluid through spaces; the act of pouring over or through.

pericarditis—inflammation of the pericardium, the covering of the heart.

pericardium—the membranous sac that covers the heart.

perineum—the region between the vagina and anus of the female and the scrotum and anus of the male.

periodic—occurring, appearing, or done again and again, at regular intervals.

periosteum—the fibrous membrane covering the bone except at the articulating surfaces.

peripheral—pertaining to a portion of the nervous system; an item attached to a computer system.

peristalsis—a progressive, wavelike muscular movement which occurs involuntarily in the urinary and digestive system.

peritoneal—pertaining to the peritoneum.

permeable—capable of being penetrated; allowing entrance.

pernicious anemia—a severe anemia characterized by progressive decrease in the production of red blood cells.

perplexing—troubling with doubt, puzzling.

persecute—treat badly; do harm to again and again; pursue to injure.

personality—the personal or individual qualities that make one person different from another.

perspective—a view of things, or facts, in which they are in the right relations.

pertinent—having to do with what is being considered; relevant or to the point.

pertussis—an acute infectious disease characterized by a paroxysmal cough, ending in a whooping inspiration.

petechiae—small, purplish, hemorrhagic spots on the skin.

petition—a written plea in which specific court action is sought.

petty—small, having little value, mean, narrow-minded.

pH—a measure of acidity or alkalinity.

phagocyte—a white blood cell that engulfs and destroys antigens.

phagocytosis—ingestion and digestion of bacteria and particles by phagocytes.

phalanges—bones of the fingers and toes.

phalanx—any one of the bones of the fingers or toes.

phantom limb—an illusion following amputation of a limb that the limb still exists.

pharmaceutical—concerning drugs or pharmacy.

pharmacist—a licensed health care provider who prepares and dispenses drugs.

pharmacology—the study and practice of compounding and dispensing medical preparations.

pharynx—the throat; that portion of the alimentary canal between the mouth and the esophagus.

phenylalanine—an amino acid of a protein.

phenylketonuria (PKU)—a genetic disorder resulting from the body's failure to oxidize an amino acid, perhaps because of a defective enzyme.

phimosis—a narrowing of the opening of the foreskin of the penis.

phlebitis—inflammation of a vein.

phlebotomist—a health care worker who specializes in obtaining blood samples.

photophobia—sensitive to light; avoiding light.

physical—pertaining to the body; also used for the examination of the body.

physical medicine—the branch of medicine dealing with the treatment of disorders and diseases with mechanical devices, as in physical therapy.

physical therapist—one who is licensed to assist in the examination, testing, and treatment of physically disabled or handicapped people through the use of special exercise, application of heat or cold, use of sonar, and other techniques.

physician's assistant—a person trained in certain aspects of the practice of medicine to provide assistance to the physician.

physiology—the study of the function of cells, tissues, and organs of the body.

pia mater—innermost of the three meninges of the brain and spinal cord.

pigment—any coloring matter.

pineal body—a small endocrine gland attached to the posterior part of the third ventricle of the brain.

pinocytosis—the process whereby a cell engulfs large amounts of liquid.

pitch—the frequency of vibrations of sound which enable one to classify sound on a scale from high to low.

pitfall—trap or hidden danger.

pituitary—a small endocrine gland attached to the base of the brain; the "master" gland.

PKU (phenylketonuria)—a genetic disorder resulting from the body's failure to oxidize an amino acid, perhaps because of a defective enzyme.

placenta—the structure through which the fetus obtains nourishment during pregnancy; the afterbirth.

planes—a flat or relatively smooth surface; points of reference by which positions or parts of the body are indicated.

plasma—the liquid part of the lymph and blood.

platelet—a type of cell found in the blood which is required for clotting.

pleura—a serous membrane which covers the lungs and lines the thoracic cavity.

pleurisy—inflammation of the pleura.

plexuses—a network of nerves.

plight—unfavorable situation or distressed condition.

pneumoconiosis—a respiratory condition due to inhalation of dust particles from mining or stone cutting.

pneumoencephalography—an X-ray examination of ventricles and subarachnoid spaces of brain following withdrawal of cerebrospinal fluid and injection of air or gas via a lumbar puncture.

pneumonia—inflammation of the lung caused primarily by microbes, chemical irritants, vegetable dust, or allergy.

pneumothorax—a collection of air or gas in the pleural cavity which displaces lung tissue.

podiatrist—(Chiropodist) a person trained to diagnose and treat diseases and disorders of the feet.

podiatry—the branch of medicine dealing with disorders of the feet.

polio—(Poliomyelitis) an acute, infectious, systemic disease which causes inflammation of the grey matter of the spinal cord.

polling—(FAX) receiving information on Fax.

polycystic disease—a condition of multiple cysts.

polycythemia—an excess of red blood cells.

polyp—a tumor with a pedicle, especially on mucous membranes such as in the nose, rectum, or intestines.

polyuria—excessive secretion and discharge of urine.

pons—a portion of the brain stem connecting the medulla oblongata and cerebellum with upper portions of the brain.

portal—pertaining to the portal circulation of blood from impaired internal organs to the liver for processing before entering the inferior vena cava.

positive—strongly affirmative.

post—to transfer charges from the day sheet to patient account records.

posterior—toward the rear or back or toward the caudal end.

postoperative (post-op)—after or following a surgical procedure.

postpartum—the period following delivery of a baby.

postscript (PS)—an addition to a letter written after the writer's name has been signed.

potential—possible; ability to develop into actuality.

Power of Attorney—a legal document authorizing a person to act as another's attorney, legal representative, or agent.

practitioner—one who practices the profession of medicine.

precancerous—a state just prior to the development of cancer.

precision—exactness, accuracy.

precordial—pertaining to that area of the chest wall over the heart for the placement of EKG chest leads.

pregnancy—the condition of being with child.

preliminary—coming before, leading up to.

premium—the amount paid or payable. For example, an insurance policy premium.

preoperative (pre-op)—the preparatory period preceding surgery.

presbycusis—impairment of acute hearing in old age.

presbyopia—a defect of vision in advancing age involving loss of accommodation.

prescribe—to lay down as a rule or direction; to order, advise, the use of.

prescription—a written direction for the preparation of a medicine.

preventive—tending to prevent or hinder. Something used to prevent disease.

primary—occurring first in time, development, or sequence; earliest.

prioritize—to arrange in order of importance.

process—to treat or prepare by some method.

proclivity—an inclination or predisposition toward something.

procrastination—intentionally delaying action of something that should be done.

proctology—the study of the rectum and anus and their diseases.

proctoscope—an instrument for the inspection of the rectum.

proctoscopy—instrumental inspection of the rectum.

procure—to get or obtain.

procurement—to obtain; acquire.

proficient—well advanced in an art, occupation, skill, or branch of knowledge; unusually knowledgeable.

profit sharing—a system by which employees receive a share of the profits of a business enterprise.

progesterone—a hormone secreted by the graafian follicle following the expulsion of the ovum.

progress notes—record of the continuing progress and treatment of a patient.

project—to produce and send forth with clarity and distinctness.

prolapse—dropping of an internal part of the body; usually refers to uterus or rectum.

prominent—conspicuous, outstanding.

prompt—to urge to action, to inspire.

prone—a position, lying horizontal with the face down.

prophylactic—warding off disease; preventive.

proprietary—referring to nonpublic educational institutions.

proprietorship—the amount by which assets exceed liabilities.

prostaglandins—a group of chemical substances secreted by mast cells or basophils that constricts smooth muscles in some organs.

prostate—a gland of the male reproductive system which surrounds the proximal portion of the urethra.

prostatectomy—excision of part or all of the prostate gland.

prosthesis—an artificial replacement of a missing body part.

pro tem—for the time being.

prothrombin—chemical substance existing in circulating blood which aids in the clotting process.

protozoan—a single-cell animal.

proximal—nearest the point of attachment.

pruritus—severe itching.

pruritus ani—itching about the anus.

psoriasis—a chronic inflammatory disease characterized by scaly patches.

psychedelics—hallucinogenic drugs.

psychiatrist—a physician specializing in the diseases and disorders of the mind, including neuroses and psychoses.

psychiatry—the branch of medicine dealing with the diagnosis, treatment, and prevention of mental illness.

psychological—of the mind; mental.

psychologist—a person specializing in the study of the structure and function of the brain and related mental processes.

psychology—the study of mental processes, both normal and abnormal, and their effects upon behavior.

psychoneuroimmunology—a science studying the connection between the brain, behavior, and immunity.

psychopathic—concerning or characterized by a mental disorder.

psychosis—mental disturbance of such magnitude that there is personality disintegration and loss of contact with reality.

psychosomatic—pertaining to interrelationship between the mind or emotions and body.

psychotherapy—the treatment of disease by hypnosis, psychoanalysis, and similar means.

ptosis—a drooping or dropping of an organ or part, for

example the eyelid or the kidney.

puberty—the period of life at which one becomes functionally capable of reproduction.

pubic—pertaining to the middle section of the lower third of the abdomen, also referred to as the hypogastric.

pulmonary—concerning or involving the lungs.

pulmonary edema—the presence of interstitial fluid in the lung tissue.

pulmonary embolism—a blockage in the pulmonary artery or one of its branches.

pulse—throbbing caused by the regular alternating contraction and expansion of an artery.

pulse deficit—the difference between the pulse rate measured radially and apically.

pulse pressure—difference between the systolic and diastolic measurements.

puncture—a hole made by something pointed.

pupil—the contractible opening in the center of the iris for the transmission of light.

purkinje—network of fibers found in the cardiac muscle which carries the electrical impulse resulting in the contraction of the ventricles.

pustule—small elevation of the skin filled with lymph or pus.

pyelonephritis—inflammation of the kidney, pelvis, and nephrons.

pyloric—pertaining to the opening between the stomach and the duodenum.

pyrogen—capable of producing fever.

QNS—quantity not sufficient.

quackery—the pretense to knowledge or skill in medicine.

quadrant—one of four regions, as of the abdomen, divided for identification purposes.

quadriceps femoris—a large muscle on the anterior surface of the thigh which is composed of four separate muscles.

R/O—rule out.

ROM—see **range of motion**

radial—referring to the radial artery or pulse taken in the radial artery.

radiation—the emission and diffusion of rays; a product of X-ray and radium.

radioactive—capable of emitting radiant energy.

radiograph—a record produced on a photographic plate, film, or paper by the action of X-ray or radium.

radiologic technologist—(X-ray technician) a person with specialized training in the techniques to prepare X-ray films to visualize the tissues and organs of the body.

radiologist—one who diagnoses and treats disease by the use of radiant energy.

radiology—the study of radiation and its uses.

radionuclides—a type of atom utilized in nuclear medicine for the diagnosis and treatment of disease.

radiopaque—impenetrable to the X-ray or other forms of radiation.

radius—a long bone of the forearm.

râles—an unusual sound heard in the bronchi on auscultation of respirations.

random—by chance; without plan.

range of motion (ROM)—refers to the degree of movement of the body's joints and extremities.

rapport—relationship characterized by harmony and cooperation.

rationalization—to explain on rational grounds, to devise plausible explanations for one's acts.

Raynaud's phenomenon—a symptom of Lupus characterized by fingers which turn white or blue in the cold.

reactivity—rate of nuclear disintegration in a reactor.

reagent—a substance involved in a chemical reaction.

realm—kingdom or empire, as used in text.

receptor—peripheral nerve ending of a sensory nerve that responds to stimuli.

reciprocity—mutual exchange, especially the exchange of special privilege.

reconcile—process to bring checkbook and bank statement into agreement.

rectal—referring to the rectum.

rectocele—the protrusion of the posterior vaginal wall with anterior wall of rectum through the vagina.

rectum—the lower part of the large intestine between the sigmoid and the anal canal.

recumbent—lying down.

recurrent—returning at intervals.

reduce—to restore the ends of a fractured bone to their usual relationship.

redundant—extra, not needed, repetitive.

reference—a source of information or authority.

reflex—an involuntary response to a stimulus.

refractive—the degree to which a transparent body deflects a ray of light from a straight path.

regimen—regulation of diet, sleep, exercise, and manner of living to improve or maintain health.

register—a formal or official recording of items, names, or actions.

regulate—control or direction.

regulatory—to control according to a rule; to adjust so as to make work accurately.

reimburse—to pay back or compensate for money spent, or losses or damages incurred.

reiterate—to say or do again.

rejuvenate—to make young again; to give youthful qualities to.

reliable—dependable, can be relied upon.

reluctant—marked by unwillingness.

rely—to depend on, to trust.

remedy—anything that relieves or cures a disease.

remission—a period that is disease- and symptom-free.

remote—from a distance; far removed in time and place; indirect.

renal—pertaining to the kidney.

renal failure—loss of function of the kidneys' nephrons.

renal threshold—the concentration at which a substance in the blood normally not excreted by the kidney begins to appear in the urine.

render—to present or to deliver, as a service or statement.

repolarization—reestablishment of a polarized state in a muscle or nerve fiber following contraction or conduction of a nerve impulse.

repression—to force painful ideas or impulses into the subconscious.

reproductive—concerning reproduction.

reputable—having a good reputation; well thought of.

res ipsa loquitur—the thing speaks for itself.

residency—physician training period in a specialty field of medicine.

residual—pertaining to that which is left as a residue.

residual barium—barium remaining in the intestinal tract following evacuation at the completion of X-ray studies.

resistance—opposition, ability to oppose.

resonance—(1) quality of the sound heard on percussion of the chest; (2) the intensification and prolongation of a sound by reflection or by vibration of a nearby object.

resource—a source of support or supply.

respiration—the taking in of oxygen and its utilization in the tissues and the giving off of carbon dioxide.

respiratory—pertaining to respiration.

respiratory therapy technician—a person trained to perform procedures of treatment which maintain or improve the ventilatory function of the respiratory tract.

respite—a temporary cessation of something that is painful or tiring; to delay, postpone.

respondeat superior—let the master answer.

retardation—slowing, delay, lag; slow in development, mental or physical.

retention—inability to void urine which is present in the bladder.

reticuloendothelial—pertaining to that group of cells which appear to aid in the making of new blood cells and the disintegration of old ones.

retina—the innermost layer of the eye which receives the image formed by the lens.

retinopathy—a degeneration of the retina due to a decrease in blood supply.

retraction—a shortening; the act of drawing backward or state of being drawn back.

retroflexed—refers to the body of the uterus being bent backward.

retrograde—refers to an X-ray procedure in which a radiopaque material is instilled by catheter into the bladder, ureters, and kidneys.

retroperitoneal—behind the peritoneum; posterior to the peritoneal lining of the abdominal cavity.

retroverted—refers to the entire uterus being tilted backward.

retrovirus—one with RNA genetic material.

revoke—to cancel, withdraw, take back.

Rh factor—an antigenic substance in human blood similar to the A and B factors which determine blood groups; apparently present only in red blood cells.

rhinitis—inflammation of the nasal mucosa.

rhythm—a measured time or movement; regularity of occurrence.

ribosome—an organelle within the cytoplasm of the cell.

rickets—a disease of the bones primarily due to the deficiency of Vitamin D.

risk—chance; hazard; chance of loss or injury; degree of probability of loss.

roentgen—refers to X-rays.

rotate—to move around; to turn on an axis.

rubella—(German measles)a mild contagious viral disease which may cause severe damage to an unborn child.

rubeola—(Measles) an acute, highly contagious disease marked by a typical cutaneous eruption.

S-A node—see **sinoatrial node**

sacrum—five fused vertebrae which lie between the coccyx and the lumbar vertebrae of the spinal column.

sagittal—refers to a plane which is made by dividing the body down the center creating a right and left side.

saliva—a digestive secretion of the salivary glands which empties into the mouth.

salivary glands—three pairs of glands that secrete the saliva which begins the digestion of food, primarily the breakdown of starch or complex carbohydrates.

salpingectomy—surgical removal of the fallopian tube or tubes.

salpingo-oophorectomy—surgical excision of the ovary and fallopian tube.

salve—an ointment.

sarcoma—malignant tumors of the connective, muscle, or bone tissue.

sartorius—a long narrow muscle of the thigh; the longest muscle of the body.

scan—to look over quickly but thoroughly.

scapula—the shoulder blade.

schedule—to arrange a timetable; to place in a list of things to be done.

sciatica—inflammation and pain along the sciatic nerve felt at back of thigh running down the inside of the leg.

sclera—the white or sclerotic outer coat of the eye.

scoliosis—lateral curvature of the spine.

screening—a preliminary or indicating procedure.

script—manuscript; type designed to look like handwriting.

scrotum—the double pouch containing the testes and part of the spermatic cord.

scurvy—a disease due to lack of fresh fruits, vegetables, and vitamin C in the diet.

sebaceous—an oily, fatty matter; glands secreting such matter.

sebum—oily secretion of the sebaceous glands of the skin.

secondary—one step removed from the first; not primary.

secretion—separation of certain materials from the blood by the activity of a gland.

sector—a section or division.

sedentary—pertaining to sitting; inactivity.

sedimentation—formation or depositing of sediment; of blood, refers to the speed at which erythrocytes settle when an anticoagulant is added to blood.

segment—a part or section of an organ or a body.

seizures—a sudden attack of pain, or disease or of certain symptoms.

semen—the mixture of secretions from the various glands and organs of the reproductive system of the male, which is expelled at orgasm.

semicircular canals—structures located in the inner ear.

semilunar—the valves of the heart located between the ventricles and the pulmonary artery and aorta.

senility—feebleness of body or mind caused by old age.

sensitivity—abnormal susceptibility to a substance.

sensorineural deafness—a loss of hearing due to transmission failure of the nerves within the inner ear or the auditory nerve.

sensory—refers to the nerves which receive and transmit stimuli from the sense organs.

septum—a membranous wall dividing two cavities, as within the heart or the nose.

sequence—order of succession.

series—a group; a set of things in the same class coming one after another.

serrated—notched, toothed.

sharps—any object which can cut, prick, stab, or scrape the skin.

sheath—a covering structure of connective tissue such as the membrane covering a muscle.

shock—a condition in which the pulse becomes rapid and weak, the blood pressure drops, and the patient is pale and clammy.

sickle cell anemia—a blood disorder in which the red blood cells are shaped like sickles.

sigmoid—an s-shaped section of the large intestine between the descending colon and the rectum.

sigmoidoscopy—an inspection of the sigmoid with an instrument.

simple—referring to a bone fracture, one without involvement of the skin surface.

simultaneous—occurring at the same time.

sinoatrial (S-A) node—the source of the nerve impulse which initiates the heartbeat; the pacemaker.

sinusitis—inflammation of the sinuses.

skeletal—pertaining to the skeleton or bony structure; also to the muscles attached to the skeleton to permit movement.

skip—a person who owes money but cannot be located.

slough—to cast off, as dead tissue.

smooth—a type of involuntary muscle tissue found in internal organs.

snap locks—metal locking devices.

Snellen chart—the chart of alphabetic letters used to evaluate distant vision.

sole—only.

solicit—to ask for.

somatic—pertaining to the body as distinguished from the mind; physical.

sonar—a device that transmits high-frequency sound waves in water and registers the vibrations reflected back from an object.

sonogram—record obtained by ultrasound.

sophisticated—not simple or natural; very refined; highly complex or developed in form, technique, etc.

spasm—an involuntary sudden movement or convulsive muscular contraction.

spastic colon—spasmodic contractions of the large intestine.

specified—named particularly; mentioned in detail.

specimen—a sample; a representative piece of the whole.

sperm—the male gamete or sex cell.

spermatozoon—a sperm cell.

sphincter—a circular muscle constricting an opening.

sphygmomanometer—a device that measures blood pressure; also called manometer.

spina bifida—a disorder characterized by a defect in the spinal vertebrae with or without protrusion of the spinal cord and meninges.

spinal—pertaining to the spinal column, canal, or cord.

spinal fusion—the surgical implanting of a bone fragment between the processes of two or more spinal vertebrae to render them immobile.

spiral—having a circular fashion.

spirometer—an apparatus which measures the volume of inhaled and exhaled air.

spleen—an oval, vascular, ductless gland below the diaphragm, in the upper left quadrant of the abdomen.

spontaneous—involuntary; produced of itself; unforced.

spores—hard capsules formed by certain bacteria which allow them to resist prolonged exposure to heat.

sports medicine—the branch of medicine dealing with the care of athletes to prevent and treat sports-related injuries.

sprain—the forcible twisting of a joint with partial rupture or other injury of its attachments.

sputum—substance ejected from the mouth containing saliva and mucus; usually refers to material coughed up from the bronchi.

standardization—process of bringing into conformity with a standard; pertaining to EKG, a mark made at the beginning of each lead to establish a standard of reference.

stapes—one of the three bones of the middle ear.

stasis ulcer—an open lesion due to stagnant or inadequate blood supply to an area.

STAT (statim)—immediately.

stature—height.

statutory—legally enacted; deriving authority from law.

stenosis—narrowing or constriction of a passage or opening.

sterile—without any organisms.

sternocleidomastoid—a muscle of the chest arising from the sternum and inner part of clavicle.

sternum—the breastbone.

stethoscope—an instrument used in auscultation to convey to the ear the sounds produced by the body.

stimulant—a substance which temporarily increases activity.

stipulations—terms of an agreement.

stomach—a dilated, saclike, distensible portion of the alimentary canal below the esophagus and before the small intestine.

stool—bowel movement, feces.

strabismus—an eye disorder caused by imbalance of the ocular muscles.

strain—injury to muscles from tension due to overuse or misuse.

stratagem—a trick or deception.

stress—to put pressure on; emphasize; urgency; tension, strained exertion. Topical; causing strain or injury to the skin.

striated—a type of muscle tissue marked with stripes or striae.

stricture—the narrowing of an opening, tube, or canal, such as the urethra or esophagus.

stylus—a pen; the EKG writer.

subarachnoid—the space between the pia mater and the arachnoid containing cerebrospinal fluid.

subcutaneous—beneath the skin.

subdural—beneath the dural mater; the space between the arachnoid and the dura mater.

subjective—relating to the person who is thinking, saying, or doing something; personal; of a disease symptom, felt by the individual but not perceptible to others.

sublimation—to express certain impulses, especially sexual, in constructive, socially acceptable forms.

sublingual—under the tongue.

subpoena duces tecum—court process initiated by party in litigation, compelling production of specific documents and other items, and material in relevance to facts in issue in appending judicial proceedings.

subsequent—coming after, following.

substantial—considerable, large.

suction—withdrawal by pressure; a sucking action.

sudden infant death syndrome (SIDS)—the sudden, unexplainable death of an infant.

superficial—on the surface.

superior—above or higher than.

supernatant—floating on the surface.

supine—lying horizontally on the back.

supplement—something added; an additional or extra section.

suppository—a medicated conical or cylindrical shaped material which is inserted into the rectum or vagina.

suppression—the shutdown of kidney function; the absence of urine excretion.

suppressor—one that holds back or stops an action.

suprapubic—above the pubic arch.

surfactant—a fatty molecule on the respiratory membranes.

surgeon—a physician with advanced training in operative procedures.

surgery—the branch of medicine dealing with manual and operative procedures for correction of deformities and defects and repair of injuries.

surrogate—a substitute; in place of another.

susceptible—having little resistance to a disease or foreign protein.

suture—to unite parts by stitching them together.

symmetry—the state in which one part exactly corresponds to another in size, shape, and position.

sympathetic—a portion of the autonomic nervous system.

symphysis pubis—the junction of the pubic bones on the midline in front.

symptom—any perceptible change in the body or its functions which indicates disease or the phase of a disease.

synapse—the minute space between the axon of one neuron and the dendrite of another.

syncope—fainting, a transient form of unconsciousness.

syndrome—the combination of symptoms with a disease or disorder.

synergism—something stimulating the action of another so that the effect of both is greater than the sum of the individual effects.

synovial—a movable joint; also called diarthroses.

syphilis—a communicable venereal disease spread by sexual contact.

system—a group of organs working together to perform a function of the body.

systematic—by a system or plan.

systole—the contraction phase of the heart; the greatest amount of blood pressure.

tachycardia—abnormal rapidity of heart action.

tact—skill in saying or doing the right thing; thoughtfulness.

tar—a sticky, brown or black carcinogenic substance.

tarsals—pertaining to the seven bones of the instep of the foot.

taut—tightly drawn; tense.

technical—relating to some particular art, science, or trade; also, requiring special skill or technique.

temperature—degree of heat of a living body; degree of hotness or coldness of a substance; usually refers to an elevation of body heat.

temporal—relating to the temporal bone on the skull.

tendon—fibrous connective tissue serving to attach muscles to bones.

tendonitis—inflammation of the tendon.

tentative—experimental, provisional, temporary.

terminal—final, end; a terminal illness, refers to a condition which cannot be reversed.

termination—ending.

testes—the male gonads of the scrotum which produce sperm.

testosterone—a male hormone secreted by the testes which causes and maintains male secondary sex characteristics.

tetanus—an acute infectious disease due to the toxins of the bacillus tetani.

tetany—intermittent tonic spasms resulting from inadequate parathyroid hormone.

thalamus—a portion of the brain lying between the cerebrum and the midbrain.

theories—beliefs not yet tested in practice; the general principles on which a science is based.

therapeutic—having medicinal or healing properties; pertaining to results obtained from treatment.

thermal—characterized by heat; heat activated.

thermography—a technique for sensing and recording on film, hot and cold areas of the body by means of an infrared detector that reacts to blood flow.

thermometer—an instrument used to measure temperature.

thesaurus—a reference book containing words and their synonyms.

third party—(Insurance) someone other than the patient, spouse, or parent who is responsible for paying all or part of the patient's medical costs.

thoracic—pertaining to the thorax or chest.

thorax—the chest; the body cavity enclosed by ribs and containing the heart and lungs.

thready—term used to describe a weak pulse which may feel like a thread under the skin surface.

thrombophlebitis—inflammation of a vein associated with the formation of a blood clot.

thrombosis—the formation of a blood clot or thrombus.

thymus—an unpaired organ located in the mediastinal cavity anterior to and above the heart.

thyroid—an endocrine gland located anteriorly at the base of the neck.

thyroidectomy—the surgical removal of the thyroid gland.

tibia—a long bone in the leg from the knee to the ankle.

tibialis anterior—a muscle of the leg.

tinnitus—a ringing or tinkling sound in the ear which is heard only be the person affected.

tissue—a collection of similar cells and fibers forming a structure in the body.

tolerance—the difference between the maximum and minimum; the amount of variation allowed from a standard.

tongue—the muscular organ of the mouth which assists in the production of speech, contains the taste buds, and provides the ability to swallow.

tonometer—instrument for measuring intraocular tension or pressure.

topical—pertaining to a specific area; local.

tort—any wrongful act, damage or injury done willfully, negligently.

torticollis—stiff neck caused by spasmotic contraction of neck muscles drawing the head to one side with the chin pointing to the other; can be congenital or acquired.

tourniquet—any constrictor used on an extremity to produce pressure on an artery and control bleeding; also used to distend veins for the withdrawal of blood or the insertion of a needle to instill intravenous injections.

toxin—poisonous substance or compound of vegetable, animal, or bacterial origin.

toxoid—a toxin treated so as to destroy its toxicity, but still capable of inducing formation of antibodies on injection.

trace—the production of a sketch by means of a stylus passing over the paper as in electrocardiography.

trachea—a cartilaginous tube between the larynx and the main bronchus of the respiratory tree.

tracheostomy—a surgically made opening in the trachea through which a person will breathe.

traction—the process of pulling; with fractures, traction is applied in a straight line to stretch the contracted muscles and permit realignment of the bone fragments.

transactions—dealings accomplished.

transcript—a copy made directly from an original record, especially an official copy of a student's educational record.

transdermal—through the skin.

transducer—a device that transforms power from one system to another in the same or different form.

transfusion—injection of the blood of one person into the blood vessels of another.

transient ischemic attack (TIA)—temporary interruption of blood flow in the brain due to small clots closing off blood vessels.

transillumination—inspection of a cavity or organ by passing a light through its walls.

transition—passing from one condition, place, or activity to another.

transmitted—sent from one person, thing, or place to another.

transpose—putting one in place of another, the accidental misplacing or words or letters.

transurethral—literally means through the urethra; refers to the removal of the prostate by going through the urethral wall.

transverse—lying across; the segment of large intestine which lies across the abdomen; a line drawn horizontally across the body or a structure.

trapezius—the large muscle of the back and neck.

traumatic—caused by or relating to an injury.

traumatize—to cause trauma or injury.

treadmill—an apparatus with a movable platform which permits walking or running in place.

Trendelenburg—a position with the head lower than the feet.

trial balance—bookkeeping strategy to confirm accuracy in debits and credits in ledger.

triceps—the posterior muscles of the arm which work as a team with the biceps; the triceps straighten the elbow.

trichomoniasis—infestation with parasitic protozoa; usually refers to vaginal involvement.

tricuspid—a valve in the right side of the heart, between the chambers; literally means three cusps or leaflets.

trimester—divided into three sections; the third segment or period.

trivial—of little value, insignificant.

tuberculosis—an infectious disease caused by the tubercle bacillus; pulmonary tuberculosis is a specific inflammatory disease of the lungs which destroys lung tissue.

tumor—a swelling or enlargement; a neoplasm; often used to indicate a malignant growth.

turbidity—flaky or granular particles suspended in a clear liquid giving it a cloudy appearance; usually refers to cloudy urine.

tympanic membrane—the eardrum.

typhoid—an acute infectious disease acquired by ingesting contaminated food or water.

URI—see **upper respiratory infection**
UTI—see **urinary tract infection**

ulcer—an open lesion on the skin or mucous membrane of the body characterized by loss of tissue and the formation of a secretion.

ulceration—suppuration of the skin or mucous membrane; an open lesion.

ulna—a long bone in the forearm from the elbow to the wrist.

ultimately—in the end, finally.

ultrasonic scanning—a process of scanning the body with sound waves to produce a picture on a screen of underlying internal structures.

umbilical—pertaining to the umbilicus or navel of the abdomen.

unemployed—the state of being without work.

unique—one of a kind, unmatched.

unit clerk—a secretarial position on the health care team of a patient care facility.

universal—relating to the universe, general or common to all.

unobtrusive—not forced upon others; not thrusted forward or pushed out.

unproductive—not productive; no accomplishment.

unstructured—without structure or order; unorganized.

upper respiratory infection (URI)—inflammatory process involving the nose and throat, may include the sinuses; refers to symptoms associated with the common cold.

uremia—a condition in which products normally found in the urine are found in the blood.

ureter—a tube carrying urine from the kidney to the urinary bladder.

urethra—a membranous canal for the external discharge of urine from the bladder.

urgency—the sudden need to expel urine or stool.

urinalysis—an analysis of the urine; a test performed on urine to determine its characteristics.

urinary meatus—the opening through which urine passes from the body.

urinary tract infection (UTI)—infection occurring within the kidneys, ureters, and/or urinary bladder.

urination—the act of urinating or voiding of urine.

urine—fluid secreted from the blood by the kidneys, stored in the bladder, and discharged from the body by voiding.

urology—the study of the urine and diseases of the urinogenital organs.

urticaria—an inflammatory condition characterized by the eruption of wheals which are associated with severe itching; commonly called hives.

uterus—a muscular, hollow, pear-shaped organ of the female reproductive tract in which a fertilized ovum develops into a baby.

utilization—to put to profitable use.

utilize—to use or make use of.

vaccine—any substance for prevention of a disease.

vagina—a musculomembranous tube which forms the passageway from the uterus to the exterior.

vaginitis—inflammation of the vagina.

vagus—the tenth cranial nerve which has both motor and sensory function, affecting the heart and stomach as well as other organs.

valve—any one of various structures for temporarily closing an opening or passageway, or for allowing movement of fluid in one direction only.

varices—enlarged, twisted veins.

varicose—pertaining to varices; distended, swollen veins, most commonly found in the legs.

vas deferens—the excretory duct of the testes.

vasectomy—the cutting out of a portion of the vas deferens.

vein—a blood vessel carrying blood toward the heart after receiving it from a venule.

vena cava—one of two large veins which empty into the right atrium of the heart.

venipuncture—the puncture of a vein; the insertion of a needle into a vein for the purpose of obtaining a blood sample or instilling a substance.

venous—pertaining to a vein.

ventilatory—that which ventilates, lets in fresh air.

ventral—pertaining to the anterior or front side of the body.

ventricle—one of the two lower chambers of the heart; also used in reference to cavities within the brain.

venule—a minute vein; a blood vessel which connects a capillary with a vein.

verify—to prove to be true; to support by facts.

veritable—actual, genuine.

vermiform appendix—the appendix; a small tube attached to the cecum.

verrucae—warts; small, circumscribed elevations of the skin formed by hypertrophy of the papillae.

vertebrae—the bones in the spinal column.

vertex—the top of the head, the crown.

vesicle—a small sac or bladder containing fluid; a small, blisterlike elevation on the skin containing serous fluid.

vested—settled; complete; absolute; continuous.

viable—capable of living.

vial—a small glass tube or bottle containing medication or a chemical.

villi—tiny projections from a surface; the villi of the small intestine which absorb nutrients during the process of digestion.

villous adenoma—a type of polyp which is invasive and malignant.

virulent—full of poison; deadly; malignant.

virus—a very simple, frequently pathogenic, microorganism capable of replicating within living cells.

visceral—pertaining to viscera, the internal organs, especially the abdomen.

vital—essential; pertaining to the preservation of life (the vital signs).

vital capacity—the total volume of air exchanged from forced inspiration and forced expiration.

vitreous humor—the substance which fills the vitreous body of the eye behind the lens.

void—to pass urine from the urinary bladder; to make ineffective or invalid.

volatile—easily changed into a gas or tending to change into a vapor; usually considered potentially dangerous.

voltage—a measure of electromotive force.

volume—the amount of space occupied by an object as measured in cubic units.

voluntary—under one's control; done by one's own choice.

vomit—to expel the contents of the stomach through the mouth.

voucher—a document that serves as proof that terms of a transaction have been met.

vulnerable—liable to injury or hurt; capable of being wounded.

vulva—the female external genitalia, including the clitoris, the labia minora, and the labia majora.

waiver—to give up; forgo; waiving of a right or claim.

warrant—to justify, to give definite assurance as to the value of; to authorize.

wart—see **verrucae**

watermark—a mark imprinted on paper that is visible when it is held to the light, usually a sign of quality.

wheals—more or less round and evanescent elevations of the skin, white in center with a pale red edge, accompanied by itching.

whorl—a type of fingerprint in which the central papillary ridges turn through at least one complete circle.

withdrawal—a removal of something that has been deposited.

womb—nonmedical name for the uterus.

writer—the person who writes; the author.

xiphoid—a process which forms the tip of the sternum.

Z-Tract—a method of injecting medication intramuscularly.

zygote—a cell produced by the union of an ovum and a sperm.

Index

Gastroenteritis, 348
Gastroenterology, 16
Gastrointestinal (GI) series, 344–45
Gastrointestinal (GI) system, *See* Digestive
    system
Gastroscopy, 345
Genetic cellular change, 215–16
Genital herpes, 401
Genitalia, 376, 500, 555
Genogram, 428
Genucubital position, 490
Genupectoral position, 489
Geriatrics, 16
Gestures, 50
Gigantism, 366
Glands. *See also* Endocrine system; main
    entries, i.e., Adrenal glands
    interrelationship of, 370–81
Glaucoma, 238–39, 497
Glomerulonephritis, 361
Glomerulus, 354
Glossitis, 243–44
Gloves, 614, 615
Glucagon, 368
Glucocorticoids, 368
Glucose
    blood screening, 531–32, 537
    in urine, 561
Glucose tolerance test (GTT), 371, 532,
    537
Gluteus maximus, 272
Glycosuria, 370
Goiter, 367
Goldsmith, Grace Arabell, 6
Golgi apparatus, 209–10
Gonadotropic hormones, 366, 562
Gonads, 370
Gonorrhea, 400–401
Good Samaritan Act, 36–37
Gout, 264
Government health plans, 164–70
Graafian follicles, 383
Graft, 357–58
Gram staining, 572–74
Granulocytes, 321–22
Grave's disease, 373–74, 580
Growth charts, 429, 432–34, 440, 441
Growth hormone (GH), 366, 368
Guaiac reagent strip test, 600–602
Guilds, medical, 3
Gunshot wound, 675
Gynecology, 16, 388, 508. *See also*
    Papanicolaou (Pap) smear

Hair, 246
    excess of, 251
    loss of, 248

Hallucinogens, 678, 709–10
Hallux valgus, 264
Hamstring group, 273–74
Hands, bones of, 258–59, 260
Handwashing, 409–11
Harvey, William, 3
Headache, 231
Head circumference (infant), 431, 436,
    439, 440, 441
Health Care Financing Administration
    (HCFA), 169, 170
Health insurance, 161–83
    claims, 180–83
    coding systems, 173–80
    government health plans, 164–70
    managed care delivery systems, 164
    private health care plans, 163–64
    terminology, 161–63
Health maintenance organizations
    (HMOs), 164
Health and personal behaviors, 695–712
Hearing, 240–41. *See also* Ear(s)
    auditory acuity, 481–86
Heart, the, 290, 499
    augmenting sound, 466
    electrical impulses, path of, 586–87
    lubb dupp sounds, 293
    rate of, 295
    rhythm disorders, 293–94
Heart attack, 667
Heart block, 293
Height, 428–31
Heimlich maneuver, 669
Hematocrit, 528–31, 533
Hematology, 16
Hematoma, 233, 545
Hematuria, 561
Hemiplegia, 232
Hemoccult sensa tests, 600–602
Hemodialysis, 357
Hemoglobin, 304, 528–31, 534
Hemoglobinometer, 534
Hemolysis, 547
Hemophilia, 216, 611, 613
Hemorrhage, 233, 306, 668
Hemorrhoids, 348
Hemothorax, 287
Henle, loop of, 354
Hepatitis, 348–49, 408, 414, 518, 656,
    662, 677
Hernia(s), 349–50, 500
Herniated disk, 264–65
Herniorrhaphy, 350
Herpes, 401
    simplex, 251, 414
    zoster, 231, 251
Heterosexual transmission (AIDS), 325

HIB vaccine, 654
Hiccough, 271, 281
Hildegarde (St.), 3
Hip dysplagia, congenital, 264
Hippocrates, 2, 3
Hippocratic oath, 2
Hirsutism, 251
Histamine(s), 318, 328, 578
Histologist, 22
Histoplasmosis, 284
History of medicine, 1–8
    ancient history, 1–3
    early leaders in American medicine, 4–5
    modern medical pioneers, 3–4
    women in medicine, 5–7
HIV/AIDS Surveillance, 326–27
Hives, 253
Hodgkins, Dorothy, 7
Holmes, Oliver Wendell, 4
Holter monitor, 307, 594, 596
Homeostasis, 214–15
Homosexual(s), 324
Hordeolum, 239
Horizontal recumbent position, 487, 488
Hormones, 365
Hornet stings, 662, 669
Hospice movement, 59
Hospitals, 4–5
House calls, 81
Human chorionic gonadotropin (HCG),
    371, 391, 396
Human immunodeficiency virus (HIV),
    324, 327, 518
Human relations, 9
Humerus, 258
Humoral immunity, 318
Humpback, 265
Hunter, John, 4
Hunter, William, 4
Hyaline membrane disease, 284
Hyde-Rowan, M. Deborah, 7
Hydrocele, 381
Hydrocephalus, 231
Hydrochloric acid, 339
Hymen, 388
Hyperglycemia, 370
Hypertension, 20, 311–12
Hyperthermia, 329
Hyperthyroidism, 367
Hyperventilation, 459
Hypnosis, 20
Hypodermic needle, 642, 740
Hypoglycemia, 370
Hypotension, 312
Hypothalamus, 225–27
Hypothyroidism, 367, 369
Hypoxia, 287

Safety
    laboratory procedures, 44, 518–20
    in the medical office, 659–60
    and security, 41–46
    universal blood and body fluid
          precautions, 408, 445, 517–18
Saf-T Clik, 549
Saliva, 336–37, 338
Salpingo-oophorectomy, 397
Sanitation, 2
Sanitization, 415
Sarcomas, 329
Sartorius, 273
Scabies, 252–53, 415
Scapula, 258
Scarlet fever (scarlatina), 415
Sciatica, 233
Scoliosis, 266
Scratch test, 580–82
Scrotum, 376
Secretarial skills
    professional recognition, 13
    word processing, 126
Security, office, 42
Semen, 378, 379
Semi-Fowler's position, 491
Seminal vesicles, 378
Senses, the, 234–44
Septum, 276, 290
Serpents, 2
Sex hormones, 368
Sex-linked disorders, 216
Sexual differentiation before birth, 377
Sexual harassment, 35–36
Sexually transmitted diseases, 400–403
Sheath(s), 271
Shingles, 231
Shippen, William (Jr.), 5
Shock, 670, 672
Sickle cell anemia, 313
Sigmoid, 343
Sigmoidoscopy, 345, 504, 510–13
Simpson, James, 4
Sims' position, 488, 490
Sinusitis, 288
Skeletal muscles, 269, 271–74
Skeletal system, 253–67. *See also* main
        entries, i.e., Skull
    bone structure, 254
    diagnostic examinations, 262
    diseases and disorders, 262–67
    functions of, 255–56
    number of bones, 254–55
Skin, 244–53
    color of, 246–47
    diagnostic tests, 247, 578–83
    diseases and disorders of, 248–53

    functions of, 245
    minor surgery, preparation for, 612,
      615
    structure of, 245–46, 247
Skin puncture test, 525–26
Sklodowska, Mary A., *See* Curie, Marie
Skull, 257, 259
    head circumference (infant), 431, 436,
      439, 440, 441
    X ray, 230
Sleep, 702
Sleep disorder, 20
Small intestine, 339–42
Smallpox vaccine, 4
Smell, 242. *See also* Nose
Smith, Theobald, 5
Smoking, 70, 710–12
    involuntary and passive, 711
Sneezing, 281
Snellen chart, 475–77, 479
Sonograms, *See* Ultrasound
Spastic colon, 352
Sperm, 376, 379, 389, 391
Spermatozoan, 375
Spermicides, 395
Sphincters, 274–75, 339
Sphygmomanometer, 462, 463–65, 496
Spina bifida, 233
Spinal column, 256
Spinal cord, 256
    defects, 233
    and PNS, 223–24
    ventricles, 228
Spinal fusion, 265
Spirometer, 282, 598
Spleen, 300–301
Splinters, 665–66
Spores, 415–16
Sports medicine, 17
Sprain(s), 266, 672, 674
Sputum, 282, 283
    specimen collection, 565–566, 567
Stab wounds, 675
Stasis ulcer, 314
Sterilization, 416, 417, 614
Sternocleidomastoid, 271
Sternum, 257
Stethoscope, 2–3, 457, 496, 497, 499
Stimulants, 678, 710
Stings (bee, wasp, and hornet), 662, 669
Stomach, 338–40
Stool specimens, 566, 568, 569
Strabismus, 240
Strains, 672, 674
Strang Clinic, 6
Strep throat, 415
Stress management, 50–53, 707

    related illness, 51–52
Stress tests, 594
Stress thallium ECG, 307
Stricture, 364
Stroke, 674
Stye, 239
Subarachnoid hemorrhage, 233
Subdural hematoma, 233
Sublimation, 54
Subluxation, 267
Substance abuse, 675–79, 704–12
    treatment, 710
Substance analysis, 563–64
Sudden infant death syndrome (SIDS),
    288
Sullivan, Louis W., 327
Sunburn, 246–47, 249, 663
Support services, 6
Suppression, urinary, 364
Surfactant, 280
Surgeon, origin of term, 3
Surgery, 17, 20, 615, 616
    assisting, 615, 616–618
    consent to, 32
    laparoscopic, 341
    minor procedures, 609–22
    ovarian tumor, removal of, 5
    scientific, 4
Suturing and removal, 618–21, 681
Sympathetic nervous system, 224
Symphysis pubis, 259
Synergism, 709
Syphilis, 402
Systemic circulation, 298
System(s) of the body, 219–20

Tachycardia, 295
Taste, 243. *See also* Tongue
Taxol, 329
Tax records, 193, 199
Teeth, 336
Telephone communications, 77–85
    angry calls, 81
    answering device and service, 83–84,
      85
    appointments, prescriptions and
      test results, 80
    business and personal calls, 81
    call monitoring, 82
    emergency calls, 80–81
    finding phone numbers, 82–83
    house calls, 81
    long distance, 82
    messages, 78–79
    patient reports, 81
    procedure, 82, 83, 84, 85
    professional calls, 81